Radiographic Positioning and Procedures

Jennifer Wagner, MS, RT(R)(M)(QM), RDMS, RVT

Director of Radiologic Technology Program
Professor of Allied Health
Fort Hays State University
Hays, Kansas

Wolters Kluwer

Philadelphia • Baltimore • New York • London
Buenos Aires • Hong Kong • Sydney • Tokyo

Acquisitions Editor: Matt Hauber
Development Editor: Eric McDermott
Editorial Coordinator: Sunmerrilika Baskar
Marketing Manager: Kirsten Watrud
Senior Production Project Manager: Catherine Ott
Manager, Graphic Arts & Design: Stephen Druding
Manufacturing Coordinator: Margie Orzech
Prepress Vendor: S4Carlisle Publishing Services

9 8 7 6 5 4 3 2 1

Printed in Mexico

Library of Congress Cataloging-in-Publication Data

ISBN-13: 978-1-9751-0827-4

Library of Congress Control Number: 2021913866

shop.lww.com

QUADM0725

DEDICATION

To my husband Eric and my children
Zachary, Lauren, and Adelyn. The
completion of this project would have
not been possible without your support,
encouragement, and patience.

Acknowledgments

I am thankful for the support of many of my colleagues in education and clinical practice that I have used as a sounding board to refine the product to be the best it could be. Thank you to Brenda Hoopingarner for supporting the scale of this project. Thank you to Christa Beiker for your confidence in me and assisting me whenever asked on many phases of this project. I cannot overemphasize my sincere gratitude to S. Katie Fulton, who has been instrumental to me on so many levels of this journey; you have a special place in this project.

I am grateful for all the support and help from my parents, Rod, Ann, in-laws Carl, and Mary Ann, and my husband, children, and many dear friends and family who helped serve as models for the photography and videography of this project. Jared Crist, your concern and stamina to ensure the perfection of many difficult photos for the text was successful. Halle Lang, I am blessed to bring you aboard with your incredible talents to help with an essential part of the product. I appreciate all the time, travel, and expertise of Mark Flanders, Ed Schultes, Freddie Patane, Lou Russo, and Holly Ray with the undertaking of the photoshoot.

I want to acknowledge R.T. program graduates Courtney, Sarah, and Mikala for their input and feedback with the initial development of this project.

I want to thank Brown's Medical Imaging, Daren Beltz, and DEL Medical Imaging for supporting this project.

Preface

Welcome to the first edition of *Radiographic Positioning and Procedures.* The text strives to educate students on the foundational knowledge of anatomy, correlative radiographic anatomy, basic pathology relative to learning examination indications, positioning steps for imaging projections, the basics of image analysis, and the recognition of positioning errors. This text is not meant to replace essential publications within the industry that cover the vast details of patient care, image production, and safety as comprehensive texts of this nature serve as an important part of a radiography student's education.

As a first edition, the goal is to prepare students for the clinical atmosphere and the American Registry of Radiologic Technologists (ARRT) Radiography examination, with the focus being on radiographic procedures. It focuses on the core elements of anatomy and correlation to radiographic anatomy, which is essential to identification of pathology and radiograph analysis. This text was laid out to align with the clinical ARRT competency requirements in order to establish foundational knowledge in the student radiographer. Realizing that each facility operates with different radiographic equipment, it is expected that protocols, technical settings, and image receptors may not align identically to what has been generalized in this text.

Features of this text:

- There is concise description of anatomy and correlation to radiographic anatomy.
- Each unit reveals details of image marking and image display.
- Each unit contains key summative points of anatomy.
- Units are enriched with art, photography, and radiographs.
- Videography of positioning for 35 standard examination protocols will serve as a helpful ancillary for lecture and laboratory instruction.
- Concise step-by-step details have been given for examination projections followed with image analysis and where possible enriched with additional radiographs with positioning errors.
- Chapter conclusion provides general and key image analysis criteria.
- Chapter conclusion provides questions with radiographic images to critically challenge the student on image acquisition results.

Design and layout of the chapters are consistent, with the exception of a few chapters. Chapters 9 and 10 are enhanced with summary protocol tables to recap the positioning pages. These protocol tables provide a quick reference to the many specific details of the more in-depth radiographic protocols. Chapters 12 and 13 are laid out differently to integrate the review of anatomy to align with elements of the different ARRT competency requirements of special and operational procedures.

Alongside this text, there is a corresponding first edition workbook that features a unique layout in each chapter to provide identification, matching, multiple choice, sequencing, critical thinking, and image critique to assess the student's knowledge and reinforce unit learnings. The workbook is organized to break down and correlate material together. For example, in the upper extremity chapter, the student can focus on the anatomy, positioning, and radiographs of the fingers, hand, and wrist. The next section of upper extremity chapter would focus on the forearm and elbow. This organization encourages a mastery of concepts by examination area. The final chapter of the workbook is comprehensive with the content arranged by chapters to provide additional questions for each unit.

Contents

CHAPTER 1 Fundamentals of Radiographic Positioning

SKELETAL SYSTEM

The skeletal system is divided into the axial and appendicular skeleton. The axial skeleton includes the head, neck, and trunk. The appendicular skeleton includes the upper and lower limbs along with the pelvic and shoulder girdles. The adult skeleton consists of 206 total bones. There are a variety of shapes of bones that fit together to build the functional skeleton (Fig. 1-1).

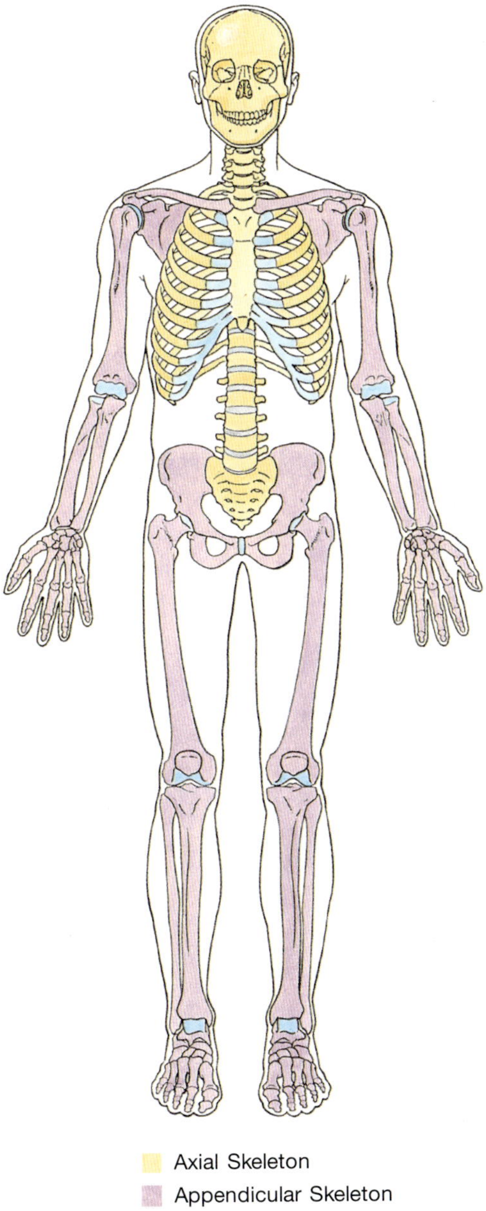

1-1 Axial and appendicular skeleton.

Bone Classification by Shape

Long Bones: Have a long shaft with two articulating ends. Examples: humerus and femur (Fig. 1-2)

Short Bones: Rectangular and square-like bones. Examples: carpals and tarsals (Fig. 1-2)

Flat Bones: Thin bone containing bone marrow. Examples: sternum and cranium (Fig. 1-2)

Irregular Bones: Bones irregularly shaped. Examples: facial and vertebral bones (Fig. 1-2)

Sesamoid Bones: Round bone(s) embedded into tendons closely associated with joints. Examples: patella and small sesamoid bones located near the head of the first metacarpal and metatarsal (Fig. 1-2)

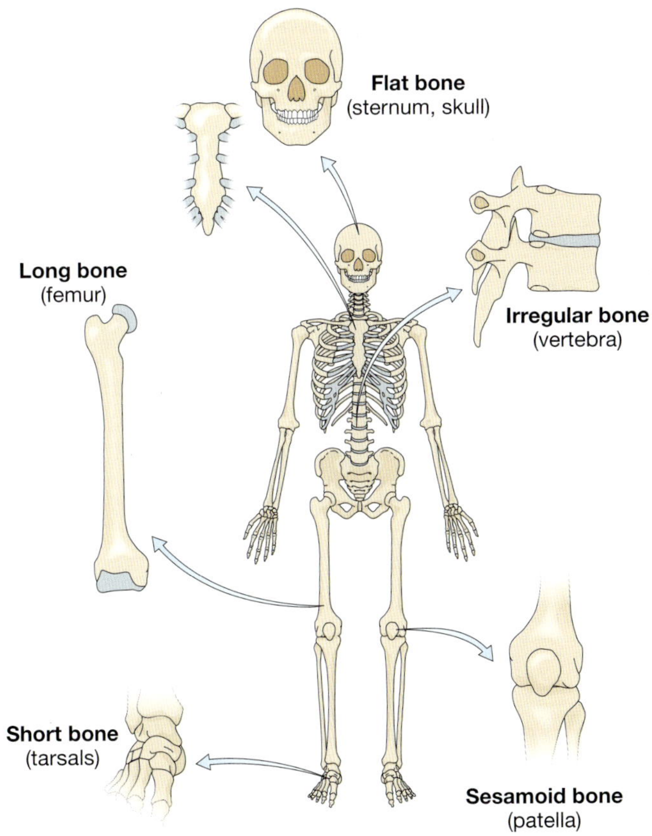

1-2 Bone classifications.

Bone Terminology

Bones have specific bone markings and features that are referenced on radiographic images. These specific features serve a purpose for tendons, ligaments, or fascia to attach to or pass through (Fig. 1-3).

Condyle: rounded articular area

Epicondyle: smaller elevated surface located superior or adjacent to a condyle

Eminence: point of elevation

Crest: ridge of bone

Facet: smooth and flat surface to allow for bone articulation

Foramen: opening or passageway through a bone

Fossa: a location that represents a depression

Notch: indentation on an edge

Protuberance: a bony projection

Sulcus: an elongated groove

Trochanter: large and blunt elevation

Tubercle: small raised bony eminence

Tuberosity: round and raised bony element

Key Anatomic Parts of Bone (Fig. 1-4)

Cortex: The outer hard shell of the bone. The cortex tends to be thicker toward the body of the bone to provide added strength.

Medullary Cavity: The hollow portion of the bone located in the body and containing the yellow bone marrow.

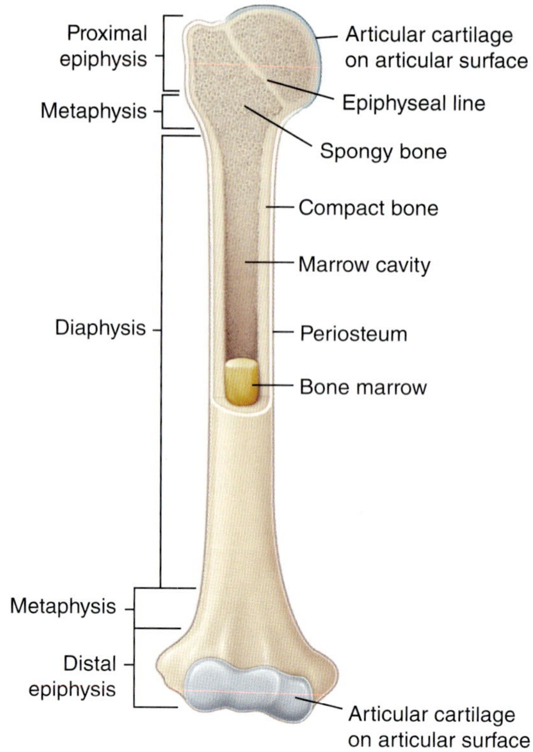

1-4 Long bone.

Cancellous Bone (Spongy): Cancellous bone is porous, contains the red bone marrow, and is located between the cortex and medullary cavity.

Periosteum: Blood vessels pass into the bone through the periosteum to nourish the bone and allow for bone growth and repair.

Articular Cartilage: Cartilage that allows connection with other bones.

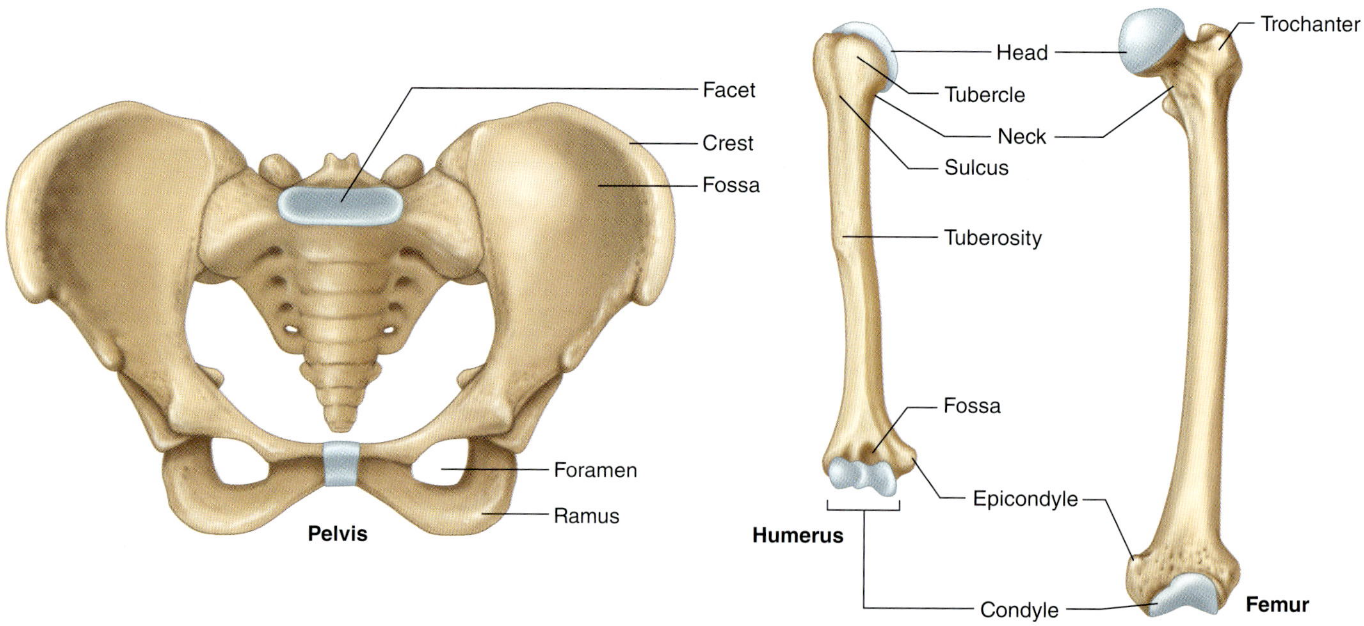

1-3 Bone markings.

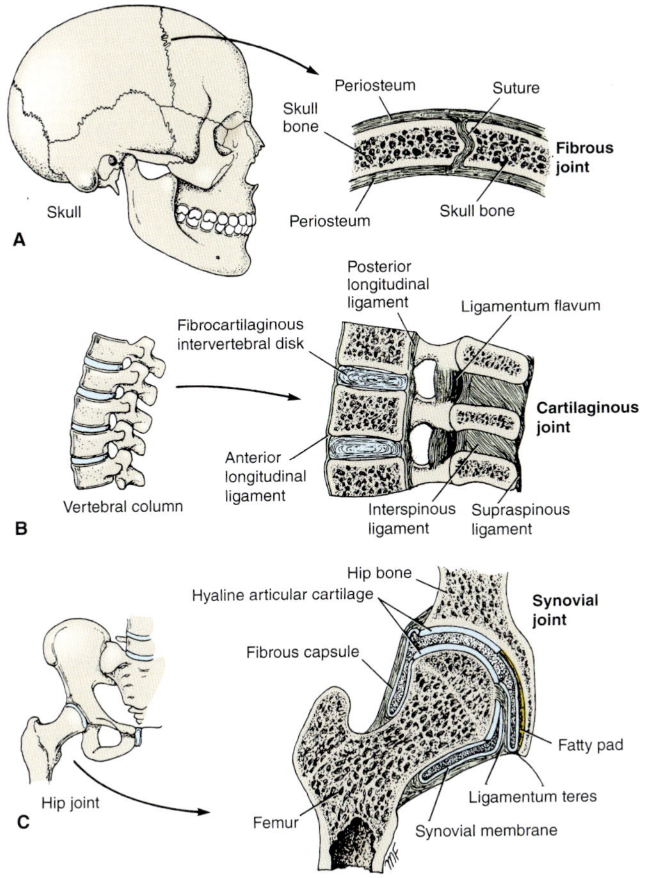

1-5 Structural classification of joints. **(A)** Fibrous joint. **(B)** Cartilaginous joint. **(C)** Synovial joint.

Joints

Joints are formed when two ends of bones articulate together. Joints have different structural classifications that influence mobility (function level) of the joint and determine what specific type of movement it has.

Structural Classification

Synovial joints surround articulating bones with a joint capsule. The joint capsule is filled with synovial fluid (Fig. 1-5).

Fibrous joints connect bones together with fibrous tissue. There is not a joint cavity (Fig. 1-5).

Cartilaginous joints connect bones together with cartilage. There is not a joint cavity (Fig. 1-5).

Mobility Type (Function Level)

Synovial joints are diarthrodial joints that are freely movable joints. These joints are further defined to have a specific type of movement (Fig. 1-6).

Plane: The articular surfaces are able to glide against one another (acromioclavicular [AC] and sternoclavicular [SC] joints and intercarpals).

Hinge: Allows flexion and extension in a plane (elbow).

Saddle: Opposing articular surfaces are concave and convex and fit together, permitting adduction, abduction, and circumduction (first carpometacarpal joint).

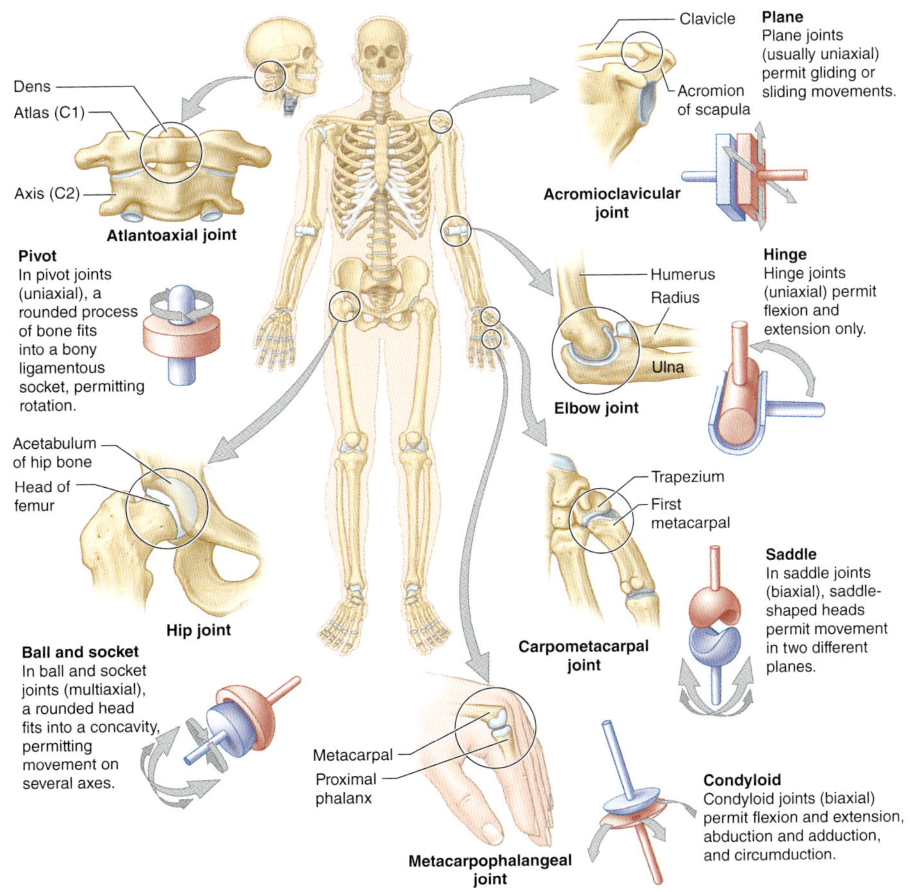

1-6 Synovial—types of synovial joint movements.

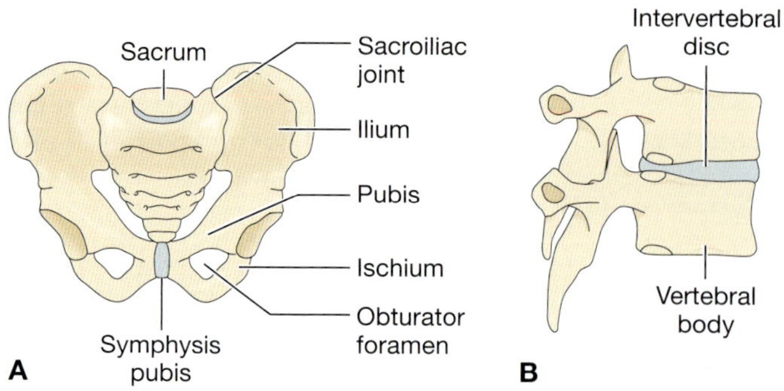

1-7 Cartilaginous: symphyses—amphiarthrodial. **(A)** Symphysis pubis. **(B)** Intervertebral disks.

Condyloid: Allows flexion and extension as well as adduction, abduction, and circumduction (2–5 metacarpophalangeal joints)

Ball and Socket: A rounded head fits into a depressed socket, providing the greatest amount of movement; stability of this joint directly influenced by the depth of the socket (shoulder and hip).

Pivot: Permits rotation around a stationary axis (C1 and C2; proximal and distal radioulnar joints)

Cartilaginous joints involve cartilage and functionally may have limited or no movement.

Symphyses: Pads of cartilage that separate flat surfaces of bone (intervertebral disks and symphysis pubis); functionally, an amphiarthrodial joint (Fig. 1-7). Amphiarthrodial joints allow for limited movement.

Synchondroses: Temporary joint associated with growth (epiphyseal) plates at the ends of long bones; these temporary joints are made of hyaline cartilage and have no movement; functionally, a synarthrodial joint (Figs. 1-8 and 1-9).

Fibrous joints connect adjacent bone segments together with connective tissue. The different identified fibrous joints will function with limited or lack of movement.

Skull Sutures: Interlocking sutures between cranial bones; adult sutures are functionally synarthrodial (Fig. 1-10). Synarthrodial joints don't allow much of any movement.

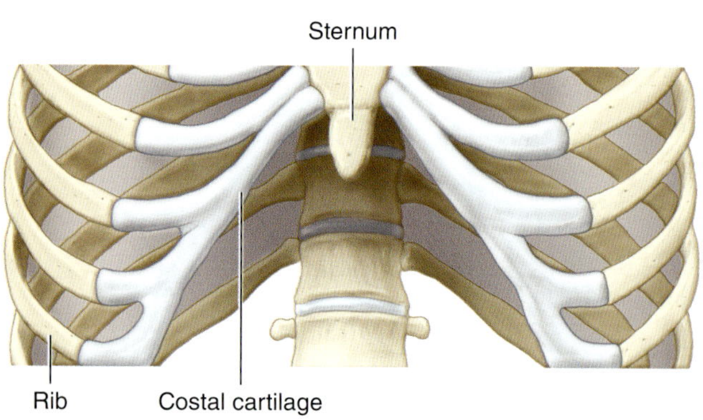

1-8 Cartilaginous: synchondroses—amphiarthrodial.

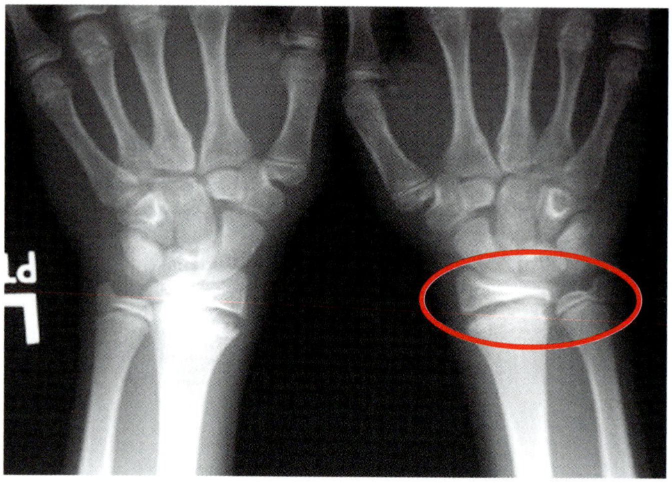

1-9 Cartilaginous: synchondroses—synarthrodial.

Gomphosis: Conical end of the tooth that fits into a socket on the maxilla and mandible; functionally, amphiarthrodial (Fig. 1-11)

Syndesmoses: Bones are connected together by way of interosseous connecting fibrous bands, allowing amphiarthrodial movement; distal tibiofibular joint and radioulnar joint (Fig. 1-12).

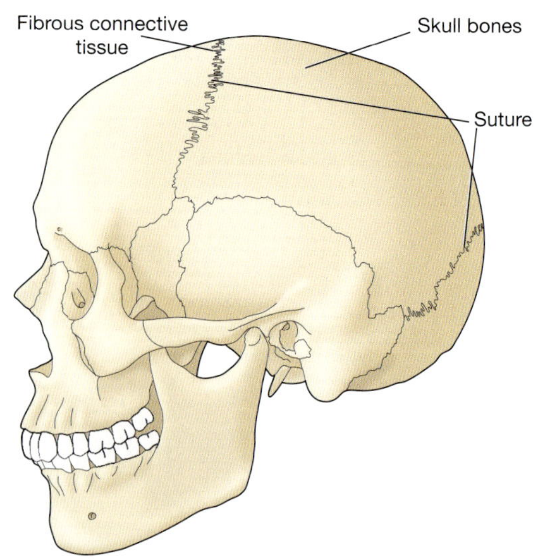

1-10 Fibrous joint: skull suture—synarthrodial.

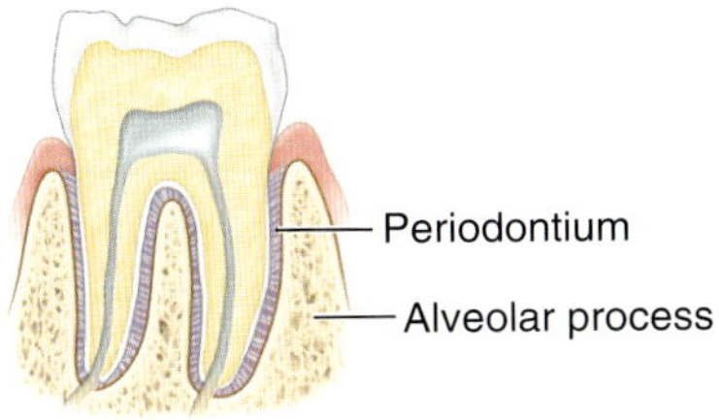

1-11 Fibrous joint: gomphosis—amphiarthrodial.

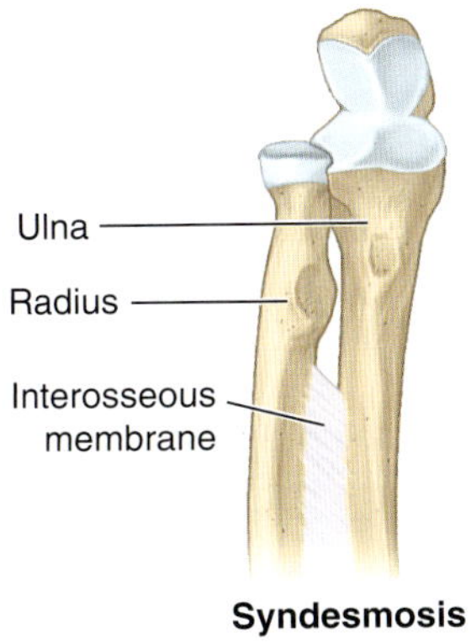

1-12 Fibrous joint: syndesmosis—amphiarthrodial.

TERMINOLOGY

Anatomic Position

The anatomic position describes a patient standing upright with the toes and palms of the hands facing forward (Fig. 1-13).

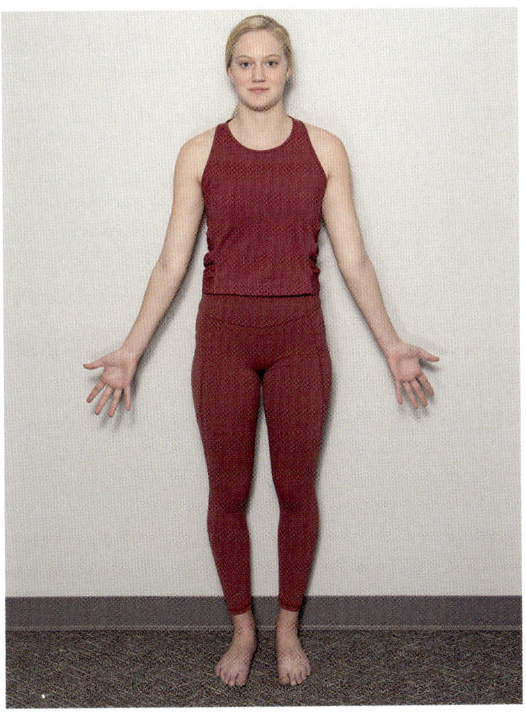

1-13 Anatomic position.

Surfaces (Fig. 1-14)

- Anterior or ventral
- Posterior or dorsal
- Dorsum—top of the foot; anterior surface
- Plantar—sole of the foot; posterior surface
- Palmar—palm of the hand; anterior surface
- Dorsal—back of the hand; posterior surface

Directional References (Fig. 1-14)

- Medial—closer to the midline
- Lateral—further away from the midline
- Superior—toward the head
- Inferior—toward the feet
- Cephalic—toward the head (Fig. 1-15)
- Caudal—toward the feet (Fig. 1-16)

Body Movements

- Medial (internal) Rotation—rotating a part toward the midline
- Lateral (external) Rotation—rotating a part away from the midline (Fig. 1-17)
- Pronation—palmar surface of the hand faces down (Fig. 1-18)
- Supination—palmar surface of the hand faces up (Fig. 1-19)
- Abduction—to move or take away from midline (Fig. 1-20)
- Adduction—to move or bring closer to midline (Fig. 1-21)
- Flexion—to reduce the angle between two parts from neutral position (Figs. 1-22 & 1-23)
- Extension—to increase the angle between two parts from neutral position (Fig. 1-24)
- Circumduction—to move in a circle (Fig. 1-25)
- Plantar Flexion—toes are pointed down from natural foot position (Fig. 1-26)
- Dorsiflexion—toes pull back toward the patient's head from natural foot position (Fig. 1-27)
- Elevation—to raise
- Depression—to lower (Fig. 1-28)
- Tilt—to tip the vertex of the head toward the shoulder (Figs. 1-29 and 1-30)
- Rotation—to turn the patient's head to the side to look right or left or to roll an extremity toward or away from the midline (Fig. 1-31)
- Radial Deviation—With the hand pronated (palm down), the wrist and the thumb of the hand are diverted toward the radius (Fig. 1-32).
- Ulnar Deviation—With the hand pronated (palm down), the wrist and fifth digit of the hand are diverted toward the ulna (Fig. 1-33).

Inversion and Eversion Stress

- Inversion Stress—stress manipulation of foot and ankle toward the midline (Fig. 1-34)
- Eversion Stress—stress manipulation of the foot and ankle away from the midline (Fig. 1-35)

Location References (Fig. 1-36)

- Proximal—closer to the source
- Distal—further from the source

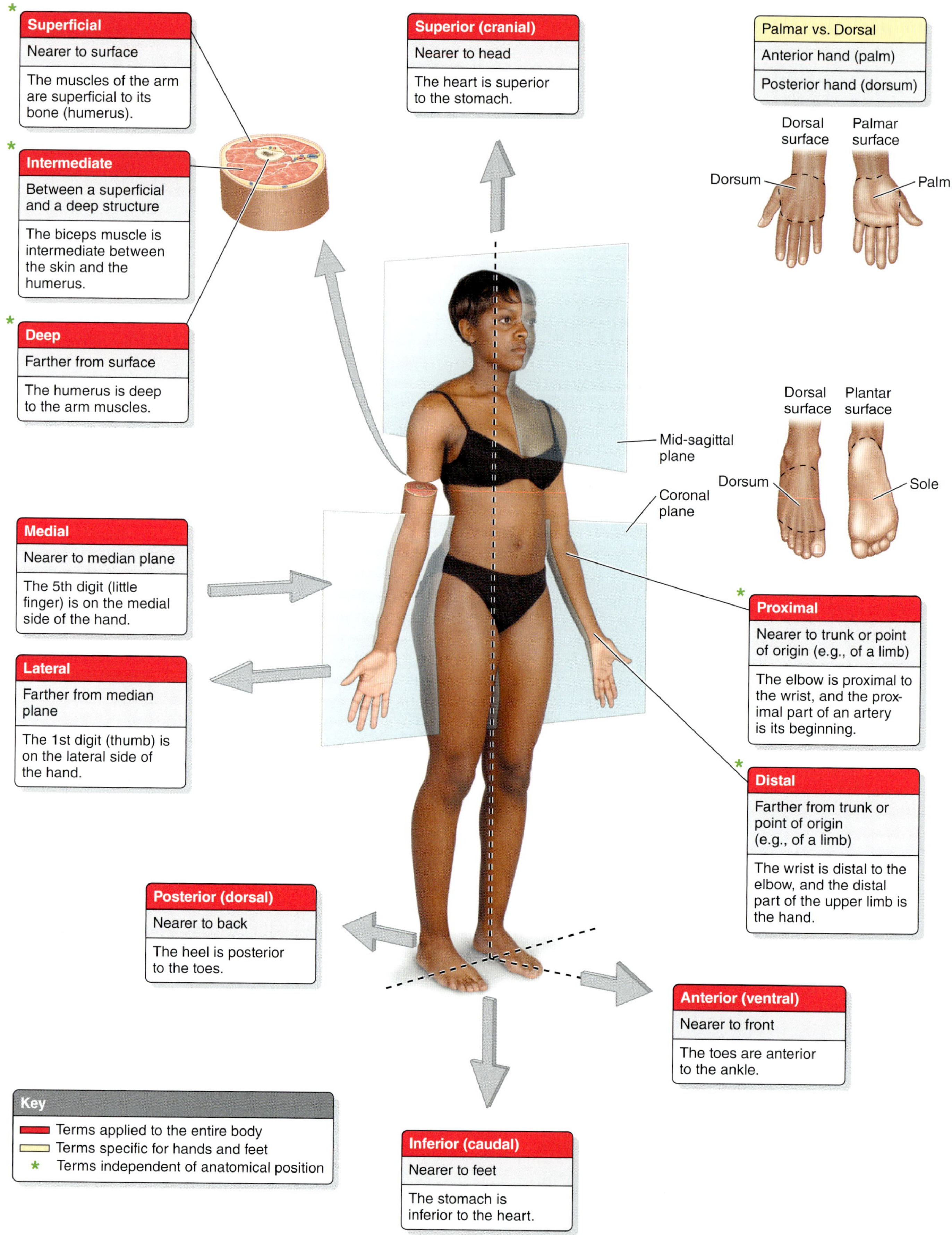

1-14 Anatomic references and surfaces of the body, hands, and feet.

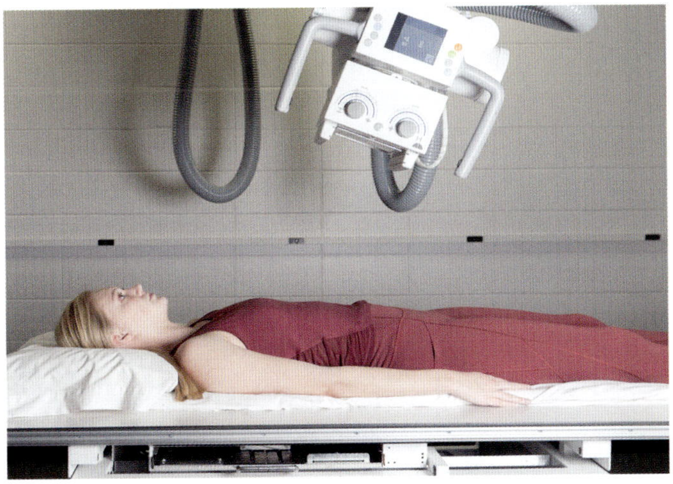

1-15 Cephalic tube angle.

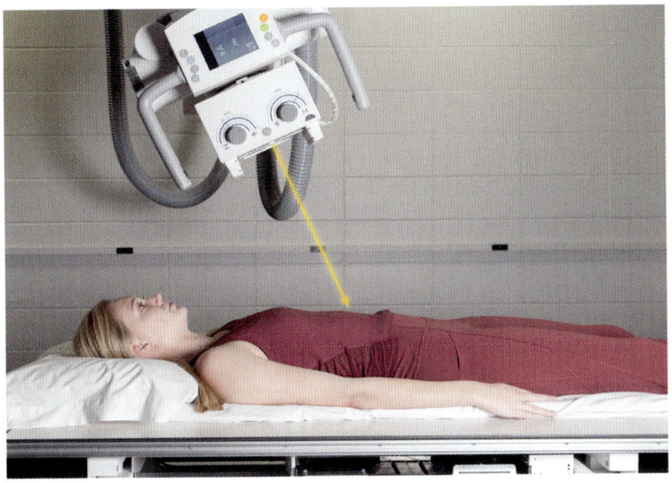

1-16 Caudal tube angle.

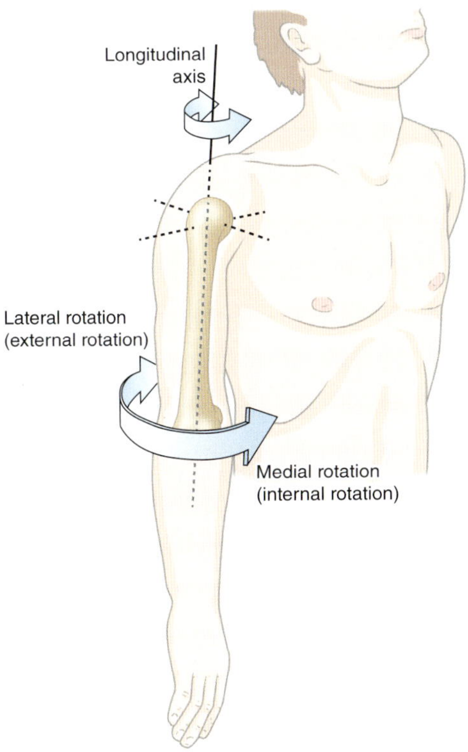

1-17 Medial versus lateral rotation.

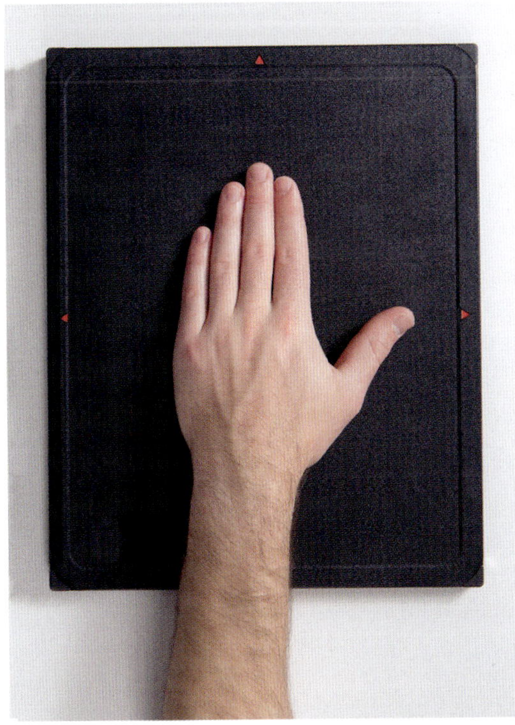

1-18 Pronation.

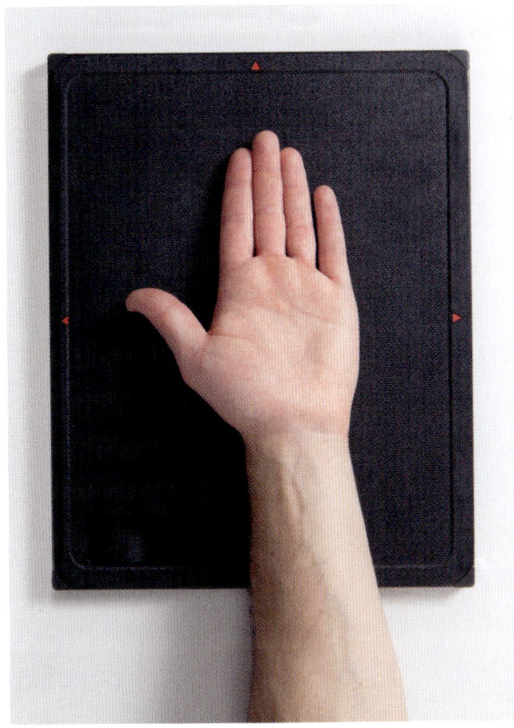

1-19 Supination.

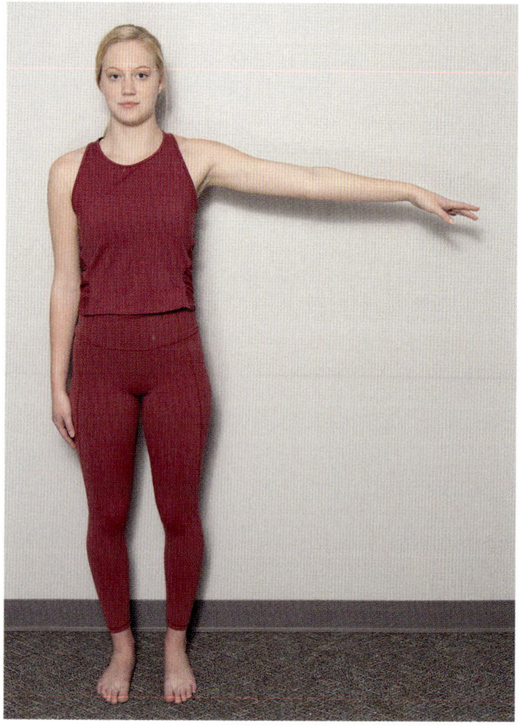

1-20 Abduction.

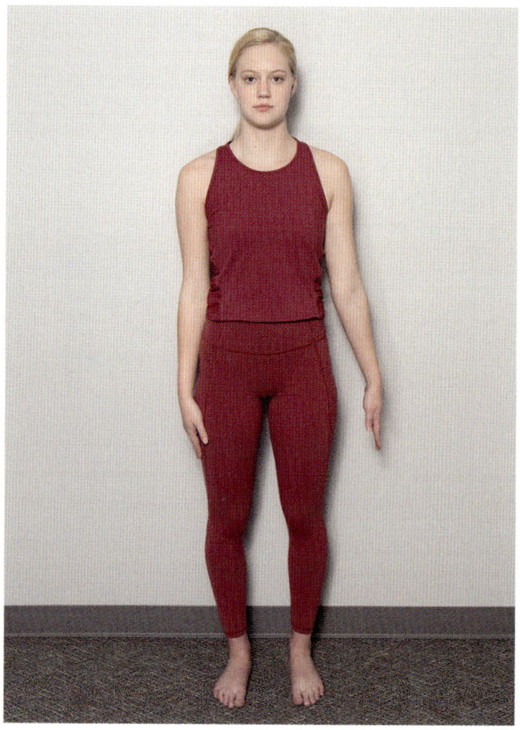

1-21 Adduction.

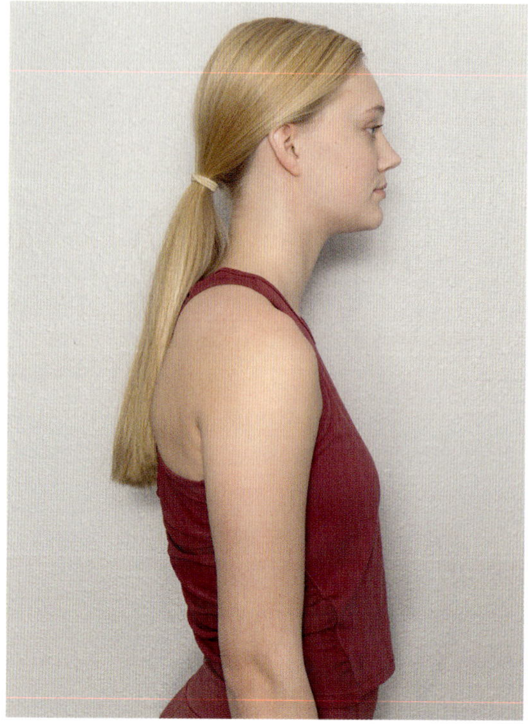

1-22 Neutral.

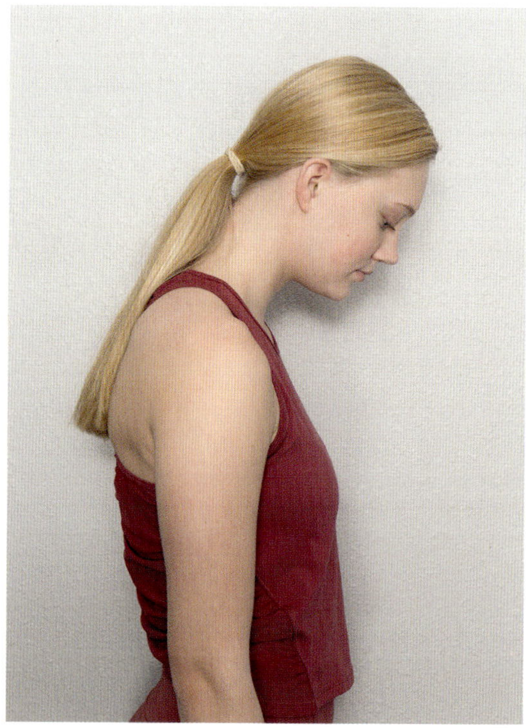

1-23 Flexion.

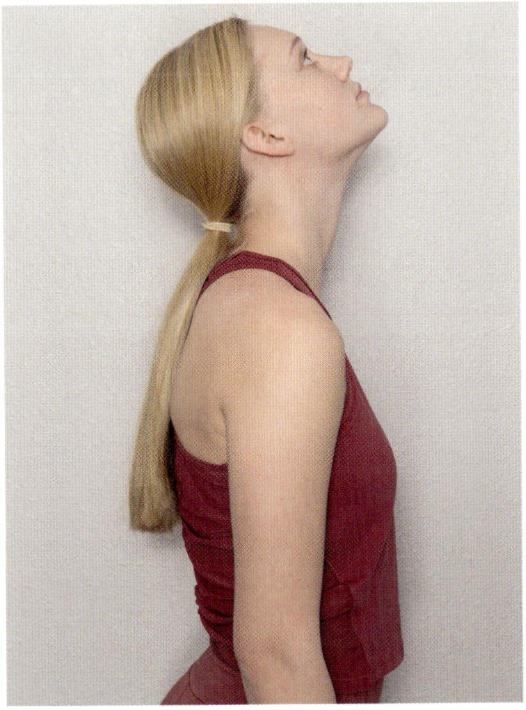

1-24 Extension.

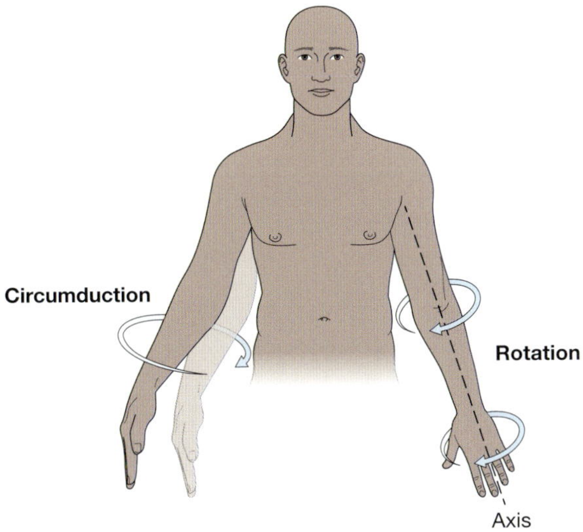

1-25 Rotation versus circumduction.

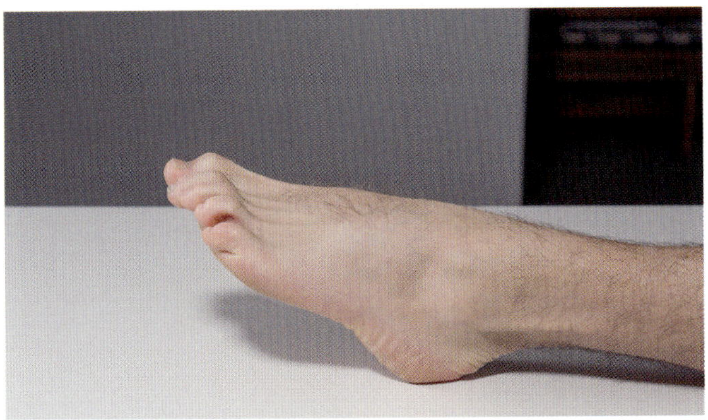

1-26 Plantar flexion.

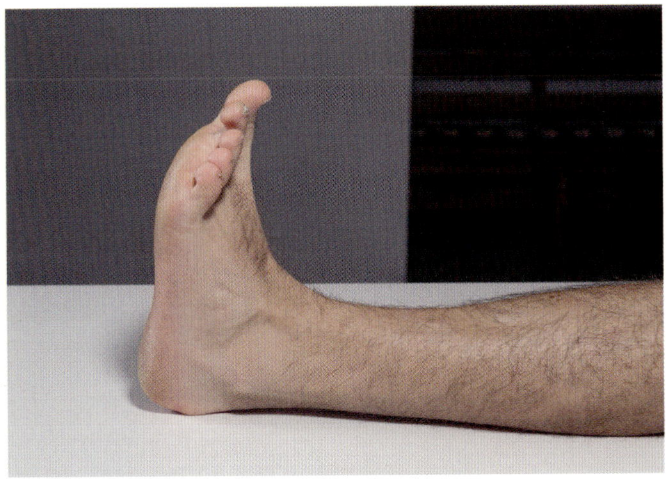

1-27 Dorsiflexion.

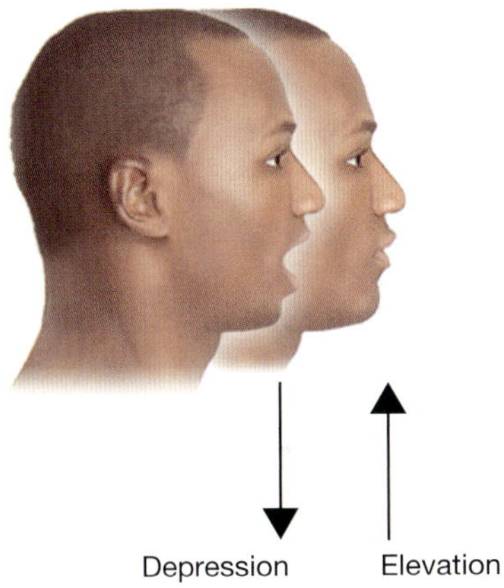

1-28 Elevation and depression.

Contralateral and Ipsilateral (Fig. 1-37)

- Contralateral—opposite side
- Ipsilateral—same side

PLANES

Midsagittal Plane (MSP)

A superior to inferior longitudinal plane that divides the body into *equal* right and left halves. (Fig. 1-38).

Sagittal Plane

A superior to inferior longitudinal plane that divides the body into right and left halves of some proportion but not into equal right and left halves (Fig. 1-38).

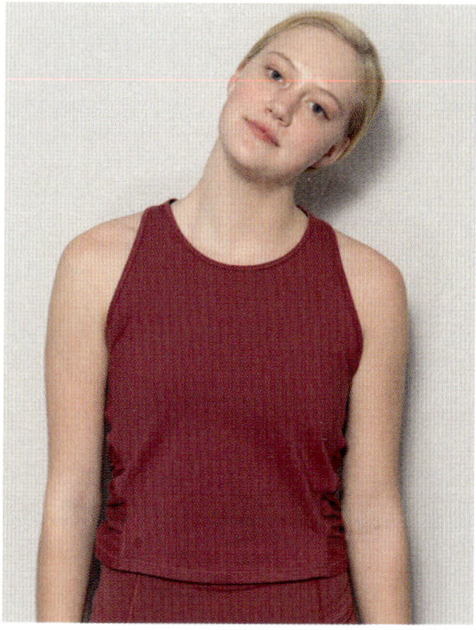

1-29 Tilt—vertex "tilt" toward the shoulder.

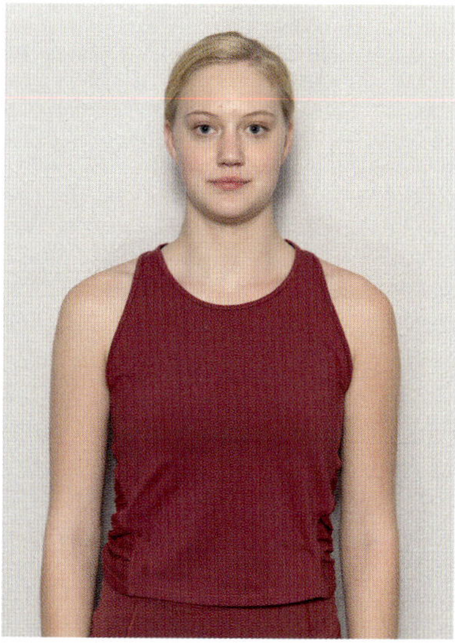

1-30 Neutral head position.

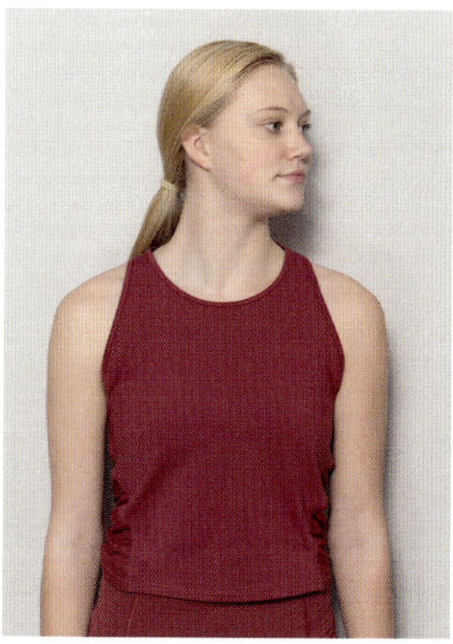

1-31 Rotate—to look toward the right or left side.

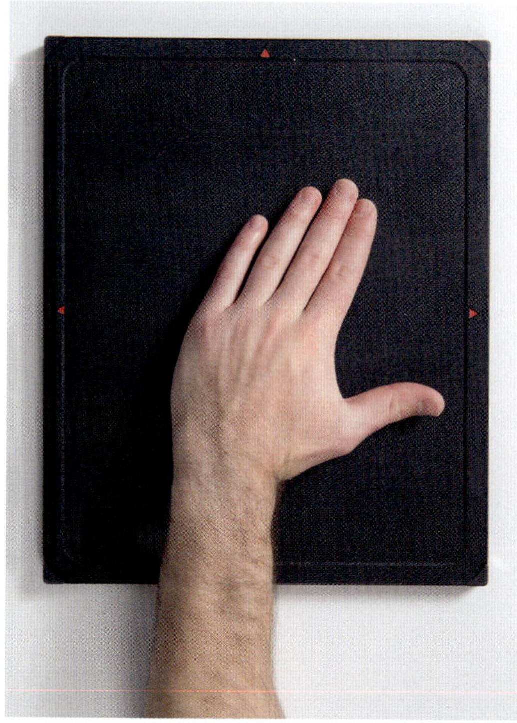

1-32 Radial deviation.

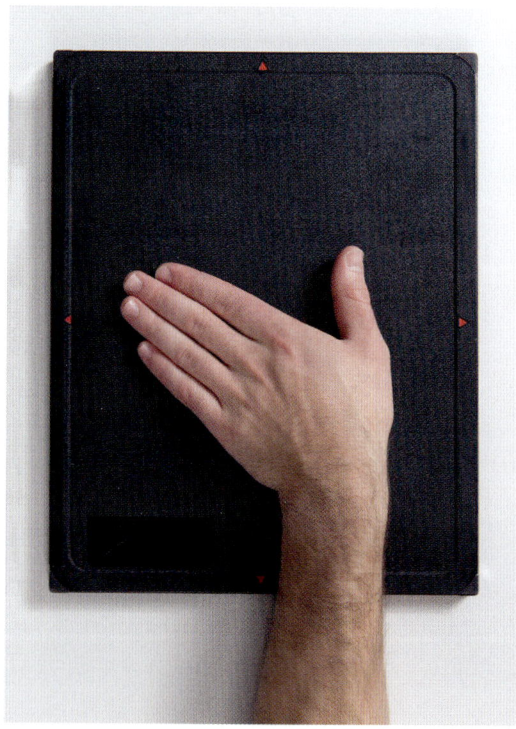

1-33 Ulnar deviation.

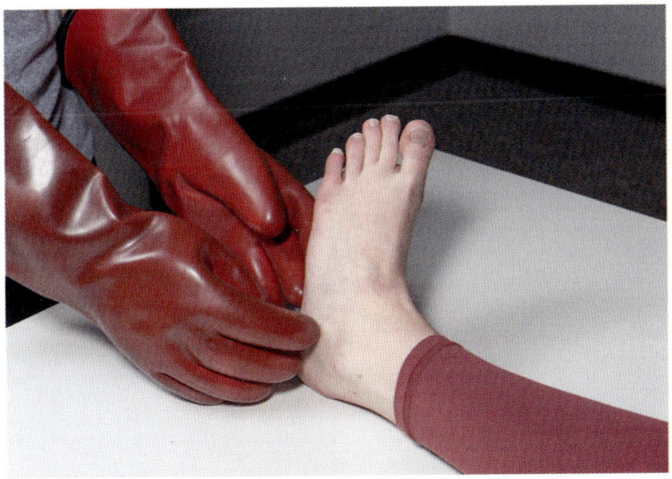

1-34 Inversion stress.

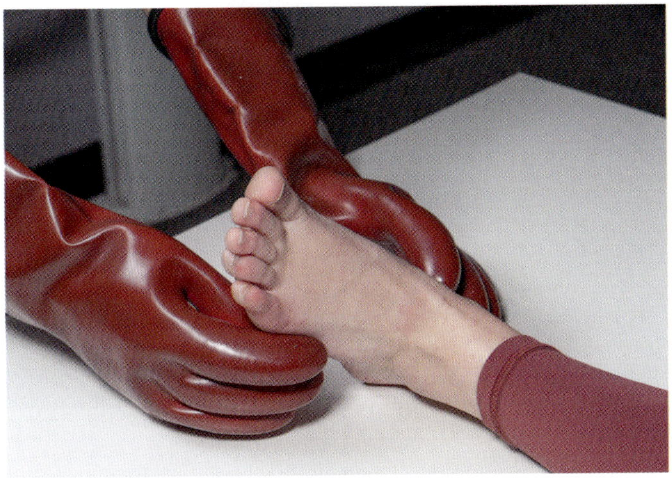

1-35 Eversion stress.

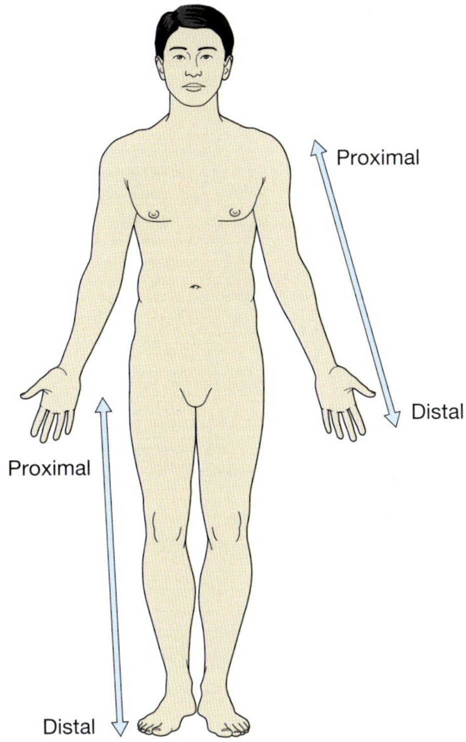

1-36 Proximal versus distal.

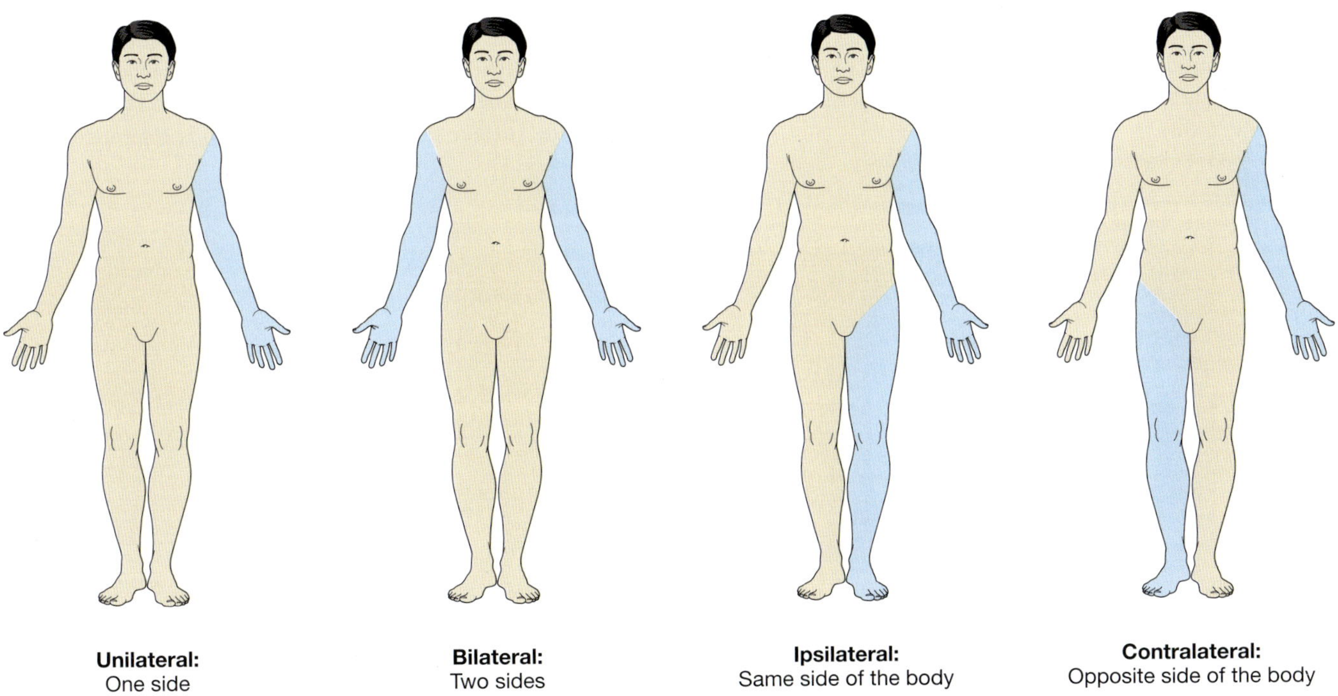

1-37 Contralateral versus ipsilateral.

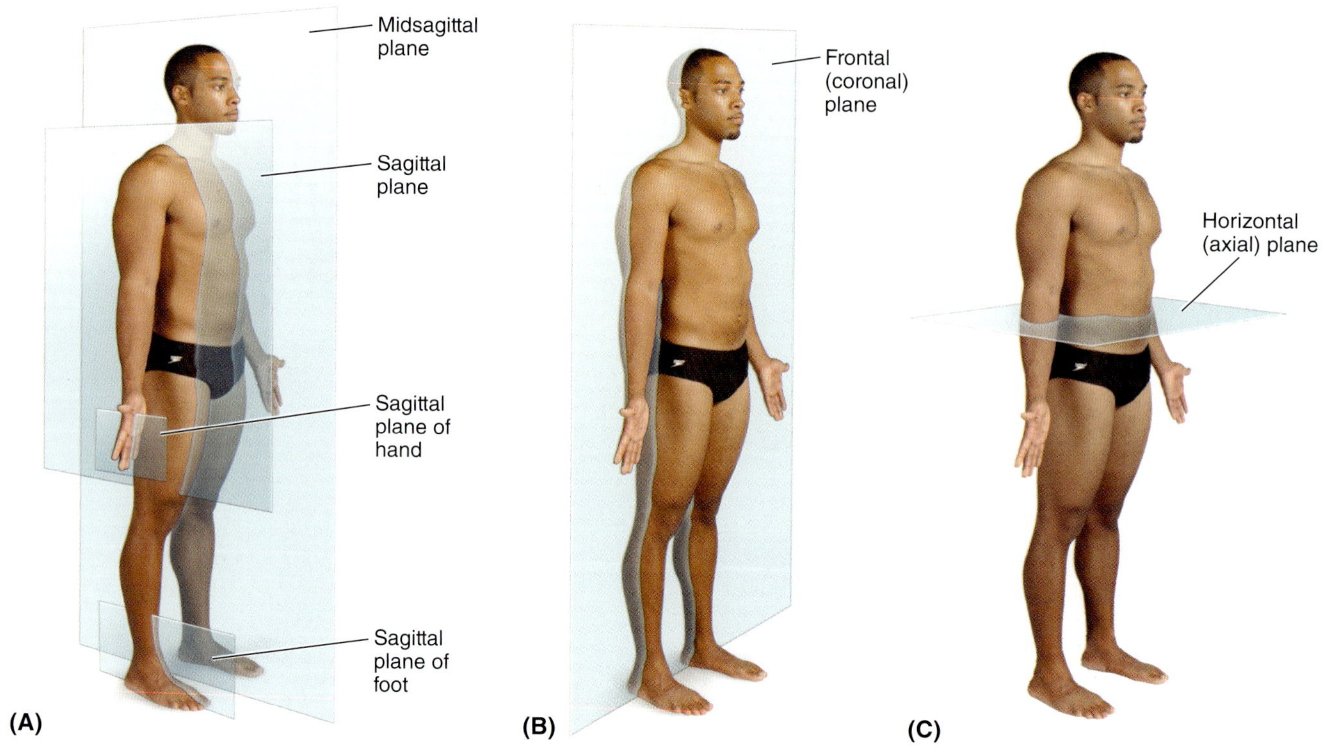

1-38 **(A)** Midsagittal plane versus sagittal plane. **(B)** Midcoronal plane versus coronal plane. **(C)** Horizontal or transverse plane.

Midcoronal Plane (MCP)

A superior to inferior longitudinal plane that divides the body into *equal* anterior and posterior halves (Fig. 1-38).

Coronal Plane

A superior to inferior longitudinal plane that divides the body into anterior and posterior halves of some proportion, but not into equal anterior and posterior halves (Fig. 1-38).

Horizontal/Axial/Transverse Plane

A 90° horizontal plane from longitudinal. The horizontal/transverse plane allows for visualization of structure in a cross section (Fig. 1-38).

POSITION

Describes the general body position of the patient. The following will cover the different positions, with focus on the more commonly used positions.

Recumbent

A general description of patient lying down, but could more accurately be referenced as:

- Supine: Patient lying down on their posterior surface (Fig. 1-39)
- Prone: Patient lying down on their anterior surface (Fig. 1-40)
- Lateral: Patient lying on their right or left lateral surface; the side surface the patient is lying on is referenced as the

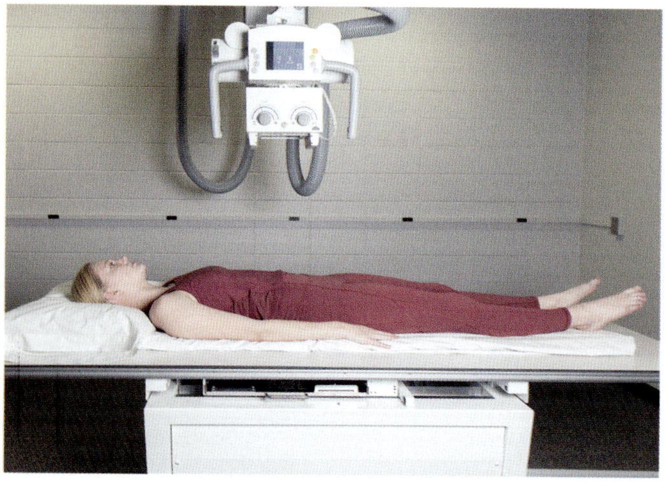

1-39 Supine position.

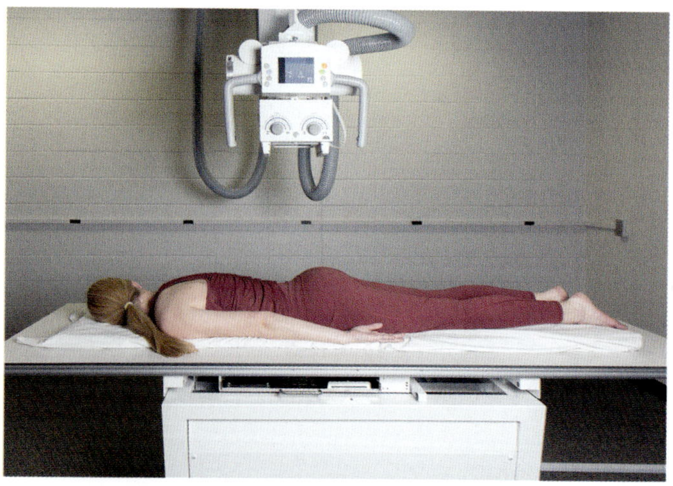

1-40 Prone position.

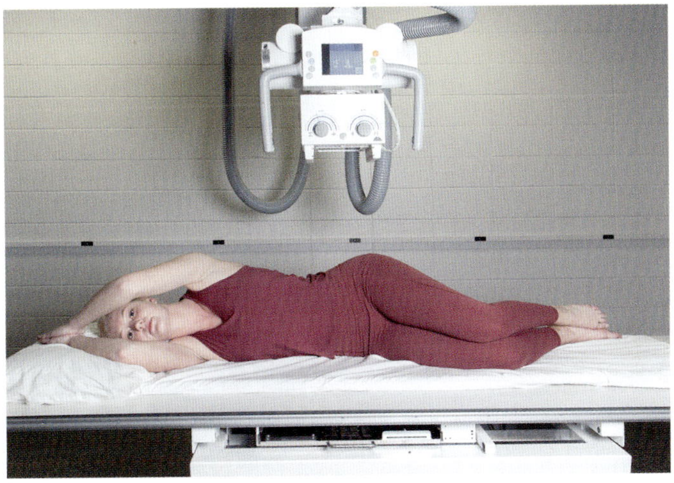

1-41 Recumbent right lateral position.

patient position. For example, a patient lying on their right-lateral side would best describe the patient position as recumbent right lateral (Fig. 1-41).

- Fowler's: The supine patient can be adjusted to position the head higher than the feet (Fig. 1-42).
- Trendelenburg: The supine patient can be adjusted to position the head lower than the feet (Fig. 1-43).

Recumbent Posterior Oblique

Right or Left Posterior Oblique (RPO or LPO) positions. The patient begins in the supine position. From supine, the patient is rotated to place either the right or the left side closer to the IR to create a RPO or LPO. The position is determined by the side and surface arranged closest to the image receptor (IR). Although various degrees of rotational oblique(s) are possible, the 45° oblique is most common (Figs. 1-44 and 1-45).

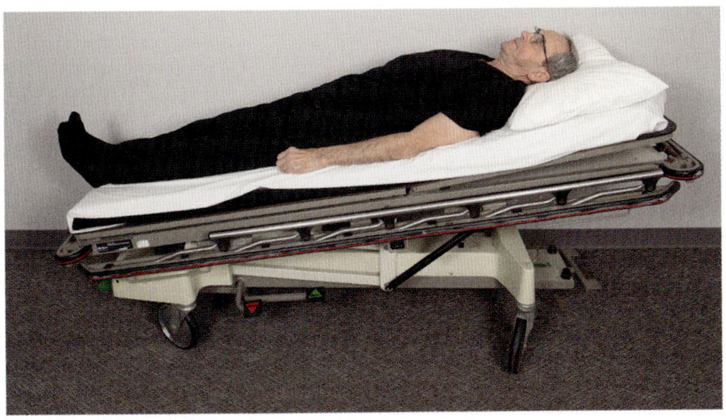

1-42 Fowler's position.

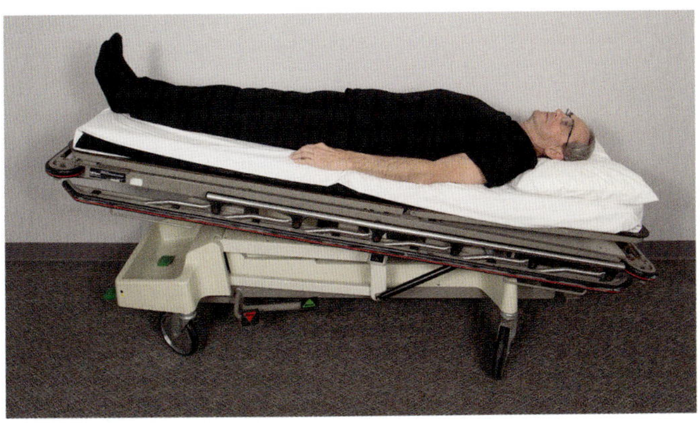

1-43 Trendelenburg position.

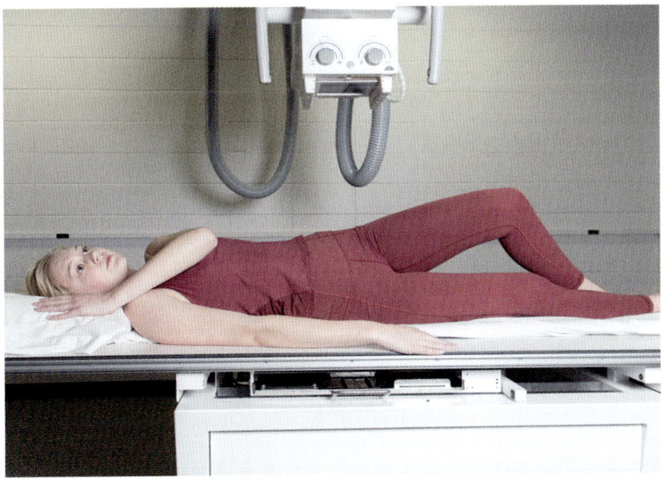

1-44 Recumbent RPO position.

Recumbent Anterior Oblique

Right or Left Anterior Oblique (RAO or LAO) positions. The patient begins in prone position. From prone, the patient rotates either the right or left side closer to the IR to create an RAO or LAO. The position is determined by the side and surface arranged closest to the image receptor (IR). Although various degrees of rotational oblique(s) are possible; the 45° oblique is most common (Figs. 1-46 and 1-47).

Upright

Patient is able to stand or sit upright. This position can prove helpful to demonstrate air–fluid levels in a particular cavity of interest.

Upright Lateral

Patient standing up with either their left or right side closest to the image receptor best describes the patient position as upright/erect left or right lateral position (Fig. 1-48).

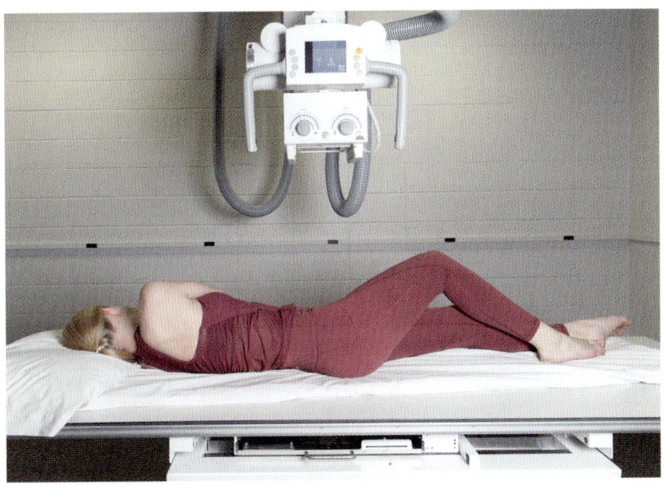

1-45 Recumbent LPO position.

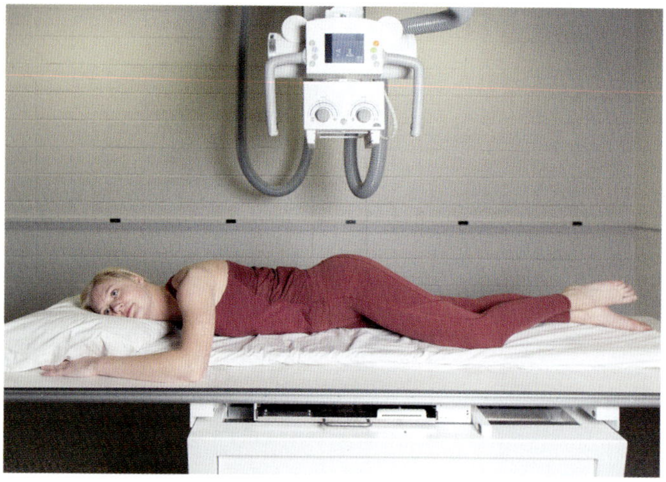

1-46 Recumbent RAO position.

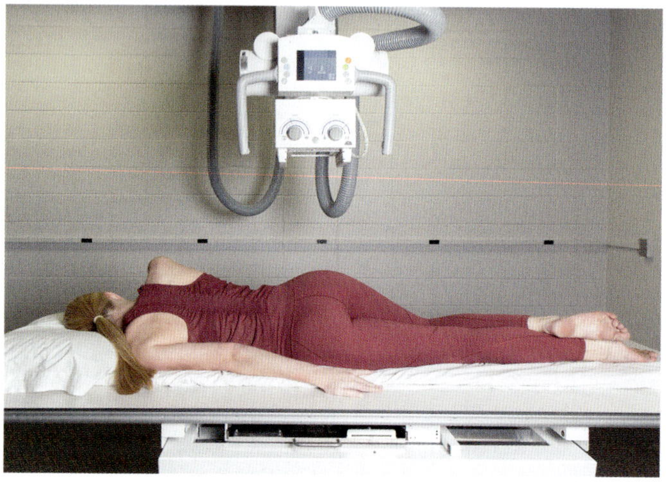

1-47 Recumbent LAO position.

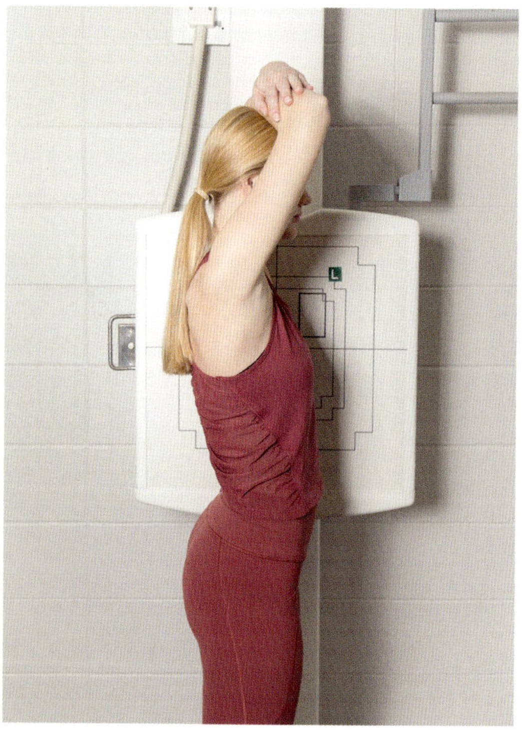

1-48 Erect left lateral position.

Upright Posterior Oblique

The patient stands to face the tube and then is rotated to place either the right or left side closer to the image receptor to create a RPO or LPO position (Figs. 1-49 and 1-50).

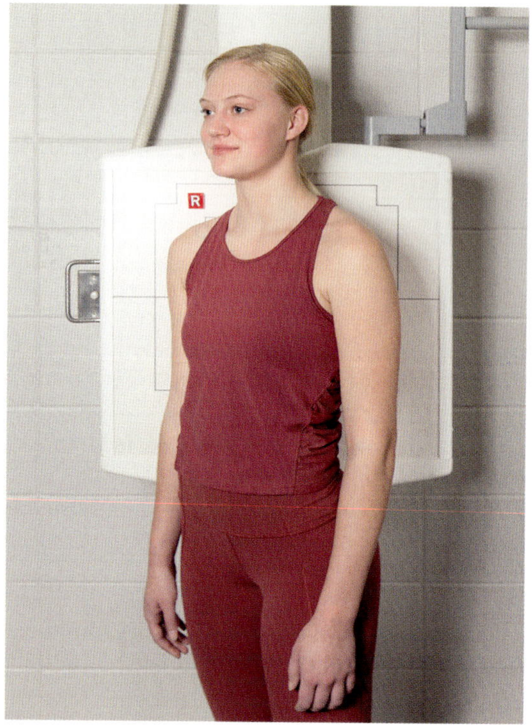

1-49 Erect RPO position.

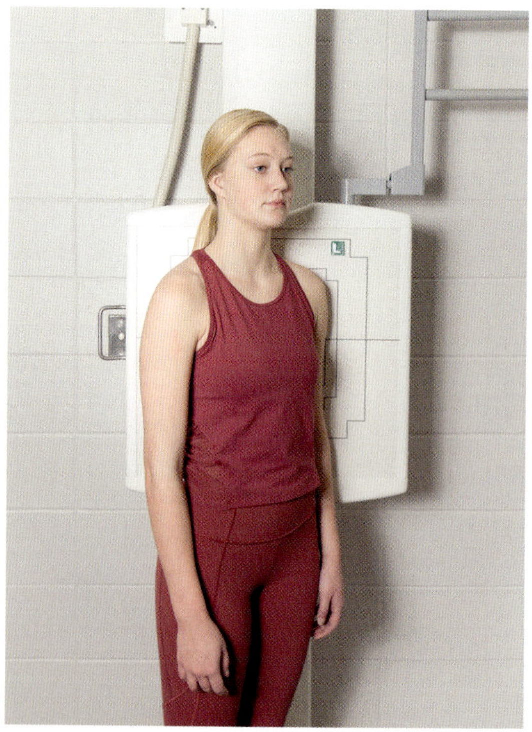

1-50 Erect LPO position.

Upright Anterior Oblique

The patient stands to face the upright Bucky and then is rotated to place either the right or left side closer to the image receptor to create a RAO or LAO position (Figs. 1-51 and 1-52).

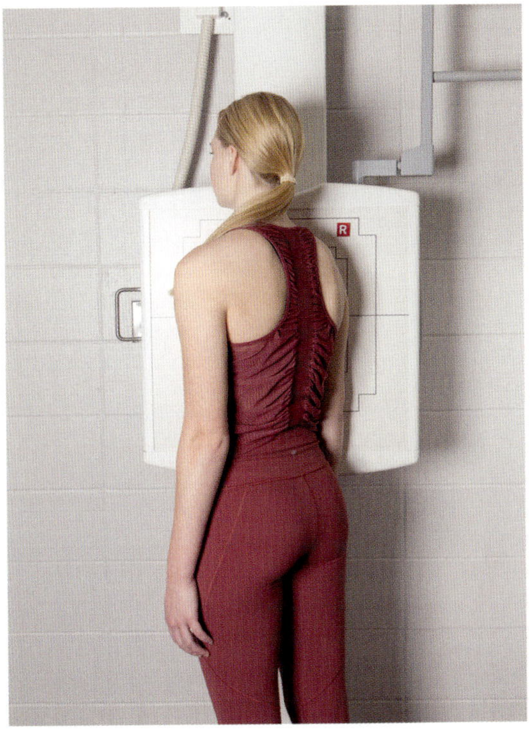

1-51 Erect RAO position.

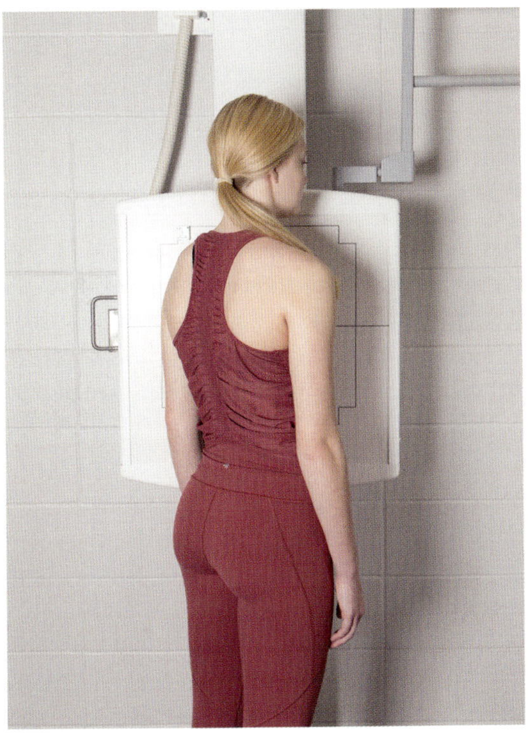

1-52 Erect LAO position.

Decubitus

This position is used in instances in which an air–fluid level is necessary to determine to a body cavity. A decubitus position could replace an upright position. The patient must lie in a decubitus position for a minimum of 5 minutes, but longer could be advantageous. Within the passing time while the patient is lying in the position, air will rise to the upside or highest point in the cavity and fluid will collect on the downside or lowest point, if free air or fluid is present. Most commonly, the right and left lateral decubitus (RLD and LLD) position(s) are used; however, a dorsal or ventral decubitus could also be implemented. In order to demonstrate the potential free air or fluid, after the patient is rotated into position, the technologist will adjust the tube head to create a horizontal beam. The beam pathway would be directed from the tube toward the patient while horizontal to the floor (Figs. 1-53 to 1-56).

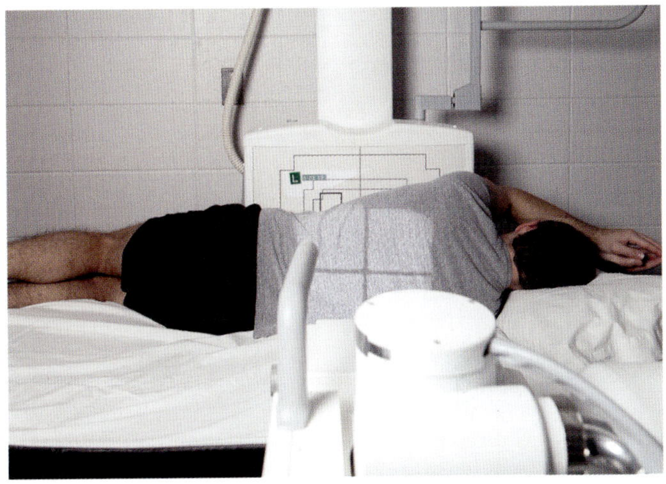

1-53 RLD position.

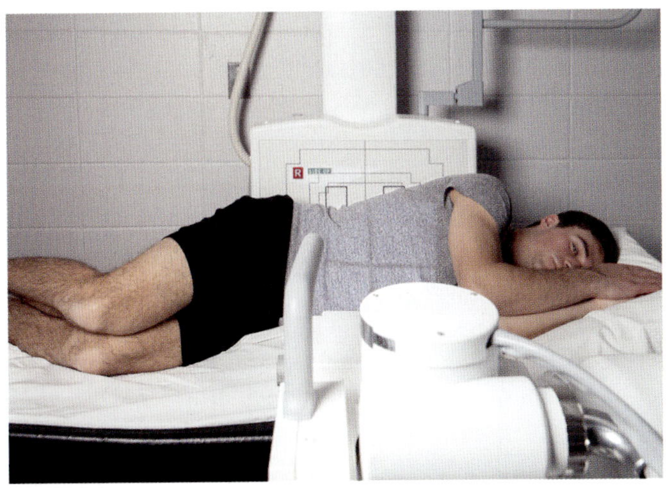

1-54 LLD position.

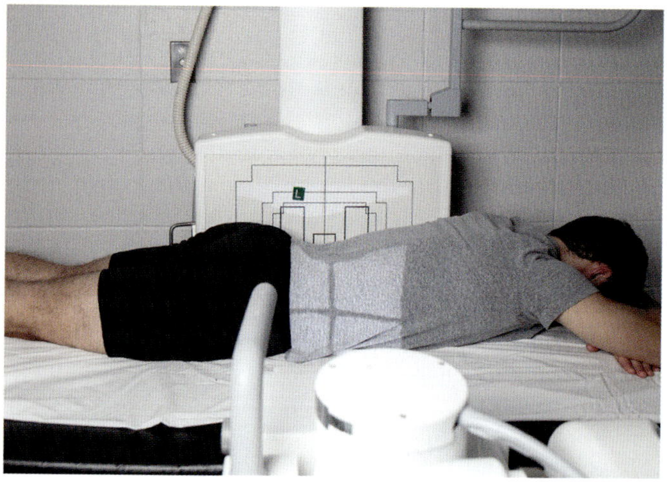

1-55 Ventral decubitus position.

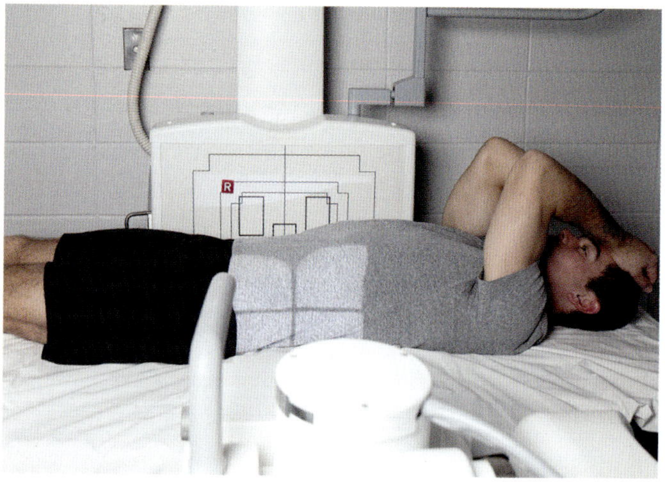

1-56 Dorsal decubitus position.

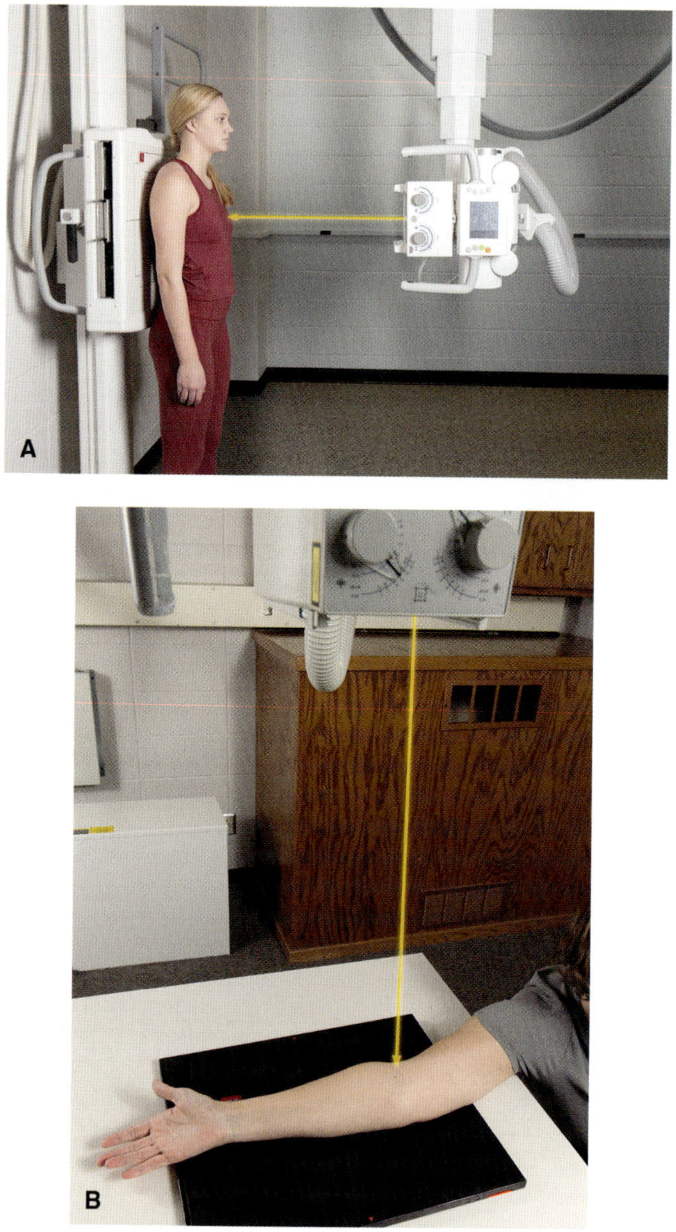

1-57 **(A)** AP projection of torso. **(B)** AP projection of elbow.

PROJECTION

Projection describes the path of the x-ray beam as it enters its first surface of the patient, exits the opposite surface, and then strikes the image receptor.

Anteroposterior (AP) Projection

The path of the beam exits the tube, enters the anterior surface, exits the posterior surface, and strikes the IR (Fig. 1-57). An AP projection could be attained with the patient seated for a tabletop extremity, supine, upright, or in a RLD or LLD position.

Posteroanterior (PA) Projection

The path of the beam exits the tube, enters the posterior surface, exits the anterior surface, and strikes the IR (Fig. 1-58). A PA projection could be attained with the patient seated for a tabletop extremity, prone, upright, or in a RLD or LLD position.

Mediolateral (ML) Projection (extremities)

Begin by identifying the medial and lateral surfaces of a limb based off anatomic position. With an ML projection, the path of the beam will exit the tube, enter the medial surface of the part, exit the lateral surface of the part, and strike the IR (Fig. 1-59).

Lateromedial (LM) Projection (extremities)

Begin by identifying the medial and lateral surfaces of a limb based off anatomic position. With an LM projection, the path of the beam will exit the tube, enter the lateral surface of the part, exit the medial surface of the part, and strikes the IR (Fig. 1-60).

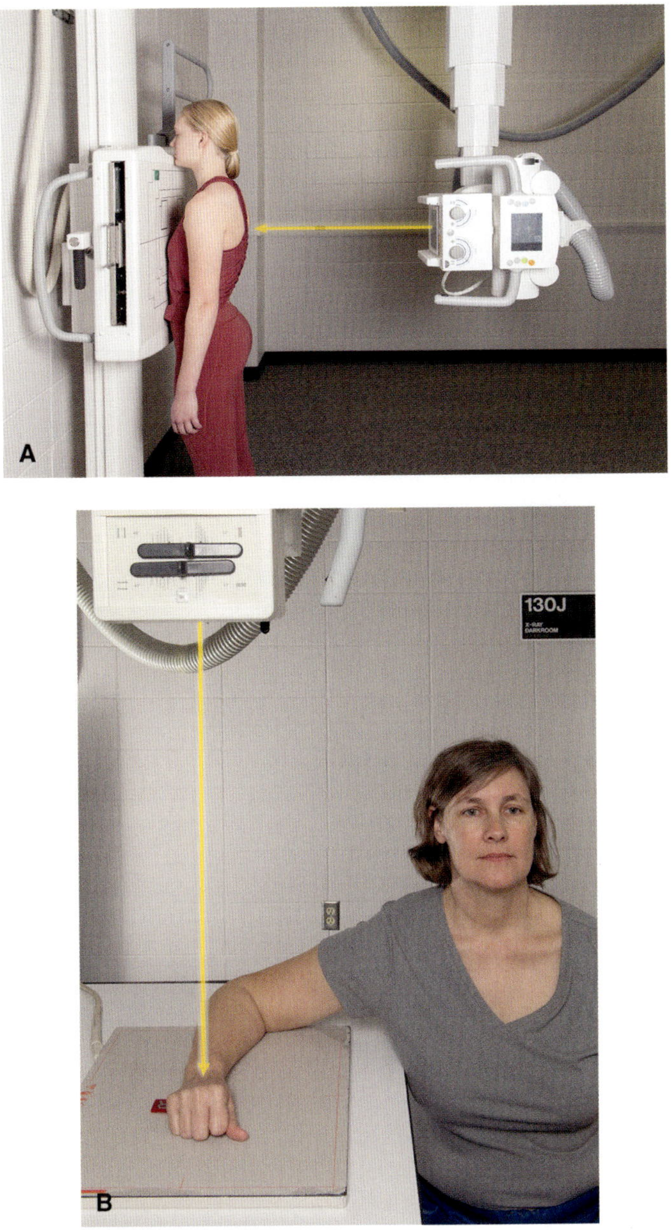

1-58 **(A)** PA projection of torso. **(B)** PA projection of wrist.

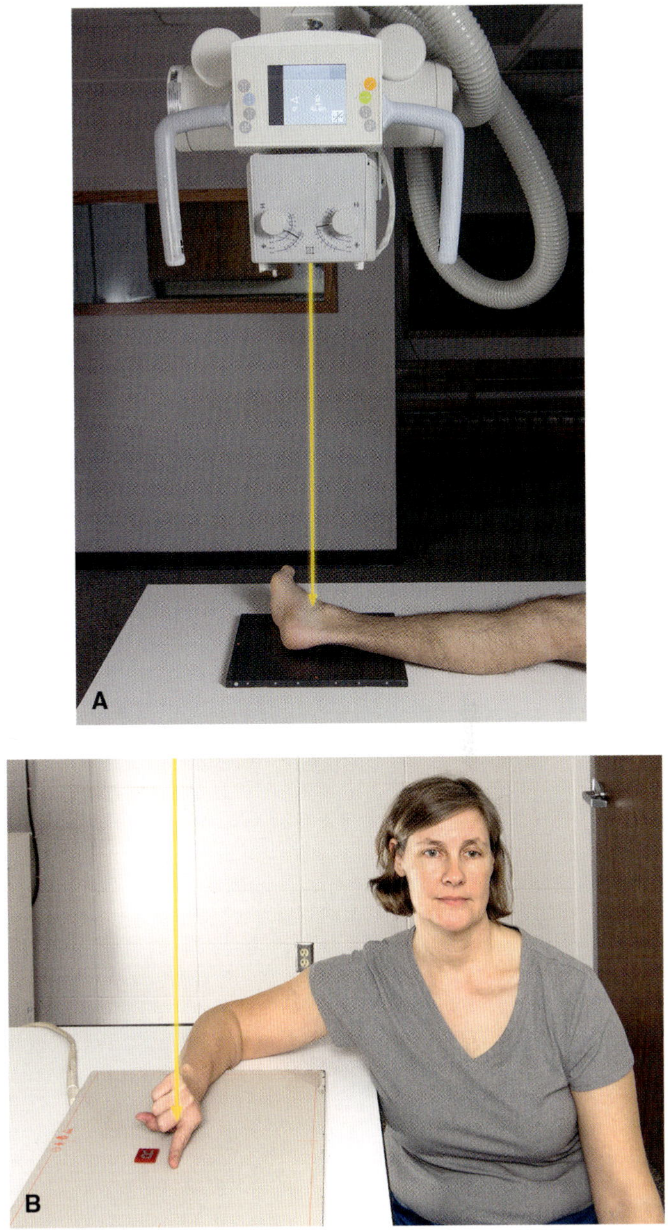

1-59 **(A)** Mediolateral projection of the ankle. **(B)** Mediolateral projection of the second digit.

AP Oblique

The patient will face the tube and will be positioned into an RPO or LPO position. When the patient is in an RPO or LPO position, the path of the beam will exit the tube, enter the anterior surface, exit the posterior surface of the part, and strike the IR. Since the part is in an oblique position, this must be identified in the projection (Fig. 1-61). The AP oblique is also referenced on the extremity.

PA Oblique

The patient will face away from the tube and will be positioned into an LAO or RAO position. When the patient is in an RAO or LAO position, the path of the beam will exit the tube, enter the posterior surface, exit the anterior surface of the part and strike the IR. Since the part is in an oblique position, this must be identified in the projection (Fig. 1-62). The PA oblique is also referenced on the extremity.

Axial Projections

The beam is angled across a part. The beam may be angled toward the head or feet. The projection must identify the projection pathway (AP or PA) and then also identify axial in the projection name to indicate a tube angle was utilized (Fig. 1-63).

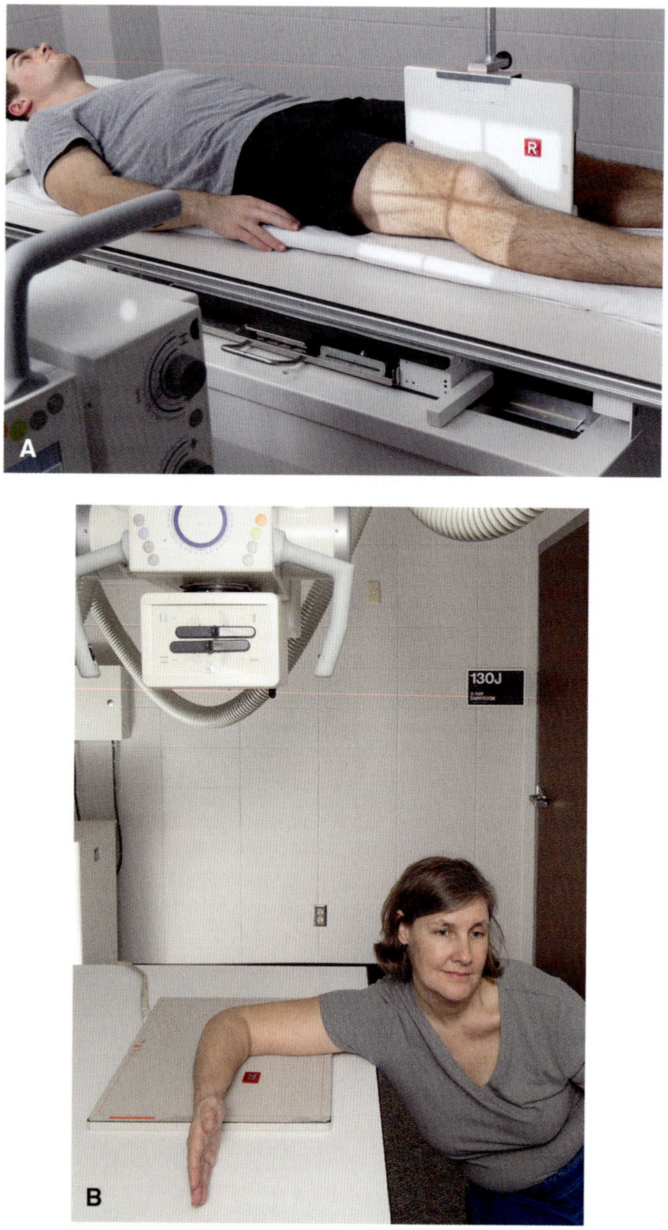

1-60 **(A)** Lateromedial projection of the knee. **(B)** Lateromedial projection of the forearm.

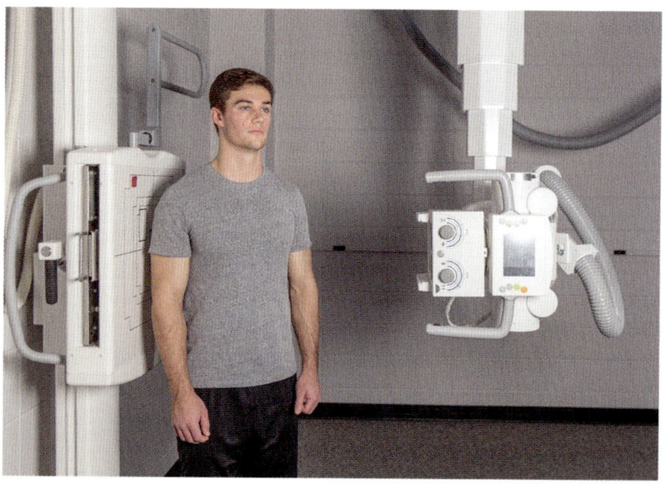

1-61 AP oblique projection.

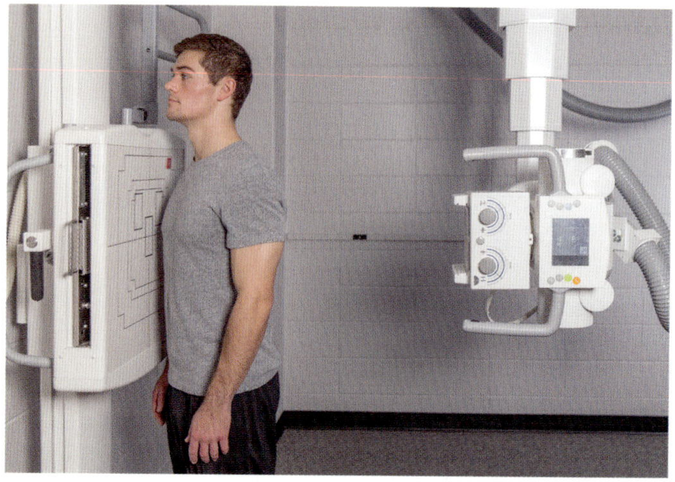

1-62 PA oblique projection.

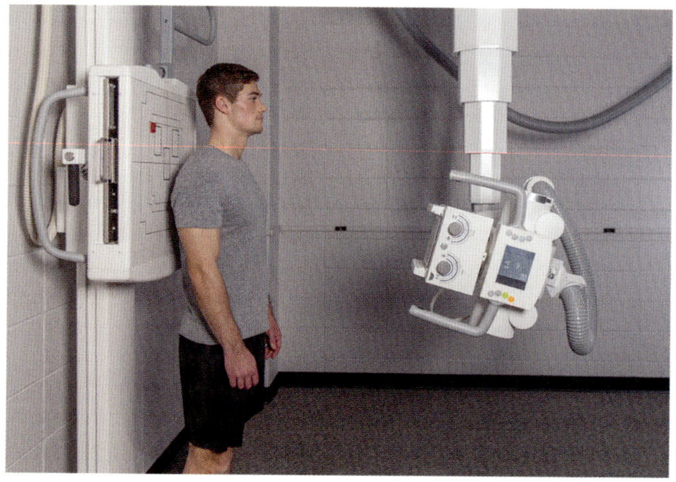

1-63 AP axial projection.

Tangential Projections

The beam skims the surface of the anatomy to produce a profile of the anatomy of interest (Fig. 1-64).

Dorsoplantar

This beam is passing through the reference surfaces of the foot. Dorsum is the top of the foot. Plantar is the sole of the foot (Fig. 1-65). In instances where the beam passes through the foot surfaces with a tube angle added, the projection becomes dorsoplantar axial.

Plantodorsal

This beam is passing through the reference surfaces of the foot. Plantar surface is the sole of the foot. Dorsum is the top of the foot (Fig. 1-66). In instances where the beam passes through the foot surfaces with a tube angle added, the projection becomes plantodorsal axial.

BODY HABITUS

There are three general types of habitus to accommodate in chest and abdominal imaging. It is important to realize that

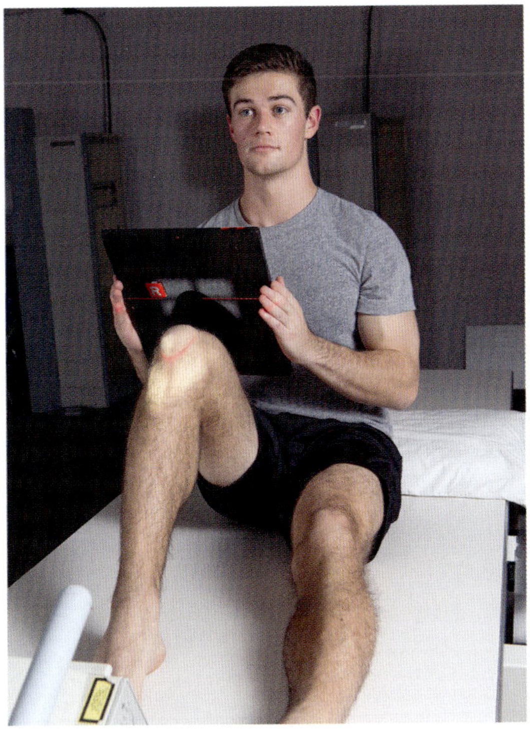

1-64 Tangential projection.

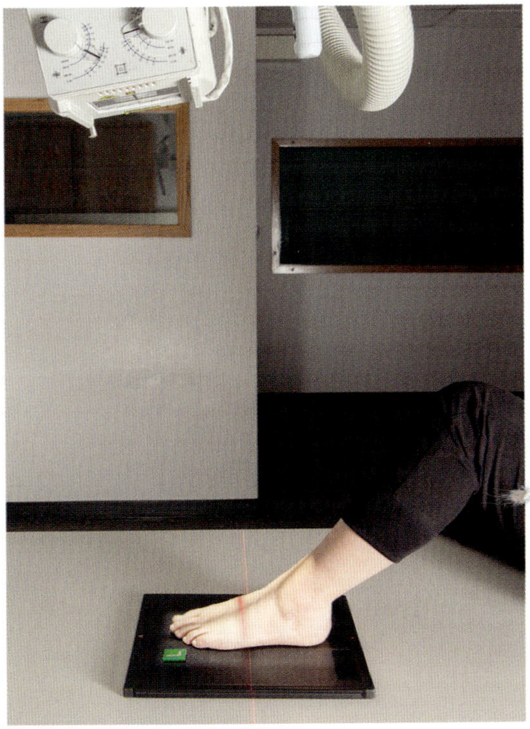

1-65 Dorsoplantar projection.

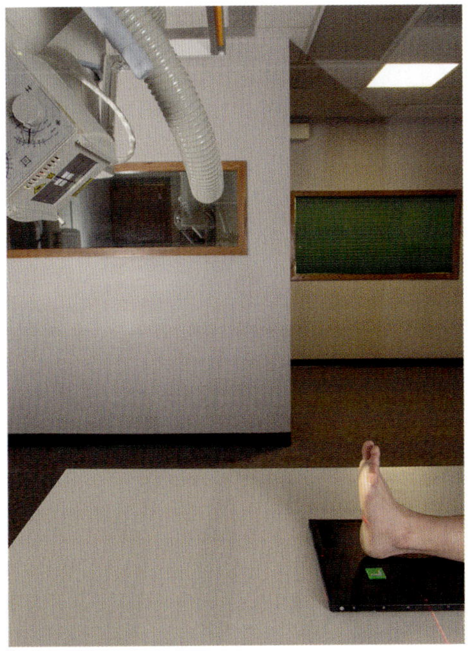

1-66 Plantodorsal axial projection.

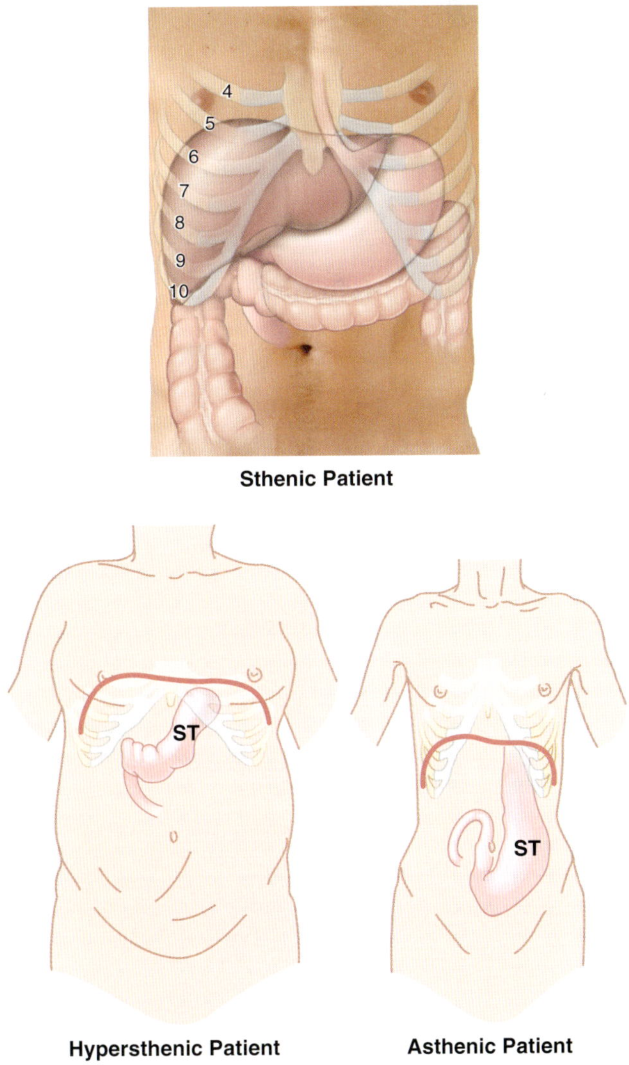

1-67 Body habitus comparison and the effect on organ placement.

a body habitus influences the location of internal structures (Fig. 1-67).

Body Habitus and Suggested Image Receptor (IR) Orientation

Sthenic Patient: This patient represents the most average size dimension in the population. The patient is of modest height

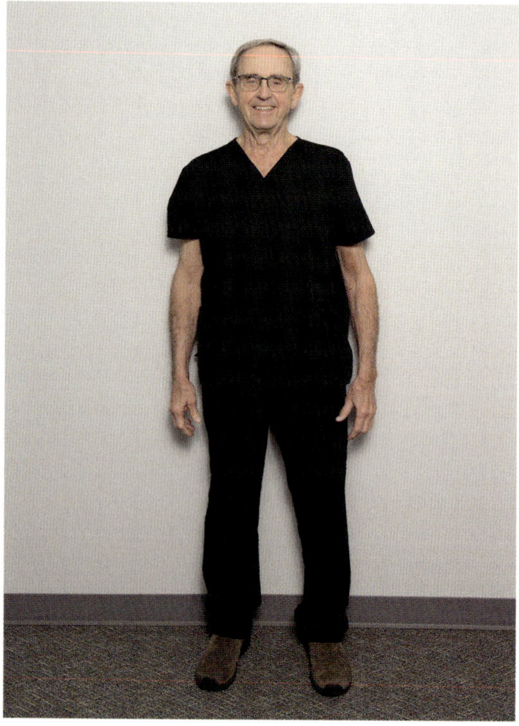

1-68 Sthenic patient.

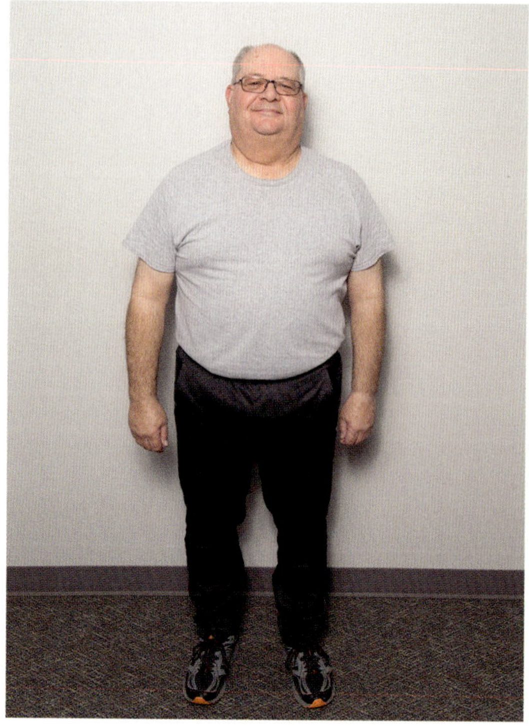

1-70 Hypersthenic patient.

and weight. The lungs are of average magnitude in vertical, width, and thickness dimensions. The abdominal structures are all located as described for that "textbook" patient (Fig. 1-68). A 14 × 17 IR will be orientated lengthwise for the chest and the abdomen (Fig. 1-69).

Hypersthenic Patient: This patient is broad through the shoulders and chest. The lungs would be expected to be wider across (transverse) and shorter vertically. The stomach will sit high within the abdominal cavity, more transverse across the abdomen beneath the diaphragm (Fig. 1-70). Therefore, it is recommended that a 14 × 17 IR be orientated crosswise (landscape) when imaging the chest. Two crosswise overlapping IRs are often necessary when imaging the abdomen (Fig. 1-71).

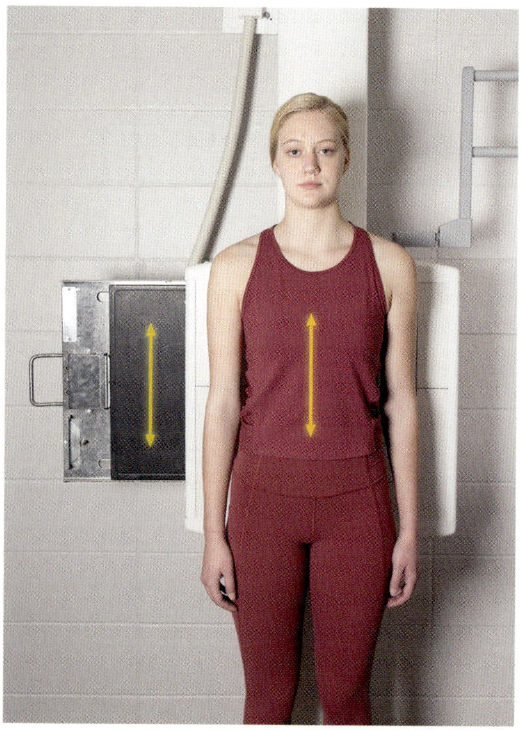

1-69 Lengthwise orientation of the IR to the patient.

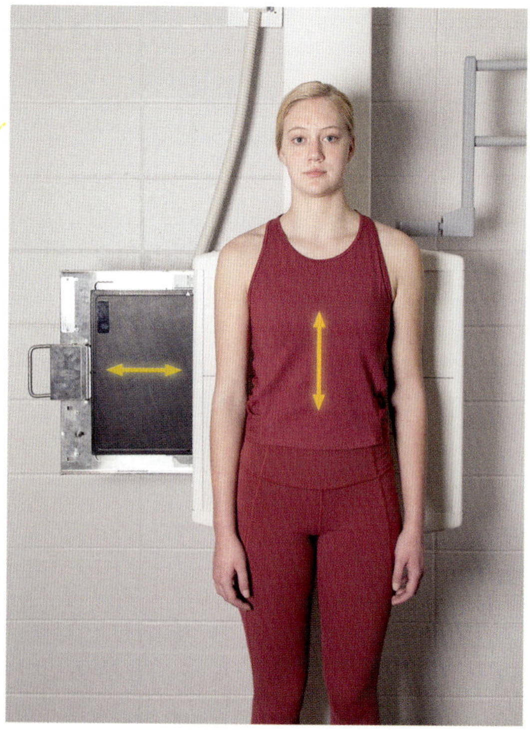

1-71 Crosswise or landscape orientation of the IR to the patient.

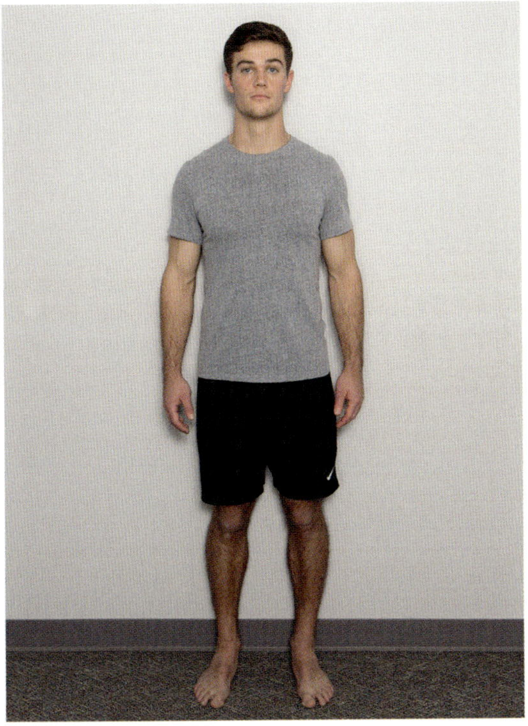

1-72 Hyposthenic patient.

Asthenic/Hyposthenic Patient: These two patient types are long and lean through the thorax and abdomen. The lungs would be expected to be longer vertically than the width across. The stomach has the appearance of an elongated "J," which will dip down deep into the pelvis. The bowel will be positioned lower in the abdomen (Fig. 1-72).

EXAM ORDER OF OPERATION

An order of operations is recommended when it comes to performing procedures to aid in exam efficiency, accuracy, and exam completeness (Table 1-1).

Review of the Exam Order

A review of the exam order before retrieving the patient is recommended before starting the imaging procedure. The technologist should be familiar with the exam ordered and the exam protocol before acquiring the patient. The technologist may have access to previous images acquired, correlative imaging studies, and/or lab values necessary for the exam ordered.

Room Setup

The imaging room should be set up for the procedure before bringing the patient in. This contributes to efficiency and organization of the exam. The technologist should ensure all supplies necessary for the exam are ready within the exam room to minimize the need to leave the patient unattended (Figs. 1-73).

Control Panel

As part of room setup, the control panel could also be initially set to designate kVp, mAs or automatic exposure control

1-1 Order of Operations

1. Review the patient order. Determine the exam, patient location, and patient transport.
2. Set up the room for the procedure.
3. Set the control panel in anticipation of an averaged sized patient.
4. Acquire the patient, introduce yourself, verify patient identification.
5. Confirm the exam ordered.
6. Patient dressed into a gown as needed for the procedure.
7. Acquire patient history and rule out potential pregnancy for a reproductive aged female.
8. Explain the procedure to the patient; acquire consent.
9. Determine recumbent or upright positioning; establish the tube detent when imaging in the Bucky.
10. Adjust the control panel if different from what was preset before beginning to position the patient.
11. Position the patient.
12. Center to the part; mark the image; apply collimation.
13. Keep a visual eye on the patient and walk to the control panel. Give breathing instructions and watch to ensure patient is following instruction.
14. Make the exposure. Tell the patient to relax.
15. Reset the control panel for the next projection. Change the image receptor out if using computed radiography.
16. Repeat the preceding steps each time.
17. Evaluate all projections ensure proper positioning and diagnostic quality.
18. Inform the patient when to expect results and how to acquire exam results.
19. Release the patient.
20. Clean and reset room for next exam.

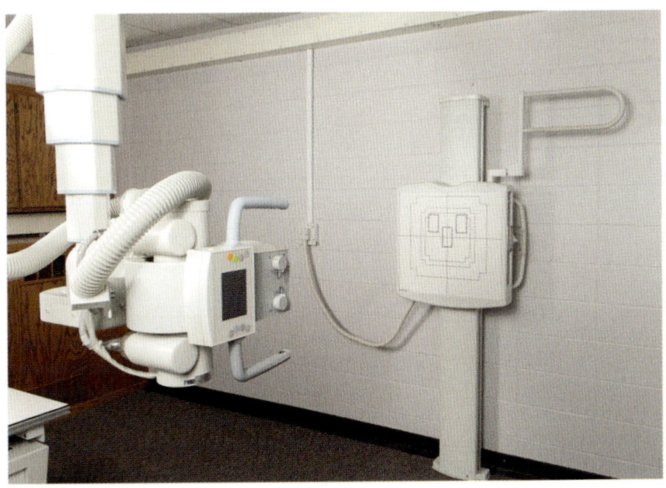

1-73 Imaging room setup with the tube directed at the upright Bucky.

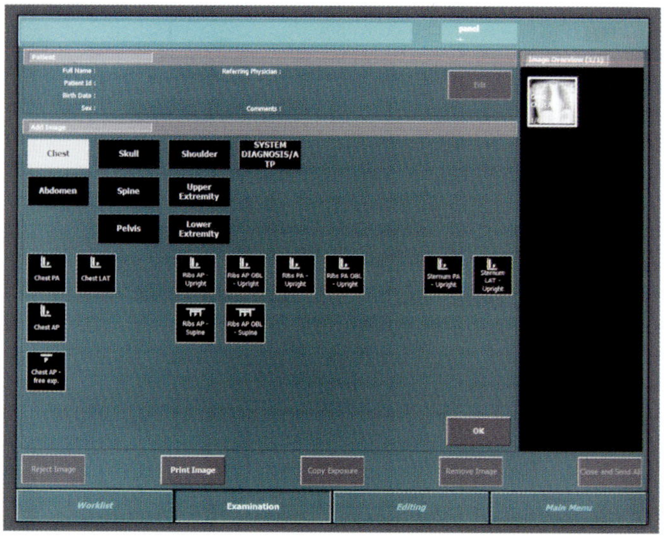

1-74 Direct radiography—exam setup.

(AEC), focal spot size, and IR location. Once the technologist brings the patient into the exam room, the control panel may still need to be adjusted according to how the technologist chooses to complete the exam and the type of patient body habitus. It is recommended that the technologist adjust the control panel as needed each time prior to positioning the patient. By setting the control panel before positioning the patient, this eliminates the need for the patient to wait and hold a position while the technologist adjusts the control panel (Figs. 1-74 and 1-75).

Source to Image Distance (SID)

The SID is commonly established at 40″, 44″, or 72″ depending on the procedure. Increasing SID will reduce structure magnification to improve image detail. Distance will also affect the quantity of photons (mAs) reaching the IR (Fig. 1-76).

Designating the Image Receptor Location

On the control panel, the technologist will identify where the exposure will be made: tabletop, table Bucky, or upright Bucky. This is extremely important, especially when AEC is activated. Failure to select the correct Bucky location could result in the

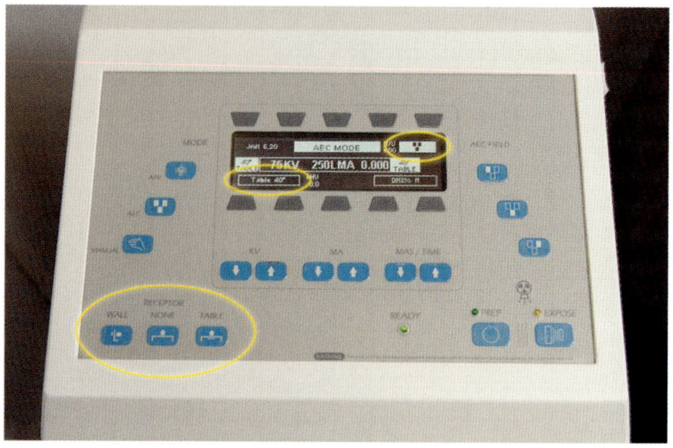

1-76 Control panel—select IR location for exposure.

selected AEC location waiting to receive exposure before it is able to terminate exposure (Fig. 1-76).

Setting a Manual Technique

A manual technique will require the radiographer to set the kVp and mAs values independently. A manual technique can be set in the imaging department, and on the mobile unit (Fig. 1-77).

Setting Technique With Automatic Exposure Control (AEC)

Optimal kVp must be set for part being imaged to achieve proper part penetration. The technologist will select the exposure cell(s) that are covered appropriately for the part of the body being imaged (Figs. 1-78 and 1-79). Exposure cells selected will control the length of the exposure, and upon exposure termination, the mAs value will appear on the control panel (Fig. 1-80). The length of the exposure and the mA station configured will determine image quality. For AEC to properly function, proper centering and collimation are essential. Excessive scatter produced from a poorly collimated exposure field may result in premature termination of the exposure. In addition, small adult anatomic parts, pediatric patients, or

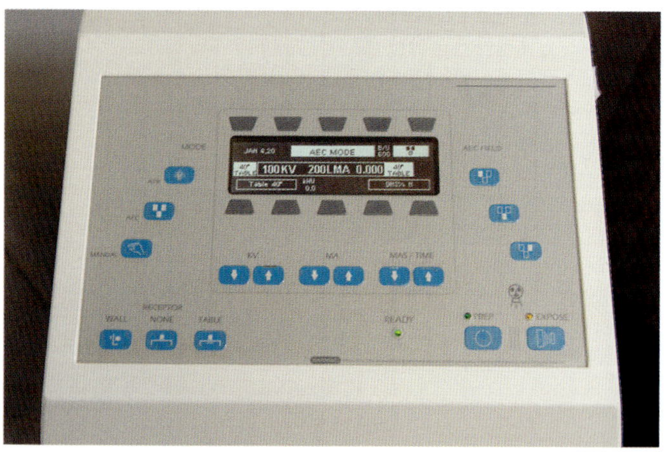

1-75 Control panel setup.

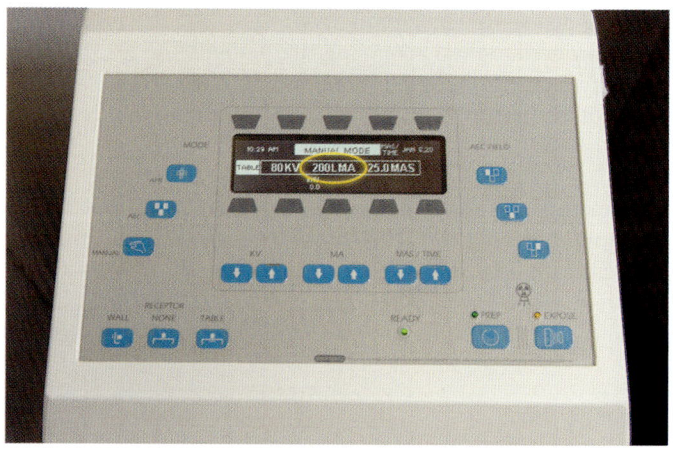

1-77 Control panel—setting a manual technique and establishing focal spot size.

patients who have surgical hardware placed within the area of centering are not good candidates to use AEC on. A backup timer should be established to avoid giving the patient excessive exposure time if the AEC circuitry fails or the incorrect Bucky is selected. The backup timer should be set at 1.5–2 times the anticipated exposure time or mAs.

AEC also has intensity settings that may be selected to increase or decrease the exposure time. However, these intensity settings are rarely applied with digital imaging. When adjusted, intensity settings may go up or down as necessary to accommodate an extreme patient size or when considering additive pathologies or destructive pathologies.

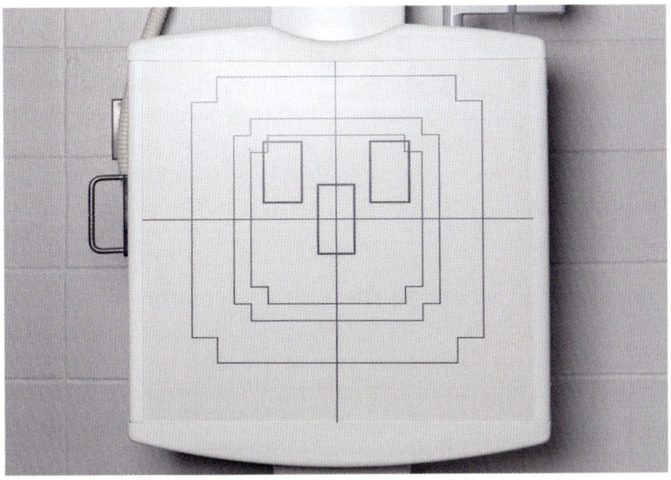

1-78 Automatic exposure ionization chambers.

Image Receptor Size

Computed radiography (CR) has a standard of two image receptor (IR) sizes, while direct radiography (DR) has a 14 × 17 or 17 × 17 digital detector (Figs. 1-81 and 1-82). With CR or DR, the technologist will only acquire one projection on the image receptor (IR) and ensure the part is centered to the IR and close collimation applied.

Acquiring the Patient

After reviewing the order, previous imaging, and setting up the imaging room, the technologist will acquire the patient from the designated location.

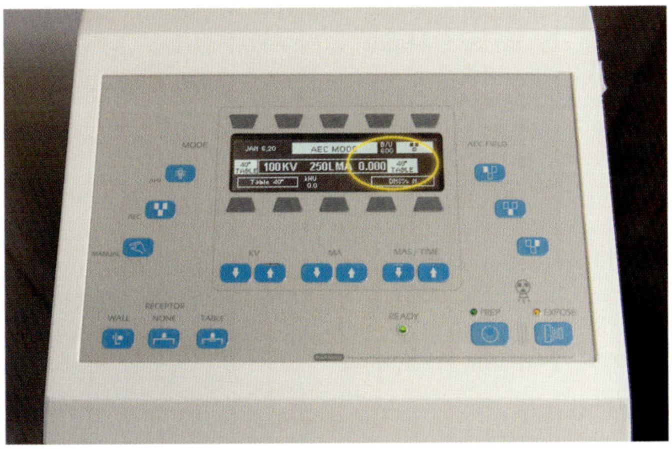

1-79 Control panel: pre-exposure. Select ionization chambers and IR location at the table Bucky or upright Bucky.

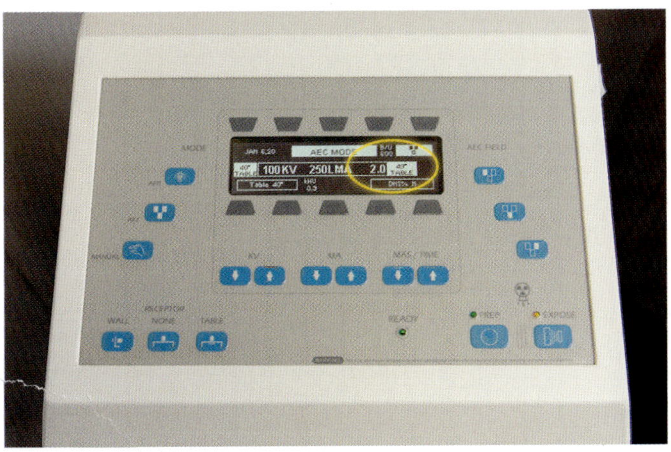

1-80 Control panel: immediately post exposure the mAs will be temporarily displayed.

1-81 CR—14 × 17 and 10 × 12 IRs.

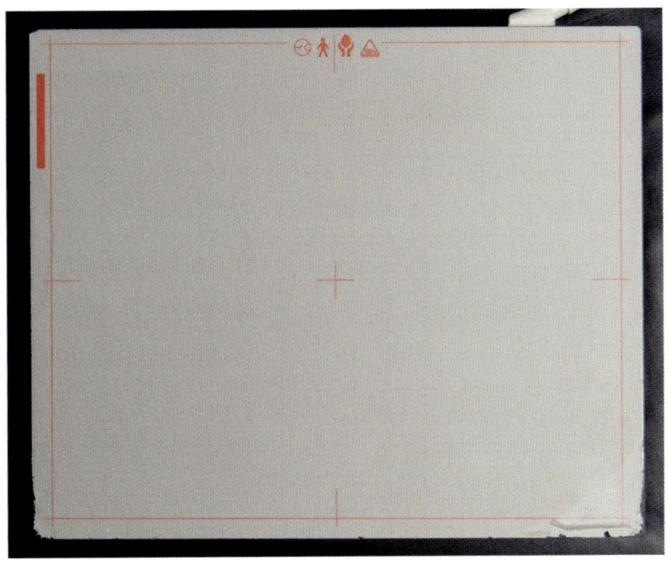

1-82 Direct imaging plate.

When acquiring the outpatient, the technologist should call the patient by name from the waiting room. The technologist should introduce themselves and the department they represent to the patient.

Example Script

"John?" (patient rises and acknowledges the address); "Hi, I am Abby. I will be your technologist from Radiology today. Are you ready to come with me?"

Once the patient is in a private location, the technologist must ensure the correct patient has been acquired. The technologist should ask the patient to state their first and last name. Often times, the birthdate is also acquired to ensure the correct patient. The technologist will ensure the patient's stated personal information matches their wrist identification and/or information on the exam order.

"John, could I ask you to state your first and last name and your birthdate?" (Technologist requests this of the patient while taking a look at their wristband identification.)

When acquiring an inpatient, the technologist will be sure to verify exam orders and patient transport orders prior to retrieving the patient. The technologist will locate the patient room, knock, and upon entering, verify the correct patient and identify themselves. The technologist should also explain what procedure they are taking them from their room to complete. It is important that the technologist verify the correct patient prior to their transport to the imaging department.

Example Script

(Technologist knocks on patient door.) "Shirlie, Hi, I am Abby, a technologist from Radiology. I have a physician order to take you to radiology for a chest x-ray today. I brought a wheelchair with me to transport you. Before we go, could you state your first and last name and your birthdate? (Technologist requests this information of the patient while taking a look at their wristband identification to ensure it matches.) Alright, if you are ready, I will assist you into the wheelchair, and we will go to the imaging department to complete the procedure."

Patient Dress

The patient, if not already appropriately dressed for the procedure, may need to be instructed and assisted to change into a gown. Even if the patient already appears dressed in a gown, the technologist should still ensure the patient has removed the necessary undergarments for the procedure and ensure the area free of artifacts (lines, jewelry, unused ECG patches, etc.).

Patient History

The technologist should obtain patient history relevant to the imaging procedure ordered. The technologist should most certainly always verify the correct exam order with the patient.

"John, it looks like we have orders to image your lower back today; does that sound correct?" (Technologist attempting to verify exam orders with the patient)

With confirmation from the patient, the technologist can begin to position the patient. While positioning the patient, the technologist can inquire about what happened, when it happened, where the pain is, level of pain, and if they have ever had any surgeries to that area. The technologist should work efficiently to acquire patient history while positioning the required projections of the patient. Once history is acquired, the technologist should resume conversation with the patient.

Example Script

"John, can you tell me a little bit about what is going on? (Allow patient to answer.) About how long ago did this happen? (Allow patient to answer.) Where is the pain at specifically? (Allow patient to answer or show you.) Is there anything that makes the pain better or worse? (Allow patient to answer.) Have you ever had any surgeries to that area?" (Allow patient to answer.)

Patient Shielding and Potential Pregnancy

All patients should be shielded for any procedures as this is considered "good practice," especially with pediatrics and reproductive aged patients as long as the shielding will not interfere with the anatomy of interest. When shielding is applied consistently, the habit will prevent inconsistent shielding practices. Female patients of reproductive age (approximately 10–52 years) should be questioned while acquiring history, prior to beginning the exam, if there is any possibility of pregnancy. Some departments now require pregnancy declarations of all females of reproductive age prior to their imaging procedure. If a patient is uncertain how to answer, the technologist should refer to the department policy and procedure to obtain orders for pregnancy testing.

Positioning the Patient

Once the technologist has determined the best means to position the patient safely and comfortably, the technologist should proceed by having the patient move toward the upright Bucky, be seated at or on the x-ray table, or laid recumbent. The IR size and orientation should be adjusted according to the patient and the projection.

Central Ray and Collimation

Central ray describes the center of the exposure field as it exits the tube (Fig. 1-83). When imaging a specific area of

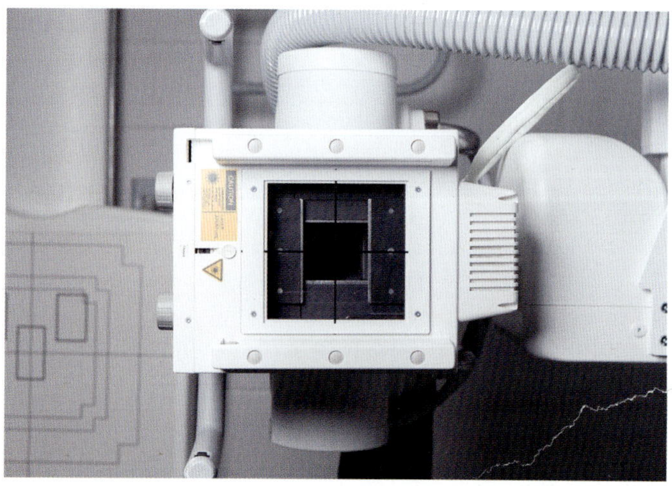

1-83 Tube window—emergence of the central ray (CR).

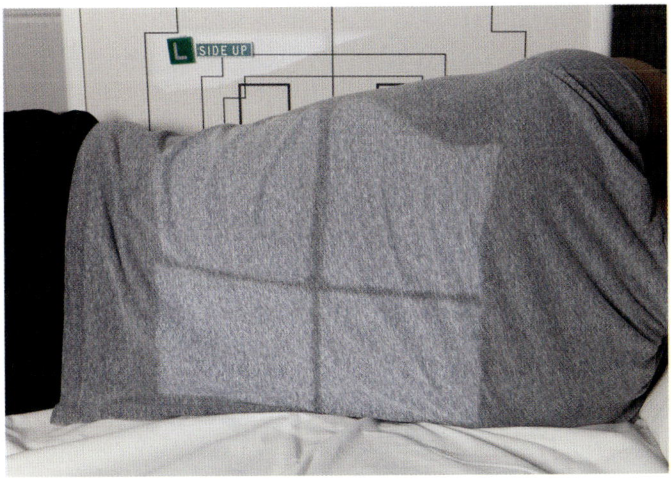

1-84 Central ray within the collimated field size.

the body, the technologist should strive to achieve the recommended centering to the part. Proper centering of the part allows for proper two- or four-sided collimation of the part (Fig. 1-84). The technologist should always collimate to the size of the IR being used or smaller.

Marking the IR

After collimation has been applied, the technologist should mark the IR with a right or left anatomic marker, according to recommendations, within the collimated exposure field.

Breathing Instructions

The patient should be instructed with proper breathing instructions necessary for the exposure. The technologists should deliver breathing instructions with a commanding voice of volume audible to the patient, especially when delivered from behind the protective barrier. While delivering breathing instructions, the technologist should watch to ensure the patient is responsive to instructions through the point of image exposure.

After exposure, the patient should be instructed to relax, the control panel reset for the next projection, and the IR switched out (unless DR) before proceeding to position the next projection.

Suggested Rules of Marking

Marking Extremities

AP or PA: The part should be marked with the right or left marker lateral to the part; furthest from the patient's midline (Figs. 1-85 and 1-86).

AP Oblique/PA Oblique: The part should be marked with the right or left marker lateral to the part; furthest from the patient's midline and placed to identify the anatomic side closest to the IR (Figs. 1-87 and 1-88).

Mediolateral or Lateromedial: The part should be marked with the right or left marker anterior to the part (Figs. 1-89 and 1-90).

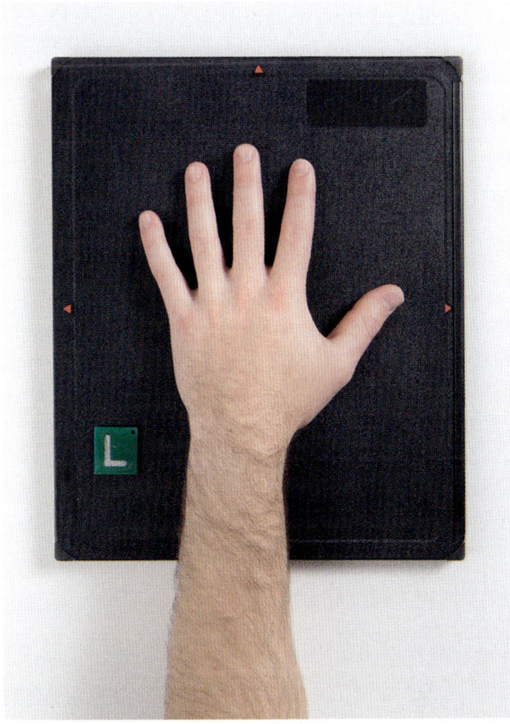

1-85 Extremity marking on the flat or oblique part—place the marker furthest away from the patient's midline.

Marking the Skull and Torso

AP or PA: The part should be marked with the right or left marker correctly depicting the side. When marking on the upright Bucky, the marker is placed on the surface of the Bucky.

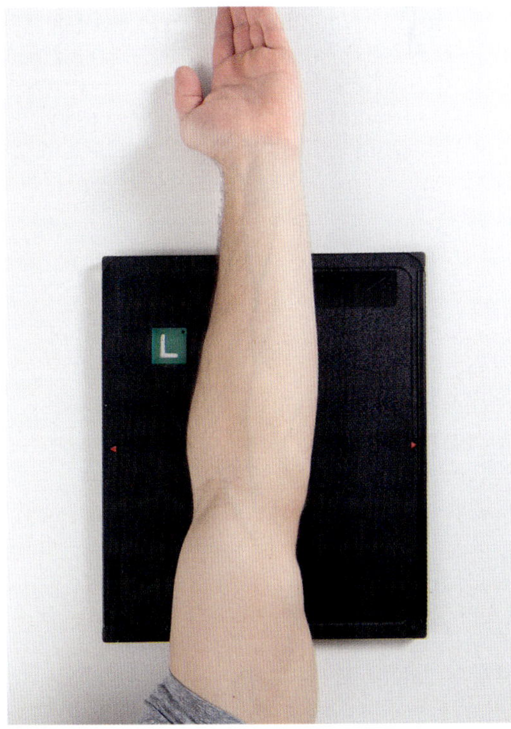

1-86 Extremity marking on the flat or oblique part—place the marker furthest away from the patient's midline.

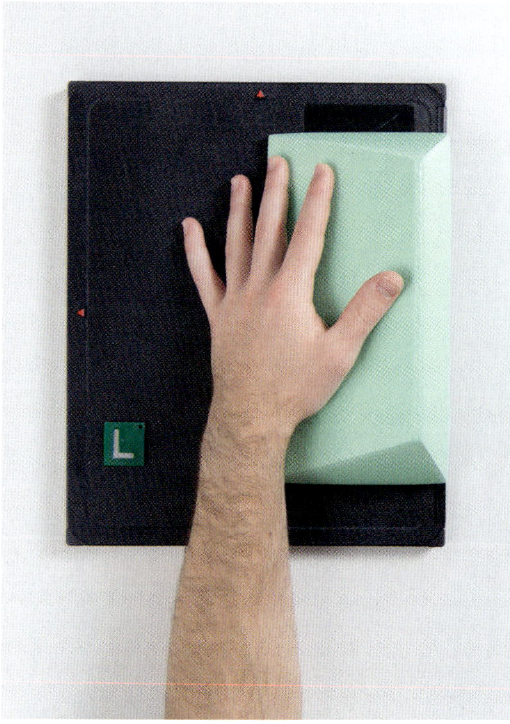

1-87 Extremity marking on the flat or oblique part—place the marker furthest away from the patient's midline.

When marking in the table Bucky, the technologist could mark the right or left side accordingly, but oftentimes will mark the side of the IR closest to where the technologist stands for ease (Figs. 1-91 and 1-92).

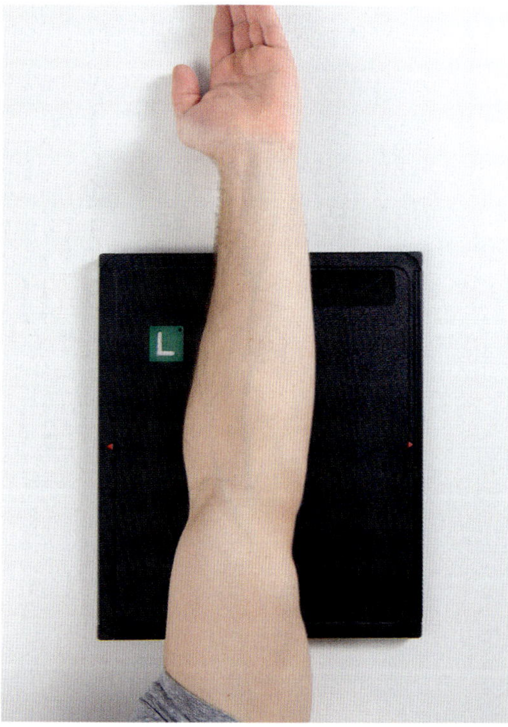

1-88 Extremity marking on the flat or oblique part—place the marker furthest away from the patient's midline.

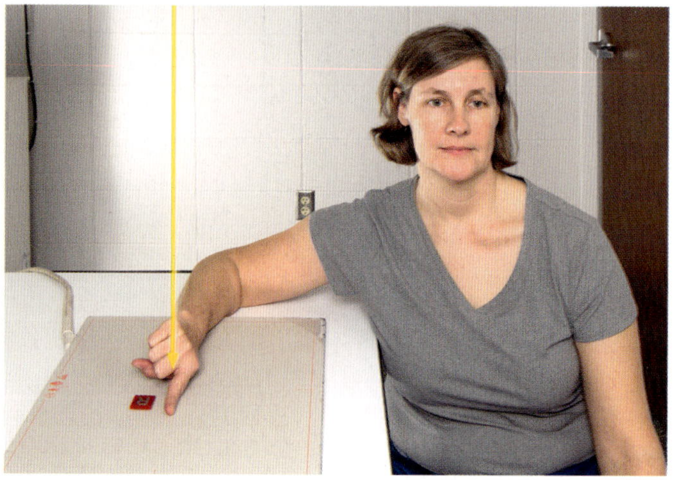

1-89 Extremity marking on a lateral position—marker is positioned along the anterior surface of the patient.

AP Oblique/PA Oblique: The anatomic side positioned closest to the IR is the side that should be marked on oblique projections (Figs. 1-93 and 1-94).

Lateral: The right or left side positioned closest to the IR is marked. The right or left side closest to the IR should be noted by placing the R/L marker anterior to the torso (Fig. 1-95).

Marking Decubitus: With RLD or LLD, the side-up "R" or "L" is most easily marked. In addition, "side up" should be added to the anatomic side marker (Figs. 1-96 and 1-97). For example, an RLD would be marked with "L" along the left lateral side of the patient along with "side up." If a dorsal or ventral decubitus is acquired, mark the lateral side of the body (right or left) that is closest to the IR, and no "side-up" marker would be added (Figs. 1-98 and 1-99). Technically, with ventral or dorsal decubitus, the patient does not have that anatomic side facing up.

Image Analysis

An exposure index (EI) is generated with each projection. Each manufactured system may have different established

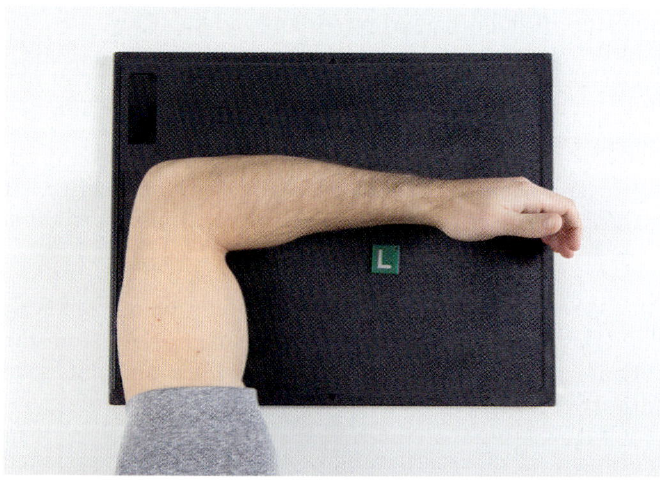

1-90 Extremity marking on a lateral position—marker is positioned along the anterior surface of the patient.

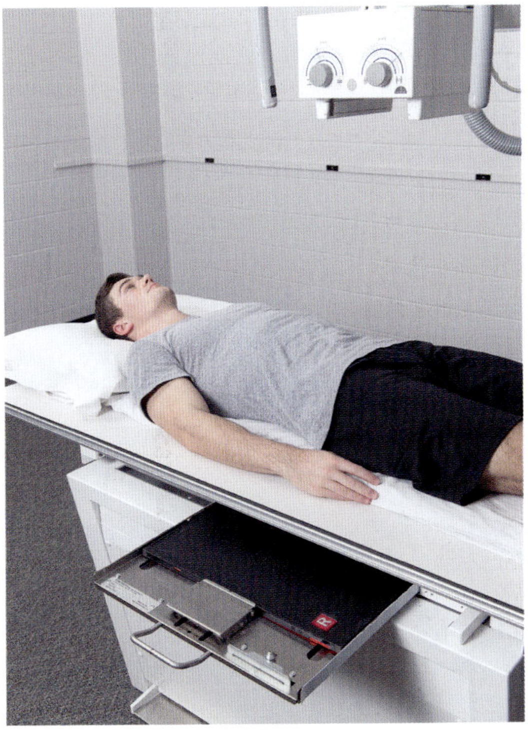

1-91 Torso marking—mark patient's true right or left by placing the anatomic marker on the IR on the corresponding right or left side of the patient.

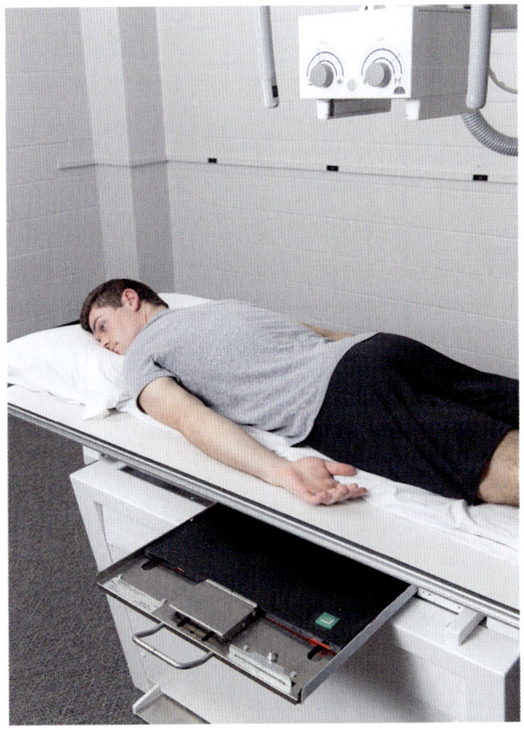

1-92 Torso marking—mark patient's true right or left by placing the anatomic marker on the IR on the corresponding right or left side of the patient.

exposure indices. The technologist should carefully analyze the control panel settings to ensure it falls within the exposure range. This evaluation is important to identify which patients are receiving too much radiation exposure and which patients are not receiving enough exposure, resulting in poor diagnostic quality. Target exposures can be identified within the range of established exposure indices. The target index would fall in the center of the range (Fig. 1-100). Numbers to the right of this center may be color coded yellow and then red, indicating the level of overexposure from the target with some systems (Figs. 1-101 and 1-102). If not color coded, values to the right of center would indicate a direct relationship correlating with the amount of exposure; values to the right of center would indicate that technical

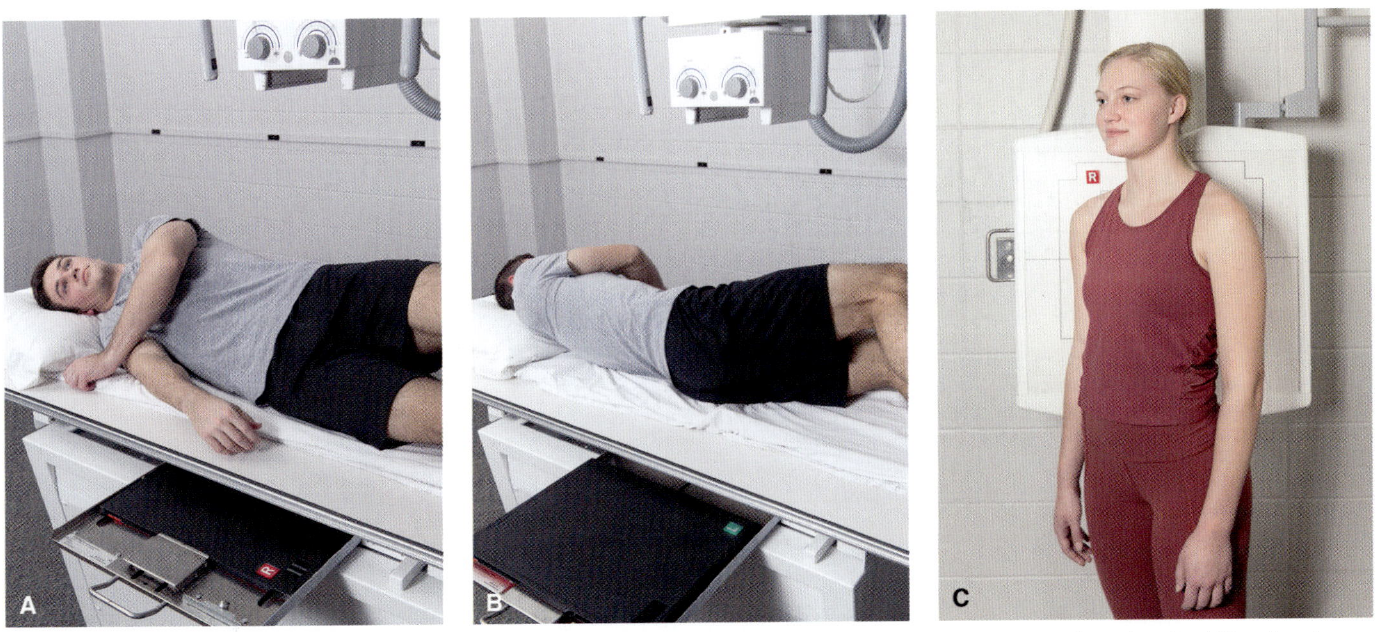

1-93 Mark oblique body positions by marking the anatomic patient side positioned closest to the IR. The anatomic side marker should be placed on the corresponding side closest to the IR **(A)** Recumbent RPO marked right. **(B)** Recumbent LPO marked left. **(C)** Upright RPO marked right.

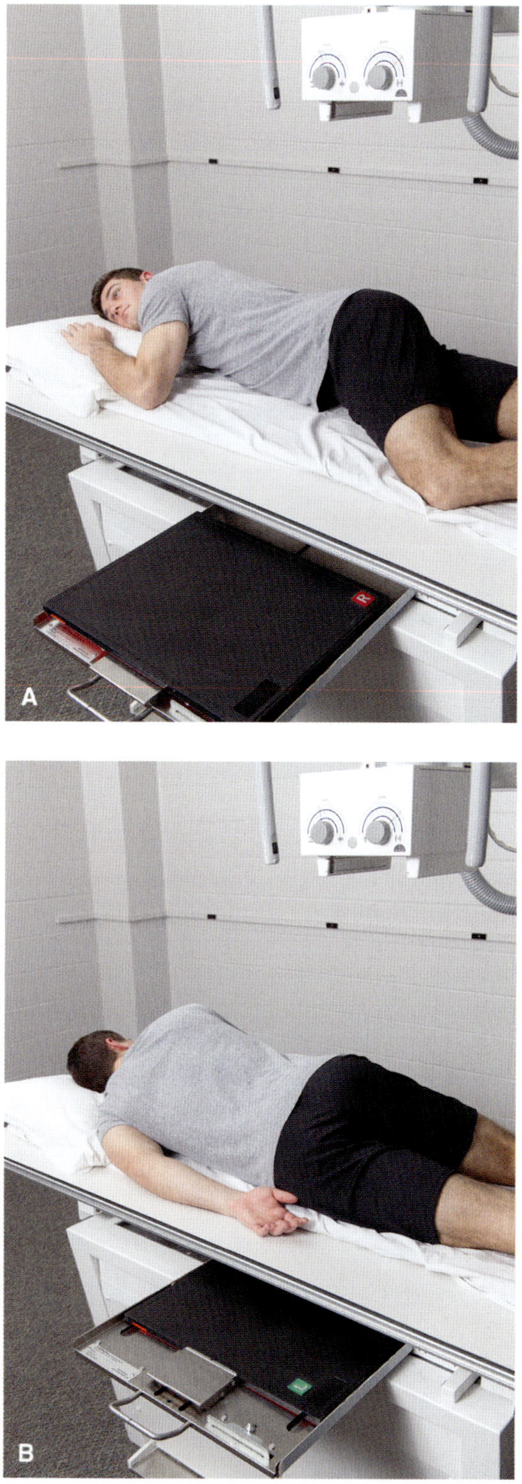

1-94 Mark oblique body positions by marking the anatomic patient side positioned closest to the IR. The anatomic side marker should be placed on the corresponding side down. **(A)** Recumbent RAO marked right to correlate to the patient's right side. **(B)** Recumbent LAO marked left to correlate to the patient's left side.

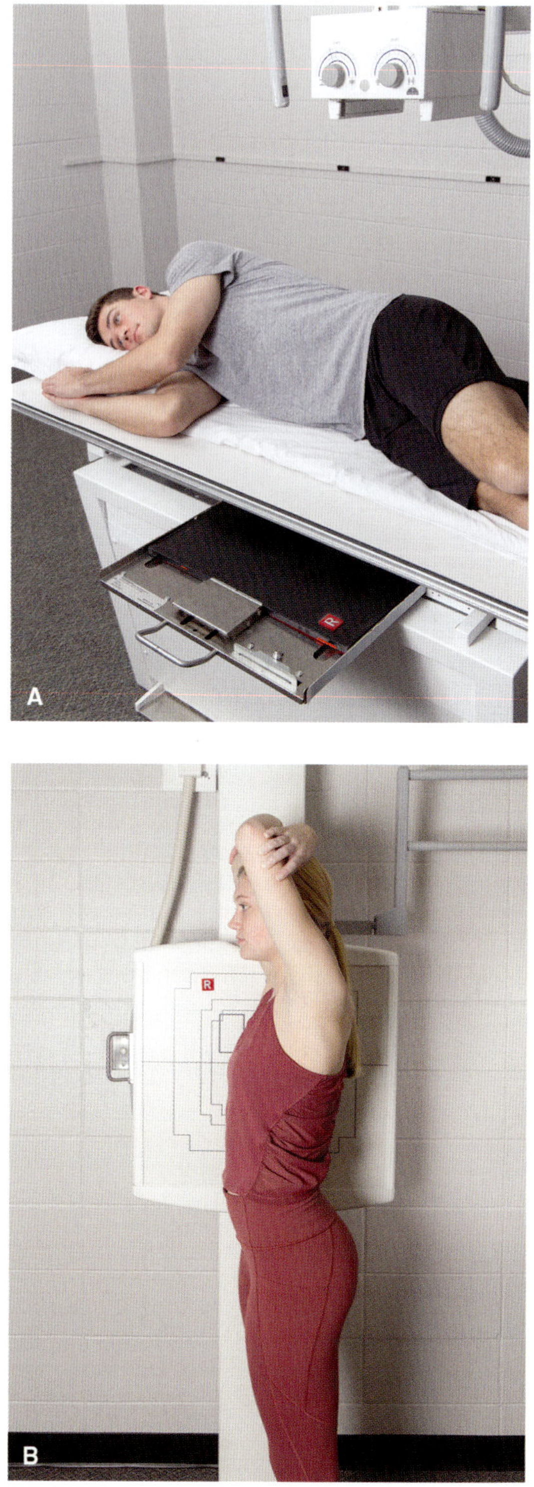

1-95 Mark lateral torso positions by designating the right or left lateral side closest to the IR. The anatomic marker should be placed along the anterior surface of the patient. **(A)** Recumbent right lateral position marked right, anterior to the torso. **(B)** Erect right lateral position marked right anterior to the torso.

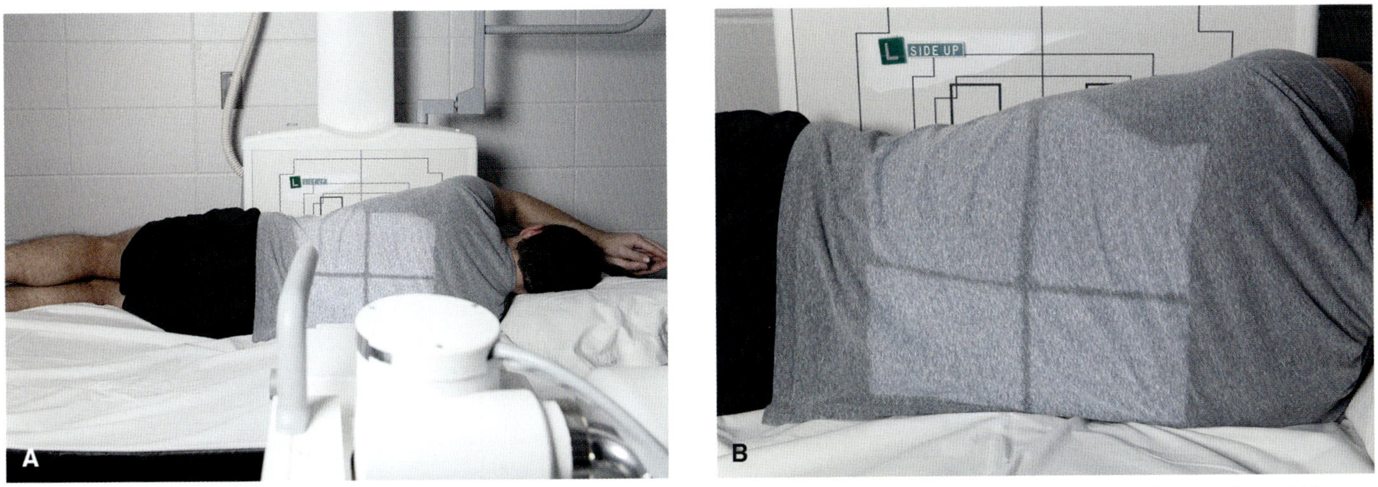

1-96 Right and left lateral decubitus positions should be marked with the anatomic side that is "up" along with a marker to indicate "side up." This patient is positioned in an RLD. The technologist should mark "L" with the "side up" along the left lateral side of the patient. **A & B:** RLD with correct image marking.

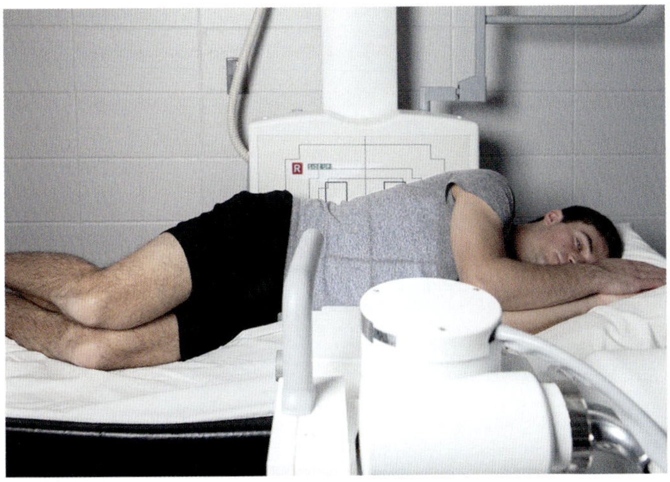

1-97 Patient is positioned in an LLD position, the "R" anatomic marker and the "side up" should be placed along the right lateral side of the patient.

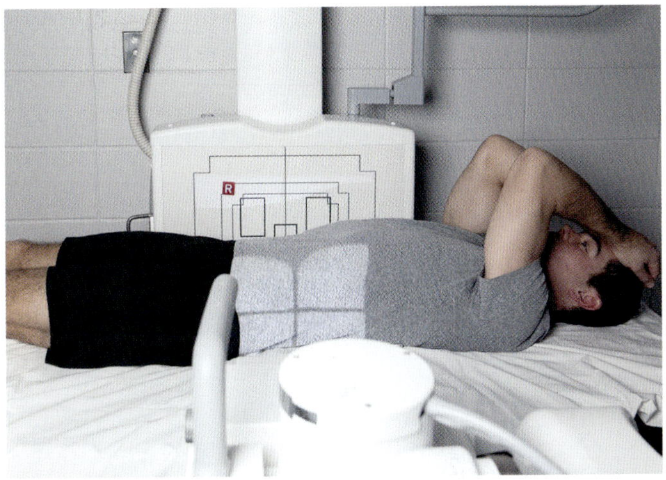

1-99 Patient is positioned in the dorsal decubitus. An "R" marker will indicate this side of the patient was closest to the IR. Technically, the left side is not facing up; no "side-up" marker is applied.

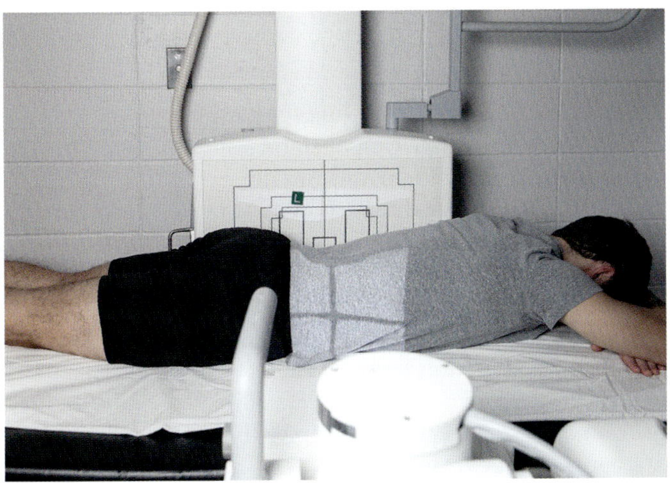

1-98 Patient is positioned in the ventral decubitus. An "L" marker will indicate this side of the patient was closest to the IR. Technically, the left side is not facing up; no "side-up" marker is applied.

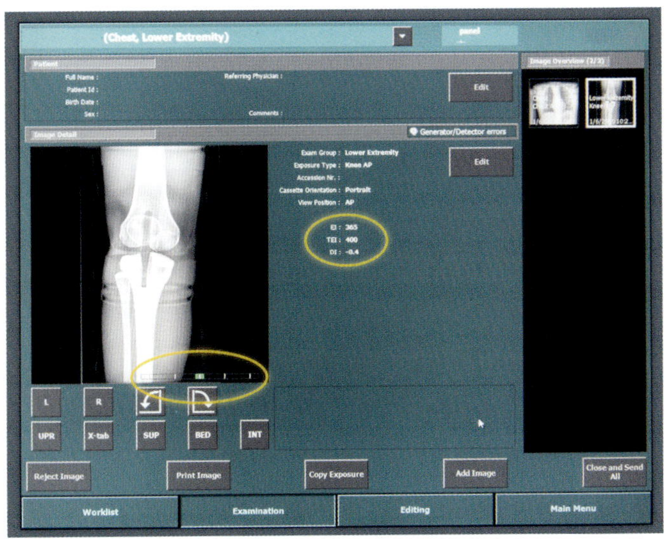

1-100 Target exposure index being displayed.

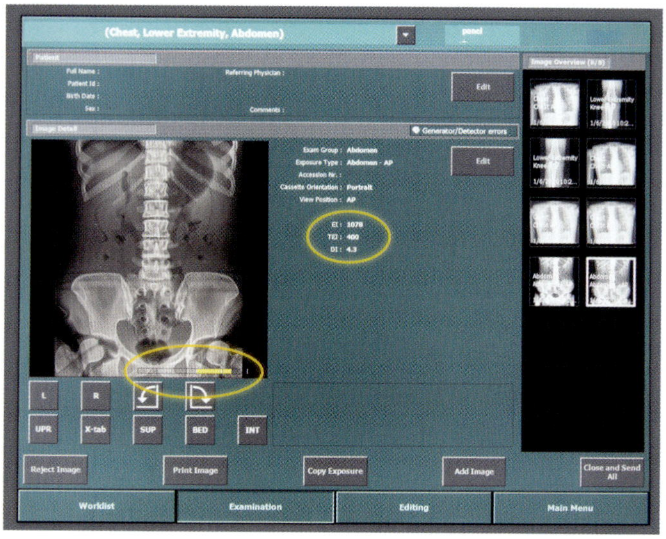

1-101 Exposure index slightly above exposure range.

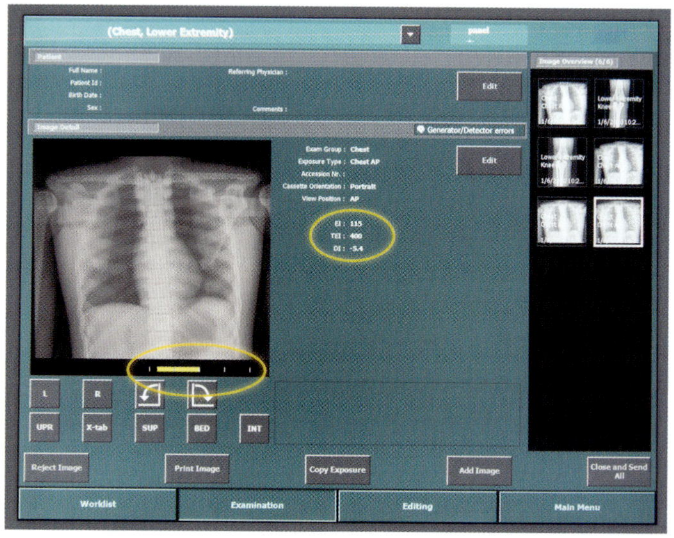

1-103 Exposure index with exposure slightly below the exposure range.

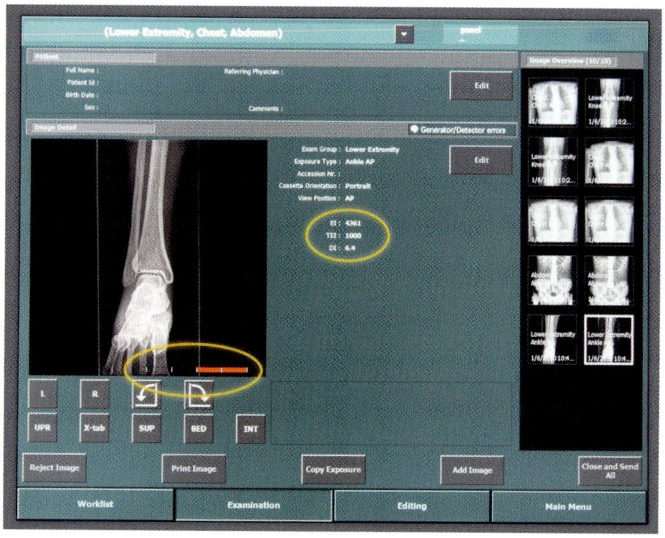

1-102 Exposure index with exposure exceeding the exposure range.

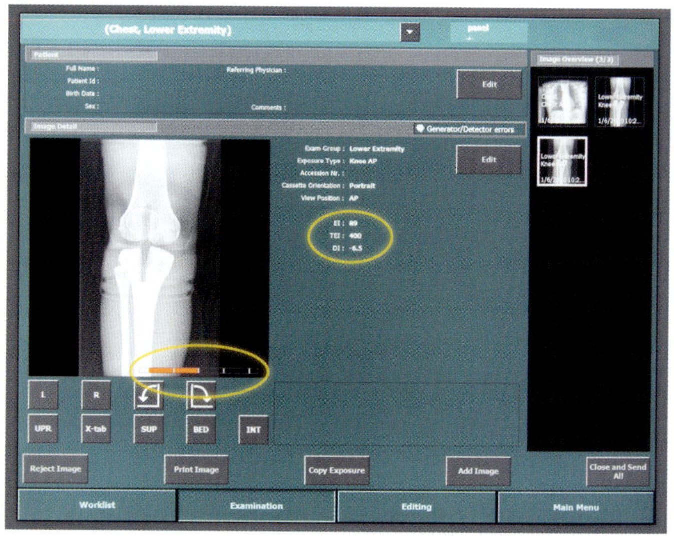

1-104 Exposure index with exposure extremely below the exposure range.

factors should be reduced. Numbers to the left of this center may also be color coded yellow and then red, indicating the level of underexposure the further away from the target exposure with some systems (Figs. 1-103 and 1-104). Again, if not color coded, values to the left of center directly indicate underexposure, which may produce a poor technical appearance, affecting image interpretation. Underexposed images should be repeated, with increased technical factors to achieve a more optimal exposure. All systems will provide either color coding or numerical value to represent the deviation index. While the preceding explanation refers to a direct relationship of the exposure amount to the target index, some systems may use an inverse relationship to represent the exposure amount to the target index. This means that below target exposures would indicate overexposure and above target exposures would indicate underexposure.

Image Post Processing

There are several postprocessing tools that could be considered. Technologists must understand which adjustments the technologist can make to the raw image before sending it to the radiologist. When a technologist adjusts the raw data and saves the image, the radiologist may not be able to make image adjustments necessary for interpretation. Departments may have a policy and procedure to establish guidelines for a technologist. Radiologic technologists should always practice four-sided collimation around the anatomy and placement of an anatomic marker within the collimated exposure field prior to the exposure. In the instance that a lead marker does not appear in the exposure field, the image may be repeated. The annotation function should be utilized to add only additional information useful to the image and should not replace the use of standardized minimum right and left markers that should be positioned within the collimated exposure field. Digital annotation of right and left markers cannot replace the need for right and left lead anatomic markers within the original collimated margins. Annotating on an image post exposure is discouraged as digital annotation could be changed or deleted.

There are a variety of other postprocessing options that are available on digital workstations. These options range from windowing, smoothing, subtraction, edge enhancement, and electronic masking. Technologists must realize that the monitor resolution at their workstation will be lower compared to the resolution of the radiologist's monitor. Additionally, if a technologist postprocesses an image and pushes it over to the department picture archiving and communication system (PACS) system, this will prevent the radiologist from being able to make any image adjustments for their interpretation. Therefore, post processing by the technologist is not advised. In addition, electronic masking should not substitute for the lack of pre-exposure collimation as this does not reduce patient exposure. The practice of electronic masking to represent the technologist's ability to collimate is discouraged. If masking is applied, it should not cover any anatomy that was obtained originally within the collimated exposure field. The radiologist is responsible for anything acquired within the original exposure field; if areas were masked by the radiologic technologist, the radiologist would not see the entire exposure field. Therefore, technologists should practice proper centering and four-sided collimation to the part ordered.

Image Review

The technologist must take time to review acquired images to ensure the anatomic area was well positioned and imaged. The technologist must have the knowledge pertinent to their role to position and care for the patient, acquire the images, and review them to determine diagnostic quality. It is left to the discretion of the radiologic technologist to determine diagnostic and nondiagnostic images and determine when an image needs to be repeated. The technologist should review each image for the following.

1. Is all of the necessary anatomy included on the image (Figs. 1-105 and 1-106)?
   - Was the central ray properly directed to the part? An "X" can be drawn to intersect within the collimated exposure field to determine if the central ray was directed to the correct location.
   - Was essential anatomy included within the collimated exposure field?
   - Is the area free of artifact(s)?
2. Is the anatomy well demonstrated?
   - Did the technologist properly position the patient to adequately demonstrate the anatomy?
   - Can the technologist recognize the anatomy best demonstrated with use of different projections? Typically, a minimum of two views 90° apart are acquired. This will demonstrate the anatomy and pathology in two planes. It will allow for determination of anatomy and/or pathology placement or displacement (Figs. 1-107 and 1-108).

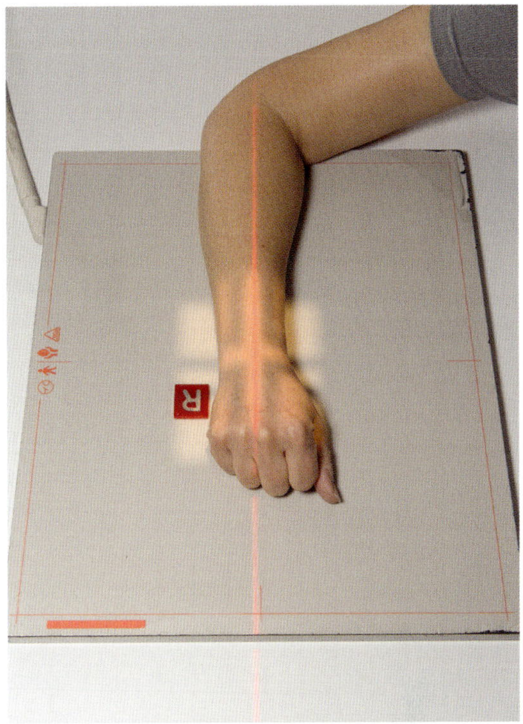

1-105 Correct CR placement with appropriate collimation to the part of interest.

3. Does the image reflect proper image markings? (Fig. 1-109)
   - Did the technologist correctly use a lead marker to identify the right or left side?
   - What additional markings or annotations could be helpful to the radiologist interpreting the exam?
   - Is the image properly displayed?

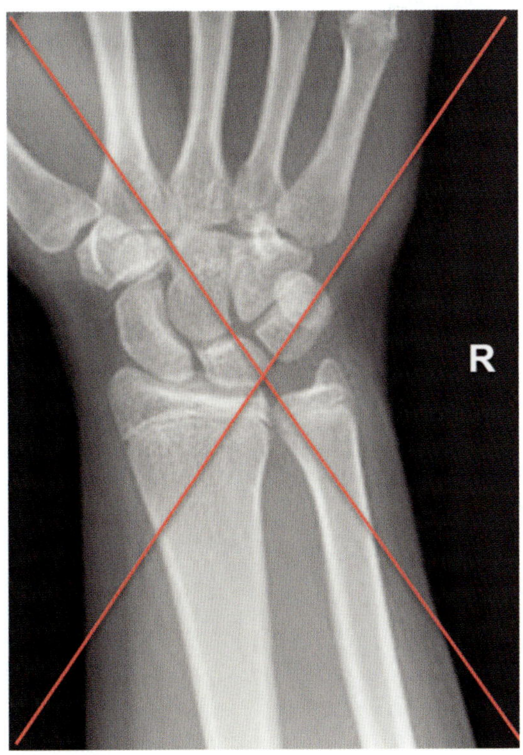

1-106 The "X" through the collimated light field ensures accurate centering to the part of interest.

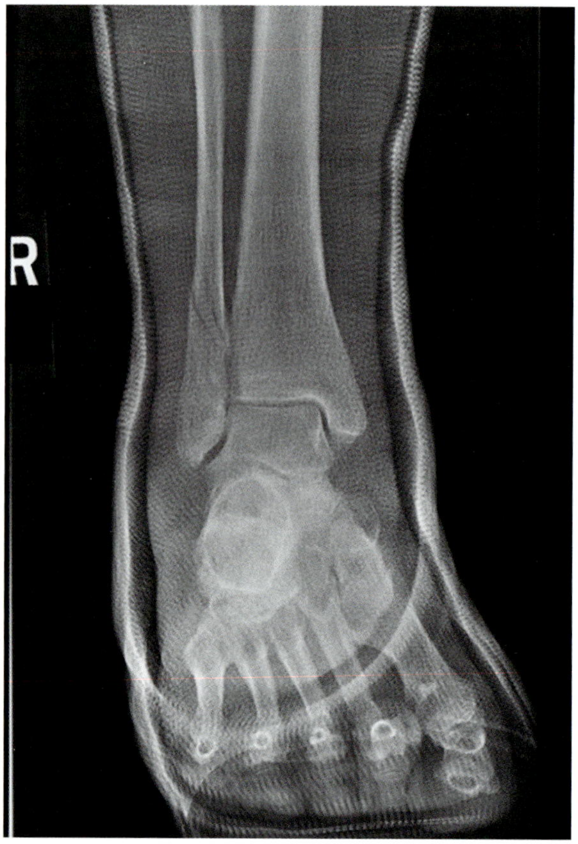

1-107 AP right trauma ankle.

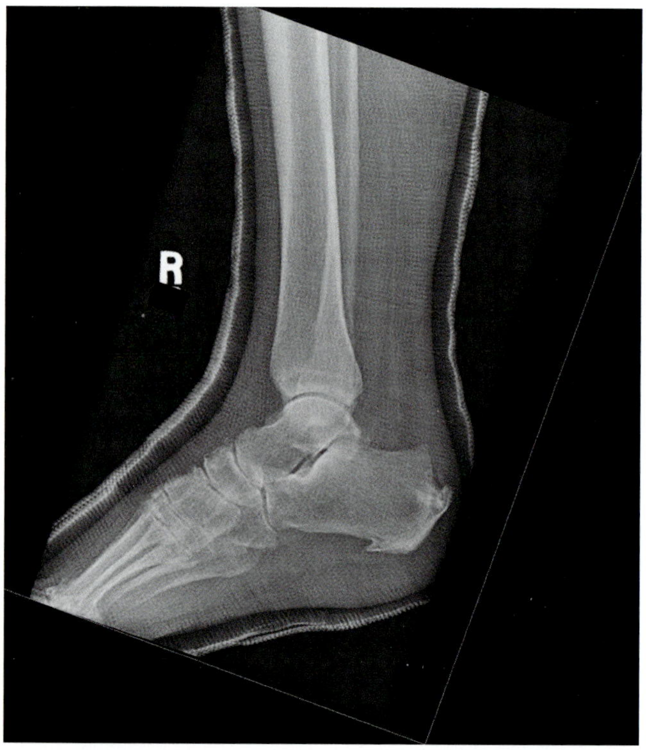

1-108 ML right trauma ankle to provide a 90° view from the AP projection.

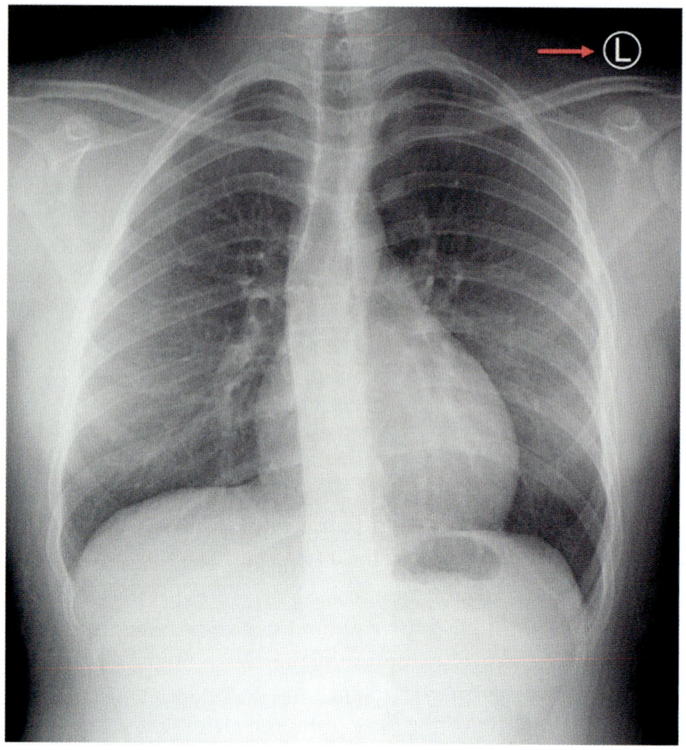

1-109 Every image, should be marked at minimum correctly with a right or left anatomic side marker.

4. Does the image prove to be technically acceptable? (Fig. 1-110)
   - Does the exposure index fall within acceptable range for the operating system? Images that are technically insufficient may appear to be of good quality if just slightly insufficient or "mottled or pixelated" if severely insufficient. Images that appear "mottled" should be repeated. Images that appear beyond optimal exposure because of higher technique may display high quality, but the patient has received more radiation dose than needed. When extreme overexposure has

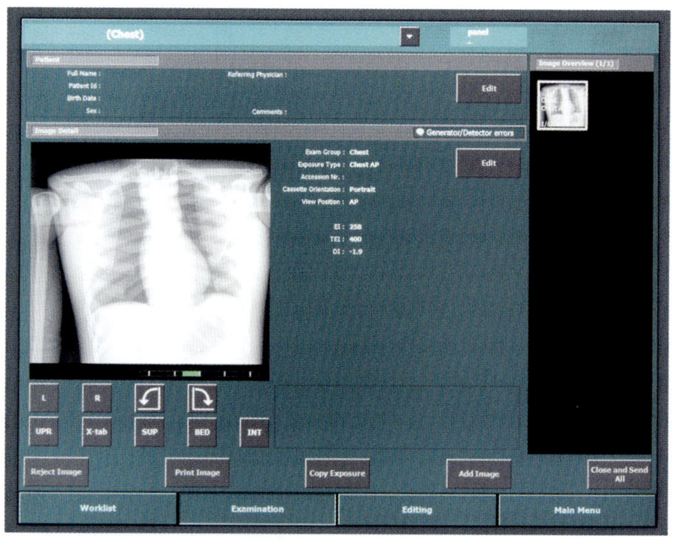

1-110 Review acquired images for correct positioning, required anatomy, and technical quality.

not been reached, these images may not necessarily need to be repeated, but, the technologist should work on reducing the amount of dose given to future patients. Extremely overexposed images result in plate saturation, which with computed radiography systems causes poor contrast and brightness and may result in a ghosting artifact. The ghosting artifact occurs with plate saturation, which prevents the image from being entirely erased from the plate, hence possibly affecting other images taken on the same plate.

Dismissal of Patient

Once the technologist acquires the exam images and determines acceptable images have been attained, the technologist will dismiss the patient. The patient should be informed of when and how they will acquire their exam results. If it is an outpatient procedure, patients will typically receive results in 24–48 hours. In the case of admitted patients or emergency department patients, turnaround results are quicker.

The technologist must escort outpatients back to the imaging waiting room and ensure they do not need assistance finding another location within the hospital. Inpatients must be transported back to their room and positioned back into their beds with bedrails up.

On returning to the imaging department, the technologist must clean up the exam room in preparation for the next technologist to use it.

HOSPITAL AREAS OF IMAGING

The radiologic technologist will work with a variety of patient types. Ambulatory patients will require little to no assistance when moving into exam positions. Nonambulatory patients will require the technologist to assess the patient and determine the level of assistance they will require to get the procedure completed. A number of patients will have exams completed with the portable/mobile radiography unit.

The technologist must review the patient orders to determine the location of the patient; for example, whether he or she is an inpatient or outpatient. Inpatient exams will require the patient to be transported, either by wheelchair or by stretcher, or if the mobile unit must be taken to their location. A wheelchair patient may require various degrees of assistance to ambulate. These patients may be able to stand upright for short periods. A stretcher patient often, but not always, aligns with a patient that lacks the strength and ability to ambulate much at all. The technologist should carefully evaluate the patient's ability to determine the safest and most diagnostic approach. Often, however, a stretcher patient should remain on the stretcher or be moved over to the imaging table for the exam. These patients may be able to sit upright on the stretcher and positioned at the upright Bucky. Transporting a patient may be accomplished by the technologist or expedited with a second person, especially if the patient has intravenous pumps and lines.

HOSPITAL DEPARTMENTS

Emergency Department (ED): Patients may be transported from the ED to the imaging department or imaged with the mobile unit in the patient's assigned room.

Intensive Care Unit (ICU): There are different types of intensive care units, and some hospitals have more than one unit to deliver a specific type of care. Patients are typically imaged with the mobile radiography unit as these patients are rarely transported out of their unit for imaging.

Operating Room (OR): The radiologic technologist could image a patient during a procedure with the mobile radiography unit or with a C-arm/O-arm unit that allows fluoroscopy to assist the surgeon during a procedure.

Post Anesthesia Care Unit (PACU): Patients post an operating procedure may require imaging with the mobile radiography unit during recovery. This could include a single view chest post a port-a-cath placement or post a pacemaker placement. Orthopedic cases will require two views 90° apart for post imaging.

CHAPTER 2 Chest

Chest imaging is the most frequent procedure performed by a radiographer and is the most commonly repeated exam. Attention to detail on these easily mastered exams is important. The technologist must take into consideration patient variables such as size, ability, and pathology while trying to attain the highest quality of images.

CLINICAL INDICATIONS

Indications are the symptomatic reasons as to why a particular exam may be ordered by the physician. The technologist should look at the clinical indications before performing a procedure. In certain circumstances, the indication may influence the need to increase or decrease the technical settings. The following briefly introduces common exam indications, but it is not an all-encompassing list.

Pneumothorax: Free air enters the pleural cavity causing the lung to be pushed away from the chest wall. The condition may result from penetrating trauma, biopsy, or surgery. A pneumothorax is identified as an area on the chest radiograph lacking lung markings (Figs. 2-1 and 2-2).

Pleural Effusion: Fluid that enters the pleural cavity. The condition may result from trauma, congestive heart failure (most common), or infection. *Hemothorax* is direct reference to blood in the pleural cavity (Fig. 2-3). *Empyema* is a purulent extension of fluid into the pleural cavity.

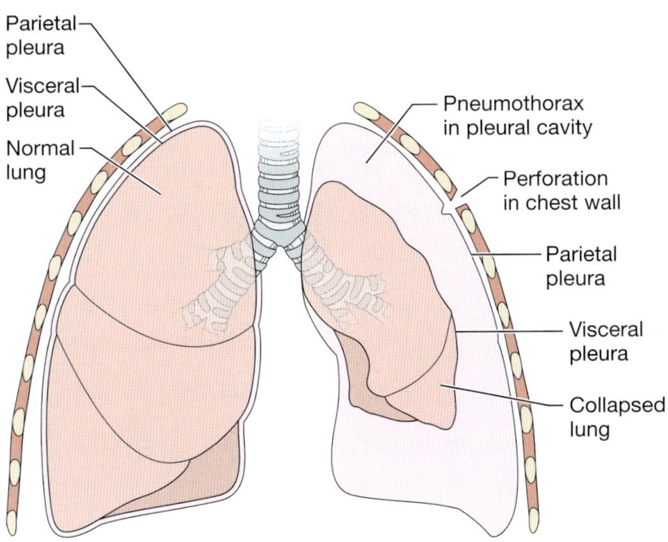

2-1 Pneumothorax.

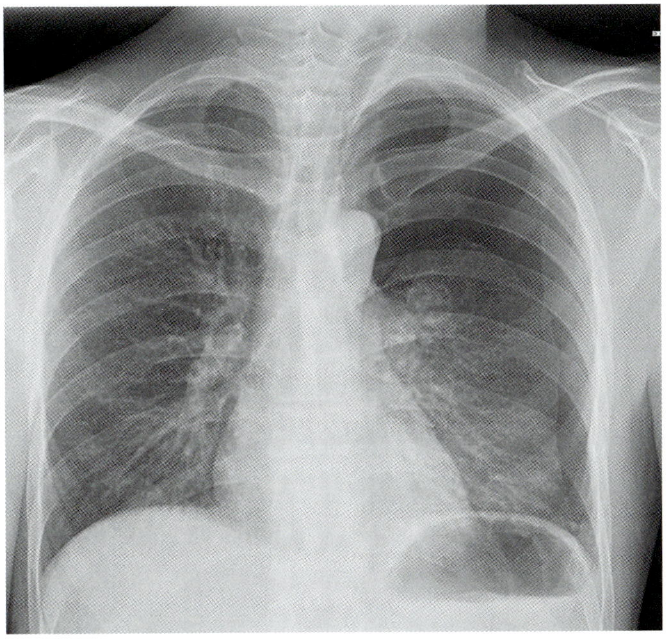

2-2 PA chest radiograph demonstrating a pneumothorax in the left lung.

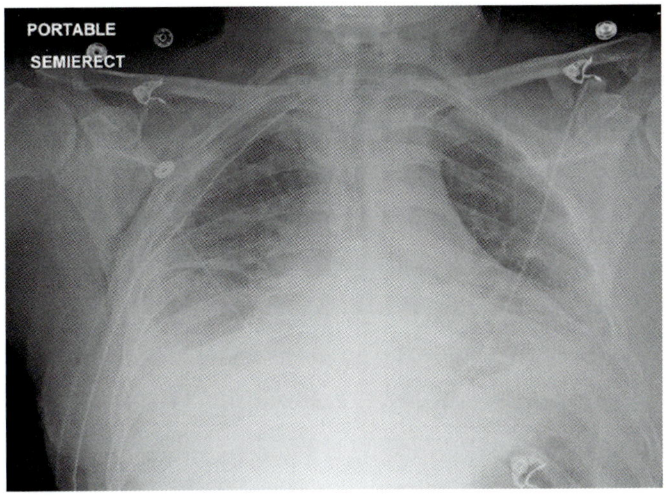

2-3 Hemothorax.

Emphysema: Damage to the alveoli in response to environmental or lifestyle factors. Alveoli lose elasticity and tend to retain air, resulting in hyperinflation of the lungs. Severely affected patients are characterized with a chest that appears barrel shaped, flattened diaphragm, and an elongated heart (Fig. 2-4).

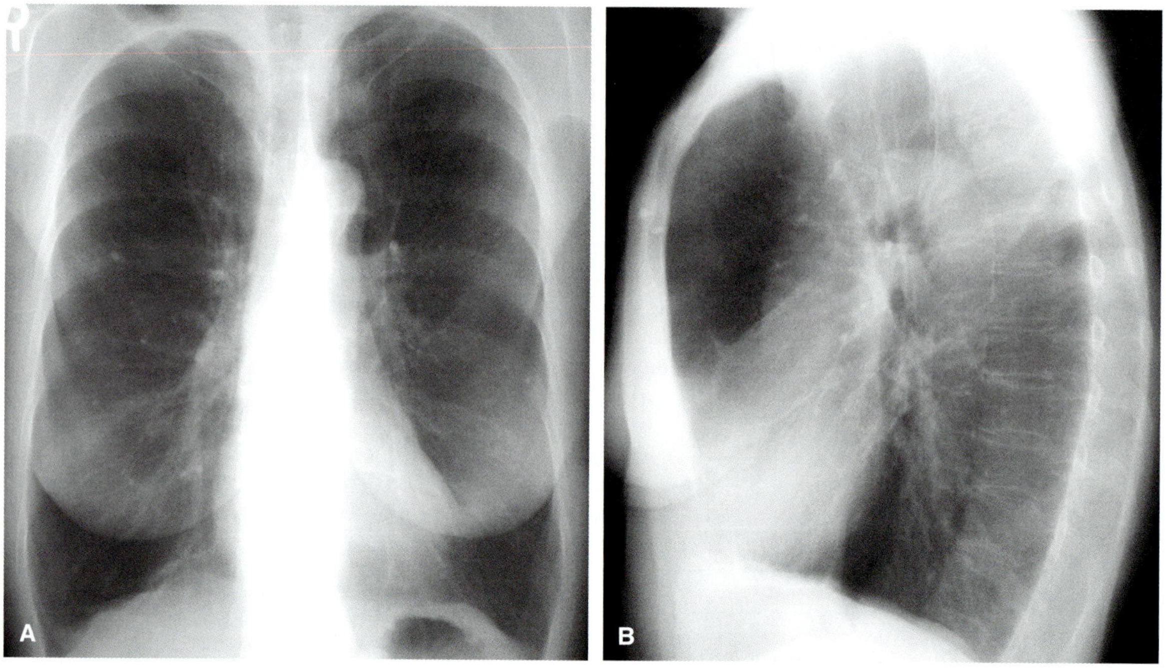

2-4 Emphysema reveals increased dimension of the thorax in the **(A)** PA chest and **(B)** lateral chest projections.

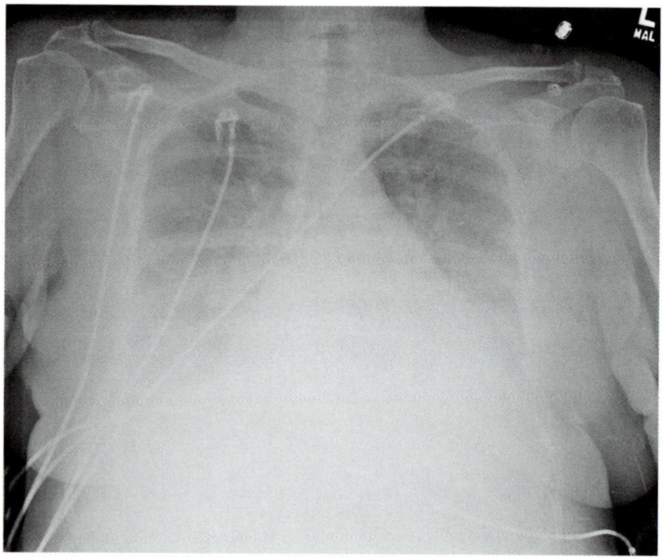

2-5 Congestive heart failure.

Congestive Heart Failure (CHF): A heart may become enlarged if it is unable to pump and supply all the needs of the tissues and organs throughout the body. The condition may result from hypertension, heart attack, cardiovascular disease, or infection. The condition may result in a patient becoming "fluid overloaded" and presenting with edema (swelling) in tissues and cavities and displaying shortness of breath (Fig. 2-5).

Line Placement: Images of the chest may be requested to verify the correct location of a placed line. It is essential that the technologist acquire an image with good positioning, good technical factors, and proper inspiration to help determine the proper placement of the line and identification of anatomy. With digital imaging technology, images acquired to verify line placement could then be adjusted with subtraction of the grayscale to better visualize the line (Fig. 2-6 and Table 2-1).

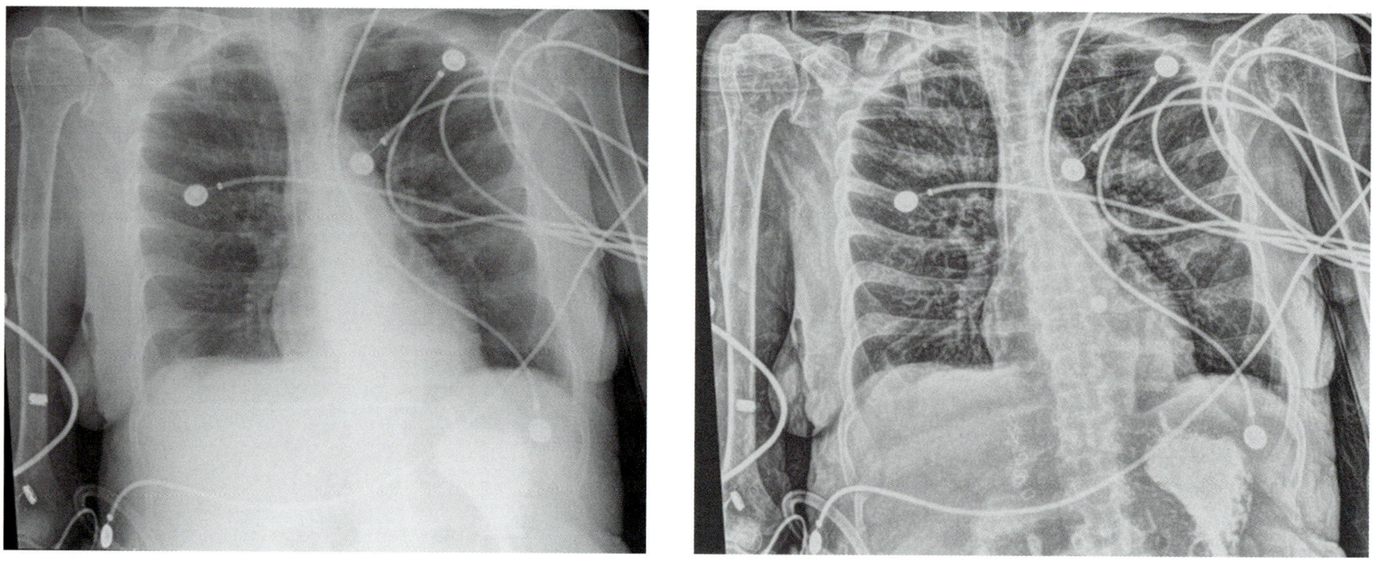

2-6 **(A)** AP portable chest. **(B)** Digital subtraction application can help with identification of a line to determine proper placement.

2-1 Chest Lines

Pacemaker

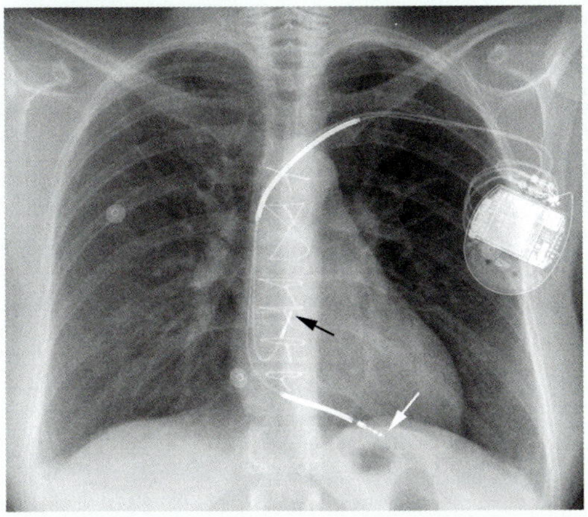

2-7 Pacemaker. *White arrow* represents lead placement in the right ventricle. *Black arrow* represents lead placement in the right atrium.

Electrical stimulus placed into the heart wall to keep pace at its programmed level. Post placement AP chest acquired to verify lead placement. Avoid elevation or movement of the arm on the side the pacemaker is placed (Fig. 2-7).

Nasogastric (NG) Tube

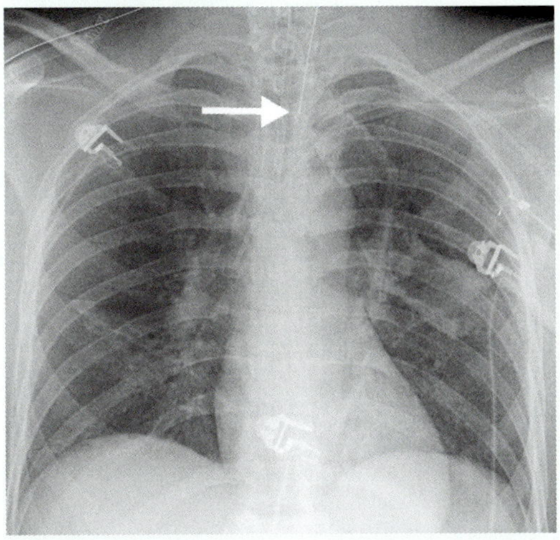

2-8 Nasogastric tube improperly placed.

Tube placed through the nose and should end with placement in the stomach. AP chest could be acquired with concern that the NG tube is positioned into the respiratory system rather than the stomach. The NG tube is used for drug and/or minimal fluid administration. The NG tube is also used for suction; especially on patients with bowel obstruction (Fig. 2-8).

Central Venous Catheters (i.e., PICC Line)

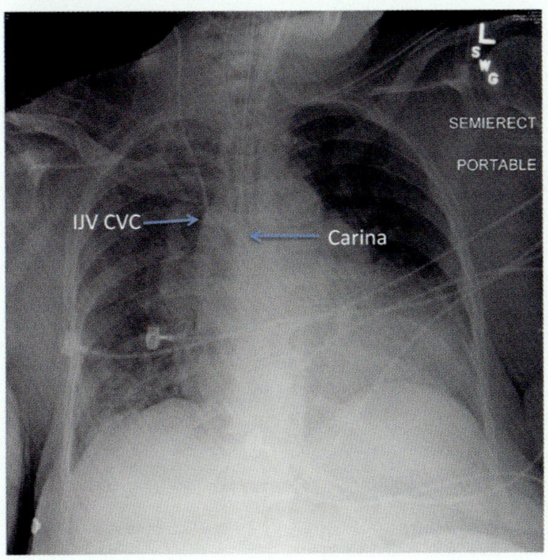

2-9 Central venous catheter.

Long catheter introduced from a peripheral location and adjusted until the end is positioned in the subclavian vein or as far as the superior vena cava. These lines are placed for patients who need long-term drug therapy. An AP chest will verify placement prior to use and rule out the presence of a pneumothorax caused from the line placement (Fig. 2-9).

(continued)

2-1 Chest Line (*Continued*)

Infusion Port

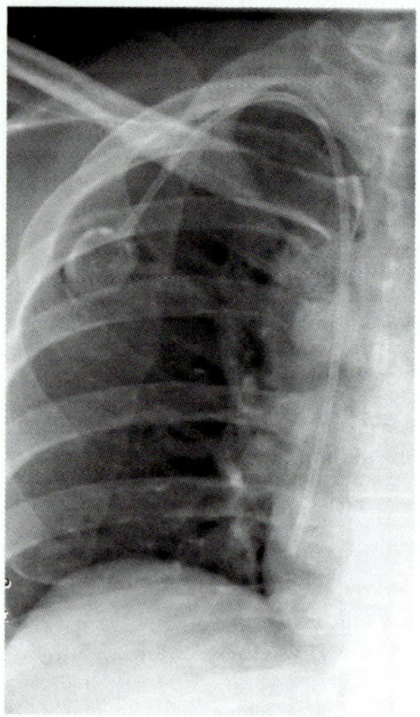

2-10 Example of a port.

Infusion ports commonly placed beneath right clavicle to access the superior vena cava. Infusion ports provide longer indwelling access to administer chemotherapy or other long-term drug therapy. During placement, fluoroscopy (live imaging) is administered by a technologist with a C-arm in the surgical suite. Post procedure, an AP chest will verify placement and rule out a potential pneumothorax caused from the line placement (Fig. 2-10).

Endotracheal Tube (ET)

Tube placed within the trachea to provide an airway. The ideal position of the tip of the tube is just above the carina. An AP chest will aid in verification of its placement (Fig. 2-11).

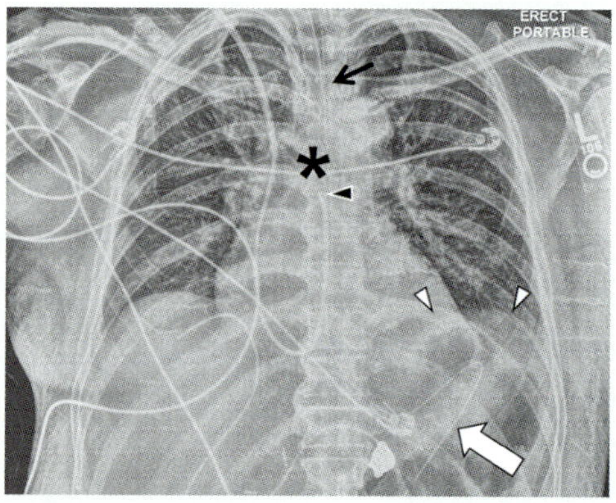

2-11 Identification of an endotracheal tube. Image reveals the end of the ET tube with the *black arrow*. The *asterisk* represents the carina. The *black arrowhead* represents the end of a Swan-Ganz catheter. The *white arrow* represents the end of a NG tube.

Chest Tube

Treatment of a pleural effusion or pneumothorax may be administered with the placement of a chest tube within the pleural space. The chest tube is often connected to a vacuum-assisted device used to help remove air, fluid, or blood from the pleural space. Chest imaging may be acquired to verify placement of the tip and monitor the progress of the patient's condition. Chest images are often acquired post removal of the chest tube to ensure maintained stability.

Internal Jugular (IJ) Catheter

Catheter placed through the IJ vein and runs down vertically to the point of the superior vena cava. This line serves to deliver fluids or to monitor venous pressure. It is a type of central venous line (Fig. 2-12).

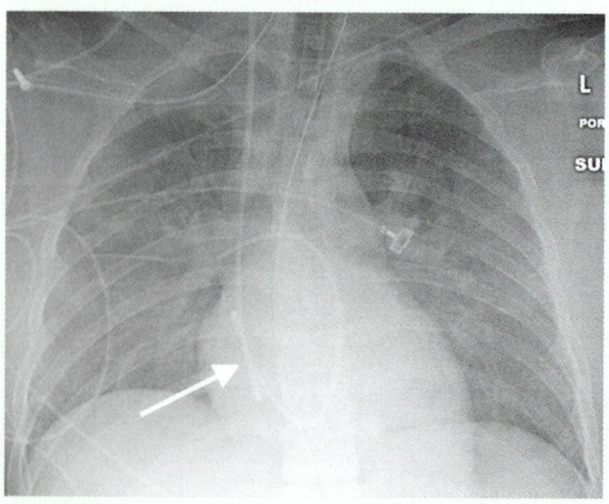

2-12 Swan–Ganz catheter is positioned into the right side of the heart and into the tip of the pulmonary trunk.

Flail Chest: A result of adjacent rib fractures in more than two places from trauma, causing concern for an unstable chest wall and underlying pulmonary injury (Fig. 2-13)

Atelectasis: A complete or partial lung collapse in response to a pathologic obstruction within the airway (Fig. 2-14)

Bronchitis: An acute or chronic condition resulting from inflammation of bronchi, causing the bronchi to produce mucous. The condition may result from lifestyle choices or environmental influences (Fig. 2-15).

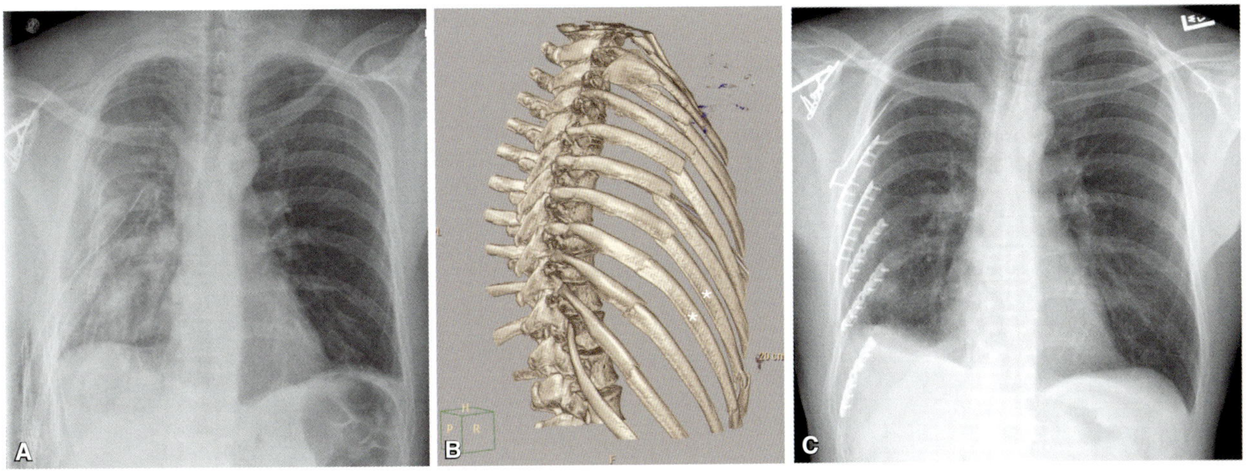

2-13 Flail chest results in instability to the chest wall due to the presence of multiple and adjacent rib fractures. **(A)** Represents multiple rib fractures to the right ribs. **(B)** The CT reconstruction image represents multiple rib fractures creating an unstable chest wall seen with flail chest. **(C)** Represents right rib fracture repair.

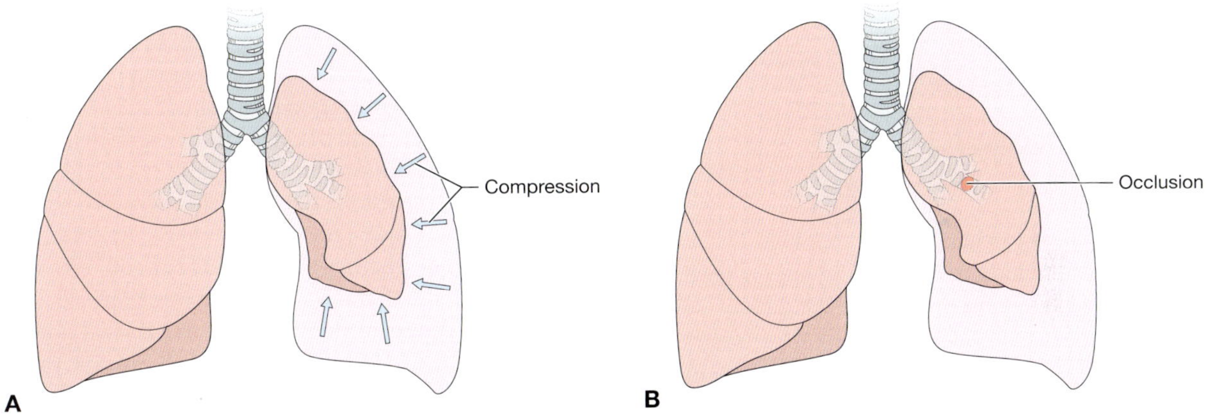

2-14 **(A)** Atelectasis caused by compression of lung tissue. **(B)** Atelectasis caused by obstruction.

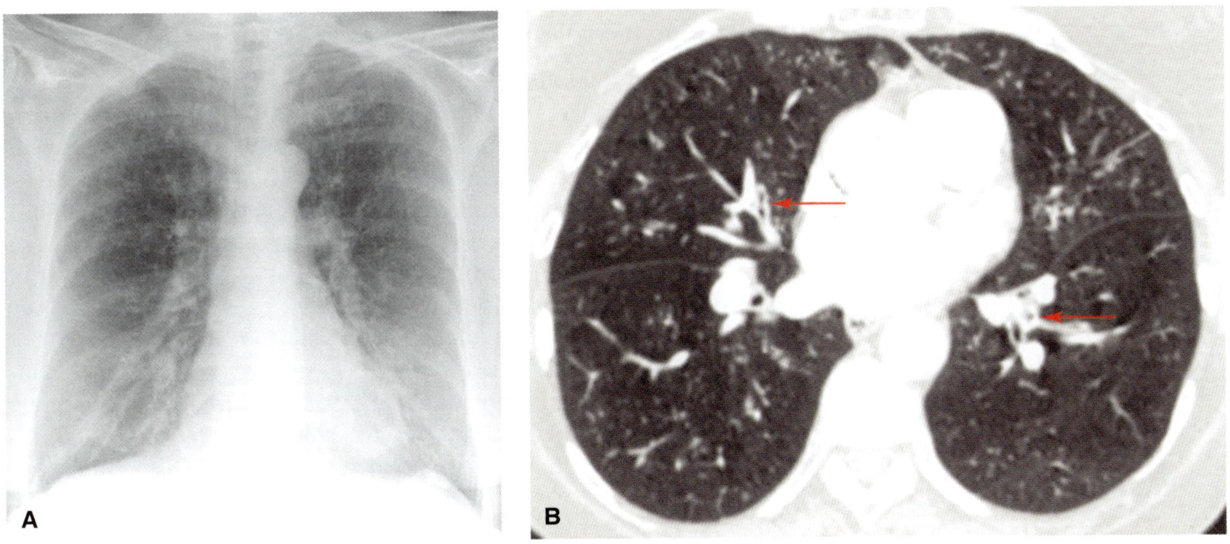

2-15 Bronchitis. **(A)** PA chest radiograph in a patient with a history of chronic bronchitis revealing hyperinflation with increased parenchymal markings. **(B)** CT scan at the level of the mid-lungs demonstrating bronchial thickening (*arrows*).

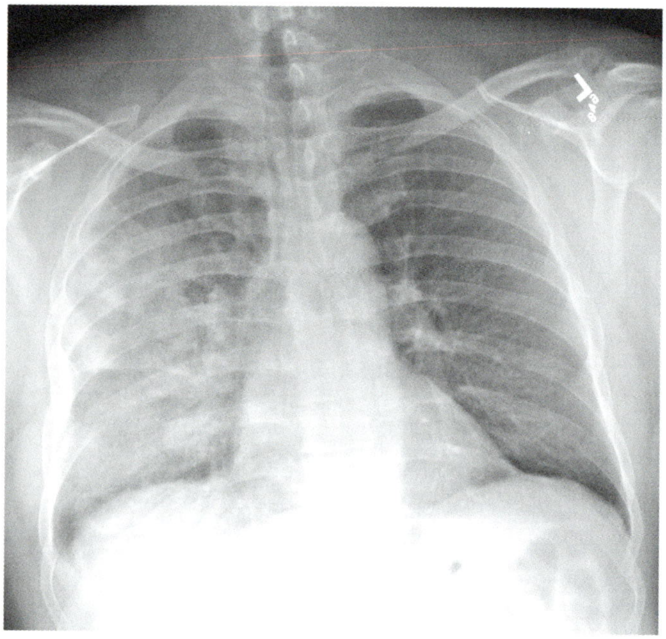

2-16 Pneumonia.

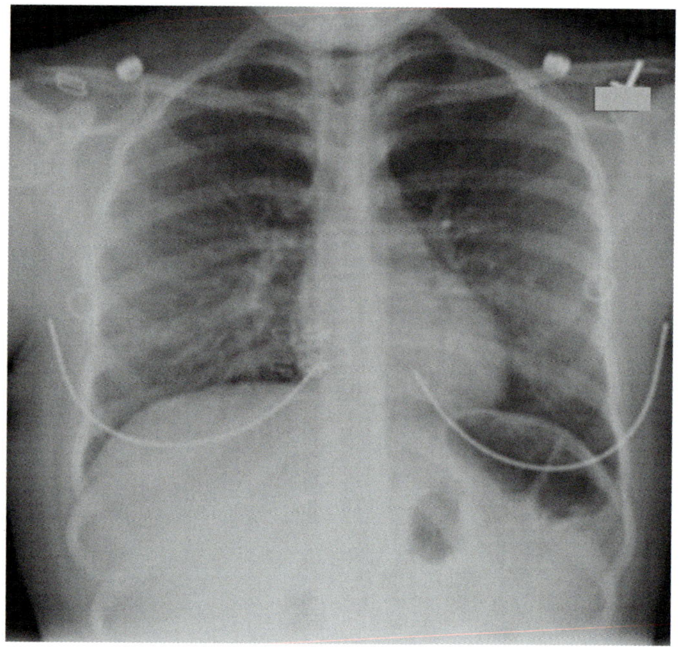

2-17 Artifact from patient clothing.

Pneumonia: An inflammation of the lungs resulting in sections filling with fluid. There are different types and locations of pneumonia (Fig. 2-16).

IMAGING CONSIDERATIONS

Patient Dress

The patient will need to change from the waist up, removing all metal or plastic objects from clothing and/or jewelry that might present as artifact on the image. The patient should be dressed into a gown. For patients already dressed in a gown, the radiographer should check the area of interest to ensure the area is free of artifact before imaging.

Artifacts

Artifacts are unwanted objects that appear on the image superimposing pertinent anatomy. This includes snaps, buttons, bras, thick banded or braided hair, and jewelry. Other artifacts that may appear could be IV lines, electrocardiogram (ECG) patches, oxygen tubing, or safety pins that may secure a line to the patient's gown. The radiographer should assess the patient's lines and tubing, pins, snaps, etc., and attempt to reposition to avoid obscuring the lung field anatomy. In cases where ECG patches are not being used, they should be removed prior to imaging. Considering the higher detail acquired with digital imaging, components such as shirt collars, pockets, and embroidering are easily identified on images and are considered artifacts that will constitute a repeat image (Fig. 2-17).

Patient Position

Erect—Will best demonstrate air–fluid levels and allow the patient to achieve a deeper inspiration.

Semierect—A tolerable height between supine and erect for the patient. Semierect is always a preferred position to supine as it will allow demonstration of air–fluid levels.

Supine—Unresponsive patients or patients on ventilators may not allow even a semierect position to be considered. Air–fluid levels will not be demonstrated.

Decubitus—The patient will lie on the right or left lateral surface for a minimum of five minutes to display a potential air–fluid level within the thoracic cavity. The choice between right and left lateral position would be determined by the consideration of whether air or fluid is of concern on the right or left side of the thoracic cavity. The position selected should ensure that the air or fluid line of concern will not collect in the region of the mediastinum. In a decubitus position, the x-ray beam will be horizontal to the floor and intersect the patient and the image receptor (IR) perpendicularly.

Ambulatory Patient Imaging

An ambulatory patient is one who can maneuver themselves and bear weight with little to no assistance. Ambulatory patients will benefit from a two-view exam, with the two views obtained ninety degrees apart. Ambulatory patients will be able to walk or come by wheelchair to the exam room to undergo a posteroanterior (PA) and lateral chest projection. Patients transported by wheelchair may still be very capable of standing for the two projections, but proper assessment of this must be made by the radiographer. If the radiographer is concerned that the patient is not strong enough to stand for two projections, he or she could consider seating the patient on a stool, thus maintaining upright positioning. Patients transported by stretcher to the department for a two-view exam, will require the assistance of a second radiographer to help carefully move the patient into position while leaving the patient on the stretcher. Upright positions are most ideal, and projections of the chest could be AP or PA.

Mobile Patient Imaging

Portable imaging is reserved for the patient that is unable to ambulate due to their condition. Mobile exams could be acquired in the emergency department, intensive care unit, PACU, surgery, and inpatient rooms. Mobile imaging will acquire a single anteroposterior (AP) projection in a supine, semierect, or nearly erect position. Semierect or nearly erect imaging is preferred over supine imaging to help with the demonstration of an air–fluid level. Depending on patient condition, the technologist should consider raising the head of the bed to a tolerable height for the patient. The technologist may want to move the patient toward the head of the bed before elevating the head to ensure the patient bends at the waist with head elevation. Unconscious or heavily sedated patients or patients connected to respiratory ventilation should remain in the position they are in for imaging. The technologist should also recognize that these patients will not respond to breathing instructions and will therefore have to carefully observe the patient's chest and expose after the inspiratory phase.

Projection(s)

- AP (Anteroposterior): The beam is directed to enter through the anterior surface, exit the posterior surface, and strikes the IR. This projection is less desirable as the heart would be a further distance from the IR, therefore causing magnification of structures.
- PA (Posteroanterior): The beam is directed to enter the posterior surface, exit the anterior surface, and strike the IR. This projection is preferred as the heart is positioned closer to the IR, reducing magnification.
- Lateral: The beam will enter the lateral thoracic surface, exit the opposite lateral surface, and strike the IR. The left lateral position is typically performed for the chest since the heart is positioned more to the left side of the thorax; thus, an attempt to reduce magnification.

ANATOMY

The bony thorax serves as the protective framework for the vital thoracic organs such as the heart and the lungs. The frame for the bony thorax is formed by 12 thoracic vertebrae, 12 pairs of thoracic ribs, and sternum (Fig. 2-18).

Sternum

A flat and irregular bone positioned anteriorly on the bony thorax. The sternum is divided into three components: manubrium, body, and xiphoid process. The manubrium contains the jugular notch, the palpable border most superiorly. The jugular notch can serve as a landmark to determine the midsagittal plane (MSP) on the patient. The jugular notch, a topographic landmark, marks the approximate location of thoracic vertebrae, T2–T3. The sternal ends of the clavicles also articulate with the manubrium, forming the right and left sternoclavicular (SC) joints. The sternal angle is the point where the manubrium and the body articulate. The body has scalloped

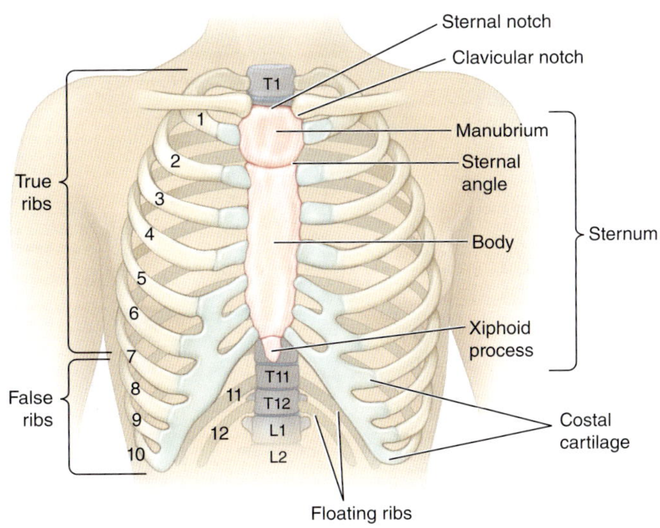

2-18 Bony thorax.

edges along the lateral margins to accept costocartilage for rib articulation. The xiphoid tip is the inferiormost portion of the sternum. The xiphoid process may also serve as a useful bony landmark to identify the patient's MSP. The xiphoid process serves as a topographic landmark, corresponding to the level of thoracic vertebrae, T9–T10 (Fig. 2-19).

Ribs

Twelve pairs of ribs articulate with the thoracic vertebrae. The head of the rib articulates with the posterior aspect of the vertebral body by way of a facet to form the costovertebral joint. Just distal to the head of the rib, the rib narrows into the neck followed by a tubercle (Fig. 2-20). The tubercle will articulate with the transverse process of the thoracic vertebrae to form the

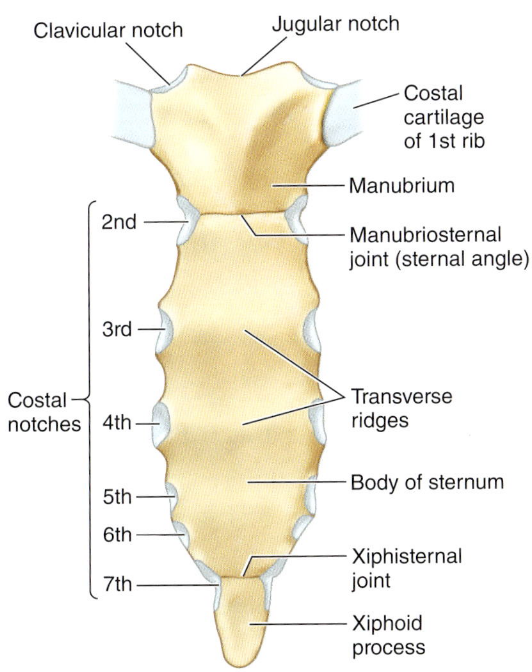

2-19 Bony landmarks.

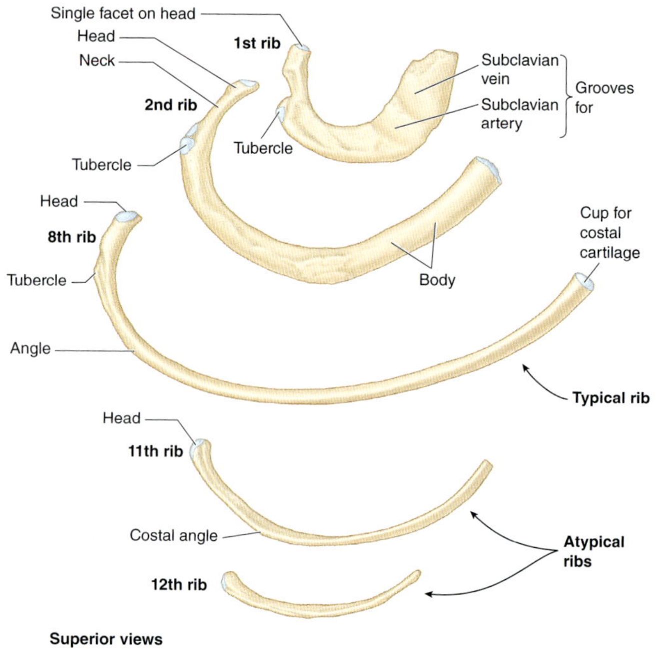

2-20 Typical rib.

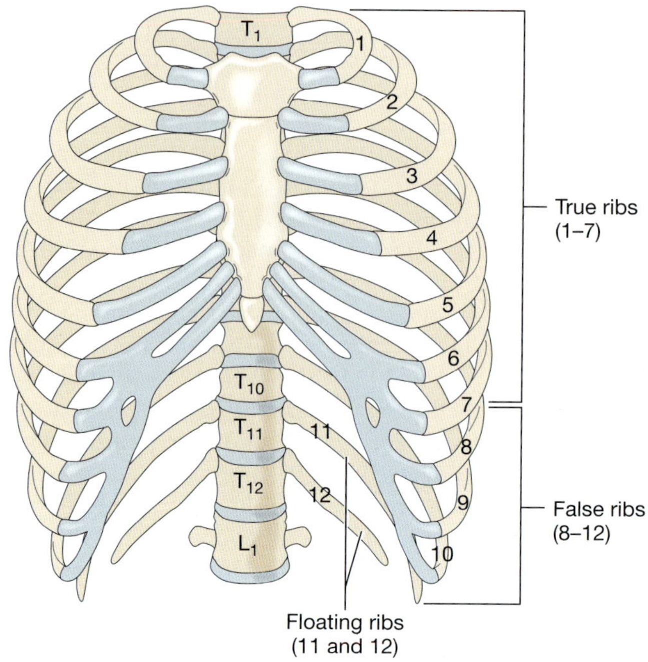

2-22 True and false ribs.

costotransverse joint (Fig. 2-21). All 12 pairs of ribs contain right and left costovertebral joints. Right and left costotransverse joints are associated only with rib pairs 1–10. Each rib has an angle that curves around the lateral aspect of the bony thorax.

The first seven rib pairs are true ribs. True ribs articulate directly with the sternum. The anterior rib is connected to the sternum with costocartilage. Rib pairs 8–12 are false ribs. False ribs do not directly articulate with the sternum. Rib pairs 8–10 do have costocartilage, but the costocartilage joins into the costocartilage of rib seven, which then connects to the lateral sternum. Rib pairs 11 and 12 are floating ribs. Ribs 11 and 12 are short, located mostly on the posterior surface, and do not articulate with any part of the bony thorax anteriorly (Fig. 2-22). The bony thorax is at its widest lateral dimension at the level of rib pairs 8–9.

It should be noted by observing a chest radiograph that the head of the rib (vertebral end) will lie superior to the anterior, sternal end of the rib (Fig. 2-23). When counting the number of ribs on a PA/AP chest radiograph, it is the posterior portion of the rib that is counted.

Lungs

The lungs are protected by the bony thorax along with the heart and great vessels. The lungs are comprised of parenchyma, spongy tissue, which allows for expansion and contraction

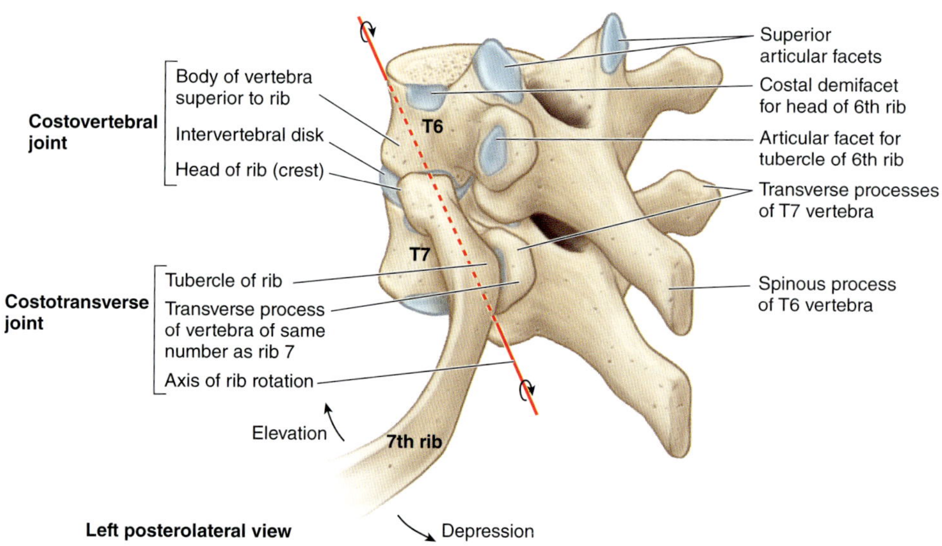

2-21 Location of the costovertebral and costotransverse joints.

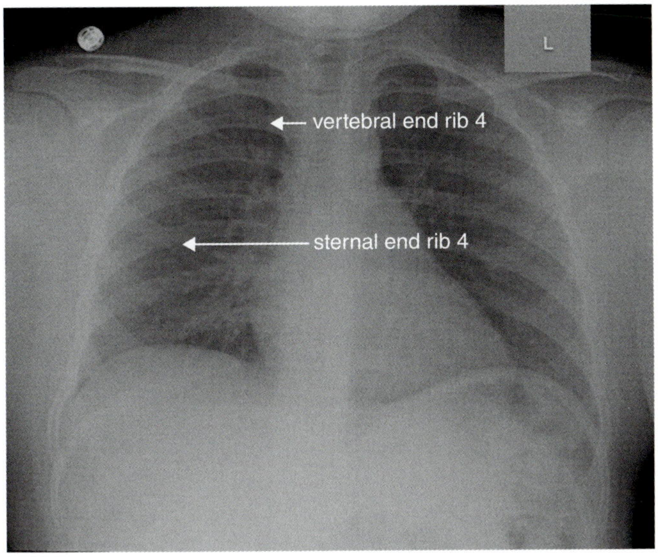

2-23 Vertebral end of the rib sits superior to the sternal end.

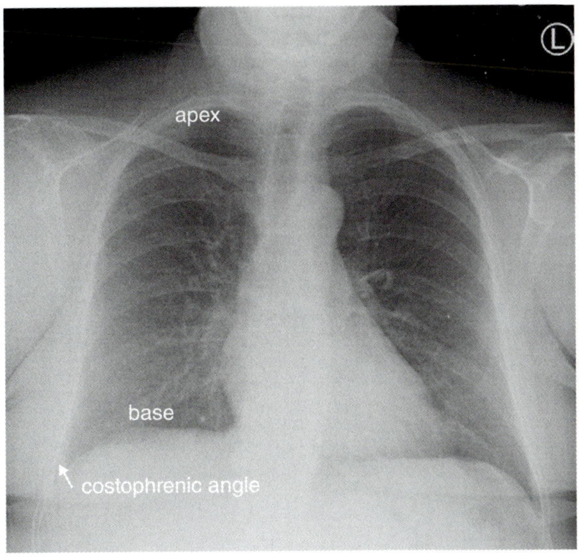

2-25 PA chest.

during the respiratory phases. The most superior portion of the lung located slightly above the clavicle is the apex. The base of the lung rests on the diaphragm. The costophrenic angle is the most inferior and lateral point of the lung formed when the lateral lung meets the chest wall and the diaphragm (Fig. 2-24).

The lungs are air filled and so will appear dark on the image compared with bone. Referring to the PA chest image (Fig. 2-25) and lateral chest image (Fig. 2-26), note the radiographic anatomy.

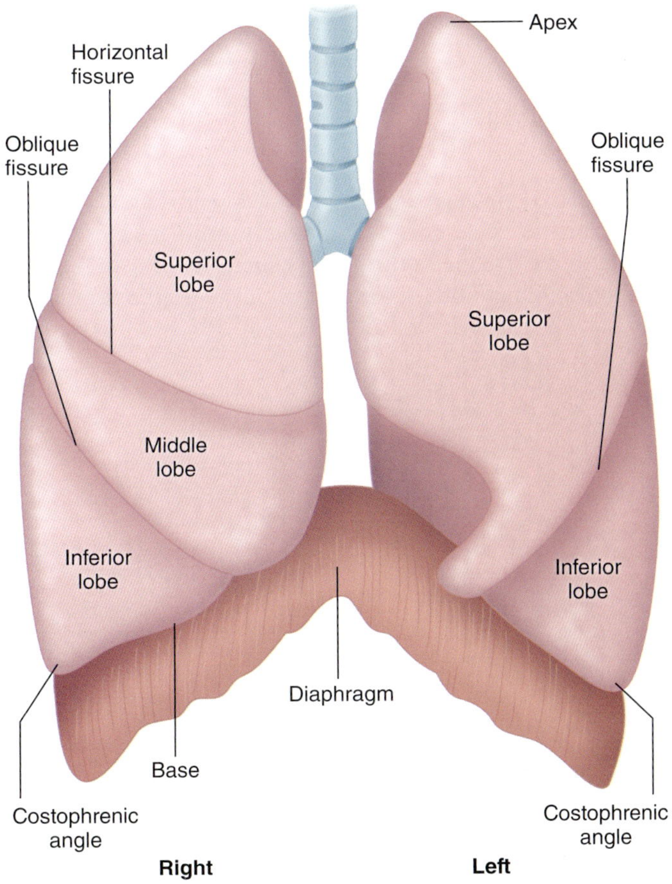

2-24 Lungs.

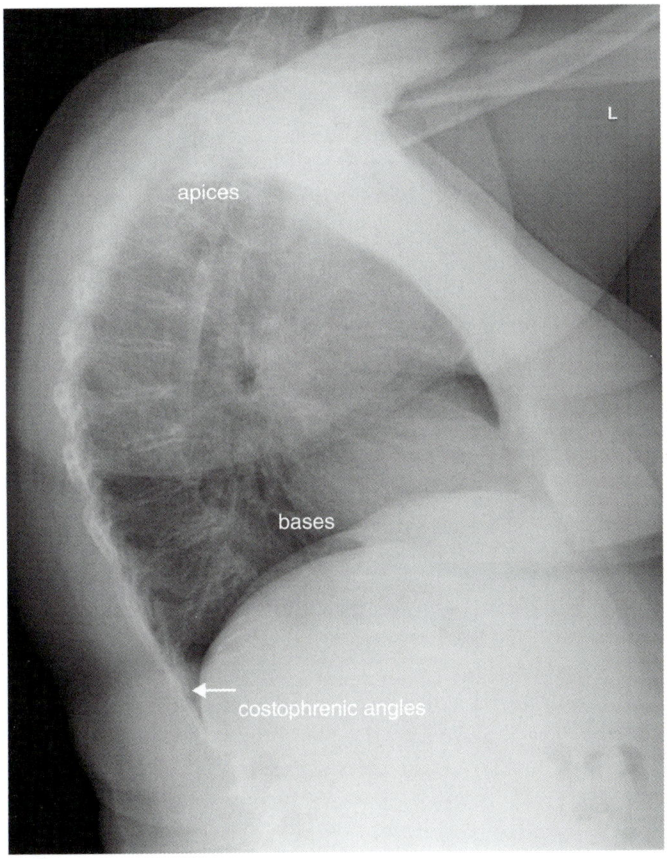

2-26 Lateral view of lungs.

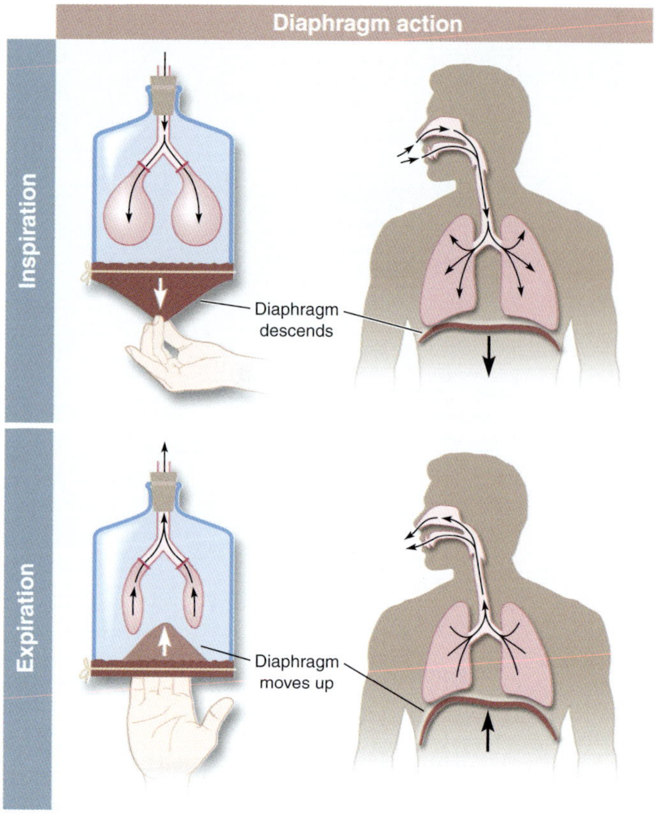

2-27 Diaphragm movements alter with inspiration and expiration respiratory phases.

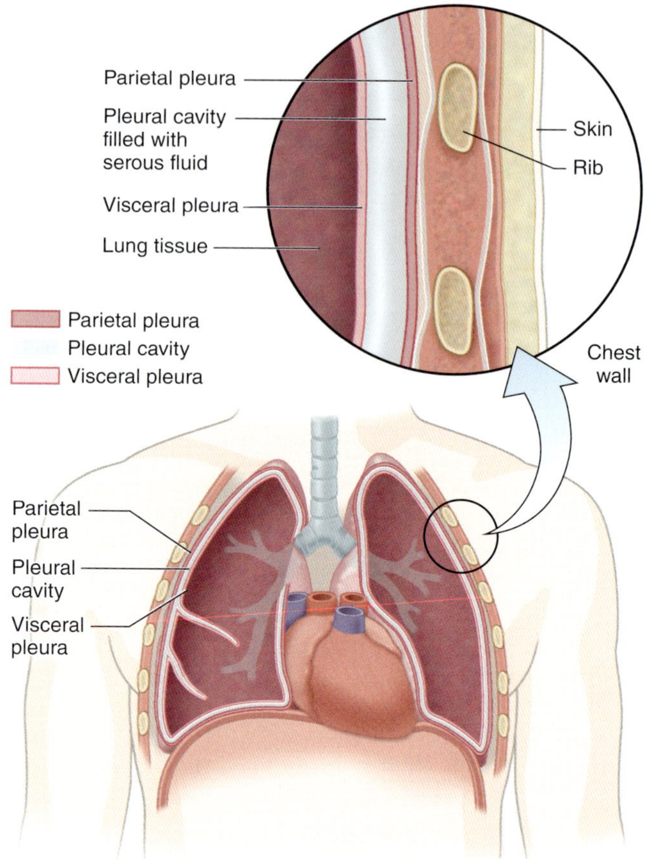

2-28 The potential space, the pleural cavity, is created by the parietal and visceral pleurae.

The diaphragm is a divisional landmark between the thoracic and abdominal cavities. The diaphragm functions to support the respiratory function. With inspiration, the diaphragm moves down to an inferior point, allowing the lungs to expand. With expiration, the diaphragm moves up to its most superior point (Fig. 2-27).

The lungs have an outer lining that covers their surface, visceral (organ) pleura. The inside of the bony thorax is lined with a protective membrane, parietal pleura. In between these two membranes, a potential space, the pleural cavity, is formed. The pleural cavity has a small amount of fluid within the space that allows the membranes to slide against one another during respiratory phases. This potential space can become a site for pathologies, such as abnormal fluid or air collection (Figs. 2-1 and 2-28).

Respiratory System Proper

The respiratory system proper allows for air passage only. The respiratory system proper includes the larynx, trachea, right and left bronchi, and their respective secondary bronchi. The pharynx will connect the oral and nasal passage to either the digestive or the respiratory tract and is therefore not considered part of the respiratory system proper. The pharynx provides a passage for food, fluid, and air. Air drawn into the respiratory system will continue passage through the larynx, trachea, and into the primary bronchi. The larynx is suspended from a "U"- shaped bone, known as the hyoid bone, located just beneath the tongue. The larynx is comprised of cartilage, membranes, and ligaments that comprise the vocal cords. The most prominent cartilage is the thyroid cartilage or the Adam's apple, which can serve as a topographic landmark for the cervical vertebra number 5, C5 (Fig. 2-29).

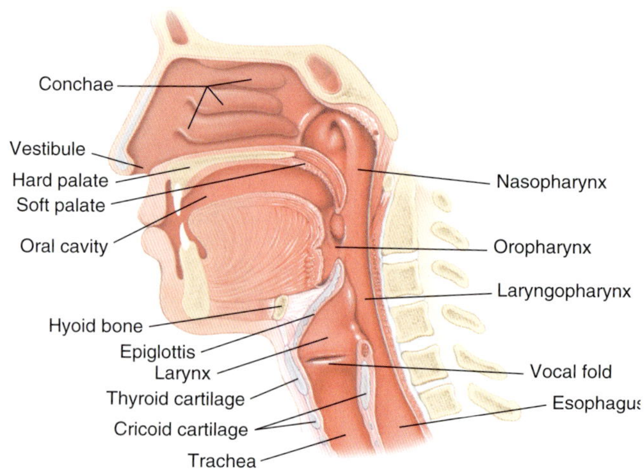

2-29 Upper airway.

At the junction between the larynx (voice box) and the superior-most trachea, the cricoid cartilage is formed. The epiglottis, a cartilage leaflet, serves to seal off the trachea while swallowing to prevent food or fluid from entering the trachea (Fig. 2-30). As the trachea continues down, the rigid and open airway is maintained by numerous "C"-shaped cartilaginous rings. The most inferior point of the trachea before bifurcation into the right and left primary bronchus is the carina (Fig. 2-31).

At the hilar region of the lung, the pulmonary artery, vein, and primary bronchus enter. The right primary bronchus is anatomically distinguished to have a wider diameter, a shorter length, and a near vertical take-off from the trachea. The left primary bronchus is anatomically distinguished to have a smaller diameter, is longer in length, and has a greater angle of divergence from midline. These anatomic differences of the right and left primary bronchus contribute to a higher likelihood of an aspirated foreign object to obstruct the right primary bronchus before the left primary bronchus (Fig. 2-32).

The right and left primary bronchi will branch even smaller. The right primary bronchus branches into three secondary bronchi—superior, middle, and inferior—to supply the respective three lobes of the right lung. The left primary bronchus branches into two secondary bronchi to supply only two lobes of the left lung, superior and inferior (Fig. 2-33). Secondary bronchi continue to branch into smaller bronchioles that terminate in microscopic alveoli. The balloon-like alveoli are the point of oxygen and carbon dioxide exchange (Fig. 2-34).

Mediastinum

Between the hilar region of both lungs and posterior to the sternum is the mediastinal. The mediastinal region contains

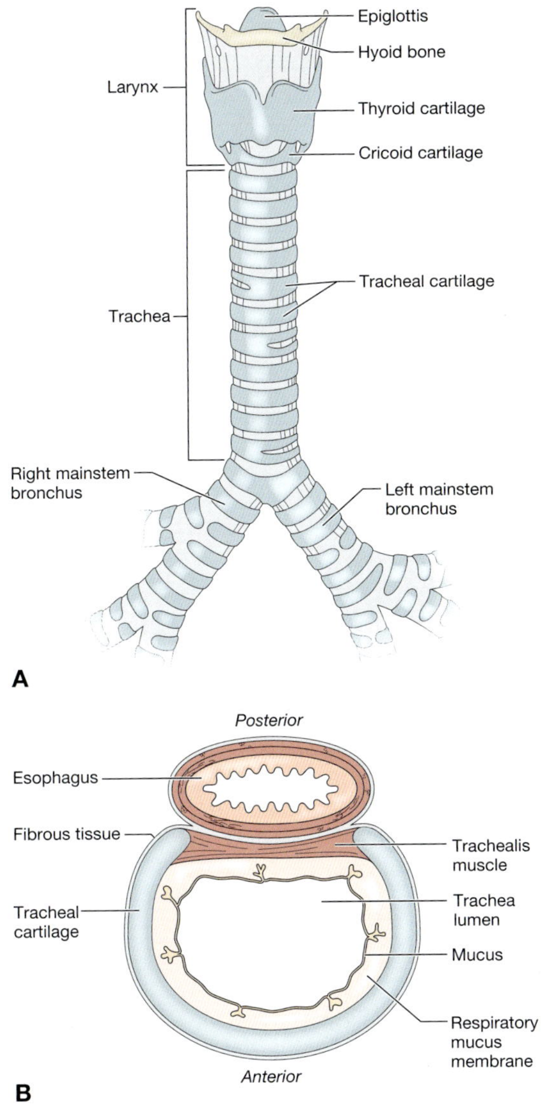

2-31 **(A)** The larynx and trachea. **(B)** Transverse view of trachea and esophagus.

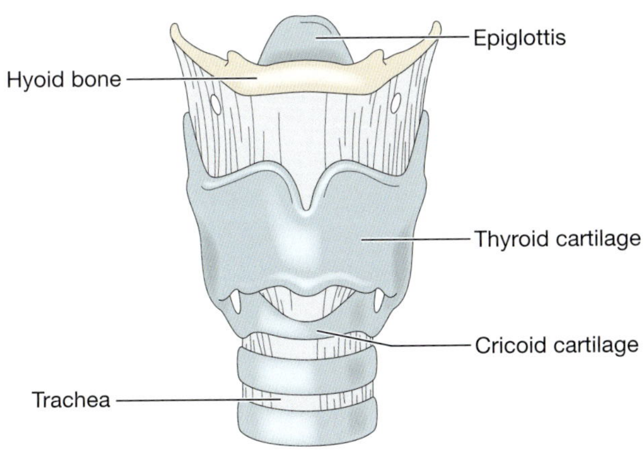

2-30 Larynx.

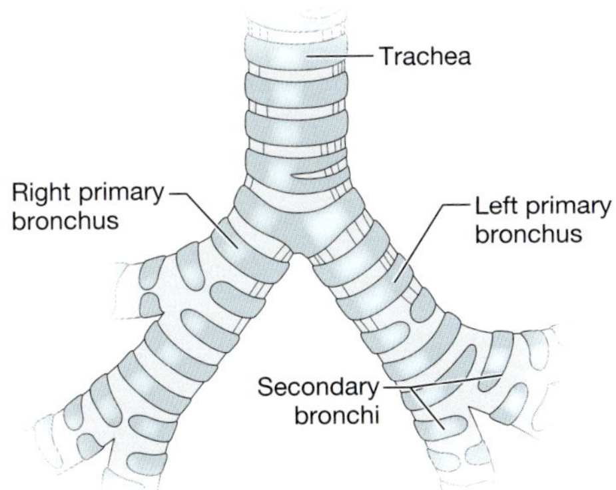

2-32 Trachea and primary bronchi.

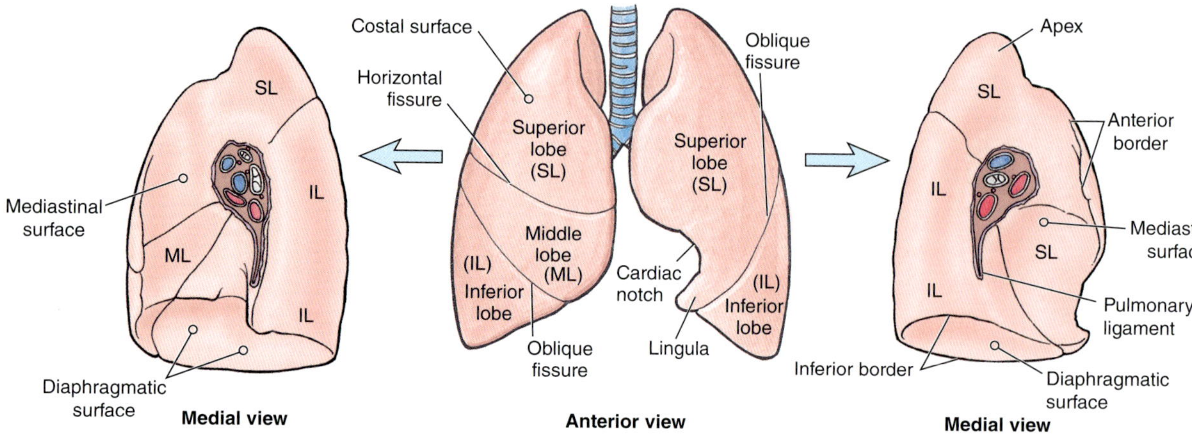

2-33 Lungs.

the heart, great vessels, thymus gland, trachea, and esophagus (Fig. 2-35). The thymus gland is most importance during childhood and adolescent years to assist with the functioning of the immune system. The size of the thymus gland may be interpreted on chest radiographs in early years (Fig. 2-36). The thymus gland is located in the superior mediastinum and below the thyroid gland located just below the larynx (Fig. 2-37).

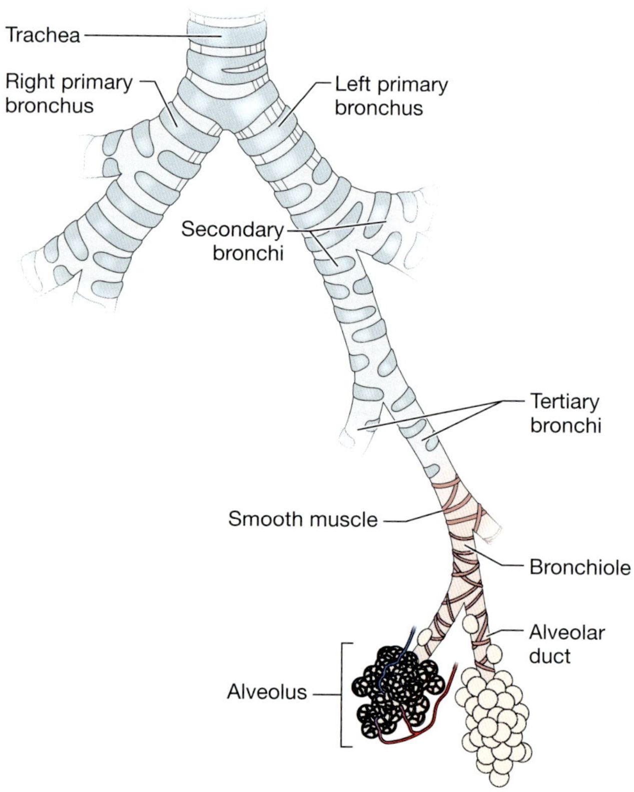

2-34 Secondary bronchi.

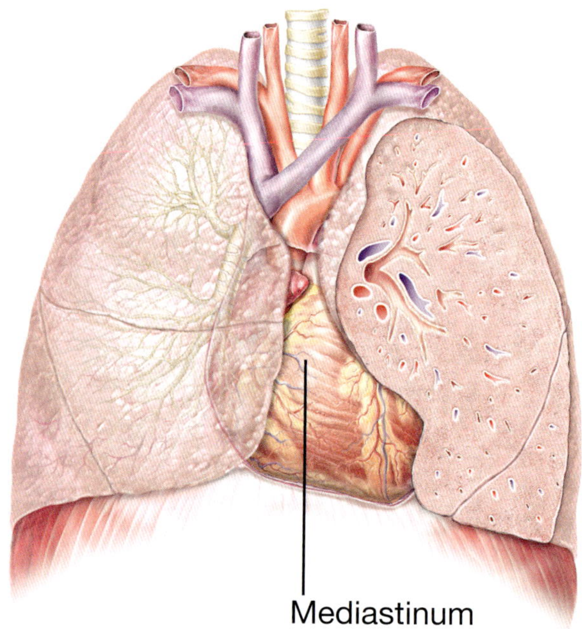

2-35 Mediastinum.

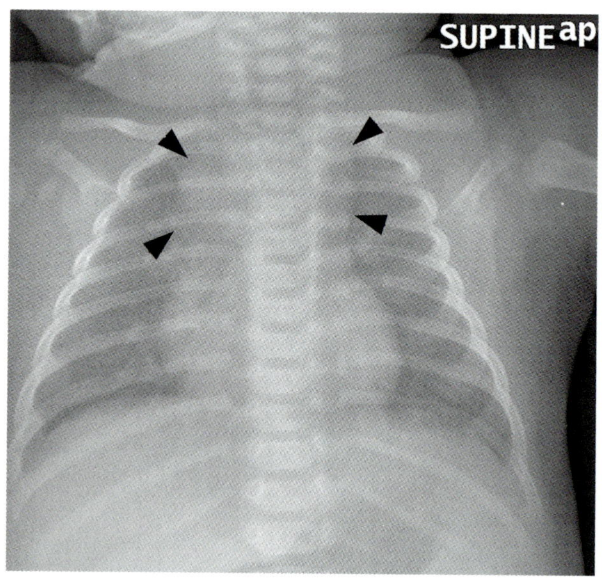

2-36 Thymus gland.

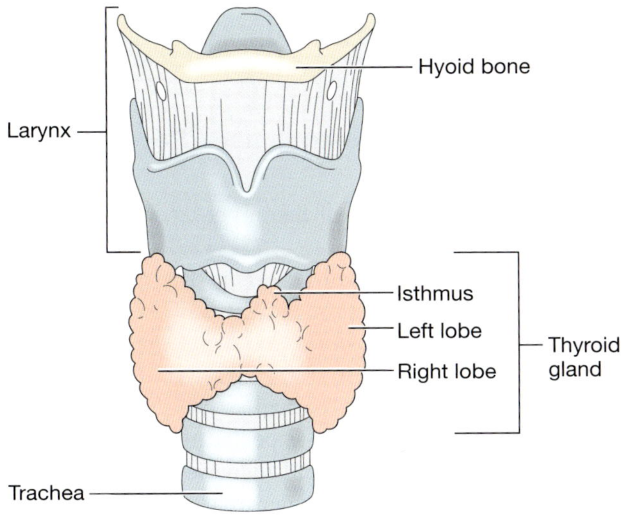

2-37 Thyroid gland.

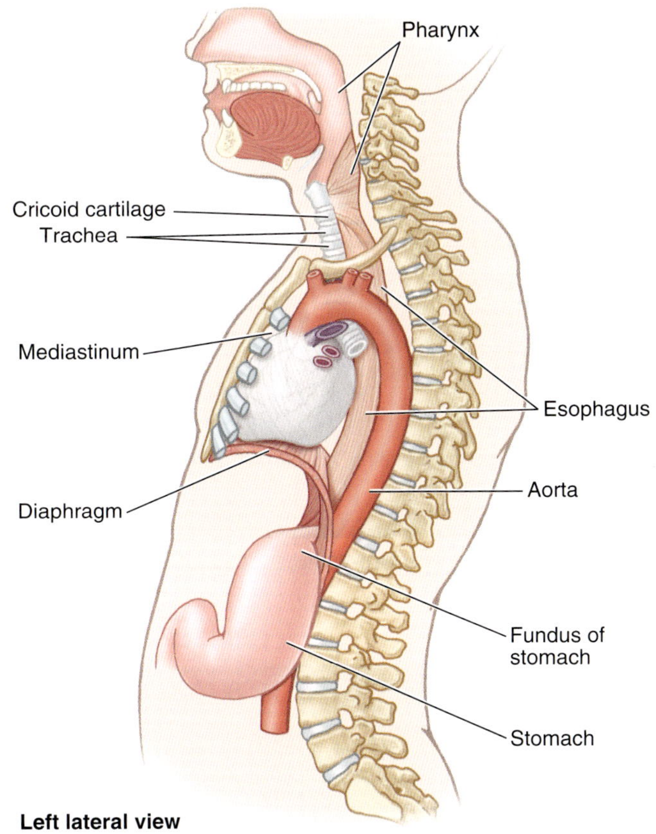

2-39 Relationship of the trachea and esophagus.

The heart is positioned more anterior in the thoracic cavity and is associated with the following great vessels posterior to it: ascending aorta, aorta arch, descending aorta, superior vena cava, inferior vena cava, and pulmonary vessels (Fig. 2-38).

The trachea, within the mediastinal area, bifurcates into the right and left primary bronchi. The esophagus, located posterior to the trachea, travels through the mediastinum and passes through the diaphragm (Figs. 2-39 and 2-40).

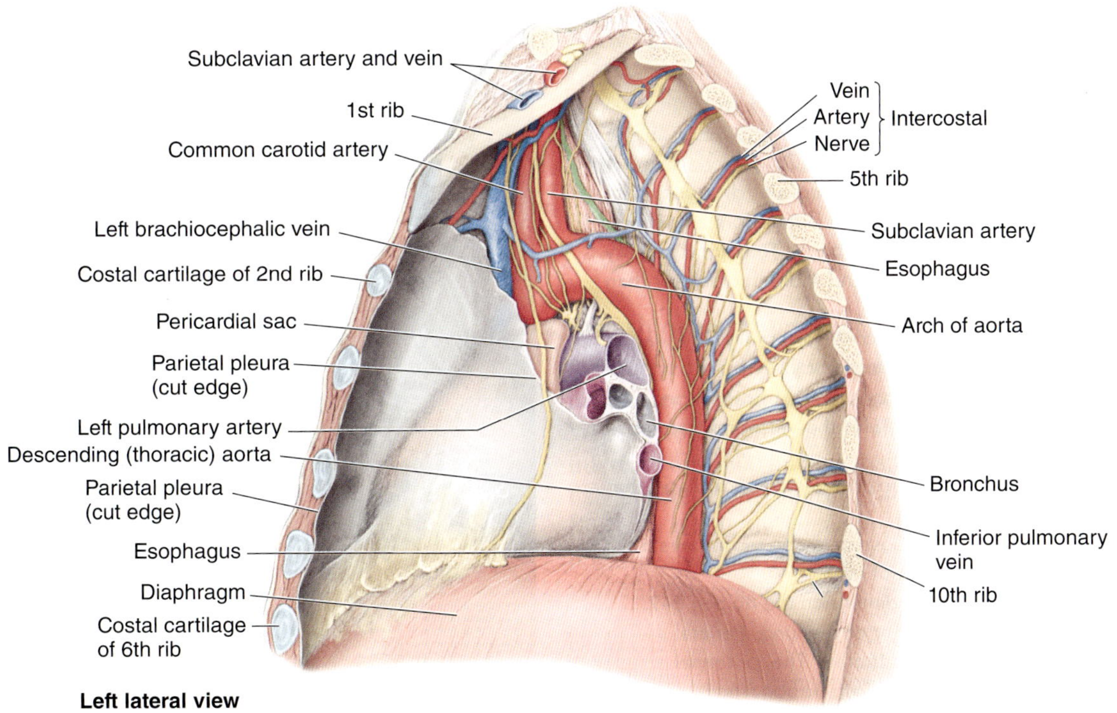

2-38 Structures within the mediastinum.

KEY ANATOMIC LANDMARKS (FIG. 2-46)

- Adam's apple corresponds to cervical vertebral level of C5.
- Vertebral prominens corresponds to cervical vertebral level of C7.
- Jugular notch corresponds to thoracic vertebral level of T2–T3.
- Xiphoid process corresponds to thoracic vertebral level of T9–T10.
- Inferior angle of scapula corresponds to thoracic vertebral level of T7.
- Jugular notch, xiphoid process, and spine would all be landmarks for MSP.

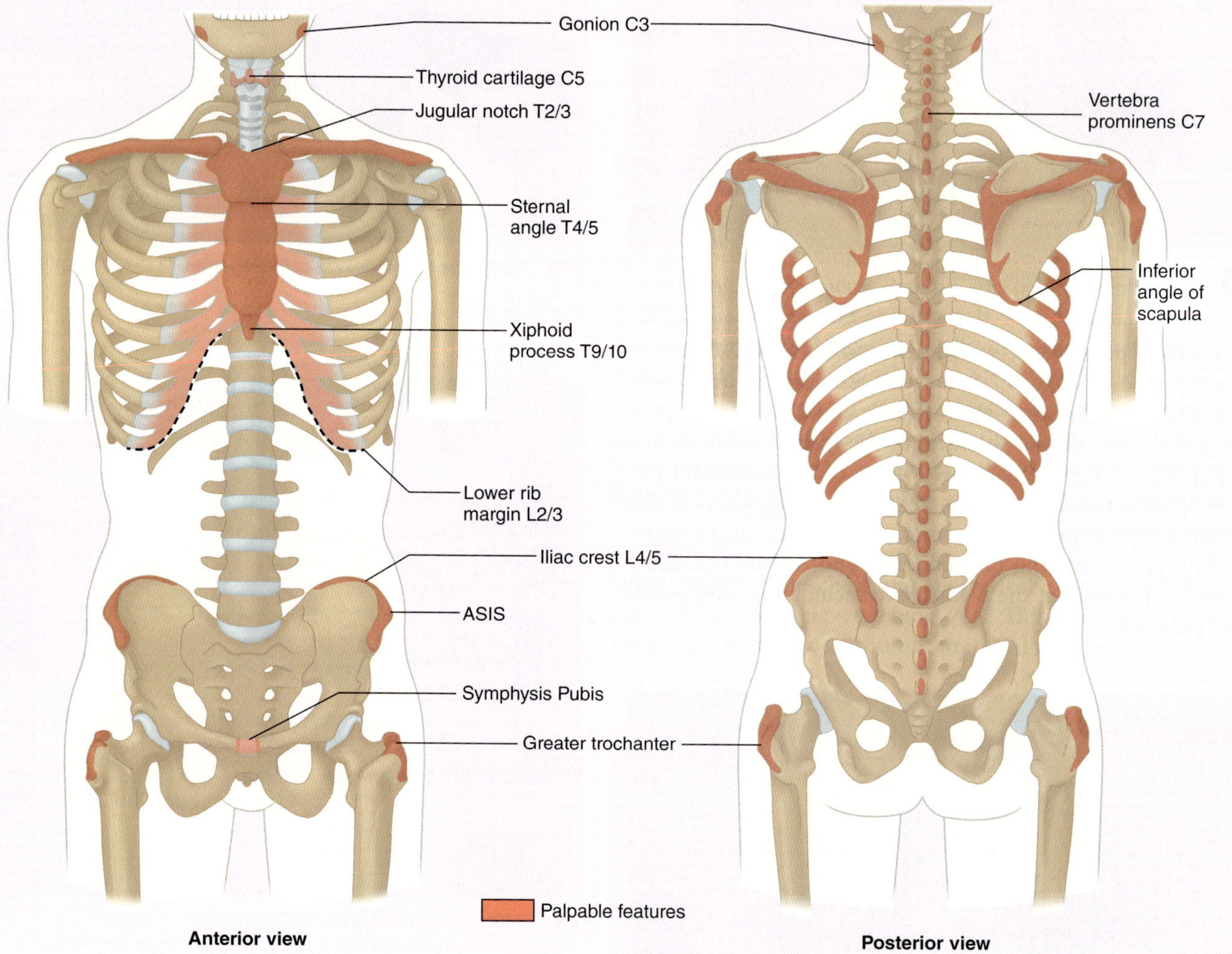

2-46 Topographic landmarks.

the diaphragm on the right side of the thorax. Counting on the right side of the thorax will avoid superimposition of ribs from the heart shadow and also take into consideration the difference in the height of the right and left hemidiaphragm. The right hemidiaphragm typically sits slightly superior to the left hemidiaphragm due to the size and presence of the liver in the right upper quadrant. Full ribs are counted above the diaphragm, but once in the region of the diaphragm, if the medial one-half of the rib above the diaphragm is identified, it can be counted as a rib (Fig. 2-47).

Number of Ribs for Ambulatory Patient

Ideally, a rib count of 10–11 ribs above the diaphragm, especially for an ambulatory patient, is desired. The radiographer should take into consideration patient conditions that may not allow the fullest inspiration and in these cases decide what is appropriate to submit to the radiologist for interpretation. The optimal 10–11 ribs visualized above the diaphragm may be attainable when considering the effects of gravity on the diaphragm, with the patient upright paired with the double inspiratory breathing instructions.

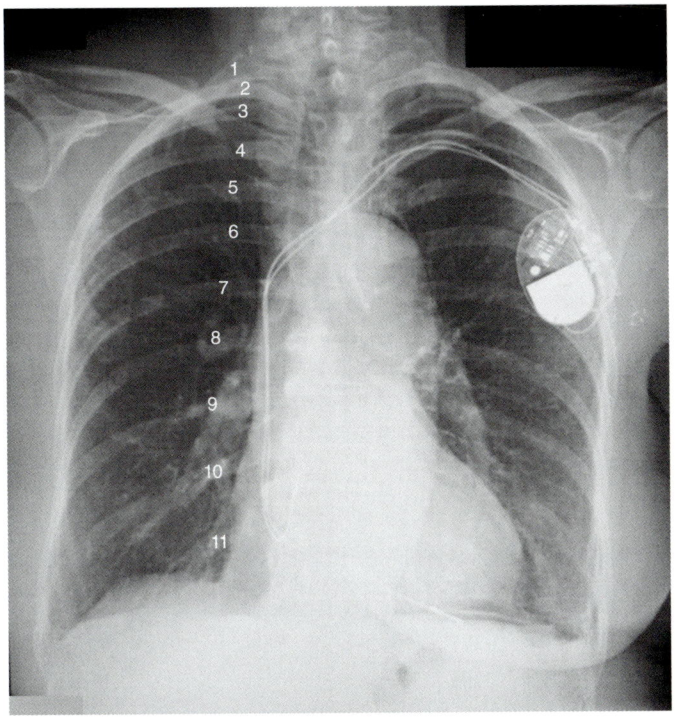

2-47 10–11 ribs above the diaphragm.

Number of Ribs for Portable Patients

In the case of a nonambulatory patient being imaged with the portable, the position and condition of the patient may not allow the maximum visualization of ribs above the diaphragm compared to that of an ambulatory patient. In these cases, a rib count of 8–9 ribs above the diaphragm is acceptable (Fig. 2-48).

Inspiration Versus Expiration Chest Imaging

Inspiration and expiration comparative images are ordered with special circumstances. Inspiration and expiration images are each acquired with a PA projection. Each projection should be additionally annotated with "inspiration" or "expiration" along with the correct anatomic marker. When comparing these two projections, a rib count above the diaphragm may differ (Fig. 2-49). With expiration, the diaphragm should ascend to its most superior point. With inspiration, the diaphragm should descend to its most inferior point. Inspiration and expiration views are reserved for the following situations:

- Suspicious area noted; but not clear if the suspicion is in the lung or rib
- Demonstration of pneumothorax
- To rule out fixation of a diaphragm (diaphragm does not move with respiratory changes)
- Determining location of a foreign object

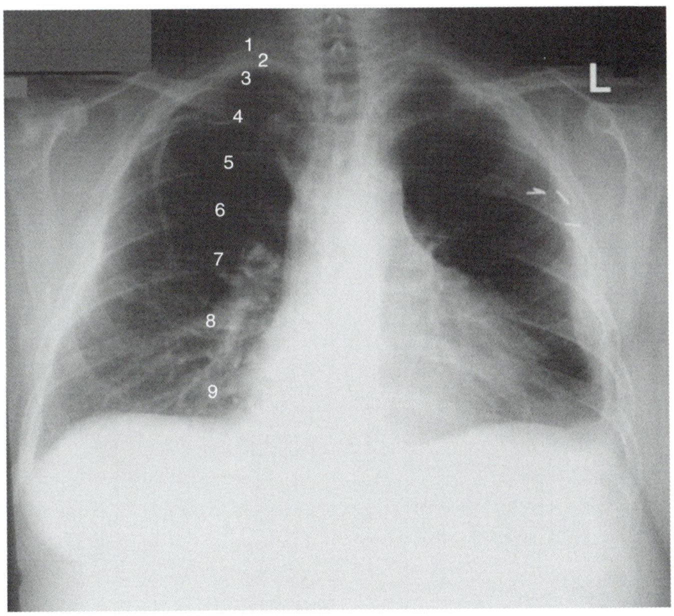

2-48 8–9 ribs above the diaphragm.

Lordotic Chest Imaging

Lordotic chest views may supplement standardized chest images to rule out or better visualize lung tissue directly beneath the clavicles. Lordotic views may also be sought when patient's chin superimposes superior lung tissue. The lordotic chest is acquired with an AP projection. The upright patient should

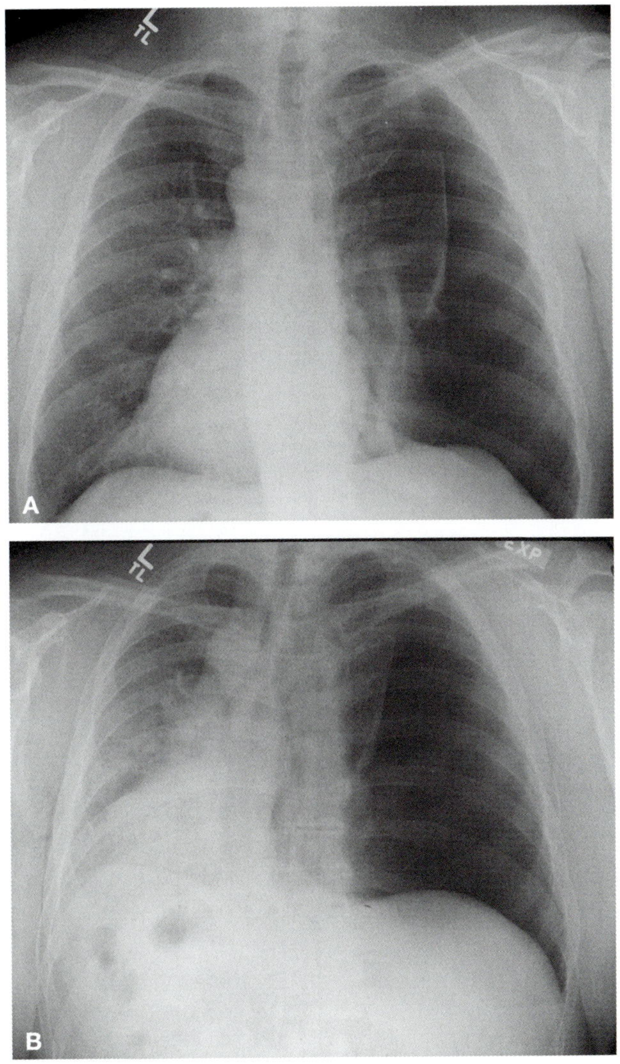

2-49 Inspiration and expiration PA chests for comparison. **(A)** Inspiration and **(B)** expiration. The radiograph reveals a right-sided pneumothorax.

step about one foot away from the upright Bucky and then lean back toward the Bucky, supporting their shoulders, neck, and head on the upright Bucky. With the patient's hands on their hips, the elbows are inverted to roll the scapulae out of the lung field (Fig. 2-50).

If a patient is unable to stand, a 15°–20° cephalic tube angle could be applied (Fig. 2-51).

A maximum distance is sought when imaging recumbent or 72″ when upright, with the central ray directed to thoracic vertebrae level 7/8 and with MSP. The clavicles should appear horizontal and superior to the apices of the lungs with the exception of the sternal ends of the clavicles, which will remain superimposed at midline (Fig. 2-52).

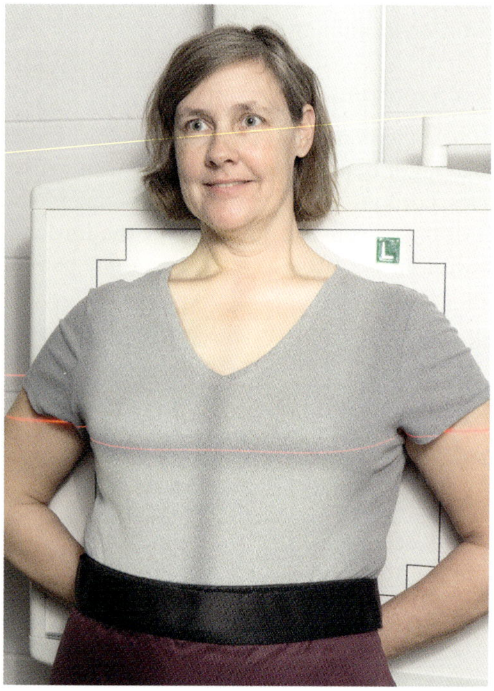

2-50 Lordotic chest view—upright patient position.

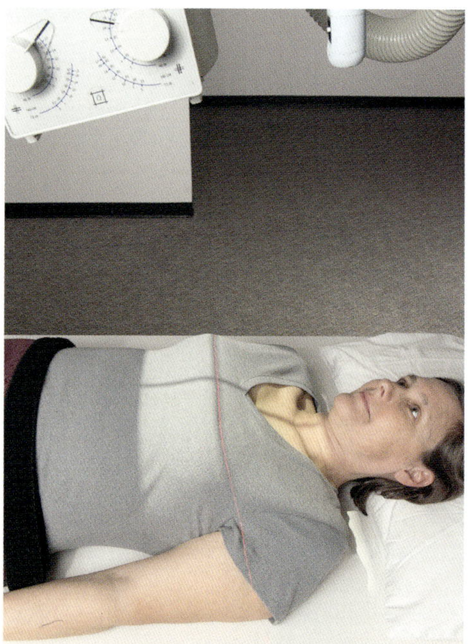

2-51 Lordotic chest view—supine patient.

Anterior Oblique Chest Projections

Oblique views of the chest may supplement standardized chest images to better visualize mediastinal structures, specifically the size and contour of the heart and great vessels. Oblique views may also be ordered to help demonstrate proper line placement and their depth in the body. The patient is positioned upright with an average of 45° with the patient in the right anterior oblique (RAO) and left anterior oblique (LAO) positions. The images will appear similar to a rib AP oblique projection, showing the chest side of interest furthest from the IR, but the technique is set as it would be for a chest. The central ray is directed to the level of thoracic level 7/8 and midway between the spine and the upside lateral most margin of the chest (Figs. 2-53 and 2-54).

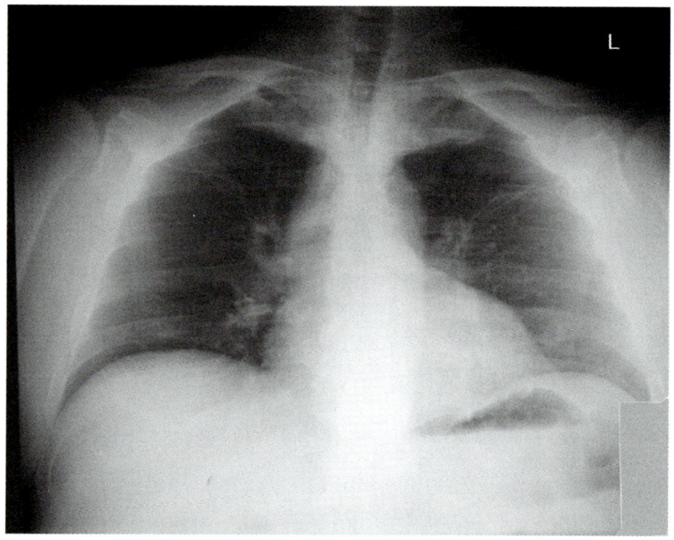

2-52 Lordotic chest view.

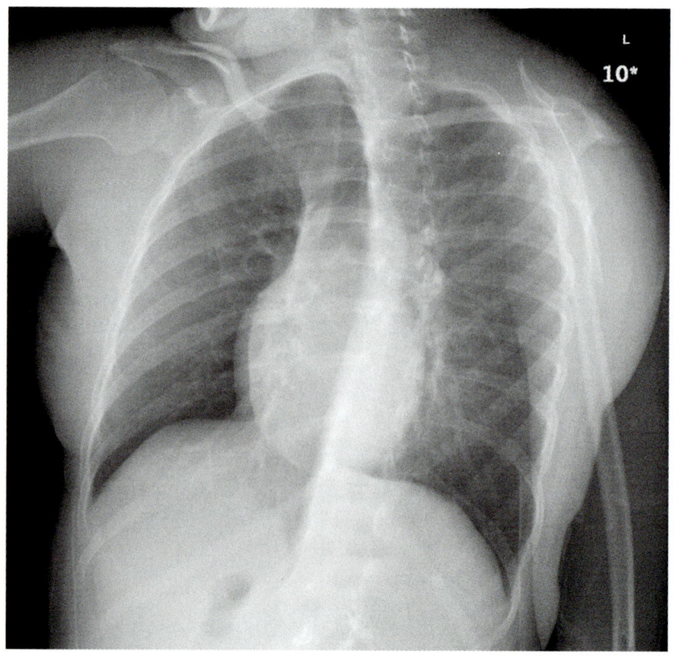

2-53 Chest oblique view.

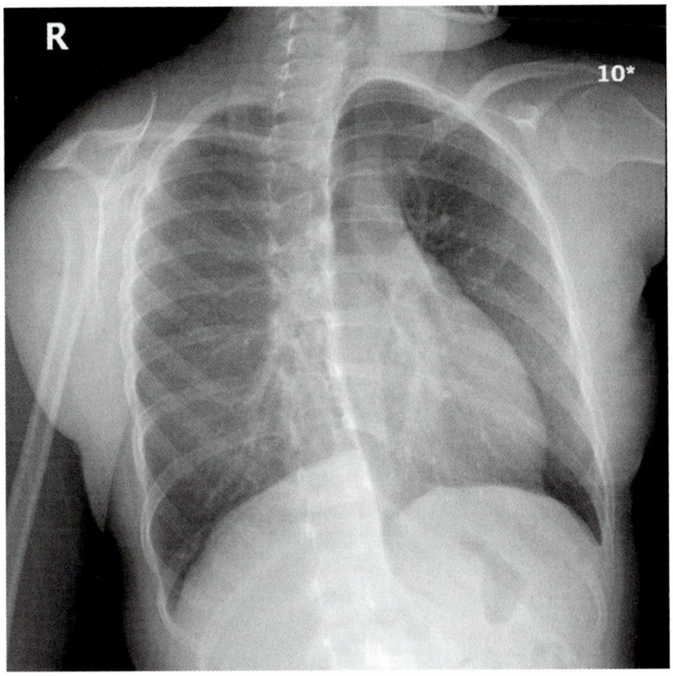

2-54 Chest oblique.

TECHNICAL CONSIDERATIONS

Setting a Manual Technique

Manual technique is defined when the radiographer sets the kVp and mAs values independently. A manual technique can be set in the imaging department and on the portable unit. Setting a manual technique will also allow the technologist to adjust the length of the exposure; something important to consider with pediatric and geriatric patients. In cases where patient motion is of concern during the length of exposure; increase the mA, which allows the exposure time to be decreased (Fig. 2-55).

Setting Technique With Automatic Exposure Control (AEC)

AEC may be an option in the imaging department. With AEC, the technologist will set the kVp, will not set an mAs, but rather must select which exposure cell(s) correspond to the anatomy centered and anatomy coverage over the cell(s) according to the projection (Fig. 2-56). The cell(s) will determine when adequate exposure has been reached according to the part thickness and composition, and then the exposure is terminated. After the exposure terminates, the radiographer will note the mAs value displayed on the control panel (Fig. 2-57).

Kilovoltage (kVp)

Kilovoltage is set to penetrate the part thickness and affects the scale of contrast seen on the image. A higher kVp for chest imaging is needed to penetrate the thickness of the chest and to penetrate through the region of heart and spine. With a higher kVp and with a thicker part, the scatter radiation produced is increased and affects the overall scale of contrast. A long or low scale of contrast (many shades of gray with slight differences) is desired for chest imaging. The long scale of contrast allows for differentiation of tissue, lung markings, heart, and pathology. It should be noted that kVp is typically the relatively constant factor when imaging, as the kVp for a specific part or region tends to be standardized within a range.

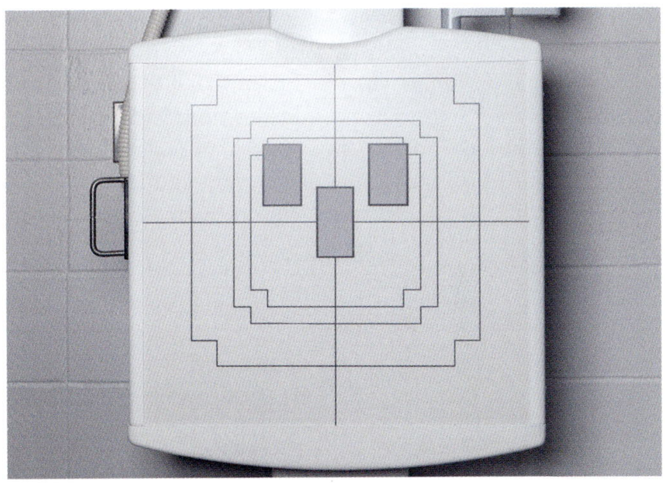

2-56 Ionization chamber locations.

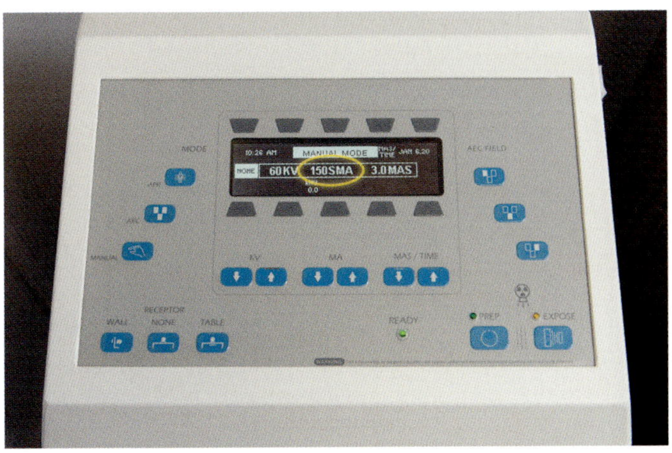

2-55 Control panel setup with manual technique selection of technical factors.

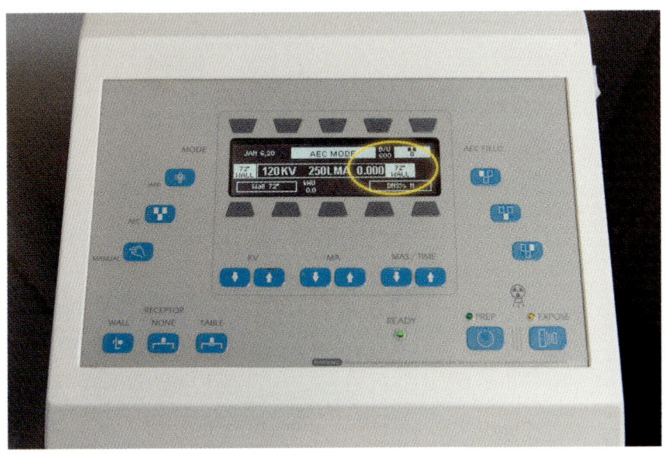

2-57 Control panel set for PA chest with AEC selection.

Source-to-Image Distance

A 72″ source-to-image distance (SID) is preferred for chest imaging as there is less divergence of the beam, specifically at the edges of the field size. Additionally, with increased SID, less magnification of structures occurs, thus improving spatial resolution. Consideration should be given to increasing the SID for chest imaging and utilizing a PA projection when possible to reduce structural magnification of the heart.

Shielding

Shielding should be applied consistently to ensure good practice among all patients when appropriate or if requested by the patient. Acceptable shielding practices include freestanding mobile shield, lap shield around the backside, lap shield to the front side, or, most ideally, a complete wrap around the waist shield for chest imaging.

Marking the Image

All images must be accurately marked with a minimum of the right or left lead marker. For AP or PA chest image, the right or left anatomic marker should be placed in the region of the shoulder to avoid superimposition with any lung tissue (Fig. 2-58). For the left lateral chest image, the left marker (indicating the side closest to the IR) should be placed "in front" of the patient or along the anterior surface of the patient up in the region of the arms (Fig. 2-59).

Additional markings, such as an arrow, could also be used to help indicate a supine or upright positioned chest. Arrows can also be used to indicate the "side up" or "side down" on a decubitus chest position. Many of the right and left anatomic markers include three lead beads within them that reposition to help identify upright or recumbent positions. When marking decubitus chest positions, it is typically best to mark in the region of the shoulders with the anatomic marker along with an "up arrow" or a "side up," indicating the patient's side positioned up (Fig. 2-60).

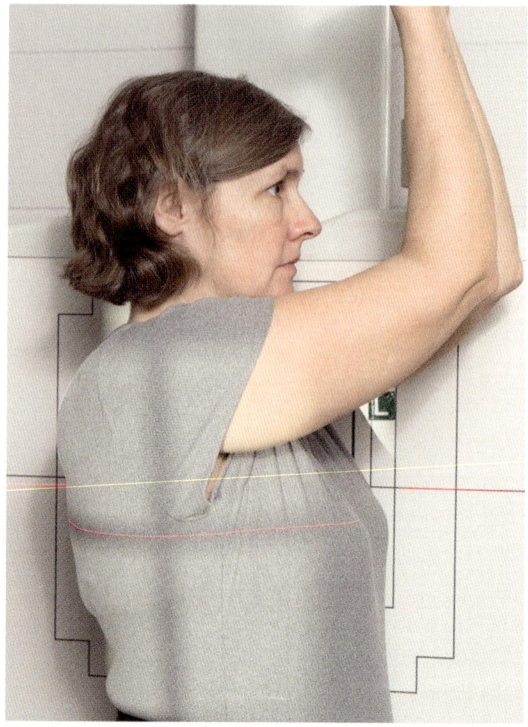

2-59 Marking the left lateral chest.

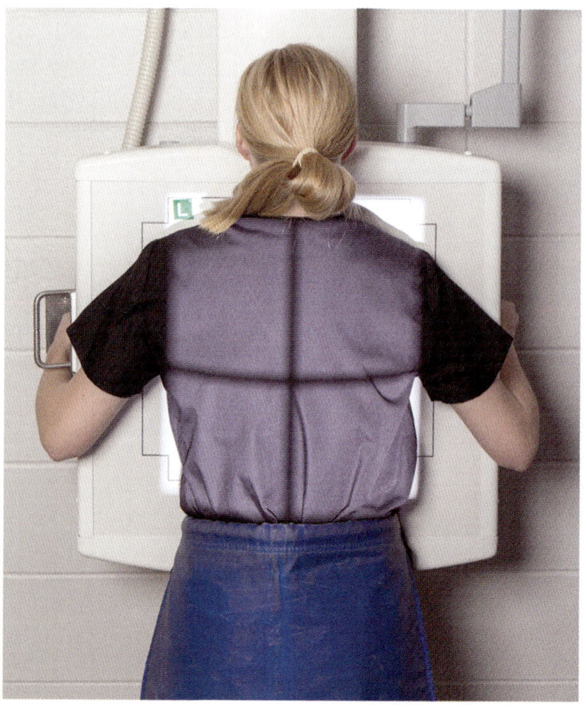

2-58 Marking the PA chest.

Image Display

Assuming the chest image was correctly marked, the image is displayed opposite of the viewer facing it, as though the image is in anatomic position. With correct marking of the left side, the heart will be displayed more predominantly slightly left of midline. In addition, the gastric bubble in the stomach that corresponds normally in the left upper quadrant may be visible (Figs. 2-61 and 2-62).

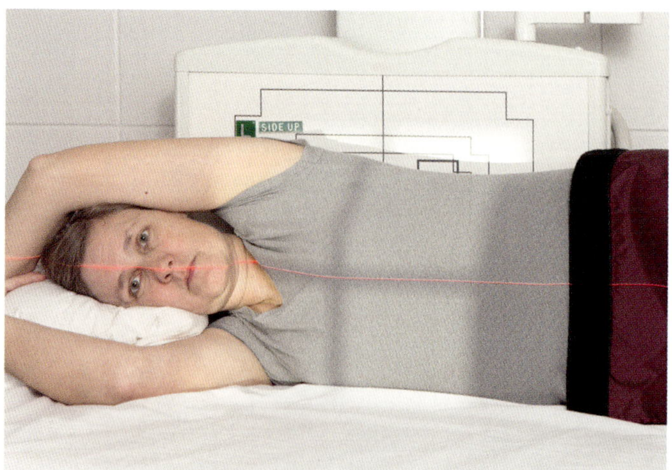

2-60 Marker placement for the right lateral decubitus chest.

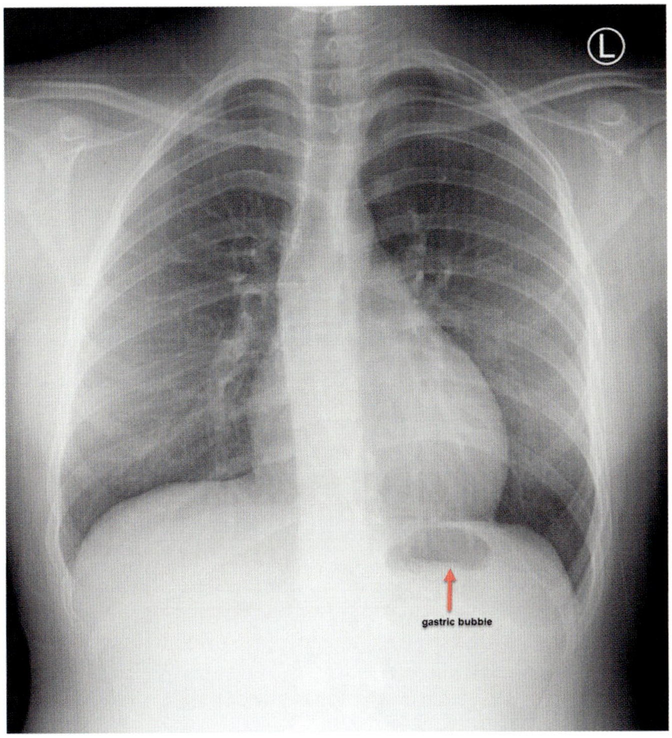

2-61 Correct PA chest display.

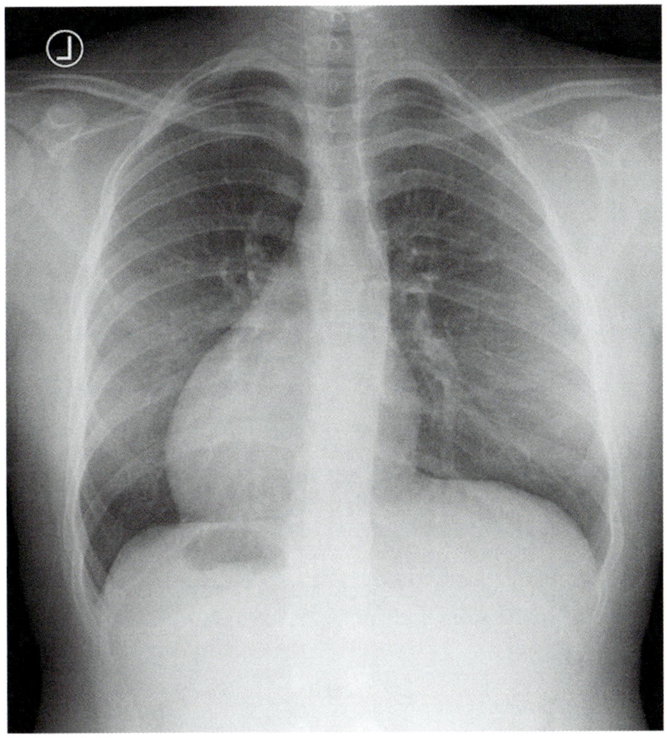

2-62 Incorrect PA chest display.

Ambulatory Chest

- Projection: PA

Ambulatory Chest Protocol
PA
Left Lateral

Technical Considerations
- kVp 110-130
- 2 outermost AEC cells selected for upright Bucky
- 72″ SID

Exposure Field Size
- 14 × 17 lengthwise for sthenic to asthenic patient
- 14 × 17 crosswise
- 17 × 17

Patient Position
- Erect and facing upright Bucky
- Shoulders relaxed. Chin elevated
- Arms wrapped around board rolling shoulders/scapulae forward
- For women with large, pendulous breasts, it may be necessary to have the patient lift their breasts up and out as they step up in contact with the upright Bucky. This may reduce additional tissue from obscuring base of the lungs and/or costophrenic angles

Centering (Figs. 2-63 and 2-64)
- Level of T7/8 and with MSP

Marking of IR
- Right or left marker up above the corresponding shoulder

Breathing
- Double inspiration and hold after second inspiration
- Watch the patient during breathing instruction and while walking away to make the exposure

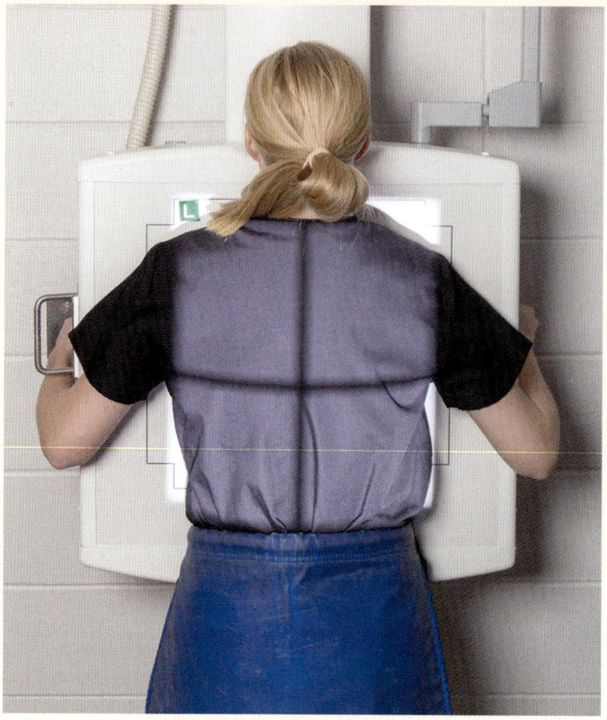

2-63 PA chest.

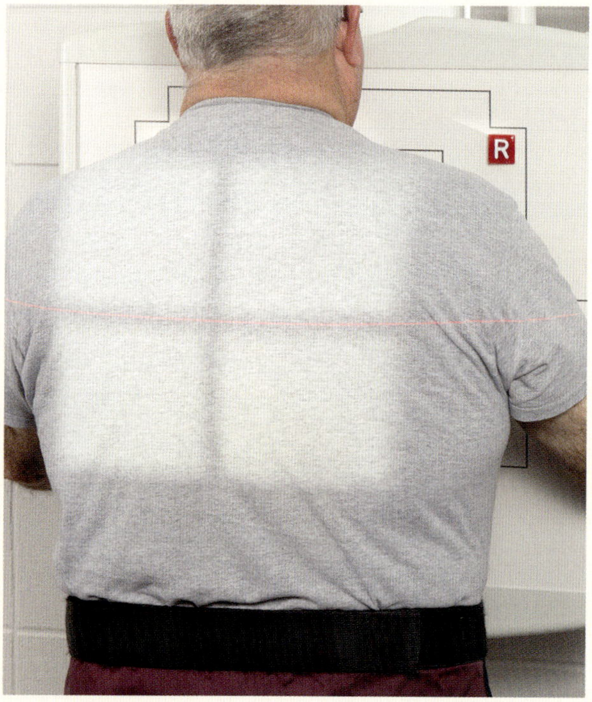

2-64 PA chest.

IMAGE CRITIQUE (FIG. 2-65)

- Entire lung fields revealing apices, bases, costophrenic angles, and lateral lung margins
- IR properly orientated, properly centered and collimated
- 10–11 ribs above the diaphragm counted on the right side of thorax
- Clavicles near horizontal. This indicates that the shoulders were relaxed
- Scapulae removed from the lung field. This indicates that the shoulders were rolled forward (Fig. 2-66)
- SC joints symmetric. This indicates the patient was not rotated; both shoulders were equal distance to the IR (Fig. 2-67)

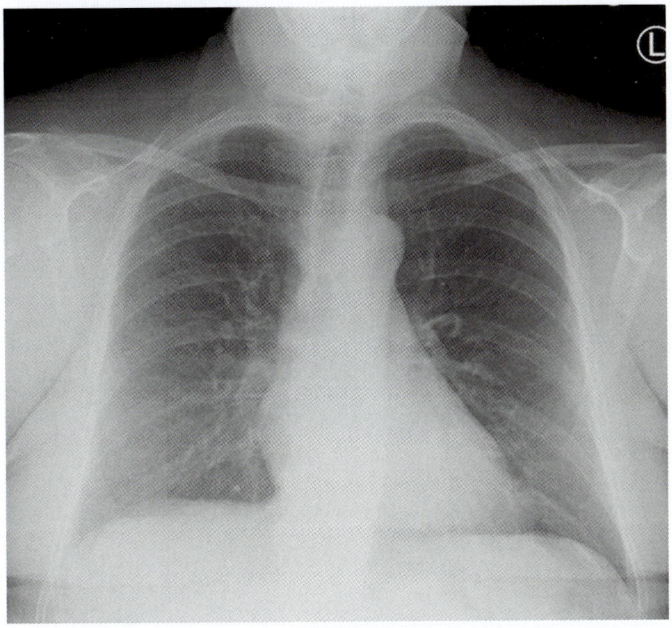

2-65 PA chest.

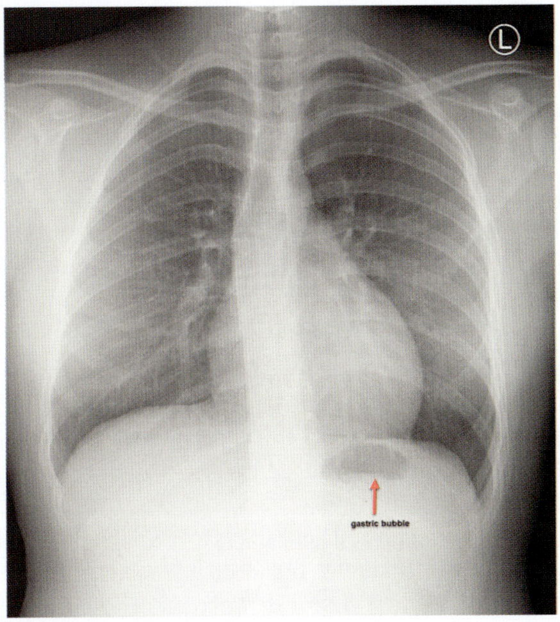

2-66 PA chest with scapulae in the lung field.

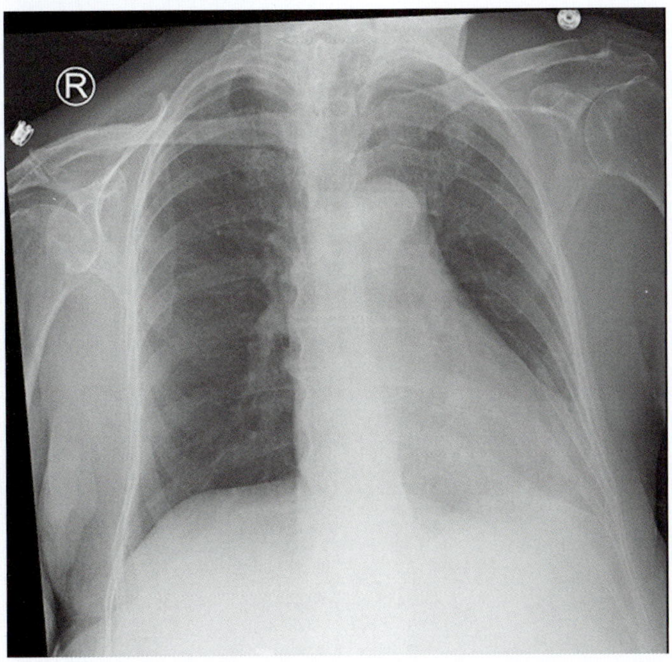

2-67 PA chest reveals rotation at the SC joints and scapulae in the lung field.

Ambulatory Chest

- Projection: Left Lateral

Ambulatory Chest Protocol
PA
Left Lateral

Technical Considerations
- kVp 110–130
- Center AEC cell selected for upright Bucky
- 72″ SID

Exposure Field Size
- 14 × 17 lengthwise for all patients
- 17 × 17

Patient Position (Figs. 2-68 and 2-69)
- Erect left lateral position
- Feet slightly separated for balance
- True lateral position of thorax with hips and shoulders aligned
- Arms elevated to hold onto chest positioning bar (proper elevation of arms is critical to remove soft tissue from the upper arms from the superior lung field)
- Chin elevated and with eyes facing forward

Centering
- Level of T7/8 and midcoronal plane (MCP) or slightly posterior to MCP

Marking of the IR
- Left marker placed on the anterior surface up in the area of the arms

Breathing
- Double inspiration and hold after second inspiration
- Watch the patient during breathing instruction and while walking away to make the exposure

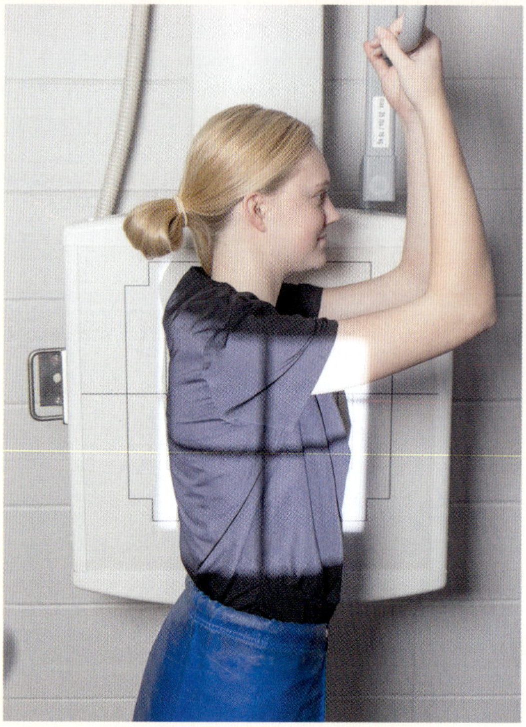

2-68 Lateral chest.

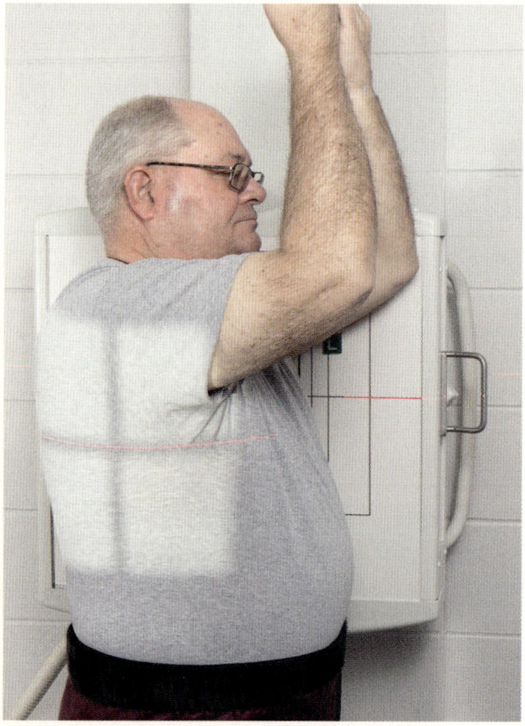

2-69 Lateral chest.

IMAGE CRITIQUE (FIG. 2-70)

- Entire lung fields revealing apices, bases, anterior to posterior lung tissue
- Properly centered and collimated
- Posterior ribs are superimposed, indicating the thorax is not rotated (Fig. 2-71). Rotation evidenced at the posterior rib margins that is <½″ or 1 cm is considered acceptable
- Arms and chin elevated insufficiently from the apical lung region (Fig. 2-72)

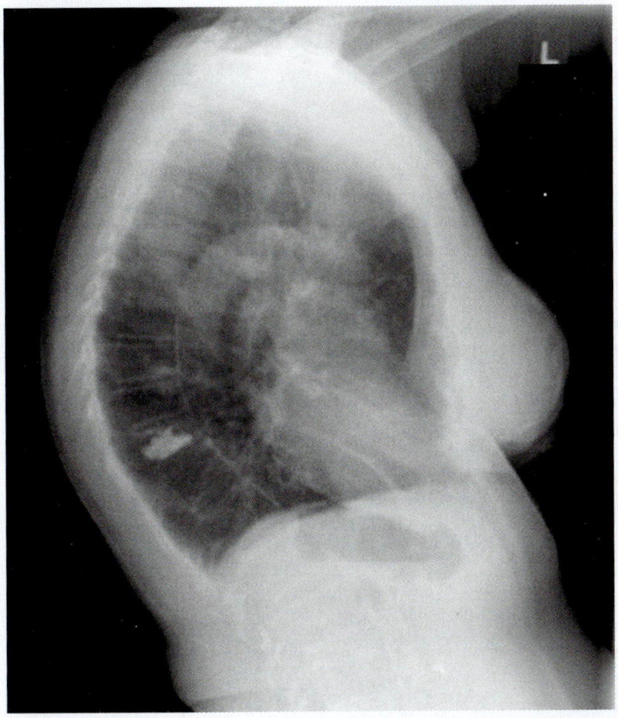

2-70 Lateral chest.

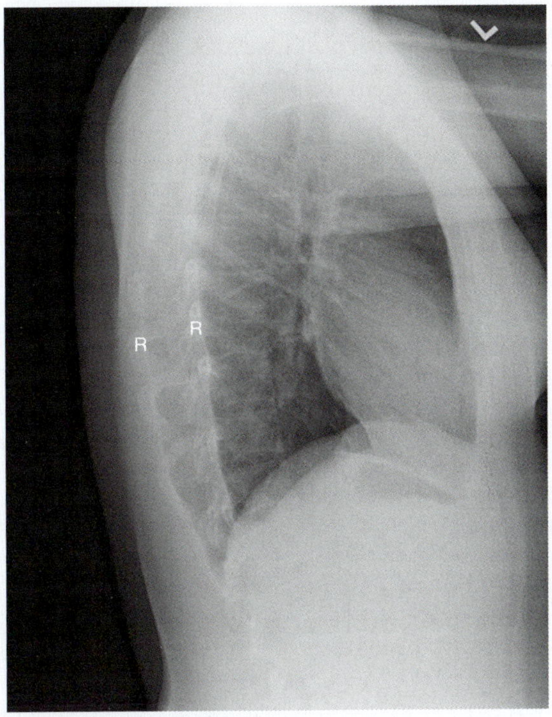

2-71 Lateral chest with rotation.

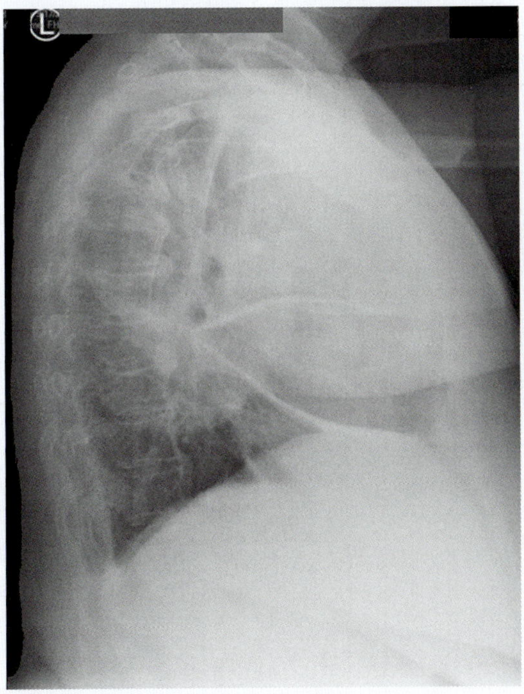

2-72 Lateral chest with arms insufficiently elevated.

Nonambulatory Chest

- Projection: PA at the Upright Bucky or AP wheelchair at the Table Bucky

Nonambulatory Chest Protocol

PA/AP

Left Lateral

Technical Considerations

- kVp 110–130
- 2 outermost AEC cells selected for upright or table Bucky
- Manual technique may be considered
- 72″ SID to the upright Bucky
- 40″ or maximum SID to the table Bucky

Exposure Field Size

- 14 × 17 lengthwise for sthenic to asthenic patient
- 14 × 17 crosswise for hypersthenic patient
- 17 × 17

Patient Position (Figs. 2-73 to 2-77)

- Erect (preferred for air–fluid levels) and facing upright Bucky to reduce magnification of mediastinal structures
- Shoulders relaxed. Chin elevated
- Arms wrapped around board rolling scapulae forward
- If patient is in a wheelchair, the back and arms of the wheelchair may be removable for imaging
- A patient not strong enough to stand for the entire exam may move to a stool for imaging
- The patient may remain on stretcher. Patient would sit up with legs over the side of the stretcher to face the upright Bucky. An alternate AP projection could be used if the patient positioning required for the PA projection is too difficult
- If a patient unable to be upright, a supine chest may be acquired

Centering (Fig. 2-78)

- Level of T7/8 and with MSP

Marking of the IR

- The right or left marker up above left shoulder

Breathing

- Double inspiration and hold after second inspiration
- Watch the patient during breathing instruction and while walking away to make the exposure

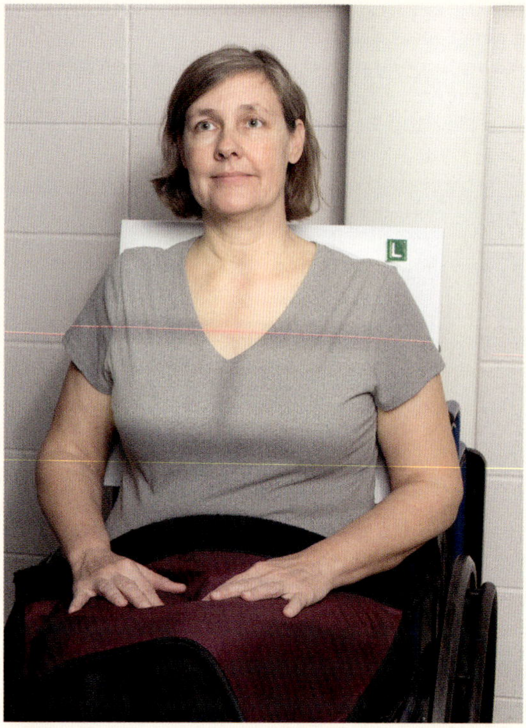

2-73 AP chest in wheelchair.

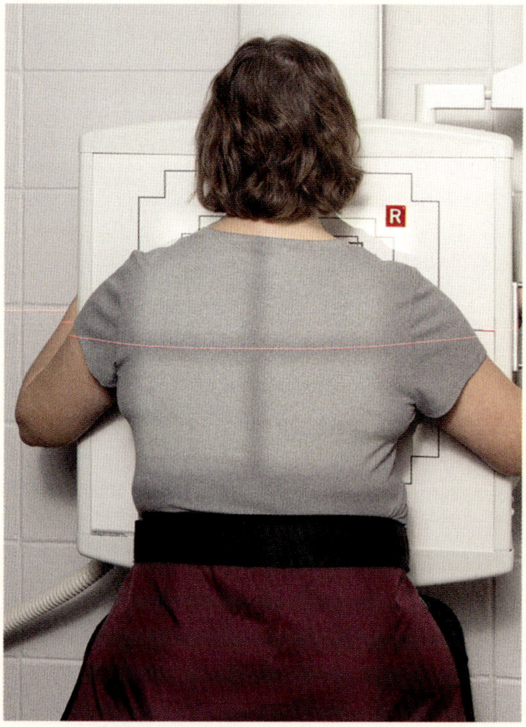

2-74 PA chest seated on stool.

(continued)

Nonambulatory Chest (*Continued*)

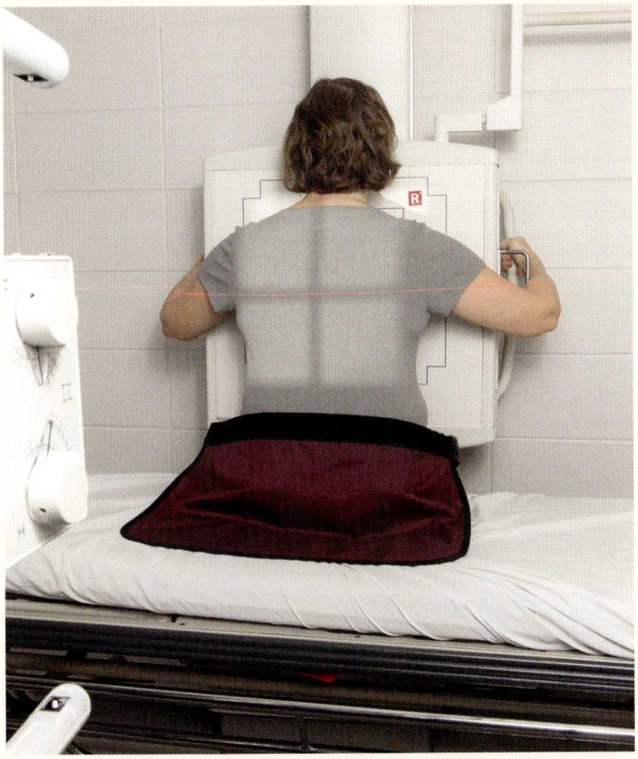

2-75 PA chest on stretcher.

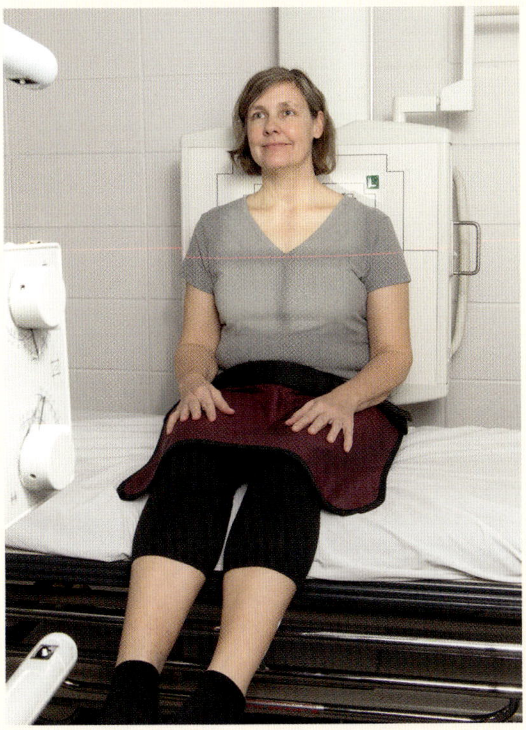

2-76 AP chest on stretcher.

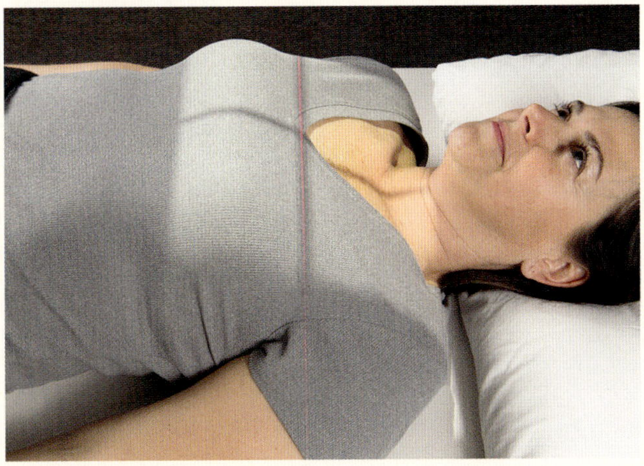

2-77 Supine AP chest.

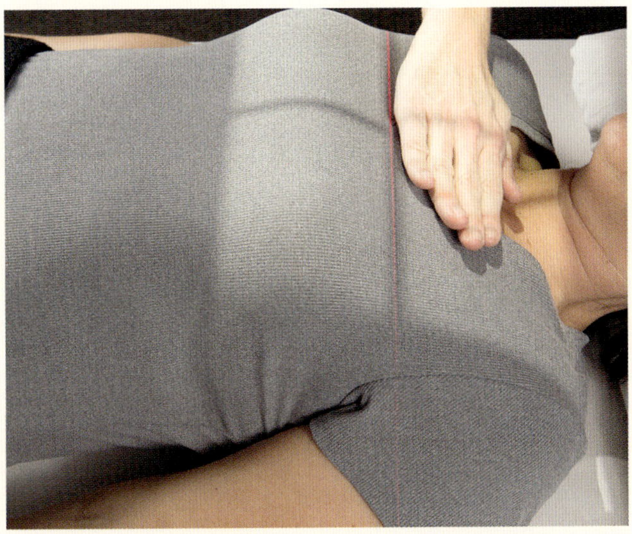

2-78 AP chest centering.

IMAGE CRITIQUE (FIG. 2-79)

- Entire lung fields revealing apices, bases, costophrenic angle, and lateral lung margins.
- Properly centered
- Ideally, 10–11 ribs above the diaphragm counted on the right side of thorax, but with health conditions and ability of the patient, this may contribute to fewer ribs being visualized
- Clavicles near horizontal. This indicates that the shoulders were relaxed
- Scapulae removed from the lung field. This indicates that the shoulders were rolled forward
- SC joints symmetric. This indicates that the patient was not rotated and the shoulders were equal distance to the IR

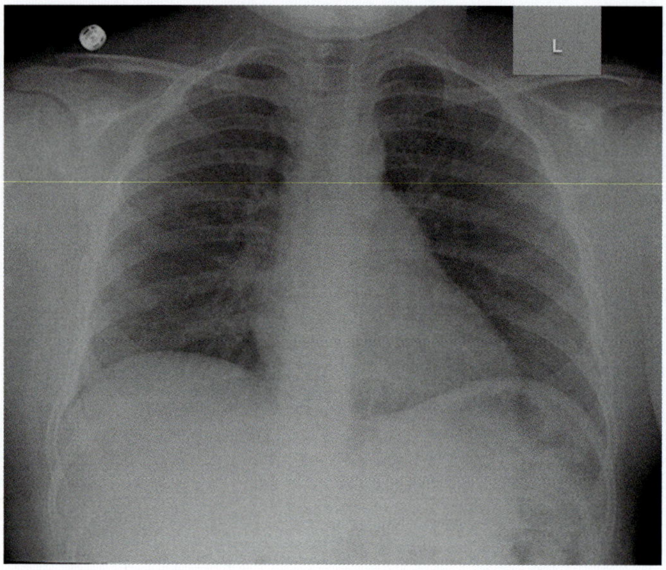

2-79 AP or PA chest.

Nonambulatory Chest

- Projection: Left Lateral

Nonambulatory Chest Protocol
PA/AP
Left Lateral

Technical Considerations

- kVp 110–130
- Center AEC cell selected for upright Bucky
- 72″ SID

Exposure Field Size

- 14 × 17 lengthwise for all patients
- 17 × 17

Patient Position (Figs. 2-80 to 2-82)

- Erect left lateral position
- True lateral position of thorax with hips and shoulders aligned
- Arms elevated to hold onto chest positioning bar
- Chin elevated with eyes facing forward
- If a patient is in a wheelchair, the wheelchair back and side arms may be removable for imaging
- A patient not strong enough to stand for the entire exam may move to a stool for imaging
- The patient may remain on the stretcher. The head of the stretcher is elevated to create a bend at the waist. A bolster may be placed behind the patient's back to build patient away from the stretcher. The patient is encouraged to reach up to grasp the chest bar to elevate the arms from the lung field

Centering

- Level T7/8 and MCP or slightly posterior to MCP

Marking the IR

- Left marker placed on the anterior surface up in the area of arms

Breathing

- Double inspiration and hold after second inspiration
- Watch the patient during breathing instruction and while walking away to make the exposure

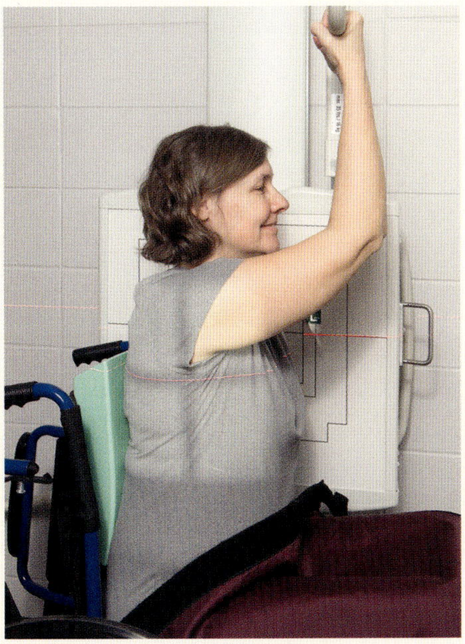

2-80 Lateral chest in wheelchair.

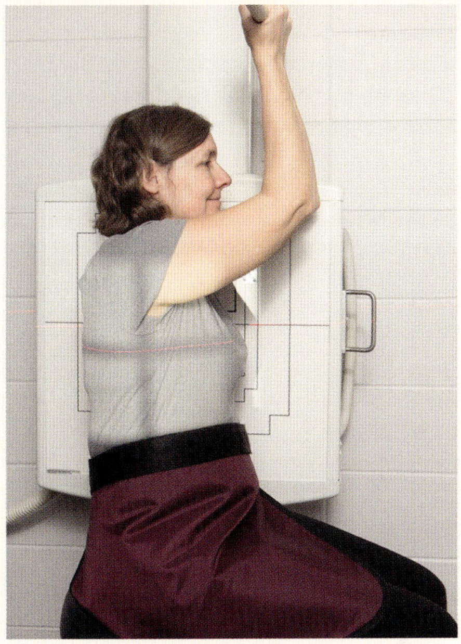

2-81 Lateral chest seated on stool.

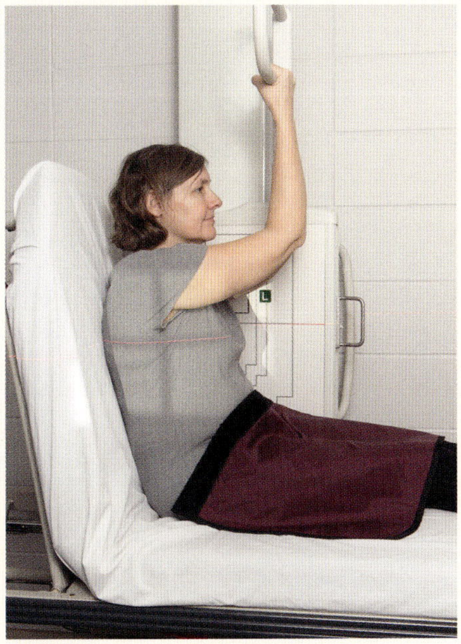

2-82 Lateral chest on stretcher.

IMAGE CRITIQUE (FIG. 2-83)

- Entire lung fields revealing apices, bases, anterior to posterior lung tissue
- Properly centered
- Posterior ribs are superimposed, indicating the thorax is not rotated. Rotation evidenced at the posterior rib margins, that is <½″ or 1 cm, is considered acceptable
- Arms and chin elevated sufficiently from the apical lung region

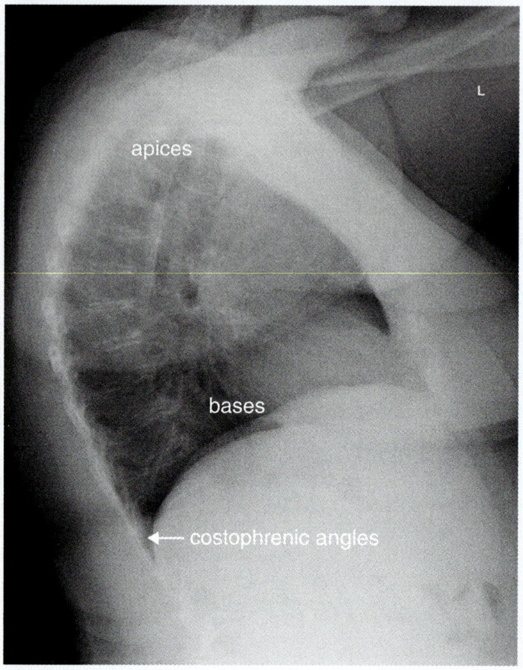

2-83 Lateral chest.

Mobile Chest

- Projection: AP

Mobile Chest Protocol
AP

Technical Considerations
- kVp for nongrid 85–90 (facility dependent)
- kVp for grid 110–115 (facility dependent
- 40″–72″ SID (depending on patient position and facility preference)

Exposure Field Size
- 14 × 17 crosswise (often used as standard consideration knowing lung capacity for ill and/or supine patients will be less compared to ambulatory upright patients)
- 14 × 17 lengthwise (considered for long lung dimensions)

Patient Position (Figs. 2-84 and 2-85)
- Supine (critically ill, ventilator patients, unconscious patient, trauma)
- Semierect to an elevation level tolerable for the patient
- Nearly erect
- Semierect/erect preferred over supine if and whenever possible to produce an air–fluid level

Centering
- Level of T7/8 and MSP—Measure 3″–4″ inferior to the jugular notch for centering level
- The tube head should be adjusted to match parallel to the angle of the IR. The central ray must be directed perpendicularly to the IR. The degree of semierect position will vary from patient to patient. A mismatch of the tube to the IR may result in distortion of the anatomy

Marking of IR
- Right or left marker up above corresponding shoulder
- Additional annotations that should be considered: SID/position/time

Breathing
- Double inspiration and hold after second inspiration if possible
- Patients unresponsive to breathing instructions will require technologist to observe and time exposure appropriately according to the respiratory phase through technologist observation

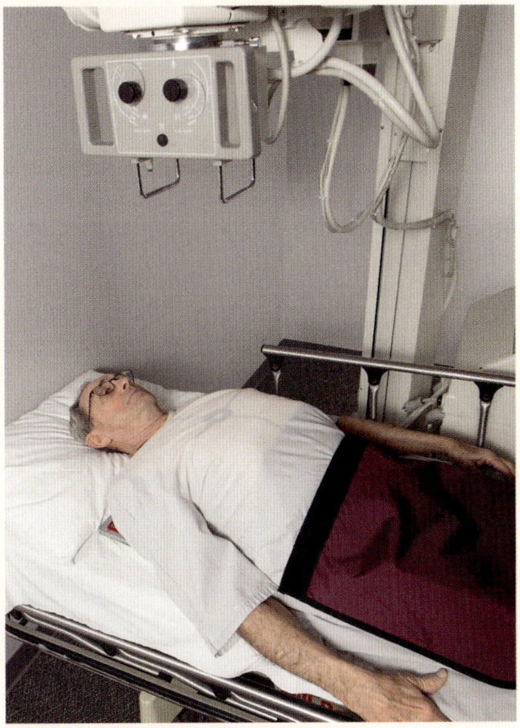

2-84 AP supine portable chest.

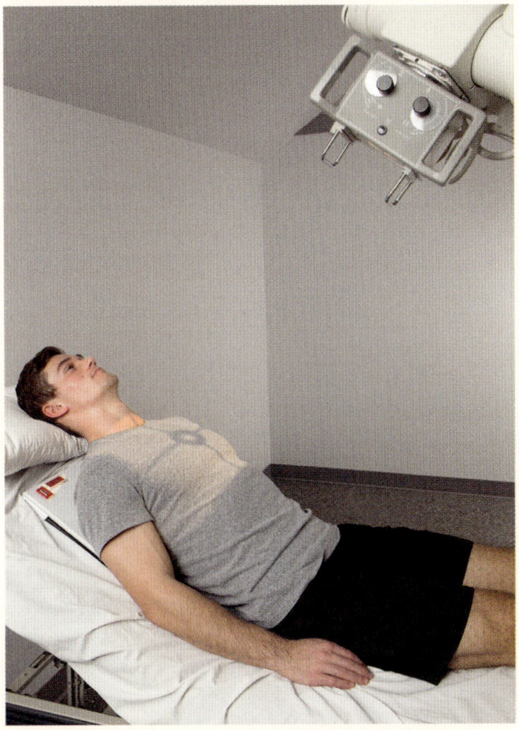

2-85 AP semierect portable chest.

IMAGE CRITIQUE (FIG. 2-86)

- Entire lung fields revealing apices, bases, costophrenic angles, and lateral lung margins
- Properly centered
- 8–9 ribs above the diaphragm counting on the right side of thorax
- Clavicles near horizontal
- Ribs free of distortion: avoiding vertical elongation of ribs or flat/horizontal ribs, indicating the tube angle set and IR were improperly matched
- SC joints symmetric, indicating the thorax was not rotated

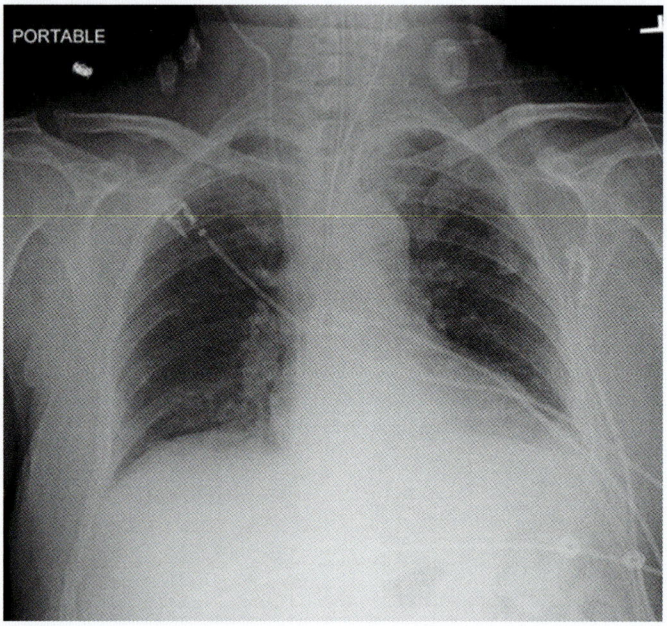

2-86 AP portable chest.

Chest Decubitus

- Projection: PA or AP
- PA would be preferred because the heart would be closer to IR decreasing magnification. AP may be easier to position and may even offer decreased object to image receptor distance (OID), considering the ability of the patient's arms to be raised high enough to place the anterior surface closest to the IR

Decubitus Chest Protocol

AP or **PA** Chest with patient positioned in a decubitus accordingly to demonstrate air or fluid

Technical Considerations

- kVp for nongrid 85–90 (facility dependent)
- kVp for grid 110–130 (facility dependent)
- mAs set manually or AEC could be considered
- 72″ SID (recommended)
- Patient can be imaged at upright Bucky, with nongrid IR or with grid IR tabletop

Exposure Field Size

- 14 × 17 lengthwise for sthenic to asthenic patient
- 14 × 17 crosswise for hypersthenic patient

Patient Position (Figs. 2-87 and 2-88)

- Position will be dependent on whether free air or fluid is of question
- Fluid levels require the affected side to be positioned down. For example, fluid suspected in the left side should be positioned with the left side down
- Free air will rise to the highest point, and suspected side of concern should then be positioned up. For example, free air suspected on the left side should be positioned with the left side up
- Patients should be positioned in the decubitus position for a minimum of five minutes to allow air or fluid to develop the air/fluid line
- Consider building patient up off table to allow the IR to drop below the level of the downside of the patient. This will be helpful in imaging entire lung field bilaterally
- A decubitus position could also be achieved with the patient positioned on a stretcher and centered at the upright Bucky
- Raise arms above head to prevent superimposition on the lung field
- Patient looks straight ahead with chin slightly elevated

Centering

- Level of T7/8 and MSP

Marking of IR

- For easy access and to prevent superimposition in the lung field, mark in the area of the shoulders
- Place the anatomic marker in the upside shoulder region and add a "side up" marker or an upward facing arrow to indicate the side up

Breathing

- Double inspiration and hold after second inspiration
- Watch the patient during breathing instruction and while walking away to make the exposure

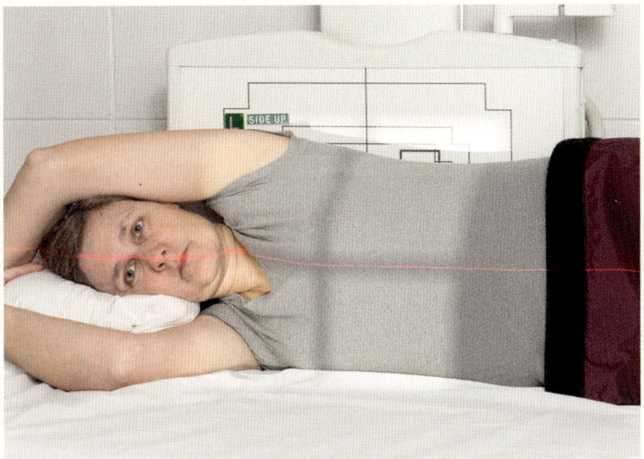

2-87 Right lateral decubitus chest at upright Bucky.

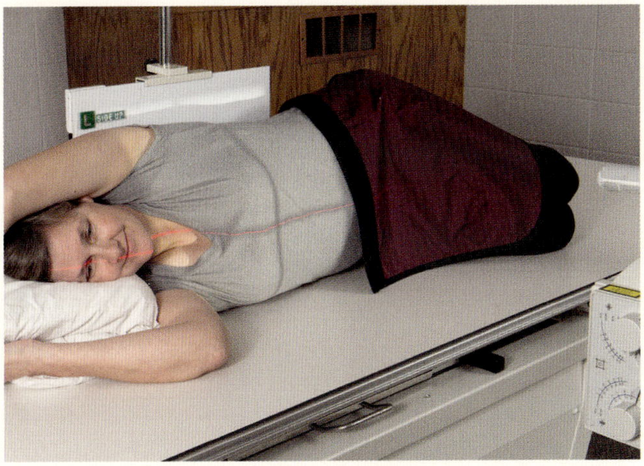

2-88 Right lateral decubitus chest on table.

IMAGE CRITIQUE (FIG. 2-89)

- Entire bilateral lung fields ideally included; side of interest with air or fluid must be well visualized
- Properly centered
- Ensure side of interest (air or fluid) is well demonstrated technically
- SC joints symmetric, indicating the thorax was not rotated

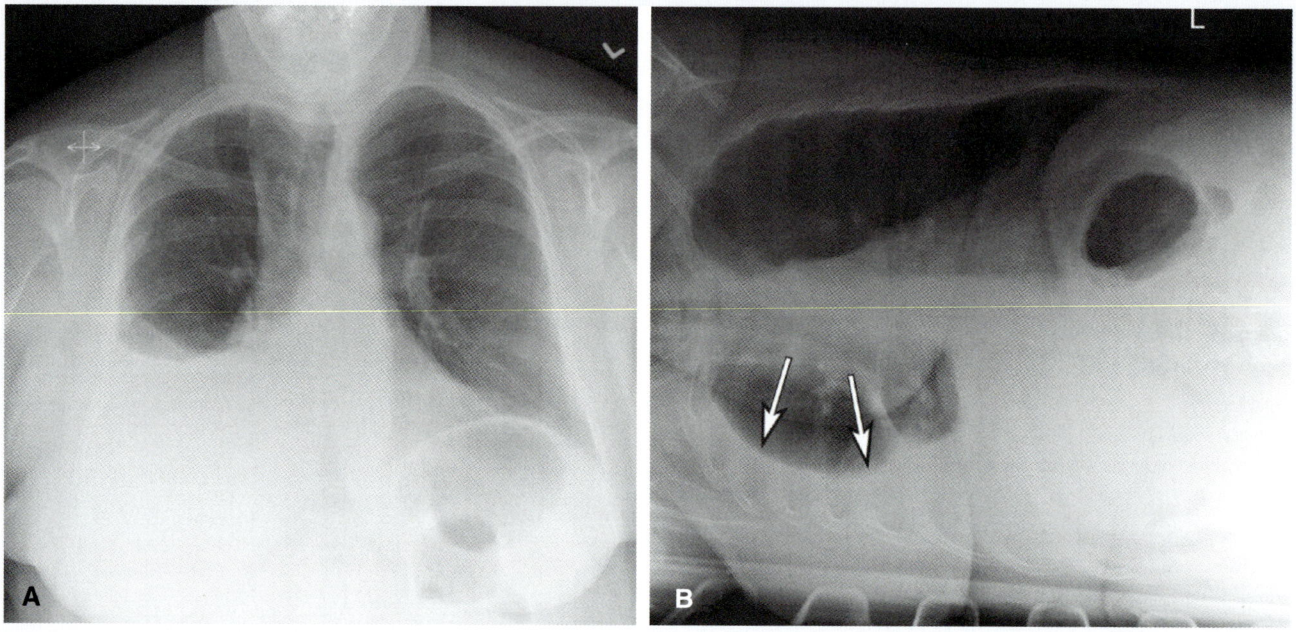

2-89 Right lateral decubitus chest. **(A)** PA chest revealing density in the base of the right lung. **(B)** Right lateral decubitus revealing the fluid level in the right lung (*arrows*).

Inspiration/Expiration Chest

- Projection: PA

Inspiration and Expiration Chest Protocol

2-PA's

1 PA with Inspiration

1 PA with Expiration

Technical Considerations
- kVp 110-130
- 2 outermost AEC cells selected for upright Bucky
- 72″ SID

Exposure Field Size
- 14 × 17 lengthwise for sthenic or asthenic patient
- 14 × 17 crosswise for hypersthenic patient
- 17× 17

Patient Position (Fig. 2-90)
- Erect and facing upright Bucky
- Shoulders relaxed. Chin elevated
- Arms wrapped around board rolling scapulae forward to remove from the lung field

Centering
- Level of T7/8 and with MSP

Marking of the IR
- Right or left marker up above the corresponding shoulder
- Inclusion of marking or annotation of "inspiration" and "expiration" required

Breathing
- Inspiration image: Double inspiration and hold after second inspiration
- Expiration image: Double breath and hold after second expiration
- Watch the patient during breathing instruction and while walking away to make the exposure

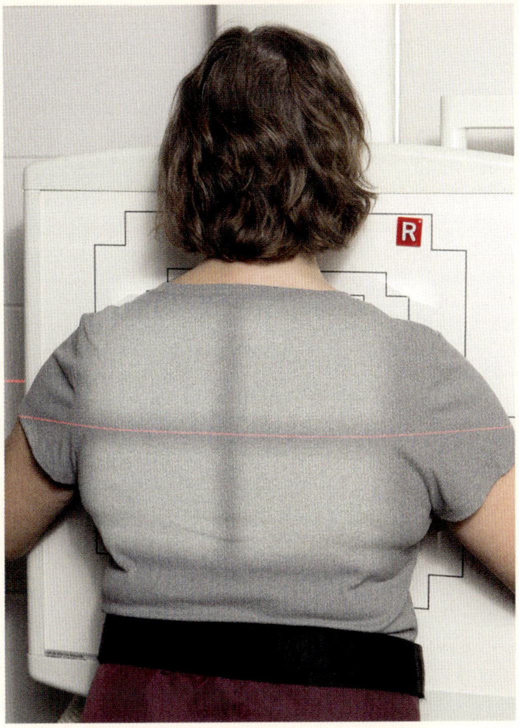

2-90 Erect PA chest.

IMAGE CRITIQUE (FIGS. 2-91 to 2-94)
- Entire lung fields revealing apices, bases, costophrenic angles, and lateral lung margins
- Properly centered
- Comparative images will ideally show a different rib count above the diaphragm
- Clavicles near horizontal. This indicates that the shoulders were relaxed
- Scapulae removed from the lung field. This indicates that the shoulders were rolled forward
- SC joints symmetric. This indicates that the patient was not rotated and the shoulders were equal distance to the IR

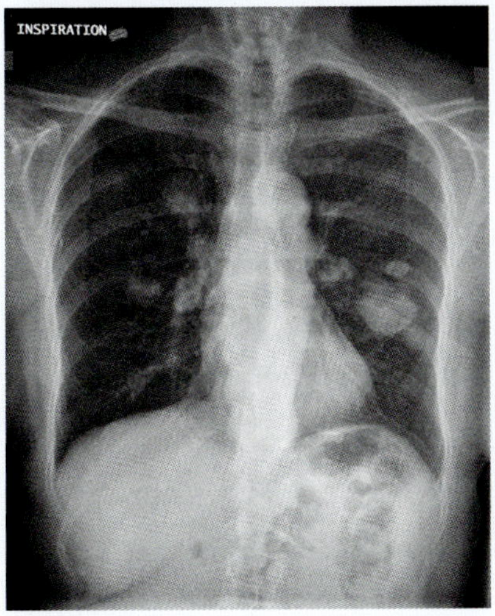

2-91 PA chest with inspiration.

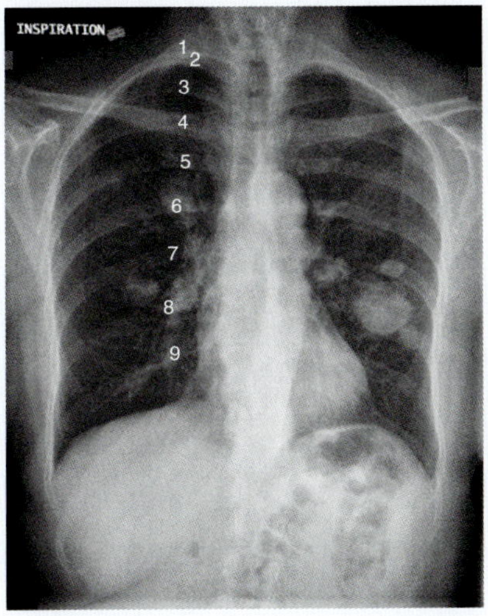

2-92 PA inspiration chest with rib count.

(continued)

IMAGE CRITIQUE (*Continued*)

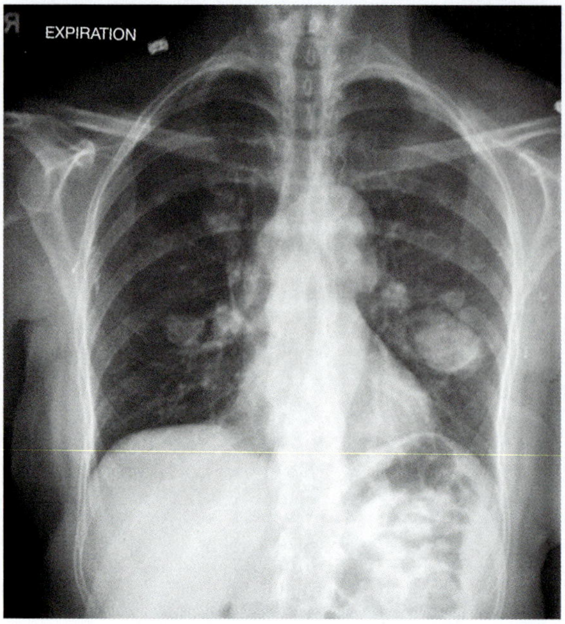

2-93 PA expiration chest.

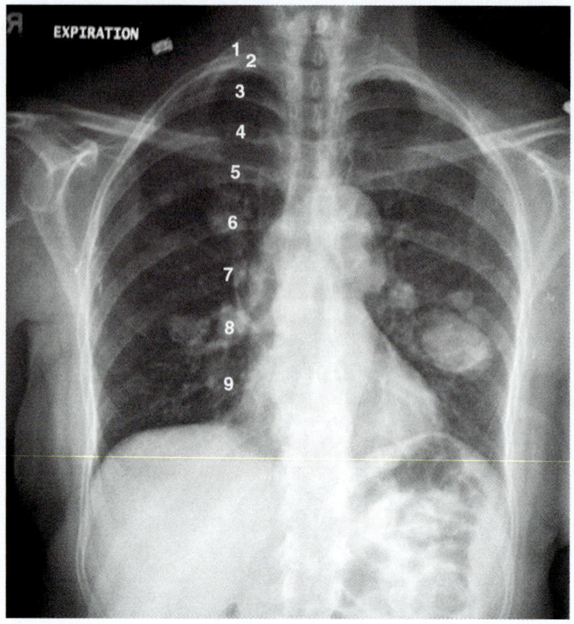

2-94 PA expiration chest with rib count.

Pediatric Chest

- Projection: AP or PA

Technical Considerations

- kVp 55+ (dependent on nongrid or grid exposure)
- mAs set manually
- Nongrid if patient's part is <10 cm
- Grid if patient's part is >10 cm
- 40″–72″ SID

> **Pediatric Chest Protocol**
>
> **Single View: AP/ PA Chest**
>
> 2 V chest order would include Left Lateral

Exposure Field Size

- 10 × 12 or 14 × 17 lengthwise or smaller according to patient size

Patient Position (Figs. 2-95 to 2-97)

- Supine for AP projection in proper restraint if patient is unable to be positioned upright
- Upright for PA projection in proper restraint if pediatric is able to support their own head and is size appropriate for a pediatric immobilization device
- Proper restraint should be considered for the safety of the child and to aid in acquisition of the highest quality image
- If patient's age and ability allow, the pediatric patient may be able to stand upright to the Bucky

Centering

- PA: Level of T7/8 (inferior scapular angle) and with MSP
- AP: Level of nipple line and with MSP

Marking of IR

- Right or left marker up above the corresponding shoulder

Breathing

- Pediatric patients (depending on age) are unable to follow breathing instructions. This will require the technologist to carefully watch and time exposure according to the respiratory phase
- Keep your eyes on the pediatric patient the entire time while walking away to take the exposure and during the exposure
- Watch the patient during breathing phase of inspiration to time the exposure

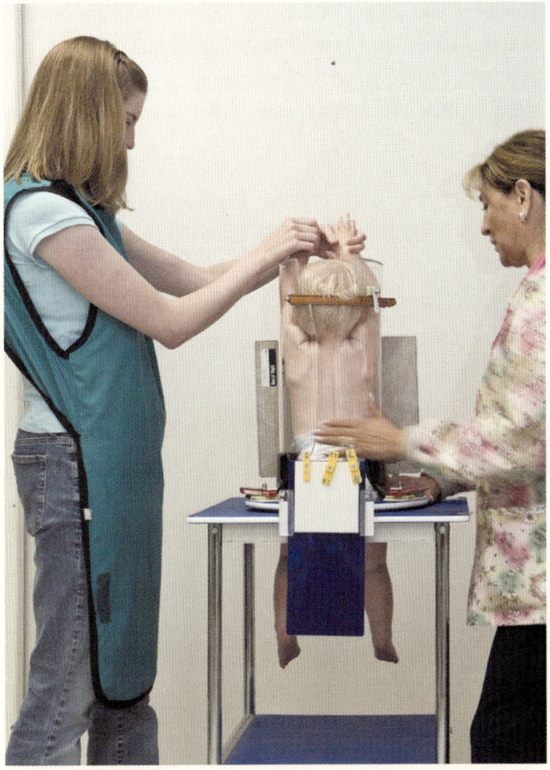

2-96 PA chest with child immobilized.

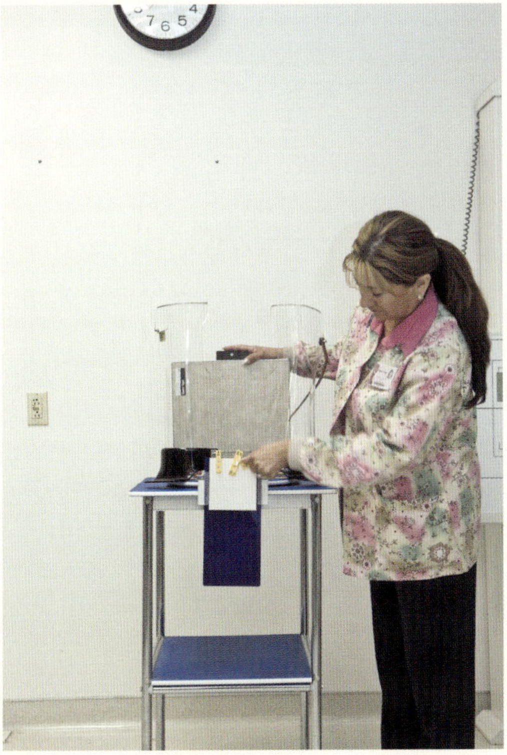

2-95 Child immobilization device.

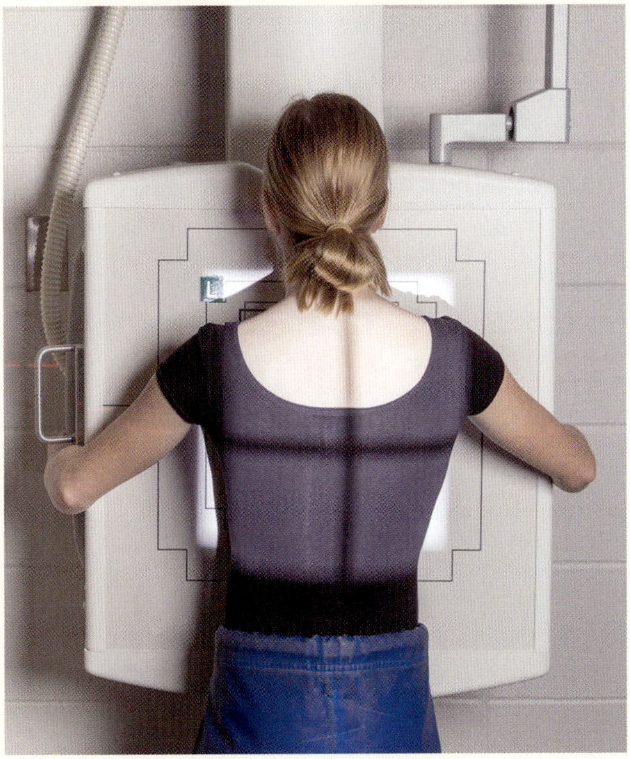

2-97 PA youth chest.

IMAGE CRITIQUE (FIG. 2-98)

- Entire lung fields revealing apices, bases, costophrenic angles, and lateral lung margins
- Properly centered
- 10–11 ribs above the diaphragm counted on the right side of the thorax is most ideal. Pediatric patient position and ability to follow respiratory instruction may influence this; therefore, visualization of 8–9 ribs above the diaphragm is acceptable
- Clavicles may not be horizontal, depending on the type of restraint. Arms restrained high and above the head will change the position of the clavicles
- Scapulae removed from the lung field
- SC joints symmetric

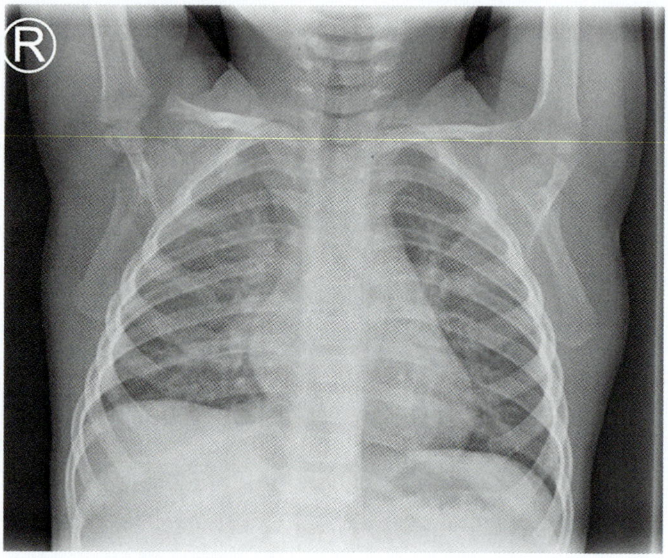

2-98 PA pediatric chest.

Pediatric Chest

- Projection: Left Lateral

Two View Pediatric Chest Protocol

AP or PA Chest

Left Lateral

Technical Considerations

- kVp 60+ (dependent on nongrid or grid exposure)
- mAs set manually
- Nongrid if patient's part is <10 cm
- Grid if patient's part is >10 cm
- 40″–72″ SID

Exposure Field Size

- 10 × 12 or 14 × 17 lengthwise (IR or collimation adjusted according to patient size)

Patient Position (Figs. 2-99 and 2-100)

- Left lateral recumbent with a patient in proper restraint if patient is unable to be positioned upright
- Upright in a lateral projection in proper restraint if pediatric is able to support their own head and are size appropriate for a pediatric immobilization device
- Proper restraint should be considered for the safety of the child and to aid in acquisition of the highest quality image
- If patient's age and ability allow, the pediatric patient may be able to stand upright to the Bucky

Centering

- Level of T7/8 (inferior scapular angle) and with MCP

Marking of IR

- Left marker placed along the anterior surface of the patient

Breathing

- Pediatrics unable to follow breathing instructions will require the technologist to watch and time exposure according to respiratory phase

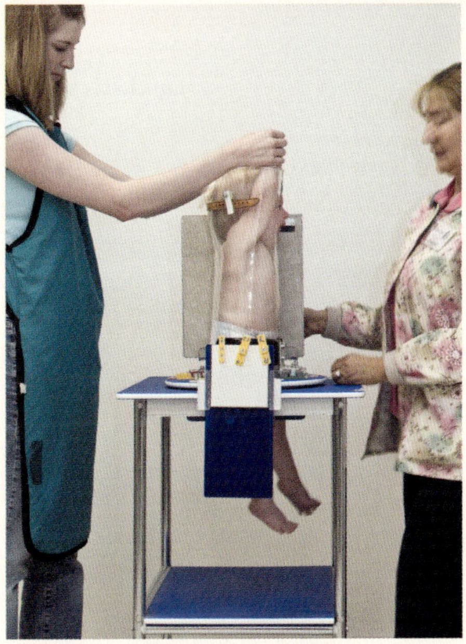

2-99 Lateral chest with child immobilized.

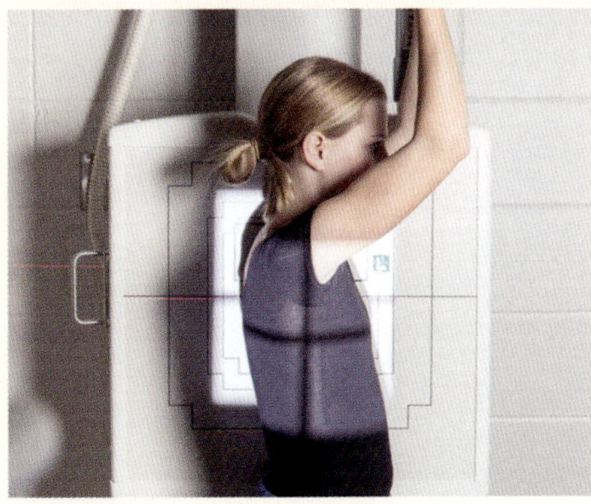

2-100 Left lateral youth chest.

IMAGE CRITIQUE (FIG. 2-101)

- Entire lung fields revealing apices, bases, anterior to posterior lung tissue
- Properly centered
- Posterior ribs are superimposed, indicating the thorax is not rotated
- Arms and chin elevated sufficiently from the apical lung region

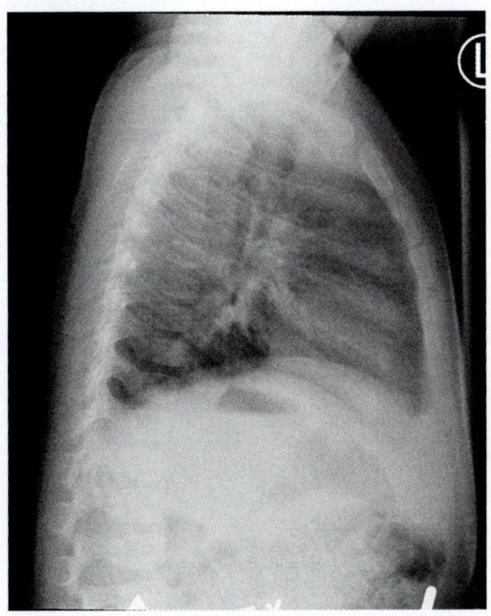

2-101 Lateral pediatric chest.

Upper Airway

- Projection: Left Lateral Upper Airway

Upper Airway Neck Protocol

Left Lateral

AP

Technical Considerations

- kVp 70
- mAs set manually for soft tissue
- 72″ SID (necessary to overcome magnification factor created from the OID between neck and IR)

Exposure Field Size

- 10 × 12 lengthwise

Patient Position (Fig. 2-102)

- Erect left lateral position
- Feet slightly separated for balance
- True lateral position of neck and thorax
- Shoulders pulled back
- Slightly elevate chin, and keep eyes looking straight ahead

Centering

- Level C6–C7 and slightly anterior to MCP
- Level of T-2 and slightly anterior to MCP if foreign body blockage is suspected lower
- Centering is dependent on location of suspected blockage. For example, if blockage is suspected due to a foreign object in the nose, the nasopharynx must be included, and centering higher would be necessary

Marking of the IR

- Left marker placed along the anterior surface

Breathing

- Expose during slow, deep inspiration
- Watch the patient during breathing instruction and while walking away to make the exposure

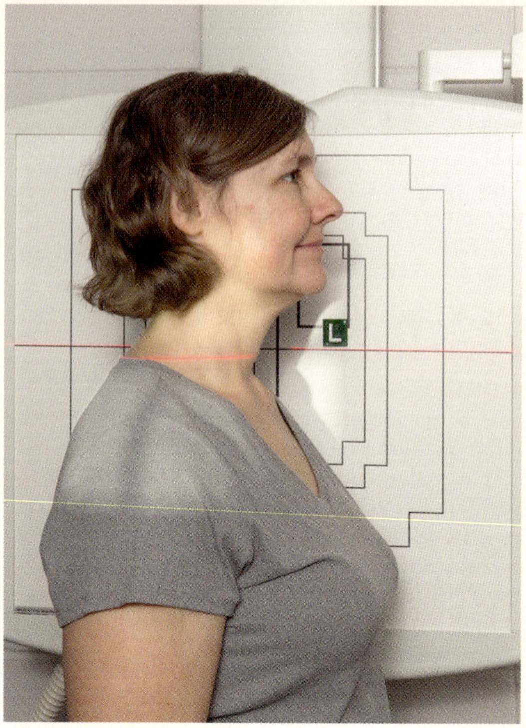

2-102 Left lateral upper airway.

IMAGE CRITIQUE (FIG. 2-103)

- Air-filled pharynx, larynx, and/or trachea to demonstrate possibly filling defects of the airway, indicating obstruction
- True lateral appearance of cervical spine, indicating no rotation of the part
- Shoulders do not appear to superimpose the airway, indicating they were pulled back during the exposure

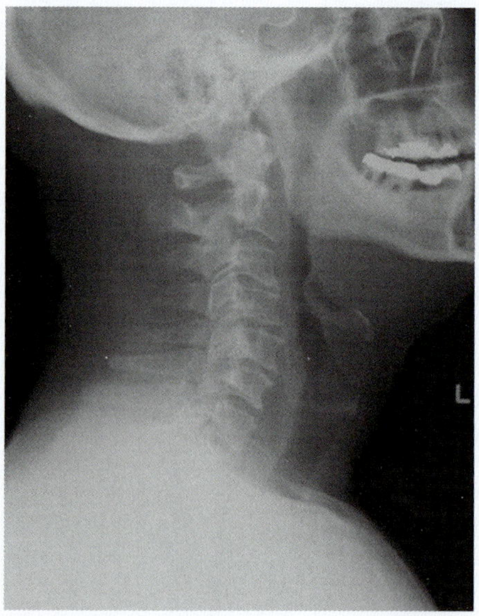

2-103 Lateral upper airway.

Upper Airway

- Projection: AP Upper Airway

Upper Airway Protocol
Left Lateral
AP

Technical Considerations
- kVp 75
- mAs set manually comparable to an AP axial C-spine
- 40″ SID

Exposure Field Size
- 10 × 12 lengthwise for all patients

Patient Position (Fig. 2-104)
- Erect
- Feet slightly separated for balance
- Slightly elevate chin and keep eyes looking straight ahead

Centering
- Level T1–T2 (move 1″ superior to the jugular notch) and MSP
- Centering is dependent on location of suspected blockage. For example, if blockage is suspected due to a foreign object in the nose, the nasopharynx must be included, and centering higher would be necessary

Marking of the IR
- Place right or left marking according to side

Breathing
- Expose during slow, deep inspiration
- Watch the patient during breathing instruction and while walking away to make the exposure

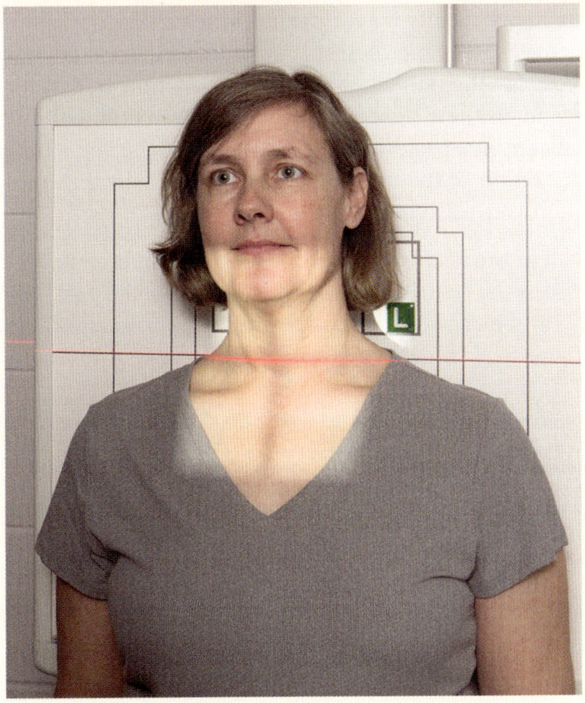

2-104 AP upper airway.

IMAGE CRITIQUE (FIG. 2-105)

- Air-filled pharynx, larynx, and/or trachea to demonstrate possibly filling defects of the airway, indicating obstruction
- SC joints are symmetric, indicating no rotation of the part

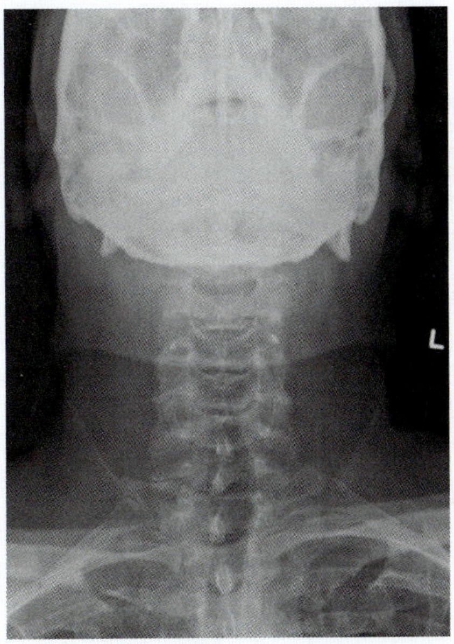

2-105 AP upper airway.

THE FINAL STEP: IMAGE REVIEW

The technologist must take time to review acquired images to ensure image quality is acceptable. The technologist must have the knowledge within their role not only to acquire the images and care for the patient, but also to know how to review the images to ensure diagnostic quality has been attained. In certain instances, a projection may need to be repeated. This is to the discretion of the radiologic technologist. The technologist should review each image for the following.

1. Is all of the necessary anatomy included on the image?
   - Was the central ray properly directed to the part? An "X" can be drawn to intersect within the collimated exposure field to determine whether the central ray was directed to the correct location.
   - Was essential anatomy in the collimated exposure field?
   - Is the area free of artifact(s)?
2. Is the anatomy well demonstrated?
   - Did the technologist properly position the patient to adequately demonstrate the anatomy?
   - Can the technologist recognize the anatomy best demonstrated with use of different projections?
3. Does the image reflect proper image markings?
   - Did the technologist correctly use a lead marker to identify the right or left side?
   - What additional markings or annotations could be helpful to the radiologist interpreting the exam?
   - Is the image properly displayed?
4. Does the image prove to be technically acceptable?
   - Does the exposure index fall within the acceptable range for the operating system? Images that are technically insufficient may appear of good quality if just slightly insufficient or "mottled or pixelated" if severely insufficient. Images that appear "mottled" should be repeated. Images that appear beyond optimal exposure owing to higher technique may display high quality, but the patient has received excessive radiation dose.

CRITICAL THINKING

1. In review of the PA chest (Fig. 2-106), the image would require a repeat for which of the following reasons?
   a. Centering is directed above T7/8, causing the right lateral lung to be clipped.
   b. Centering is directed to below T7/8, causing the right lateral lung to be clipped.
   c. Centering is not directed to the MSP, causing the right lateral lung to be clipped, but CR is to the correct level.
   d. Overcollimation caused the right lateral lung to be clipped.

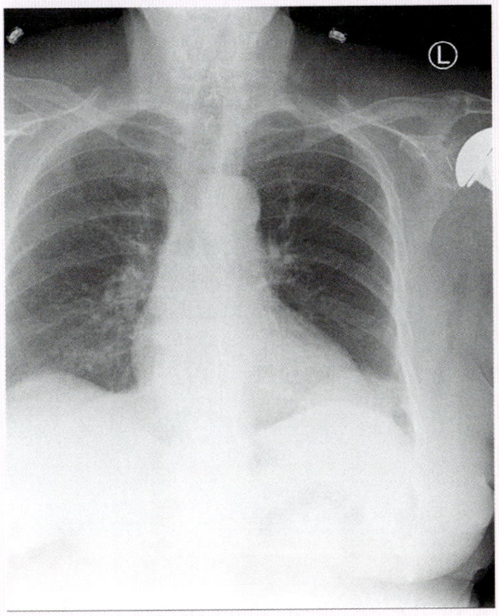

2-106

2. In review of the AP Chest (Fig. 2-107), which of the following would be the reason(s) for a repeat image?
   1. The CR directed to include all essential anatomy.
   2. The costophrenic angles are clipped.
   3. The thorax shows evidence of excessive rotation.
   4. The shoulders were not rolled forward.
      a. 1 only
      b. 2 and 3
      c. 2 and 4
      d. 2, 3, and 4

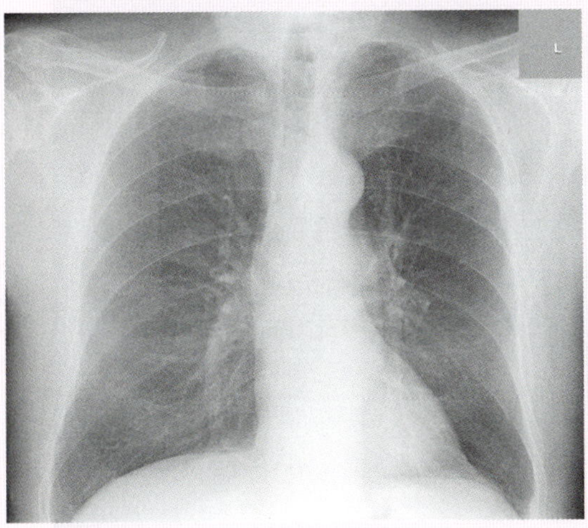

2-107

3. In review of the lateral chest (Fig. 2-108), the image would be repeated for which of the following reasons?
   a. Scapulae in lung fields
   b. The centering is too low, causing the apices to be clipped.
   c. Rotation of the part
   d. The centering is too high, causing the costophrenic angles to be clipped.

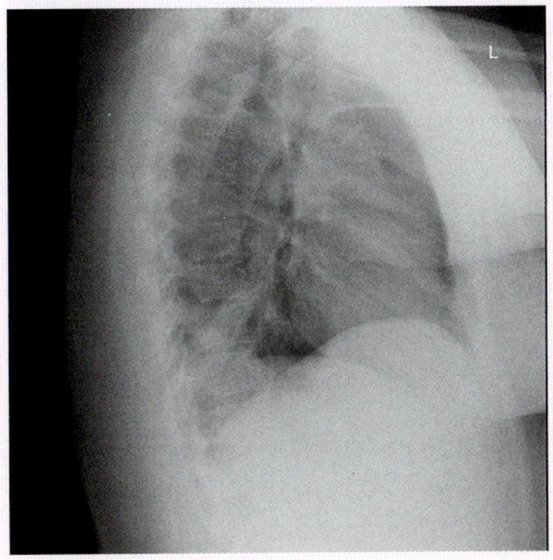

2-108

4. In review of the lateral chest taken on an elder patient with one side of the body suffering paralysis following a stroke (Fig. 2-109), the image would fail for which of the following reasons?
   a. Arms were potentially elevated to their best.
   b. The centering is directed to anterior to MCP, causing the posterior lungs to be clipped.
   c. The centering is directed to posterior to MCP, causing the posterior lungs to be clipped.
   d. Considering the condition of the patient, the image would not need to be repeated.

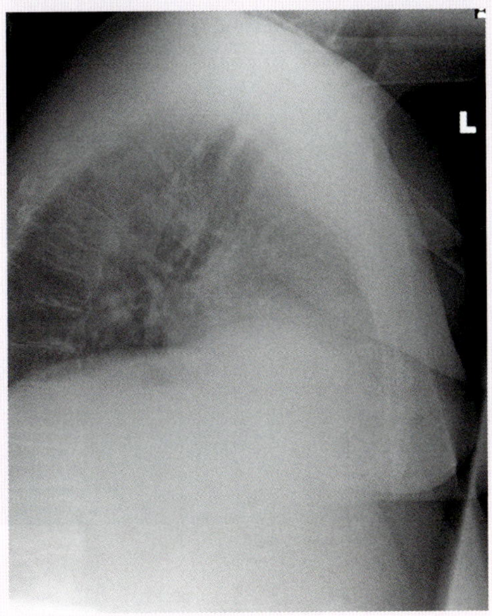

2-109

CHAPTER 3 Bony Thorax

Imaging of the bony thorax is necessary when the patient sustains trauma to the chest. Imaging of the bony thorax will determine the presence and extent of injury to the bony framework. Imaging of the bony thorax may also be combined with chest imaging to rule out the possibility of chest pathology resulting from a rib fracture.

CLINICAL INDICATIONS

Indications are the symptomatic reasons as to why a particular exam may be ordered by the physician. The technologist should look at the clinical indications before performing a procedure. The following briefly introduces common exam indications, but it is not an all-encompassing list.

Rib Fracture: Fracture resulting from trauma or potential underlying bone disease. Rib fracture can cause concern for resultant lung or organ injury (Fig. 3-1).

Flail Chest: A result of adjacent rib fractures in more than two places from trauma, affecting the stability of the chest wall and could result in pulmonary injury (Fig. 3-2).

Pneumothorax: Free air enters the pleural cavity, causing the lung to be pushed away from the chest wall. The condition may result from penetrating trauma, biopsy, or surgery. Pneumothorax is identified when an area on the chest radiograph fails to reveal lung markings (Fig. 3-3).

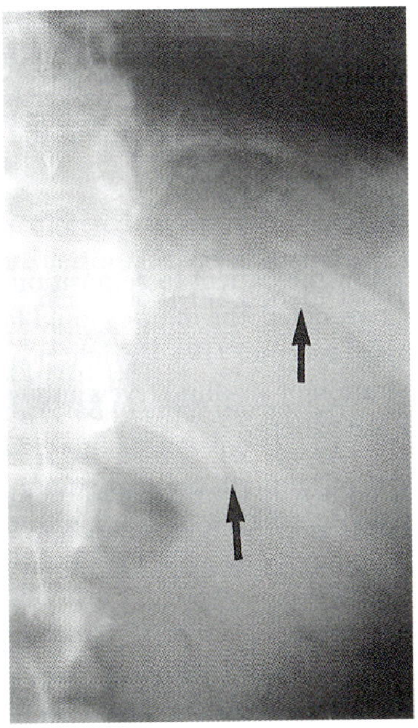

3-1 Rib fracture.

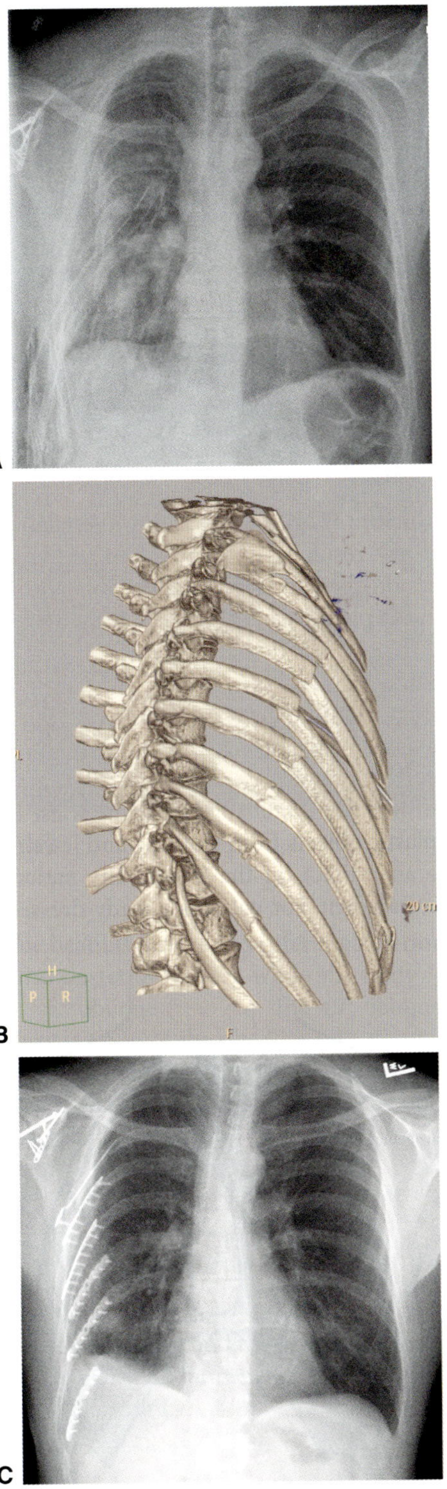

A

B

C

3-2 Flail chest. **(A)** Represents multiple rib fractures to the right ribs. **(B)** Represents multiple rib fractures creating an unstable chest wall seen with flail chest. **(C)** Image to represent right rib fracture repair.

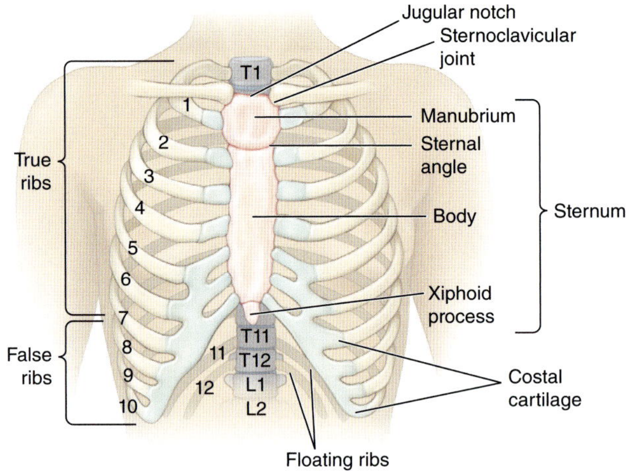

3-9 Bony thorax.

contains the jugular notch, the palpable border most superiorly. The jugular notch can serve as a landmark to determine the midsagittal plane (MSP) on the patient. The jugular notch, a topographic landmark, marks the approximate location of thoracic vertebrae, T2–T3. The sternal ends of the clavicles also articulate with the manubrium, forming the right and left sternoclavicular (SC) joints. The sternal angle is the division point where the manubrium and the sternal body articulate. The body has scalloped edges along the lateral margins to accept costocartilage for rib articulation. The xiphoid process is the inferiormost portion of the sternum. The xiphoid process may also serve as a useful bony landmark to identify the patient's MSP. The xiphoid process serves as a topographic landmark, corresponding to the level of thoracic vertebrae T9–T10 (Fig. 3-10).

Ribs

Twelve pairs of ribs articulate with the thoracic vertebrae. The head of the rib articulates with a facet on the posterior vertebral body to form the costovertebral joint (Fig. 3-11). The costovertebral joint is a diarthrodial joint with gliding type movement. Just distal to the head of the rib, the rib narrows into the neck, followed by a tubercle. The tubercle will articulate with the transverse process of the thoracic vertebrae to form the costotransverse joint (Fig. 3-11). The costotransverse joint is also a diarthrodial joint with gliding type movement. All 12 rib pairs possess right and left costovertebral joints. Right and left costotransverse joints are only associated with rib pairs 1–10.

Each rib has an angle that curves around the lateral aspect of the bony thorax. Within the angle of the rib, the costal groove helps to protect nerves and vessels. Rib fractures may sever vessels and nerves, causing the patient pain.

The first seven rib pairs are true ribs. True ribs articulate directly with the sternum when a short piece of costocartilage connects the sternal end of the rib to the lateral sternum. Rib pairs 8–12 are false ribs. False ribs do not directly articulate with the sternum. Rib pairs 8–10 possess costocartilage. The costocartilage of these rib pairs join into the costocartilage of rib 7. Rib pairs 11 and 12 are floating ribs. Ribs 11 and 12 are short, located mostly on the posterior surface, and do not articulate with any part of the bony thorax anteriorly. The widest transverse diameter of the bony thorax is at the level of rib pairs 8 and 9 (Fig. 3-12).

It should be noted by observing a chest radiograph that the head of the rib (vertebral end) will lie superior to the anterior (sternal end) of the rib (Fig. 3-13). This is important to realize when counting the number of ribs above the diaphragm.

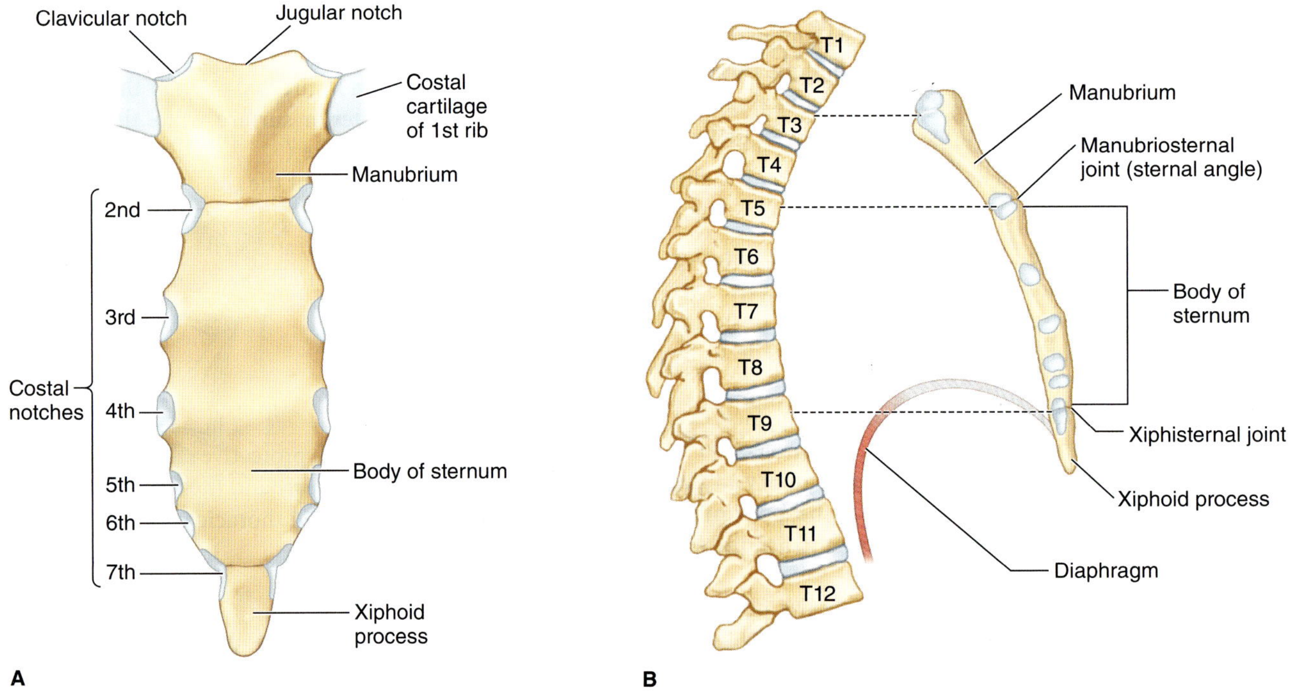

3-10 Frontal and lateral view sternum. **A:** Anterior view. **B:** Lateral view.

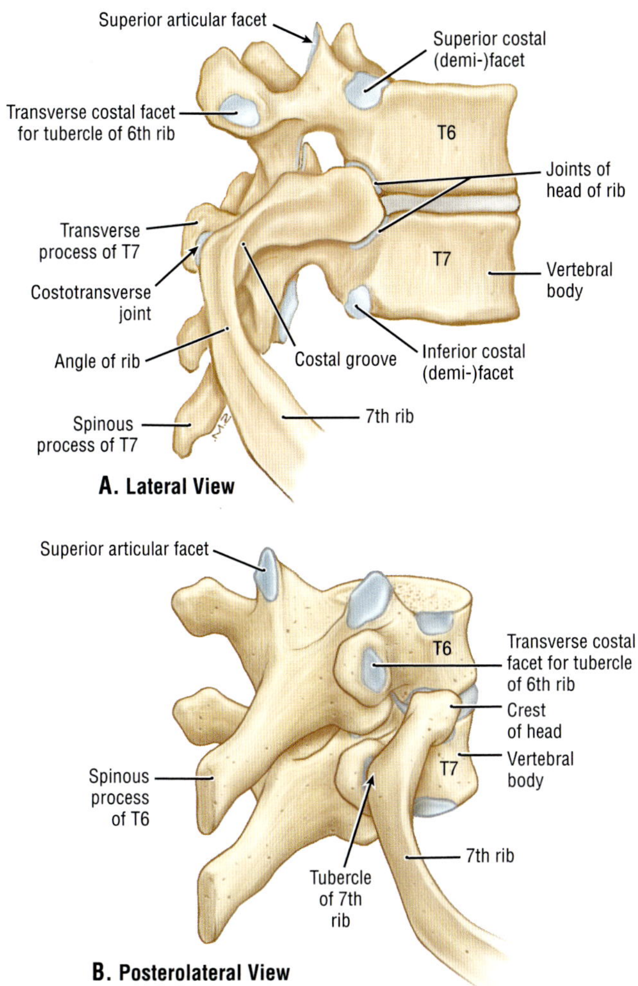

3-11 Costovertebral and costotransverse joints. **A:** Lateral view. **B:** Posterolateral view.

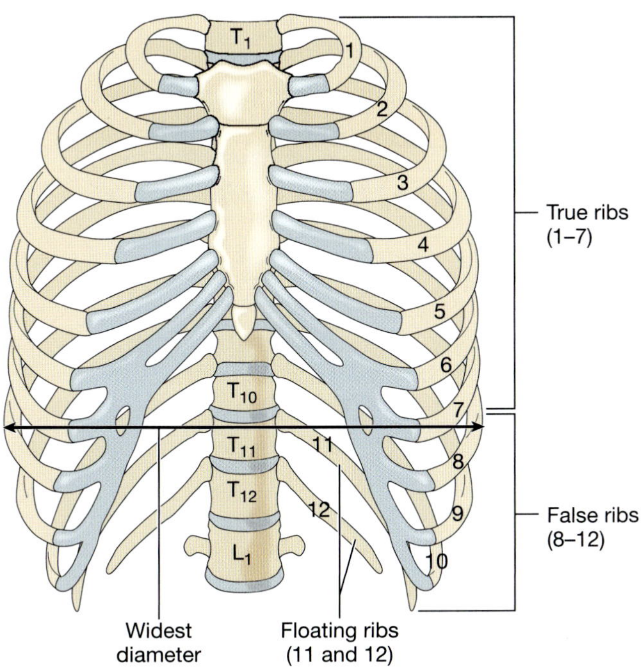

3-12 True and false rib divisions.

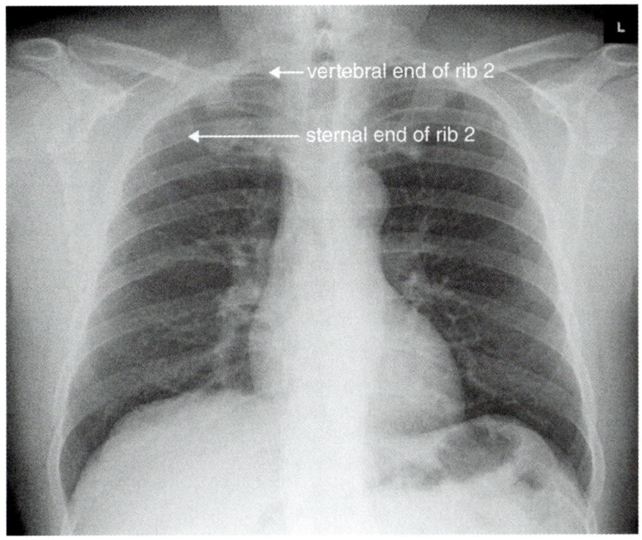

3-13 The vertebral end of the rib is positioned superior to the sternal end of the rib.

KEY SUMMATION POINTS OF ANATOMY

- All 12 thoracic vertebrae possess a costovertebral joint (head of the rib articulates with the vertebral body).
- First 10 thoracic vertebrae possess a costotransverse joint (tubercle of the rib articulates with the vertebral transverse process).
- Rib pairs 1–7 are true ribs. Each rib has costocartilage that articulates to the sternum.
- Rib pairs 8–12 are false ribs. Costocartilage of rib pairs 8–10 connects to the costocartilage of rib 7.
- Rib pairs 11 and 12 are floating ribs. Ribs are short and located on the posterior surface.
- Bony thorax is at its widest dimension at the rib pair level of 8–9.
- The vertebral end of the rib sits superior to the sternal (anterior) end of the rib.

POSITIONING AND TECHNICAL CONSIDERATIONS

General Rib Positioning Considerations

Generally, patients with a rib injury will be more comfortable if they are allowed to remain upright for the imaging examination. If a patient, in the instance, is unable to assume an upright position, supine imaging can be implemented.

Upright positioning:

1. Better descension of diaphragm (with the influence of gravity), maximizing the number of ribs above the diaphragm. This is especially important for high rib visualization.

2. Patient's surface of injury can be accommodated by being positioned closer to the image receptor improving the structure detail.
3. Less patient discomfort; patient is not lying upon a rib injury.
4. Ideal for the PA chest if acquired with the rib protocol to reveal potential air-fluid levels.

Supine positioning:

1. Better ascension of the diaphragm (gravity has less influence), maximizing the number of ribs below the diaphragm. This may be the best consideration for low rib visualization.
2. The patient is imaged in the supine and oblique positions when the patient is unable to tolerate upright positioning. AP and AP oblique projections are acquired.

Body Habitus and Suggested Image Receptor Orientation

There are three general types of habitus to accommodate in chest imaging. A posteroanterior (PA) chest could be incorporated into a standard rib imaging protocol. The PA chest will provide a comparison of right ribs to left ribs. Second, the PA chest will provide evaluation for secondary injury beyond the point of pain for the patient. Lastly, and most importantly, the PA chest will evaluate for any lung pathology resulting from a rib injury.

Sthenic Patient: This patient represents the most average size dimension in the population. Patient is of modest height and weight. The lung dimensions would not expectedly fall outside of a 14 × 17 lengthwise IR for the PA chest.

Hypersthenic Patient: This patient is broad through the shoulders and chest. The lungs would be expected to be wider across and shorter vertically, and it is therefore recommended that a 14 × 17 IR be oriented crosswise for the PA chest or a 17 × 17 IR if available.

Asthenic/Hyposthenic Patient: This patient is long and lean through the thorax and abdomen. The lungs would be expected to be longer vertically than the width across, and a 14 × 17 lengthwise IR should therefore be utilized for the PA chest or a 17 × 17 IR if available.

When imaging high ribs, regardless of body habitus, the 14 × 17 IR will always be oriented lengthwise as the centering is directed to a unilateral side.

Centering for Ribs

When imaging the high ribs, the central ray (CR) will be directed to the level of thoracic vertebrae 7–8 (location found as it was for AP/PA chest) and centered between midline and the lateral rib margin of the affected side. If centering on the posterior bony thorax, this can be measured down with a pinky finger to thumb stretch down from the point of vertebra prominens, or this location could also be closely determined by locating the inferior angle of the scapula (Fig. 3-14). If centering on the anterior surface, 3"–4" below the jugular notch can be measured, similar to the AP chest (Fig. 3-15).

When imaging low ribs, the technologist will work up from the level of the iliac crest, thus ensuring that high and low ribs overlap.

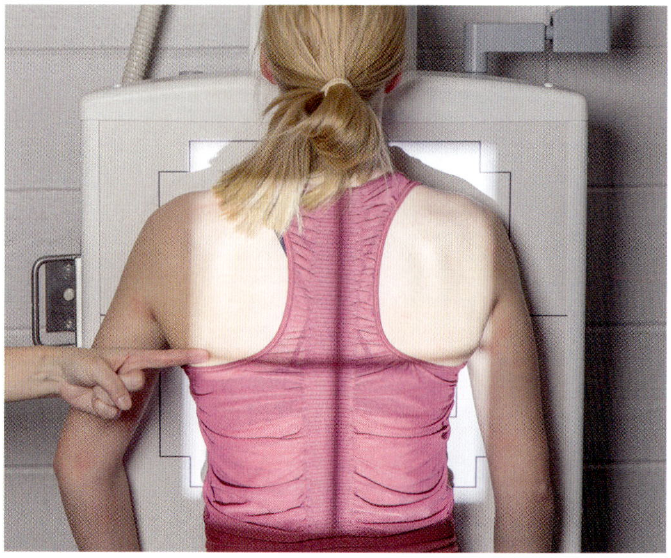

3-14 Centering technique to locate the T7 location on the posterior surface.

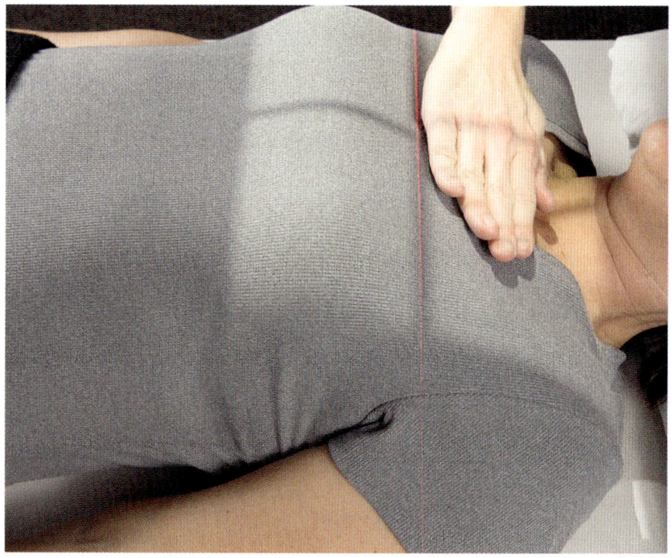

3-15 Centering technique to locate the T7 location on the anterior surface.

Centering for Sternum

The sternum is a flat bone situated anteriorly on the bony thorax and anterior to the thoracic vertebrae. When centering to the midsternum, the landmarks of the jugular notch and the xiphoid process are helpful.

KEY ANATOMIC LANDMARKS (FIG. 3-16)

- Vertebral prominens corresponds to cervical vertebral level of C7.
- Jugular notch corresponds to thoracic vertebral level of T2–T3.
- Xiphoid process corresponds to thoracic vertebral level of T9–T10.
- Inferior angle of scapula corresponds to thoracic vertebral level of T7.
- Lower rib margin corresponds to the lumbar vertebrae level of L2–L3.
- Jugular notch, xiphoid process, and spine would all be landmarks for MSP.

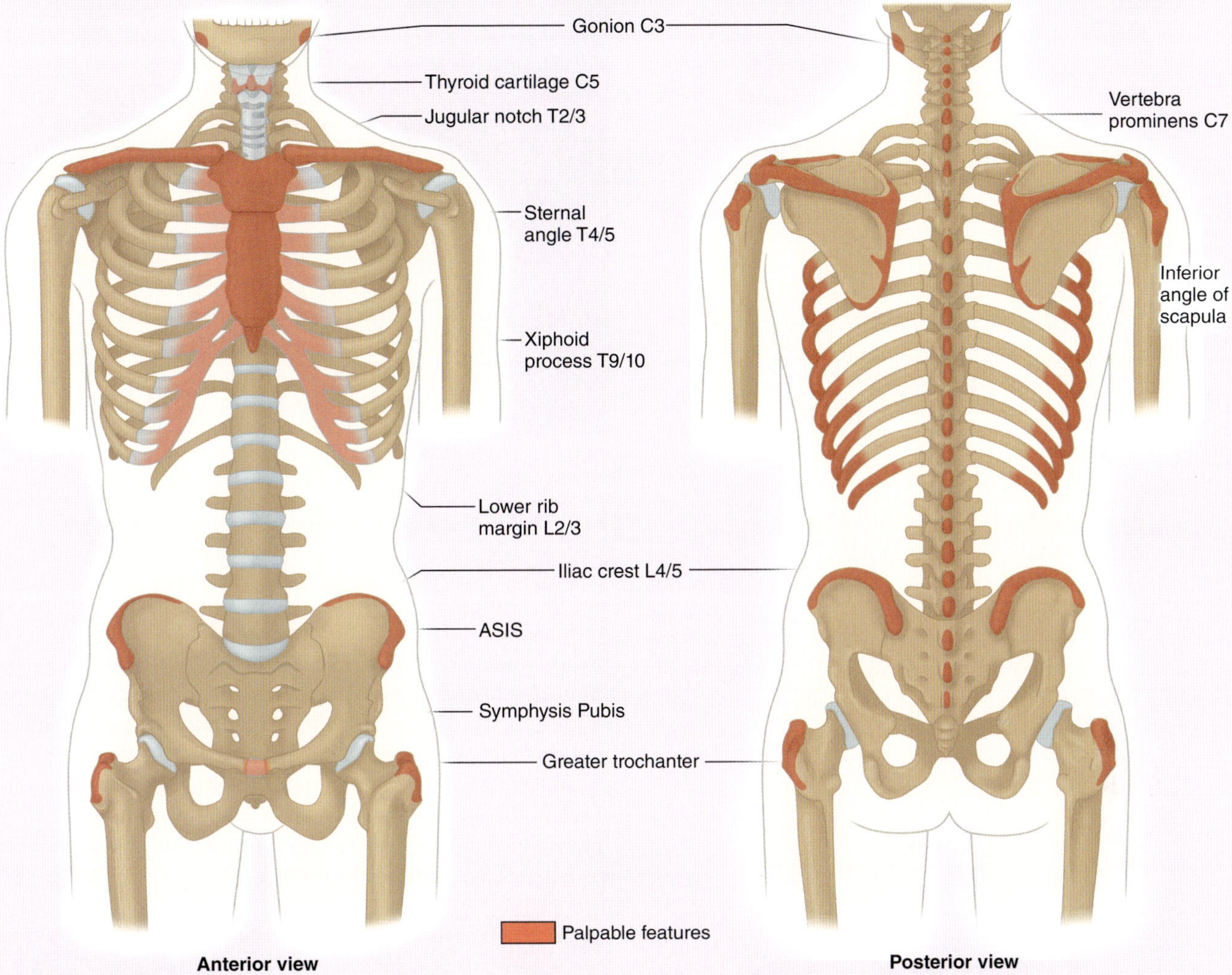

3-16 Topographic landmarks.

Breathing Instructions for Ribs

The patient must be instructed to suspend breath in different respiratory phases during rib imaging to alter the location of the diaphragm to better visualize ribs. On inspiration, the diaphragm will descend inferiorly. On expiration, the diaphragm will ascend superiorly (Fig. 3-17). Between high and low rib exposures, breathing instructions are administered to change the position of the diaphragm to help demonstrate all 12 ribs.

High Ribs

It is recommended that the image exposure for the high ribs be made after holding in the second breath after deep inspiration. With a good inspiration, the diaphragm will move to its most inferior point, maximizing the lung capacity and increasing the number of ribs visible above the diaphragm. For patients with a rib injury, the second inhalation may be better than the first and should be implemented in order to maximize rib visualization (Fig. 3-18).

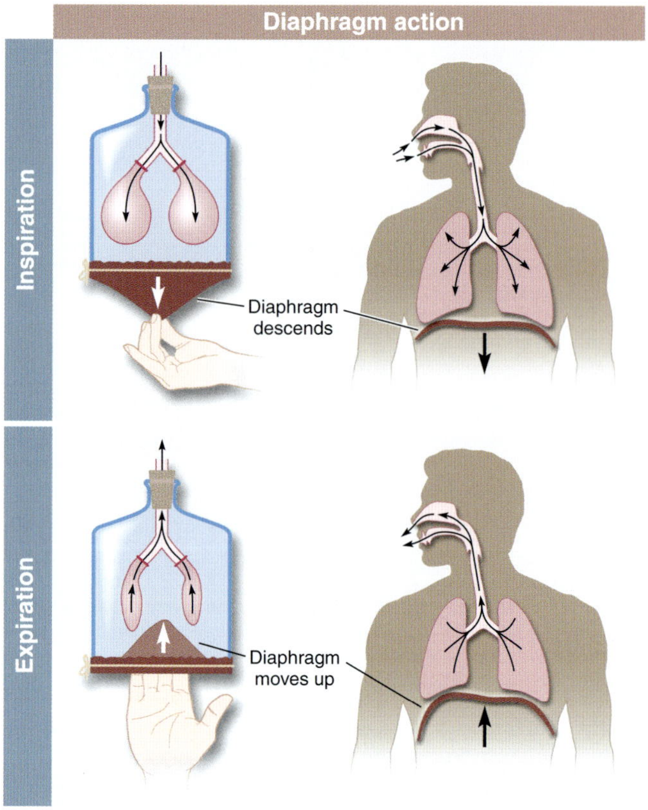

3-17 Diaphragm movements with inspiration and expiration respiratory phases.

Low Ribs

It is recommended that the image exposure for the low ribs be made after expiration. With expiration, the diaphragm will move up to a more superior point, allowing ribs below the diaphragm to be visible (Fig. 3-19).

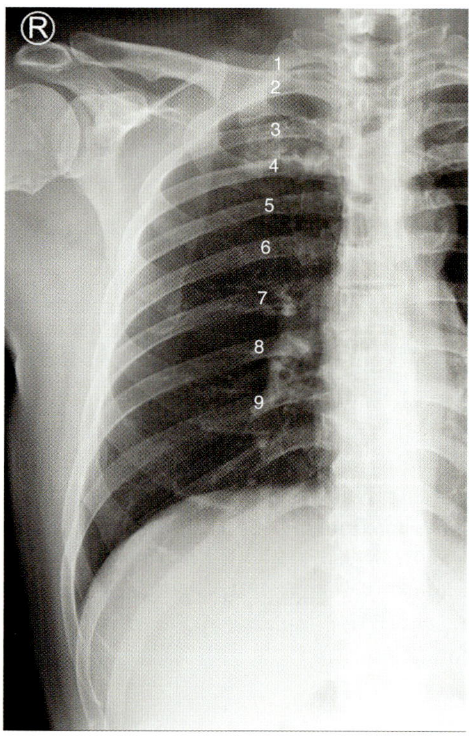

3-18 Rib count for the AP high rib projection.

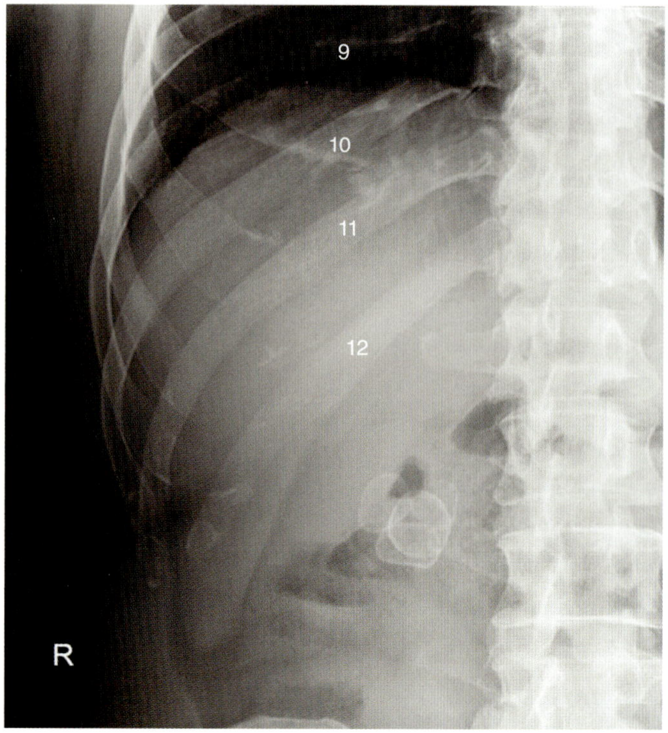

3-19 Rib count for the AP low rib projection.

Breathing Instructions for Sternum

RAO Sternum

For the right anterior oblique (RAO) sternum, there are two options for breathing. The first would be suspension of the breath. The second, and offering the best visibility of the sternum, is a breathing technique. The breathing technique will require the control panel to be set with a kVp, an mA station, and an exposure time of 3–4 seconds (Fig. 3-20). The patient should be instructed to take short, shallow breaths throughout the length of the exposure. The breathing motion will optimally blur out overlying ribs and lung markings to allow better visualization of the sternum (Fig. 3-21).

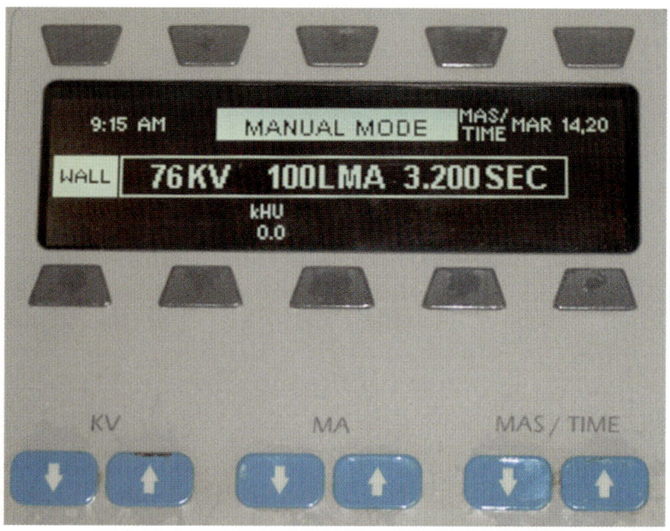

3-20 Setting one example of a breathing technique on the control panel.

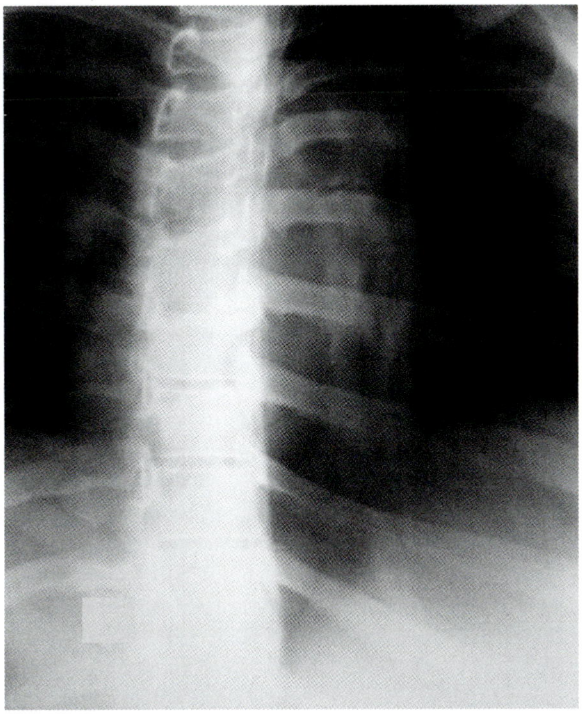

3-21 RAO sternum acquired with the breathing technique.

Lateral Sternum

The lateral sternum will require the exposure to be taken after deep inspiration. Deep inspiration will push the sternum out and away from superimposition of the anterior ribs.

TECHNICAL CONSIDERATIONS

Setting a Manual Technique

A manual technique is defined when the radiographer sets the kVp and mAs values independently. Manual techniques are recommended for rib imaging over the use of automatic exposure control (AEC), but AEC could be applied. Rib imaging often poses challenges technically when contending with patients of poor bone health and/or lung pathologies. Attaining bony thorax images with even exposure density can be difficult.

Kilovoltage is set to penetrate the part thickness and affects the scale of contrast seen on the image. A lower kVp is used for rib and sternum imaging, compared to chest imaging. It is desired that a short scale of contrast on images be attained, demonstrating more blacks and whites as desired for bony structures.

Rib injuries leave concern of associated pathologies such as pneumothorax, hemothorax, and flail chest. Rib protocols often include a PA chest to evaluate for secondary injury to the bony thorax and to evaluate for any lung pathology. The single chest view will require the kVp to be set to 110–130. A higher kVp for chest imaging is needed to penetrate the thickness of the chest and to penetrate through the region of heart and spine. With a higher kVp and a thicker part, the scatter radiation produced is increased, affecting the overall scale of contrast. A long scale of contrast (many shades of gray with slight differences) is desired for chest imaging. The long scale of contrast allows for differentiation of tissues, lung markings, the heart, and pathology.

Setting a manual technique will also allow the technologist to adjust the length of the exposure, something important to consider with pediatric and geriatric patients. In cases where motion can be detrimental to image quality, the technologist can increase the mA station, thus allowing a decrease in the exposure time, to minimize the chance of patient motion. In consideration of pediatric and geriatric patients, a decrease in the kVp may be necessary to accommodate the patient's size. In addition, to compensate for the overall loss in bone density seen in geriatric patients, the kVp may be slightly decreased.

Source-to-Image Distance

40" source-to-image distance (SID) is employed for a singular view of the oblique sternum and all rib images.

72" SID is preferred for the PA chest as there is less divergence of the beam, specifically at the edges of the field size, which improves recorded detail. Additionally, with increased SID, less magnification of structures occurs, thus improving detail. An increase in the SID for the PA chest should be considered to reduce structural magnification of the heart. The lateral projection of the sternum will also employ a 72" SID to compensate for the increased object to distance between the sternum and the image receptor.

Marking the Image

When marking high ribs, the respective right or left lead marker identifies the correct side, and the marker is placed up in the region of the shoulder (Fig. 3-22). This placement will avoid superimposition over the ribs. When marking oblique high ribs, the respective right or left lead marker identifies the side of the patient closest to the image receptor and should be placed up in the region of the shoulder (Fig. 3-23). When marking low ribs, the respective right or left lead marker identifies the correct side, and the marker should be placed down in the region of the iliac crest. This placement will avoid superimposition over the ribs (Fig. 3-24).

Image Display

Assuming the bony thorax image was correctly marked, the image is displayed opposite the viewer facing it, as though the image is in anatomic position. Therefore, the side of the image marked "right" is opposite the viewer's left (Figs. 3-25 and 3-26).

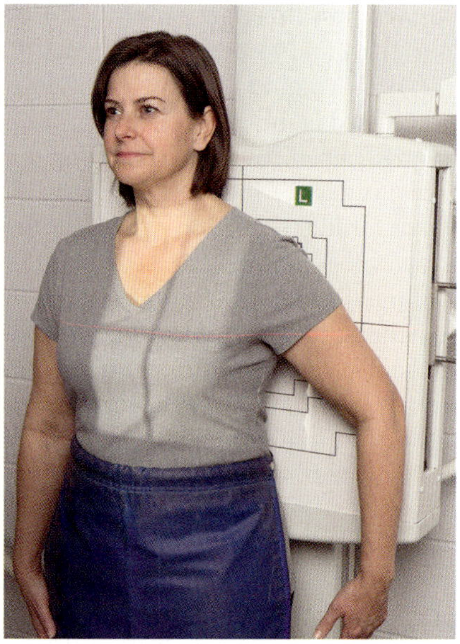

3-22 AP high rib marker placement.

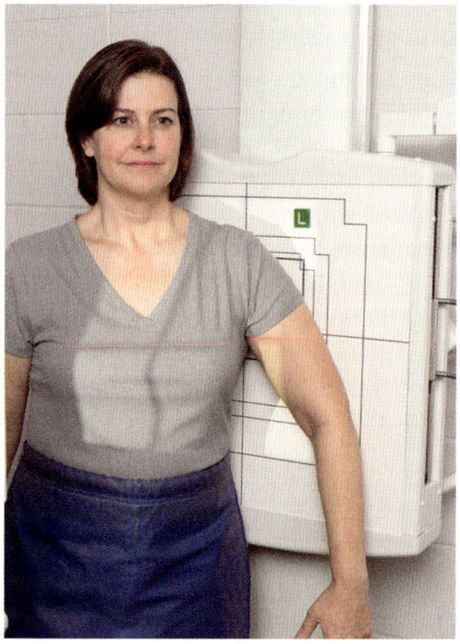

3-23 AP oblique high rib marker placement.

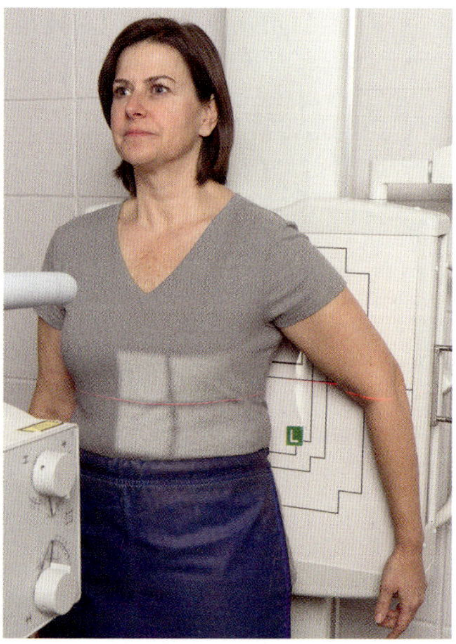

3-24 AP low rib marker placement.

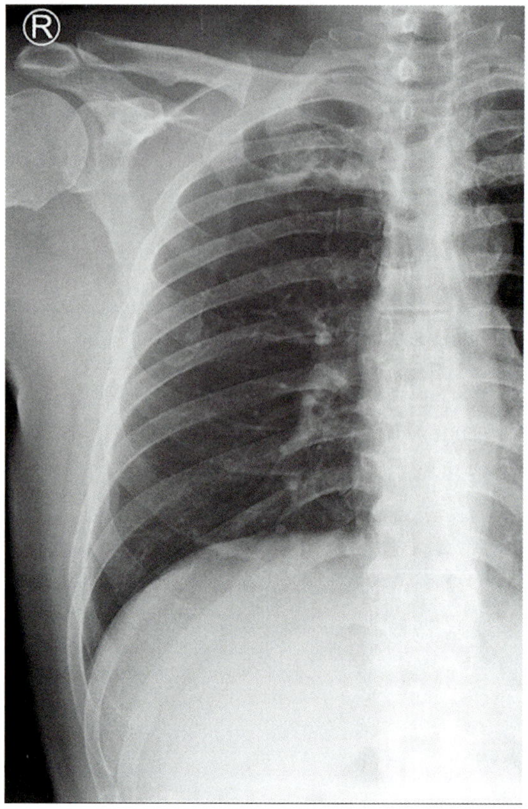

3-25 Correct anatomic display of the right high ribs.

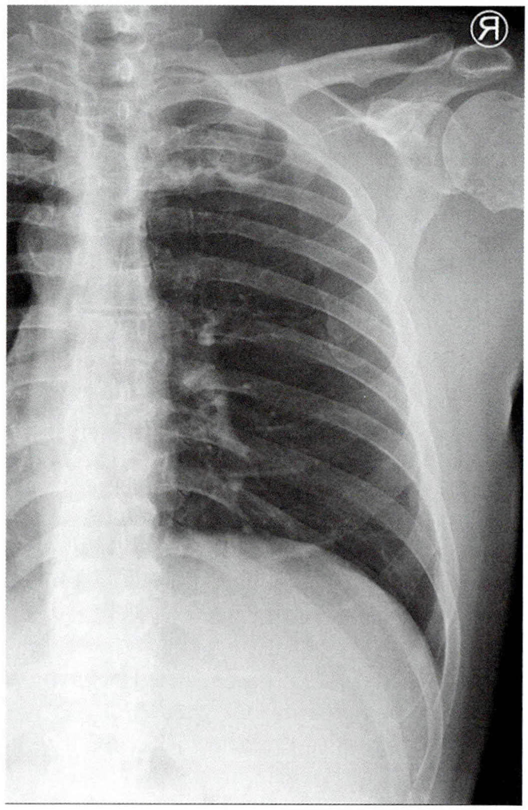

3-26 Incorrect anatomic display of the right high ribs.

Ambulatory Chest

- Projection: PA
- *Chest imaging may or may not be incorporated into a rib protocol. When imaging ribs, it is essential to ask the patient if they are experiencing any difficulty breathing*

Ambulatory Ribs Protocol

PA Chest

AP/PA High

AP Low

AP Oblique/PA Oblique High

Technical Considerations

- kVp 110–130
- 2 outermost AEC cells selected for upright Bucky
- 72" SID

Exposure Field Size

- 14 × 17 lengthwise for sthenic to asthenic patient
- 14 × 17 crosswise for hypersthenic patient
- 17 × 17

Patient Position (Fig. 3-27)

- Erect and facing upright Bucky
- Shoulders relaxed. Chin elevated
- Arms wrapped around upright Bucky rolling scapulae forward

Centering

- Level of T7/8 and with MSP

Marking of IR

- Anatomic side marker R or L up in the region above the shoulder correctly identifying side

Breathing

- Double inspiration and hold after second inspiration
- Watch the patient during breathing instruction and while walking away to make the exposure

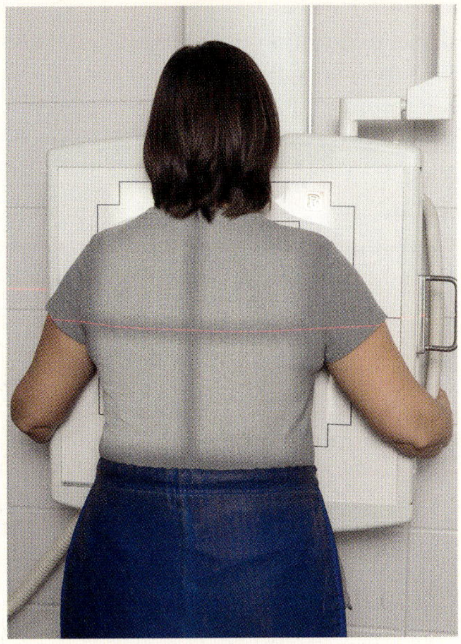

3-27 Erect PA ambulatory chest.

IMAGE CRITIQUE (FIG. 3-28)

- Entire lung fields revealing apices, bases, costophrenic angles, and lateral lung margins
- PA chest provides comparison of the right to left sides of the bony thorax
- PA chest provides an image to rule out any lung pathology resulting from rib fracture
- Properly centered
- 10–11 ribs above the diaphragm counted on the right side of thorax. The degree of inspiration may be dependent on trauma to the chest and potential rib fracture. Patients with rib fracture may be unable to take a deep inspiration, hence achieving fewer ribs above the diaphragm
- Clavicles near horizontal. This indicates that the shoulders were relaxed
- Scapulae removed from the lung field. This indicates that the shoulders were rolled forward
- SC joints symmetric. This indicates that the patient was not rotated; shoulders were equal distance from the IR

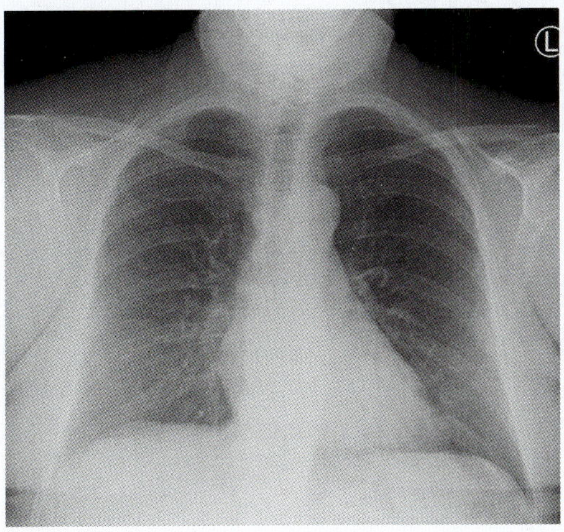

3-28 PA chest.

High Ribs

- Projection: AP or PA
- *Be certain to question the patient as to which surface they are experiencing pain in order to utilize the best projection*

Ambulatory Ribs Protocol

PA Chest

AP/PA High

AP Low

AP Oblique/PA Oblique High

Technical Considerations

- kVp 65–80
- mAs set manually
- 40" SID

Exposure Field Size

- 14 × 17 lengthwise for all patients

Patient Position (Figs. 3-29 and 3-30)

- Erect will be most comfortable for patients with rib fracture
- Erect will also improve the patient's degree of inspiration
- To attain the best detail of the region of pain, that surface should be positioned closest to the IR
- Patients with posterior injury will face the tube and therefore an AP projection is acquired
- Patients with anterior injury will face the upright Bucky and therefore a PA projection is acquired
- Shoulders relaxed. Chin elevated
- Arm of the affected side should be slightly abducted

Centering

- Level of T7/8 and midway between MSP and the lateral rib margin. Collimate down to unilateral ribs according to patient ensuring costovertebral joints and the axillary rib margin are included

Marking of IR

- Anatomic side marker R or L up in the region above the shoulder correctly identifying side

Breathing

- Double inspiration and hold after second inspiration. The second breath will likely be deeper than the first, helping the rib count above the diaphragm
- Watch the patient during breathing instruction and while walking away to make the exposure

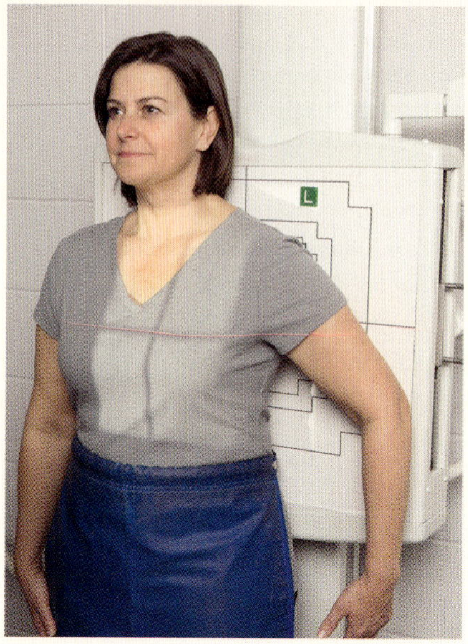

3-29 Erect AP high ribs for posterior rib injury.

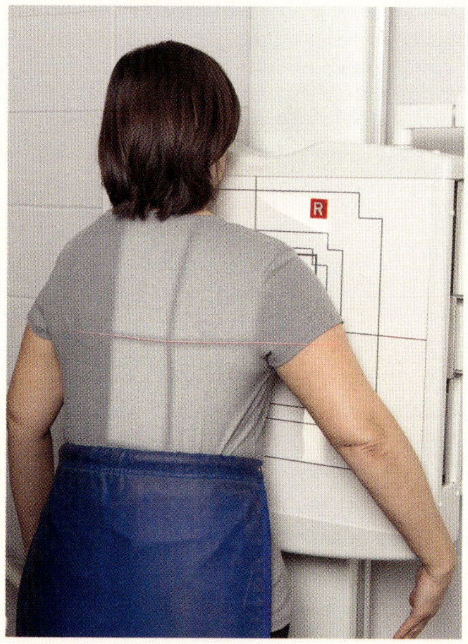

3-30 Erect PA high ribs for anterior rib injury.

IMAGE CRITIQUE (FIGS. 3-31 and 3-32)

- Entire first rib (pay special attention to include the entire head of the first rib)
- Count down to determine the number of full ribs above the diaphragm
- Ideally, ribs 1–8/9 visible above the diaphragm. The majority of the rib must be visualized above the diaphragm in order to count it as a rib above the diaphragm
- Properly centered with evidence of, at minimum, lateral collimation
- Costovertebral joints to the axillary margin included within the collimated exposure field
- Clavicle appears near horizontal
- SC joint aligned with midline, indicating no rotation of the thorax

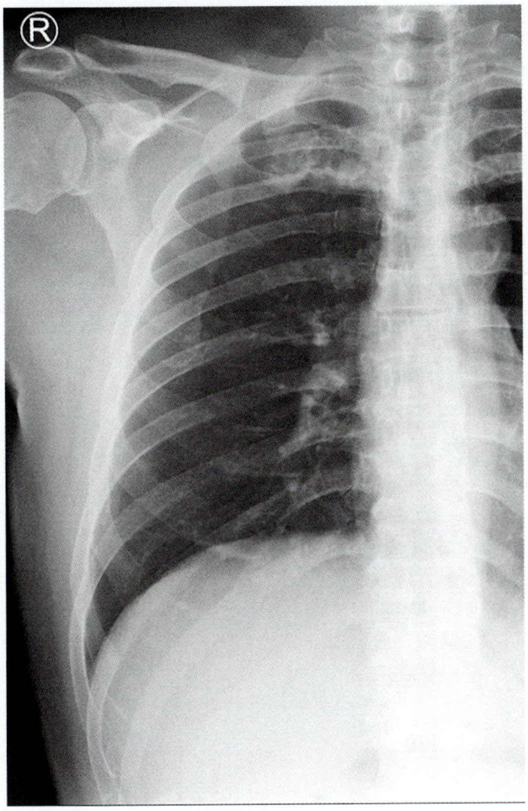

3-31 High ribs.

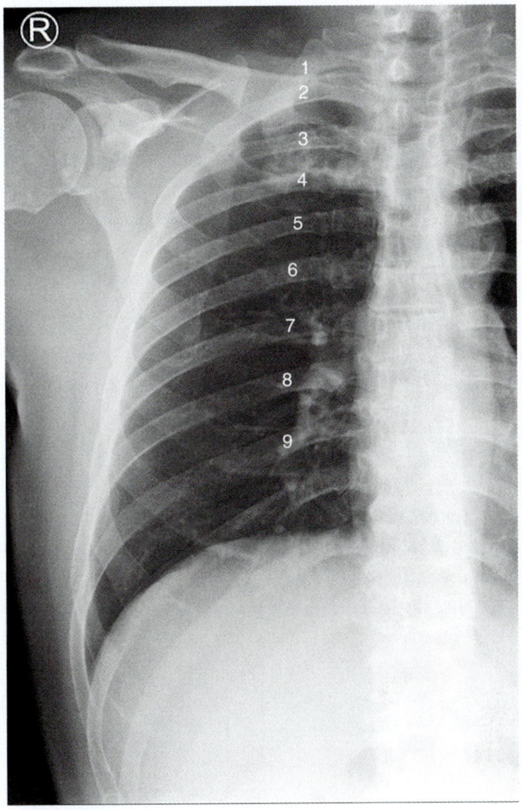

3-32 High ribs with rib count.

Low Ribs

- Projection: AP

Technical Considerations
- kVp 70–80
- mAs set manually (consider abdominal thickness)
- 40" SID

Exposure Field Size
- 10 × 12 crosswise

Patient Position (Fig. 3-33)
- Erect will be most comfortable for patients with rib fracture
- *Low ribs may be better demonstrated with the patient in a supine position to lessen the effects of gravity upon the diaphragm*
- All patients are positioned facing the tube. Ribs 11 and 12 are short and posteriorly positioned ribs on the bony thorax. AP projection is necessary to better image the lower ribs closer to the IR
- Arm of the affected side should be slightly abducted

Centering
- Bottom of the IR positioned at the top of the iliac crest
- Central ray directed midway between MSP and the lateral rib margin. Collimate down to unilateral ribs according to patient ensuring costovertebral joints and the axillary rib margin are included

Marking of IR
- Anatomic side marker R or L down in the region of the iliac crest correctly identifying side

Breathing
- Patient is instructed to take a deep breath in and then to exhale and hold air out
- Expiration will position the diaphragm superiorly
- Watch the patient during breathing instruction and while walking away to make the exposure

Ambulatory Ribs Protocol

PA Chest

AP/PA High

AP Low

AP Oblique/PA Oblique High

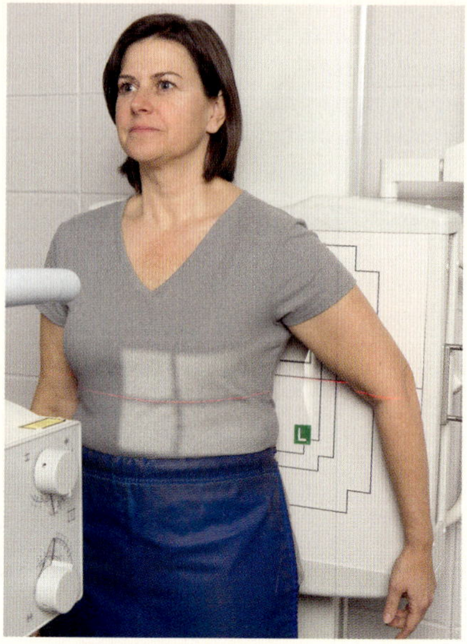

3-33 Erect AP low ribs.

IMAGE CRITIQUE (FIGS. 3-34 and 3-35)

- Ribs 8/9–12 visualized
- Ribs 10–12 ideally free of superimposition from the diaphragm
- Between the AP/PA high rib and AP low rib, one rib should overlap between the two projections
- Low ribs of interest and their respective costovertebral joints must be visualized

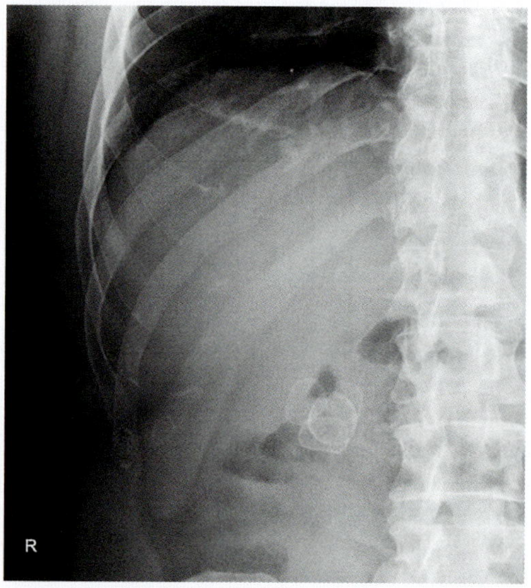

3-34 Low ribs.

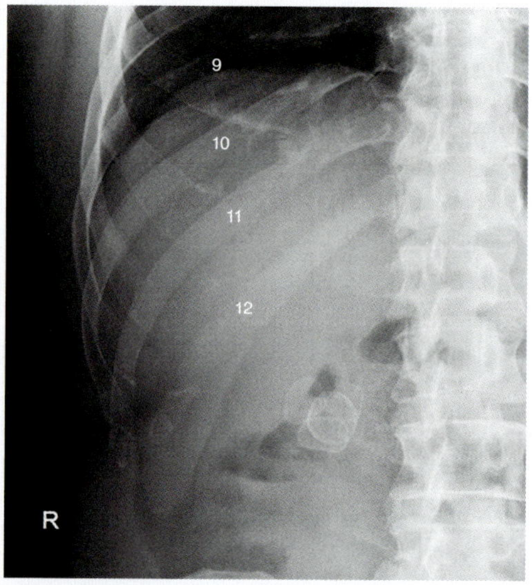

3-35 Low ribs.

High Oblique Ribs

- Projection: AP Oblique or PA Oblique
- *Be certain to question the patient as to which surface they are experiencing pain in order to utilize the best projection*

Ambulatory Ribs Protocol
PA Chest
AP/PA High
AP Low
AP Oblique/PA Oblique High

Technical Considerations
- kVp 70–80
- mAs set manually
- 40" SID

Exposure Field Size
- 14 × 17 lengthwise for all patients

Patient Position (Figs. 3-36 and 3-37)
- Erect will be most comfortable for patients with rib fracture
- Erect will also improve the patient's inspiration; gravity will help lower the level of the diaphragm
- To attain the best detail of the region of pain, that surface should be positioned closest to the IR
- Patient is rotated 45° into an anterior or posterior oblique position
- Patients with posterior injury will face the tube and therefore an AP oblique projection is acquired. The patient's affected side should be positioned closest to the IR. For example, a patient with a right posterior injury would be positioned into the right posterior oblique (RPO)
- Patients with anterior injury will face the upright Bucky and therefore a PA oblique projection is acquired. The patient's affected side should be positioned further away from the IR. Rotating the affected side away from the IR will prevent the vertebral column from superimposing the rib side of interest. For example, a patient with a right anterior injury would be positioned into a left anterior oblique (LAO) position
- Shoulders relaxed. Chin elevated
- Arm of the affected side should be slightly abducted, and patient's hand could be secured on the lower corner of the upright Bucky

Centering
- Level of T7/8 and midway between MSP and the lateral rib margin. Collimate down to unilateral ribs according to patient ensuring costovertebral joints and the axillary rib margin are included

Marking of IR
- Anatomic side marker R or L up in the region above the shoulder correctly identifying side
- Oblique positions should be marked with R or L to indicate patient's side closest to the IR

Breathing
- Double inspiration and hold after second inspiration. The second breath will likely be deeper than the first, helping the rib count above the diaphragm
- Watch the patient during breathing instruction and while walking away to make the exposure

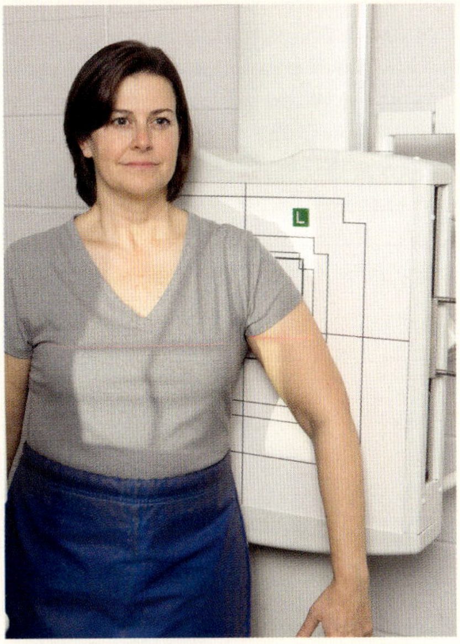

3-36 Erect AP oblique high ribs for the left posterior surface rib injury.

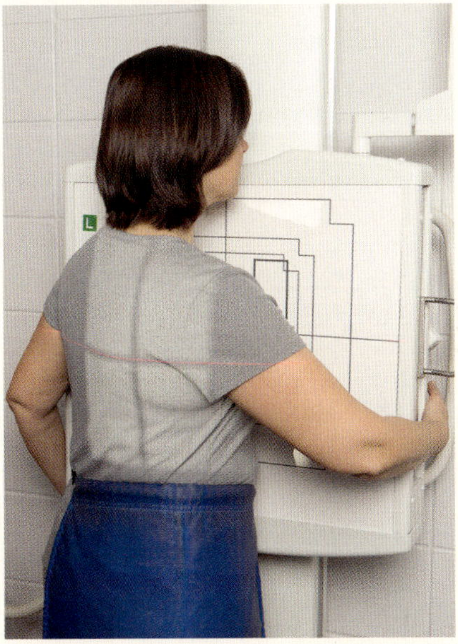

3-37 Erect PA oblique high ribs for the right anterior surface rib injury.

IMAGE CRITIQUE (FIG. 3-38)

- Entire first rib (pay special attention to include the entire head of the first rib)
- Ideally, ribs 1–8/9 visible above the diaphragm
- Properly centered with evidence of, at minimum, lateral collimation
- Costovertebral joints visualized
- The axillary/angle portion of the rib should appear elongated for visualization

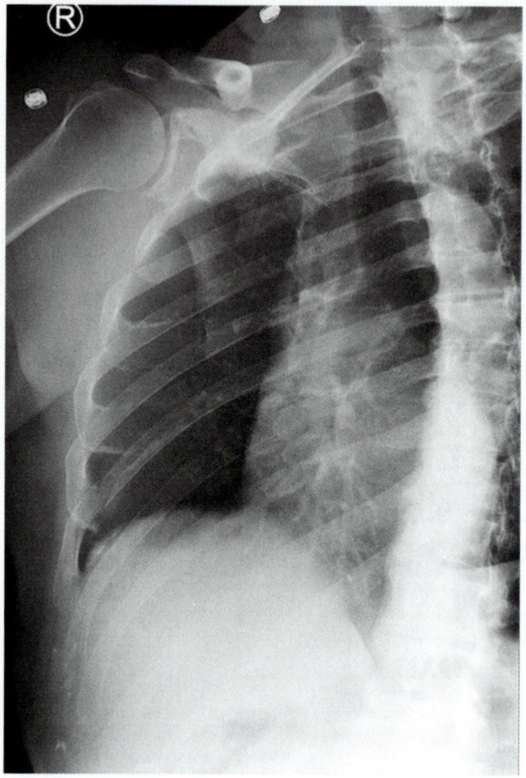

3-38 Oblique ribs.

Supine Chest

- Projection: AP (Perform chest upright if possible)
- *Chest imaging may or may not be incorporated into a rib protocol. When imaging ribs, it is essential to ask the patient if they are experiencing any difficulty breathing. Supine imaging will not display potential air-fluid levels*

Nonambulatory Ribs Protocol

AP Chest
AP High
AP Low
AP Oblique High Ribs

Technical Considerations

- kVp 100–120
- 2 outer AEC cells selected for table Bucky
- 40" or maximum SID (depending on suspension of overhead tube and facility preference)

Exposure Field Size

- 14 × 17 crosswise (often used as standard consideration, knowing lung capacity for ill and/or supine patients will be less compared to ambulatory upright patients)
- 14 × 17 lengthwise can be considered and applied

Patient Position (Fig. 3-39)

- Supine; ensure no rotation
- Chin elevated

Centering

- Level of T7/8 and MSP—Measure 3"–4" inferior to jugular notch for centering level
- Measuring approximately with one hand width down from the jugular notch for adult patients should closely achieve the T7/8 location

Marking of IR

- Anatomic side marker R or L up in the region above the shoulder correctly identifying side

Breathing

- Double inspiration and hold after second inspiration
- Watch the patient during breathing instruction and while walking away to make the exposure

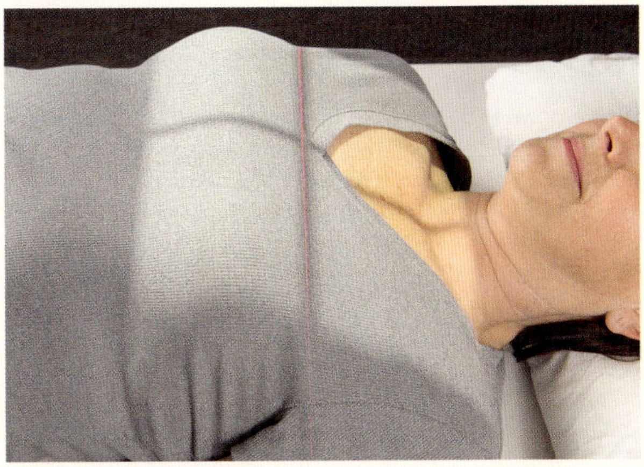

3-39 Supine AP chest.

IMAGE CRITIQUE (FIG. 3-40)

- Entire lung fields revealing apices, bases, costophrenic angles, and lateral lung margins
- AP chest provides comparison of the right to left sides of the bony thorax
- AP chest provides an image to rule out any lung pathology as a result of rib fracture; however, will not show evidence of air–fluid levels if a supine position was implemented
- Properly centered
- 8–9 ribs above the diaphragm counting on the right side of thorax
- Clavicles near horizontal
- SC joints symmetric, indicating the thorax was not rotated

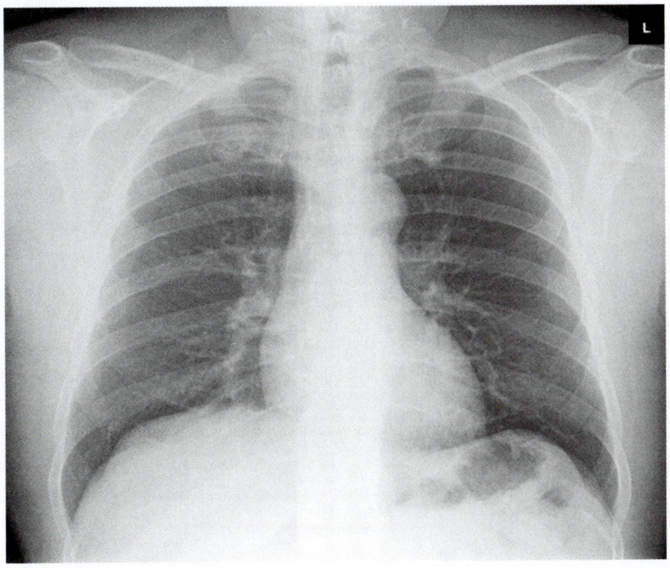

3-40 AP supine chest.

High Ribs

- Projection: AP

Nonambulatory Ribs Protocol

AP Chest

AP High

AP Low

AP Oblique High Ribs

Technical Considerations

- kVp 65–80
- mAs set manually
- 40" SID

Exposure Field Size

- 14 × 17 lengthwise for all patients

Patient Position (Fig. 3-41)

- Patient will lie supine regardless of the patient's surface of injury
- Shoulders relaxed. Chin elevated
- Arm of the affected side should be slightly abducted

Centering

- Level of T7/8 and midway between MSP and the lateral rib margin. Collimate down to unilateral ribs according to patient ensuring costovertebral joints and the axillary rib margin are included
- Measuring approximately with one hand width down from the jugular notch for adult patients should closely achieve the T7/8 location

Marking of IR

- Anatomic side marker R or L up in the region above the shoulder correctly identifying the side

Breathing

- Double inspiration and hold after second inspiration. The second breath will likely be deeper than the first, which will improve the rib count above the diaphragm
- Watch the patient during breathing instruction and while walking away to make the exposure

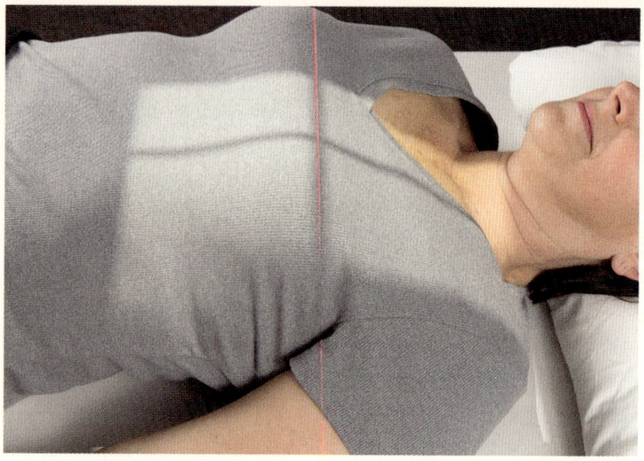

3-41 Supine AP high ribs.

IMAGE CRITIQUE (FIG. 3-42)

- Entire first rib (pay special attention to include the entire head of the first rib)
- Count down to determine the number of full ribs above the diaphragm
- Ideally, ribs 1–8/9 visible above the diaphragm, but could be less with a supine position
- Properly centered with evidence of, at minimum, lateral collimation
- Costovertebral joints to the axillary rib margin included within the collimated exposure field
- Clavicle appears near horizontal
- SC joint aligned with midline, indicating no rotation of the thorax

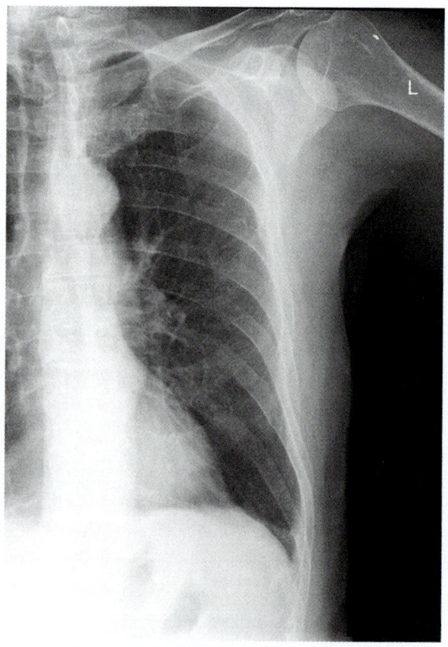

3-42 AP supine high ribs.

Low Ribs

- Projection: AP

Nonambulatory Ribs Protocol
AP Chest
AP High
AP Low
AP Oblique High Ribs

Technical Considerations
- kVp 70–80
- mAs set manually (consider abdominal thickness)
- 40" SID

Exposure Field Size
- 10 × 12 crosswise

Patient Position (Fig. 3-43)
- Patient remains supine
- Arm of the affected side should be slightly abducted

Centering
- Bottom of the IR positioned with the top of the iliac crest
- Central ray directed midway between MSP and the lateral rib margin. Collimate down to unilateral ribs according to patient ensuring costovertebral joints and the axillary rib margin are included

Marking of IR
- Anatomic side marker R or L down in the region of the iliac crest

Breathing
- Patient is instructed to take a deep breath in and then to exhale and hold their air out
- Expiration will position the diaphragm superiorly
- Watch the patient during breathing instruction and while walking away to make the exposure

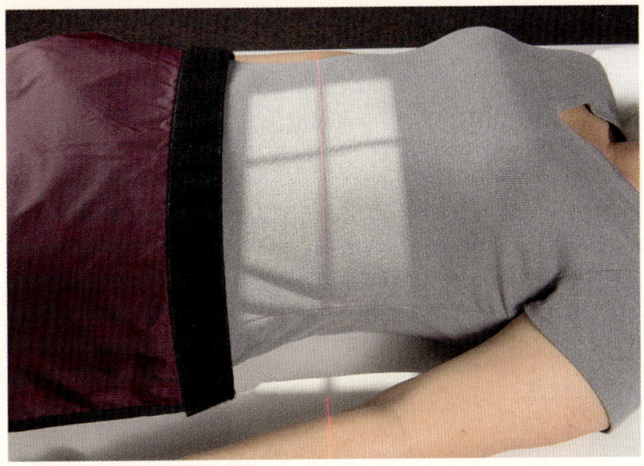

3-43 Supine AP low ribs.

IMAGE CRITIQUE (FIG. 3-44)

- Ribs 8/9–12 visualized
- Ribs 10–12 are, ideally, free of superimposition from the diaphragm
- Between the AP high rib and AP low rib, 1 rib should overlap between the two projections
- Low ribs of interest and their respective costovertebral joints must be visualized

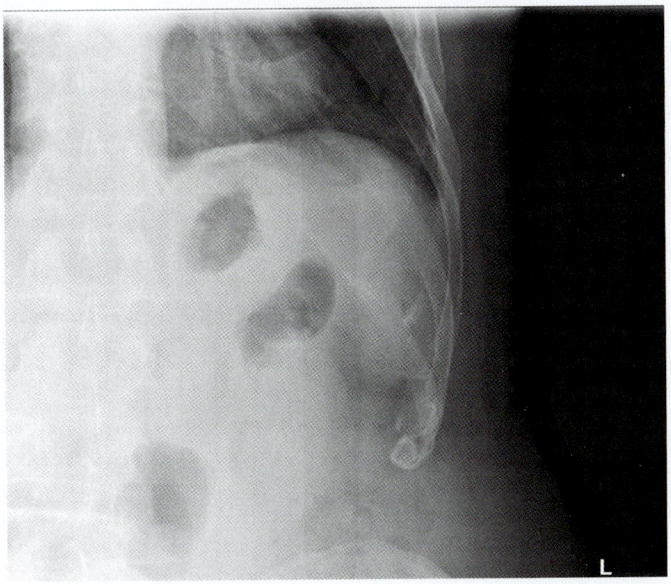

3-44 AP supine low ribs.

High Oblique Ribs

- Projection: AP Oblique

Technical Considerations:
- kVp 70–80
- mAs set manually
- 40" SID

Exposure Field Size
- 14 × 17 lengthwise for all patients

Nonambulatory Ribs Protocol
AP Chest
AP High
AP Low
AP Oblique High Ribs

Patient Position (Fig. 3-45)
- From supine position, rotate the patient 45° toward the affected side into a posterior oblique position, and provide a wedge sponge under the patient for support
- Arm of the affected side should be slightly abducted

Centering
- Level of T7/8 and midway between MSP and the lateral rib margin. Collimate down to unilateral ribs according to patient ensuring costovertebral joints and the axillary rib margin are included

Marking of IR
- Anatomic side marker R or L up in the region above the shoulder correctly identifying the side
- Oblique positions should be marked with R or L to indicate the patient's side closest to the IR

Breathing
- Double inspiration and hold after second inspiration. The second breath will likely be deeper than the first, which will improve the rib count above the diaphragm
- Watch the patient during breathing instruction and while walking away to make the exposure

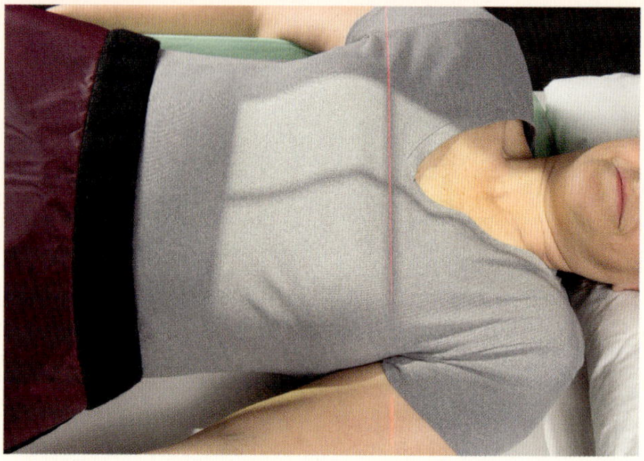

3-45 Supine AP oblique high ribs.

IMAGE CRITIQUE (FIGS. 3-46 and 3-47)

- Entire first rib (pay special attention to include the entire head of the first rib)
- Ideally ribs 1–8/9 visible above the diaphragm
- Properly centered with evidence of, at minimum, lateral collimation
- Costovertebral joints visualized
- The axillary/angle portion of the rib should appear elongated for better visualization

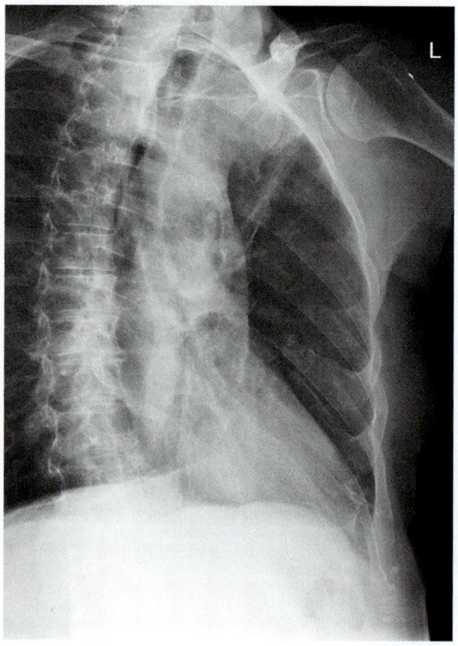

3-46 AP oblique high ribs.

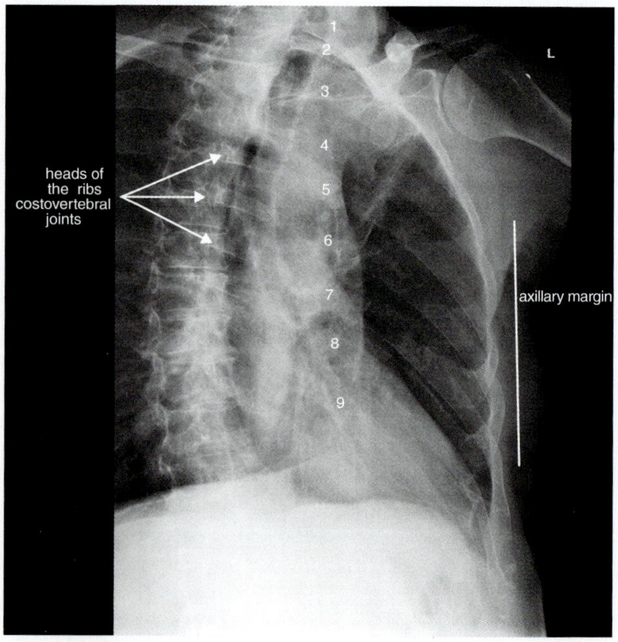

3-47 AP oblique high ribs.

PA Oblique (RAO) Sternum

- Projection: PA Oblique

Sternum Protocol
PA Oblique (RAO)
Lateral

Technical Considerations

- kVp 70–80
- Breathing Technique: lowest mA setting with a minimum of 3–4 seconds set for time
- Manual technique could also be considered
- 40" SID

Exposure Field Size

- 10 × 12 lengthwise for all patients

Patient Position (Figs. 3-48 and 3-49)

- Patient will start by facing the upright Bucky
- Patient rotated into a 15°–20° RAO position. A patient with a thinner thorax will require more rotation than the patient with a deep and broad thorax. A thinner patient has less distance between the spine and the sternum, therefore requiring more rotation (closer to 20°) to shift the sternum and thoracic spine off of one another. Proper rotation is critical to position the sternum within the heart shadow and free of superimposition of the thoracic spine
- *A patient unable to stand could be alternatively imaged supine with the tube angled 15°–20°* (Fig. 3-50)

Centering

- Midsternum (easiest to find this location by placing the top of the 10 × 12 IR 1½" above the jugular notch)
- Align the tube with the height of the Bucky (set the top of the 10 x 12 exposure field margin 1½" above part first and then adjust the tube to line up with the Bucky)
- Adjust the CR entrance 2-3 fingers width to the left of the spine
- It should be noted that there should not be visible light above the top of the shoulders. If so, the height of the upright Bucky is not set to the level of the midsternum or exposure field exceeds 10 × 12 lengthwise

Marking of IR

- Right marker corresponding to the right side of the patient
- Oblique position should be marked with R to indicate patient's side closest to the IR

Breathing

- A breathing technique is an optimal setting as it will blur overlying ribs and lung markings due to the motion created during the lengthened exposure time. Once the control panel has been set and the patient has been positioned, the patient should be instructed to take short shallow breaths until instructed to stop
- Alternative breathing: Suspend respiration

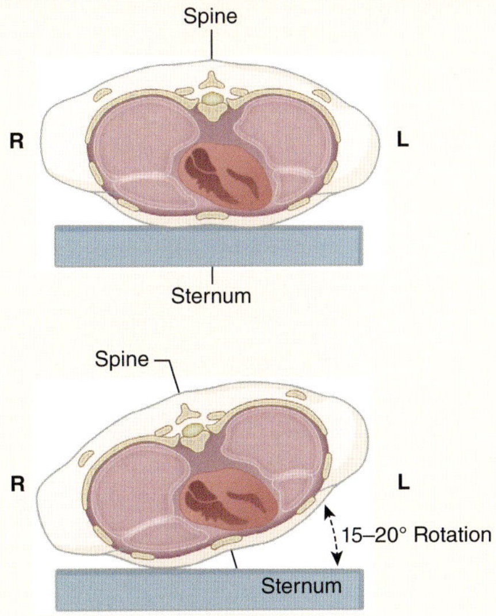

3-48 Torso rotation affects spine and sternum placement.

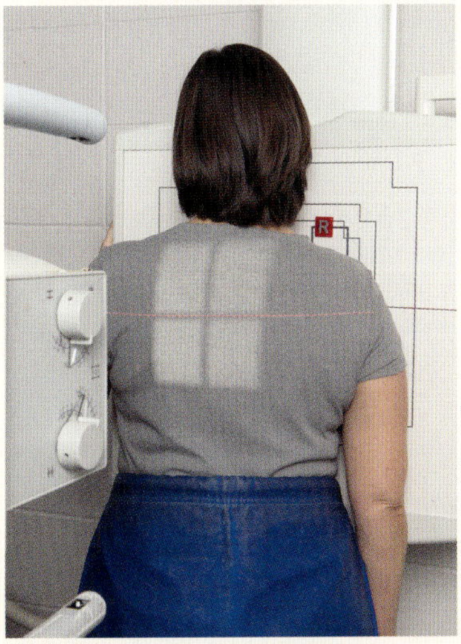

3-49 Erect RAO sternum.

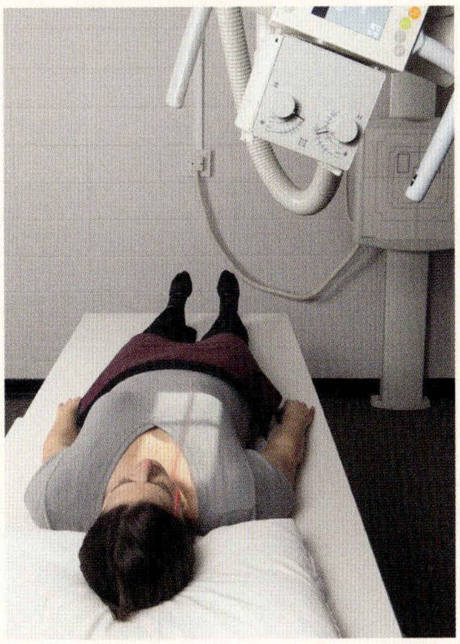

3-50 Recumbent alternate LPO sternum.

IMAGE CRITIQUE (FIGS. 3-51 and 3-52)

- Proper obliquity of the patient will position the sternum within the heart shadow. The heart shadow will provide a homogeneous background to allow better visualization of the thin sternum. This is why the RAO/LPO position is optimal
- Underrotation of the thorax will display the sternum with vertebral superimposition
- Overrotation of the thorax will display the sternum lateral to the heart shadow and into the density of the lungs
- Entire sternum visualized (Figs. 3-53 and 3-54)

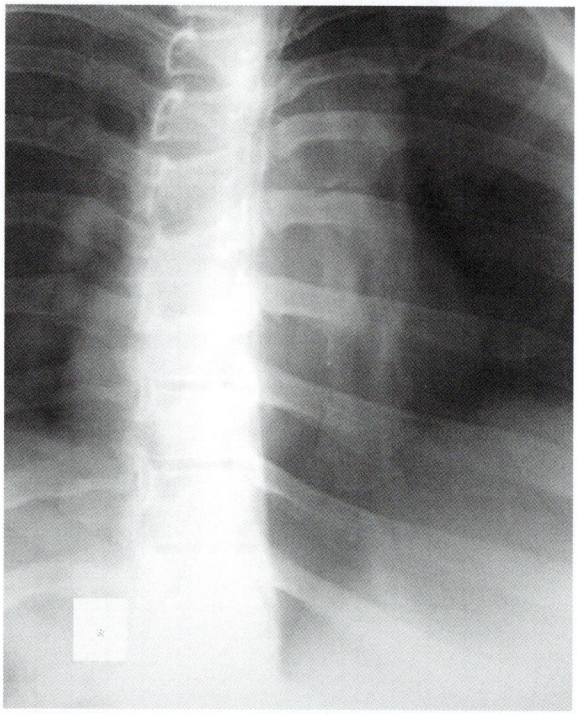

3-51 RAO sternum.

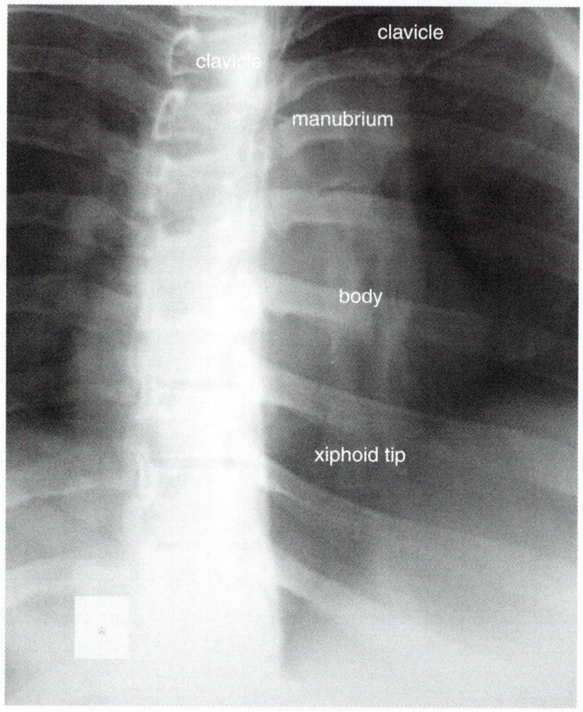

3-52 RAO sternum.

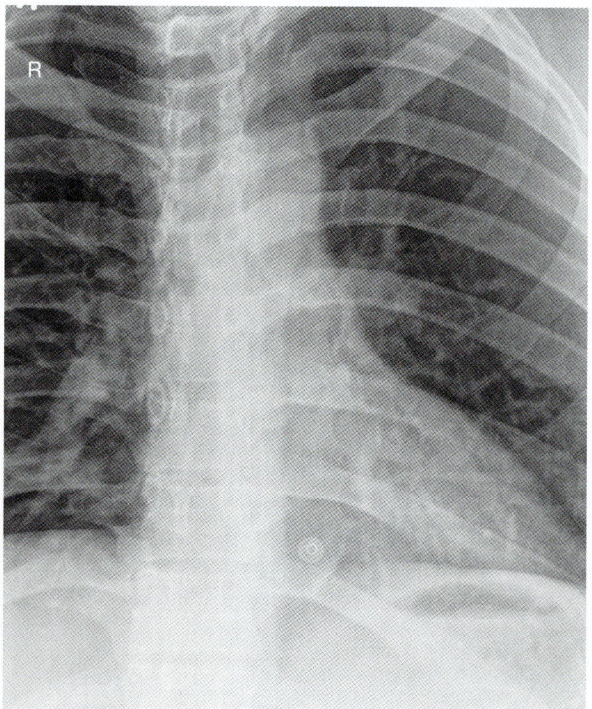

3-53 RAO sternum underrotated.

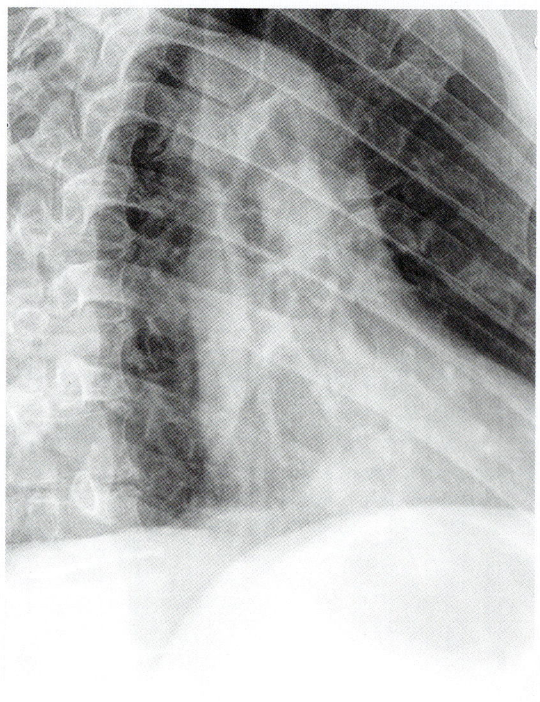

3-54 RAO sternum overrotated.

Lateral Sternum

- Projection: Lateral

Sternum Protocol
PA Oblique (RAO)
Lateral

Technical Considerations
- kVp 70–80
- mAs manually set
- 72" SID

Exposure Field Size
- 10 × 12 lengthwise

Patient Position (Fig. 3-55)
- Erect left lateral position
- Ensure a true lateral position of the thorax
- Patient should be instructed to clasp hands behind waist and pull their shoulders back and project their chest out
- A patient unable to stand could be alternatively imaged supine with a horizontal beam (Fig. 3-56)

Centering (Fig. 3-57)
- Midsternum (easiest to find this by placing the top of the 10 × 12 IR 1½" above the jugular notch)
- Align the tube with the height of the Bucky
- Adjust the CR entrance anterior to MCP. Collimate the exposure field smaller than 10 X 12 if needed

Marking of IR
- Anatomic side marker L along the anterior border of the patient

Breathing
- Patient is instructed to take in a deep breath and hold it. The exposure is acquired after the deep inspiration. Deep inspiration will project the sternum out anteriorly from the ribs
- Watch the patient during breathing instruction and while walking away to make the exposure

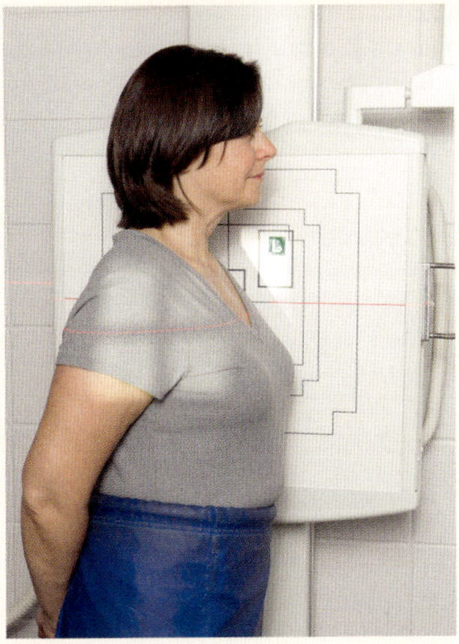

3-55 Erect lateral sternum.

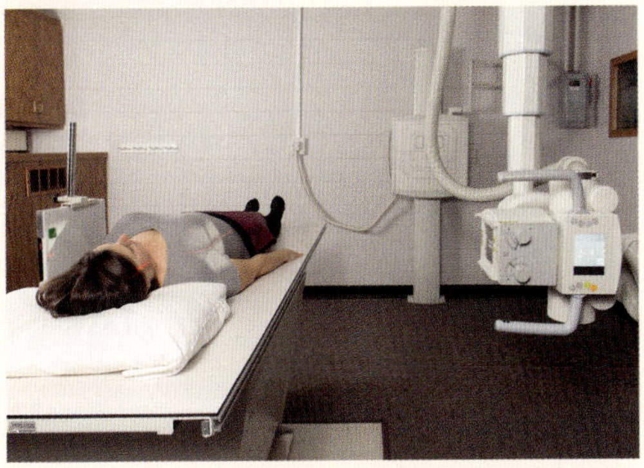

3-56 Horizontal beam established to achieve a lateral sternum with 72″ SID.

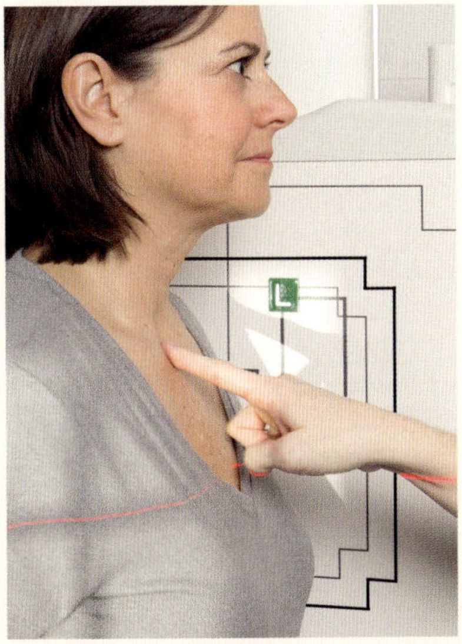

3-57 Palpate the level of the jugular notch to help position the top of the IR superior to the level of the sternum to accommodate the superior movement of the sternum with inspiration.

IMAGE CRITIQUE (FIGS. 3-58 and 3-59)

- Entire sternum visualized from the jugular notch to include the xiphoid tip
- The sternum should be in a true lateral and with a profile appearance
- The humeral heads should not superimpose the sternum

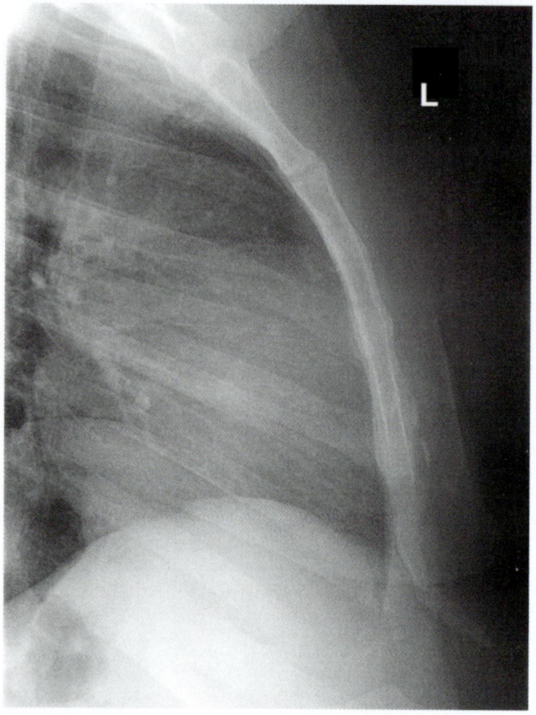

3-58 Lateral sternum.

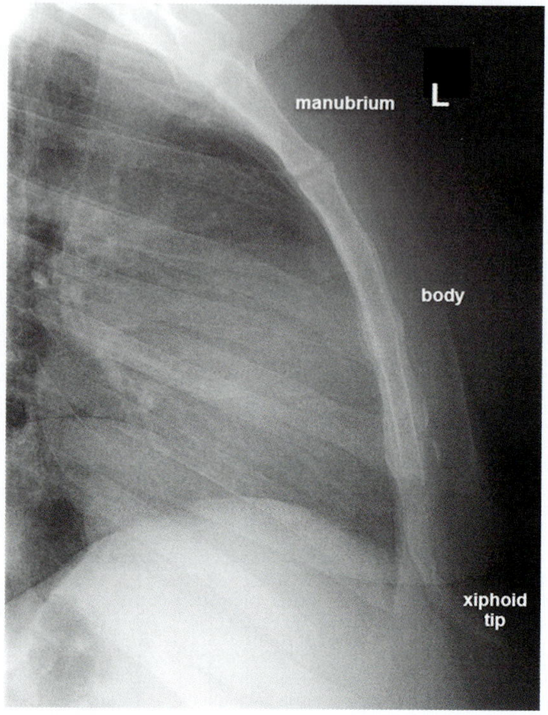

3-59 Lateral sternum.

THE FINAL STEP: IMAGE REVIEW

The technologist must take time to review acquired images to ensure image quality is acceptable. The technologist must have the knowledge within their role not only to acquire the images and care for the patient, but also to know how to review the images to ensure diagnostic quality has been attained. In certain instances, a projection may need to be repeated. This is to the discretion of the radiologic technologist. The technologist should review each image for the following.

1. Is all of the necessary anatomy included on the image?
   - Was the central ray (CR) properly directed to the part? An "X" can be drawn to intersect within the collimated exposure field to determine whether the CR was directed to the correct location.
   - Was essential anatomy in the collimated exposure field?
   - Is the area free of artifact(s)?
2. Is the anatomy well demonstrated?
   - Did the technologist properly position the patient to adequately demonstrate the anatomy?
   - Can the technologist recognize the anatomy best demonstrated with use of different projections?
3. Does the image reflect proper image markings?
   - Did the technologist correctly use a lead marker to identify the right or left side?
   - What additional markings or annotations could be helpful to the radiologist interpreting the exam?
   - Is the image properly displayed?
4. Does the image prove to be technically acceptable?
   - Does the exposure index fall within acceptable range for the operating system? Images that are technically insufficient may appear of good quality if just slightly insufficient or "mottled or pixelated" if severely insufficient. Images that appear "mottled" should be repeated. Images that appear beyond optimal exposure owing to higher technique may display high quality, but the patient has received excessive radiation dose.

CRITICAL THINKING

1. In review of the PA chest acquired for a right rib series (Fig. 3-60), how should the technologist proceed?
   a. Repeat the image as the inspiration is insufficient.
   b. Repeat the image for the left-sided artifact.
   c. Repeat the image as the right axillary ribs are not entirely included due to off-centering.
   d. The PA chest sufficiently meets the criteria as needed for a rib series.

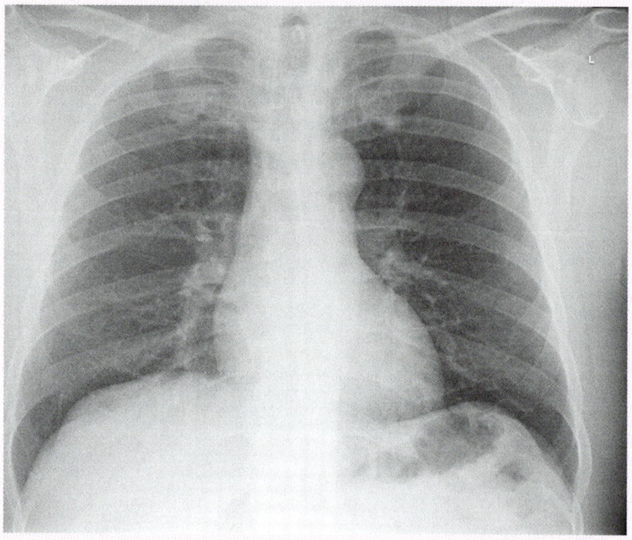

3-60

2. If this oblique high rib (Fig. 3-61) is acquired as an AP oblique projection, what is the position of the patient?
   a. LAO
   b. RAO
   c. LPO
   d. RPO

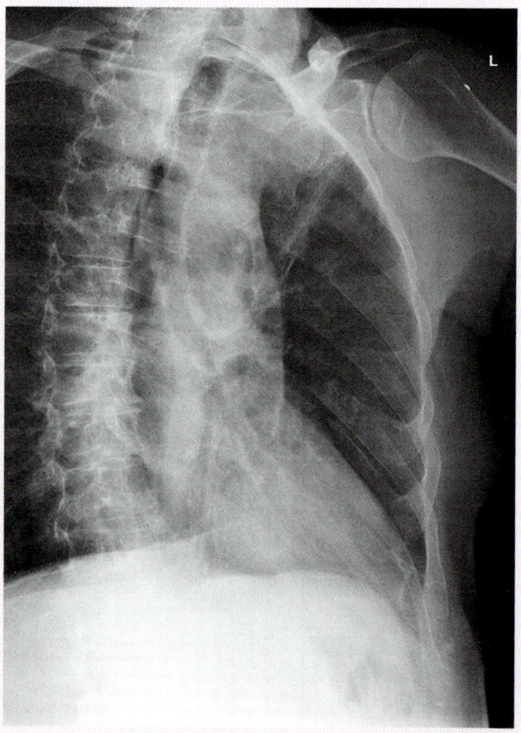

3-61

3. In review of the AP high rib image (Fig. 3-62), how should the technologist proceed?
   a. Image represents good centering and all essential anatomy.
   b. Image represents good centering, but poor collimation.
   c. Image represents centering that is directed too inferior, failing to include all essential anatomy.
   d. Image represents centering that is directed too superior, failing to include all essential anatomy.

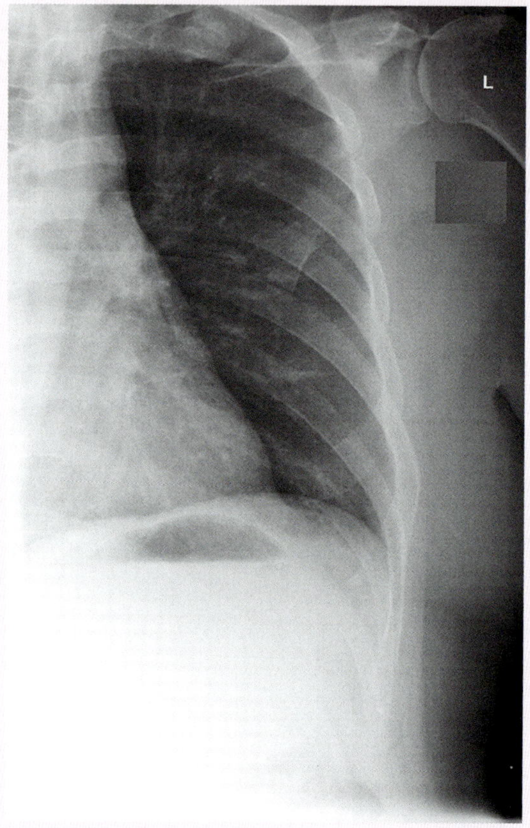

3-62

4. In review of the AP oblique high rib image (Fig. 3-63), characterize the positioning.
   a. The image represents good positioning and all essential anatomy.
   b. The image appears underrotated and should be repeated.
   c. The image fails to include the entire first rib and should be repeated.
   d. The image fails to include costovertebral joints.

5. In review of the lateral sternum image (Fig. 3-64), characterize the results.
   a. The image represents good positioning and all essential anatomy.
   b. The image appears rotated and should be repeated.
   c. The image fails to include the entire sternum and should be repeated.
   d. The image represents that the humeral heads were not pulled back posteriorly enough and should be repeated.

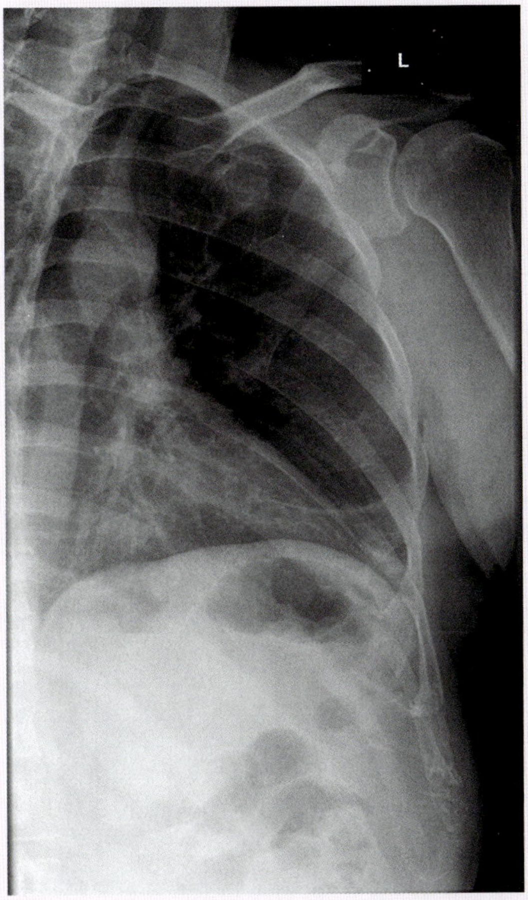

3-63

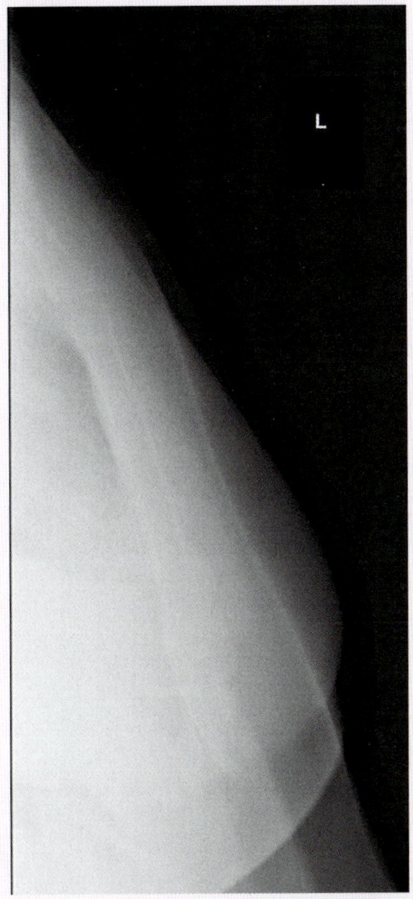

3-64

ANSWERS TO THE CRITICAL THINKING QUESTIONS

1. d
2. c
3. c
4. d
5. c

CHAPTER 4 Abdomen

Abdominal imaging is a frequent exam and is not unusual to be paired with chest imaging orders. Abdominal images will be centered to include the diaphragm or the symphysis pubis. These anatomic structures mark the superior and inferior boundaries of the abdominal cavity. The patient may be positioned either recumbent or upright in efforts to display pathology or according to the requirements of a procedure. The technologist must take into consideration patient variables such as size, ability, and pathology while trying to attain images of the highest quality.

CLINICAL INDICATIONS

Indications are the symptomatic reasons as to why a particular exam may be ordered by the physician. The technologist should look at the clinical indications before performing a procedure. In certain circumstances, the indication may influence the need to increase or decrease the technical settings. The following briefly introduces common exam indications, but it is not an all-encompassing list.

Pneumoperitoneum: Free air within the peritoneal cavity as a result of visceral perforation of stomach or bowel. Upright and/or decubitus imaging of the abdomen will be necessary for diagnosis (Figs. 4-1 and 4-2).

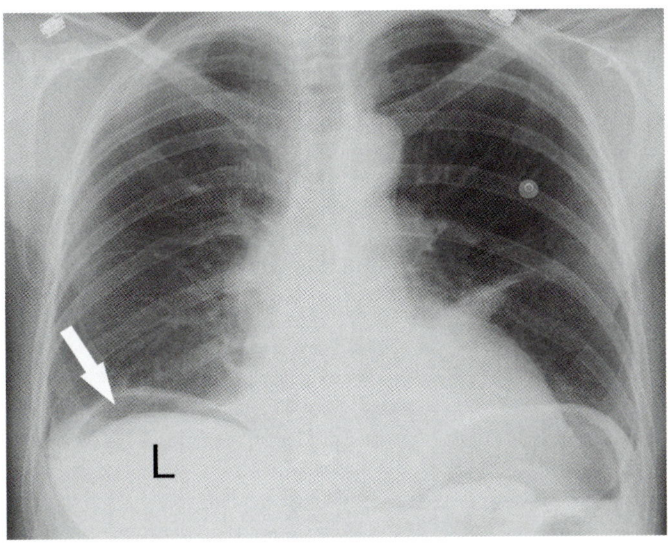

4-1 Pneumoperitoneum identified below the right hemidiaphragm.

Ascites: An abundant accumulation of serous fluid within the peritoneal cavity. The condition may be a result of malignancy, congestive heart failure, cirrhosis, or peritonitis. Excessive volumes of fluid may be reduced through an ultrasound-guided paracentesis procedure. With ultrasound guidance, fluid volumes are drained and reduced (Figs. 4-3 to 4-5).

Ileus: Bowel obstruction categorized into two types. *Mechanical obstruction* defines a physical blockage caused by fibrous adhesions, a mass, twisted bowel (volvulus), or telescoping bowel (intussusception). Air is seen distending the small bowel. *Paralytic ileus* is a result of inactive bowel. A paralytic ileus may result from extensive operative procedures with anesthesia or from use of certain types of medication. A bowel obstruction will result in small and large bowel dilation. The patient will present with a distended, rigid, and painful abdomen (Fig. 4-6).

Crohn Disease: A disease process of unknown origin affecting a regional portion of the small bowel, but may extend to include the cecum and ascending colon. Chronic inflammation will result in bowel wall thickening and potential narrowing of the lumen. The terminal ileum is most often affected (Fig. 4-7).

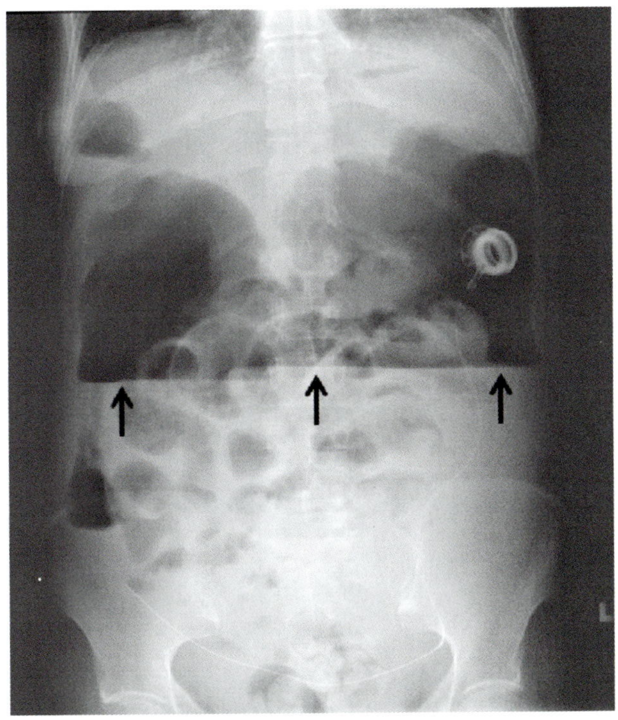

4-2 Upright abdomen with black arrows denoting the presence of air rising in the loops of bowel.

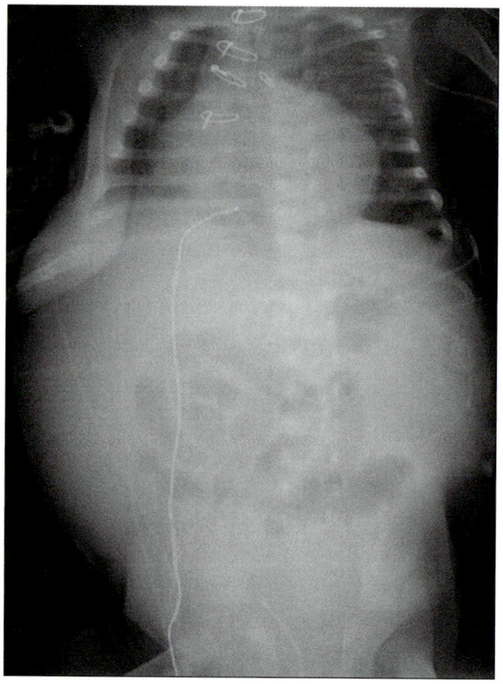

4-3 Pediatric ascites—distention of the abdominal wall denoted by the contour of the abdomen.

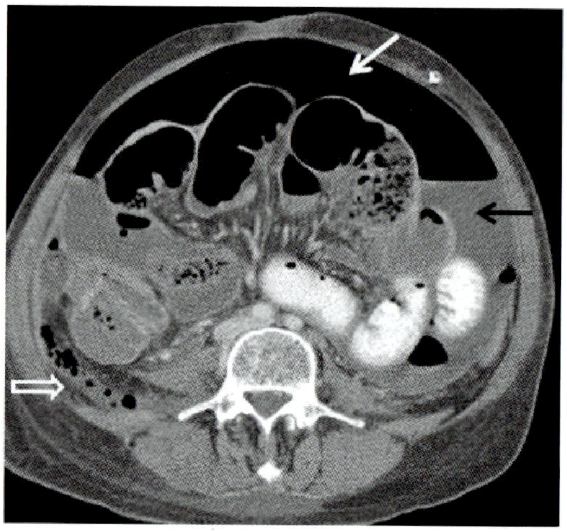

4-4 White arrow denotes free intraperitoneal air. Black arrow denotes ascites. Open white arrow denotes gas collection.

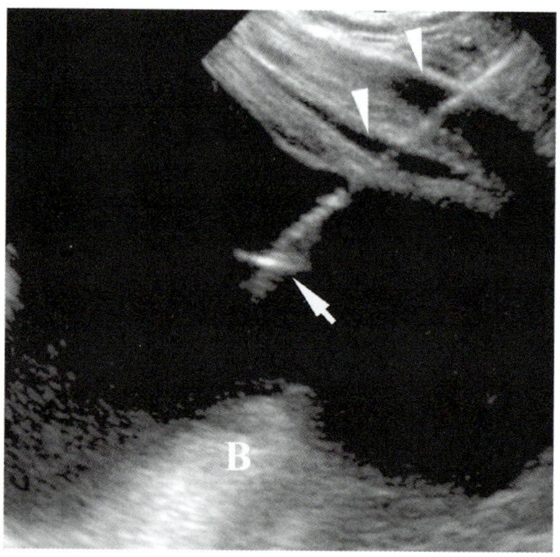

4-5 Ultrasound-guided paracentesis. White arrow denotes tip of needle positioned within a pocket of fluid (anechoic-black).

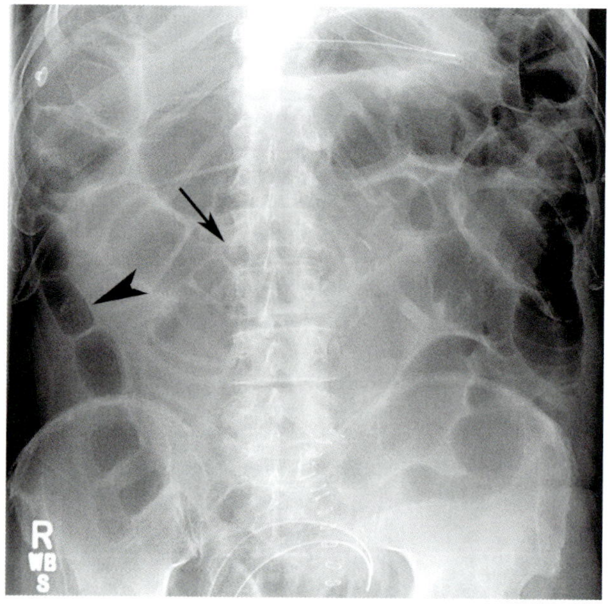

4-6 Radiographic appearance of an ileus. *Small arrow* denotes air distention in the small intestine. *Large arrow* denotes air distention in the colon.

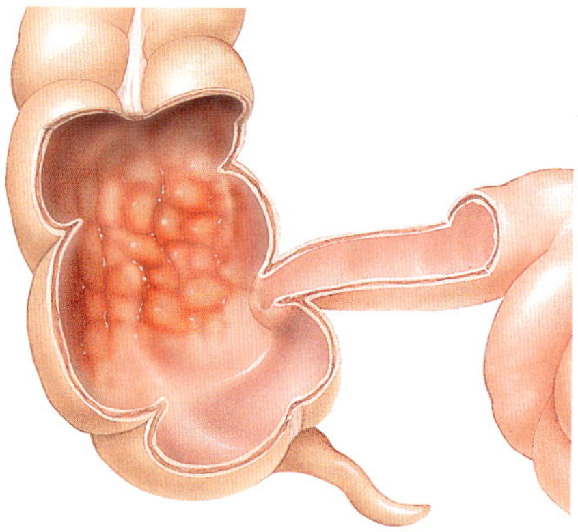

4-7 Crohn disease.

Volvulus: A result of a segment of bowel twisting upon itself, causing an obstruction. It can affect the small or large bowel (Figs. 4-8 and 4-9).

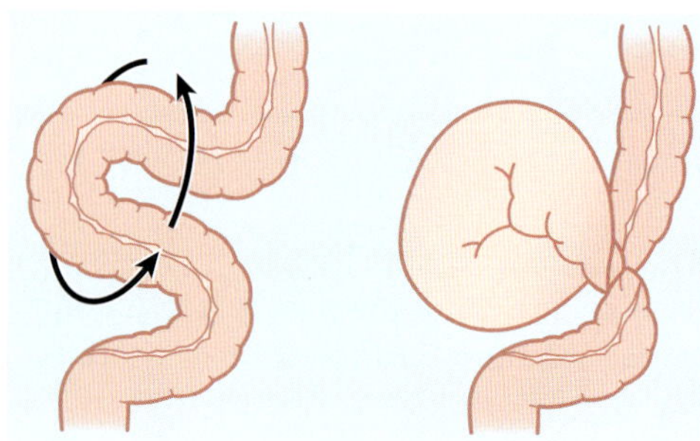

4-8 Volvulus.

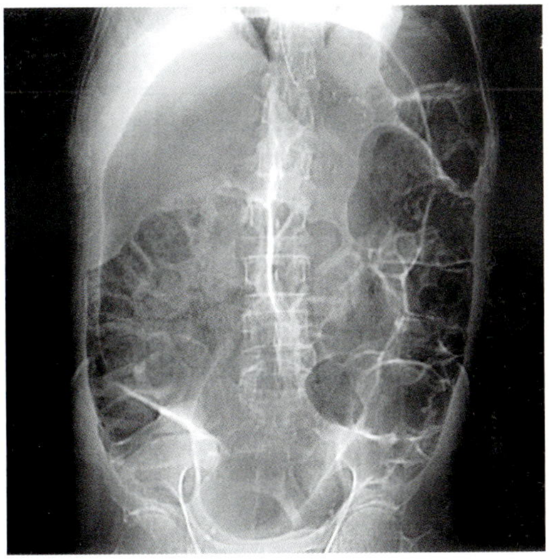

4-9 Volvulus radiographic appearance.

Intussusception: A portion of bowel that telescopes into another segment. The condition most predominantly affects infants and toddlers; rarely adults (Figs. 4-10 to 4-12).

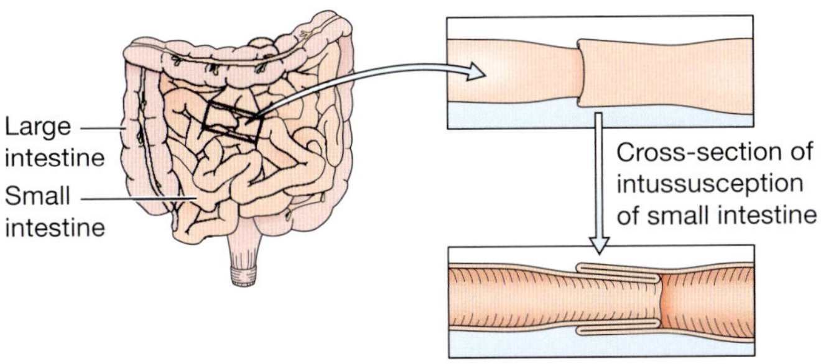

4-10 Intussusception.

Renal Calculi: A variety of minerals contribute to the formation of calcified stones. The size of the stone and its location as it passes from the kidney into the bladder can cause obstruction in the ureter or urethra. Based on the size of the stone, the patient may not manifest any symptoms until it passes into the ureter (Fig. 4-13).

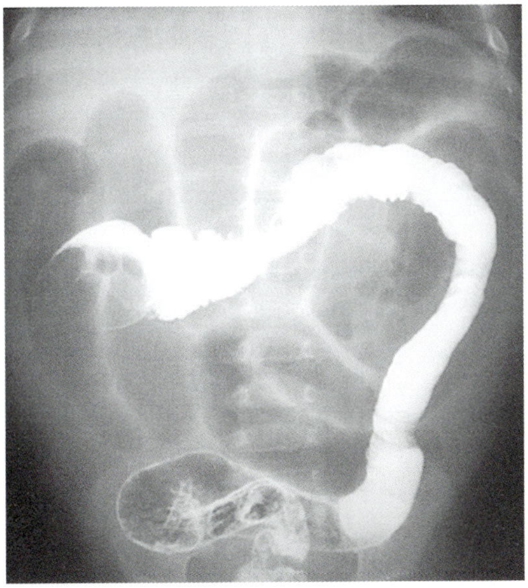

4-11 Barium enema may be a therapeutic attempt to correct a case of intussusception.

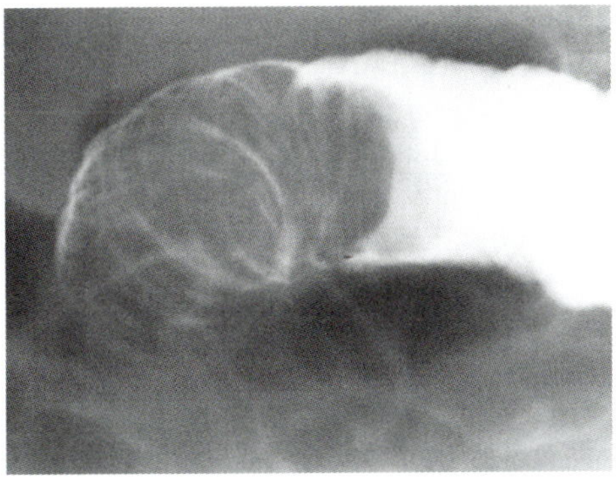

4-12 Classic spring coil appearance of an intussusception.

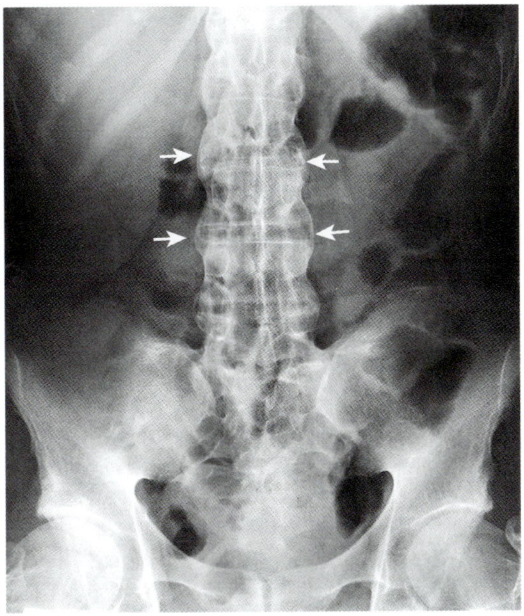

4-13 Arrow denotes a stone present within the left kidney.

Foreign Bodies: Swallowing a foreign object may be tracked through the gastrointestinal (GI) tract with abdominal imaging to verify the presence of a foreign body, track passage through the GI tract, and, hopefully, avoid obstruction (Fig. 4-14).

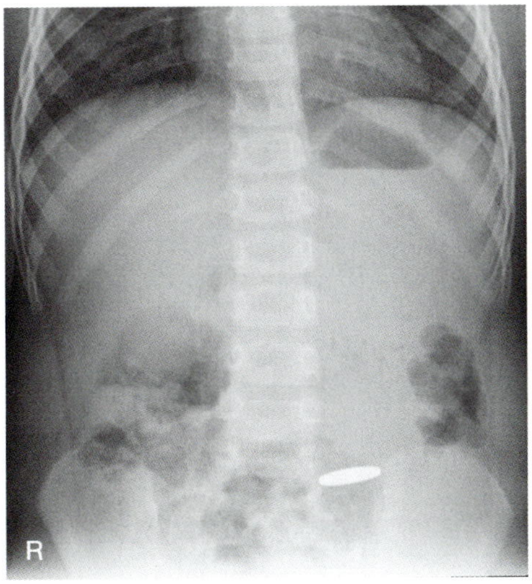

4-14 Abdominal image to reveal the location of an ingested foreign object.

Line Placement: Images of the abdomen may be requested to verify correct location of a placed line. It is essential that the technologist acquire an image with proper positioning and technical settings to help determine proper placement of the line and identification of anatomy. Centering may be adjusted to show the distal point of the line and the area proximal (above) it. Therefore, it is essential know which line has been placed to allow for adjusted centering from the standard expectation if necessary. With digital imaging technology, images acquired to verify line placement could then be adjusted with subtraction of grayscale to better view the line (Table 4-1).

4-1 Abdominal Lines

Nasogastric (NG) tube

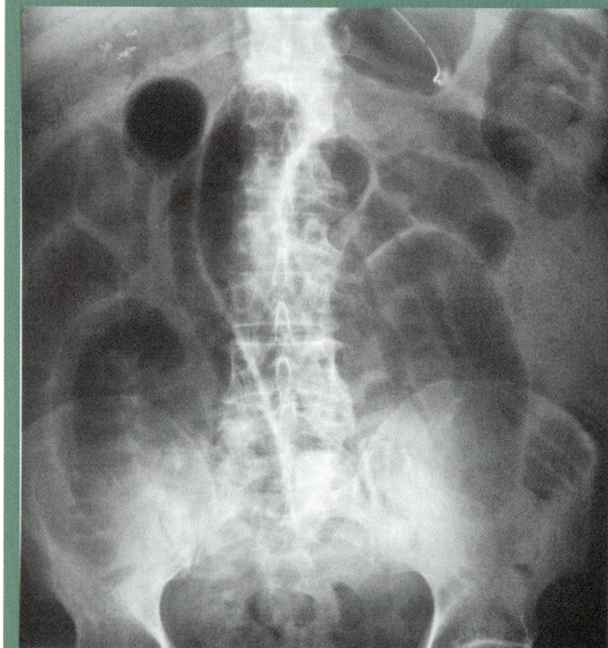

4-15

Tube placed through the nose and should end with placement in the stomach. A radiograph can be acquired to ensure the NG tube is properly positioned in the stomach and not the respiratory system. Centering in this case scenario may be higher than normally directed for a KUB. The NG tube is used for drug and/or minimal fluid administration. The NG tube is also used for suction, especially on patients with bowel obstruction (Fig. 4-15).

Ureteric stents

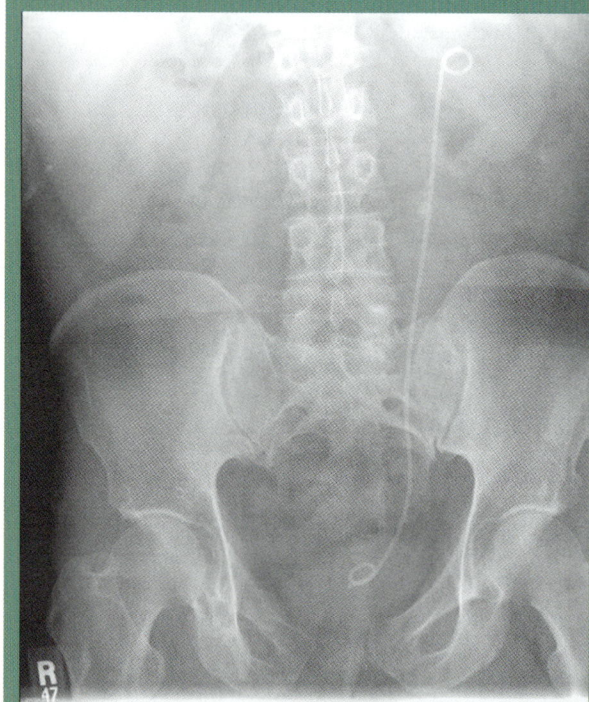

4-16

A stent that creates an open lumen from the renal pelvis to the bladder for urine drainage. Placement of a stent could be verified with a KUB (Fig. 4-16).

4-1 Abdominal Lines (*Continued*)

Ventriculoperitoneal shunts

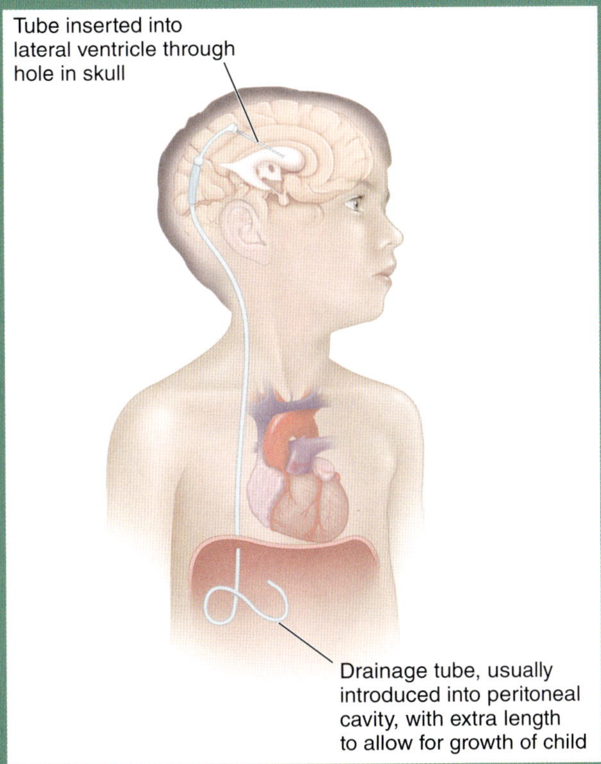

4-17

In cases where excessive cerebrospinal fluid is produced in the lateral ventricle, a shunt or tube can be placed to begin in the lateral ventricle and to end within the peritoneal cavity. Imaging of the head, neck, chest, and abdomen (Shunt Series) will confirm proper placement of a shunt (Fig. 4-17).

Feeding tube

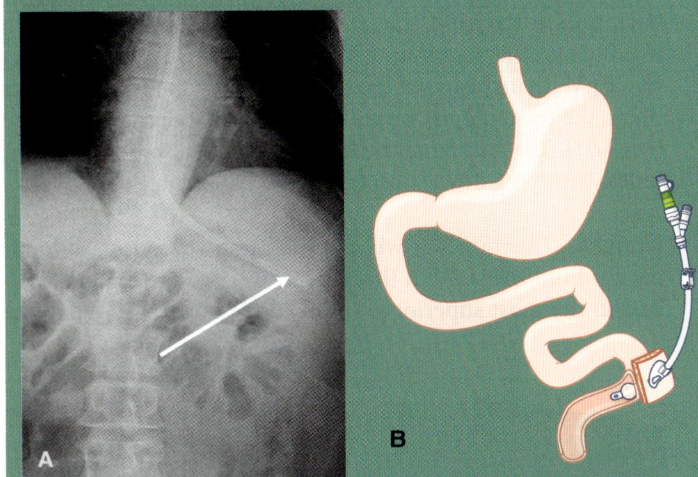

4-18

There are various types of feeding tubes that could be placed. The tube enters through the nose and ends within the proximal small bowel (Fig. 4-18A). Imaging of the chest or abdomen would confirm correct placement within the GI tract and not within the respiratory tract. Fluoroscopy (live x-ray) also often involved for guided placement. Gastro-enteric feeding tubes can also be directly placed through the abdominal wall and into the stomach (G-Tube) and into the jejunum (J-Tube, Fig. 4-18B).

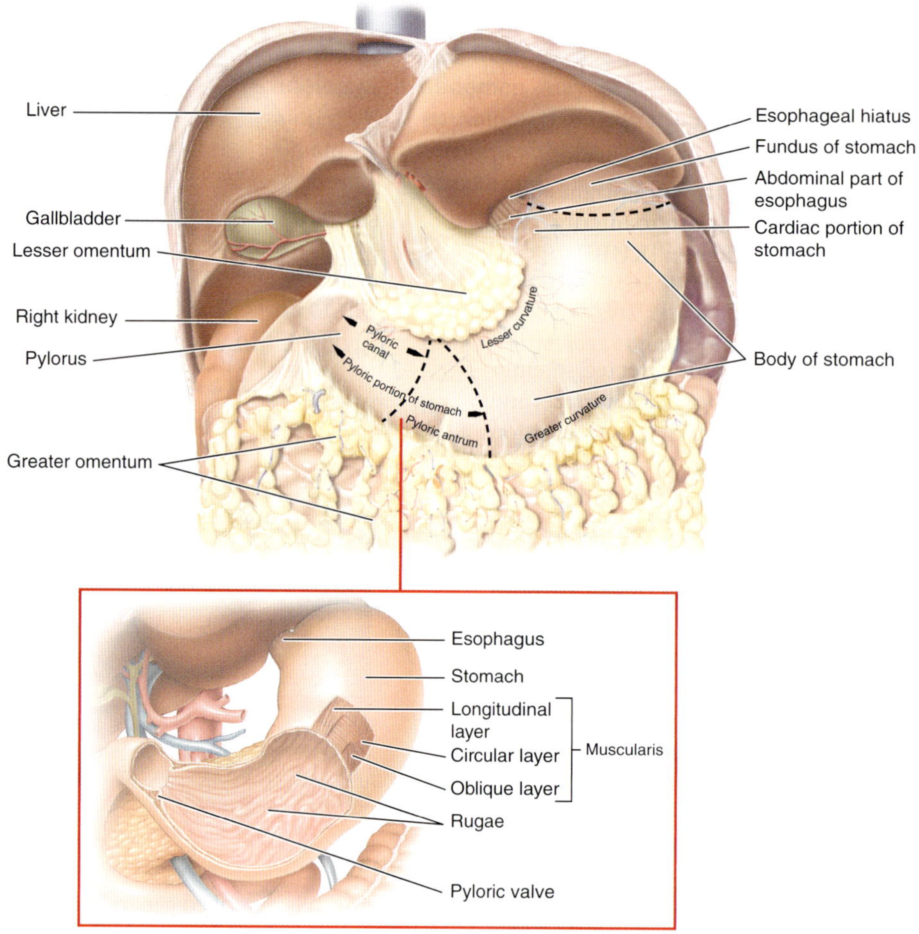

4-31 Stomach.

Small Intestines

The small intestine is divided into three segments. The first segment is the duodenum. The duodenum is distinguished by its c-loop appearance and is located in the right upper quadrant (Fig. 4-32). The c-loop surrounds the head of the pancreas. The second segment is the jejunum. The jejunum begins at the Ligament of Treitz (a ligament that secures the proximal jejunum to the posterior abdominal wall) (Fig. 4-33). The jejunum occupies a large amount of space in the left upper quadrant and left lower quadrant. The third segment is the ileum. The ileum may occupy the left lower quadrant, central, and right lower quadrants of the abdomen. The ileocecal valve is positioned in the right lower quadrant and regulates digestive contents into the cecum (Fig. 4-34).

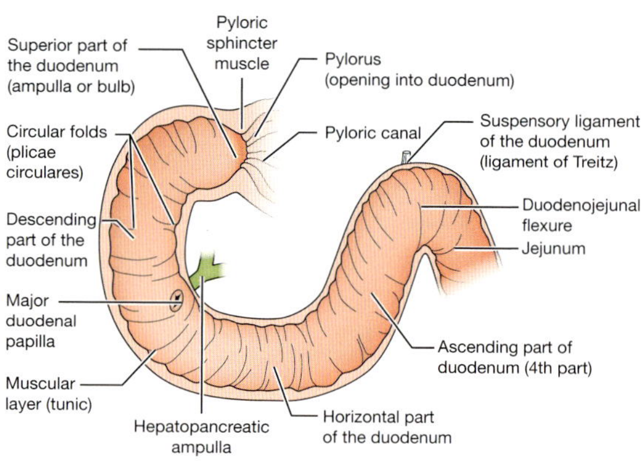

4-32 Duodenum.

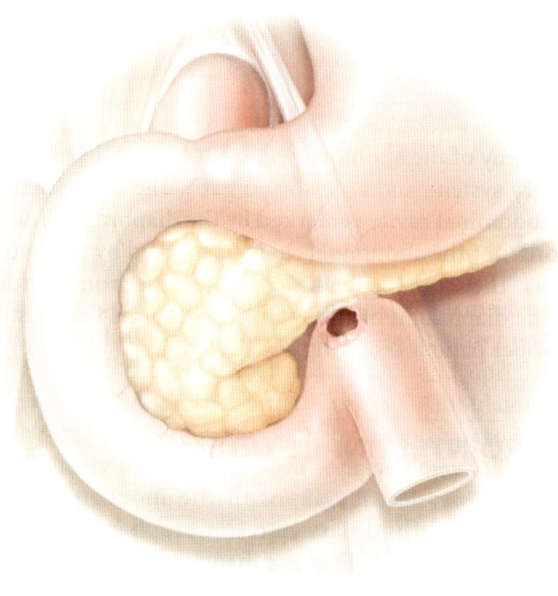

4-33 Ligament of Treitz.

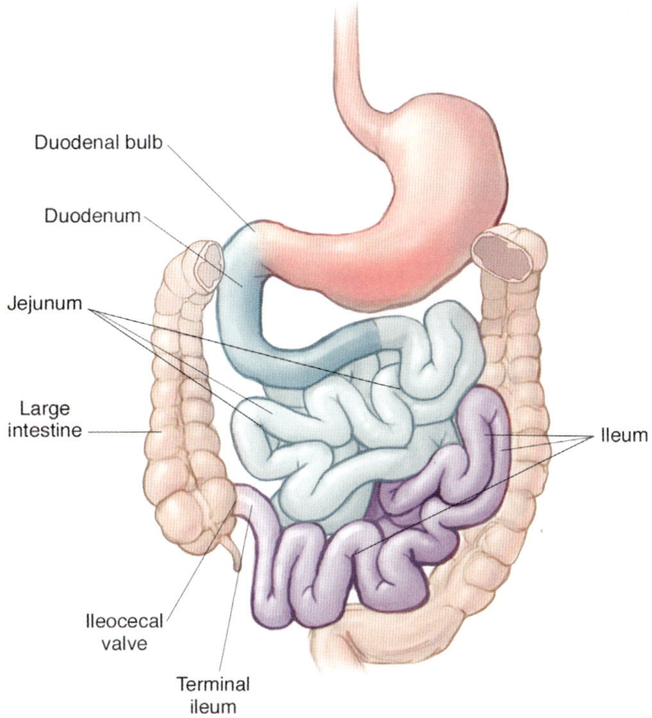

4-34 Divisions of the small bowel.

Large Intestines

The large intestine surrounds the small intestines and lies around the outside edge of the abdominal cavity. The divisions of the large intestine describe its travel path around the periphery of the small bowel. The cecum is located in the right lower quadrant and is the proximal portion of the large intestine. The appendix extends off the cecum (Fig. 4-35). The ascending colon ascends up the right side and toward the liver in the right upper quadrant. The colon will bend beneath the liver and is referenced as the right colic flexure or hepatic flexure.

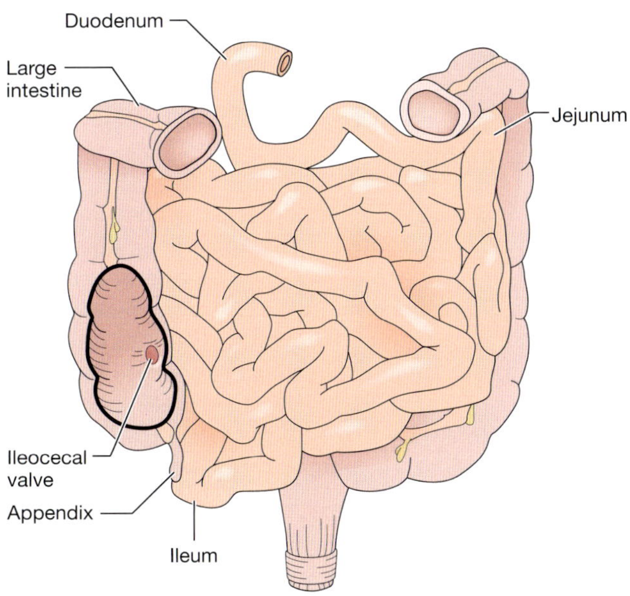

4-35 Large bowel surrounds the small bowel.

The transverse colon courses across the superior abdomen. The transverse colon will bend beneath the spleen and is referenced as the left colic flexure or splenic flexure. The descending colon descends down the left side of the abdomen toward the iliac crest. In the region of the iliac crest, the sigmoid colon courses back to midline, which contributes to its classic "S" shape. The rectum follows the curvature of the sacrum, and, finally, the large intestine terminates with the anus (Fig. 4-36).

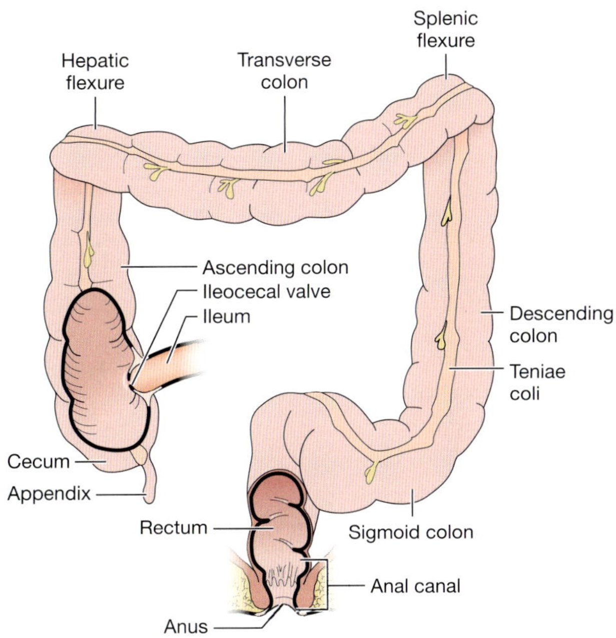

4-36 Divisions of the large bowel.

The large intestines may take on a variable position based on body habitus that should be considered by the technologist when centering. The hypersthenic patient tends to have a high and transverse stomach and a transverse colon that lies high within the abdominal cavity. The asthenic patient tends to have an elongated stomach that drops down toward the pelvis and a transverse colon that sits lower toward the pelvis (Fig. 4-37).

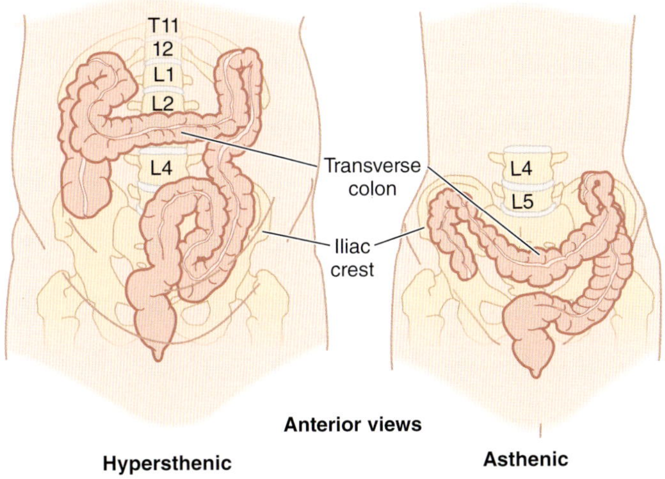

4-37 Body habitus and the effect on colon position.

ACCESSORY DIGESTIVE ORGANS

Liver

The liver is a large organ that occupies the right upper quadrant (Fig. 4-29). The liver is responsible for filtering received blood and creating bile from expiring red blood cells. The bile produced by the liver is drained by the right and left hepatic ducts, which will unite to form the common hepatic duct. The common hepatic duct will anastomose with the cystic duct (from the gallbladder) and form the common bile duct, which courses inferiorly and through the head of the pancreas (Fig. 4-38).

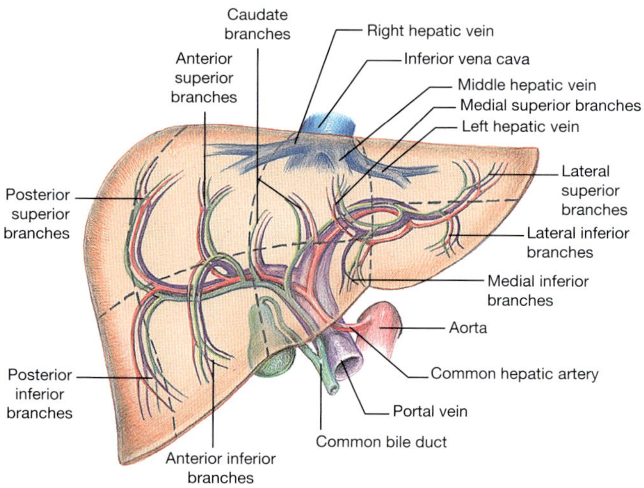

4-38 Liver. Liver segments visceral view with biliary draining areas.

Gallbladder

The gallbladder stores and concentrates bile until needed by the body. The gallbladder is located on the inferior surface of the right lobe of the liver (Fig. 4-38). The gallbladder will distend with collected bile until contraction of the gallbladder is stimulated by the release of the CCK (cholecystokinin) hormone. The concentrated bile will travel down the common bile duct and will be regulated into the c-loop of the duodenum to aid in the digestive process (Fig. 4-39). The common bile duct travels down through the head of the pancreas and anastomoses with the main pancreatic duct. The digestive enzymes are transported into the c-loop of the duodenum. The Ampulla of Vater is the opening in which the digestive enzymes enter the c-loop. Digestive enzymes are regulated through the Ampulla of Vater by the hepatopancreatic sphincter/Sphincter of Oddi.

Pancreas

The pancreas consists of a head, neck, body, and tail. The head of the pancreas is cradled into the c-loop of the duodenum. This relationship creates the reference of "romance of the abdomen" (Fig. 4-39). The pancreas functions as part of the exocrine system as it produces digestive enzymes that are transported through the main pancreatic duct. The main pancreatic duct joins the common bile duct before entering into the c-loop of the duodenum. The pancreas also functions as part of the endocrine system as it produces insulin for the body.

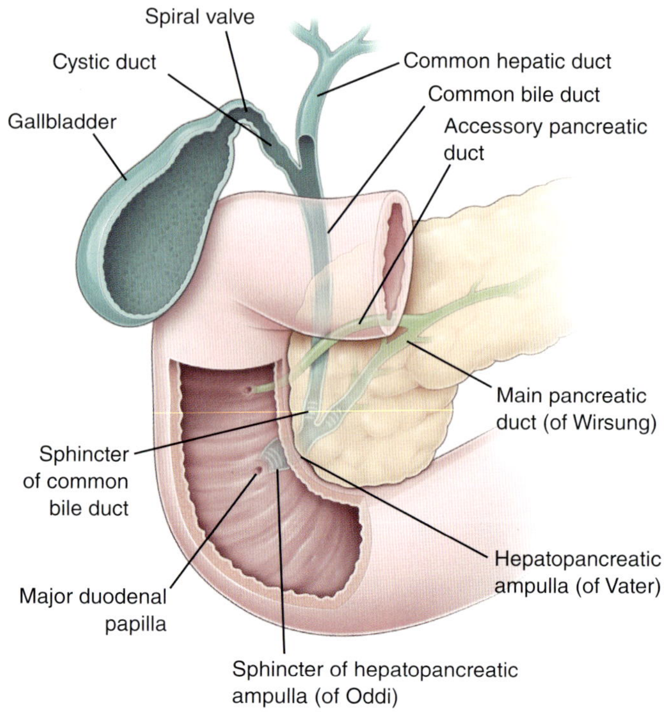

4-39 Biliary system.

LYMPHATIC SYSTEM

The spleen serves as part of the lymphatic system. It filters blood and helps the body fight infection. The spleen is not as large as the liver and sits in the left upper quadrant of the abdomen under the protection of the ribs (Fig. 4-40).

URINARY SYSTEM

The urinary system consists of two kidneys, their respective ureters, that connect to the bladder and finally the urethra. The kidneys function to filter the blood, produce urine, and help maintain blood pressure. The kidneys are typically paired and sit lateral to the lumbar vertebra (L1 and L2); with the right slightly lower than the left owing to the size of the liver in the right upper quadrant. Each ureter comes off the renal pelvis and courses inferiorly to the bladder. The ureters insert inferiorly on the bladder. The urethra will serve as the exit point from the bladder (Fig. 4-41).

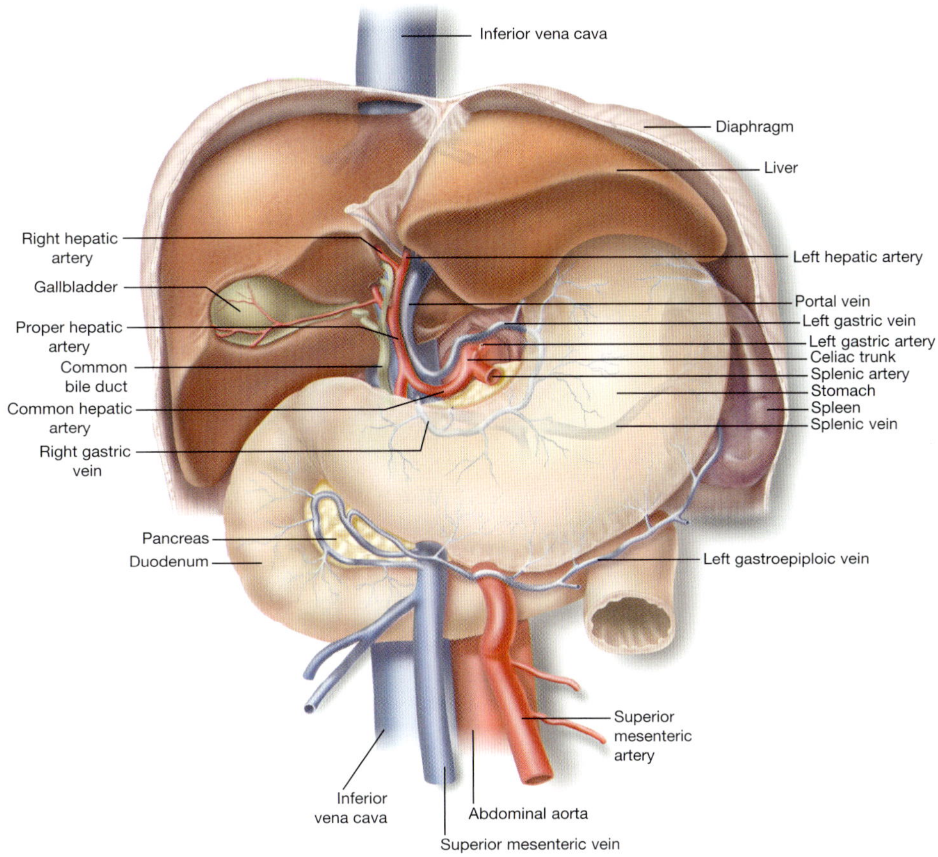

4-40 Organ relationships of the liver, duodenum, pancreas, kidneys, and spleen in the RUQ and LUQ.

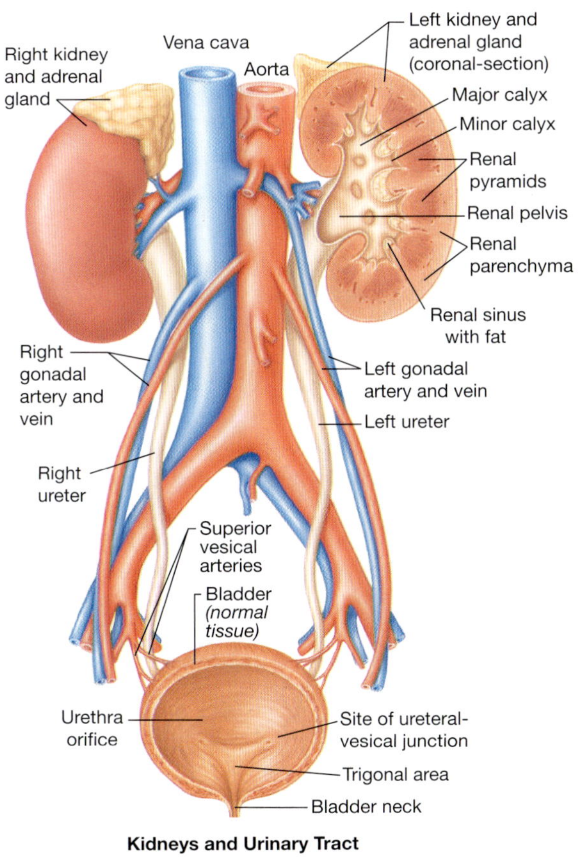

4-41 Urinary system.

ABDOMINAL CAVITY

The abdominal cavity is lined with a double-walled sac referenced as the peritoneum. The outermost wall is the parietal peritoneum as it lines the inside of the abdominal wall. The innermost wall is called the visceral peritoneum as it covers the surfaces of some organs. The potential space created in between the two walls contains a small amount of serous fluid and is known as the peritoneal cavity (Fig. 4-42). The serous fluid within the peritoneal space allows the surfaces of structures to move against each other. Abdominal structures will be categorized as intraperitoneal (within the peritoneal cavity), retroperitoneal (posterior to the peritoneal cavity), and infraperitoneal (below the peritoneal cavity) (Fig. 4-43 and Table 4-2).

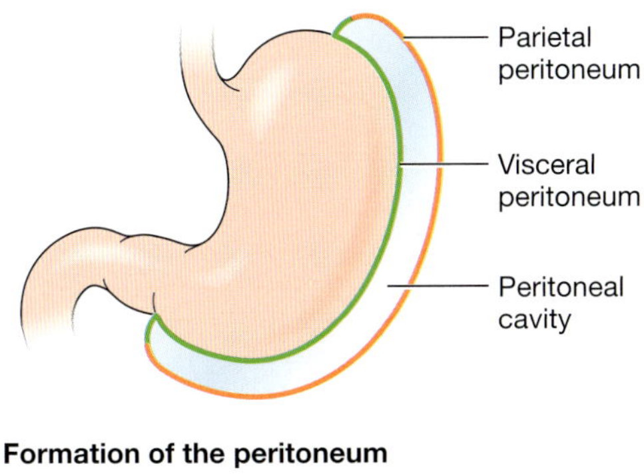

4-42 Visceral peritoneum, parietal peritoneum, and peritoneal cavity.

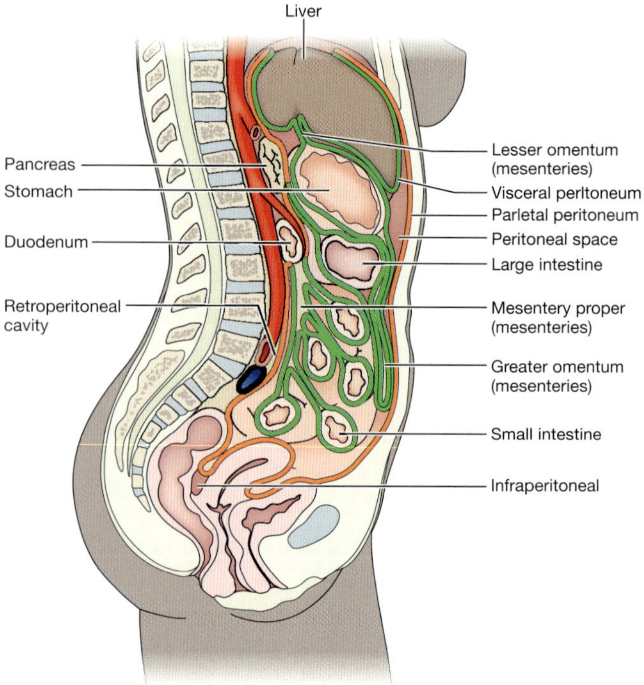

4-43 Retroperitoneal, Intraperitoneal, and Infraperitoneal locations.

4-2 Organ Placement in Abdominal Cavities

Intraperitoneal Organs	Retroperitoneal Organs	Infraperitoneal Organs
All organs are covered by visceral peritoneum	**Organs sit behind the parietal peritoneum and in front of the posterior abdominal wall**	**Organs sit below the peritoneal cavity and down in the pelvic cavity**
Stomach	Kidneys	Urinary bladder
Jejunum	Adrenal glands	Rectum
Ileum	Ureters	Reproductive organs
Cecum	Duodenum	
Transverse colon	Ascending colon	
Sigmoid colon	Descending colon	
Liver	Aorta	
Spleen	Inferior vena cava	
Gallbladder	Pancreas	

The folding of the peritoneum provides support to structures. Different parts of the peritoneum connect organs to other organs or to the abdominal wall. Peritoneum will fold back upon itself, creating a double-fold, which extends from one point to another. *Mesentery*, is a double-fold of peritoneum that completely encases a section of small bowel and anchors it to the posterior abdominal wall. *Omentum*, also a double-fold of peritoneum, extends off the stomach and connects to another structure. The lesser omentum connects the lesser curvature of the stomach to the liver. The greater omentum descends in the abdomen from the greater curvature of the stomach and folds back up to connect at the transverse colon; it resembles a waist-like apron (Fig. 4-44). *Mesocolon* is a double-fold of the peritoneum that encases a segment of the colon and anchors it to the posterior abdominal wall. There are four different segments of mesocolon, referenced by which colon section is encased: ascending, transverse, descending, or sigmoid (Fig. 4-45).

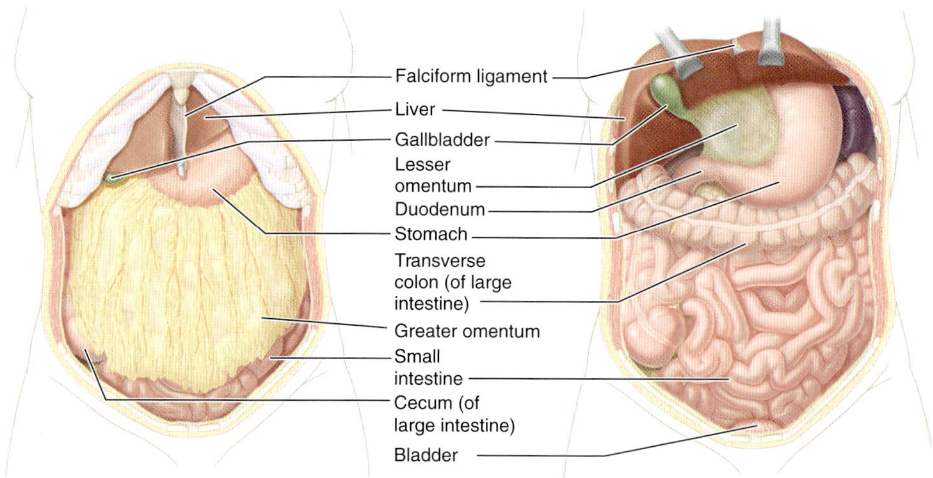

4-44 Omentum.

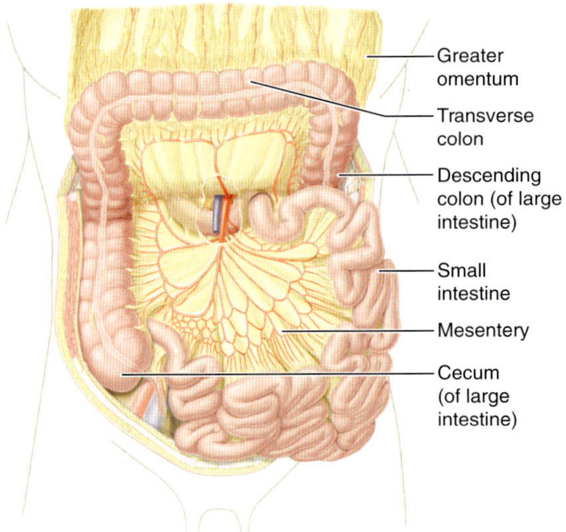

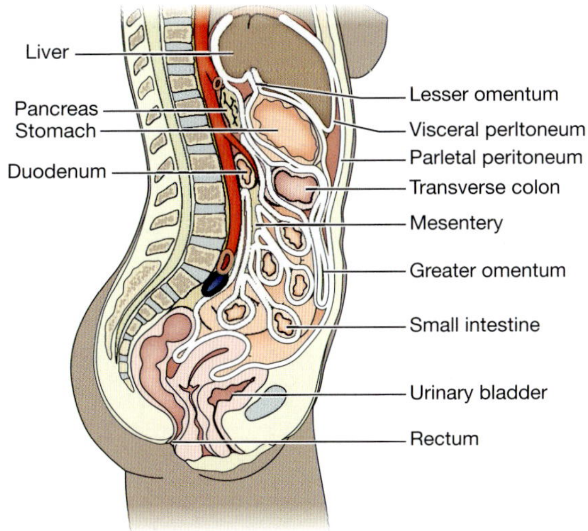

4-45 Mesentery and mesocolon.

KEY SUMMATION POINTS OF ANATOMY

- Pharynx serves as part of the respiratory system and digestive system.
- Stomach contents that are exposed to gastric juices and churning create a substance called chyme.
- The c-loop of the duodenum cradles the head of the pancreas.
- The Ampulla of Vater is the opening into the c-loop of the duodenum. The Hepatopancreatic Ampulla or the Ampulla of Vater is surrounded by the Sphincter of Oddi that regulates the release of biliary enzymes into the small intestines.
- The Ligament of Treitz secures the proximal jejunum to the posterior abdominal wall, creating the most secure portion of the small intestines.
- The ileum terminates in the right lower quadrant and into the cecum.
- The digestive contents of the small bowel are regulated into the large bowel through the ileocecal valve.
- The small intestine is more central in location, while the large intestine is located around its outside edge.
- The double-walled membrane, known as the peritoneum, in the abdomen will create spaces such as intraperitoneal, retroperitoneal, and infraperitoneal, which each contain different abdominal structures.
- Omentum is a double-fold of peritoneum that connects a side of the stomach to another structure. Lesser omentum is the peritoneum extending from the lesser curvature of the stomach to the liver. Greater omentum is the peritoneum that extends down like an apron from the greater curvature of the stomach to the lower abdomen and wraps back up to connect to the transverse colon.
- Mesentery is a double-fold of peritoneum that encases small bowel and anchors it to the posterior abdominal wall.
- Mesocolon is a double-fold of the peritoneum that encases segments of the colon and anchors it to the posterior abdominal wall.
- Location of key anatomy into four Abdominal Quadrants (Table 4-3 and Fig. 4-46).

4-3 Organ Placement in the Four Abdominal Quadrants

RUQ	LUQ	RLQ	LLQ
Liver	Spleen	Cecum	Portion of descending colon
Gallbladder	Stomach	Appendix	Sigmoid colon
Duodenum	Jejunum	Terminal ileum	
Head of pancreas	Left colic flexure	Ileocecal valve	
Right colic flexure	Left Kidney	Portion of ascending colon	
Right Kidney	Tail of Pancreas		

(*continued*)

KEY SUMMATION POINTS OF ANATOMY (*Continued*)

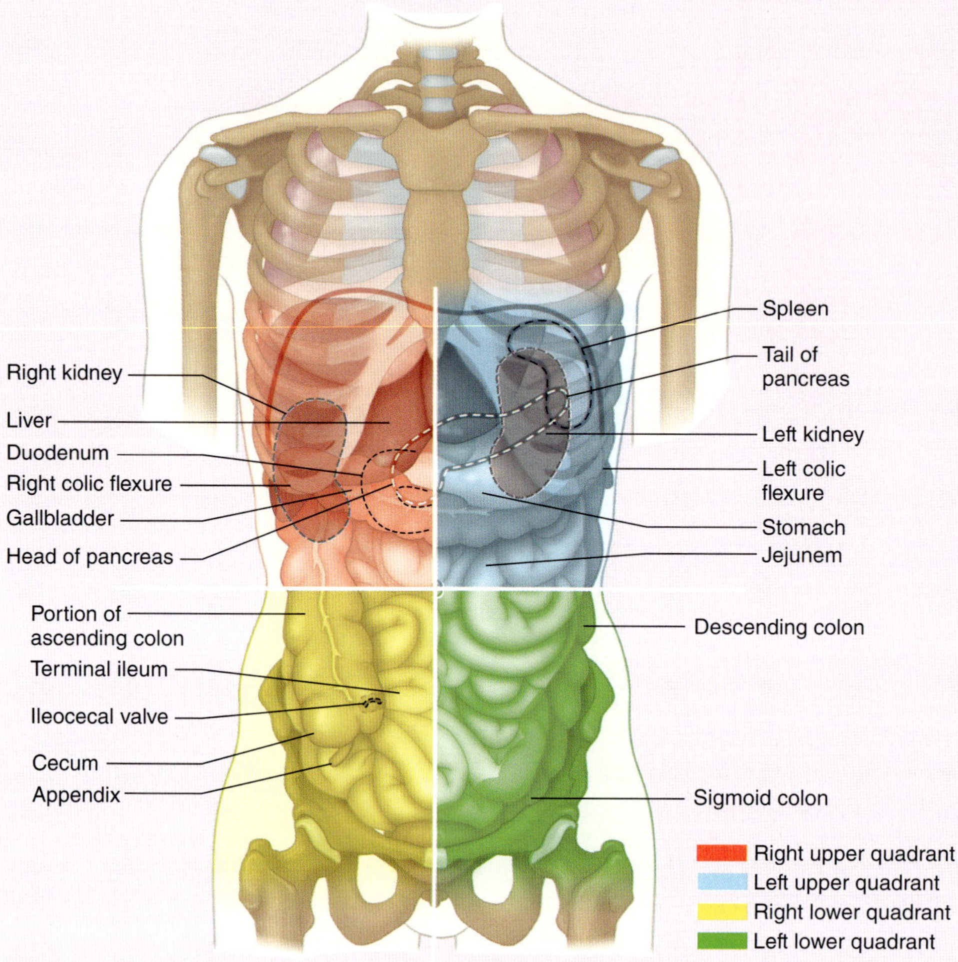

4-46 Abdominal quadrants.

POSITIONING AND TECHNICAL CONSIDERATIONS

Body Habitus and Suggested Image Receptor Orientation

In consideration of different body types among the population, there are three general types to accommodate in abdominal imaging.

Sthenic Patient: This patient represents the most average size dimension in the population. Patient is of modest height and weight. Abdominal organs are located in their predictable quadrants. Lengthwise image receptor orientation will be suitable for the patient's anatomy (Fig. 4-47).

Hypersthenic Patient: This patient is broad through the chest and abdomen. The stomach typically sits high and underneath the diaphragm in a transverse orientation. The large intestines are found at the periphery of the abdomen. To adequately image the entire abdomen, two 14 × 17 crosswise (CW) images set to overlap are recommended (Fig. 4-48).

Asthenic/Hyposthenic Patient: This patient is long and lean through the thorax and abdomen. Abdominal structures tend to sit lower in the abdomen and extend down into the pelvis. Lengthwise image receptor orientation will be the best fit for the patient. Certain patients may need two images set to overlap to include all necessary anatomy.

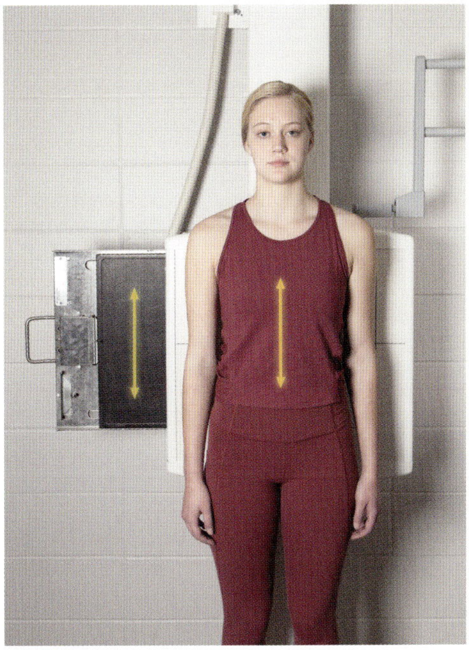

4-47 Lengthwise IR orientation.

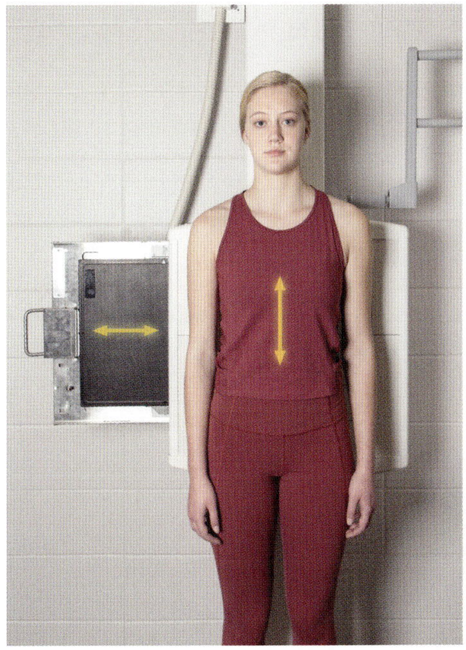

4-48 Crosswise IR orientation.

Centering for Abdomen

When imaging the abdomen, the centering will be set to include the symphysis pubis or the diaphragm. Centering will also be influenced by differing body habitus types while taking into consideration the anatomy that needs to be included on the exposure. The central ray for the supine abdomen on a sthenic patient will be directed to the level of the iliac crest (L4–L5) to ensure the symphysis pubis is included on the image.

The central ray for the upright abdomen on the sthenic patient will be directed 2" superior to the iliac crest to ensure the diaphragm is included on the image. In the case of hypersthenic patients, and sometimes asthenic/hyposthenic patients, two crosswise (CW) images may be necessary to include the essential anatomy. The images should include 1"–2" of overlapping anatomy. When imaging the *supine abdomen* with two crosswise image receptors, it is advisable to position the bottom of the first image receptor even with the symphysis pubis (required anatomy) and then overlap the second image receptor with the first image receptor to include the kidneys. When imaging the *upright abdomen* with two crosswise image receptors, it is advisable that the top of the first image receptor be positioned at the level of the axilla (ensures diaphragm is included) and that the second image receptor overlap to include the lower abdomen and, quite possibly, include the symphysis pubis.

With extreme patient variables for abdominal images, such as pediatrics, it is important to center according to topographic landmarks to allow for proper collimation of the exposure field (Fig. 4.49). With extreme patient variables such as bariatric patients, it is important to center according to landmarks and use overlapping high and low techniques or four-quadrant imaging to ensure the lateralmost borders of the abdomen are included. When centering on any type of patient, the technologist will have to palpate the patient to locate the bony landmarks. It is important that the technologist inform the patient of necessary palpation.

KEY ANATOMIC LANDMARKS (FIG. 4-49)

- Xiphoid tip corresponds to thoracic vertebral level of T9–T10.
- Iliac crest corresponds to lumbar vertebral level of L4–L5.
- Jugular notch, xiphoid tip, and spine would all be landmarks for midsagittal plane (MSP).
- Symphysis pubis
- Greater trochanter may serve as an alternative landmark for the symphysis pubis.

(continued)

KEY SUMMATION POINTS OF ANATOMY (*Continued*)

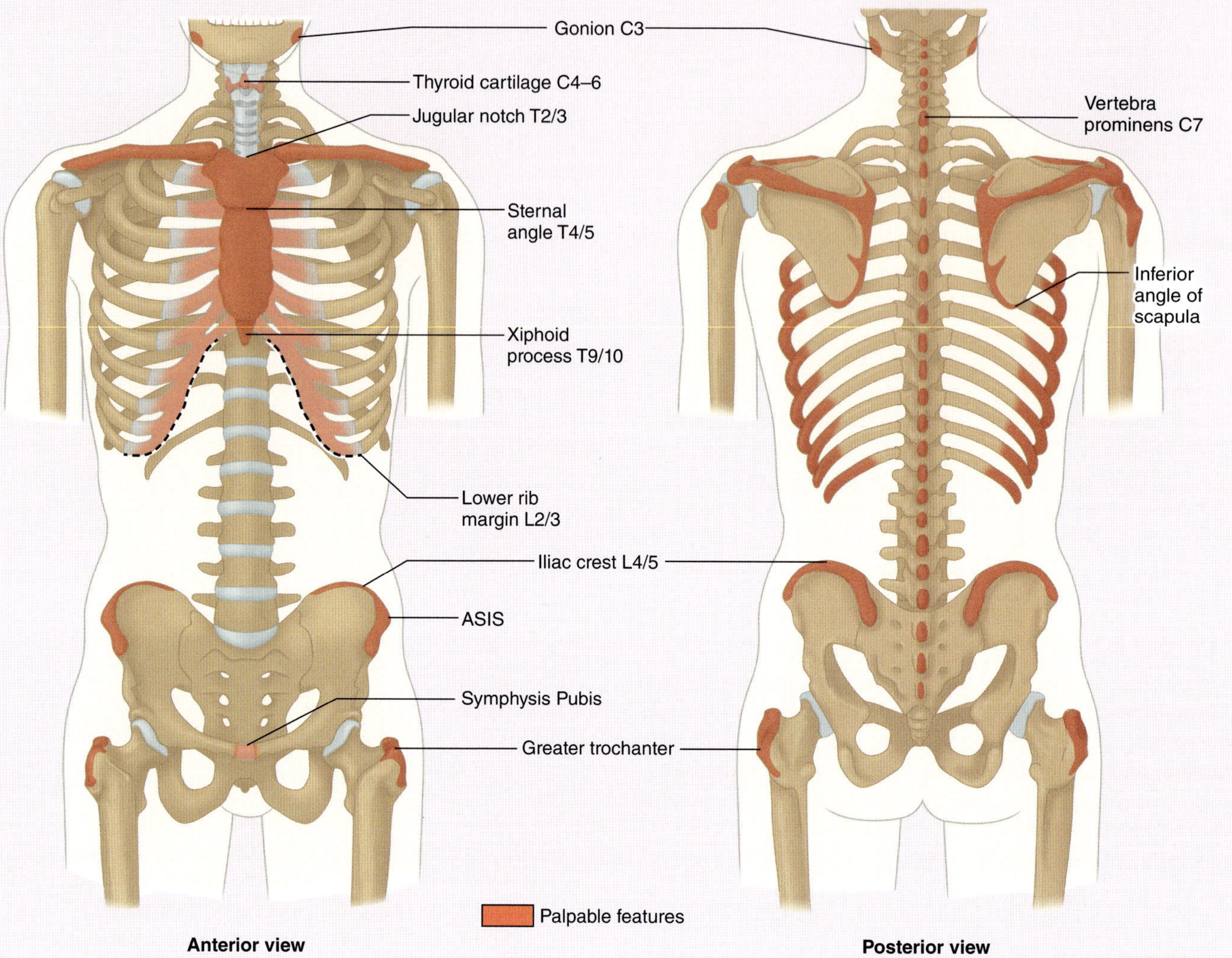

4-49 Topographical landmarks.

Breathing Instructions for Abdomen

It is recommended that the image exposure for the abdomen be made after the patient exhales. With expiration, the diaphragm moves up or ascends to its most superior point and avoids compression of abdominal structures. To avoid voluntary patient motion (patient can control), the technologist should give breathing instructions and wait to administer the technical exposure until the patient suspends breathing.

TECHNICAL CONSIDERATIONS

Setting a Manual Technique

Manual technique is defined when the radiographer sets the kVp and mAs values independently. A manual technique can be set in the department and as well on a mobile imaging unit.

Kilovoltage is set to penetrate the part thickness and affects the scale of contrast seen on the image. A mid-level kVp, 70–85 is used for abdominal imaging. Visualization of the outline of the psoas muscles and abdominal organs such as the kidneys and liver, will aid in determination if an appropriate contrast scale has been achieved for the abdomen. The determination of mAs would be influenced by part size, considering the amount of abdominal tissue. In situations of known potential additive pathologies (ascites) or destructive pathologies (ileus), a manual technique will allow appropriate modifications of kVp and/or mAs levels.

Setting a manual technique will also allow the technologist to adjust the length of the exposure (something important to consider with pediatric and geriatric patients), but also reduces the chances of involuntary motion (patient cannot control) such as bowel peristalsis. In cases where motion can be detrimental to image quality, the technologist can increase the mA station, thus allowing the exposure time to be decreased to minimize the chance of motion.

Setting Technique With Automatic Exposure Control

Automatic Exposure Control (AEC) may be an option in the imaging department. With AEC, the technologist will set the kVp value, will not set a mAs, but rather must select which exposure cell(s) correspond to the anatomy centered and anatomy coverage over the cell(s) according to the projection. The cell(s) will determine when adequate exposure has been reached according to the part thickness and composition, and then the exposure is terminated. After the exposure terminates, the radiographer can see the mAs value displayed on the control panel. When imaging the abdomen, the center cell must be selected along with one or both outer cells (Figs. 4-50 and 4-51).

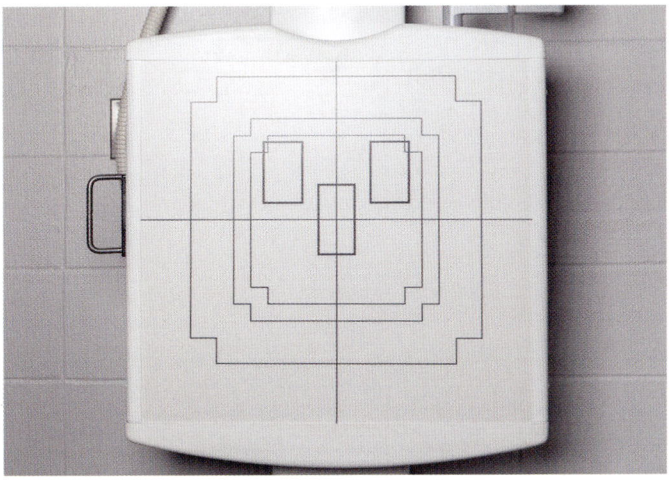

4-50 Upright Bucky to display placement of ionization chambers.

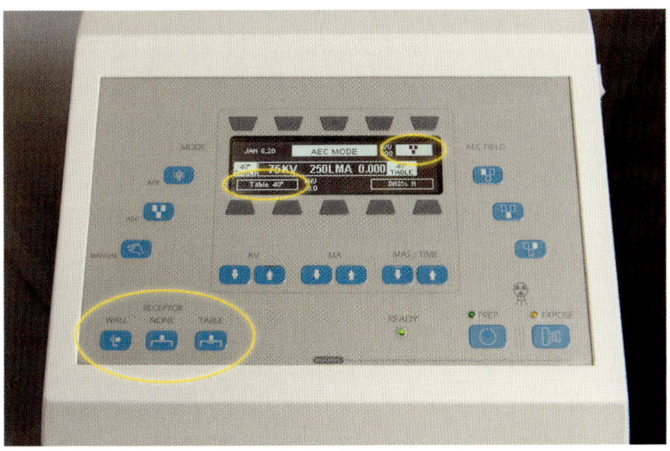

4-51 Setting the AEC for an abdomen.

Source-to-Image Distance

40" source-to-image distance (SID) is employed for all abdominal images.

Marking the Image

At minimum, when marking abdominal images, the right or left anatomic side lead marker should be placed down low and lateral in the region of the hip (Fig. 4-52). This placement ensures the marker is not placed in the region of the diaphragm, bowel, abdominal tissue, or kidney. Arrows may also be used to delineate upright images. Anatomic markers with the lead BB's will gravitate to signify an upright position.

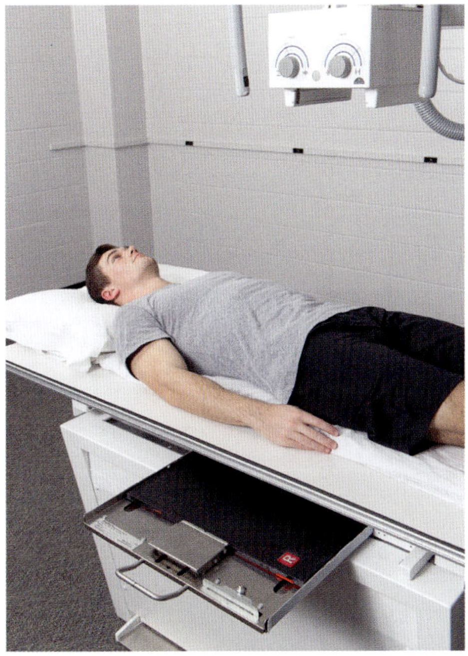

4-52 Suggested anatomic marker placement for supine abdomen.

Viewing the Image

Assuming the abdomen image was correctly marked, the image is displayed opposite the viewer facing it, as though the image is in anatomical position (Figs. 4-53 and 4-54).

PROTOCOL CONSIDERATIONS FOR ABDOMEN

Single-View Abdomen

The single view is acquired with the patient supine and includes abdominal anatomy of kidneys down to the entire bladder (KUB). The outline of both kidneys and the superior margin of the symphysis pubis should be included on one lengthwise image or between two crosswise images.

Two-View Abdomen

The two views will include a supine abdomen (KUB) and an upright abdomen. The supine image should display the

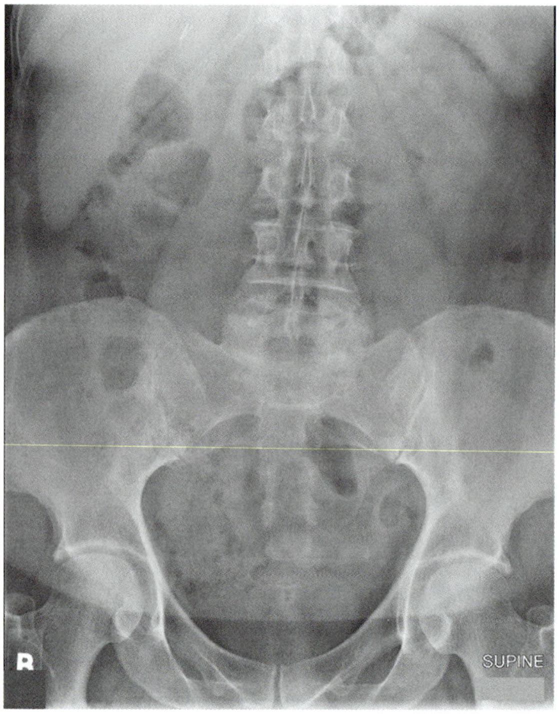

4-53 Correct display of supine abdomen.

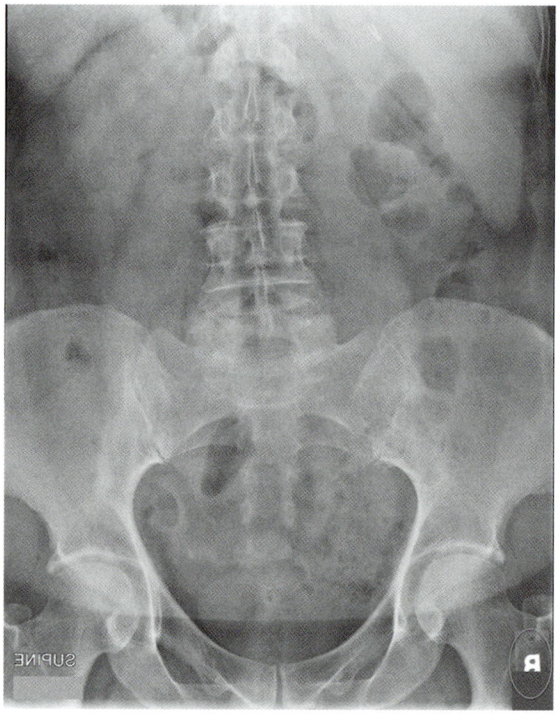

4-54 Incorrect display of supine abdomen.

outline of both kidneys superiorly and include the superior margin of the symphysis pubis. The upright image is centered superior to the iliac crest to allow for inclusion of the entire diaphragm. In cases of a suspected pneumoperitoneum, the free air will rise up and collect beneath the diaphragm. If the patient is ambulatory or has been transported by wheelchair, the upright image should be acquired before the supine abdomen. In cases of an ambulatory or wheelchair patient, consider the patient has been in an upright position for a minimum of 5 minutes and likely longer, and, therefore, a pneumoperitoneum may be revealed. For a patient unable to stand or sit for the upright abdomen, an left lateral decubitus is the substitute position.

Acute Abdominal Series

Three views will be acquired to include a PA chest along with two views of the abdomen. The contrast scale created on the chest image will allow demonstration of a potential pneumoperitoneum beneath the diaphragm. If the patient is ambulatory or has been transported by wheelchair, the PA chest should be acquired first at 72" SID, then the upright abdomen at 40" SID, and, finally, the supine abdomen.

Ambulatory Acute Abdominal Series—PA Chest

- Projection: PA

Ambulatory Acute Abdominal Series Protocol
PA Chest
Upright Abdomen
Supine Abdomen

Technical Considerations
- kVp 110–130
- Two outermost AEC cells selected for upright Bucky
- 72" SID

Exposure Field Size
- 14 × 17 lengthwise for sthenic to asthenic patient
- 14 × 17 crosswise for hypersthenic patient
- 17 × 17 available with same systems

Patient Position (Figs. 4-55 and 4-56)
- Erect and facing upright Bucky
- Shoulders relaxed. Chin elevated
- Arms wrapped around board rolling shoulders and scapulae forward

Centering
- Level of T7/8 and with MSP

Marking of IR
- Anatomic side right or left marker up above corresponding shoulder

Breathing
- Double inspiration and hold after second inspiration
- Ensure you watch the patient the entire time while breathing them and walking away to make the exposure

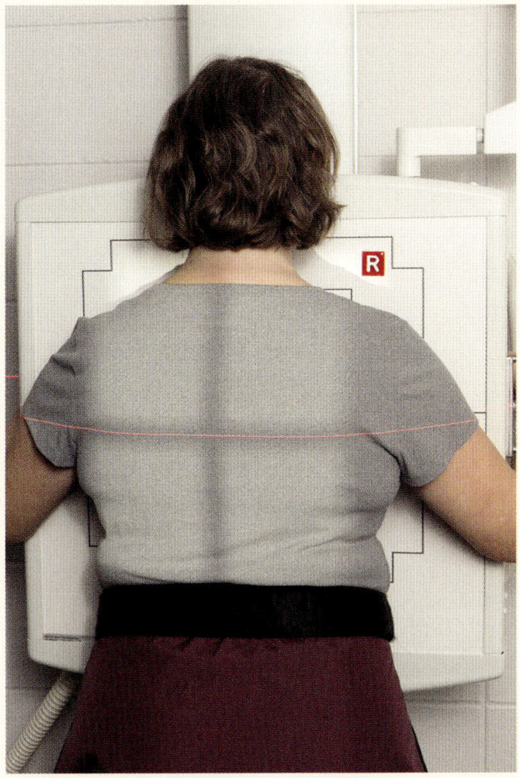

4-55 PA sthenic chest.

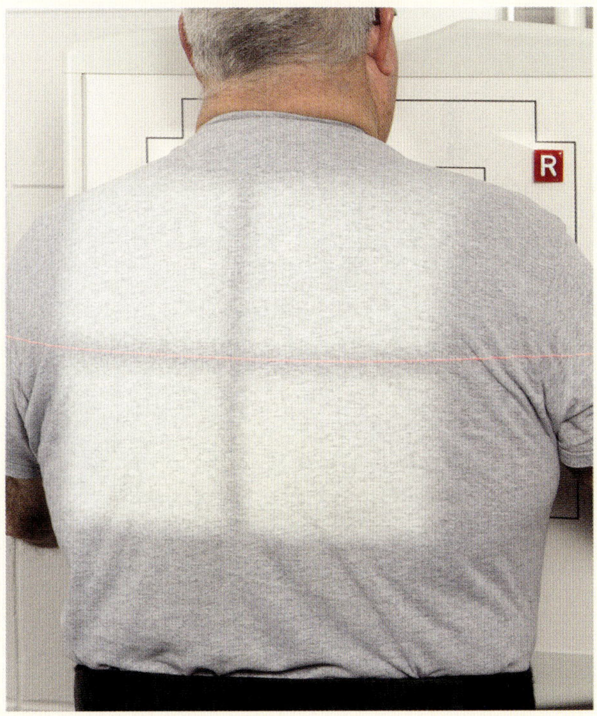

4-56 PA hypersthenic chest.

IMAGE CRITIQUE (FIG. 4-57)

- Entire lung fields revealing apices, bases, costophrenic angles, and lateral lung margin
- Properly centered to ensure inclusion of all essential anatomy
- 10–11 ribs above the diaphragm counted on the right side of thorax
- Clavicles near horizontal. This indicates that the shoulders were relaxed
- Scapulae removed from the lung field. This indicates that the shoulders were rolled forward
- SC joints symmetrical. This indicates that the patient was not rotated; shoulders were equal distance to the image receptor

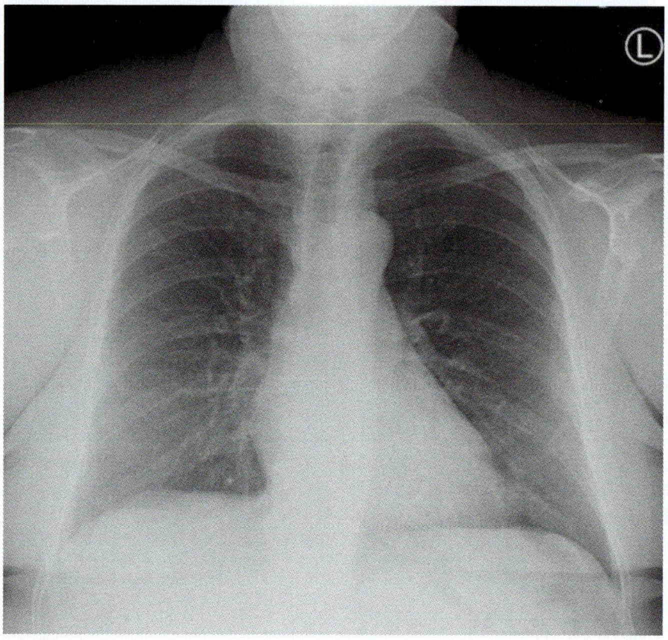

4-57 PA chest. Image may reveal a pneumoperitoneum beneath the diaphragm.

Ambulatory Acute Abdominal Series—Upright Abdomen

- Projection: AP

Ambulatory Acute Abdominal Series Protocol
PA Chest
Upright Abdomen
Supine Abdomen

Technical Considerations
- kVp 75–85
- All three AEC cells selected for upright Bucky
- 40" SID

Exposure Field Size
- One 14 × 17 lengthwise for sthenic patient
- Two 14 × 17 crosswise for hypersthenic patient

Patient Position
- Erect with patient's back to the upright Bucky (image should be taken before or after PA chest. The patient's upright position will allow time for a potential pneumoperitoneum to collect beneath the diaphragm.)
- Arms slightly abducted from patient's sides

Centering (Figs. 4-58 to 4-60)
- When the tube is directed toward the upright Bucky, the central ray will align horizontally with the floor and intersect the IR perpendicularly; essential to demonstrate an air–fluid level. Use of a true horizontal beam is necessary to reveal an air–fluid level, even in cases where the patient may be able to attain only a semierect position
- 2" superior to the iliac crest and to MSP (it is essential that both hemidiaphragms are included)
- Centering for hypersthenic patient will require (2-CW images) a high and low image working down from the diaphragm to include the lower abdominal region
- Method of acquiring two 14 × 17 CW images of the upright abdomen. The technologist will place the top of the first 14 × 17 CW even with the level of the axilla and MSP to ensure the diaphragm is included. For the second 14 × 17 CW image, the technologist will mark the bottom 1½"–2" of the first light field, and place the top of the second CW IR to overlap with the first light field to include down to the lower abdominal region
- *Some radiologists may prefer the upright abdomen to include all anatomy between the diaphragm and the symphysis pubis, for which a high and low image will need to be acquired or an alteration of increased SID*

Marking of IR
- Anatomic side marker R or L down in the lowest corner margin of the IR
- An upright arrow could also be considered. Lead markers that possess the lead BB's will indicate the upright position as they will settle to the bottom of the "circle" on the marker

Breathing
- The patient is instructed to take in a breath, exhale, and hold their breath out
- The image is acquired after expiration

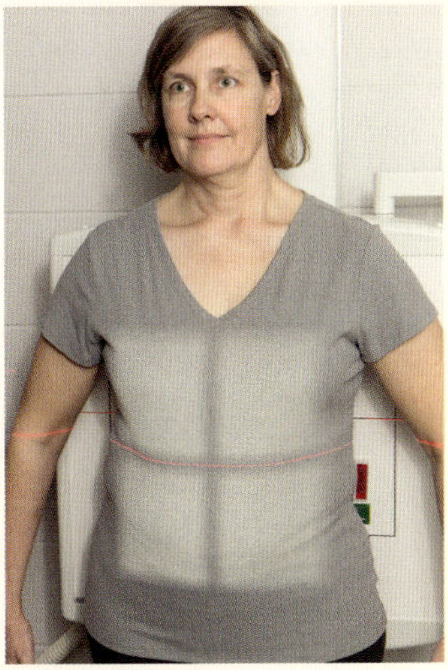

4-58 Upright sthenic abdomen.

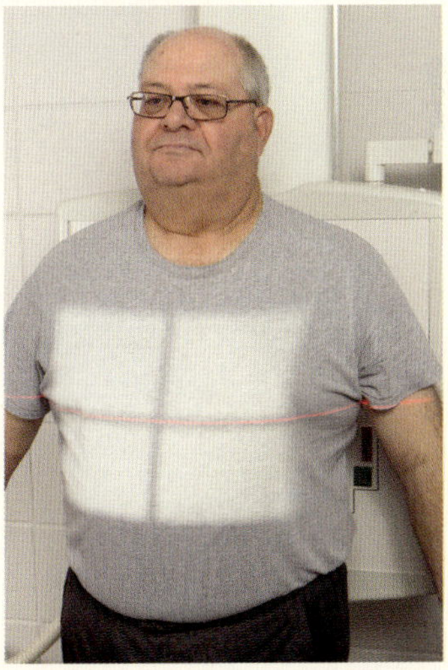

4-59 Upright hypersthenic abdomen with high crosswise IR.

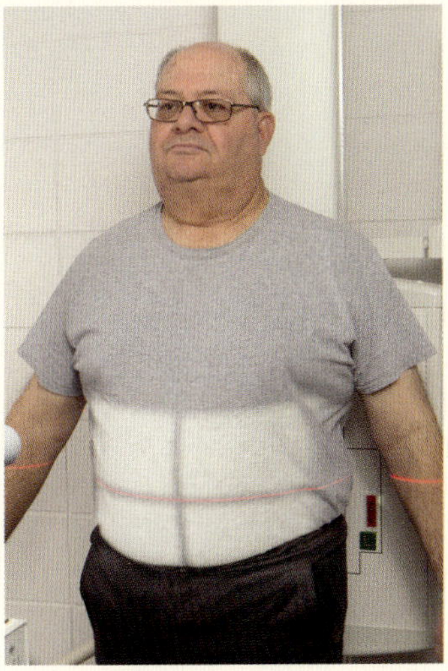

4-60 Upright hypersthenic abdomen with low crosswise IR.

IMAGE CRITIQUE (FIGS. 4-61 to 4-63)

- Both hemidiaphragms and down to the midpelvic region included. The diaphragm will mark the highest point of the abdominal cavity. When the patient is upright, a potential pneumoperitoneum will rise up to the highest point of the abdominal cavity
- Symmetry of the vertebral column and iliac wings. This ensures no rotation of the part
- Properly centered to ensure inclusion of all essential anatomy
- Air may be seen within superior portions/loops of bowel as the air is rising to the highest point within each loop
- Air may be seen within the gastric fundus

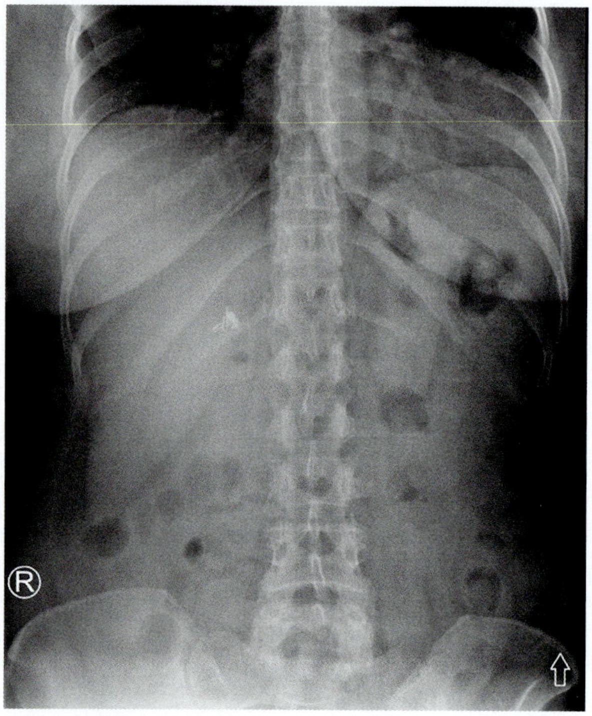

4-61 Upright abdomen.

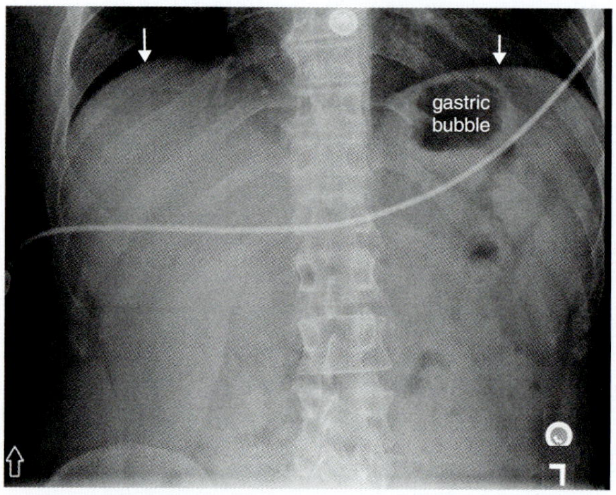

4-62 Upright abdomen with high crosswise IR.

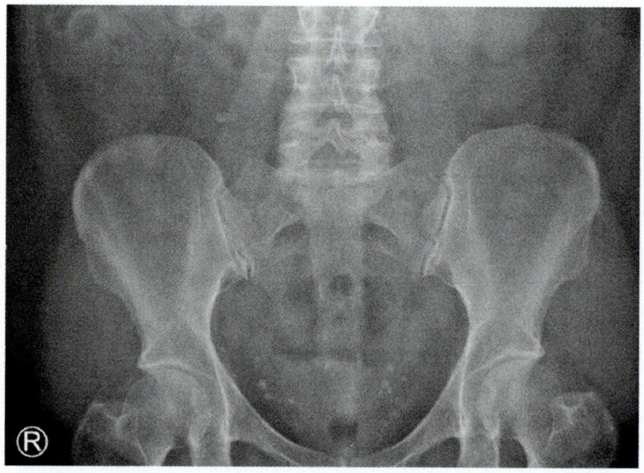

4-63 Overlap low crosswise IR.

Ambulatory Acute Abdominal Series—Supine Abdomen (KUB)

- Projection: AP

Ambulatory Acute Abdominal Series Protocol
PA Chest
Upright Abdomen
Supine Abdomen

Technical Considerations
- kVp 70–85
- All three AEC cells selected for table Bucky
- 40" SID

Exposure Field Size
- One 14 × 17 lengthwise for sthenic patient
- Two 14 × 17 crosswise for hypersthenic patient

Patient Position
- Supine support could be provided under the patient's knees and patient covered with a blanket
- Arms slightly abducted from patient's sides

Centering (Figs. 4-64 to 4-66)
- Level of the iliac crest and to MSP (it is essential that the symphysis pubis be included)
- Crosswise imaging required for a hypersthenic patient will require a low and high image to be acquired to include the majority of the abdomen working up from the symphysis pubis. The first image would include the symphysis pubis and lower abdomen. The second overlapped higher image would include the kidneys
- Method of acquiring two 14 × 17 CW images of the supine abdomen. The technologist will place the bottom of the first 14 × 17 CW even with the level of the symphysis pubis and MSP. For the second 14 × 17 CW image, the technologist will mark the top 1½"–2" of the first light field and then place the bottom of the second CW IR to overlap with the first light field
- Some radiologists may prefer the KUB to include all anatomy between the diaphragm and the symphysis pubis, which will require a low and high image to be acquired
- In cases of a bariatric patient, the technologist may take four images, one to represent each abdominal quadrant

Marking of IR
- Anatomic side marker R or L down in the lowest corner margin of the IR (down in the area of the greater trochanter)

Breathing
- The patient is instructed to take in a breath, exhale, and hold their breath out
- The image is acquired after expiration

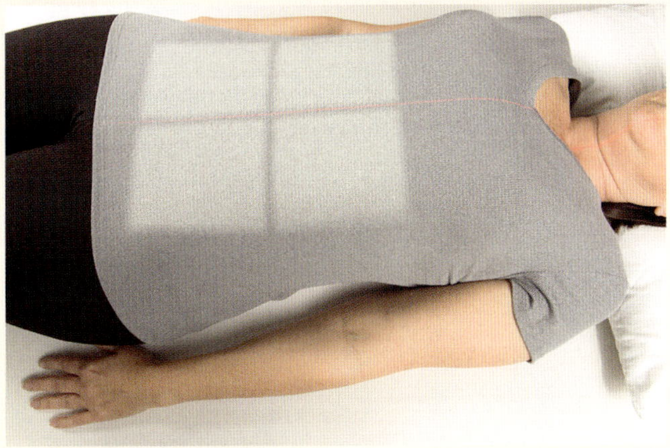

4-64 Supine abdomen position.

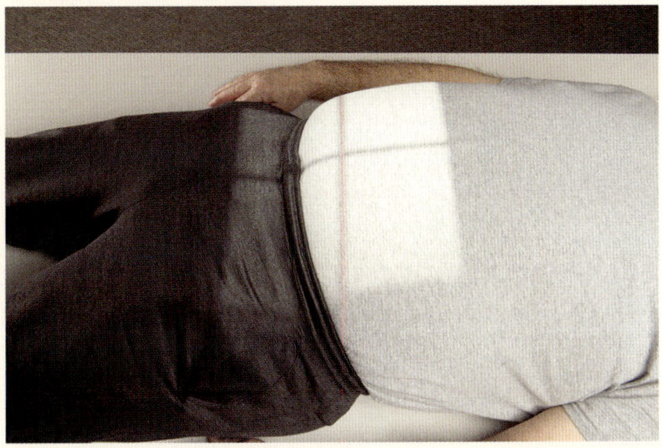

4-65 Supine low CW IR abdomen.

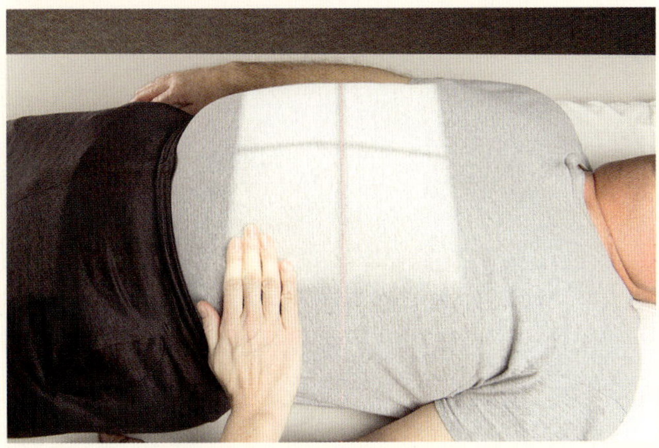

4-66 Supine high CW IR abdomen.

IMAGE CRITIQUE (FIGS. 4-67 to 4-69)

- Symphysis pubis must be included. Inclusion of the symphysis ensures the bladder was included on the image
- Outline of the kidneys included, which could potentially reveal the presence of renal calculi
- Bowel pattern can be observed
- Symmetry of the vertebral column and iliac wings. This ensures no rotation of the part
- Properly centered for inclusion of all essential anatomy

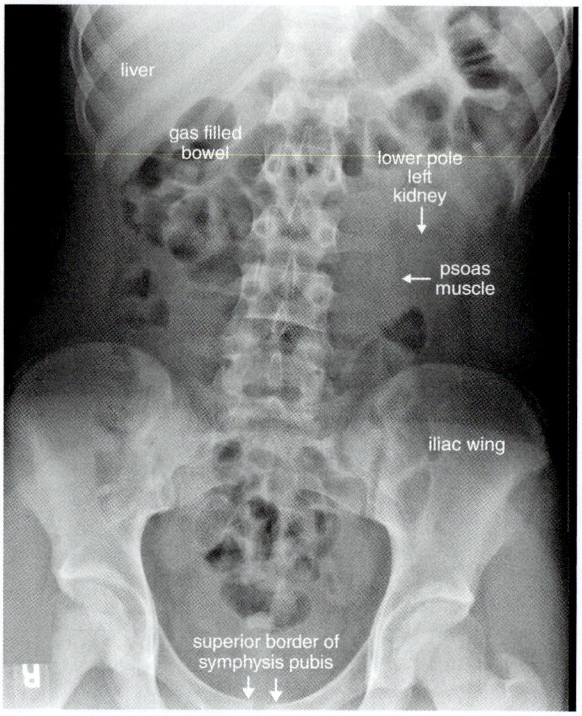

4-67 Supine abdomen.

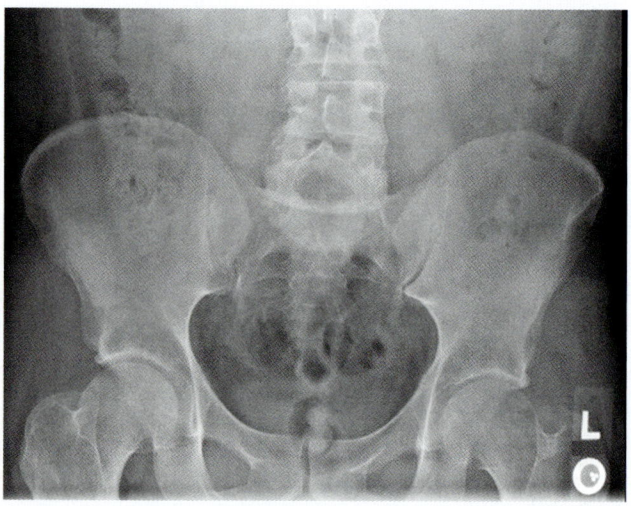

4-68 Supine low crosswise abdomen.

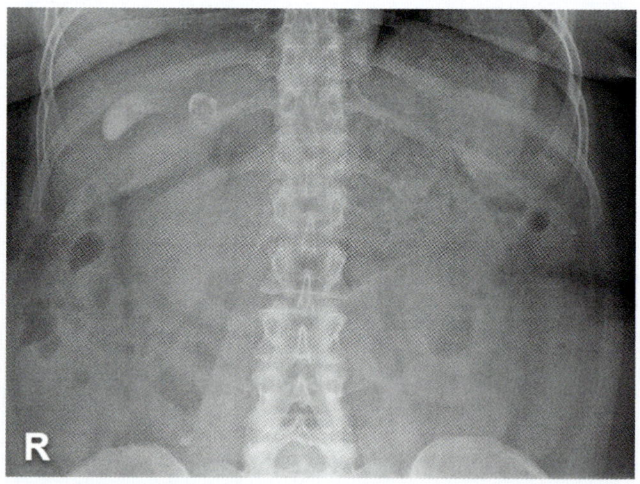

4-69 Supine high crosswise abdomen.

Nonambulatory Acute Abdominal Series—Left Lateral Decubitus Abdomen

- Projection: AP (most preferred if kidneys are of interest)

Nonambulatory Acute Abdominal Series Protocol
AP/PA Chest
Supine Abdomen
LLD Abdomen

Technical Considerations
- kVp 75–85
- mAs manually set
- Grid
- 40" SID

Exposure Field Size
- One 14 × 17 lengthwise for sthenic patient
- Two 14 × 17 crosswise for hypersthenic patient

Patient Position
- Patients should be positioned in LLD position for a minimum of 5 minutes to allow air or fluid to develop the air/fluid line. It is recommended that the patient remain in the LLD position longer than the minimum 5 minutes when a small pneumoperitoneum is of concern. It may take longer for a small pneumoperitoneum to work around the loops of bowel to present itself on the upside. The LLD is implemented on the abdomen to keep the gastric bubble more to the patient's left and away from the potential upside (right side of patient) where the potential pneumoperitoneum will display
- Consider building patient up off table to allow the IR to drop below the level of the downside of the patient. This will be helpful to image entire abdominal cavity. The patient could also be imaged at the upright Bucky
- Raise arms above head to prevent superimposition on the lung field
- Patient looks straight ahead with chin slightly elevated

Centering (Figs. 4-70 to 4-73)
- 2" superior to the iliac crest and to MSP (it is essential that both hemidiaphragms are included)
- When the tube is directed toward the IR, the central ray will align horizontally with the floor and intersect the IR perpendicularly; essential to demonstrate an air–fluid level
- Crosswise imaging required for a hypersthenic patient will require a high and low image to be acquired to include the lower abdominal region
- Method of acquiring two 14 × 17 CW images of the decubitus abdomen. The technologist will place the top of the first 14 × 17 CW even with the level of the axilla and MSP. For the second 14 × 17 CW image, the technologist will mark the bottom 1½"–2" of the first light field and then place the top of the second CW IR to overlap with the first light field. If the overlap method is necessary, this method mirrors that used for the upright abdomen on the hypersthenic patient

Marking of IR
- Anatomic right side marker placed in the lowest corner margin of the IR in the region of the upside hip
- A "side up" marker or upright arrow should also be considered to indicate this special position

Breathing
- The patient is instructed to take in a breath, exhale, and hold their breath out
- The image is acquired after expiration

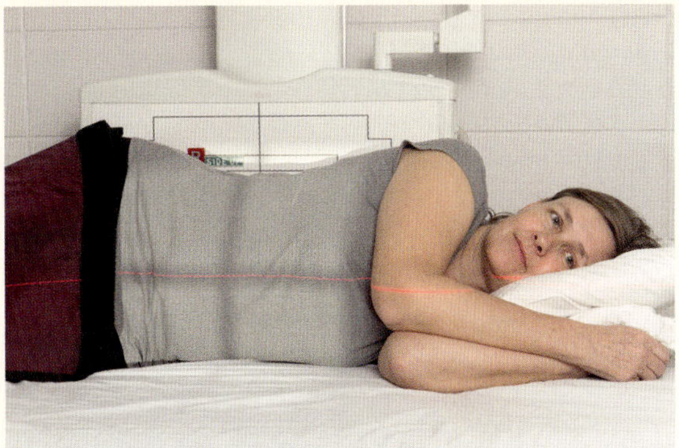

4-70 LLD abdomen position with AP projection.

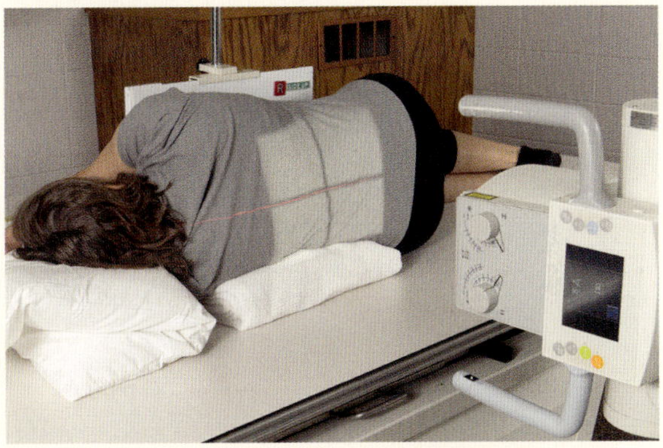

4-71 LLD abdomen position with PA projection.

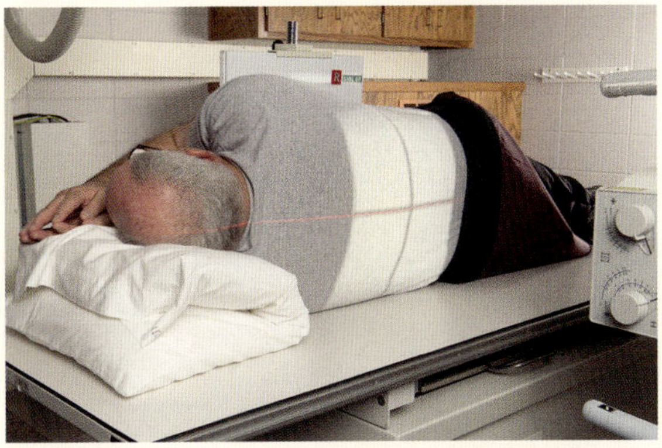

4-72 LLD abdomen with high CW IR.

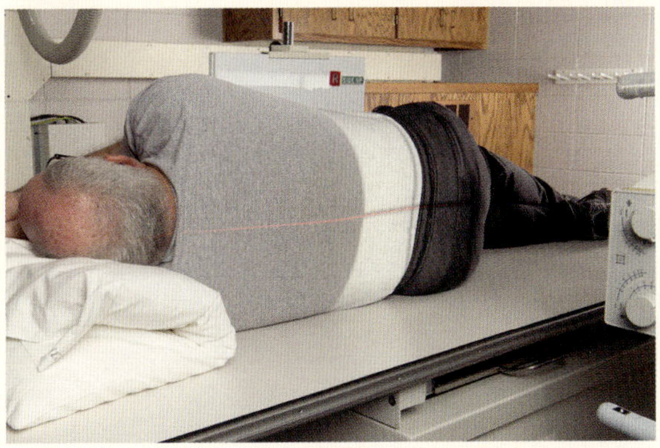

4-73 LLD abdomen with low CW IR.

IMAGE CRITIQUE (FIG. 4-74)

- Both hemidiaphragms down to midpelvic region included. The diaphragm will mark the highest point of the abdominal cavity. When the patient is in an LLD, a potential pneumoperitoneum will rise up to the highest point of the abdominal cavity, which will be on the patient's right side in the region of the liver (highest point)
- Symmetry of the vertebral column and iliac wings. This ensures no rotation of the part
- Properly centered to ensure inclusion of all essential anatomy
- Air may be seen within superior portions/loops of bowel as the air is rising to the highest point within each loop
- Air may be seen within the gastric fundus. The gastric bubble will be contained in the stomach around the point of midline

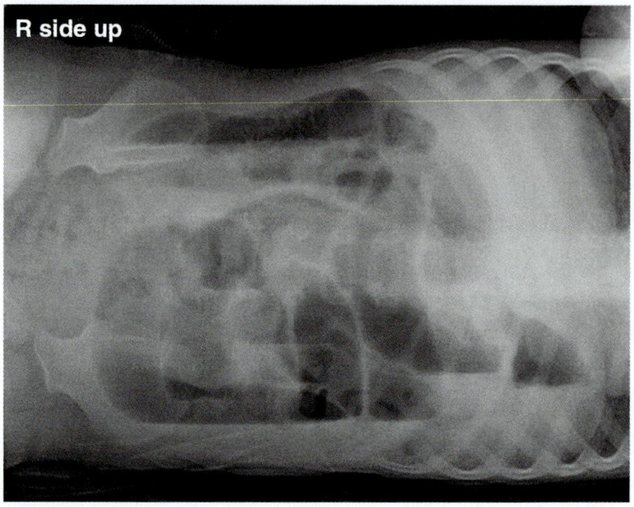

4-74 LLD abdomen.

Pediatric Abdomen—Supine Abdomen (KUB)

- Projection: AP

Pediatric Abdomen Protocol

Supine Abdomen

with potential to include

Upright Abdomen

Technical Considerations

- 60 kVp with nongrid if abdomen measures <10 cm
- 70 kVp with grid if abdomen measures >10 cm
- mAs set manually
- 40" SID

Exposure Field Size

- 10 × 12 or 14 × 17 lengthwise (IR or collimation adjusted accordingly to patient size)

Patient Position (Figs. 4-75 to 4-77)

- Supine without rotation of the part
- Immobilization of the patient as needed
- If the parent is assisting with the immobilization, ensure no possible pregnancy for the mother and secure proper protective shielding

Centering

- Level of the iliac crest and with MSP

Marking of IR

- Anatomic side marker R or L placed low and lateral in the region of the hip

Breathing

- On expiration if possible
- Keep your eyes on the pediatric patient the entire time while walking away to take the exposure and during the exposure. Ensure the safety of the pediatric patient. Imaging may require use of the guardian and/or the technologist to immobilize the patient if a restraint mechanism is not utilized or available

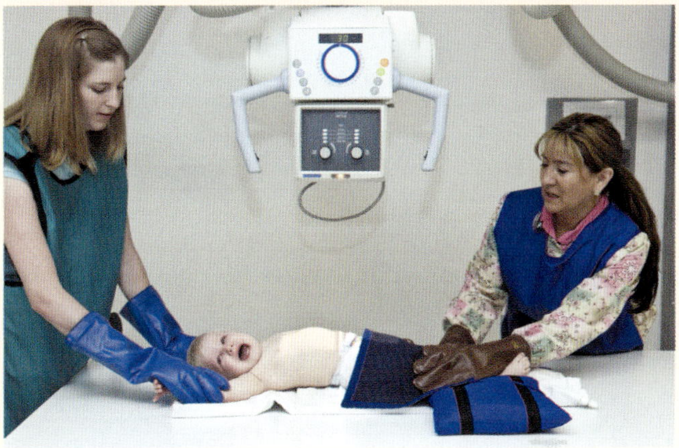

4-75 Supine abdomen.

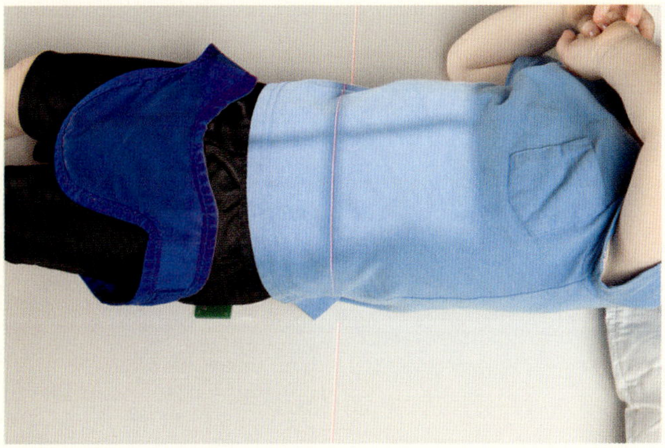

4-76 Supine abdomen.

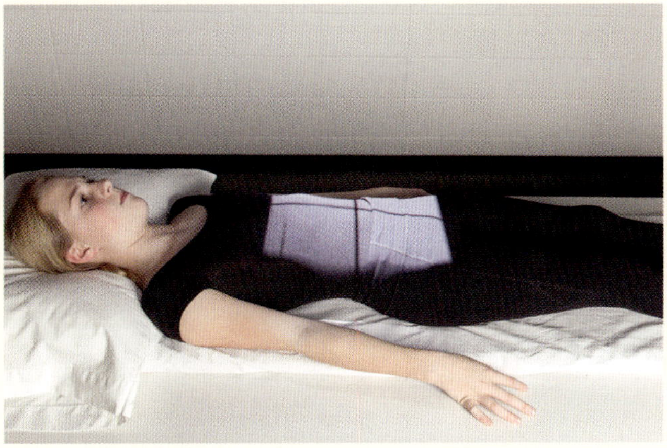

4-77 Supine abdomen.

IMAGE CRITIQUE (FIG. 4-78)

- Symphysis pubis must be included. Inclusion of the symphysis ensures the bladder was included on the image
- Outline of the kidneys included
- Bowel pattern can be observed
- Symmetry of the vertebral column and iliac wings. This ensures no rotation of the part
- Properly centered to ensure inclusion of all essential anatomy

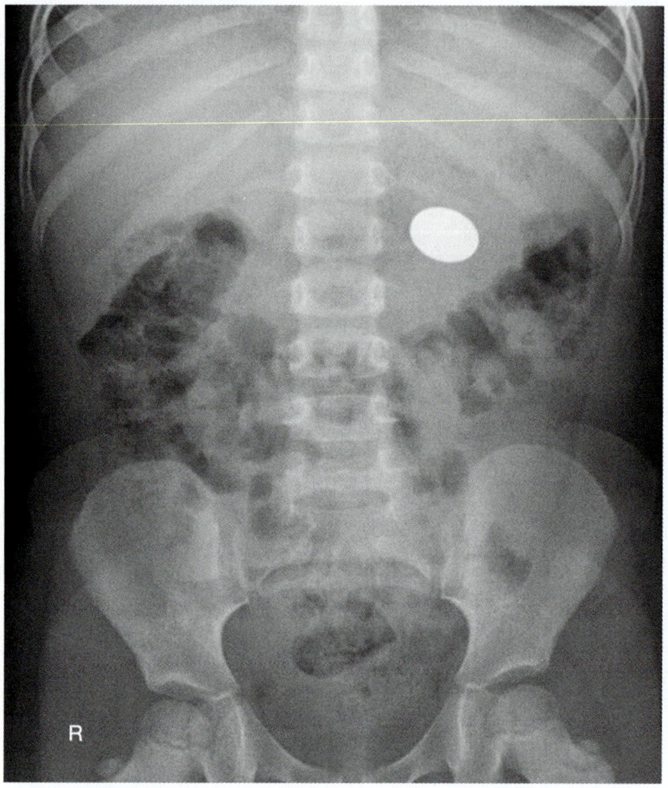

4-78 Supine abdomen.

Pediatric Abdomen—Upright Abdomen

Projection: AP

Pediatric Abdomen Protocol
Supine Abdomen
with potential to include
Upright Abdomen

Technical Considerations

- 60 kVp with nongrid if abdomen measures <10 cm
- 70 kVp with grid if abdomen measures >10 cm
- mAs set manually
- 40" SID

Exposure Field Size

- 10 × 12 or 14 × 17 lengthwise (IR or collimation adjusted according to patient size)

Patient Position (Fig. 4-79)

- Upright without rotation of the part
- Immobilization, such as with an upright immobilization device, of the patient as needed based on size and development
- If the parent is assisting with the immobilization, ensure no possible pregnancy for the mother and secure proper protective shielding

Centering

- Level of the iliac crest and with MSP

Marking of IR

- Anatomic side marker R or L placed low and lateral in the region of the hip
- An upright arrow could also be considered. Lead markers that possess the lead BB's, will indicate the upright position as they will settle to the bottom of the "circle" on the marker

Breathing

- Upon expiration if possible
- Keep your eyes on the pediatric patient the entire time while walking away to take the exposure and during the exposure. Ensure the safety of the pediatric patient. Imaging may require use of the guardian and/or the technologist to immobilize the patient if a restraint mechanism is not utilized or available

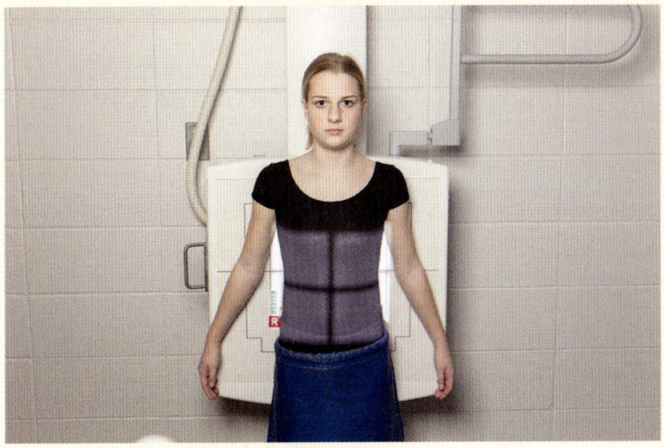

4-79 Upright abdomen.

IMAGE CRITIQUE (FIG. 4-80)

- Both hemidiaphragms to midpelvic region must be included
- Bowel pattern can be observed
- Symmetry of the vertebral column and iliac wings. This ensures no rotation of the part
- Properly centered to ensure inclusion of all essential anatomy

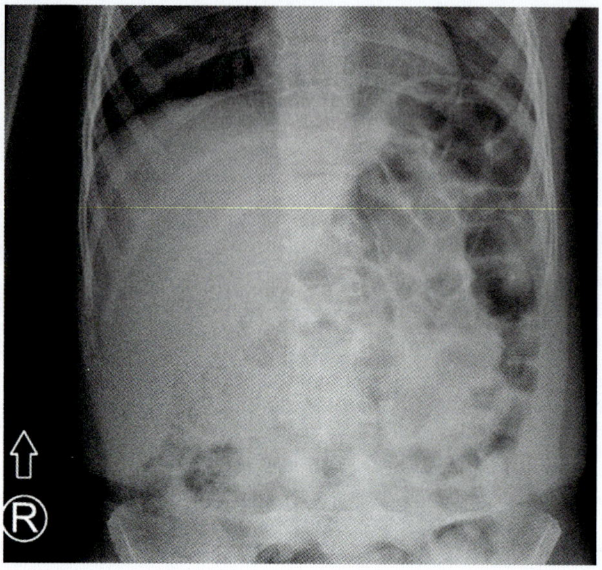

4-80 Upright abdomen.

Mobile Supine Abdomen (KUB)

- Projection: AP

Technical Considerations
- kVp 70–85
- Grid
- mAs set according to patient size
- 40" SID

Exposure Field Size
- One 14 × 17 lengthwise for sthenic patient
- Two 14 × 17 crosswise for hypersthenic patient

Patient Position
- Adjust patient in bed so they are flat, supine with no rotation
- Arms slightly abducted from patient's sides

Centering (Figs. 4-81 and 4-82)
- Place grid underneath patient by having the patient roll up toward one side. Be sure the bottom of the grid is set to the level of the symphysis pubis before rolling the patient up. Once the grid is placed halfway underneath the patient, lay the patient flat and then have the patient roll toward the other side to pull the grid the rest of the way under the patient's abdomen. Ensure the patient's abdomen is centered on the grid
- Level of the iliac crest and with MSP (it is essential that the symphysis pubis is included)
- Crosswise imaging required for a hypersthenic patient will require a low and high image to be acquired to include the majority of the abdomen working up from the symphysis pubis. The first image would include the symphysis pubis and lower abdomen. The second overlapped higher image would include the kidneys

Marking of IR
- Anatomic side marker R or L down in the lowest corner margin of the IR (down in the area of the greater trochanter)

Breathing
- The patient is instructed to take in a breath, exhale, and hold their breath out. Ensure the technologist has a six feet distance with a portable exposure and is able to see the patient
- The image is acquired after expiration

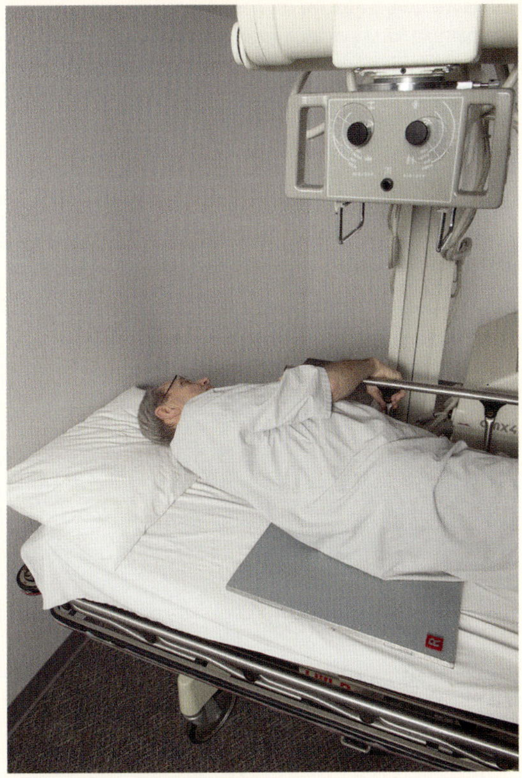

4-81 Roll method for grid placement for portable abdomen.

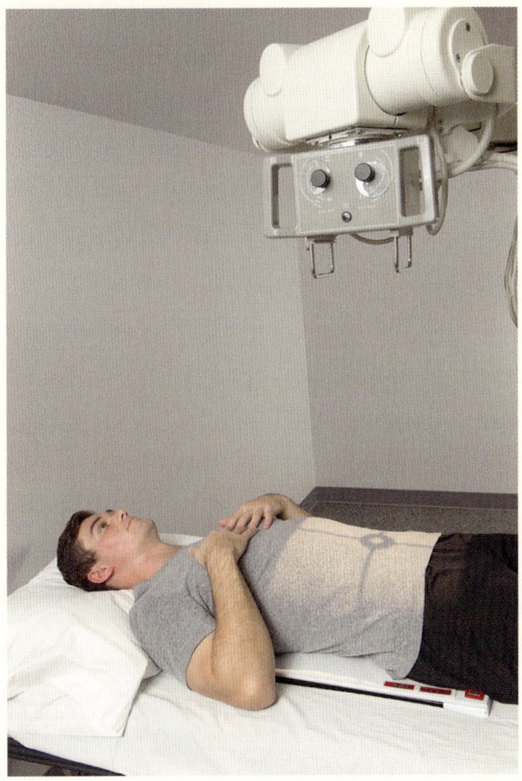

4-82 Portable supine abdomen.

IMAGE CRITIQUE (FIG. 4-83)

- Symphysis pubis must be included. Inclusion of the symphysis ensures the bladder was included on the image
- Outline of the kidneys included, which could potentially reveal the presence of renal calculi
- Bowel pattern can be observed
- Symmetry of the vertebral column and iliac wings. This ensures no rotation of the part
- Properly centered for inclusion of all essential anatomy

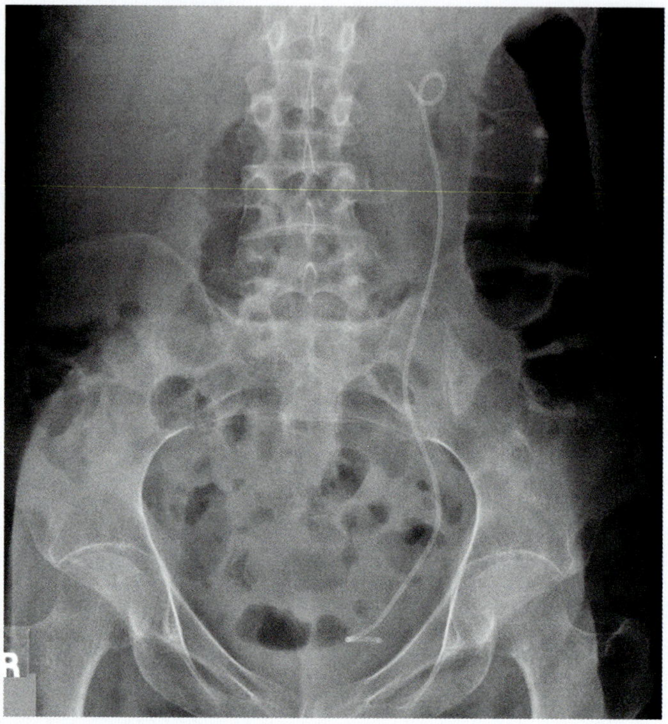

4-83 Portable supine abdomen.

THE FINAL STEP: IMAGE REVIEW

The technologist must take time to review acquired images to ensure image quality is acceptable. The technologist must have the knowledge within their role not only to acquire the images and care for the patient, but also to know how to review the images to ensure diagnostic quality has been attained. In certain instances, a projection may need to be repeated. This is to the discretion of the radiologic technologist. The technologist should review each image for the following.

1. Is all of the necessary anatomy included on the image?
   - Was the central ray (CR) properly directed to the part? An "X" can be drawn to intersect within the collimated exposure field to determine whether the CR was directed to the correct location.
   - Was essential anatomy in the collimated exposure field?
   - Is the area free of artifact(s)?
2. Is the anatomy well demonstrated?
   - Did the technologist properly position the patient to adequately demonstrate the anatomy?
   - Can the technologist recognize the anatomy best demonstrated with use of different projections?
3. Does the image reflect proper image markings?
   - Did the technologist correctly use a lead marker to identify the right or left side?
   - What additional markings or annotations could be helpful to the radiologist interpreting the exam?
   - Is the image properly displayed?
4. Does the image prove to be technically acceptable?
   - Does the exposure index fall within acceptable range for the operating system? Images that are technically insufficient may appear of good quality if just slightly insufficient or "mottled or pixelated" if severely insufficient. Images that appear "mottled" should be repeated. Images that appear beyond optimal exposure owing to higher technique may display high quality, but the patient has received excessive radiation dose.

CRITICAL THINKING

1. In review of the supine abdomen (Fig. 4-84), characterize the results.
   a. Image passes; all image criteria met.
   b. Image fails; patient needs to undergo bowel prep.
   c. Image fails; image is technically insufficient.
   d. Image fails; required anatomy is not demonstrated.

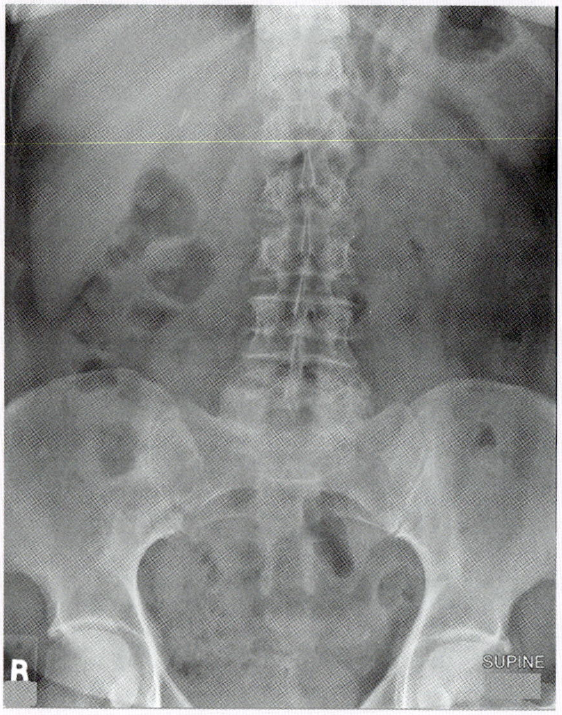

4-84

2. In review of the upright abdomen (Fig. 4-85), characterize the results.
   a. Image displays all appropriate anatomy.
   b. Image displays appropriate technical settings for potential free air.
   c. The image is incorrectly marked.
   d. Image fails to display required anatomy entirely.

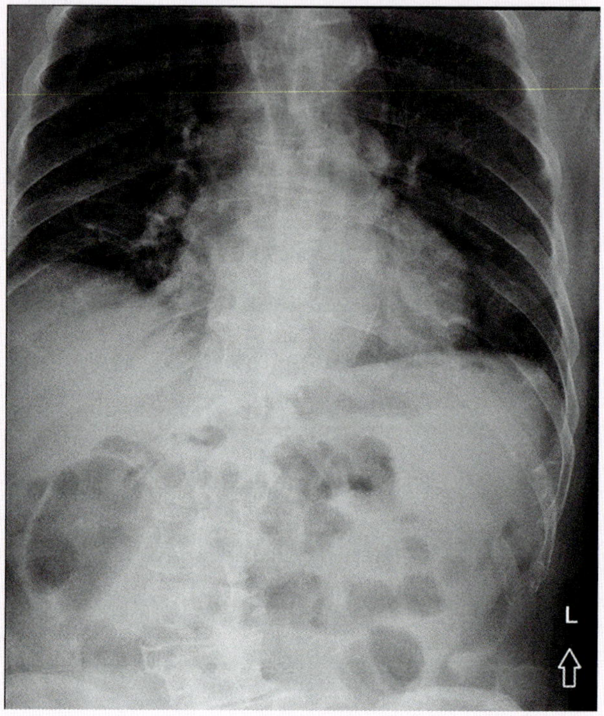

4-85

3. In review of the upright abdomen (Fig. 4-86), characterize the results.
   a. Image is technically insufficient.
   b. Central ray appears correctly directed.
   c. Centering fails to include the entire diaphragm.
   d. Image should be repeated for the artifact in the field of view.

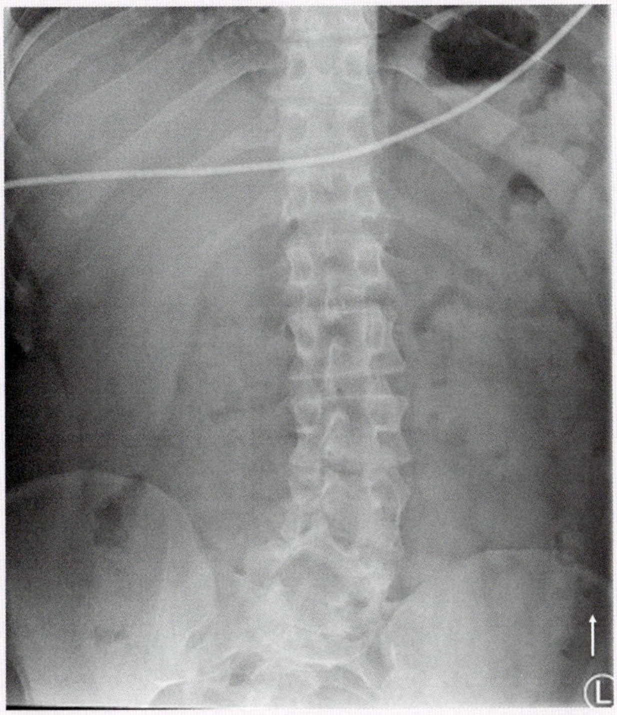

4-86

4. In review of the decubitus abdomen (Fig. 4-87), what could have been considered to fulfill the general purpose of acquiring an abdominal decubitus?
   a. Increase the technical factors.
   b. Ensure the patient is not rotated.
   c. Build the patient up evenly from shoulders to hips.
   d. Centering

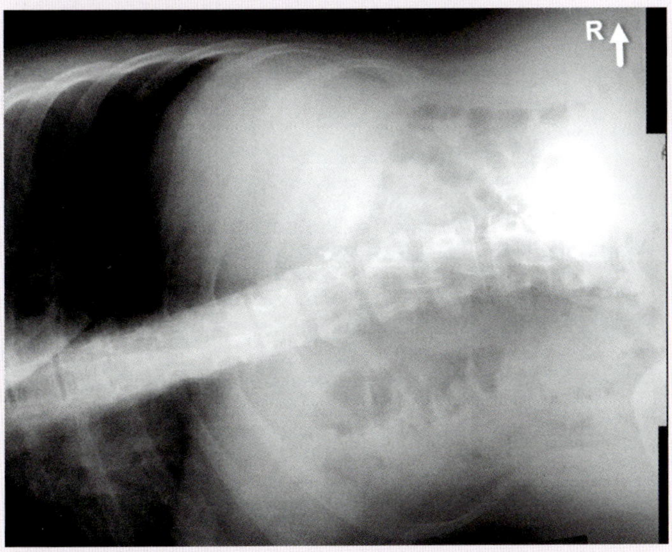

4-87

5. In review of the upright abdomen (Fig. 4-88), what does the arrow signify?
   a. Pneumoperitoneum
   b. Gastric bubble
   c. Pneumothorax
   d. Bowel loop

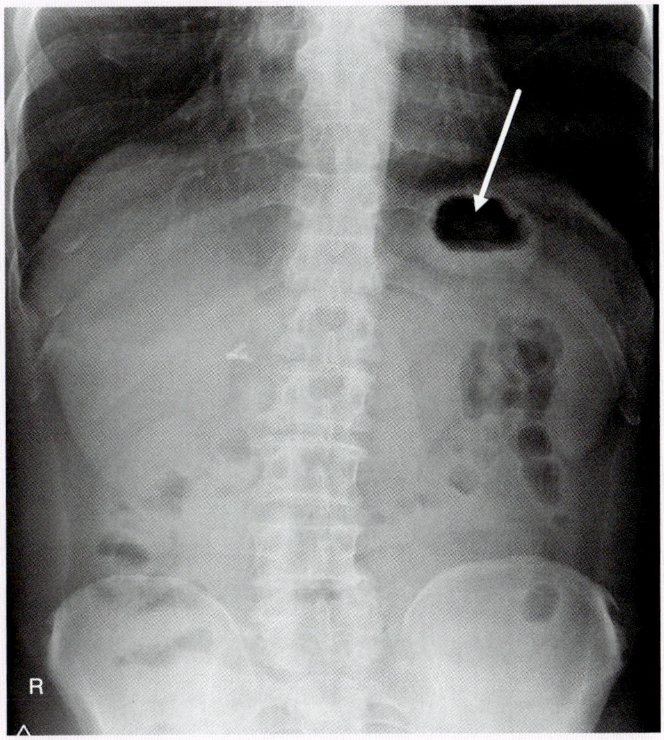

4-88

ANSWERS TO THE CRITICAL THINKING QUESTIONS

1. d
2. d
3. c
4. c
5. b

CHAPTER 5 Upper Extremity

Imaging of the upper extremity will include nontrauma and trauma patient situations. The technologist will need a proficient understanding of nontrauma protocols and be able to critically think and modify protocols in instances of patient trauma. Imaging of the trauma extremity may involve imaging the patient while in the emergency department, surgical suite and/or post anesthesia settings.

CLINICAL INDICATIONS

Indications are the symptomatic reasons as to why a particular exam may be ordered by the physician. The technologist should look at the clinical indications before performing a procedure. The following briefly introduces common exam indications but is not an all-encompassing list.

Boxer Fracture: Transverse fracture in the region of the metacarpal neck on the fifth metacarpal. Fracture could potentially include the fourth metacarpal as well. The direct force of striking an object with a fisted hand is a common cause (Figs. 5-1 and 5-2).

Colles Fracture: Transverse fracture to the distal radius with a posterior displacement of the radial fragment. It is possible that an avulsion (chip) fracture may also be identified to the ulnar styloid process (Figs. 5-3 to 5-5).

Smith Fracture: Transverse fracture to the distal radius with radial fragment displaced anteriorly (Figs. 5-6 and 5-7).

Scaphoid Fracture: Commonly fractured carpal bone with or without displacement. Additional imaging with stress views of the wrist may be necessary in certain cases to identify discrete fractures (Figs. 5-8 and 5-9).

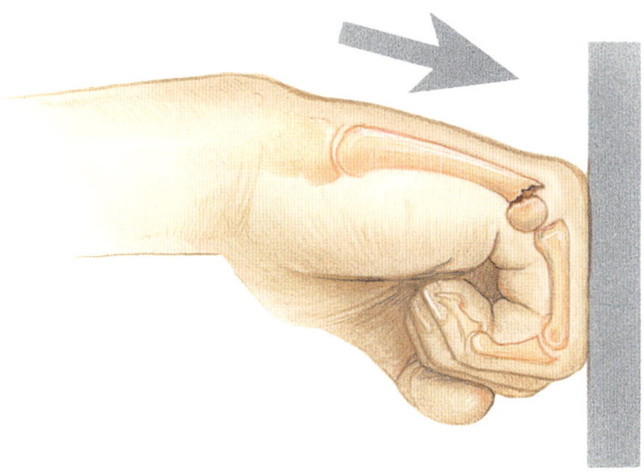

5-1 Boxer fracture.

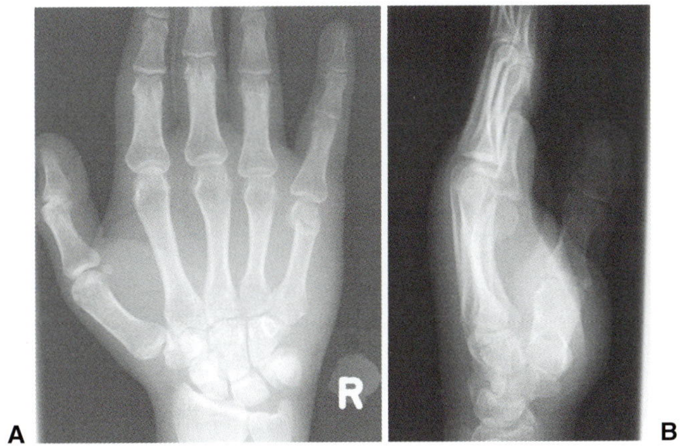

5-2 Boxer fracture. **(A)** PA hand. **(B)** Lateromedial hand.

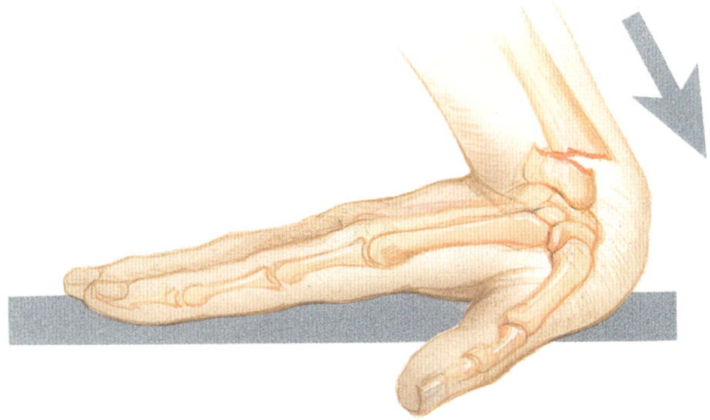

5-3 Colles fracture.

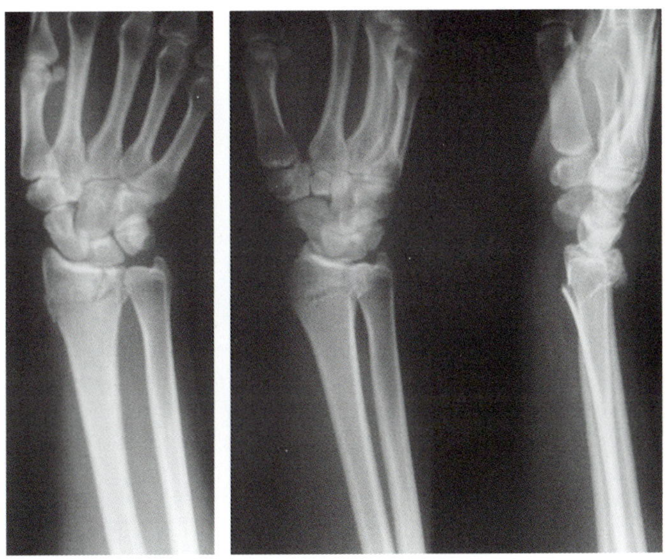

5-4 Three view wrist to display the position of the distal radius.

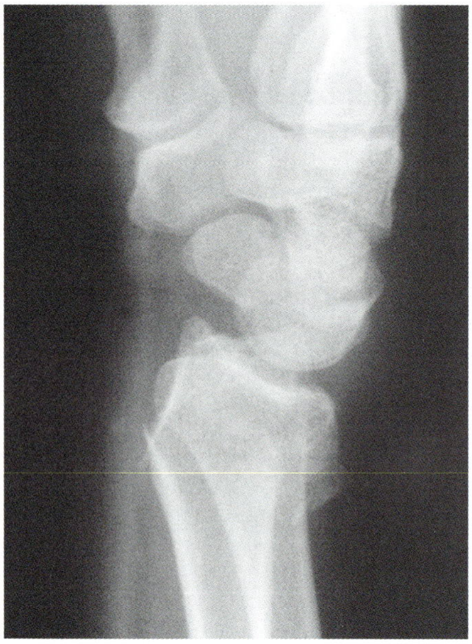

5-5 Posterior displacement of the distal radius.

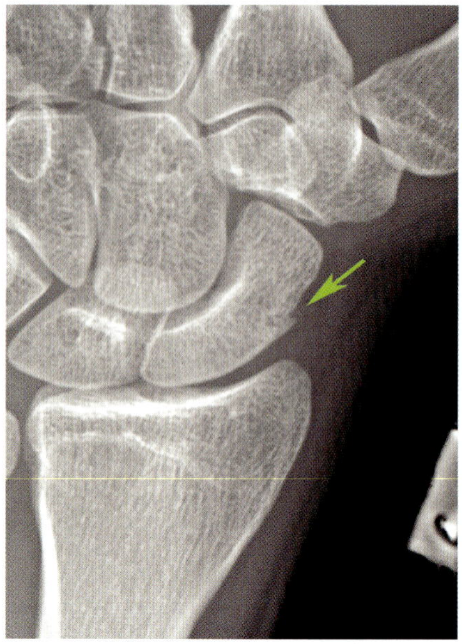

5-8 Scaphoid fracture.

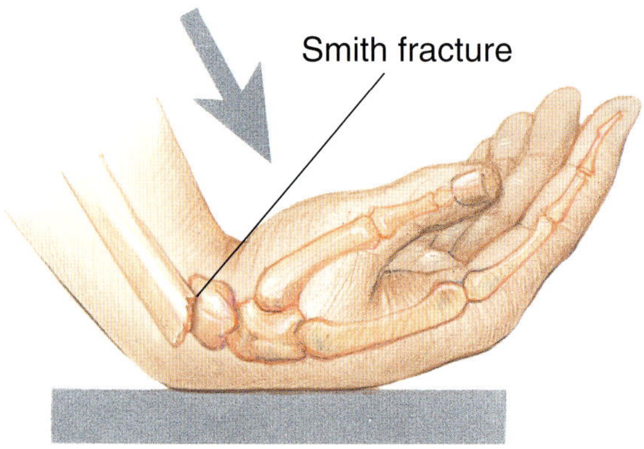

5-6 Smith fracture.

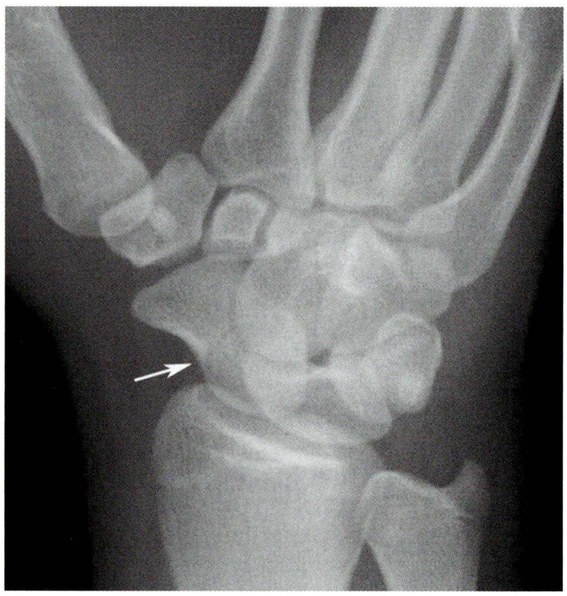

5-9 PA oblique wrist to reveal scaphoid fracture.

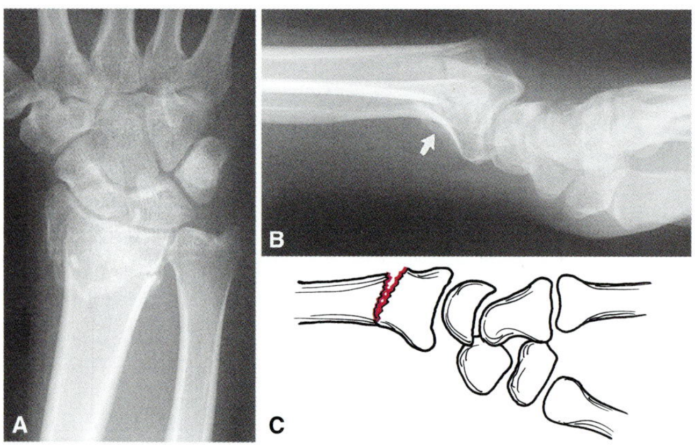

5-7 Anterior displacement of the distal radius. **A:** PA hand. **B:** Lateral wrist. **C:** Fracture to distal radius with anterior displacement.

Bennett Fracture: Fracture to the base of the first metacarpal, which may be complicated with fracture extending into the first carpometacarpal (CMC) joint and/or include subluxation (partial dislocation) of the part (Figs. 5-10 and 5-11).

Dislocation: Displacement of a bone from a joint. Pre- and postreduction imaging may be necessary to acquire with two views ninety degrees apart.

Foreign Body: Presence of wood, glass, or metal in the extremity. The foreign object must be determined to be within the soft tissue only or to have penetrated the bone.

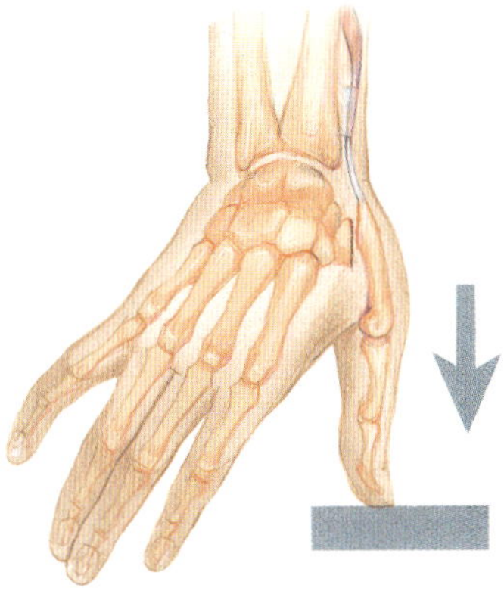

5-10 Bennett's fracture.

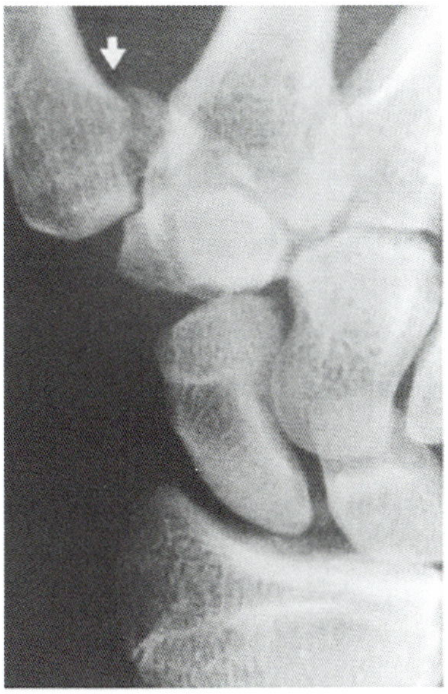

5-11 Bennett's fracture evident at the base of the first metacarpal.

Using a soft tissue technique by decreasing the kilovoltage will be important when trying to locate glass or wood. In some cases, a lead BB marker can be placed relative to the entrance wound and exit wound if applicable to call attention to the specific area. Two views ninety degrees from one another should be acquired.

IMAGING CONSIDERATIONS

Patient Dress

The patient may remain in their clothes as long as the sleeves do not create clothing artifact over the region of interest. Patients need to remove all jewelry from the area of interest. When imaging the region of the humerus, it may be necessary to have the patient change into a gown and remove undergarments that may create artifact.

Artifacts

Artifacts are unwanted objects that appear on the image, superimposing pertinent anatomy. Failure to have the patient remove rings, watches, or bracelets will appear as an

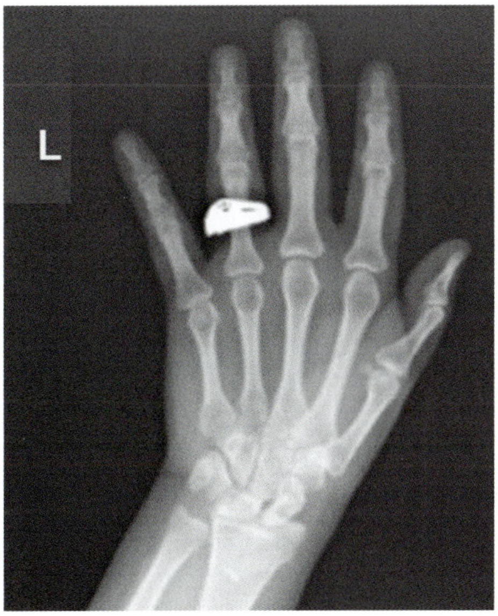

5-12 Patient artifact.

artifact and potentially obscure essential anatomy. Repeat imaging may be necessary when artifact obscures the area of interest (Fig. 5-12).

Patient Position

The General Position of the Patient or Part

Seated on Stool—Will allow the patient's extremity to be positioned easily by placing the extremity on the tabletop. Tabletop imaging is common when imaging fingers, hands, wrist, forearm, and elbow (Fig. 5-13). When patient is seated on a stool, ensure the body is turned to avoid the legs and waist being positioned beneath the tabletop to reduce patient exposure from scatter radiation.

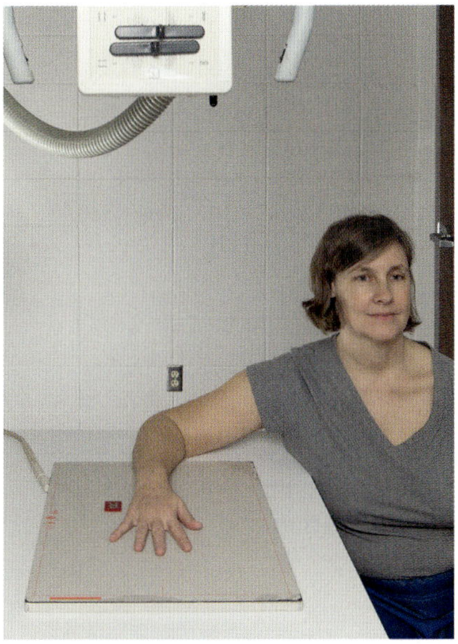

5-13 Upper extremity tabletop setup.

Upright—Relative to this chapter, this position could be considered when imaging the entire humerus. This will allow centering to include both joints, shoulder and elbow.

Supine—May be implemented when the patient is in trauma and is unable or unwilling to sit or stand upright.

Ambulatory Patient Imaging

An ambulatory patient is one who can maneuver themselves and bear weight with little to no assistance. Ambulatory patients may be able to stand upright for images or easily transfer to a stool. Ambulatory patients will be able to walk or may come by wheelchair to the exam room. Patients transported by wheelchair may be able to remain in the wheelchair for necessary tabletop imaging, eliminating the need to transfer them to a stool.

Projection(s)

How the X-Ray Beam Passes Through the Part

- AP (Anteroposterior): The beam is directed to enter through the anterior surface, exit the posterior surface, and strike the image receptor (IR) (Fig. 5-14).
- PA (Posteroanterior): The beam is directed to enter the posterior surface, exit the anterior surface, and strike the image receptor.
- PA Oblique: The beam is directed to enter the posterior surface and exit the anterior surface while the part is positioned in a particular degree of obliquity (Fig. 5-15).
- AP Oblique: The beam is directed to enter the anterior surface and exit the posterior surface while the part is positioned in a particular degree of obliquity.
- Mediolateral: The beam will enter the anatomic medial surface and exit the anatomic lateral surface that is closest to the image receptor (Fig. 5-16).
- Lateromedial: The beam will enter the anatomic lateral surface and exit the anatomic medial surface that is closest to the image receptor (Fig. 5-17).

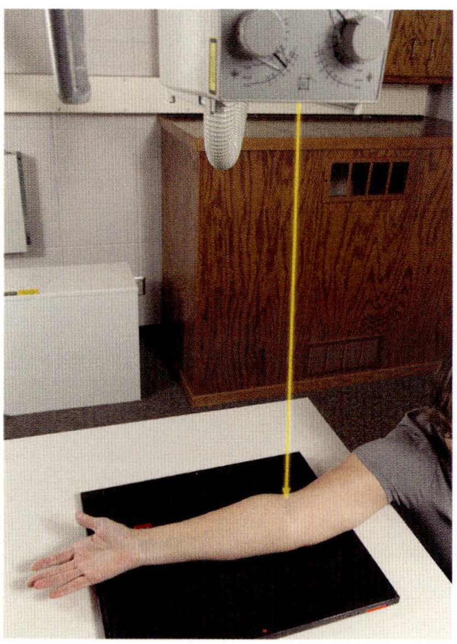

5-14 AP projection of the forearm.

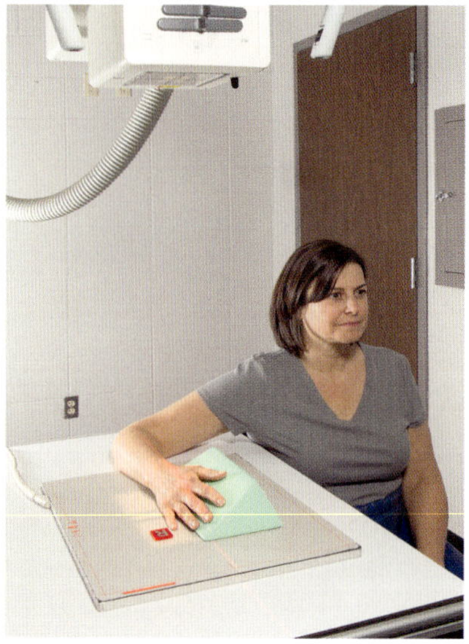

5-15 PA oblique projection of the wrist.

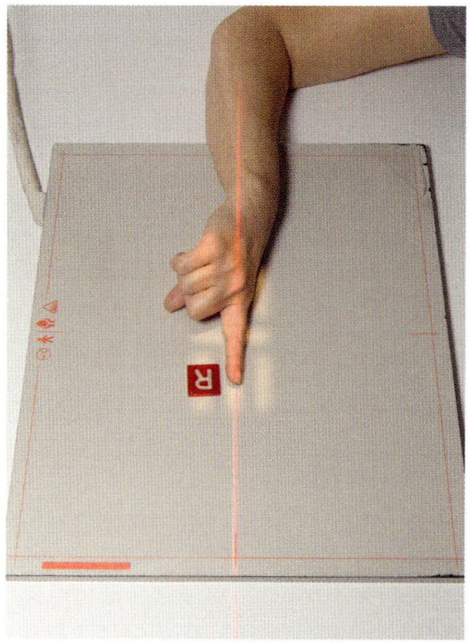

5-16 Mediolateral projection of the second digit.

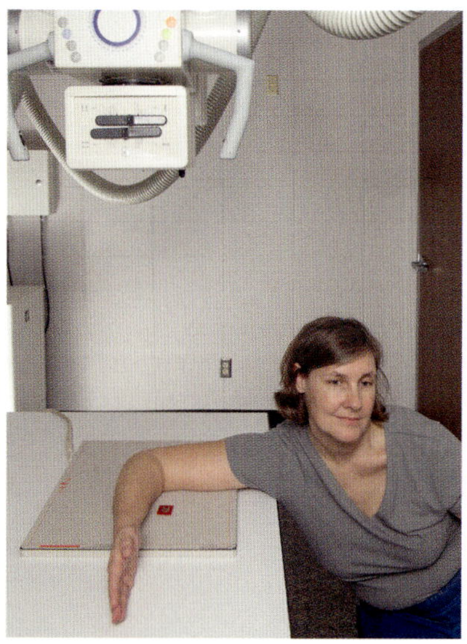

5-17 Lateromedial projection of the elbow.

ANATOMY

Imaging the upper extremity includes the anatomy of the fingers, hand, wrist, forearm, elbow, and humerus (Fig. 5-18).

Fingers

A finger can also be referred to as a digit. The thumb is digit one. Each digit is comprised of two or three articulated smaller phalanges (phalanx if singular). The thumb only has a proximal and distal phalanx. In between the thumb's proximal and distal segments, the articulating joint is the interphalangeal (IP) joint. Digits 2–5 have a proximal, middle, and distal phalanx (Fig. 5-19). In digits 2–5, the articulating joint between the distal and middle segment is the distal interphalangeal (DIP) joint. The articulating joint between the middle and proximal segment is the proximal interphalangeal (PIP) joint (Fig. 5-20). The technologist should attempt to position the digits with full extension and align parallel to the plane of the image receptor (IR) to better ensure these small joint spaces can be evaluated for small avulsion (chip) fractures (Fig. 5-21). All IP joints are of synovial and diarthrodial type with ginglymus or hinge-like movement.

Hand

The palm of the hand is comprised of five metacarpals. Each metacarpal is numbered respectably to align with the digits. Each metacarpal, similarly to each phalangeal segment in the fingers, has a head (rounded and most distal), a shaft, and a base (expanded and most proximal) component (Fig. 5-20). Located distal to the head of each metacarpal, a metacarpophalangeal (MCP) joint exists. MCP joints are of the synovial and diarthrodial type with condyloid type movement. Located

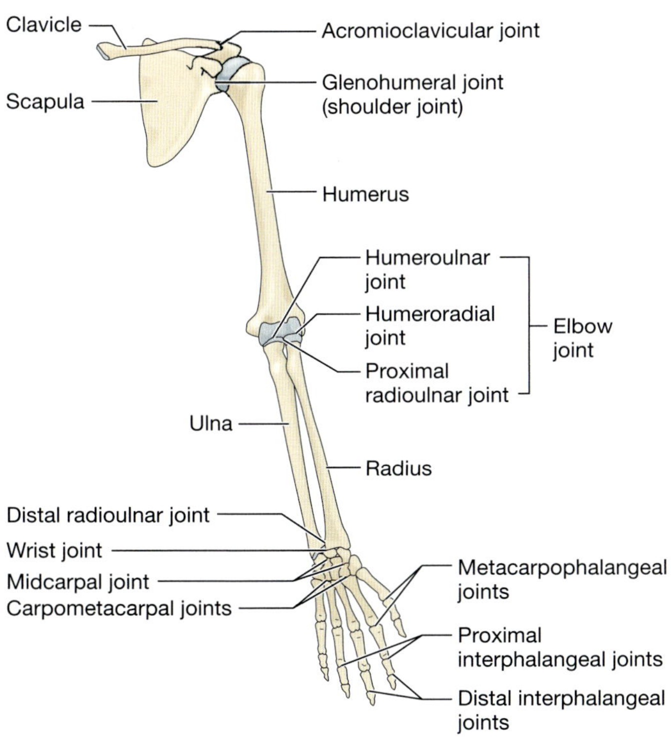

5-18 Upper extremity.

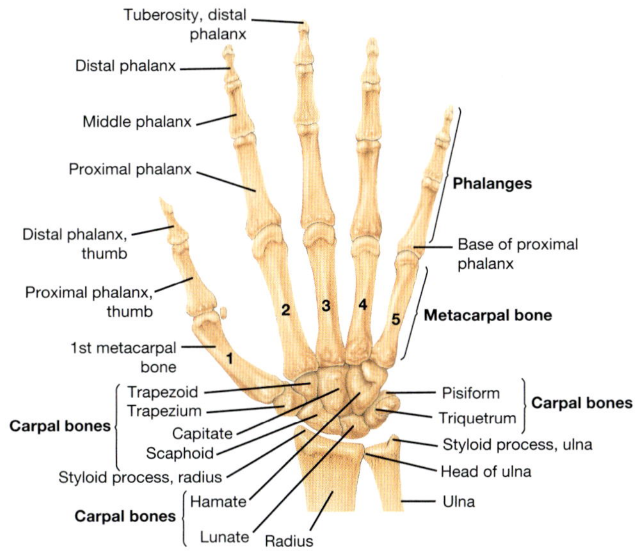

5-19 Hand.

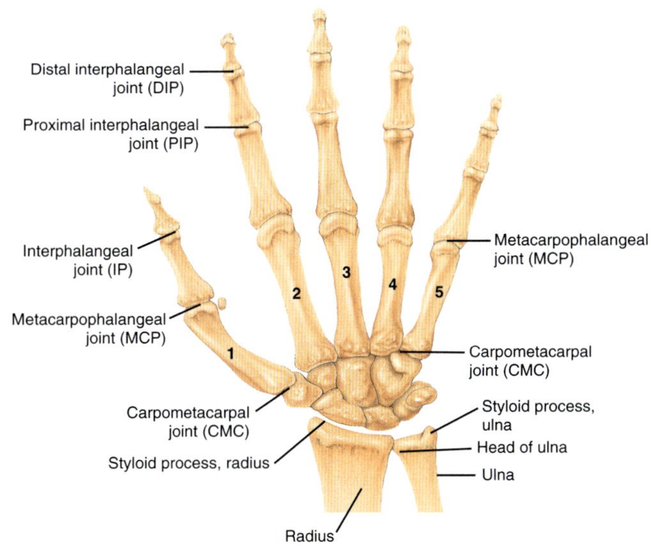

5-20 Joints of the hand.

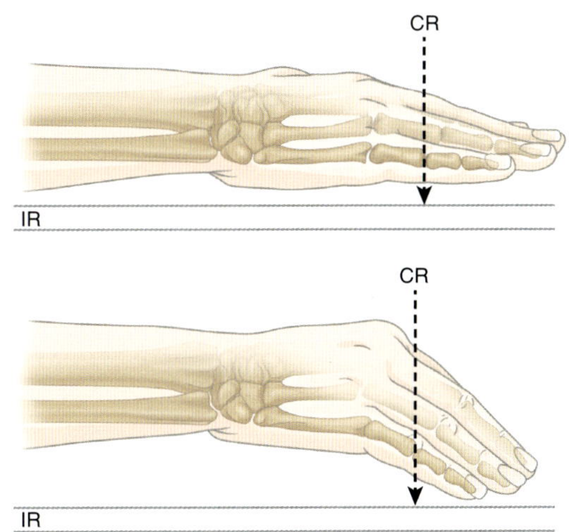

5-21 Ideally, CR intersects perpendicularly with the part and the IR.

proximal to the base of each metacarpal, a carpometacarpal joint (CMC) exists (Figs. 5-20 and 5-22). The CMC joints 2–5 are of the synovial and diarthodial type with plane or gliding type movement. Distinctively different, the first CMC joint is a saddle-type joint as the articulating surfaces oppose each other in order to fit together. This articulation allows for a greater range of movement compared to the other CMC joints.

Wrist (Carpals)

The carpals are divided into two rows, a proximal and a distal row (Fig. 5-23). The proximal row of carpals includes the scaphoid, lunate, triquetrum, and the pisiform. The scaphoid, being the largest carpal in the proximal row, is located on the thumb side of the wrist. The scaphoid will articulate with the distal radius. The scaphoid is known to most frequently incur fracture. Adjacent to the scaphoid is the lunate. The lunate also articulates with the distal radius. The triquetrum is the third carpal over from the scaphoid, and just anterior to the triquetrum sits a small, round carpal known as the pisiform.

The distal row of carpals includes the trapezium, trapezoid, capitate, and hamate (Fig. 5-23). In the distal row of carpals, referencing from the thumb side of the wrist, the carpal that directly articulates with the base of the first metacarpal is the trapezium. Adjacent to the trapezium is the trapezoid, which primarily articulates with the base of the second metacarpal. The capitate, the largest carpal in the distal row, articulates with the base of the third metacarpal. Finally, the hamate, which articulates with metacarpals four and five, has a distinctive hook-like extension (hamulus) that extends off the anterior surface (Figs. 5-24 and 5-25). The intercarpal joints or spaces in

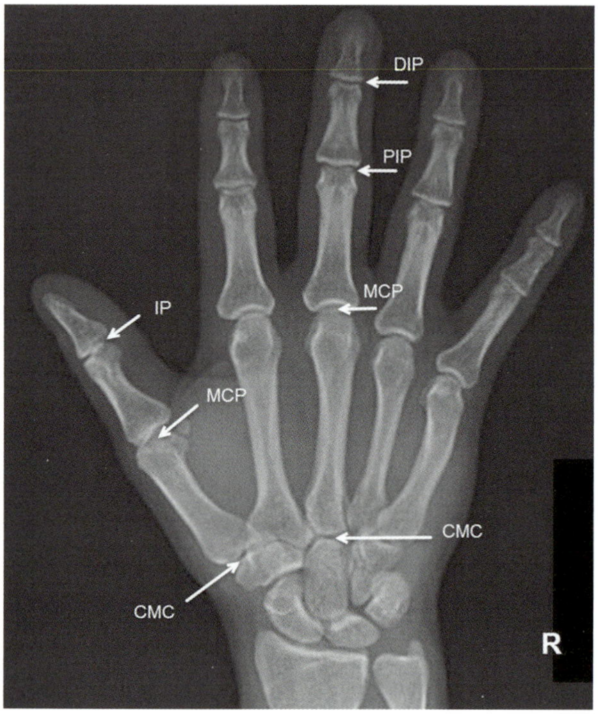

5-22 Joints of the hand.

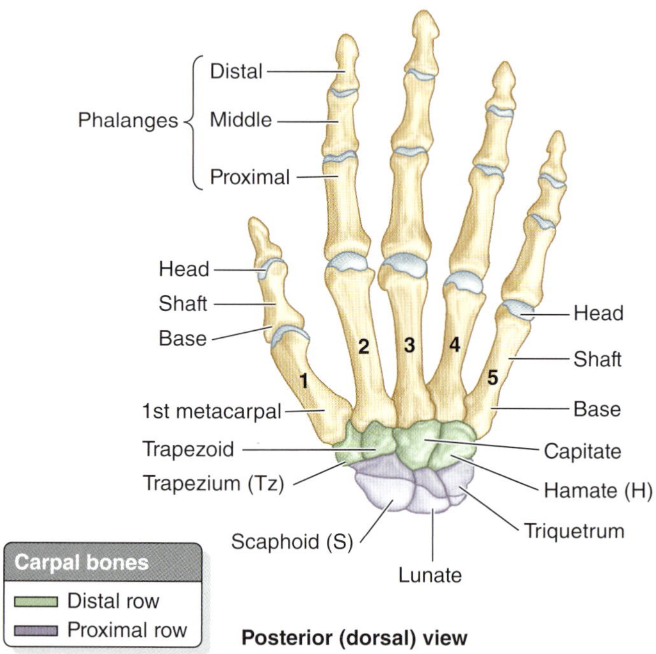

5-23 Proximal and distal rows of carpals.

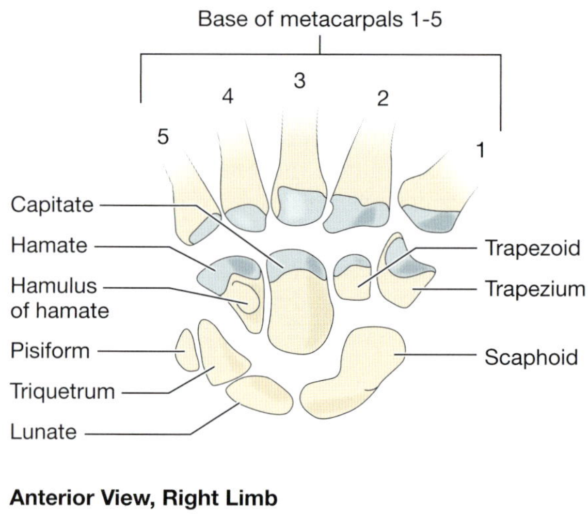

5-24 Carpal articulation.

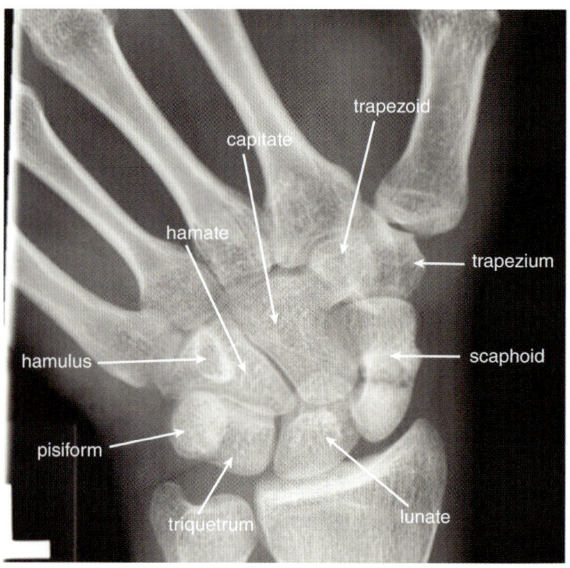

5-25 Carpals.

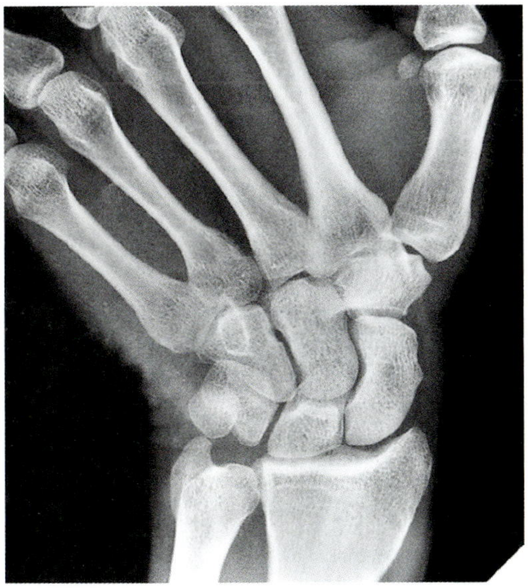

5-26 Ulnar deviation.

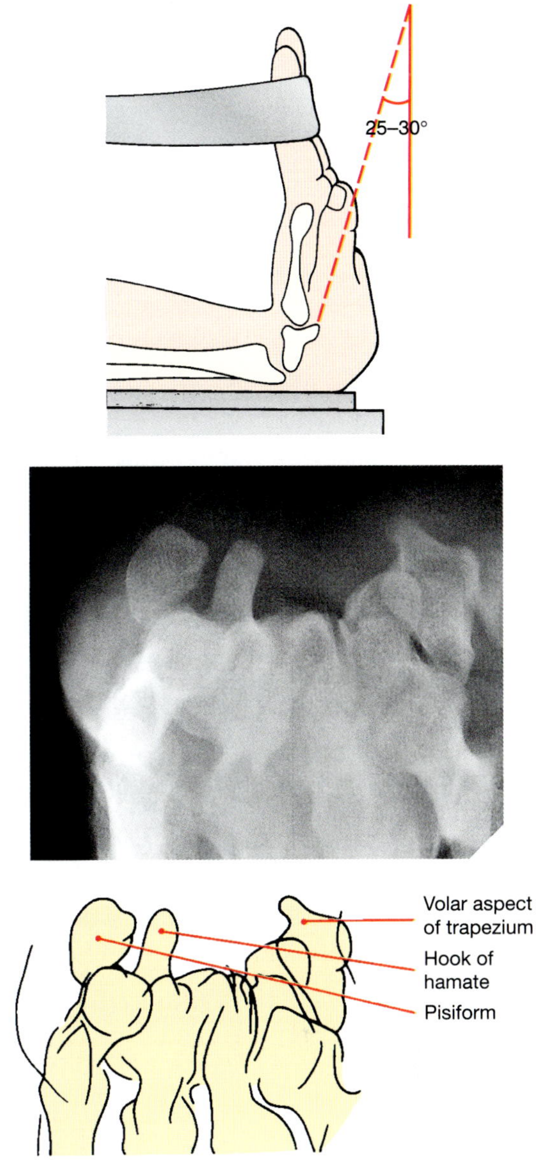

5-27 Carpal canal.

between the carpals are of synovial and diarthrodial type with a plane or a gliding movement. The radiocarpal joint (wrist joint) displays condyloid or ellipsoidal movement.

Specialty views are implemented to demonstrate certain carpals. One specialty view, in particular, that is more common for the wrist is ulnar deviation. The patient will be positioned with the hand pronated, and the fifth digit diverted toward the ulna (Fig. 5-26). This position will open up the carpal interspaces around the scaphoid and the carpals on the radial side. If carpal interspaces on the ulnar side of the wrist are of interest, the first digit is diverted toward the radius or radial deviation. Patients who suffer from carpal tunnel symptoms may have images taken specifically of the tunnel formed by the carpals. The carpal tunnel, the concave canal area within the palm of the hand, is demonstrated with the patient's hand hyperextended through which a tangential beam is directed. In particular, the pisiform and the hamulus of the hamate are of interest (Fig. 5-27).

Forearm

The forearm is comprised of the radius and ulna, which articulate with one another through distal and proximal radioulnar joints. The ulna remains stationary as it articulates with the distal humerus. The radius is able to pivot around the stationary ulna by way of the distal and proximal radioulnar joints. The radius and ulna lie parallel to one another when the arm is positioned in anatomic position or when the hand is supinated. With pronation of the hand, the proximal radius will cross over near the upper one-third of the ulna (Fig. 5-28).

The radius is the shorter of the two bones in the forearm. Distally, the radius broadens out and will articulate with the scaphoid and the lunate. A styloid process is noted on the distal most radius. From anatomic reference, the medial aspect of the distal radius has a depression known as the ulnar notch. The ulnar notch accepts the head of the ulna and forms the distal radioulnar joint (Fig. 5-29). Proximally, the radius has a flattened, broad, round head. The radial head will articulate with the capitulum of the distal humerus, forming the humeroradial joint. The proximal radius contains the radial head, narrows into a neck, and a tuberosity is noted on the anteromedial aspect (Fig. 5-30).

The ulna is the longer and stationary bone in the forearm. Most distally, a small conical extension, a styloid process extends off the ulnar head (Fig. 5-29). Proximally, the ulna appears similar to an ice cream scoop. The olecranon process is the most superior, pointed end on the scoop. The olecranon process will fit within the olecranon fossa, a deep posterior depression on the distal humerus, when the arm is full extended. The more inferior, pointed process is the coronoid process. With anatomic reference, a coronoid tubercle is located medial from the coronoid process (Fig. 5-30). The radial notch is located lateral from the coronoid process. The radial notch on the ulna will accept the radial head to form the proximal radioulnar joint. In between the olecranon process and coronoid process, the large concave depression, known as the trochlear

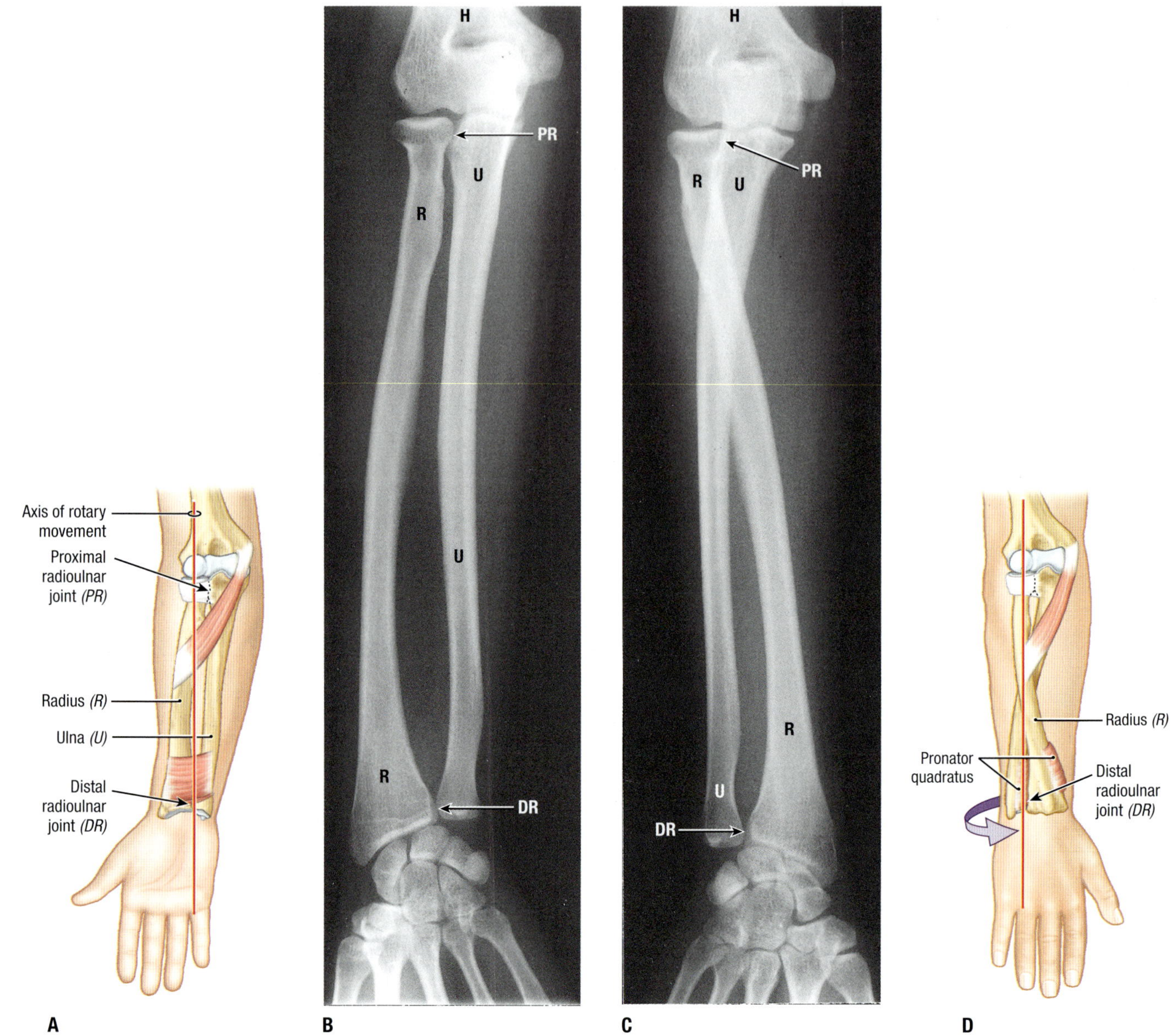

5-28 Rotational movements of the forearm. A: Anterior view, supination. B: Anteroposterior radiograph, supination. C: Anteroposterior radiograph, pronation. **D:** Anterior view, pronation.

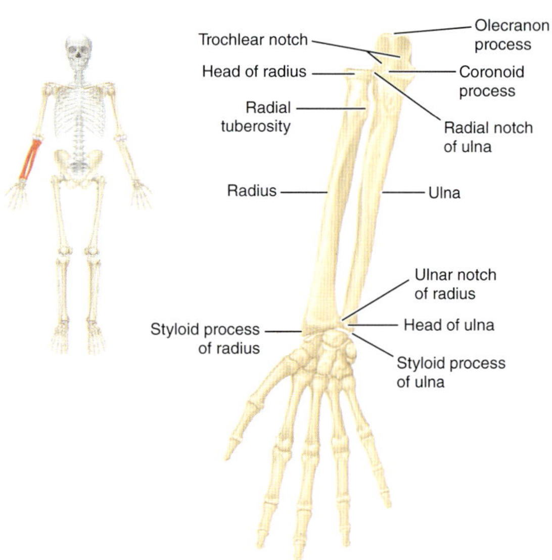

5-29 Anatomic reference of the radius and ulna.

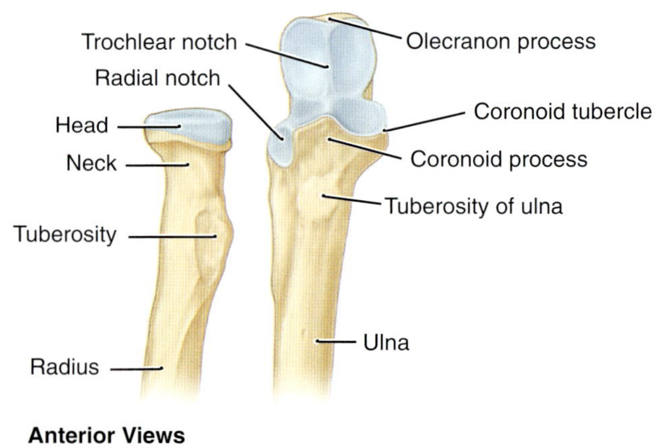

5-30 Proximal radius and ulna.

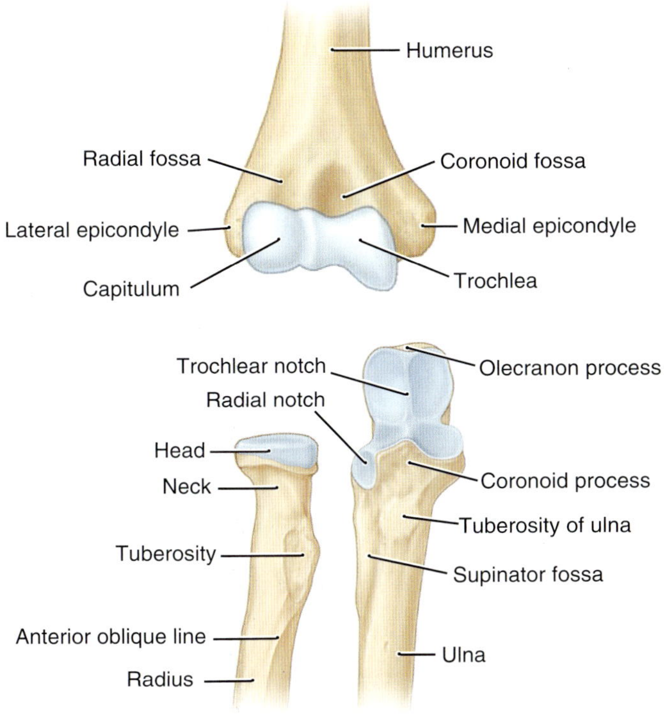

5-31 Anterior view of the distal humerus, radius, and ulna.

notch, will fit around the rounded trochlea located on the medial and distal humerus (Fig. 5-31). The proximal ulna hinges around the trochlea.

Elbow

The elbow joint is formed between the proximal radius, proximal ulna, and distal humerus. Visualizing the correct anatomy that comprises the elbow joint is important when imaging an elbow, a forearm, or a humerus. It is essential that the technologist use proper positioning techniques when the patient is capable of doing so. Best practices when imaging the forearm or elbow include the following: (1) full extension of the upper limb when imaging AP and AP oblique projections (Fig. 5-32), (2) 90° flexion of the elbow for lateral forearm and elbow exams, (3) the shoulder is dropped down or the part built up to ensure forearm and humerus are on the same imaging plane, and (4) the thumb is rotated "up" when the forearm is in a lateral position (Fig. 5-33).

Humerus

The distal humerus is directly involved with formation of the elbow joint. On the distal and lateral humerus is the capitulum (Fig. 5-34). The capitulum, which is round in shape, will articulate with the radial head, forming the humeroradial joint. On the proximal ulna, the trochlear notch will fit and hinge around the trochlea, located on the medial and distal humerus. The trochlea is shaped somewhat like a cylinder, with the two outer edges rounded and broad and the center of the trochlea marked by a depression; the trochlear sulcus (Fig. 5-34). The trochlea is larger than the capitulum. Medial to the trochlea, the prominent and palpable medial epicondyle is located. The

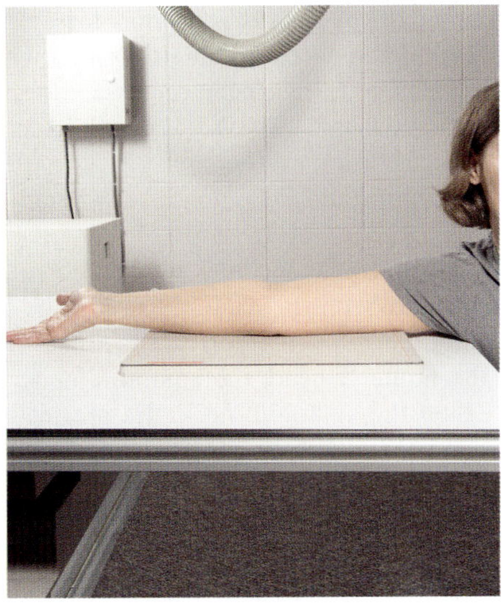

5-32 Upper extremity tabletop positioning.

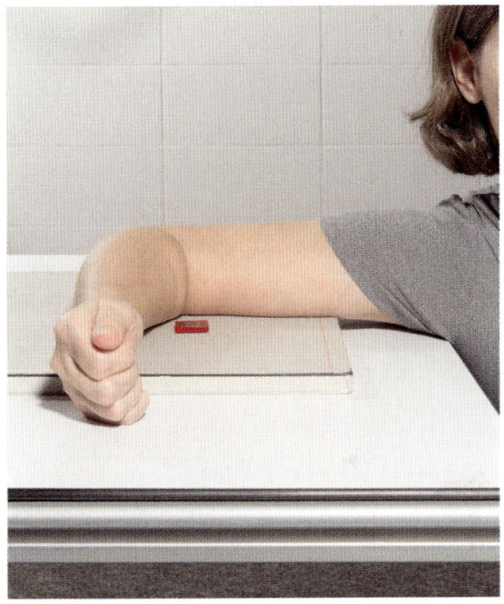

5-33 Upper extremity tabletop positioning.

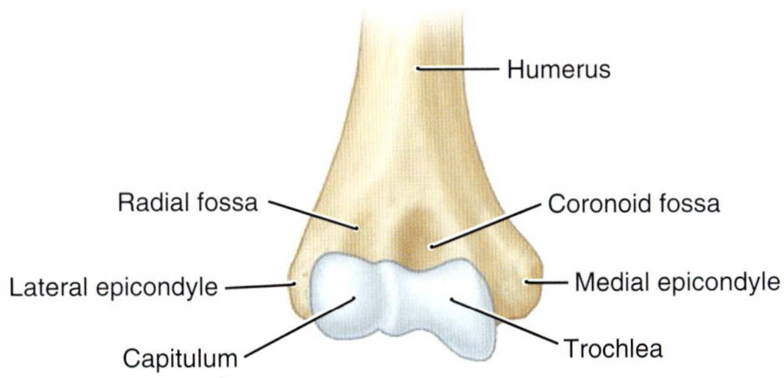

5-34 Anterior view of the distal humerus.

lateral epicondyle (significantly smaller than the medial epicondyle) sits just superior and lateral to the capitulum.

The distal humerus contains two anterior depressions and one posterior depression. On the anterior surface, two shallow depressions are present (Fig. 5-34). The radial fossa sits superior to the capitulum and will accept the radial head when the elbow is flexed in position. The coronoid fossa sits superior to the trochlea and accepts the coronoid process when the elbow is flexed in position. The olecranon fossa is located on the posterior, distal humerus (Fig. 5-35). It is deep and pronounced, allowing it to be visible on radiographs (Fig. 5-36). The olecranon process sits within the olecranon fossa when the elbow is in full extension (Figs. 5-37 and 5-38).

The proximal humerus includes the prominent, rounded head that articulates with the glenoid fossa of the scapula to form the glenohumeral (shoulder) joint. Adjacent and just inferior to the humeral head, the anatomic neck is located (Fig. 5-39). Below the anatomic neck, the greater and lesser tubercles are located, which provide the attachment sites for muscles. The greater and lesser tubercles are separated by the intertubercle groove (Fig. 5-39).

The greater and lesser tubercles are demonstrated separately with positional changes of the arm, which may also allow the intertubercle groove to be seen. With the hand and arm in anatomic position and palpating the humeral epicondyles to ensure they are parallel to the imaging plane behind, the greater tubercle is seen most lateral on the humeral head, while the lesser tubercle is located anteriorly and superimposed upon the humerus (Fig. 5-40). With internal rotation of

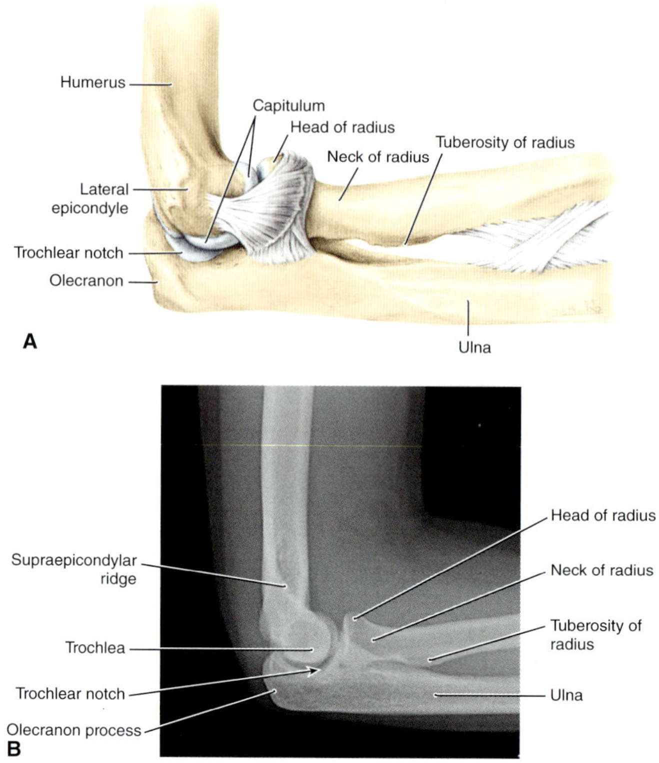

5-37 Lateral elbow. **A:** Lateral view. **B:** Lateral view.

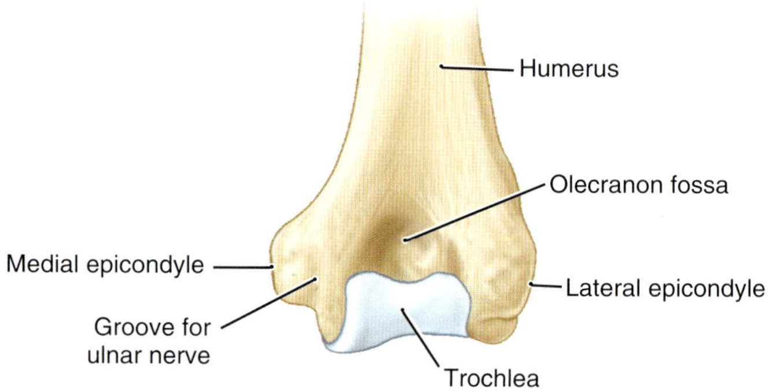

5-35 Posterior view of the distal humerus.

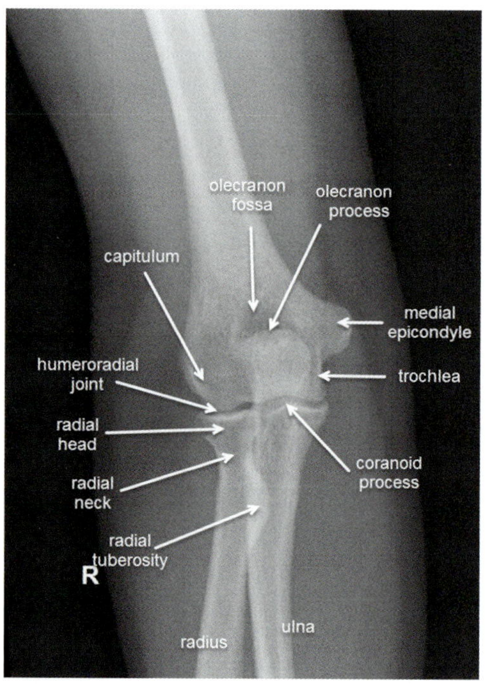

5-36 AP elbow.

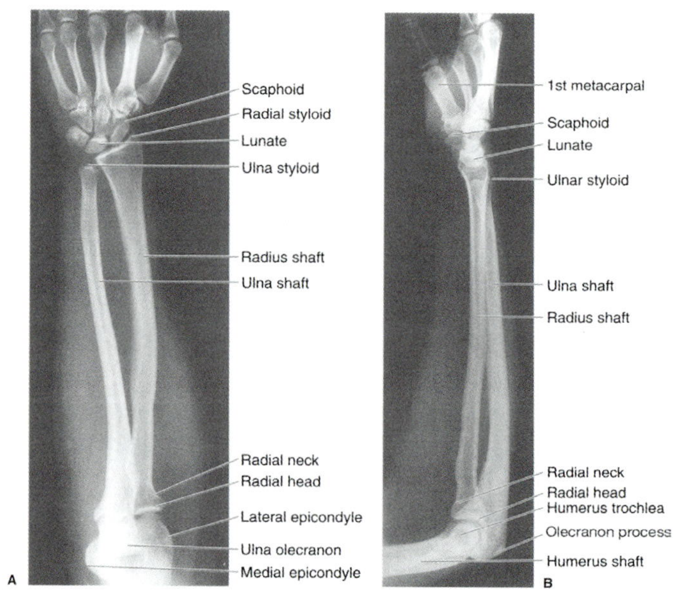

5-38 **A:** AP right forearm. **B:** Lateral right forearm.

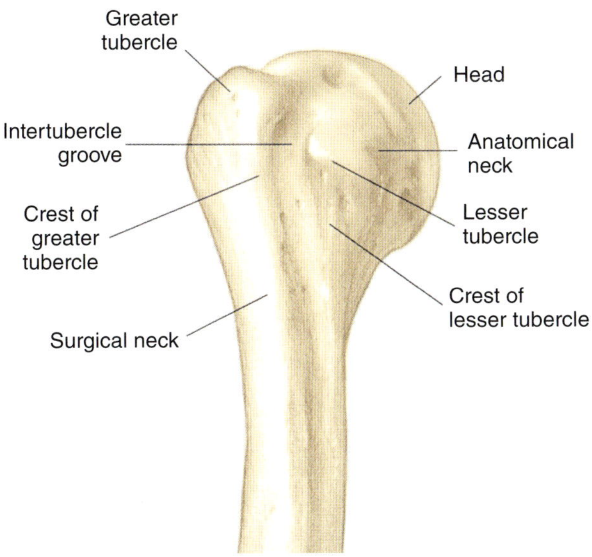

5-39 Proximal humerus.

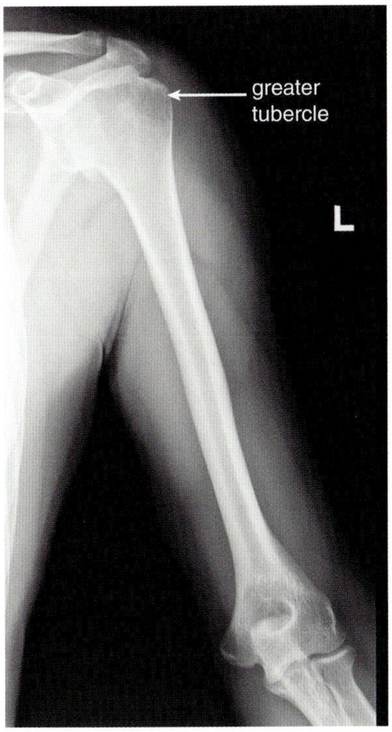

5-40 AP humerus.

the arm, the humeral epicondyles are palpated and adjusted to intersect perpendicularly with the imaging plane behind; the lesser tubercle will rotate medially and appear adjacent to the glenohumeral joint creating a profile perspective. With internal rotation of the humerus, the greater tubercle moves from its lateral position on the humerus to an anterior position superimposed upon the humerus (Fig. 5-41).

The surgical neck of the humerus is the narrowed area on the proximal-most portion of the humeral shaft, just below the humeral head and tubercle region. It is not uncommon to see a fracture to the surgical neck (Fig. 5-42). This often requires

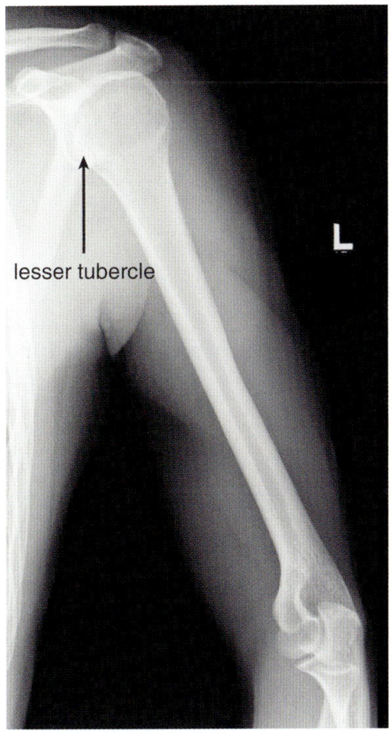

5-41 Rotational lateral humerus.

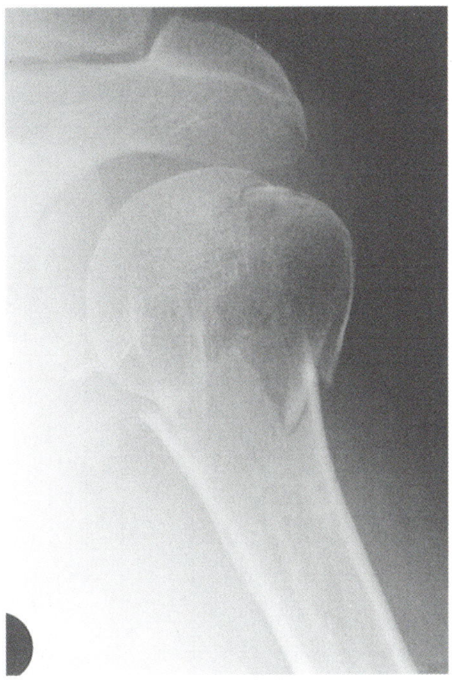

5-42 Fracture to the surgical neck.

surgical repair. The shoulder joint is of synovial and diarthrodial type with a ball and socket movement. The ball and socket joint of the shoulder lacks stability compared to the ball and socket joint of the hip. The glenoid fossa provides a shallow socket, which increases mobility, but subjects the joint to easier dislocation even with added reinforcement of the rotator cuff (Figs. 5-43 to 5-46).

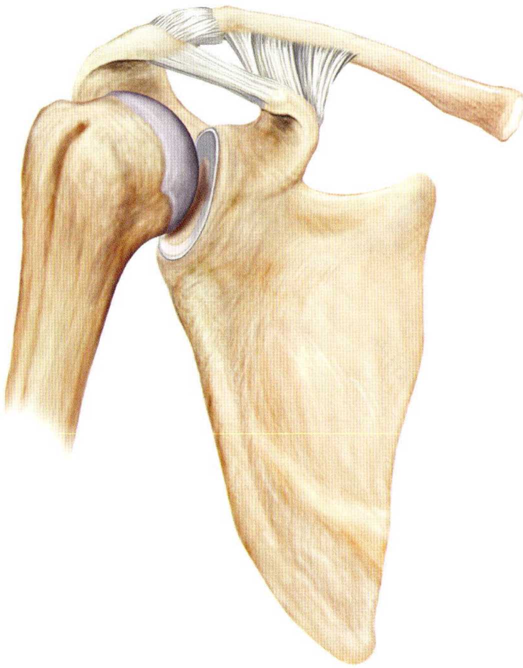

5-43 Shoulder joint.

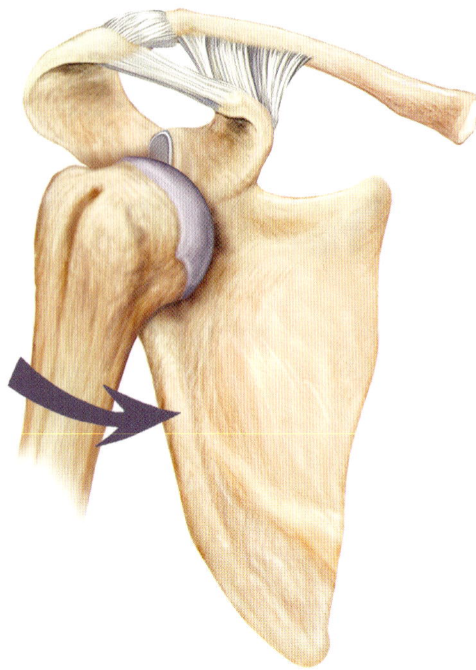

5-45 Anterior dislocation of the humeral head from the glenoid fossa.

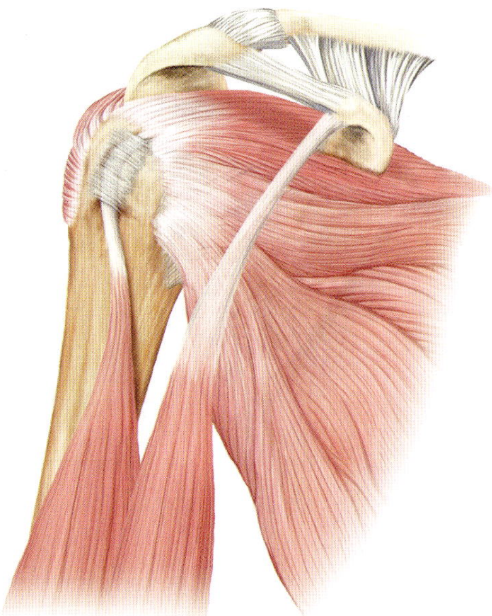

5-44 Shoulder joint with the added security of the rotator cuff.

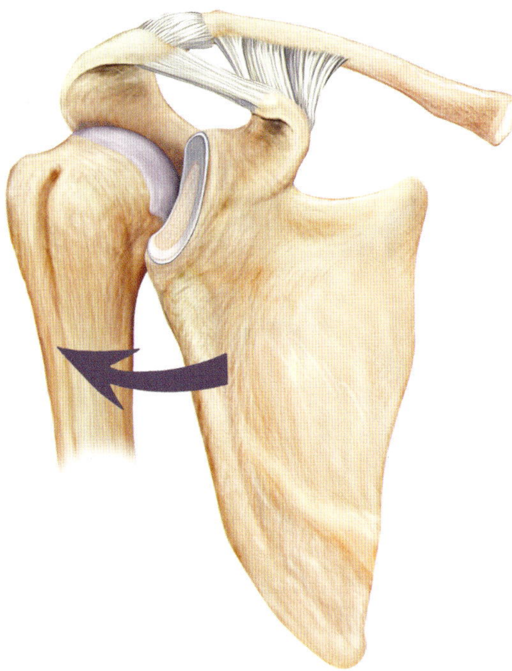

5-46 Posterior dislocation of the humeral head from the glenoid fossa.

KEY SUMMATION POINTS OF ANATOMY

- The first digit contains only an IP joint in between the proximal and distal phalanges. Digits 2–5 contain a DIP joint and a PIP joint.
- The scaphoid is the most commonly fractured carpal bone and may be better imaged with a PA projection of the wrist with the hand positioned in ulnar deviation.
- The distal row of carpals primarily articulates respectively with the metacarpal bases. The trapezium articulates with the first metacarpal. The trapezoid articulates with the second metacarpal. The capitate articulates with the third metacarpal. The hamate articulates with the fourth and fifth metacarpals.
- The scaphoid and the lunate are the only carpals to articulate with the radius and form the radiocarpal (wrist) joint.
- The radius and ulna lie parallel to one another with supination of the hand. With pronation of the hand, a crossover of the radius and ulna appears at the proximal one-third of the forearm.
- The radius pivots around the stationary ulna through the proximal and distal radioulnar joints.
- The medial epicondyle of the humerus is palpable and prominent on the medial and distal humerus.
- The trochlea is larger than the capitulum and contains a small depression within it that is the trochlear sulcus.
- Articulation of the capitulum and the radial head form the humeroradial joint.
- The proximal ulna is shaped like an ice cream scoop. The olecranon process is the most superior point, and the coronoid process is the more inferior point. The trochlear notch is concave between the two processes and hinges around the trochlea on the distal humerus.
- With full extension of the elbow, the olecranon process will seat itself within the deep olecranon fossa on the posterior and distal humerus.
- With full flexion of the elbow, the radial head will position within the radial fossa, a shallow depression just superior to the capitulum. The coronoid process will position within the coronoid fossa, a shallow depression just superior to the trochlea.
- The greater and lesser tubercles of the proximal humerus are visualized in profile (lateral or medial) with positional changes (external and internal rotation) of the arm.
- All joints in the upper extremity contain synovial fluid and are diarthrodial (freely movable). Each joint displays a different type of movement (Table 5-1).

5-1 Joints of the Upper Extremity

Joint	Classification	General Movement	Specific Movement
Interphalangeal joints	Synovial	Diarthrodial	Ginglymus or hinge
Metacarpophalangeal joints	Synovial	Diarthrodial	Ellipsoidal or condyloid
First carpometacarpal joint	Synovial	Diarthrodial	Saddle
Second to fifth carpometacarpal joints	Synovial	Diarthrodial	Plane or gliding
Intercarpal joints	Synovial	Diarthrodial	Plane or gliding
Radiocarpal (wrist) Joints	Synovial	Diarthrodial	Ellipsoidal or condyloid
Radioulnar joints	Synovial	Diarthrodial	Trochoidal or pivot
Elbow	Synovial	Diarthrodial	Ginglymus or hinge
Glenohumeral (shoulder) Joint	Synovial	Diarthrodial	Spheroidal or ball and socket

POSITIONING CONSIDERATIONS

Patient Part Size and Suggested Image Receptor Orientation

Imaging the upper extremity most commonly includes imaging a part size <10 cm in thickness allowing for tabletop and nongrid imaging. Once a part measures >10 cm, the part is typically imaged with a grid. In the upper extremity, the consideration of grid versus nongrid occurs at the humerus. With digital radiography, one exposure is taken on the imaging plate at a time. With one projection per image receptor, the length of the image receptor is orientated with the length of the part. The part should be positioned in the center of the image receptor.

Centering and Collimation

The central ray should be directed to the proper and suggested centering locations. With proper centering, four-sided collimation can be applied to ensure good radiation safety practices, ensure all essential anatomy is included, allow digital imaging systems ideal processing and configuration of accurate exposure indices.

Breathing Instructions

Specific breathing instructions need not be given to the patient as the extremities are not affected by the respiratory motions. However, as imaging approaches the thorax as with the humerus, breathing instructions may be given. It is important that once the technologist gives the instructions to the patient to hold still for the exposure. The technologist should ensure there is alteration of position of the part.

Identification of Arm Position in Nontrauma Versus Trauma Situations

Patients with potential and suspected fracture to a limb should be handled carefully the by the technologist. The technologist may have to deviate from normal protocol to image a dislocated or fractured part. The technologist certainly does not want to risk worsening an injury or cause additional and unnecessary pain to the patient. If the patient presents with potential fracture, the technologist should proceed with caution and leave the arm in the neutral or presenting position while acquiring a minimum of two views 90° apart (Figs. 5-47 and 5-48).

The position of the arm can be determined on humerus images by identifying the placement position of the greater and lesser tubercles on the proximal humerus. When the arm is positioned in external rotation, and the epicondyles are aligned parallel with the imaging plane behind, the greater tubercle is seen laterally in profile. The lesser tubercle is not visualized in this arm position as it is superimposed on the proximal humerus due to its anterior location with anatomic position (Figs. 5-49 and 5-50). With internal rotation of the arm, the arm and palm of the hand are rotated until the humeral epicondyles are perpendicular to the imaging plane behind. The internal rotation position displays the lesser tubercle in profile medially, toward the glenohumeral joint. The greater tubercle shifts from the anatomic lateral position to the anterior position and superimposes upon the humerus and therefore is not well visualized (Figs. 5-51 and 5-52). When the arm is in neutral position, the humeral epicondyles may be at an approximate 45° angle to the image receptor; therefore, neither the greater nor the lesser

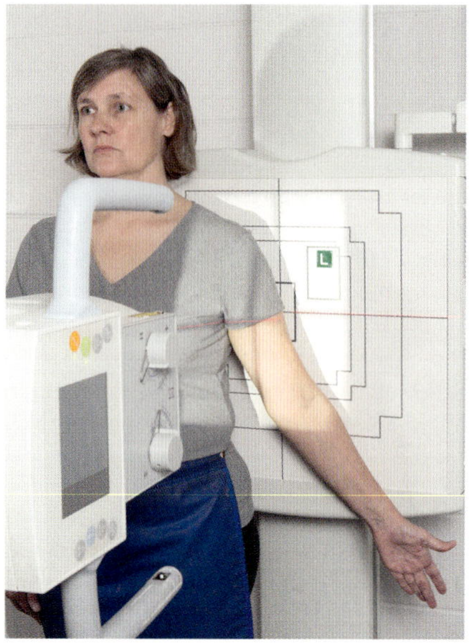
5-49 AP with external arm position.

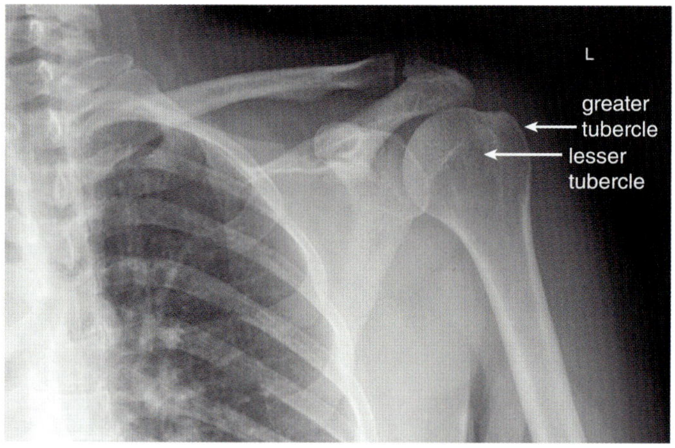

5-50 AP projection with external rotation of the arm.

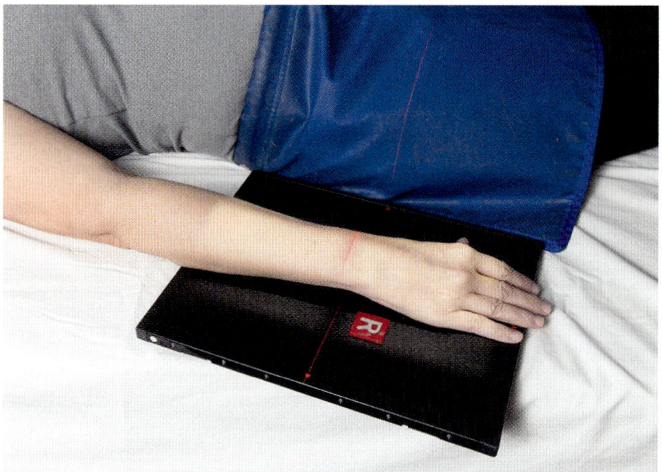
5-47 PA trauma wrist.

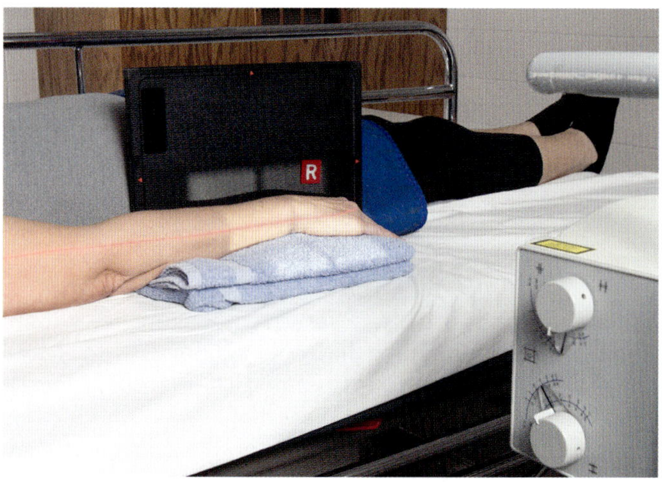
5-48 Horizontal beam lateral trauma wrist.

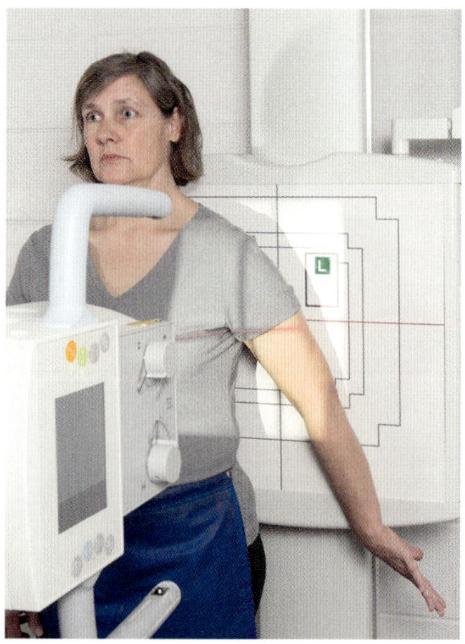
5-51 AP with internal arm position.

tubercle will be seen in profile, as both are superimposed upon the humerus (Figs. 5-53 and 5-54).

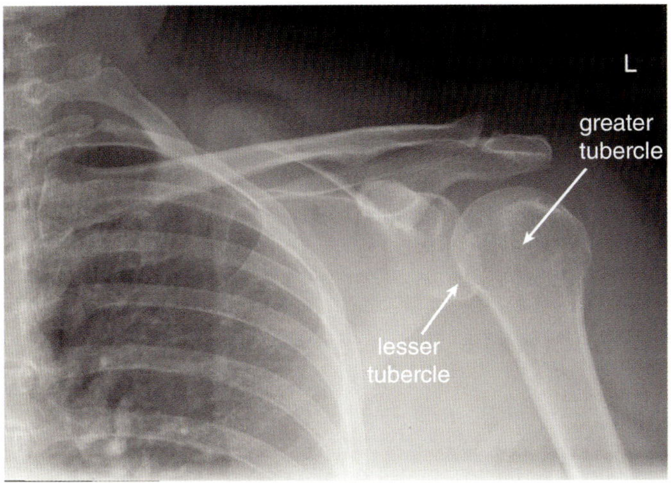

5-52 AP projection with internal rotation of the arm.

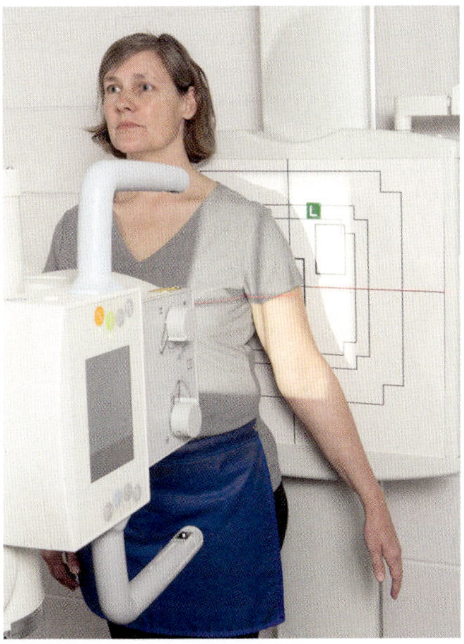

5-53 AP with neutral arm position.

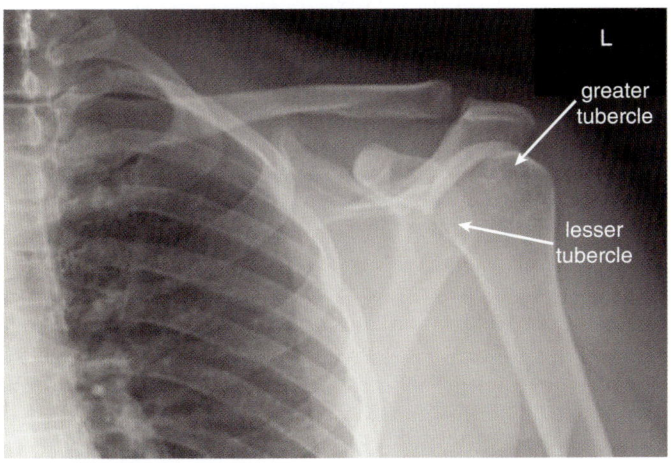

5-54 AP projection with neutral position of the arm.

TECHNICAL CONSIDERATIONS

Setting a Manual Technique

Manual techniques are set for all extremity imaging. Tabletop imaging requires use of manual technique. Kilovoltage is set to penetrate the part thickness and affects the scale of contrast seen on the image. A lower kVp is used for extremity set appropriately to penetrate the part thickness. A lower kVp will produce a high scale of contrast, demonstrating more black and white shades, and this is desirable when imaging the extremities. If imaging a patient in a cast, the kVp must increase in order to penetrate the thickness and the material of the cast. A plaster cast may require a 5–10 kVp increase, whereas fiberglass may need only half the kVp increase of the plaster cast. A small focal spot setting is encouraged when imaging extremities in an effort to improve detail, especially of the small bones and joints (Fig. 5-55).

Setting a manual technique will also allow the technologist to adjust the length of the exposure—something important to consider with any patient, but especially with pediatric and geriatric patients. In cases where motion can be detrimental to image quality, the technologist can increase the mA station, thus allowing the exposure time to decrease in order to minimize the chance of voluntary patient motion.

Source-to-Image Distance (SID)

40″ source-to-image distance is employed for all extremity imaging.

Shielding

Acceptable shielding practices include a lap shield at minimum, but a full lead shield could also be considered. Double shielding around the front and back of the waist should be considered when imaging declared pregnant patients.

Marking the Image

When marking an extremity positioned flat or obliquely, the anatomic marker should be placed within the collimated exposure field furthest away from the patient's midline or lateral to the part (Figs. 5-56 to 5-58). When marking the lateral position, the anatomic marker is placed along the anterior surface of the part or "in front" of the part and within the collimated exposure field (Fig. 5-59).

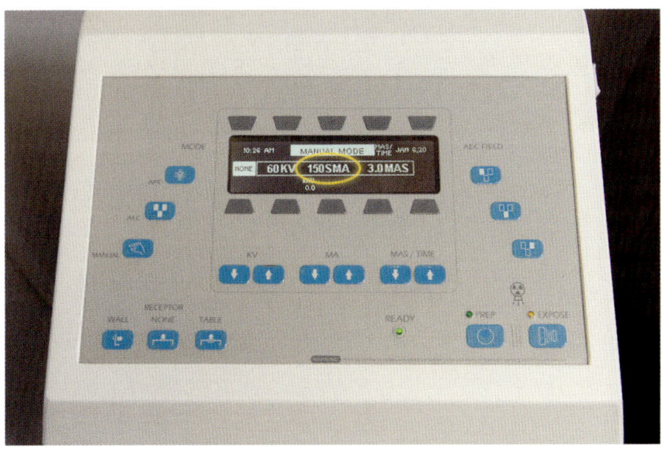

5-55 Control panel considerations for the upper extremity.

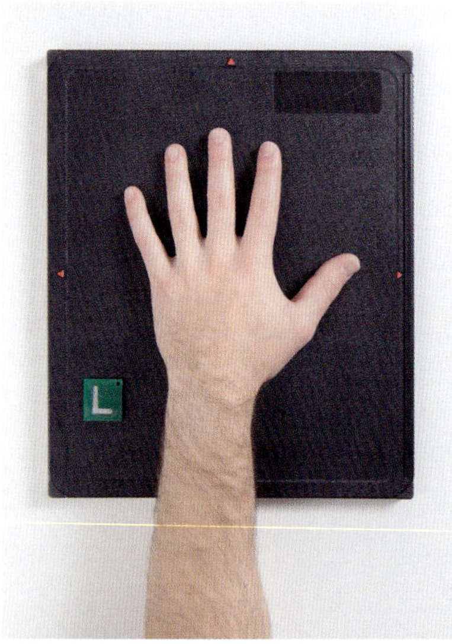

5-56 Suggested anatomic marker placement for flat or oblique part positions.

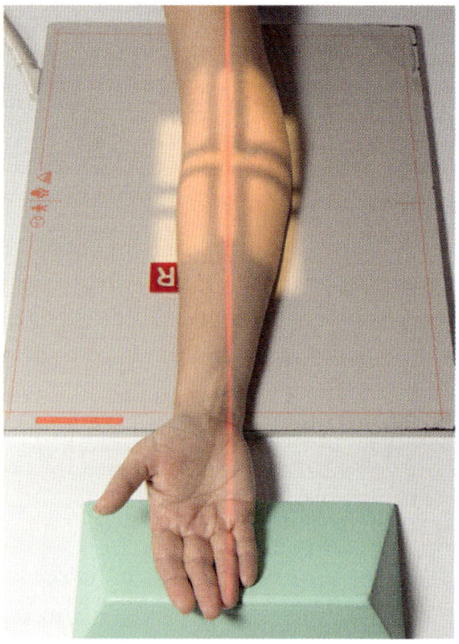

5-57 Suggested anatomic marker placement for flat or oblique part positions.

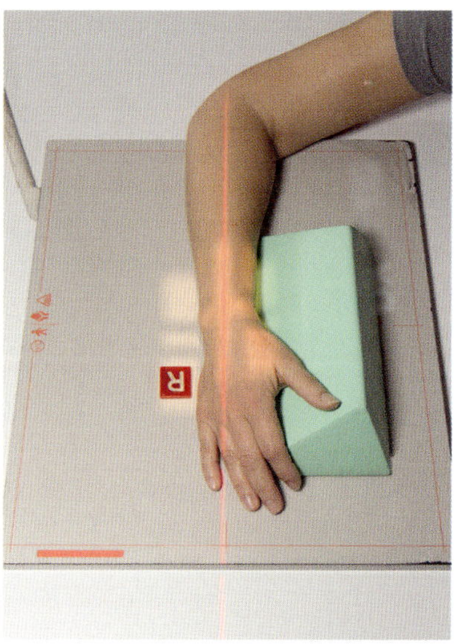

5-58 Suggested anatomic marker placement for flat or oblique part positions.

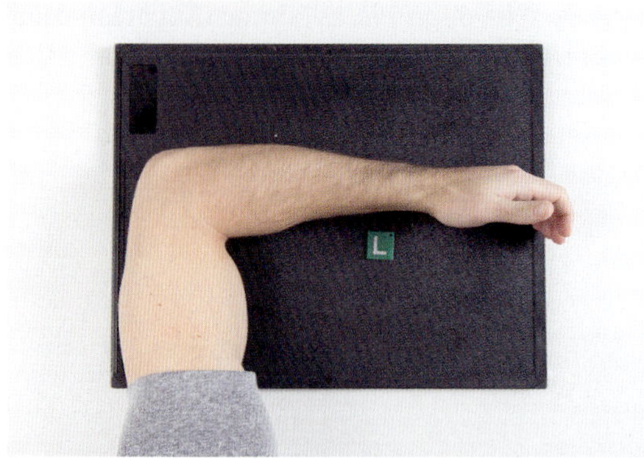

5-59 Suggested anatomic marker placement for a lateral part position.

Viewing the Image

When viewing the upper extremities such as digits, hand, wrist, and forearm, the image is displayed with the finger tips "up," and as though the viewer's part is directly overlying the image to replicate how the part was positioned (Figs. 5-60 to 5-63).

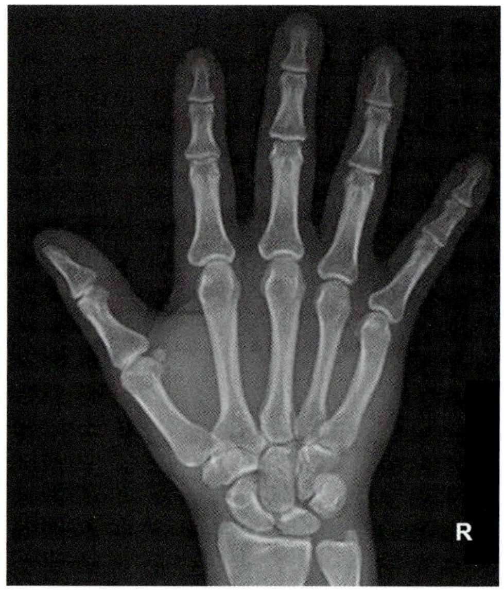

5-60 Proper display of the right PA hand.

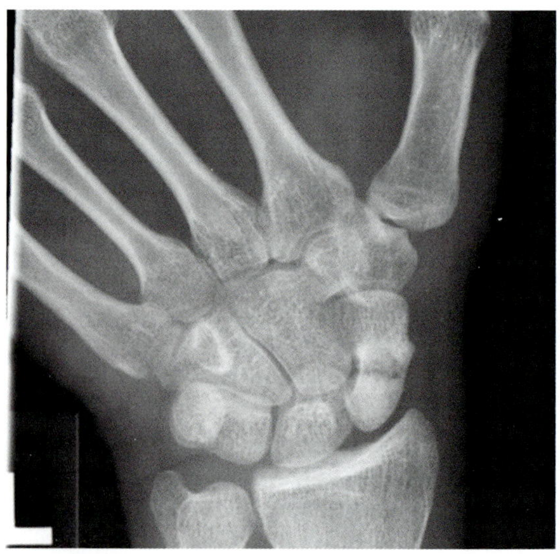

5-61 Proper display of the left PA wrist with ulnar deviation.

Once at the elbow, the image is hung to represent anatomic position, displayed with the shoulder "up" and as though the fingers would be down. Images of the elbow and humerus are displayed opposite the viewer facing it, as though the image is in anatomic position (Figs. 5-64 and 5-65).

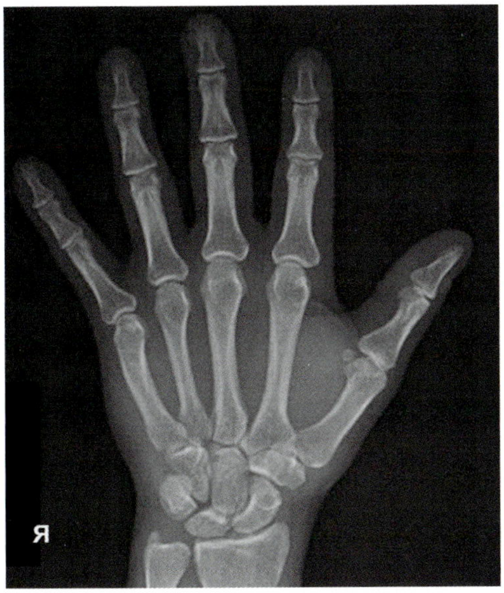

5-62 Incorrect display of the right PA hand.

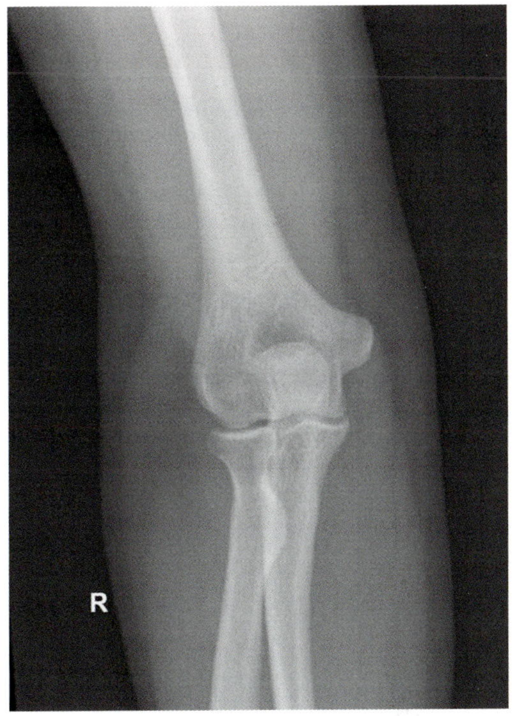

5-64 Correct display of the right AP elbow.

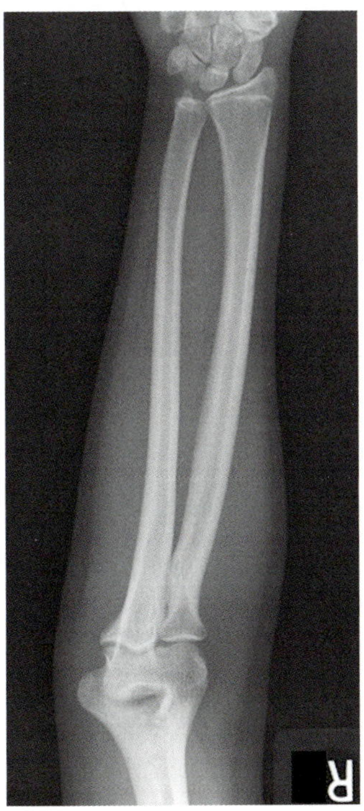

5-63 Correct display of the right AP forearm.

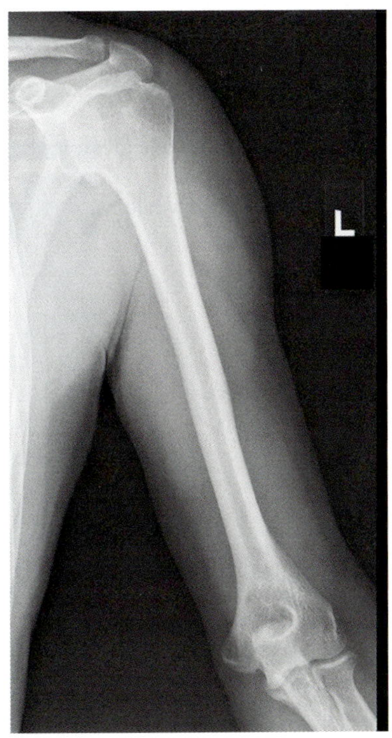

5-65 Correct display of the left AP humerus.

Fingers 2–5

- Projection: PA Oblique of the finger

Fingers 2–5 Protocol
PA Hand or Finger
PA Oblique
Lateromedial/ Mediolateral

Technical Considerations
- kVp 50–60
- mAs set manually
- 40″ SID

Exposure Field Size
- 10 × 12 lengthwise with collimation down to the digit of interest

Patient Position (Figs. 5-72 and 5-73)
- Erect and seated on a stool
- Ensure patient's legs and waist are not positioned directly under the table and beam
- From the pronated hand position, rotate the hand and forearm laterally or medially 45°
- Direction of medial or lateral rotation is determined by rotating the part in the direction that will keep it closest to the image receptor. Typically, the second digit is rotated medially from a pronated position, and digits 3–5 are rotated laterally from a pronated position
- Stabilization of the part could be considered
- Digit positioned should remain extended and parallel to the image receptor

Centering
- PIP joint on the digit in question. Collimate to the digit to include the distal one-third of the metacarpal

Marking of IR
- Anatomic side marker R or L placed furthest from the patient's midline or lateral to the part

Breathing
- No specific breathing instructions given to the patient. Instruct the patient to hold still
- Ensure patient holds position while walking away to make the exposure

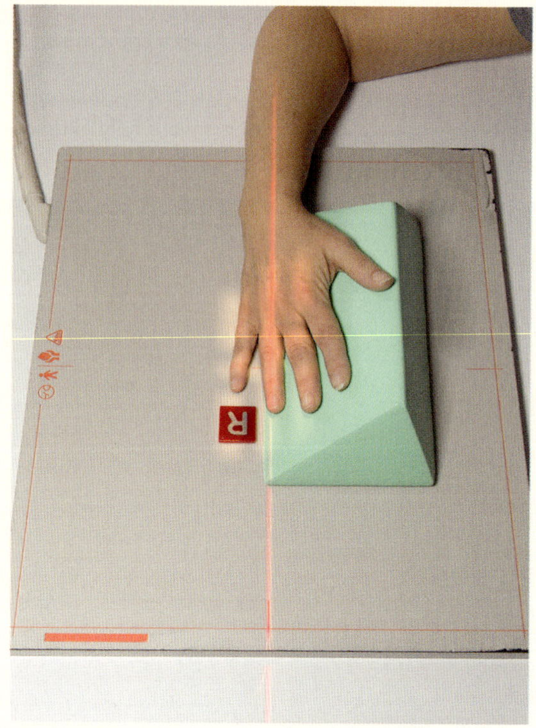

5-72 PA oblique fourth digit—lateral rotation.

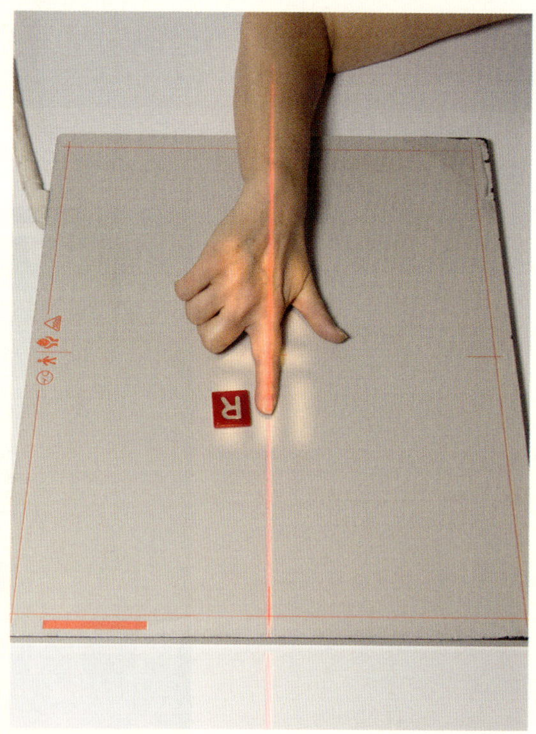

5-73 PA oblique second digit—medial rotation.

IMAGE CRITIQUE (FIGS. 5-74 and 5-75)

- Distal, middle, and proximal phalanx and the distal one-third of the metacarpal in question are demonstrated within the collimated exposure field
- IP joints may appear open if the finger was fully extended and positioned parallel to the IR, allowing the beam to intersect the joint space perpendicularly
- Properly centered with four-sided collimation

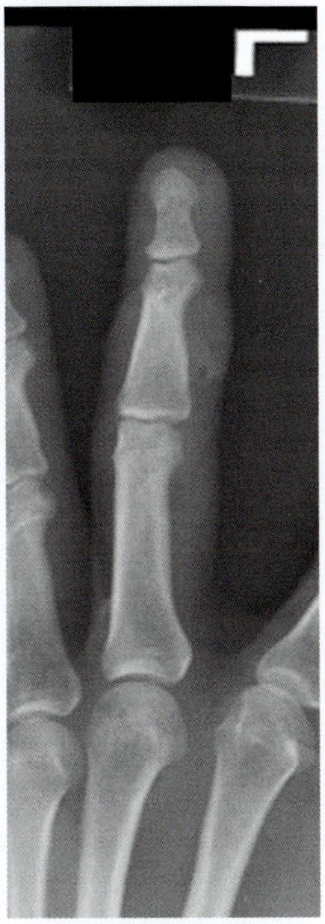

5-74 PA oblique digit.

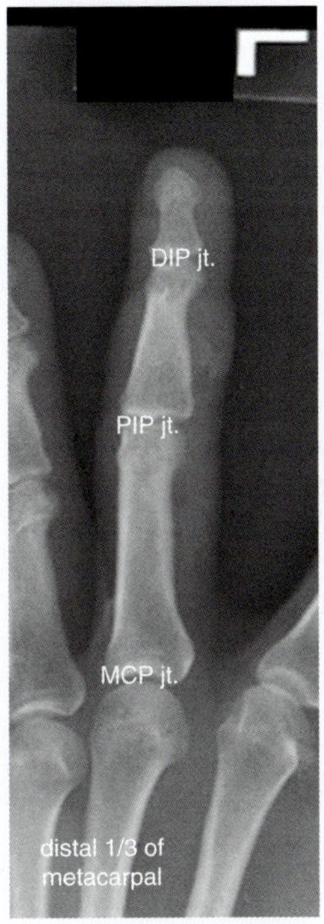

5-75 PA oblique digit.

Fingers 2–5

- Projection: Lateromedial or Mediolateral of Finger

Fingers 2–5 Protocol
PA Hand or Finger
PA Oblique
Lateromedial/ Mediolateral

Technical Considerations
- kVp 50–60
- mAs set manually
- 40″ SID

Exposure Field Size
- 10 × 12 lengthwise with collimation down to the digit of interest

Patient Position (Figs. 5-76 and 5-77)
- Erect and seated on a stool
- Ensure patient's legs and waist are not positioned directly under the table and beam
- From the pronated hand position, rotate the hand and forearm laterally or medially until the digit of interest is in a true lateral position
- Direction of medial or lateral rotation is determined by rotating the part in the direction that will keep it closest to the image receptor. Typically, the second digit is rotated medially from a pronated position, and digits 3–5 are rotated laterally from a pronated position
- Stabilization of the part could be considered
- Digit positioned should remain extended and parallel to the image receptor

Centering
- PIP joint on the digit in question. Collimate to the digit of interest to include the distal one-third of the metacarpal

Marking of IR
- Anatomic side marker R or L placed along the anterior surface or "in front" of the part

Breathing
- No specific breathing instructions given to the patient. Instruct the patient to hold still
- Ensure patient holds position while walking away to make the exposure

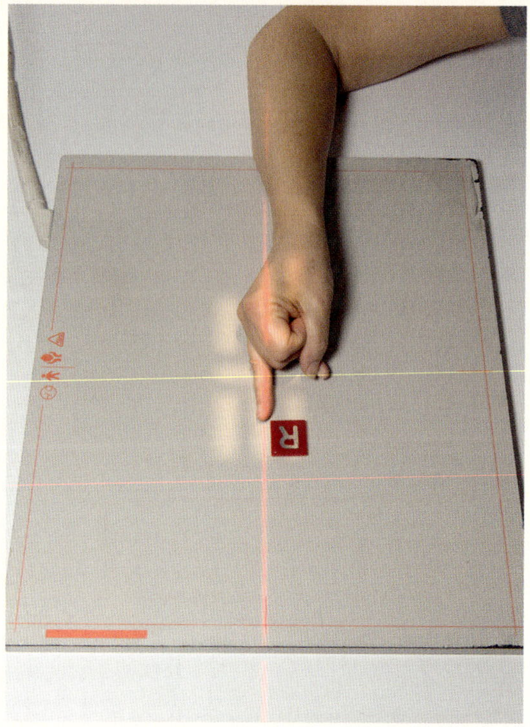

5-76 Lateromedial projection of the fourth digit.

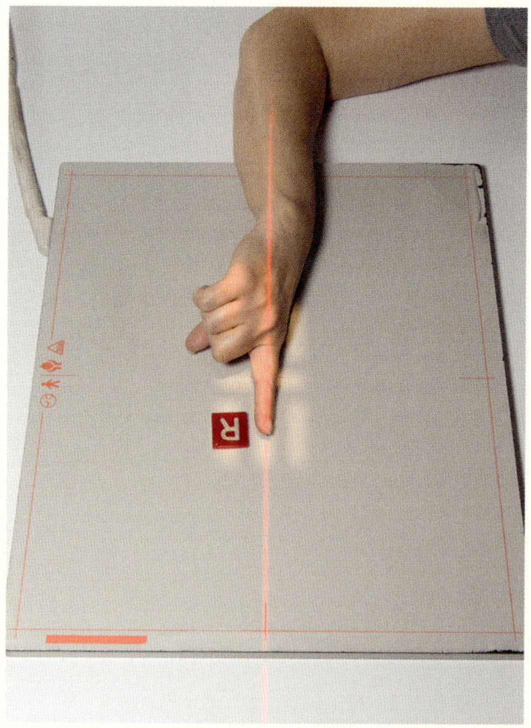

5-77 Mediolateral projection of the second digit.

IMAGE CRITIQUE (FIGS. 5-78 and 5-79)

- Distal, middle, and proximal phalanx and the distal one-third of the metacarpals in question are demonstrated within the collimated light field. The metacarpal will appear with superimposition
- Interphalanageal joints may appear open if the finger was fully extended and positioned parallel to the image receptor, allowing the beam to intersect the joint space perpendicularly
- Properly centered with four-sided collimation

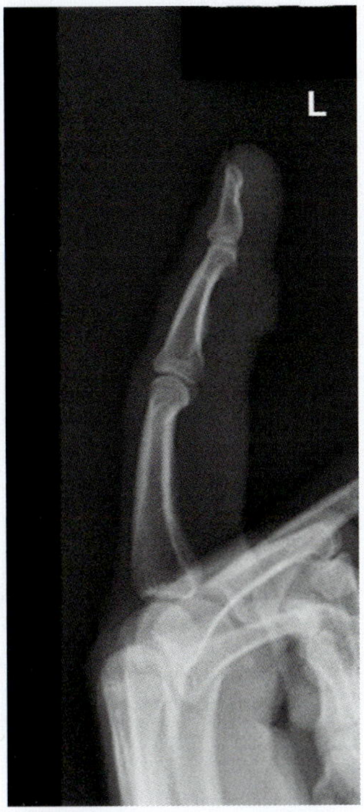

5-78 Lateral digit.

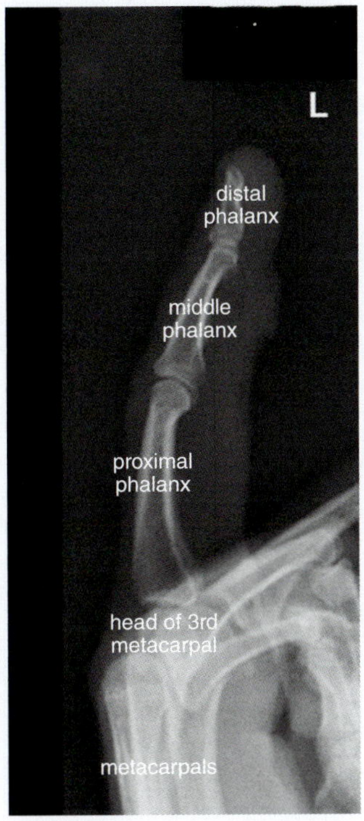

5-79 Lateral digit.

Thumb

- Projection: PA of the Hand

Thumb
PA Hand
Lateral
AP

Technical Considerations

- kVp 50–60
- mAs set manually
- 40″ SID

Exposure Field Size

- 10 × 12 lengthwise

Patient Position (Fig. 5-80)

- Erect and seated on a stool
- Ensure patient's legs and waist are not positioned directly under the table and beam
- Position hand in a pronated (palm down) position with fingers extended and slightly separated
- *Thumb is in an oblique position when the hand is pronated. Therefore, the remaining projections in the protocol of the thumb will be the lateral and AP projections*

Centering

- Third MCP joint when the entire hand is acquired
- First MCP joint when only the thumb is acquired

Marking of IR

- Anatomic side marker R or L placed furthest from the patient's midline or lateral to the part

Breathing

- No specific breathing instructions given to the patient. Instruct the patient to hold still
- Ensure patient holds position while walking away to make the exposure

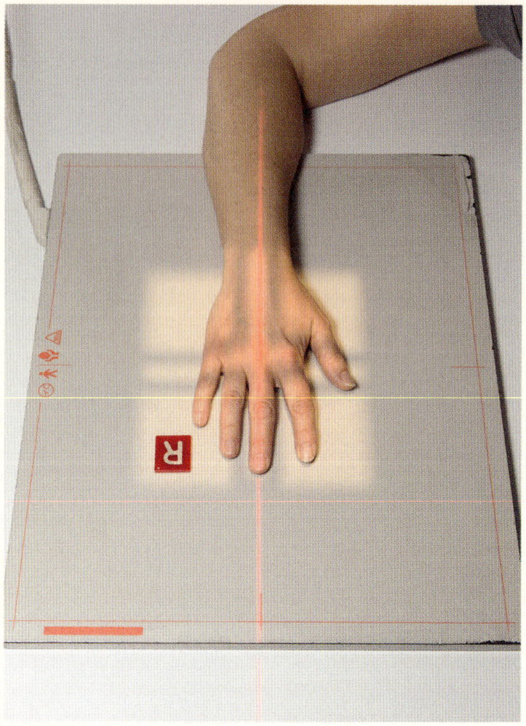

5-80 PA hand—positions the thumb in an oblique position.

IMAGE CRITIQUE (FIG. 5-81)

- Entire hand to include distal phalanges, metacarpals, carpals, and distal radius and ulna. When a complete hand is acquired, the other digits can serve as a comparison to the injured digit. An entire hand will also allow a secondary injury in the hand to be revealed
- Shafts of phalanges and metacarpals 2–5 appear with equal concavity on both sides of the shafts
- The PA projection of the hand will display the oblique position of the thumb. If the only the thumb is acquired, the image must include the distal phalanx, proximal phalanx, first metacarpal, the CMC joint, and the trapezium
- Properly centered with four-sided collimation

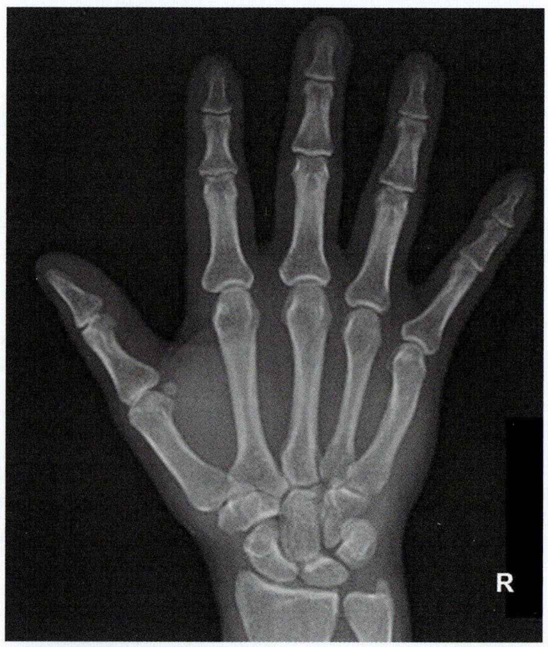

5-81 PA hand.

Thumb

- Projection: Lateral

Thumb
PA Hand
Lateral
AP

Technical Considerations
- kVp 50–60
- mAs set manually
- 40″ SID

Exposure Field Size
- 10 × 12 lengthwise with collimation down to the digit

Patient Position (Fig. 5-82)
- Erect and seated on a stool
- Ensure patient's legs and waist are not positioned directly under the table and beam
- From a pronated hand position, evert digits 2–5 away from the thumb, and use digits 2–5 to push thumb from the oblique position up into a true lateral position

Centering
- First MCP joint

Marking of IR
- Anatomic side marker R or L placed along the anterior surface or "in front" of part

Breathing
- No specific breathing instructions given to the patient. Instruct the patient to hold still
- Ensure patient holds position while walking away to make the exposure

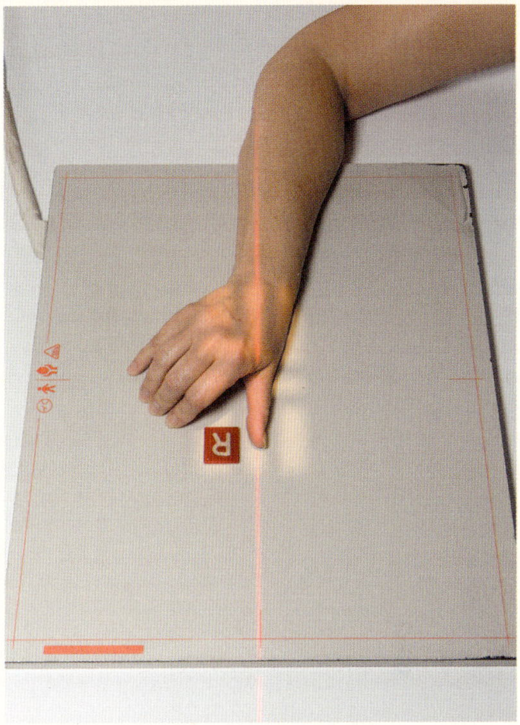

5-82 Lateral thumb.

IMAGE CRITIQUE (FIGS. 5-83 and 5-84)

- Distal phalanx, proximal phalanx, the entire first metacarpal, the CMC joint, and trapezium are included within the collimated light field
- It is imperative that the base of the first metacarpal and CMC joint are well demonstrated to rule out a Bennett's fracture
- Ensure sufficient eversion of the second metacarpal has been attained to avoid superimposition of the first and second metacarpal bases
- Properly centered with four-sided collimation. Proper centering to the MCP joint will allow the collimation to extend just beyond the distal phalanx and will include the CMC joint and trapezium

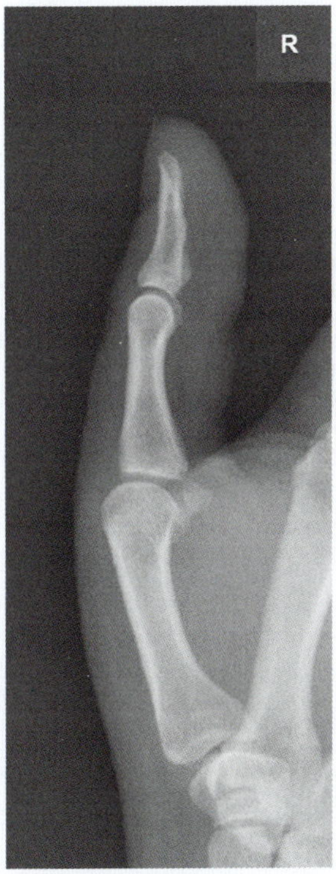

5-83 Lateral thumb.

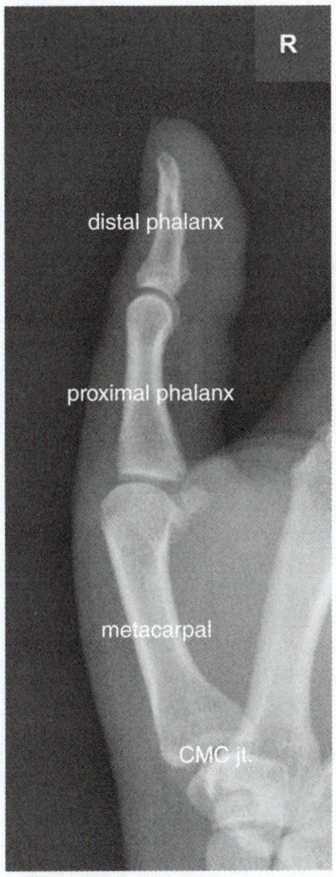

5-84 Lateral thumb.

Thumb

- Projection: AP

Thumb
PA Hand
Lateral
AP

Technical Considerations

- kVp 50–60
- mAs set manually
- 40″ SID

Exposure Field Size

- 10 × 12 lengthwise with collimation down to the digit

Patient Position (Fig. 5-85)

- Erect and seated on a stool
- Ensure patient's legs and waist are not positioned directly under the table and beam
- From the lateral thumb position, continue to rotate digits 2–5 internally (toward the midline) until the thumb is flat and in a true AP

Centering

- First MCP joint

Marking of IR

- Anatomic side marker R or L placed furthest away from the patient's midline

Breathing

- No specific breathing instructions given to the patient. Instruct the patient to hold still
- Ensure patient holds position while walking away to make the exposure

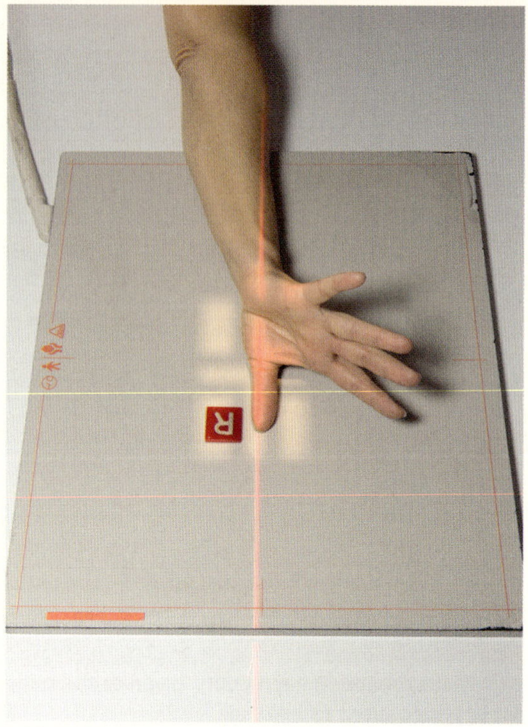

5-85 AP thumb.

IMAGE CRITIQUE (FIGS. 5-86 and 5-87)

- Distal phalanx, proximal phalanx, the entire first metacarpal, CMC joint, and trapezium are included within the collimated light field
- It is imperative that the base of the first metacarpal and CMC joint are well demonstrated to rule out a Bennett's fracture
- Ensure digits 2–5 are extended away from the thumb to prevent superimposition over the base of the first metacarpal
- Properly centered with four-sided collimation. Proper centering to the MCP joint will allow the collimation to extend just beyond the distal phalanx and will include the CMC joint and trapezium

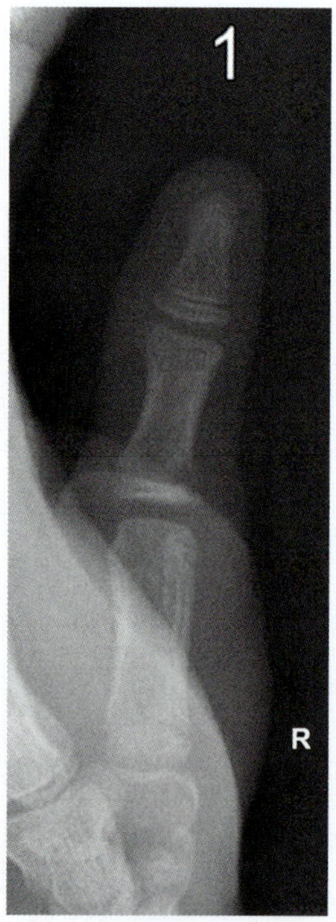

5-86 AP thumb.

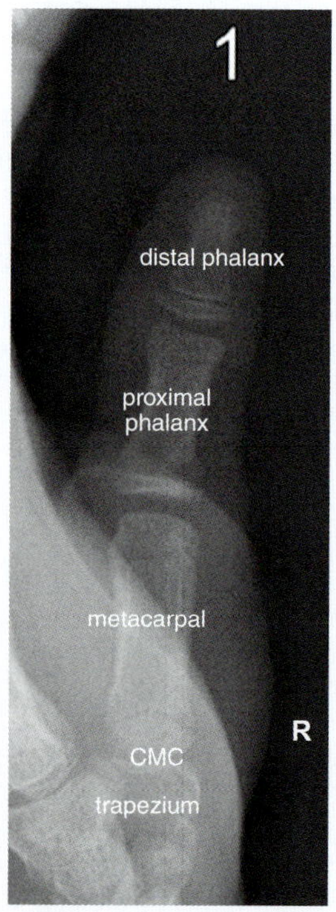

5-87 AP thumb.

Hand

- Projection: PA

Hand Protocol
PA
PA Oblique
Lateromedial

Technical Considerations
- kVp 50–60
- mAs set manually
- 40″ SID

Exposure Field Size
- 10 × 12 lengthwise

Patient Position (Fig. 5-88)
- Erect and seated on a stool
- Ensure patient's legs and waist are not positioned directly under the table and beam
- Position hand in a pronated (palm down) position with fingers extended and slightly separated

Centering
- Third MCP joint. Collimate down to the region of interest including all fingertips and the distal radius and ulna

Marking of IR
- Anatomic side marker R or L furthest from the patient's midline or lateral to the part

Breathing
- No specific breathing instructions given to the patient. Instruct the patient to hold still
- Ensure patient holds position while walking away to make the exposure

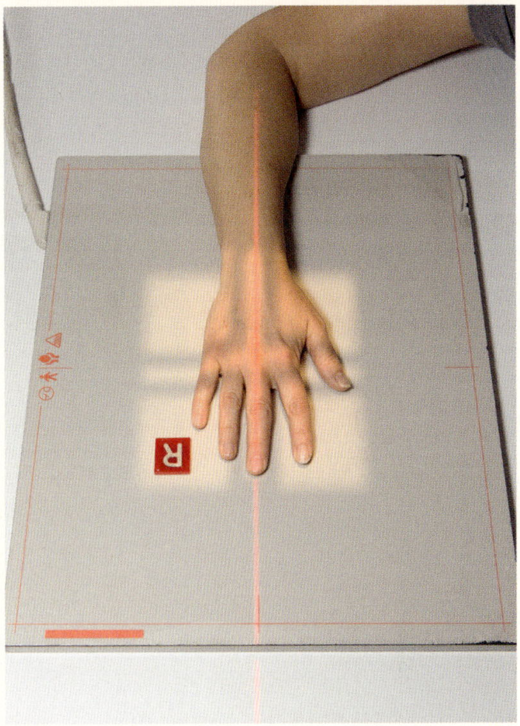

5-88 PA hand.

IMAGE CRITIQUE (FIG. 5-89)

- Entire hand to include distal phalanges, metacarpals, carpals, and distal radius and ulna included within the collimated light field
- Shafts of phalanges and metacarpals appear with equal concavity on both sides of the shafts
- Properly centered with four-sided collimation

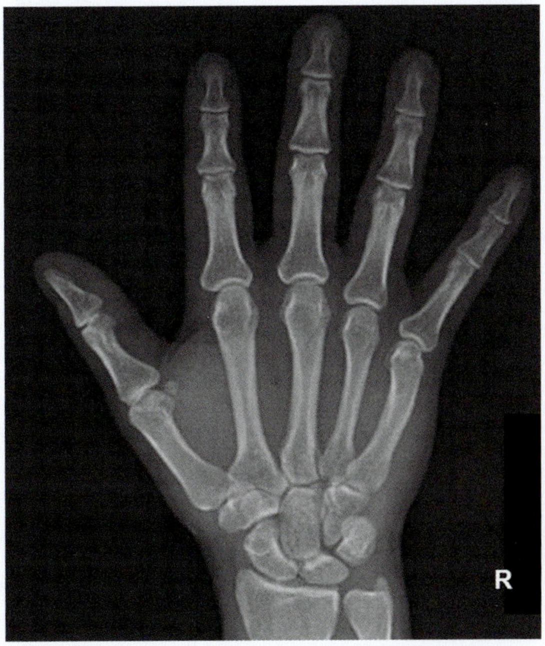

5-89 PA hand.

EXAM ORDER VARIATION: BONE AGE (FIG. 5-90)

Bone Age imaging may be acquired for pediatric patients to evaluate the development of carpals and evaluation of growth plates to determine pediatric patients that may be lagging behind in growth. If a bone age exam is requested, a single PA projection of the left hand is acquired. Utilizing the left hand provides a standardization of the protocol and provides consistency for image interpretations, especially in cases where serial images are compared. The image allows for observation of growth plates and development of carpal bones according to the child's age compared to what has been established for the normal growth/development for a child of that same age.

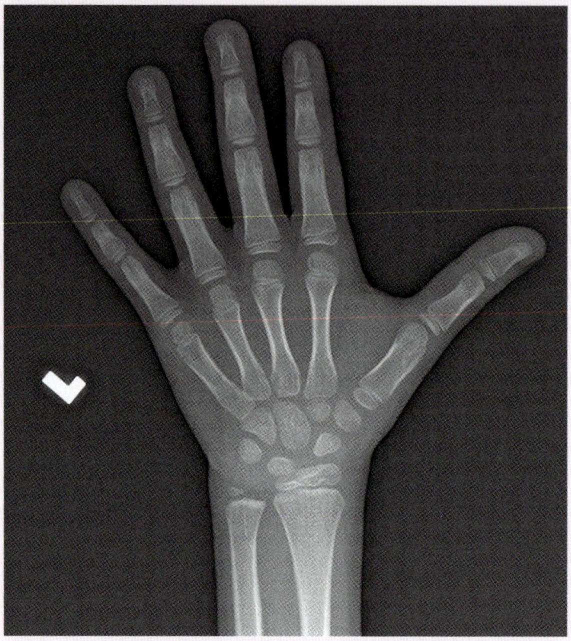

5-90 Bone age.

Hand

- Projection: PA Oblique

Hand Protocol
PA
PA Oblique
Lateromedial

Technical Considerations

- kVp 50–60
- mAs set manually
- 40″ SID

Exposure Field Size

- 10 × 12 lengthwise

Patient Position (Fig. 5-91)

- Erect and seated on a stool
- Ensure patient's legs and waist are not positioned directly under the table and beam
- From the pronated hand position, rotate the hand and forearm laterally 45°
- Fingers should remain extended and parallel to the plane of the IR. This ensures the imaging beam to intersect the joints perpendicularly to demonstrate open joint spaces
- Stabilization of the part could be considered

Centering

- Third MCP joint. Collimate down to the region of interest including all fingertips and the distal radius and ulna

Marking of IR

- Anatomic side marker R or L placed furthest from the patient's midline or lateral to the part

Breathing

- No specific breathing instructions given to the patient. Instruct the patient to hold still
- Ensure patient holds position while walking away to make the exposure

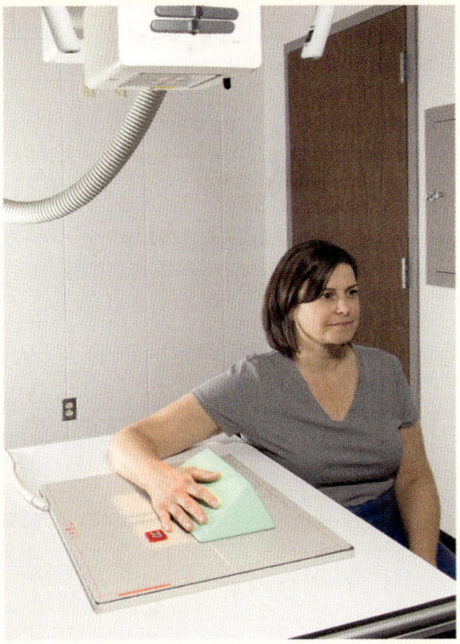

5-91 PA oblique hand—45° lateral rotation.

IMAGE CRITIQUE (FIGS. 5-92 to 5-94)

- Entire hand to include distal phalanges, metacarpals, carpals, and distal radius and ulna within the collimated exposure field
- Correct 45° obliquity is noted when the metacarpal shafts 3–5 have space between them and the heads slightly superimpose one another
- Overrotation of the part will display the shafts of metacarpals 3–5 superimposed
- Underrotation of the part may resemble a PA hand
- IP joints may appear open if fingers remained extended and parallel to the plane of the IR
- Properly centered with four-sided collimation

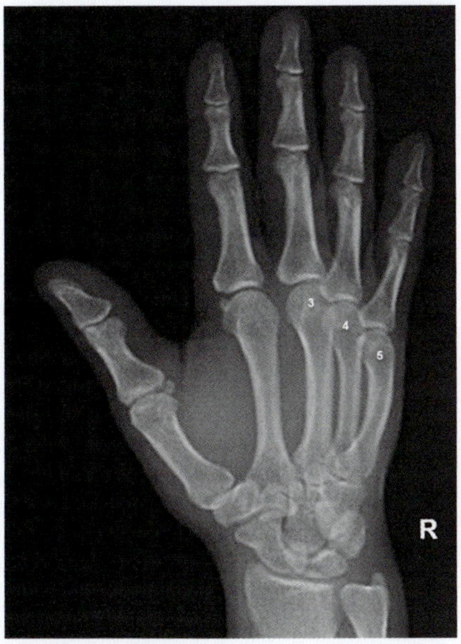

5-92 PA oblique hand—45° lateral rotation.

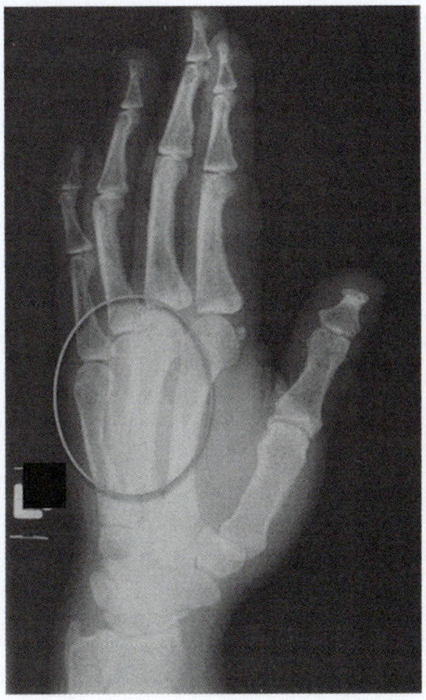

5-93 PA oblique hand—overrotation.

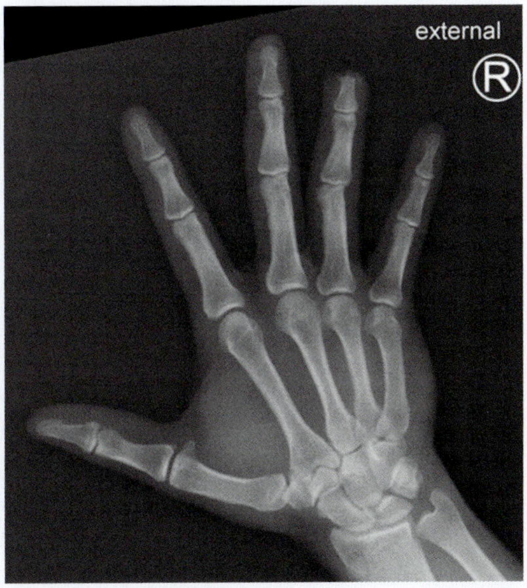

5-94 PA oblique hand—underrotation.

Hand

- Projection: Lateromedial

Hand Protocol
PA
PA Oblique
Lateromedial

Technical Considerations
- kVp 50–60
- mAs set manually
- 40″ SID

Exposure Field Size
- 10 × 12 lengthwise

Patient Position (Fig. 5-95)
- Erect and seated on a stool
- Ensure patient's legs and waist are not positioned directly under the table and beam
- Position hand with the thumb side "up," leaving the medial surface (refer to anatomic position) closest to the IR
- Ensure the hand, distal radius, and ulna are superimposed
- Separate the phalanges, by fanning apart, but trying to keep the fingers fully extended

Centering
- Second MCP joint. Collimate down to the region of interest including all fingertips and the distal radius and ulna

Marking of IR
- Anatomic side marker R or L placed anterior or "in front" of the part

Breathing
- No specific breathing instructions given to the patient. Instruct the patient to hold still
- Ensure patient holds position while walking away to make the exposure

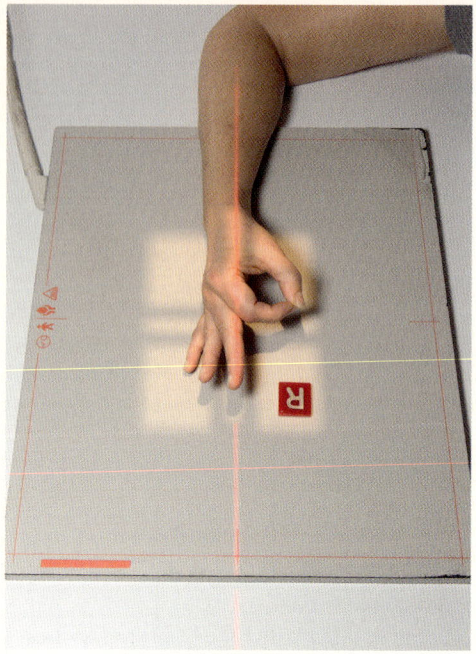

5-95 Lateromedial hand.

IMAGE CRITIQUE (FIGS. 5-96 and 5-97)
- Entire hand to include distal phalanges, metacarpals, carpals, and distal radius and ulna within the collimated exposure field
- Distal radius and ulna should appear superimposed
- Anterior to posterior displacement of anatomy can be determined
- Metacarpals are of primary interest and should be superimposed
- IP joints open, indicating the digits were parallel to the IR and central ray intersected the digit(s) perpendicularly
- Properly centered with four-sided collimation

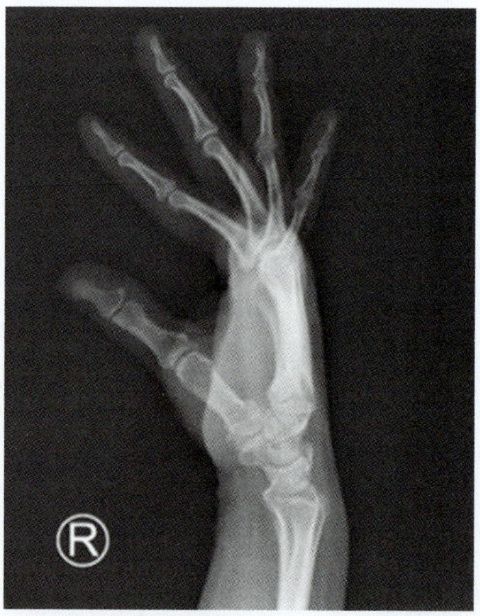

5-96 Lateromedial hand.

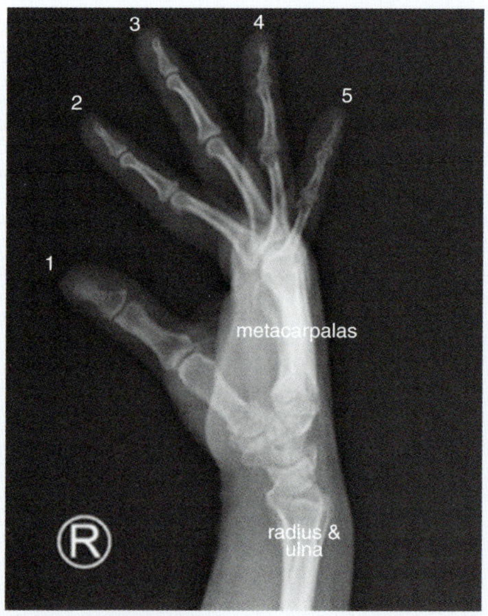

5-97 Lateromedial hand.

POSITION VARIATION: FLEXION AND EXTENSION LATERALS (FIGS. 5-98 and 5-99)

Upon request, the patient's lateral hand position could be varied to supplement with additional views. Comparative lateral projections are acquired with the hand in full extension and flexion positions. These comparative views may assist with determination of foreign body placement or metacarpal fracture displacement. If acquired for foreign body localization, the technical settings, specifically kVp, may need to be decreased to avoid overpenetration if wood or glass is the foreign object.

- The hand extension lateral position will stack digits 2–5 fully extended and in line with the metacarpals and distal radius and ulna.
- The hand flexion lateral will stack digits 2–5 fully extended, and flexion is then added at the MCP joints.

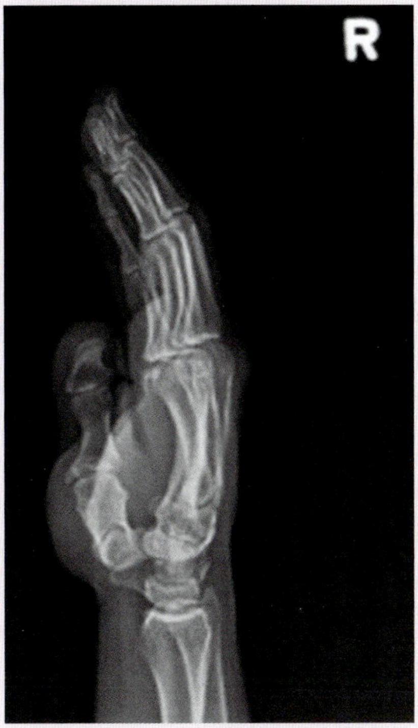

5-98 Lateral hand in extension.

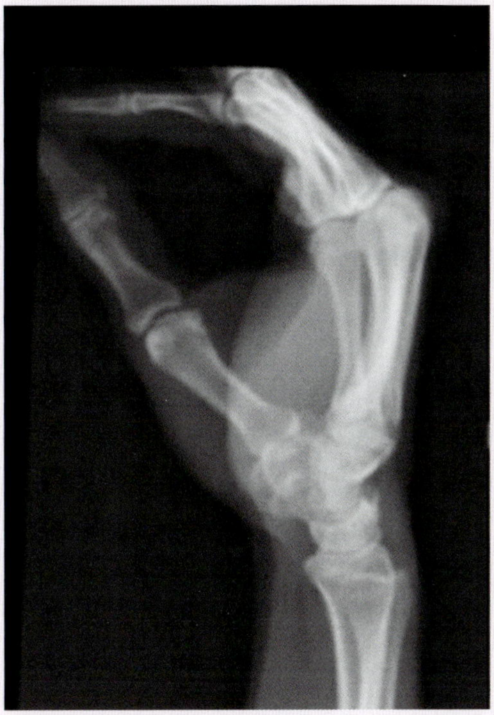

5-99 Lateral hand in flexion.

Wrist

- Projection: PA

Wrist Protocol
PA
PA Oblique
Lateromedial

Technical Considerations
- kVp 50–60
- mAs set manually
- 40″ SID

Exposure Field Size
- 10 × 12 lengthwise with collimation down to the wrist

Patient Position (Fig. 5-100)
- Erect and seated on a stool
- Ensure patient's legs and waist are not positioned directly under the table and beam
- Position hand in a pronated (palm down) position with fingers slightly cuffed under
- *Slight cuffing of the fingers will drop the carpals closer to the IR (reduced object to image distance [OID]), providing improved spatial resolution*

Centering
- Midcarpal region (bend of the wrist). Collimate to include mid-metacarpals and the distal radius and ulna

Marking of IR
- Anatomic side marker R or L placed furthest from the patient's midline or lateral to the part

Breathing
- No specific breathing instructions given to the patient. Instruct the patient to hold still
- Ensure patient holds position while walking away to make the exposure

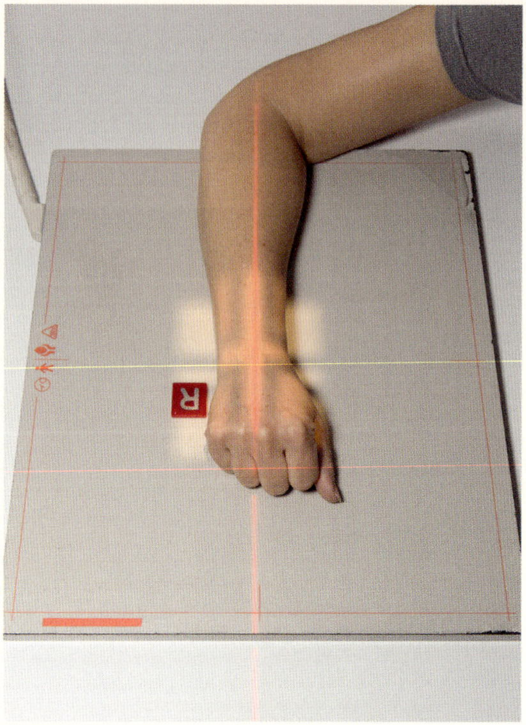

5-100 PA wrist.

IMAGE CRITIQUE (FIG. 5-101)

- Mid metacarpals, carpals, and distal radius and ulna are of interest within the collimated exposure field
- The radius and ulna will be parallel to one another
- Metacarpal shafts 2-5 will show equal concavity
- Properly centered with four-sided collimation

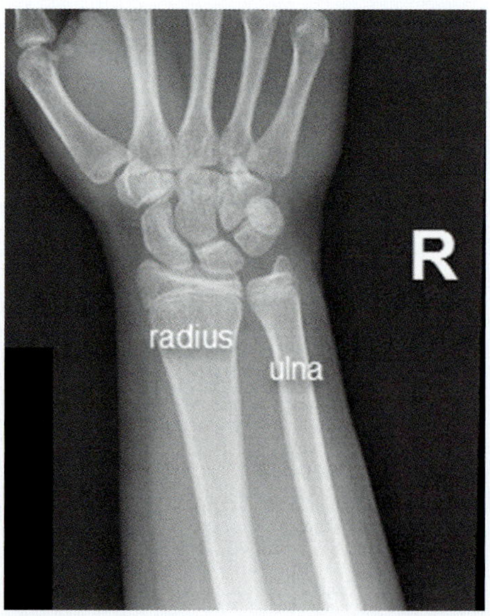

5-101 PA wrist.

Wrist

- Projection: PA Oblique

Wrist Protocol
PA
PA Oblique
Lateromedial

Technical Considerations

- kVp 50–60
- mAs set manually
- 40″ SID

Exposure Field Size

- 10 × 12 lengthwise with collimation down to the wrist

Patient Position (Fig. 5-102)

- Erect and seated on a stool
- Ensure patient's legs and waist are not positioned directly under the table and beam
- From the pronated position, rotate the hand, wrist and forearm laterally (away from midline) 45°
- Stabilize part if necessary

Centering

- Midcarpal region (bend of the wrist) and toward the "upside" of the part to allow even collimated light field on each side of the part to include mid-metacarpals and distal radius and ulna

Marking of IR

- Anatomic side marker R or L placed furthest from the patient's midline or lateral to the part

Breathing

- No specific breathing instructions given to the patient. Instruct the patient to hold still
- Ensure patient holds position while walking away to make the exposure

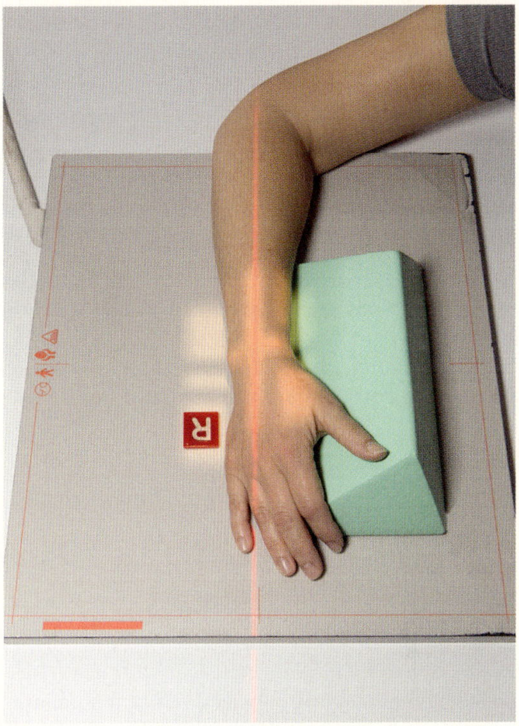

5-102 PA oblique wrist with 45° lateral rotation.

IMAGE CRITIQUE (FIGS. 5-103 and 5-104)

- Mid metacarpals, carpals, and distal radius and ulna are of interest within the collimated exposure field
- The radius and ulna will be parallel to one another but represent some superimposition due to the obliquity
- Scaphoid and trapezium are carpal bones of primary interest
- Carpal superimposition should be observed on the ulnar side of the wrist
- Metacarpal heads of 3–5 will superimpose
- Properly centered with four-sided collimation

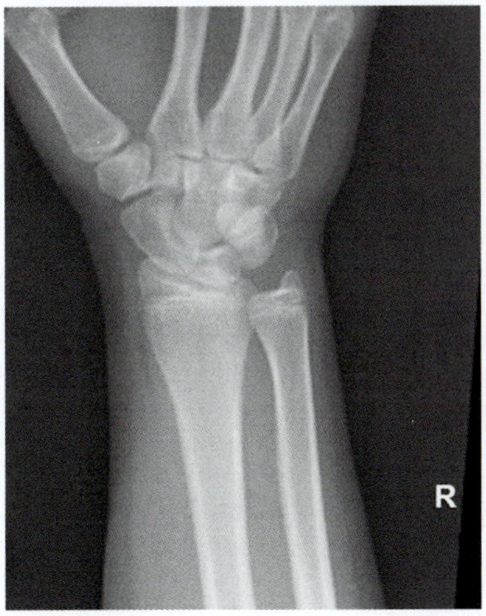

5-103 PA oblique wrist.

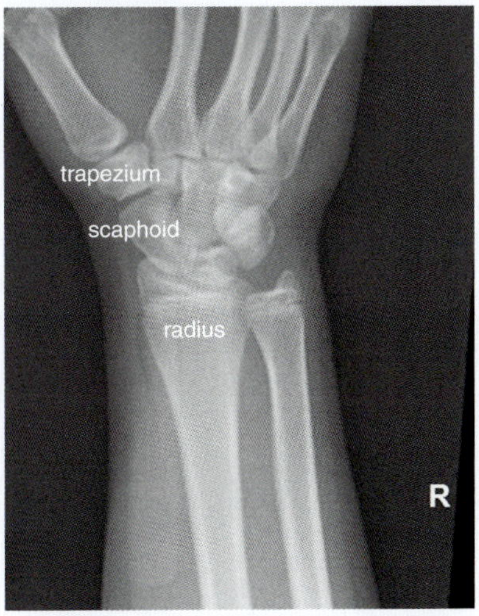

5-104 PA oblique wrist.

Wrist

- Projection: Lateromedial

Wrist Protocol
PA
PA Oblique
Lateromedial

Technical Considerations
- kVp 55–60
- mAs set manually
- 40″ SID

Exposure Field Size
- 10 × 12 lengthwise with collimation down to the wrist

Patient Position (Fig. 5-105)
- Erect and seated on a stool
- Ensure patient's legs and waist are not positioned directly under the table and beam
- From the 45° lateral oblique position, rotate the thumb up until the radius and ulnar are in a true lateral position

Centering
- Midcarpal region (bend of the wrist) to enter upon the lateral surface. Collimate to include mid-metacarpals and the distal radius and ulna

Marking of IR
- Anatomic side marker R or L placed along the anterior surface or "in front" of the part

Breathing
- No specific breathing instructions given to the patient. Instruct the patient to hold still
- Ensure patient holds position while walking away to make the exposure

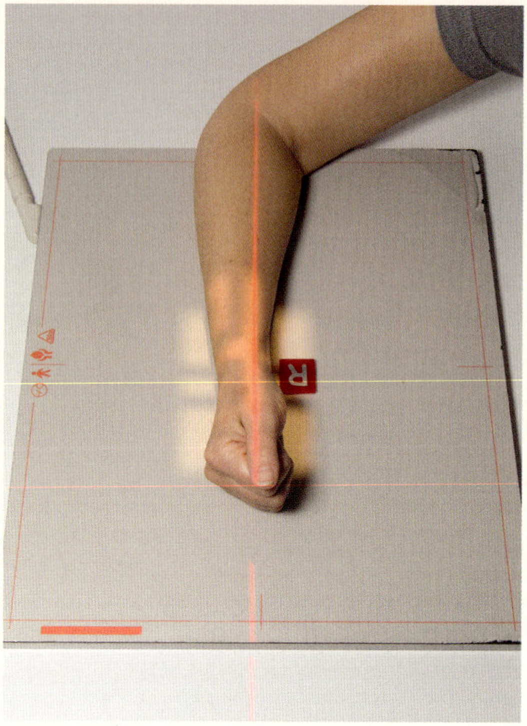

5-105 Lateromedial wrist.

IMAGE CRITIQUE (FIG. 5-106)

- Mid metacarpals, carpals, and distal radius and ulna are of interest within the collimated exposure field
- The radius and ulna should be directly superimposed
- Anterior to posterior displacement of the radius and ulna will be displayed
- Thumb may appear magnified owing to the OID
- Properly centered with four-sided collimation

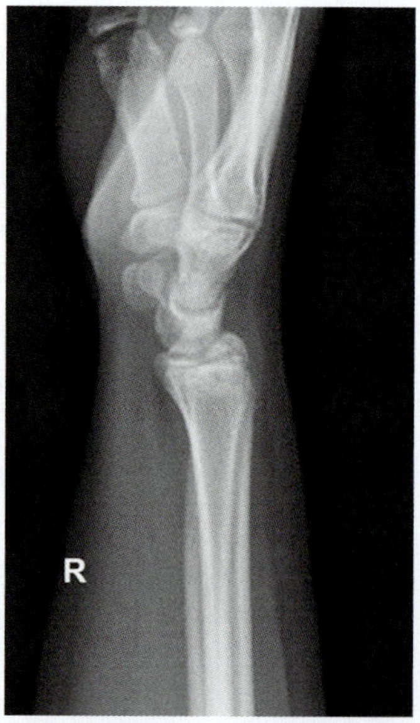

5-106 Lateromedial wrist.

Wrist

- Projection: PA or PA Axial with wrist in ulnar deviation position
- Patient should undergo a prior routine wrist series in order to rule out possible fracture

Technical Considerations

- kVp 55–60
- mAs set manually
- 40″ SID

Exposure Field Size

- 10 × 12 lengthwise with collimation down to the carpals

Patient Position (Fig. 5-107)

- Erect and seated on a stool
- Ensure patient's legs and waist are not positioned directly under the table and beam
- Position hand in a pronated (palm down) position with fingers extended
- Have the patient divert their hand away from midline as far as tolerable. The fifth digit should be directed toward the ulna
- The carpals on the radial side of the wrist, specifically the scaphoid should open up. This stress position may reveal a subtle fracture within the scaphoid

Centering (2 options to consider)

- Perpendicular beam directed to the scaphoid (just distal to the bend of the wrist and toward the thumb side)
  OR
- Direct a 10°–15° cephalic angle (toward the elbow joint) directed to the scaphoid

Marking of IR

- Anatomic side marker R or L placed furthest from the patient's midline or lateral to the part

Breathing

- No specific breathing instructions given to the patient. Instruct the patient to hold still
- Ensure patient holds position while walking away to make the exposure

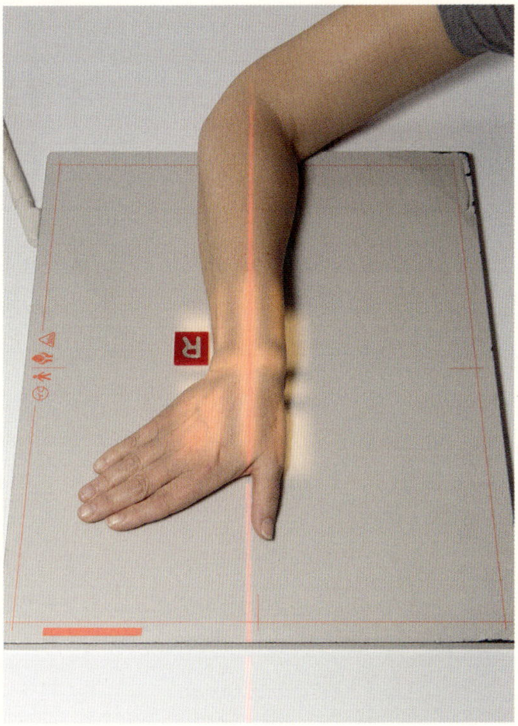

5-107 PA wrist projection with the hand positioned in ulnar deviation.

IMAGE CRITIQUE (FIGS. 5-108 and 5-109)

- Carpals on the radial side, specifically the scaphoid, are of interest within the collimated exposure field
- Scaphoid should be free of superimposition
- Midmetacarpals, carpals, and distal radius and ulna are included
- Properly centered with four-sided collimation

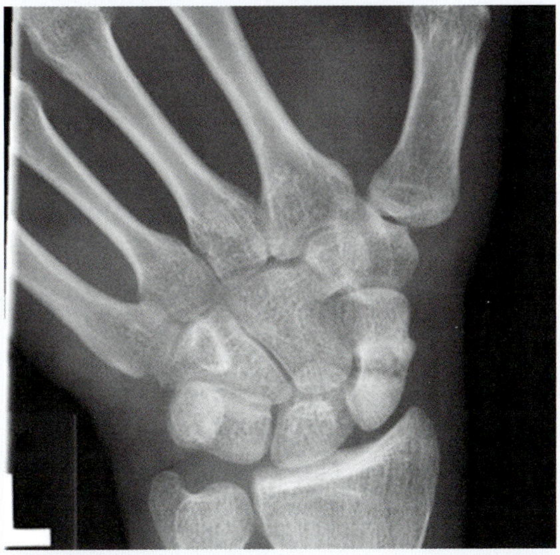

5-108 PA wrist with ulnar deviation.

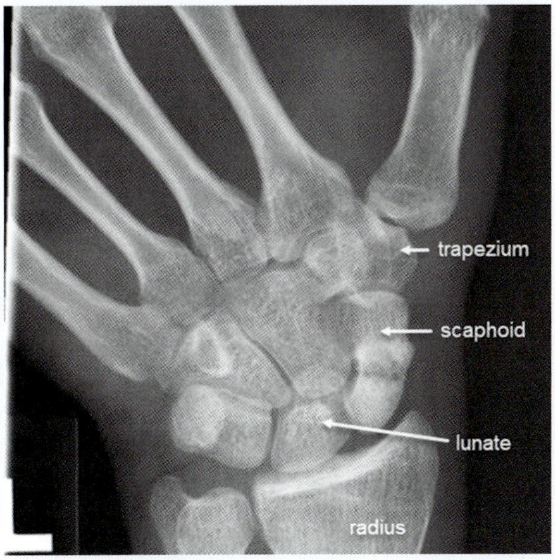

5-109 PA wrist with ulnar deviation.

POSITION VARIATION: MODIFIED STECHER METHOD (FIGS. 5-110 and 5-111)

Modified Stecher method suggests the PA scaphoid with ulnar deviation be acquired with the patient's forearm and hand to be inclined on a 20° wedge sponge. With incline of the part, the scaphoid will align parallel to the IR. With part elevation, the central ray will be directed perpendicularly.

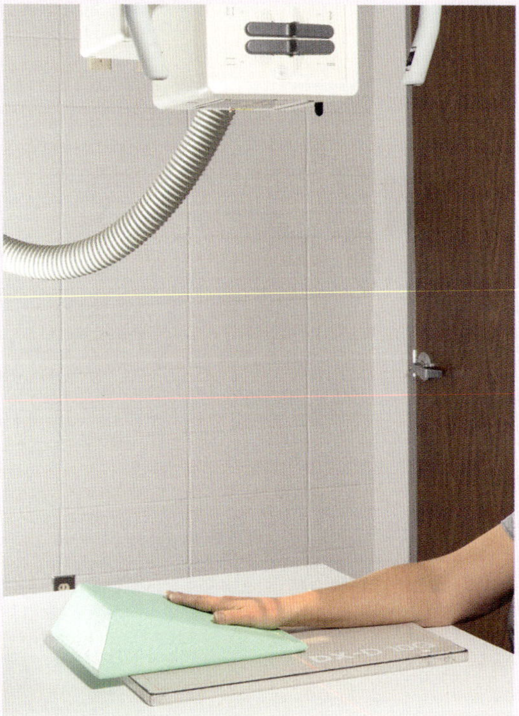

5-110 Modified Stecher.

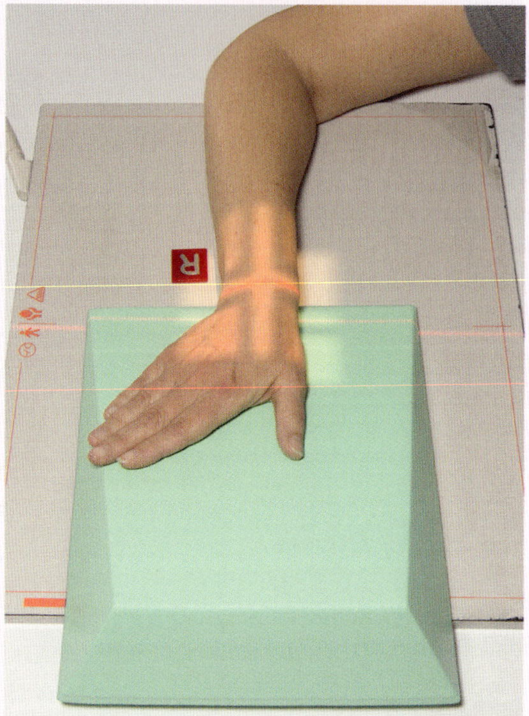

5-111 Modified Stecher.

Wrist

- Projection: Inferosuperior Axial Tangential for Carpal Canal
- Gaynor–Hart method
- Patient should undergo a prior routine wrist series in order to rule out possible fracture

Technical Considerations

- kVp 55–60
- mAs set manually
- 40″ SID

Exposure Field Size

- 10 × 12 lengthwise with collimation down to the carpals

Patient Position (Figs. 5-112 and 5-113)

- Erect and seated on a stool
- Begin with patient's forearm outstretched and hand pronated
- Hyperextend the fingers back toward the shoulder to a point of maximum tolerance by the patient or until the metacarpals are near vertical. Patient can pull back on fingers or use a band to stabilize
- Internally rotate the hand and wrist approximately 10°

Centering

- Begin with the tube in vertical position or at 0° and then angle the tube 25°–30° toward the elbow
- Central ray should be directed to the center of the palm of the hand

Marking of IR

- Anatomic side marker R or L placed furthest from the patient's midline or lateral to the part

Breathing

- No specific breathing instructions given to the patient. Instruct the patient to hold still
- Ensure patient holds position while walking away to make the exposure

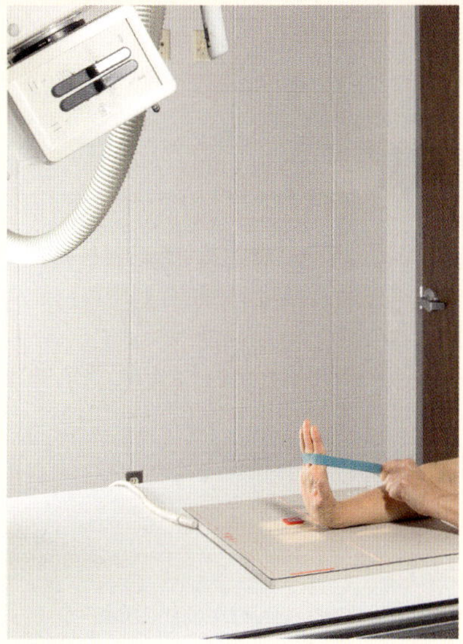

5-112 Inferosuperior axial tangential carpal canal.

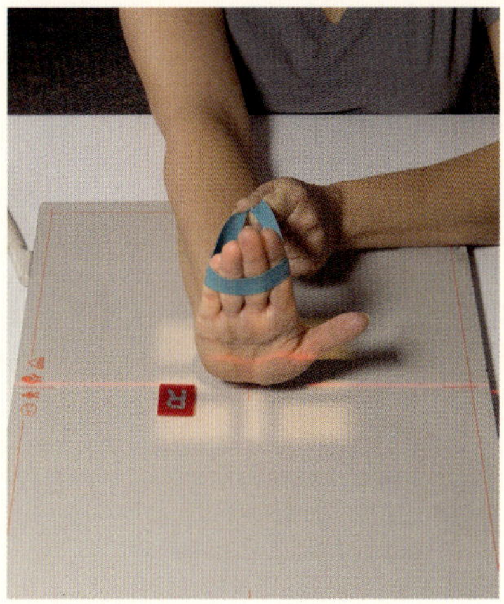

5-113 Inferosuperior axial tangential carpal canal.

IMAGE CRITIQUE (FIG. 5-114)

- Carpals will arrange into an arched appearance within the collimated exposure field
- The pisiform and the hamulus free of superimposition of one another, indicating the wrist and hand were slightly internally rotated
- Properly centered with four-sided collimation

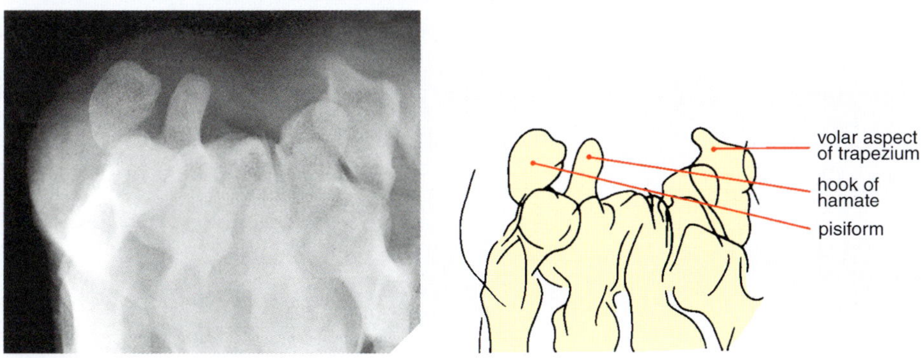

5-114 Inferosuperior axial tangential carpal canal.

Trauma Wrist

- A minimum of two views 90° apart are required
- Trauma extremity routine described here is an example that can be applied similarly to other upper extremities
- Projection: PA

Trauma Wrist Protocol
PA
Mediolateral

Technical Considerations
- kVp 55–60
- mAs set manually
- Technical changes in consideration of a cast. A 3–10 increase in kVp can be considered
- 40″ SID

Exposure Field Size
- 10 × 12 lengthwise with collimation down to the wrist

Patient Position (Fig. 5-115)
- Patient ability and condition may be variable
- Erect and seated on a stool
- Patient may be recumbent on a table or stretcher
- Position hand in a pronated (palm down) position with fingers slightly cuffed under if the patient's condition allows
- If the patient is in the operating room, the IR(s) will be given to the nurse to drop into a sterile covering. The operating room physician and/or nurse will touch the sterile IR and place under the patient's part. The technologist, being very aware of the sterile field, will center to the part and keep the collimation open to include all of the part. Center where designated by the surgeon

Centering
- Midcarpal region (bend of the wrist) unless designated differently by the surgeon. Leave collimation open more than usual

Marking of IR
- Anatomic side marker R or L placed furthest from the patient's midline or lateral to the part
- Marking the IR when imaging in a sterile field (operating room) is not possible

Breathing
- No specific breathing instructions given to the patient. Instruct the patient to hold still. Breathing instructions are not necessary while imaging the patient in the operating room

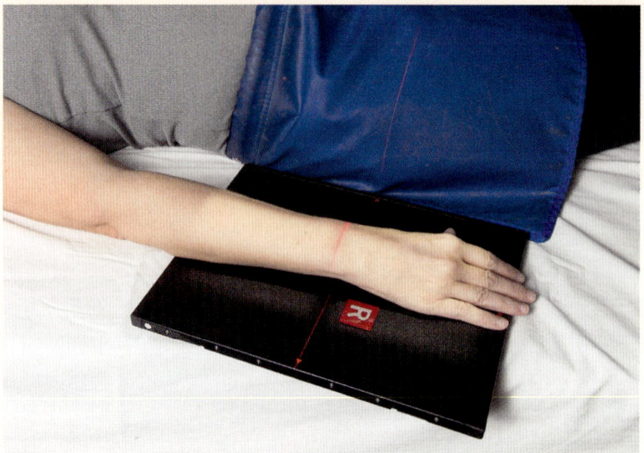

5-115 PA trauma wrist.

IMEDIOLATERALMAGE CRITIQUE (FIGS. 5-116 and 5-117)

- Mid metacarpals, carpals, and distal radius and ulna are of interest within the collimated exposure field.
- The radius and ulna will be parallel to one another
- Properly centered with four-sided collimation
- Images acquired in the OR suite or postoperatively, the collimated exposure field must include surgical metal implants in their entirety
- Patients that are post ORIF (open reduction internal fixation) will require the all-metal plates, wires, pins, and/or screws to be included on the image

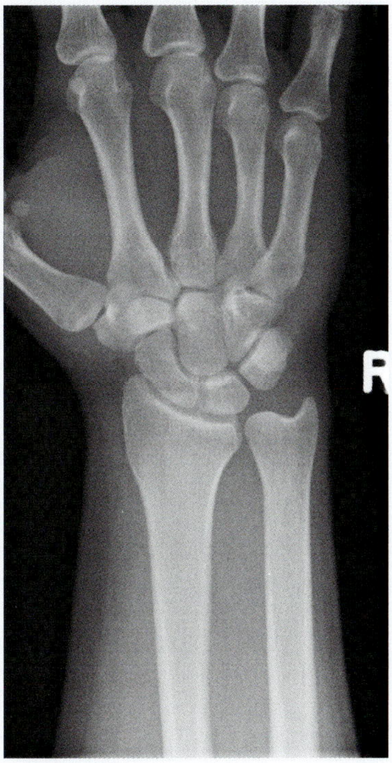

5-116 PA wrist.

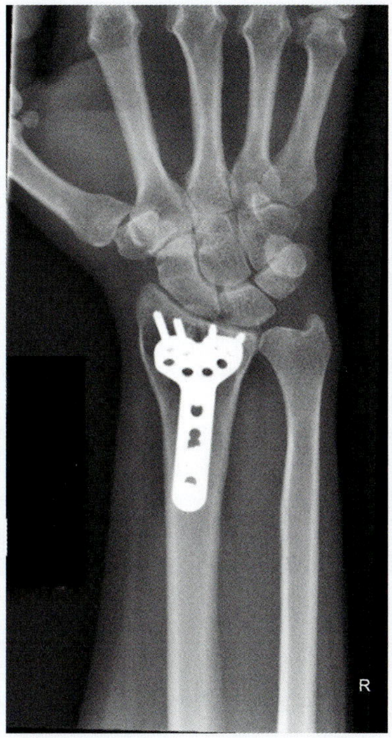

5-117 PA wrist repaired with internal fixation.

Trauma Wrist

- A minimum of two views 90° apart are required
- Trauma extremity routine described here is an example that can be applied similarly to other upper extremities
- Projection: Mediolateral

Trauma Wrist Protocol
PA
Mediolateral

Technical Considerations
- kVp 55–60
- mAs set manually
- Technical changes in consideration of a cast. A 3–10 increase in kVp can be considered
- 40″ SID

Exposure Field Size
- 10 × 12 lengthwise with collimation down to the wrist

Patient Position (Fig. 5-118)
- Patient condition may be variable
- Erect and seated on a stool
- Patient may be recumbent
- Position hand in the best lateral position, rotating the thumb side up or a horizontal beam can be utilized if patient is unable to move the part
- If the patient is in the operating room, the IR(s) will be given to the nurse to drop into a sterile covering. The operating room physician and/or nurse will touch the sterile IR and place under the patient's part. The technologist, being very aware of the sterile field, will center to the part and keep the collimation open to include all of the part. If the part is not positioned lateral, the technologist may have to use a horizontal beam approach to acquire an image 90° from the first image

Centering
- Midcarpal region (bend of the wrist) to enter the lateral surface

Marking of IR
- Anatomic side marker R or L placed along the anterior surface or "in front" of the part
- Marking the IR when imaging in a sterile field (operating room) is not possible

Breathing
- No specific breathing instructions given to the patient. Instruct the patient to hold still. Breathing instructions are not necessary while imaging the patient in the operating room

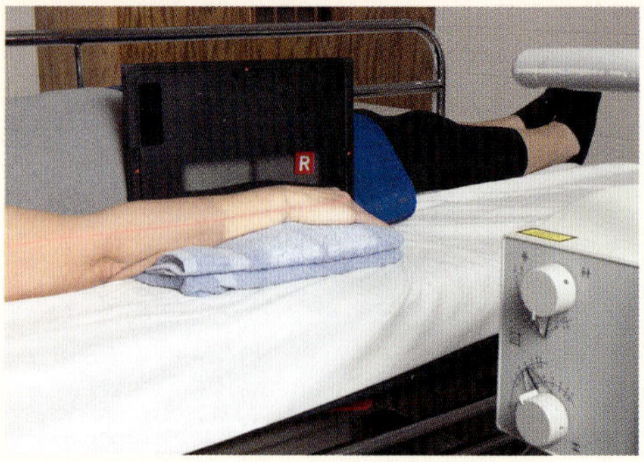

5-118 Horizontal beam lateral wrist.

IMAGE CRITIQUE (FIGS. 5-119 and 5-120)

- Mid metacarpals, carpals, and distal radius and ulna are of interest within the collimated exposure field
- Ideally, the lateral position would demonstrate the radius and ulna superimposed
- Anterior to posterior displacement of the radius and ulna will be displayed
- Properly centered with four-sided collimation
- Patient that are post ORIF will require the all-metal plates, wires, pins, and/or screws to be included on the image

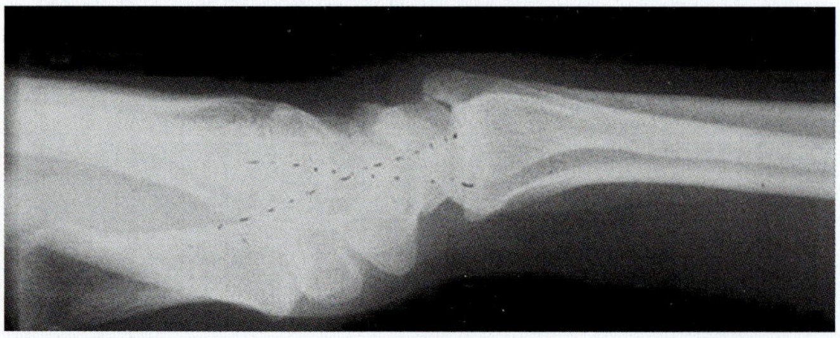
5-119 Horizontal beam lateral wrist.

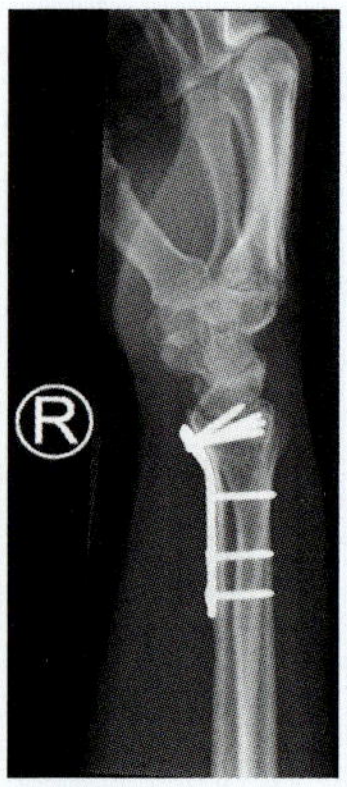

5-120 Lateral wrist with internal fixation.

Forearm

- Projection: AP

Forearm Protocol
AP
Lateromedial

Technical Considerations

- kVp 60–65
- mAs set manually
- 40″ SID

Exposure Field Size

- 14 × 17 lengthwise with collimation down to forearm

Patient Position (Figs. 5-121 and 5-122)

- Erect and seated on a stool
- Ensure patient's legs and waist are not positioned directly under the table and beam
- Fully extend the arm and drop the patient's shoulder down
- Humerus and forearm should both be on the same plane
- Supinate the hand
- *Hand supination is critical in positioning the patient as the radius and forearm will position parallel to one another. Failure to supinate the hand will result in radial and ulnar crossover at the proximal one-third of the forearm*
- Palpate the humeral epicondyles and adjust to align parallel to the plane of the IR

Centering

- Midshaft of the forearm. Collimate to include distal humerus, radius, ulna, and carpals

Marking of IR

- Anatomic side marker R or L placed furthest away from midline

Breathing

- No specific breathing instructions given to the patient. Instruct the patient to hold still
- Ensure patient holds position while walking away to make the exposure

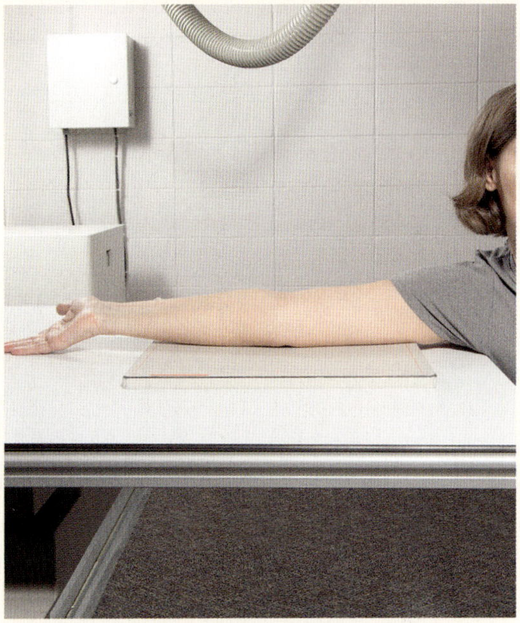

5-121 AP forearm.

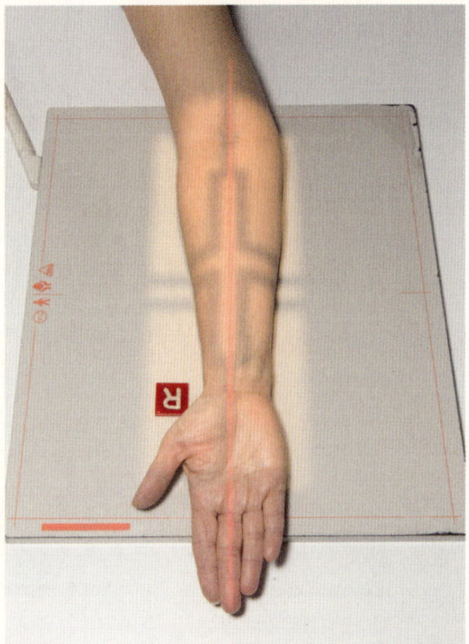

5-122 AP forearm.

IMAGE CRITIQUE (FIGS. 5-123 and 5-124)

- Entire radius and ulna are included along with visualization of both the wrist and elbow joints within the collimated exposure field. Ensure that sufficient distal humerus is visualized to ensure the most proximal end of the ulna is included within the collimated exposure field
- Radius and ulna should appear parallel to one another. Failure to supinate the hand will cause the proximal radius and ulna to cross over
- The humeroradial joint may appear open if the forearm and the humerus were truly positioned on the same plane
- Properly centered with four-sided collimation

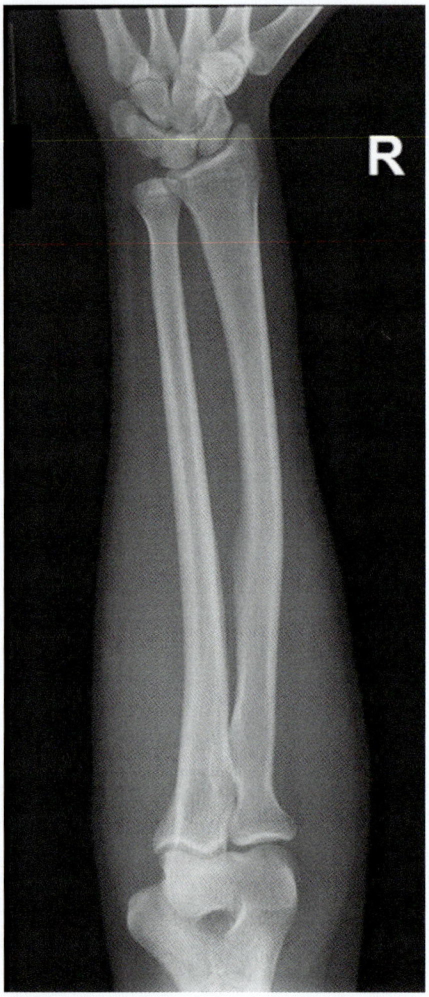

5-123 AP forearm.

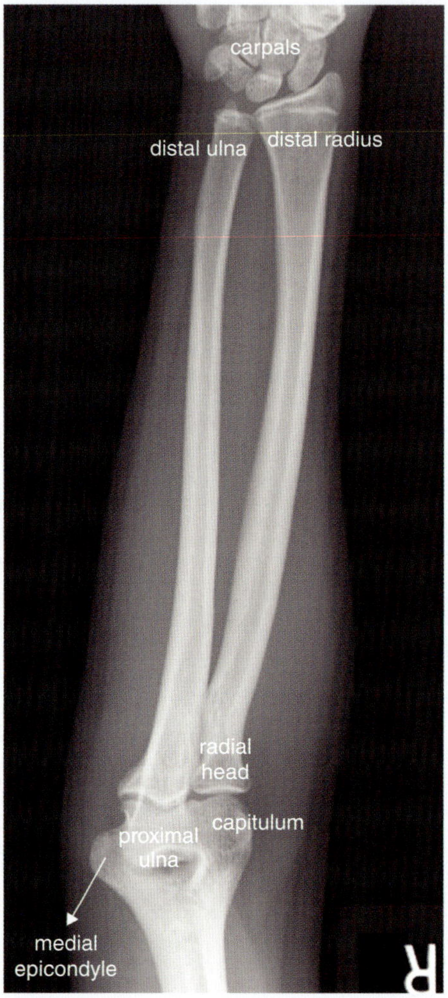

5-124 AP forearm.

Forearm

- Projection: Lateromedial

Forearm Protocol
AP
Lateromedial

Technical Considerations
- kVp 60–65
- mAs set manually
- 40″ SID

Exposure Field Size
- 14 × 17 lengthwise with collimation down to the forearm

Patient Position (Fig. 5-125)
- Erect and seated on a stool
- Ensure patient's legs and waist are not positioned directly under the table and beam
- Bend the elbow 90°
- Position the thumb "up."
- Drop the patient's shoulder down so the forearm and humerus are on the same plane

Centering
- Midshaft of the forearm. Collimate to include distal humerus, radius, ulna, and carpals

Marking of IR
- Anatomic side marker R or L placed along the anterior surface or "in front" of the part

Breathing
- No specific breathing instructions given to the patient. Instruct the patient to hold still
- Ensure you watch the patient the entire time while walking away to make the exposure

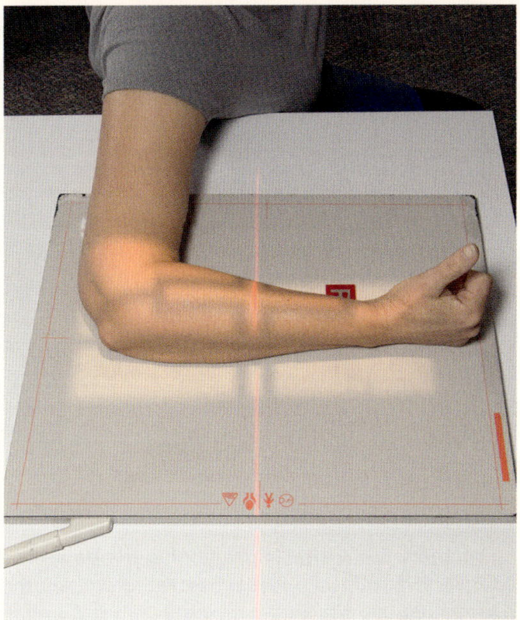

5-125 Lateromedial forearm.

IMAGE CRITIQUE (FIGS. 5-126 and 5-127)
- Radius and ulna will superimpose one another at the wrist. The radius and ulna will separate toward the elbow joint. The radial head will superimpose the coronoid process
- The entire radius and ulna are included along with visualization of the wrist and elbow joint within the collimated exposure field
- Anterior to posterior displacement of the part can be determined
- Properly centered with four-sided collimation

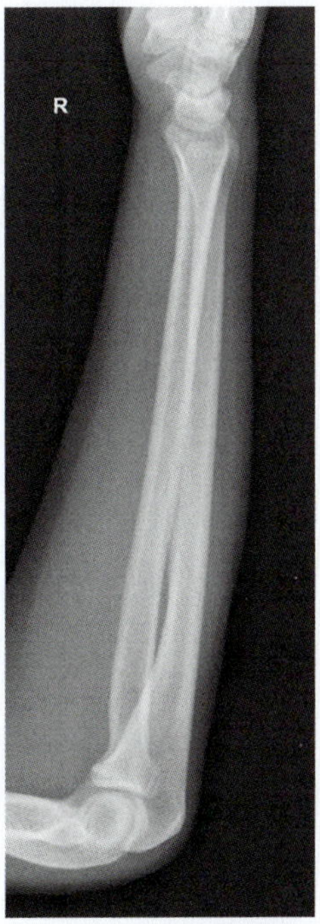

5-126 Lateromedial forearm.

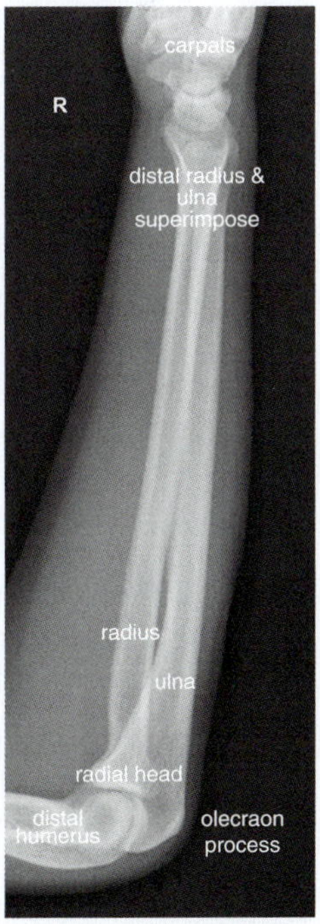

5-127 Lateromedial forearm.

Elbow

- Projection: AP

Elbow Protocol
AP
AP Oblique
Lateromedial

Technical Considerations
- kVp 60–65
- mAs set manually
- 40″ SID

Exposure Field Size
- 10 × 12 lengthwise with collimation down to elbow

Patient Position (Fig. 5-128)
- Erect and seated on a stool
- Ensure patient's legs and waist are not positioned directly under the table and beam
- Fully extend the arm and drop the patient's shoulder down
- Humerus and forearm should both be on the same plane
- Supinate the hand
- *Hand supination is critical in positioning the patient as the radius and forearm will position parallel to one another. Failure to supinate the hand will result in radial and ulnar* crossover at the proximal one-third of the forearm
- Palpate the humeral epicondyles and ensure that they are aligned parallel to the plane of the IR

Centering
- Midelbow joint (bend of the elbow). Collimate to include distal humerus and the proximal radius and ulna

Marking of IR
- Anatomic side marker R or L placed furthest away from midline

Breathing
- No specific breathing instructions given to the patient. Instruct the patient to hold still
- Ensure patient holds position while walking away to make the exposure

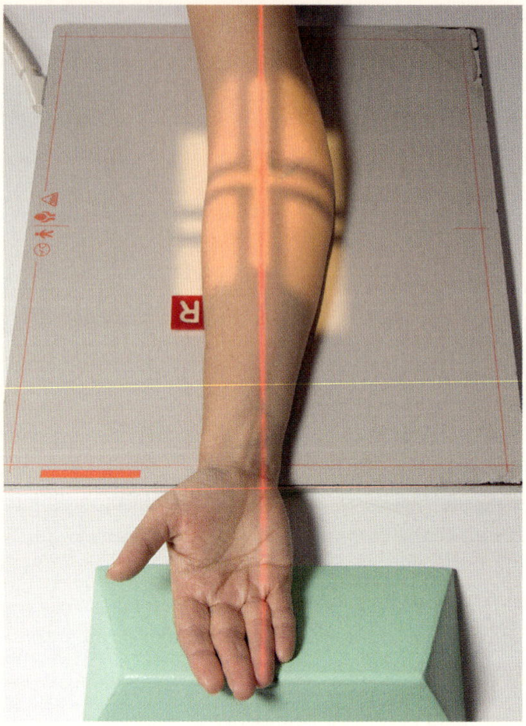

5-128 AP elbow.

IMAGE CRITIQUE (FIGS. 5-129 and 5-130)

- Proximal radius, ulna, and distal humerus are included within the collimated exposure field
- Radius and ulna should appear parallel to one another
- The radial head, neck, and tuberosity will display slight superimposition upon the ulna
- The humeroradial joint is, ideally, open if the forearm and the humerus were truly positioned on the same plane
- The olecranon process will be positioned within the olecranon fossa on the distal and posterior humerus
- Properly centered with four-sided collimation

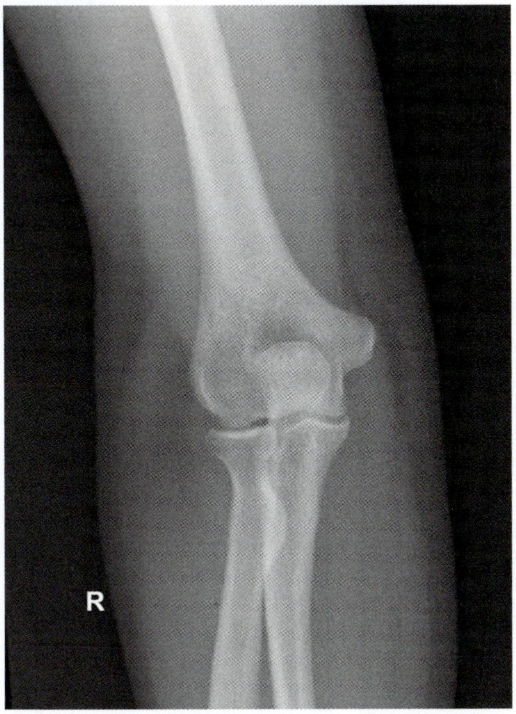

5-129 AP elbow.

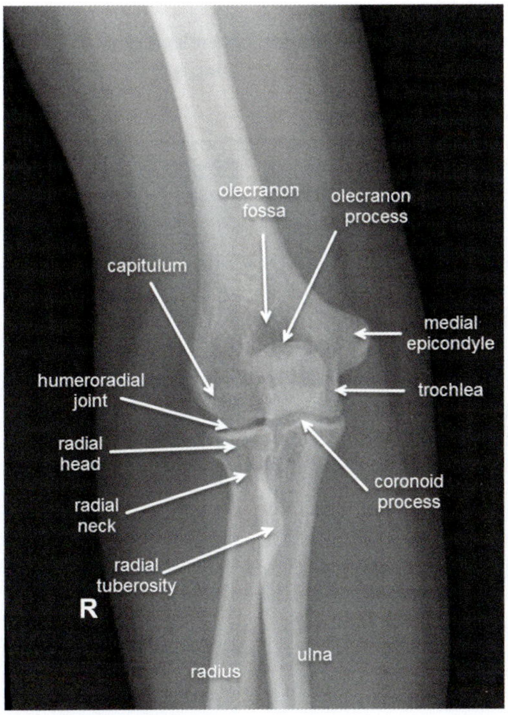

5-130 AP elbow.

Trauma Elbow

- Projection: Axial Lateromedial and Mediolateral
- Coyle method
- Two lateral projections may aid in demonstration of the radial head and coronoid process in a trauma circumstance. These projections can substitute the oblique projections of the elbow when they are unattainable

Technical Considerations

- kVp 60–65
- mAs set manually
- 40″ SID

Exposure Field Size

- 10 × 12 lengthwise with collimation down to the elbow

Patient Position (Figs. 5-155 and 5-156)

- Erect and seated on a stool if patient is able
- Patient may be recumbent if unable to ambulate
- Attempt to drop the patient's shoulder so the forearm and humerus are on the same plane
- *Lateral position to demonstrate the radial head:*
  - Patient's elbow flexed 90° with the hand placed in pronation
  - Axial tube angle of 45° directed toward the shoulder is applied
- *Lateral position to demonstrate the coronoid process*:
  - Patient's elbow flexed 80° with the hand placed in pronation
  - Axial tube angle of 45° directed down from the shoulder

Centering

- Midelbow joint

Marking of IR

- Anatomic side marker R or L placed along the anterior surface or "in front" of the part

Breathing

- No specific breathing instructions given to the patient. Instruct the patient to hold still
- Ensure patient holds position while walking away to make the exposure

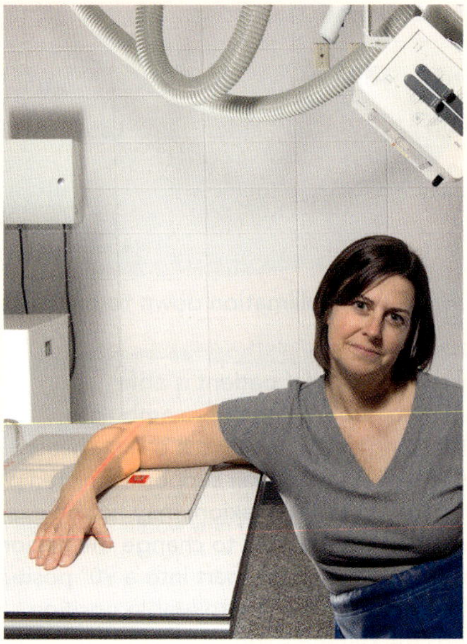

5-155 Coyle method to visualize the coronoid process.

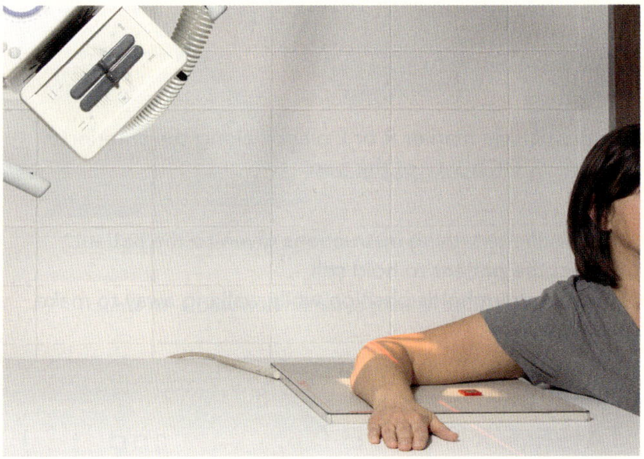

5-156 Coyle method to visualize the radial head.

Humerus

- Projection: Lateromedial or Mediolateral

Technical Considerations

- kVp 65–70
- mAs set manually
- Grid or nongrid could be dependent on exposure location and part thickness
- 40″ SID

Exposure Field Size

- 14 × 17 lengthwise with collimation c

Patient Position (Figs. 5-163 to 5-165)

- Erect or seated on a stool
- Patient may be recumbent
- If the patient is upright, bend the elbc across the abdomen, positioning the I IR. Have the patient face the upright E acquire the humerus with a *mediolate*
- If the patient is upright or recumbent arm from the side of the body. With f arm, internally rotate the hand and ar epicondyles are perpendicular to the Palpate the epicondyles to ensure pr would acquire the humerus with a *lat* (Fig. 5-163)

Centering

- Midhumeral shaft. Collimate to incluc shoulder joint, and elbow joint

Marking of IR

- Anatomic side marker R or L placed f midline

Breathing

- Hold breath and instruct the patient
- Ensure patient holds position while w the exposure

IMAGE CRITIQUE (FIGS. 5-157 and 5-158)

- Axial lateromedial projection with the elbow flexed 90° will demonstrate the radial head and visualize the humeroradial joint space open. The radial head will still have superimposition with the coronoid process. The radial head, neck, and tuberosity will be seen in profile. This axial projection resembles display of the anatomy as seen in the 45° lateral oblique of the elbow (Fig. 5-157)
- Axial mediolateral projection with the elbow flexed 80° will demonstrate the coronoid process. The radial head will superimpose the ulna. The coronoid process will be seen in profile. This axial projection resembles display of the anatomy as seen in the 45° medial oblique of the elbow (Fig. 5-158)
- Midelbow joint properly centered with four-sided collimation

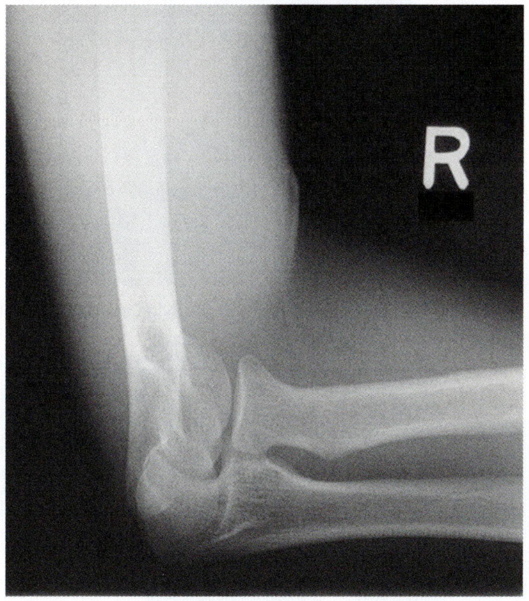

5-157 Coyle method to visualize the radial head.

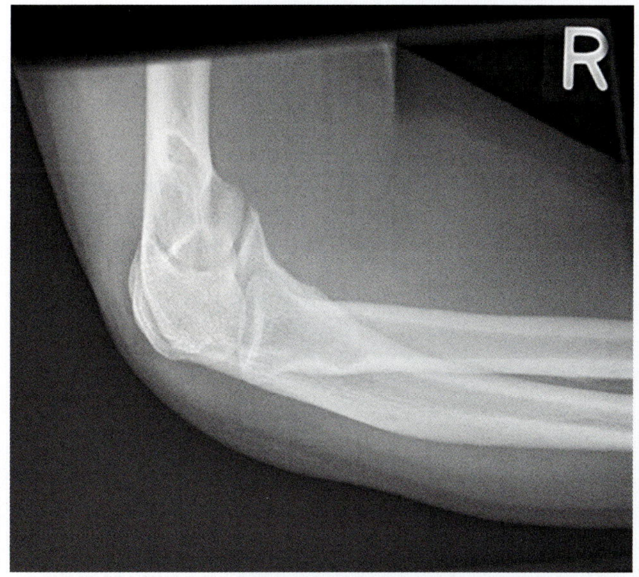

5-158 Coyle method to visualize the coronoid process.

Humerus

- Projection: AP

Technical Considerations

- kVp 65–70
- mAs set manually
- Grid or nongrid could be considered for part thickness
- 40″ SID

Exposure Field Size

- 14 × 17 lengthwise with collimation dc

Patient Position (Figs. 5-159 and 5-160)

- Erect or seated on a stool
- Patient may be recumbent
- Slightly abduct affected arm from the s
- Supinate the hand, create anatomic pc palpate humeral epicondyles to ensure the plane of the IR

Centering

- Midhumeral shaft. Collimate to include shoulder joint, and elbow joint

Marking of IR

- Anatomic side marker R or L placed fu midline

Breathing

- Hold breath and instruct the patient tc
- Ensure patient holds position while wa the exposure

IMAGE CRITIQUE (FIGS. 5

- Entire humerus to include both elbow joint within collimated exposure field
- Greater tubercle visualized laterally ar proper positioning of the humeral epi tubercle will not be visualized as it is s the proximal humerus
- The humeral epicondyles will both be AP elbow appearance
- Properly centered with four-sided coll

IMAGE CRITIQUE (FIGS. 5-166 to 5-168)

- Entire humerus to include both elbow joint and shoulder joint within collimated exposure field
- Lesser tubercle visualized medially adjacent to the glenohumeral joint and in profile with proper positioning of the humeral epicondyles. Greater tubercle will not be visualized as it is shifted from profile laterally and superimposed on the proximal humerus
- The humeral epicondyles will be nearly superimposed with or without a 90° flexion of the elbow
- Properly centered with four-sided collimation

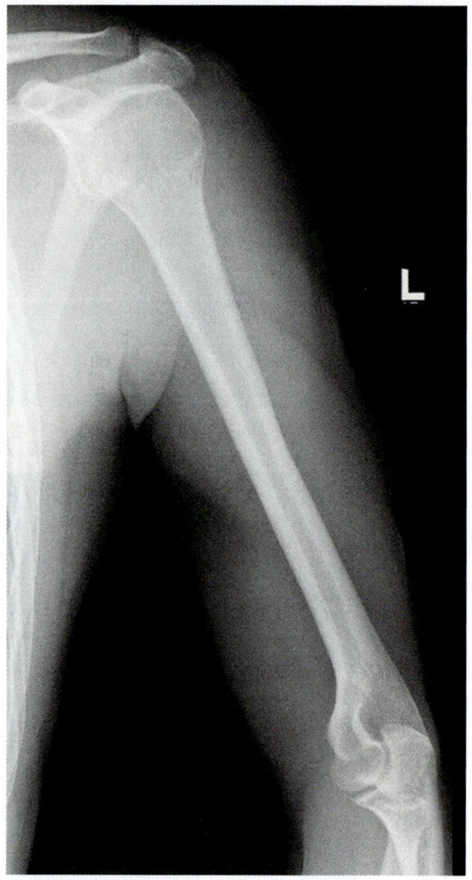

5-166 Lateromedial humerus.

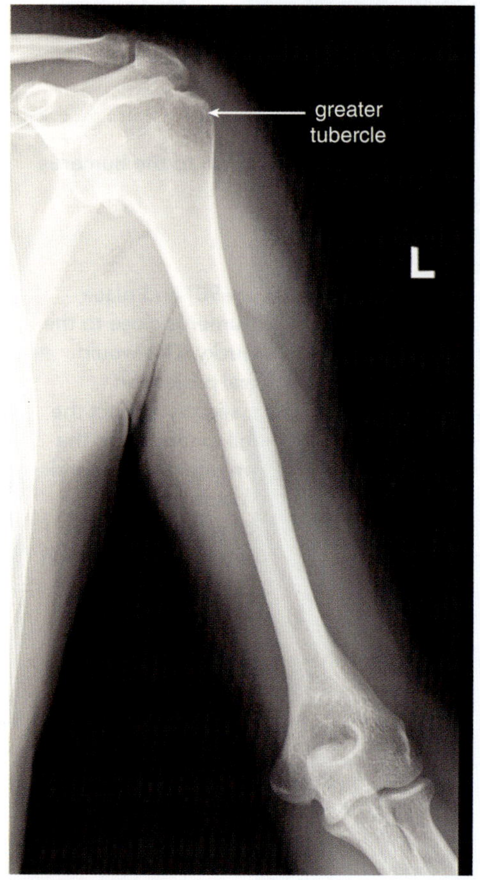

5-167 Lateromedial humerus.

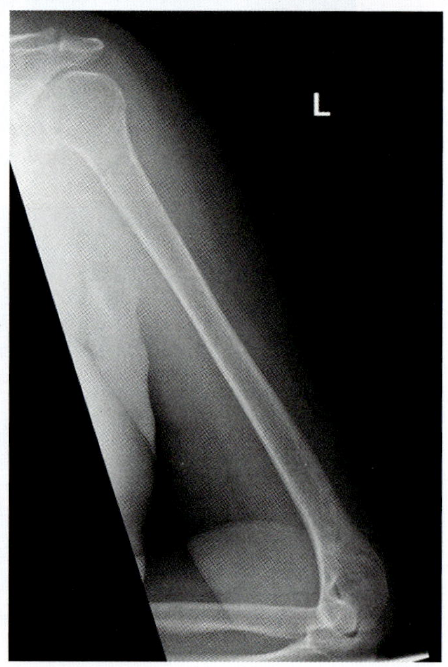

5-168 Mediolateral humerus.

Trauma Humerus

- Projection: AP

Trauma Humerus Protocol
AP
Transthoracic Lateral
Lateromedial

Technical Considerations
- kVp 65–70
- mAs set manually
- Grid or nongrid could be dependent on exposure location and part thickness
- 40″ SID

Exposure Field Size
- 14 × 17 lengthwise with collimation down to the humerus

Patient Position (Figs. 5-169 to 5-171)
- Erect or seated on a stool
- Patient may be recumbent
- Patient's arm should remain in neutral position (presenting position); this will likely create the humeral epicondyles to be positioned at about a 45° oblique with the plane of the IR

Centering
- Midhumeral shaft. Collimate to include entire humerus, shoulder joint, and elbow joint

Marking of IR
- Anatomic side marker R or L placed furthest away from midline

Breathing
- Hold breath and instruct the patient to hold still
- Ensure patient holds position while walking away to make the exposure

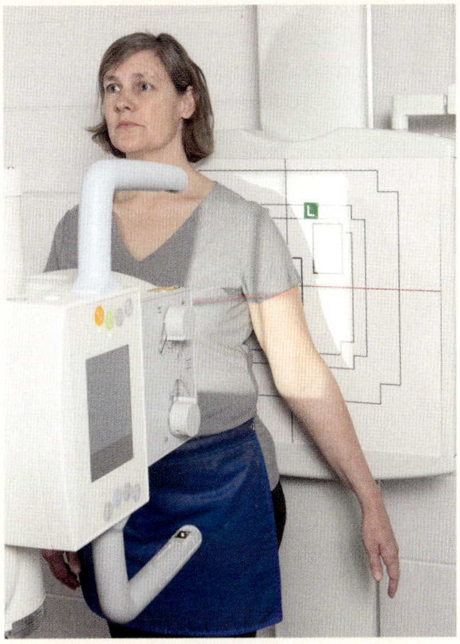

5-169 AP humerus—humeral epicondyles are in neutral position.

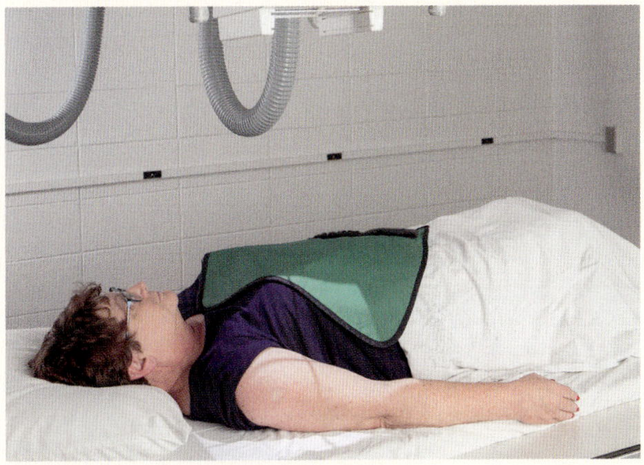

5-170 AP humerus—humeral epicondyles are in neutral position.

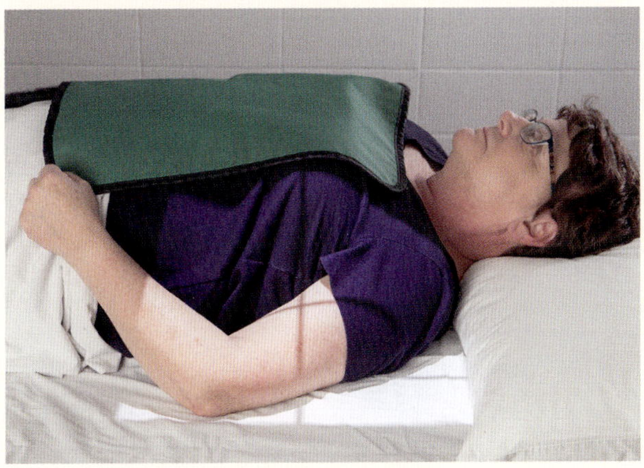

5-171 AP humerus—humeral epicondyles are in neutral position.

IMAGE CRITIQUE (FIG. 5-172)

- Entire humerus to include both elbow joint and shoulder joint within collimated exposure field
- Greater tubercle nor the lesser tubercle will be seen in profile owing to position of the humeral epicondyles. The humeral epicondyles when the arm is in neutral position, will be in an oblique relationship with the image receptor
- Properly centered with four-sided collimation

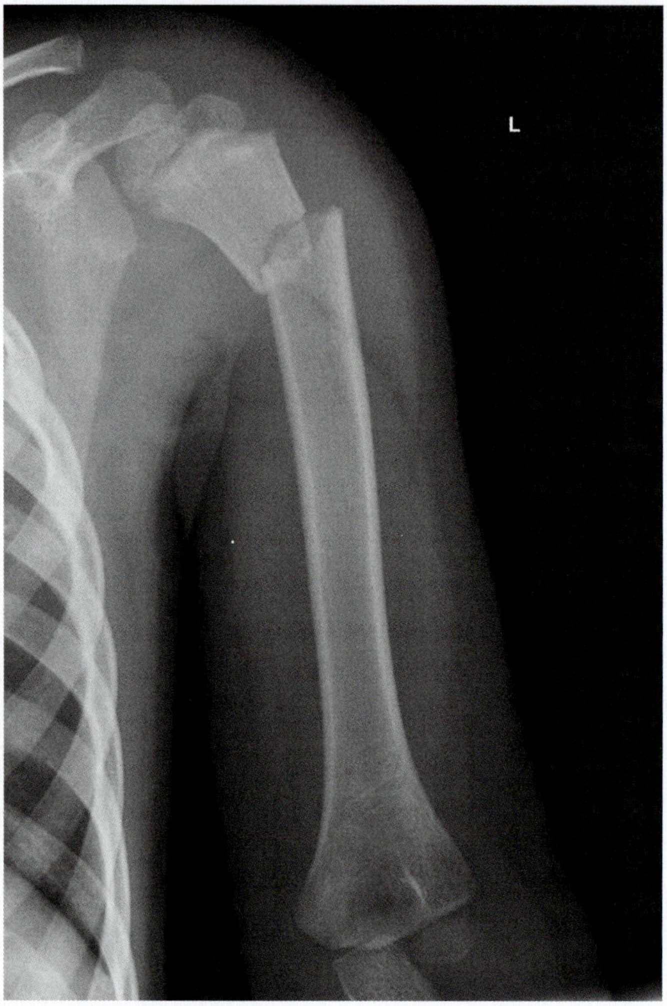

5-172 AP neutral humerus.

Trauma Humerus

- Projection: Transthoracic Lateral
- Lawrence method

Trauma Humerus Protocol
AP
Transthoracic Lateral
Lateromedial

Technical Considerations

- kVp 70-80
- mAs set manually
- Breathing technique is most optimal
- 40″ SID

Exposure Field Size

- 10 × 12 lengthwise for proximal humerus
- 14 × 17 lengthwise for entire humerus

Patient Position (Figs. 5-173 to 5-175)

- Erect or seated on a stool
- Patient may be recumbent. Horizontal beam is implemented
- True lateral position of the thorax
- Patient's affected arm should remain in neutral position (presenting position); this will likely create the humeral epicondyles to be positioned at about a 45° oblique with the plane of the IR
- Unaffected arm elevated above the patient's head in an attempt to separate the shoulders as much as possible

Centering

- To achieve the best penetration of the proximal humerus, direct CR to the surgical neck of the affected humerus. The center of the IR should be set to this level with the 10 × 12 collimated light field
- The central ray is lined up to the IR
- The beam will enter the midcoronal plane or slightly posterior on the side that is closest to the tube
- Alternate centering to midshaft of the humerus (14 × 17), to include both joints, can be used, but may cause technical challenge in visualizing both the shoulder and elbow joint in one exposure

Marking of IR

- Anatomic side marker R or L, indicating affected side closest to the IR. The marker should be placed anterior to the part

Breathing

- Hold breath and instruct the patient to hold still.
- Breathing technique is also an option. The breathing technique will require a longer exposure time while the patient purposely breathes to blur out lung markings and ribs overlying the stationary humerus. The transthoracic lateral directs the beam through the entire thorax before reaching the affected humerus
- Ensure patient holds position while walking away to make the exposure

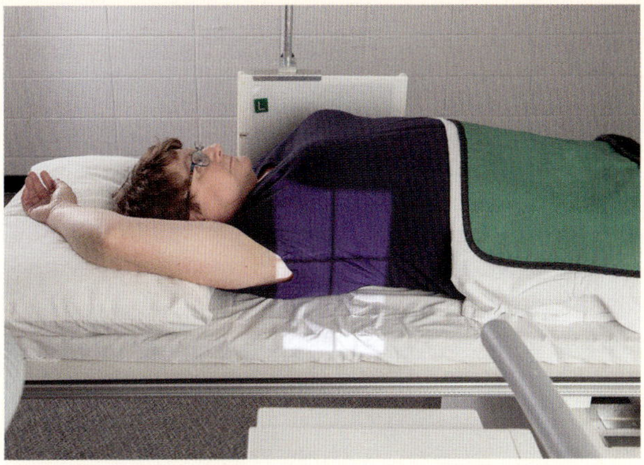

5-173 Recumbent transthoracic lateral for proximal humerus.

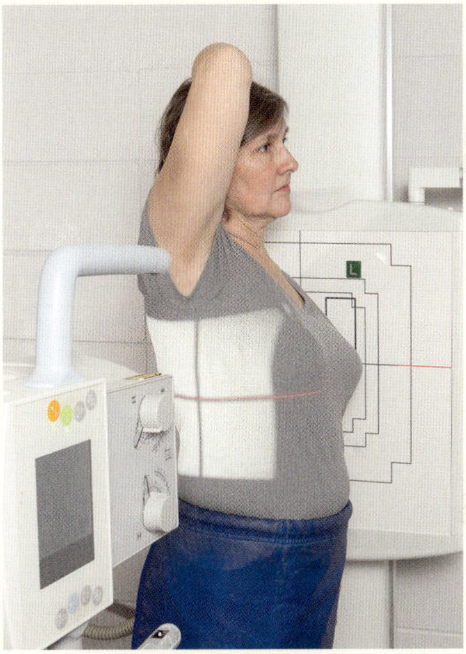

5-174 Upright transthoracic lateral for proximal humerus.

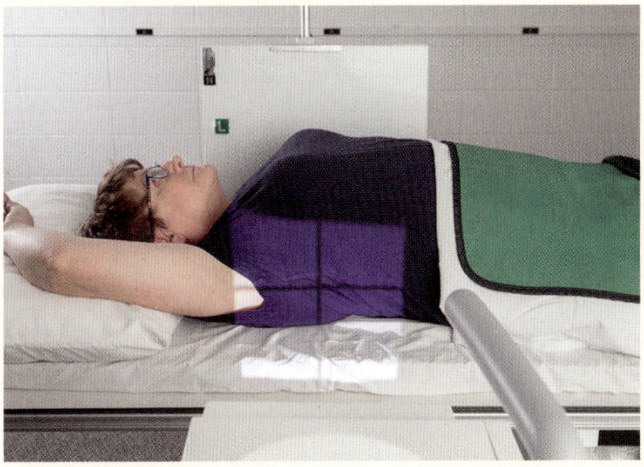

5-175 Recumbent transthoracic lateral for entire humerus.

IMAGE CRITIQUE (FIGS. 5-176 to 5-178)

- The relationship of the humeral head to the glenoid fossa is demonstrated. Anterior to posterior displacement of the part determined
- Proximal humerus and the glenohumeral joint are within the collimated exposure field. To achieve good technical appearance and diagnostic quality, center to the proximal humerus
- The humeral head and upper portion of the humeral shaft visualized anterior to the thoracic spine
- Properly centered to display the proximal one-third of the humerus or entire humerus with four-sided collimation is ideal

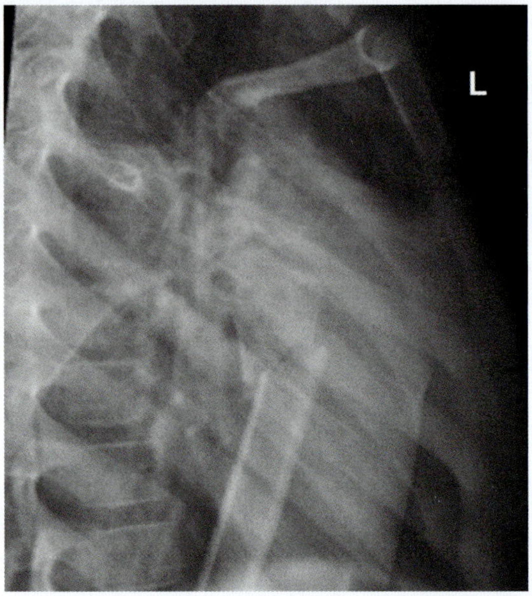

5-176 Transthoracic lateral for proximal humerus.

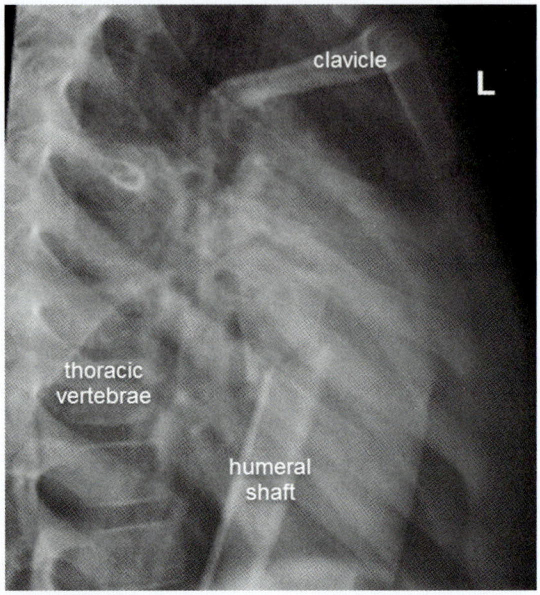

5-177 Transthoracic lateral for proximal humerus.

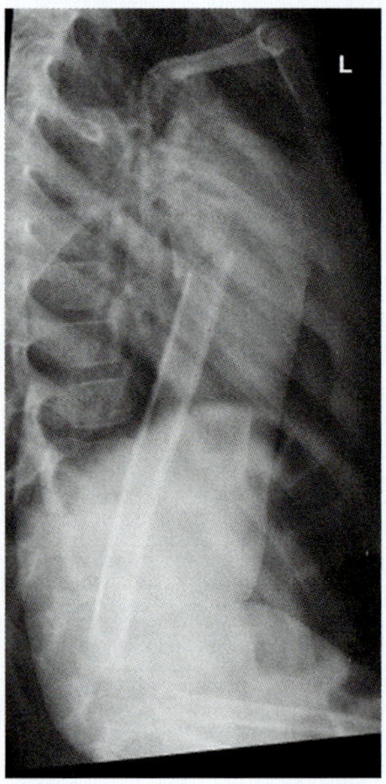

5-178 Transthoracic lateral for entire humerus.

Trauma Humerus

- Projection: Lateromedial for distal humerus

Trauma Humerus Protocol
AP
Transthoracic Lateral
Lateromedial

Technical Considerations
- kVp 60–65
- mAs set manually
- 40″ SID

Exposure Field Size
- 10 × 12 (nongrid) lengthwise

Patient Position (Fig. 5-179)
- Recumbent.
- Patient's arm should remain in neutral position (presenting position)
- Patient's arm may need slightly built up off the surface to allow the IR to drop below the level of the part

Centering
- A horizontal beam will be created ensuring the tube head is parallel with the plane of the IR
- Midway between midhumeral shaft and elbow joint
- Ensure the elbow joint is included and as much as the humeral shaft to include some overlap of the humeral shaft with the transthoracic lateral

Marking of IR
- Anatomic side marker R or L placed anterior to the part

Breathing
- Hold breath and instruct the patient to hold still
- Ensure patient holds position while walking away to make the exposure

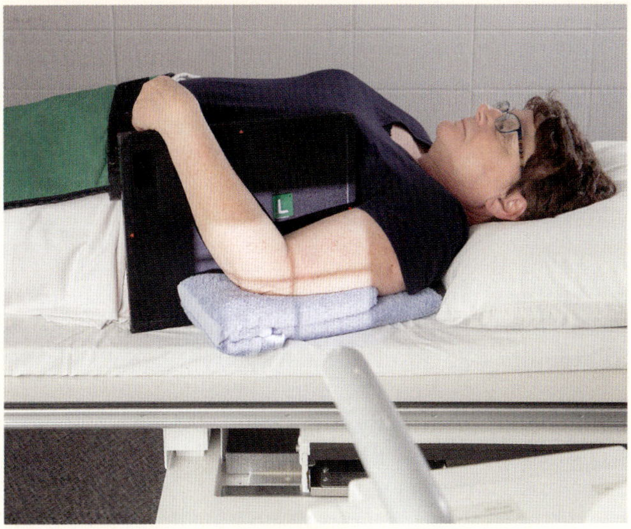

5-179 Lateromedial distal humerus.

IMAGE CRITIQUE (FIG. 5-180)

- Mid- to distal humerus as well as proximal radius and ulna within collimated exposure field
- Humeral epicondyles may not be truly perpendicular to the IR owing to patient injury
- It is critical to ensure that between the transthoracic lateral acquired for the proximal humerus and the lateromedial for the distal humerus that the entire humerus and both the shoulder and elbow joints are visualized
- Properly centered with four-sided collimation

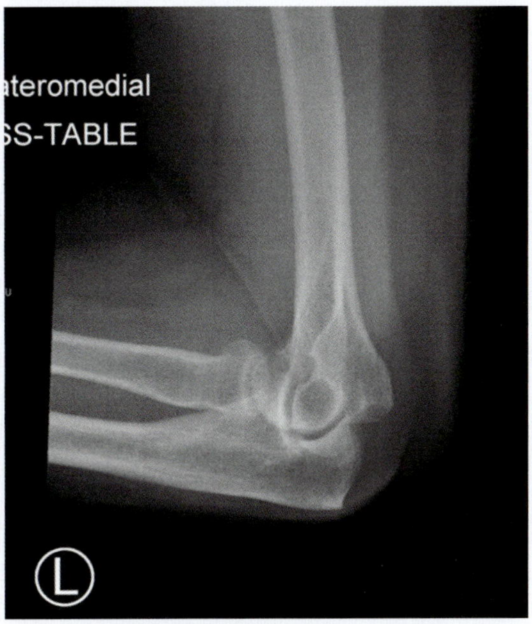

5-180 Lateromedial distal humerus.

THE FINAL STEP: IMAGE REVIEW

The technologist must take time to review acquired images to ensure image quality is acceptable. The technologist must have the knowledge within their role not only to acquire the images and care for the patient, but also to know how to review the images to ensure diagnostic quality has been attained. In certain instances, a projection may need to be repeated. This is to the discretion of the radiologic technologist. The technologist should review each image for the following.

1. Is all of the necessary anatomy included on the image?
   - Was the central ray (CR) properly directed to the part? An "X" can be drawn to intersect within the collimated exposure field to determine whether the CR was directed to the correct location.
   - Was essential anatomy in the collimated exposure field?
   - Is the area free of artifact(s)?
2. Is the anatomy well demonstrated?
   - Did the technologist properly position the patient to adequately demonstrate the anatomy?
   - Can the technologist recognize the anatomy best demonstrated with use of different projections?
3. Does the image reflect proper image markings?
   - Did the technologist correctly use a lead marker to identify the right or left side?
   - What additional markings or annotations could be helpful to the radiologist interpreting the exam?
   - Is the image properly displayed?
4. Does the image prove to be technically acceptable?
   - Does the exposure index fall within acceptable range for the operating system? Images that are technically insufficient may appear of good quality if just slightly insufficient or "mottled or pixelated" if severely insufficient. Images that appear "mottled" should be repeated. Images that appear beyond optimal exposure owing to higher technique may display high quality, but the patient has received excessive radiation dose.

CRITICAL THINKING

1. According to the image of the lateral thumb (Fig. 5-181), characterize its results.
   a. Image represents proper positioning and demonstration of essential anatomy.
   b. Image represents poor positioning, which affects demonstration of essential anatomy.
   c. Image represents poor centering, clipping essential anatomy.
   d. Image represents poor technical quality.

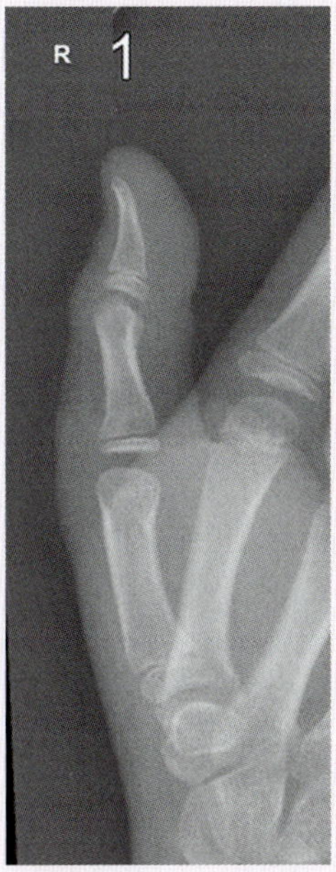

5-181

2. According to the image of the AP oblique elbow with internal rotation (Fig. 5-182), characterize its results.
   a. Image represents proper positioning.
   b. Image represents underrotation.
   c. Image represents overrotation.

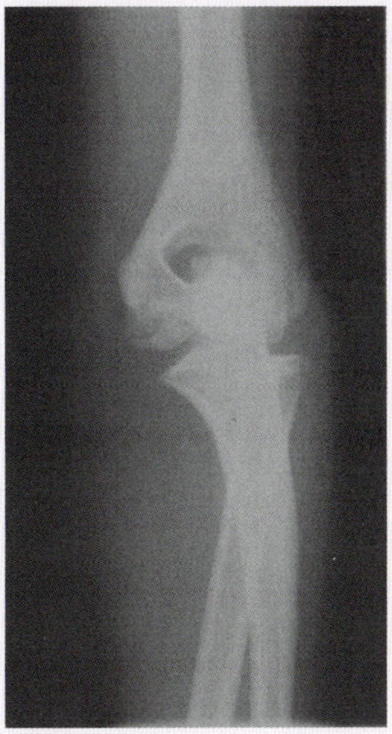

5-182

3. According to the image of the AP elbow (Fig. 5-183), characterize its results.
   a. Image represents proper positioning, centering, and essential anatomy.
   b. Image represents the hand positioned in supination.
   c. Image represents the hand positioned in pronation.
   d. Image represents the hand positioned with the thumb up.

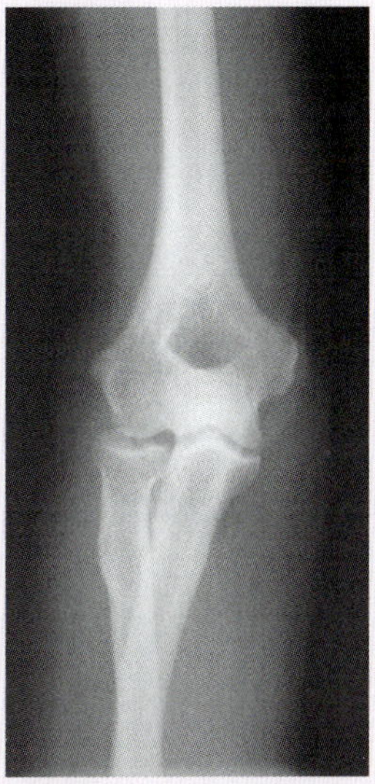

5-183

4. According to the image of the transthoracic lateral humerus (Fig. 5-184), characterize its results.
   a. Image represents proper centering and positioning to demonstrate essential proximal anatomy and will complement with a distal lateromedial humerus.
   b. Image represents centering directed to inferiorly but demonstrates all essential proximal anatomy and will complement with a distal lateromedial humerus.
   c. Image represents centering directed to superiorly but demonstrates all essential proximal anatomy and will complement with a distal lateromedial humerus.
   d. Image represents an inadequate overall technical appearance.

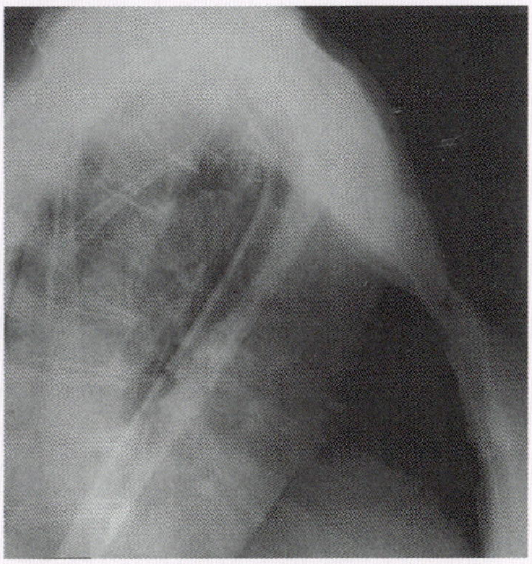

5-184

5. According to the image of the PA oblique hand (Fig. 5-185), characterize its results.
   1. Image represents perfect rotation of the part.
   2. Image represents underrotation of the part.
   3. Image represents overrotation of the part.
   4. Image fails to include all essential anatomy.
   5. Image includes all essential anatomy:
      a. 1 and 4
      b. 2 and 4
      c. 3 and 4
      d. 3 and 5

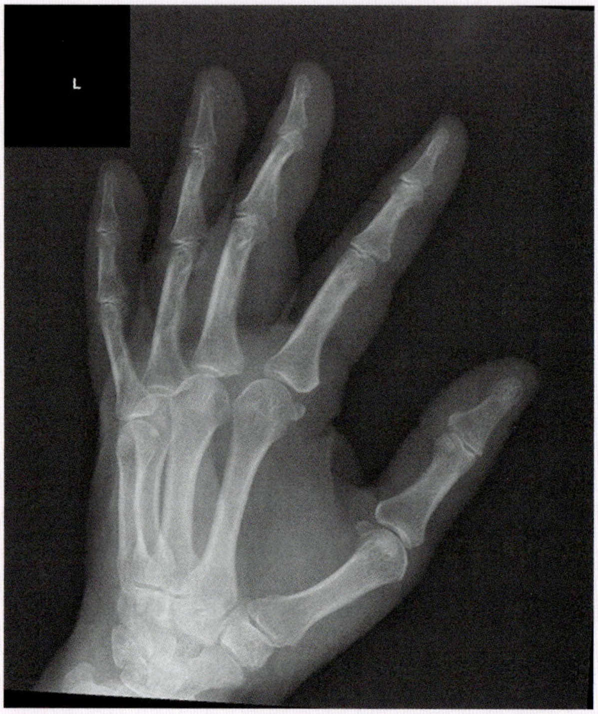

5-185

6. According to the image of the AP forearm (Fig. 5-186), characterize its results.
   1. Image is properly displayed.
   2. Image is improperly displayed.
   3. Image represents good centering and includes all essential anatomy.
   4. Image represents good centering but fails to include all essential anatomy.
      a. 1 and 3
      b. 1 and 4
      c. 2 and 3
      d. 2 and 4

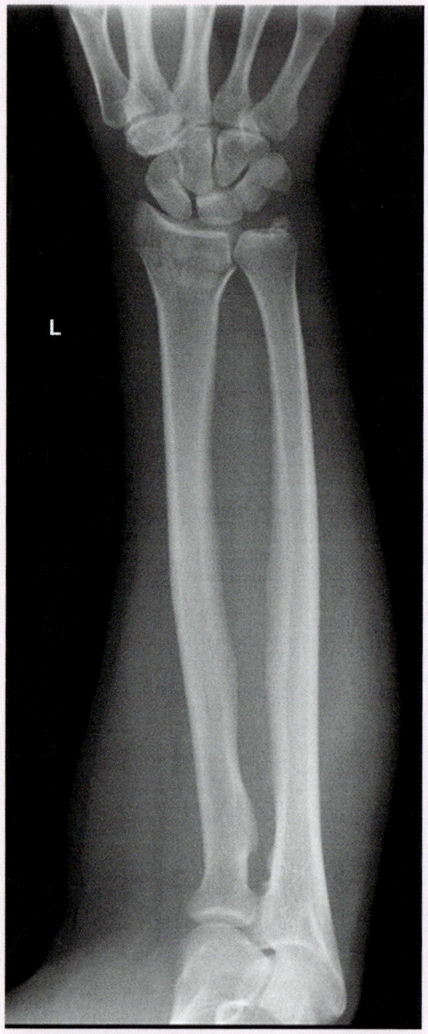

5-186

ANSWERS TO THE CRITICAL THINKING QUESTIONS

1. b
2. b
3. c
4. b
5. c
6. b

CHAPTER 6 Shoulder Girdle

Imaging of the shoulder girdle will include nontrauma and trauma patient situations. The technologist will need a profound understanding of nontrauma protocols and should also be able to think critically and modify protocols in instances of patient trauma. Situationally based, a basic protocol may be extended to include specialty views based on physician preference or request. Imaging of the trauma extremity will involve the technologist to image the patient while in the emergency department, surgical suite, and/or post anesthesia settings.

CLINICAL INDICATIONS

Indications are the symptomatic reasons as to why a particular exam may be ordered by the physician. The technologist should look at the clinical indications before performing a procedure. The following briefly introduces common exam indications, but it is not an all-encompassing list.

Dislocation: Displacement of a bone from a joint. Imaging the part on initial assessment and then potentially again post reduction will require two views 90° apart. The shoulder joint is prone to dislocation owing to the shallow depth of the ball and socket articulation. The shoulder joint most commonly dislocates anteriorly. The lateral projection is essential to determine the direction of the dislocation (Fig. 6-1).

Bursitis: Inflammation of the fluid-filled sacs that line the joint. Bursitis could be a result of repetitious movement, but could also be a result of injury or arthritis (Fig. 6-2).

Rotator Cuff: Injury to one or more of the muscles that form the rotator cuff around the shoulder. Patients will experience pain and have limited range of movement in the affected shoulder. MRI, musculoskeletal sonography, or shoulder arthrogram may be considered for diagnosis (Figs. 6-3 and 6-4).

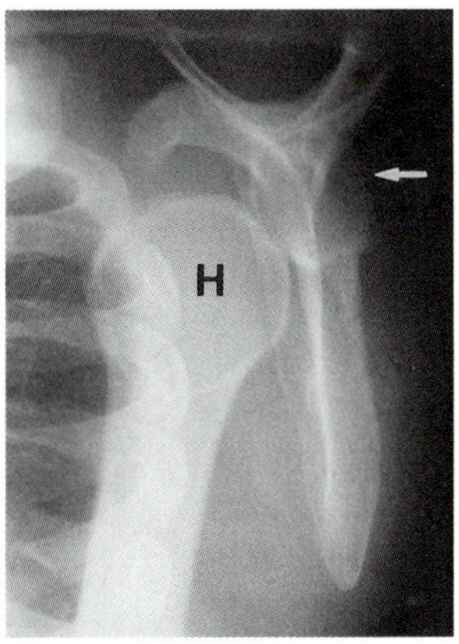

6-1 Dislocation of the humerus from the glenohumeral joint.

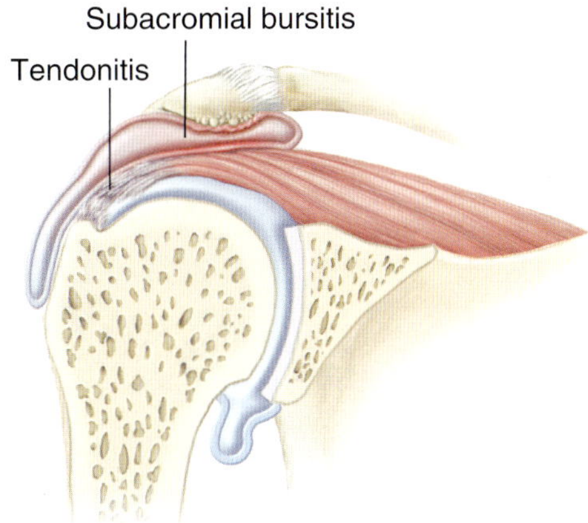

6-2 Bursitis.

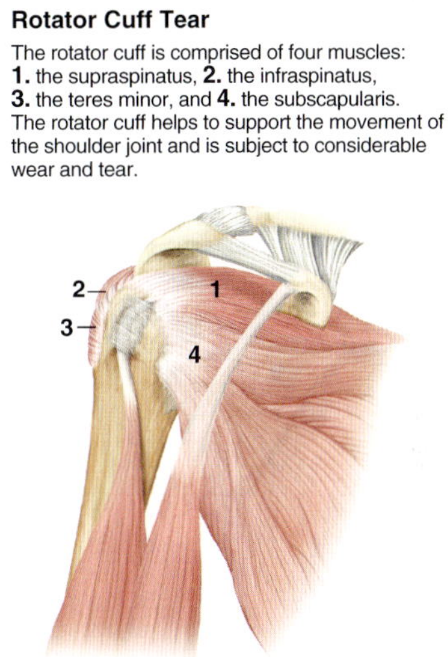

6-3 Rotator cuff.

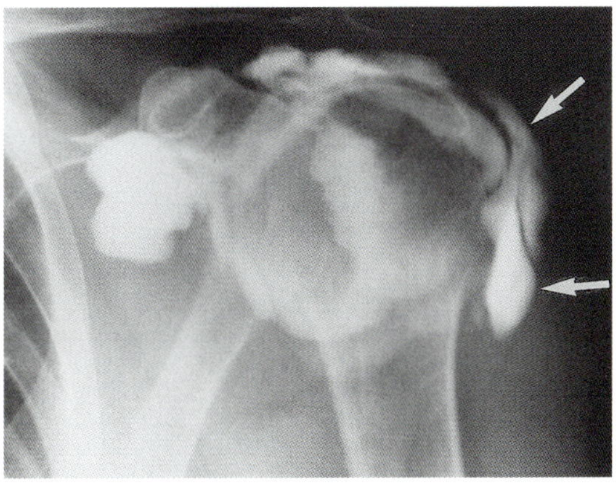

6-4 White arrows highlight extravasation of contrast media, indicating a tear in the rotator cuff.

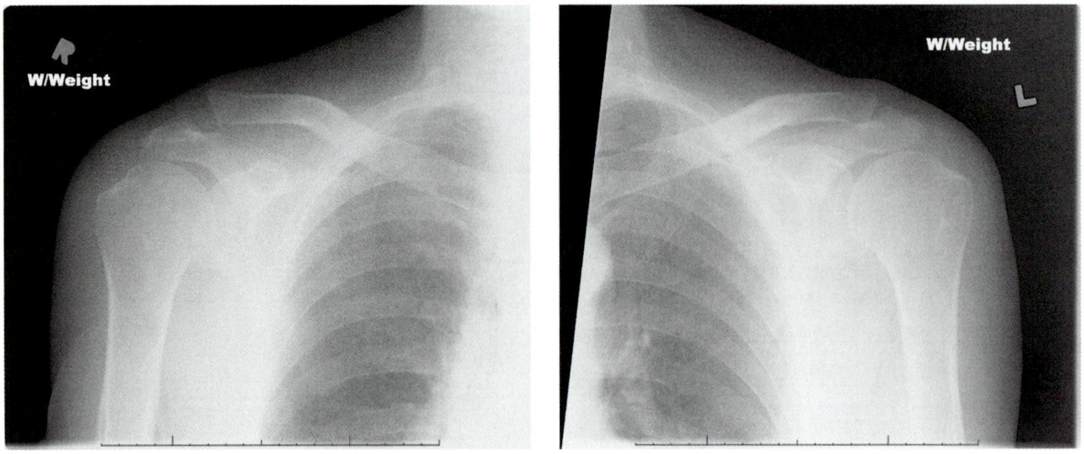

6-5 Comparative right and left AC joints with stress.

Acromioclavicular Joint Separation: A separation at the acromioclavicular (AC) joint caused by a sprain or ligamental tears. Comparative AC joint imaging is necessary, and clavicular fracture should be ruled out (Fig. 6-5).

Osteoarthritis: A common, noninflammatory degenerative form of arthritis that typically affects joints of aging patients, joints with overuse, and weight-bearing joints (Fig. 6-6).

Osteoporosis: Loss of bone density that may result in bone fracture. This condition is more prevalent with postmenopausal aged women and aged men (Fig. 6-7). Reduction in technical factors will be necessary.

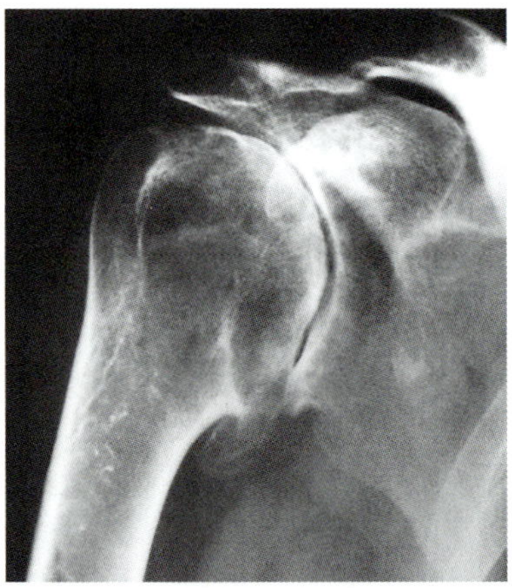

6-6 Osteoarthritis.

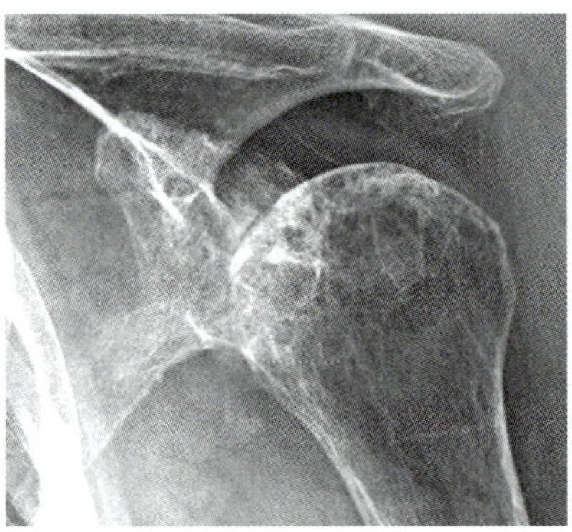

6-7 Osteoporosis.

IMAGING CONSIDERATIONS

Patient Dress

The patient will likely need to remove clothing from the waist up and change into a gown. Patients need to remove all jewelry from the area of interest. Digital imaging is sensitive to text writing, embroidery stitching, or imprinted text or logos from the clothing garment appear on the radiograph. Similarly, thickened, elastic bands on a sports bra may be seen.

Artifacts

Artifacts are unwanted objects that appear on the image superimposing pertinent anatomy. Failure to have the patient remove earrings, necklaces, hair ties, long braids, bras, sports bras, shirts with buttons, and clothing with imprinted or embroidery stitching may result in the appearance of artifacts. Repeat imaging may be necessary when artifact obscures the area of interest (Fig. 6-8).

Patient Position

The general position of the patient or part.

Upright—Relative to this chapter, this position could be considered and preferred when imaging the clavicle, shoulder, and AC joints.

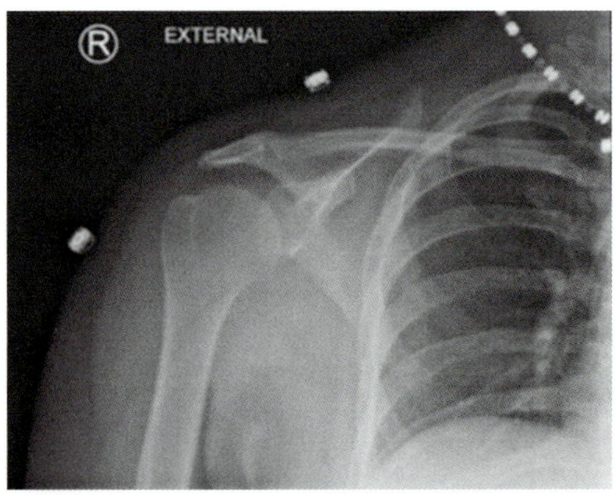

6-8 Jewelry artifact.

Supine—May be implemented when the patient is in trauma and is unable to sit or stand upright. Additionally, certain specialty views may require the patient to lie recumbent.

Posterior Oblique—The patient will be rotated into a right or left posterior oblique (RPO or LPO). The beam is directed to enter the anterior surface and exit the posterior surface while the body is positioned into a particular degree of obliquity.

Anterior Oblique—The patient will be rotated into a right or left anterior oblique (RAO or LAO). The beam is directed to enter the posterior surface and exit the anterior surface while the body is positioned into a particular degree of obliquity.

Ambulatory Patient Imaging

An ambulatory patient is one who can maneuver themselves and bear weight with little to no assistance. Ambulatory patients may be able to stand upright for images necessary in their series or easily transfer to a stool. Ambulatory patients will be able to walk or may come by wheelchair to the exam room. Patients transported by wheelchair may still be able to stand. The technologist needs to make a proper assessment of the patient's ability in determining the best and safest way to complete their imaging study.

Projection(s)

How the x-ray beam passes through the part.

- AP (Anteroposterior): The beam is directed to enter through the anterior surface, exit the posterior surface, and strike the image receptor.
- PA (Posteroanterior): The beam is directed to enter the posterior surface, exit the anterior surface, and strike the image receptor.
- PA Oblique: The beam is directed to enter the posterior surface and exit the anterior surface while the part is positioned into a particular degree of obliquity (Fig. 6-9).

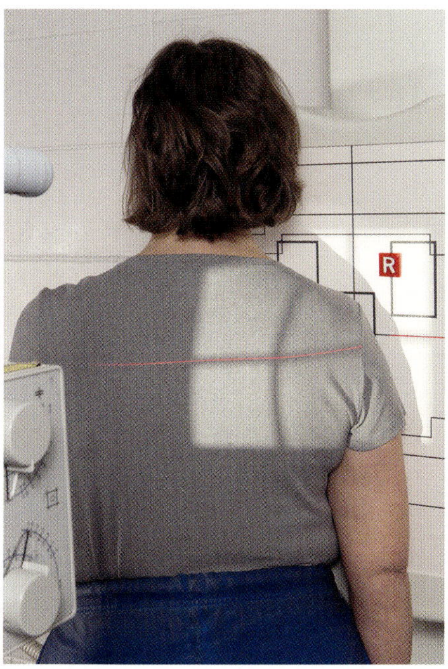

6-9 PA oblique projection.

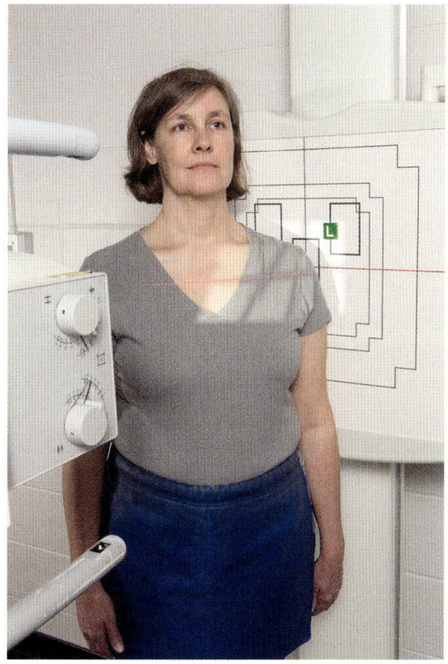

6-10 AP oblique projection.

- AP Oblique: The beam is directed to enter the anterior surface and exit the posterior surface while the part is positioned into a particular degree of obliquity (Fig. 6-10).
- AP or PA Axial: The beam directs anterior to posterior (AP) or posterior to anterior (PA), with an added specified tube (axial) angle directed to the part.
- Inferosuperior Axial: The beam is directed inferiorly to superiorly on a part with an angle applied to the beam.

ANATOMY

Imaging the shoulder girdle includes the proximal humerus, glenohumeral/scapulohumeral (shoulder) joint, scapula, clavicle, and AC joints (Fig. 6-11). The shoulder girdle consists of the clavicle and scapula to secure the upper extremity to the trunk of the body.

Proximal Humerus

The proximal humerus includes the prominent, rounded head that articulates with the glenoid fossa of the scapula to

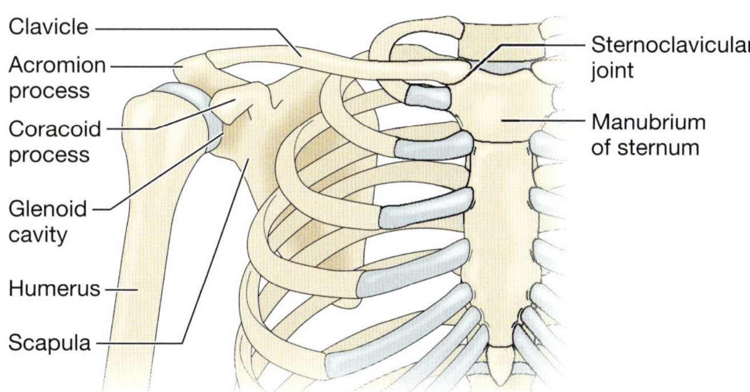

6-11 Shoulder girdle.

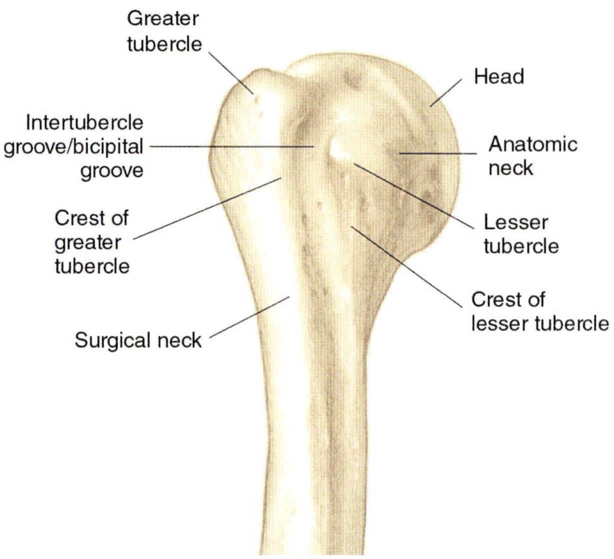

6-12 Proximal humerus.

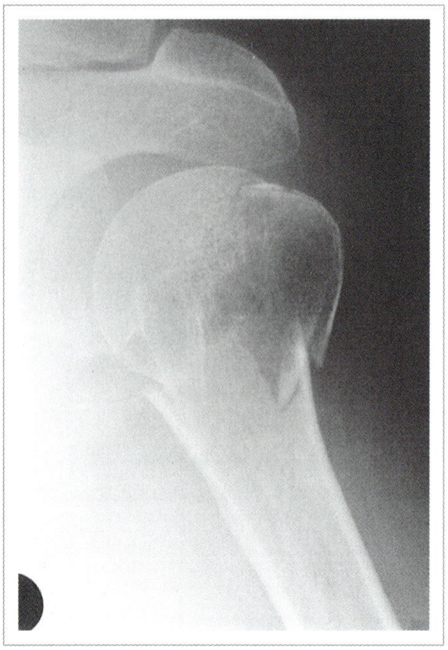

6-14 Fracture of the surgical neck.

form the glenohumeral or scapulohumeral (shoulder) joint. Adjacent to the humeral head, the anatomic neck narrows and surrounds the humeral head. Below the anatomic neck lie the greater and lesser tubercles, which provide attachment for muscles. The greater and lesser tubercles are separated by the intertubercle groove or the bicipital groove (Fig. 6-12). The greater and lesser tubercles are demonstrated during imaging with positional changes of the arm. With the hand and arm in anatomic position and palpating the humeral epicondyles to adjust parallel to the imaging plane behind, the greater tubercle is seen most laterally on the humeral head, whereas the lesser tubercle is located anteriorly and superimposed upon the humerus (Fig. 6-13). The surgical neck of the humerus narrows on the proximal-most portion of the humeral shaft, just below the humeral head and tubercle region. It is not uncommon to see fracture to the surgical neck; hence requiring potential surgery (Fig. 6-14). The shoulder joint is of synovial and diarthrodial type, with ball and socket movement. The ball and socket joint in the shoulder lacks stability compared to the ball and socket joint in the hip. The glenoid fossa provides a shallow socket, which increases mobility, but subjects the joint to easier dislocation even with added reinforcement of the rotator cuff (Figs. 6-15 and 6-16).

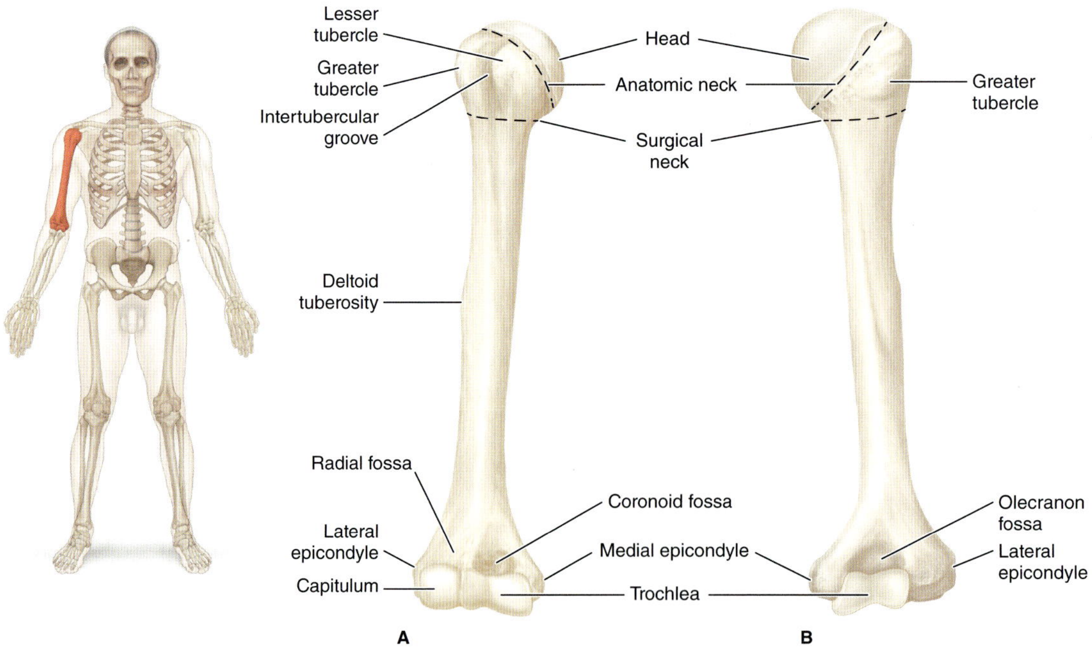

6-13 Humerus. **A:** Anterior view of right humerus. **B:** Posterior view of right humerus.

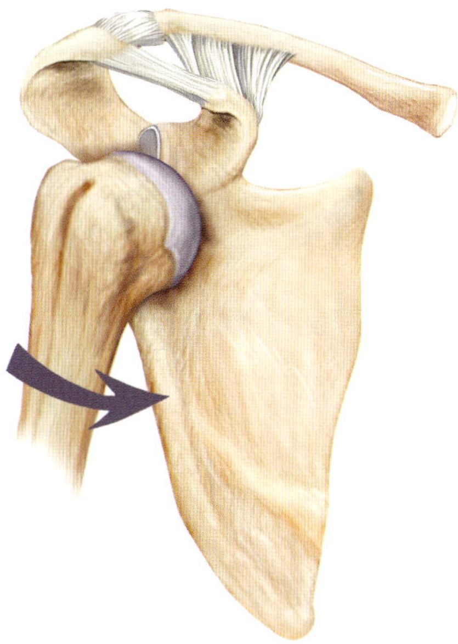

6-15 Anterior dislocation of the shoulder joint.

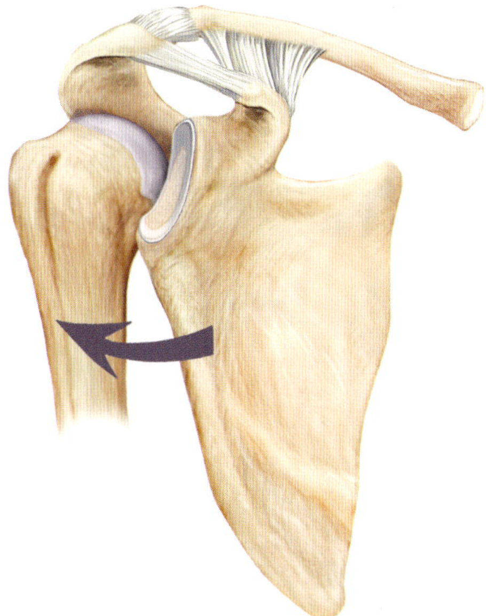

6-16 Posterior dislocation of the shoulder joint.

Clavicle

The clavicle consists of a body/shaft and two articulating ends (Fig. 6-17). The sternal end, triangularly shaped, articulates with the manubrium (superior-most portion of the sternum) and forms a diarthrodial joint with gliding movement, known as the sternoclavicular (SC) joint. The acromial end, rectangularly shaped, articulates with the acromion of the scapula and forms a diarthrodial joint with gliding movement, known as the acromioclavicular (AC) joint (Fig. 6-18). The clavicle has slight curvature between the two ends. Curvature may be more pronounced in male

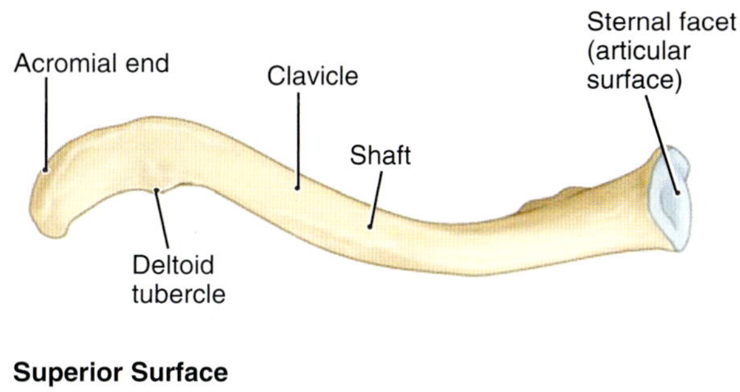

6-17 Clavicle.

patients, especially those that are extremely muscular. The curvature of the clavicle and the thickness of the upper thorax will influence the amount of axial tube angle necessary when imaging the clavicle.

Scapula

The scapula is essential to attaching the upper limb to the trunk of the body along with the help of the clavicle. The scapula sits on the posterior and upper region of the bony thorax (Fig. 6-19). The superior border of the scapula corresponds to the second posterior rib and extends down to the seventh posterior rib (T7), where the inferior angle of the scapula is palpable. In general, the scapula has two surfaces, three borders, and three angles. The detail of the scapular anatomy will be presented from an anterior, a posterior, and lateral perspective.

Anterior Surface

The anterior surface may also be referred to as the costal surface. The scapula is positioned posteriorly on the bony thorax, allowing the anterior surface of the scapula to have close proximity to the posterior ribs (costa). The scapula has a curvature or arch to the body that provides added strength to this paper-thin section of the bone. The center depression or concavity on the anterior surface is the subscapular fossa (Fig. 6-20). Along the superior border, the coracoid process extends out anteriorly. The coracoid process may be palpable, but this is influenced by body habitus. Just medial to the base of the coracoid process, a small scapular notch is located. Where the superior border meets with the medial or vertebral border, the superior angle is formed. The vertebral border descends adjacent to the thoracic vertebrae and meets up with the lateral or axillary border and forms the inferior angle. The inferior angle of the scapula serves as a palpable landmark for T7. The axillary border referenced by the proximity to the axilla (armpit) is notably thicker than the vertebral border (Fig. 6-20). The thickness difference in the borders may be helpful in distinguishing between the two borders when evaluating lateral scapula images for rotational errors. The axillary border also contains the scapular head, which gives rise to the lateral angle. The glenoid fossa is seen most laterally to accept the humeral head.

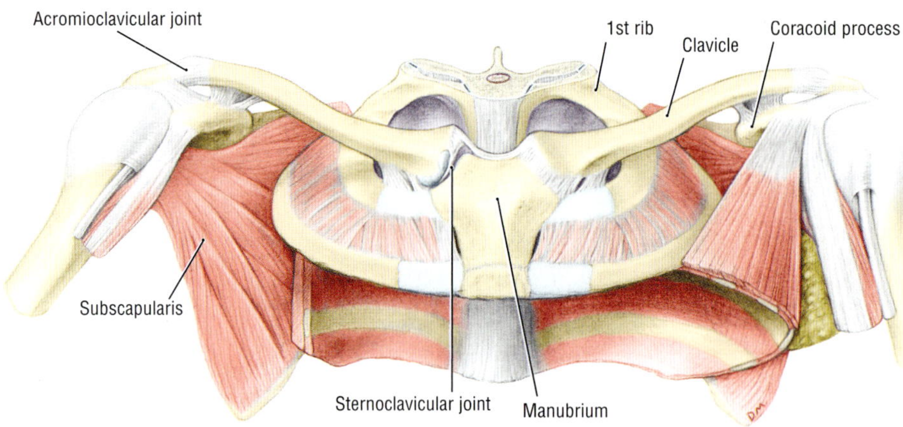

6-18 AC and SC joints.

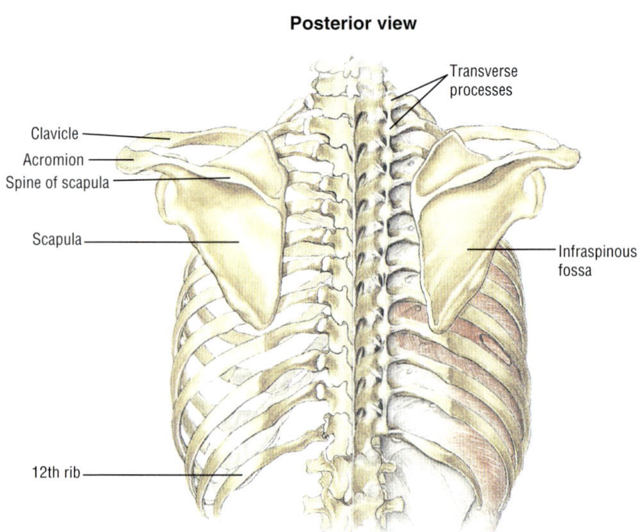

6-19 Scapula position on the posterior rib cage.

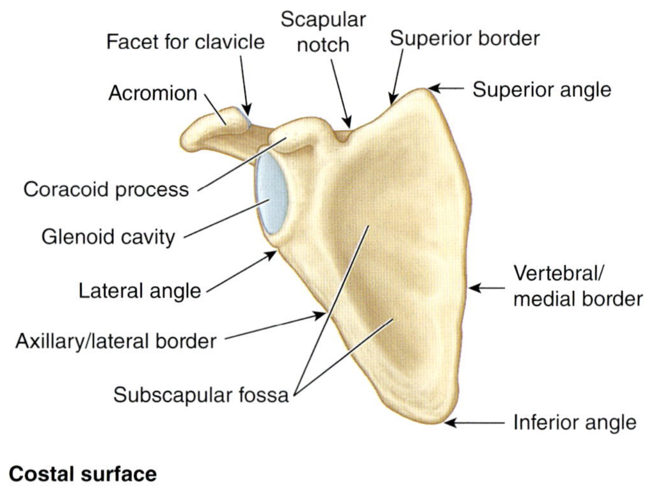

6-20 Anterior view of the scapula.

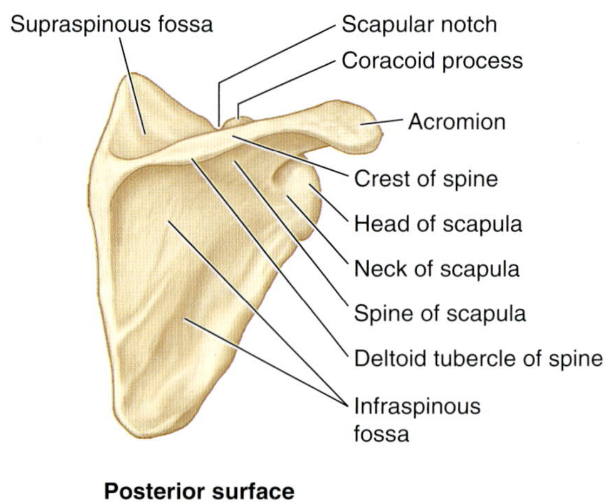

6-21 Posterior view of the scapula.

Posterior Surface

The posterior surface of the scapula still reveals the superior, axillary, and vertebral borders as well as the superior angle, inferior angle, and lateral angle. The scapular spine originates from the vertebral border and traverses laterally across the upper one-third of the scapula. The scapular spine thickens as it courses laterally from the vertebral border and is identified as the crest of the spine (Fig. 6-21). The spine terminates with the extension of the acromion. The acromion has an angle before it terminates into a broadened process that sits posterior to the humeral head. Superior to the scapular spine, the supraspinous fossa is located, and inferior to the scapular spine the infraspinous fossa is located (Fig. 6-21). Shoulder muscles attach at the superior and inferior scapular fossae.

Lateral View

In a lateral perspective, the scapula resembles a "Y." The acromion and the coracoid processes are superiorly located, whereas the body is represented with superimposed axillary and vertebral borders and the body terminates inferiorly with the inferior angle (Fig. 6-22). When the scapula is positioned into a true lateral, the relationship of the humeral head to the glenoid fossa can be determined. Fracture fragments or joint dislocation can be evaluated for anterior or posterior displacement.

KEY SUMMATION POINTS OF ANATOMY

- The clavicle and scapula form the shoulder girdle and provide attachment of the upper extremity to the trunk of the body.
- The most commonly fractured location on the humerus is the surgical neck and may require surgical attention.
- The greater tubercle is seen in profile laterally when the humeral epicondyles are aligned parallel to the plane of the image receptor.
- The lesser tubercle is seen in profile medially (closest to the glenoid fossa) when the humeral epicondyles are aligned perpendicular to the plane of the image receptor.
- The intertubercle groove, also known as the bicipital groove, separates the greater tubercle from the lesser tubercle.
- The greater and lesser tubercles on the proximal humerus serve as sites for muscle attachment.
- The coracoid is an anterior, beak-like extension off the superior border of the scapula.
- The acromion is an extension off the scapular spine that sits posterior to the humeral head.
- The male clavicle has increased curvature between the sternal and acromial ends compared to the female clavicle, especially in the muscular male.
- The supraspinous and infraspinous fossae are located on the posterior surface of the scapula above and below the scapular spine. The fossae are sites for muscle attachment.
- The axillary or lateral border of the scapula is anatomically thicker than the vertebral or medial border of the scapula.
- The anterior surface of the scapula is also known as the costal surface owing its close proximity to the posterior ribs.
- The lateral "Y" view of the scapula will demonstrate the coracoid process closest to the ribs, extending toward the anterior surface of the patient.
- All joints within the shoulder girdle have a joint capsule (synovial) and have a general movement of diarthrodial. Each diarthrodial joint will have a more specified movement (Table 6-1).

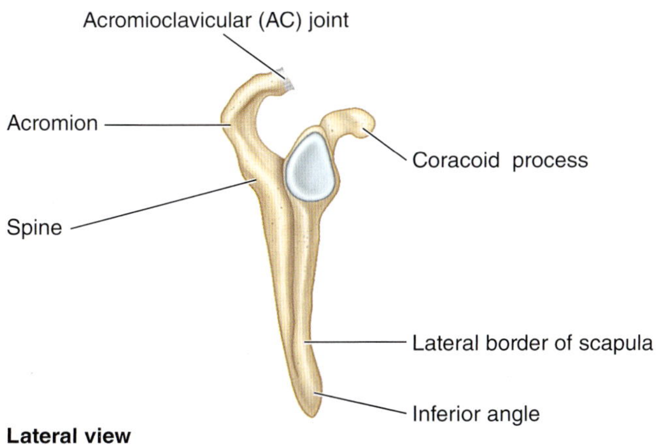

6-22 Lateral view of the scapula.

6-1 Joints of the Shoulder Girdle

Joint	Classification	General Movement	Specific Movement
Glenohumeral joint	Synovial	Diarthrodial	Spheroidal or ball and socket
Acromioclavicular joint	Synovial	Diarthrodial	Plane or gliding
Sternoclavicular joint	Synovial	Diarthrodial	Plane or gliding

POSITIONING CONSIDERATIONS

Patient Part Size and Suggested Image Receptor Orientation

Imaging the shoulder girdle on adult patients generally has a part thickness of >10 cm and, therefore, grid imaging is recommended. Exceptions could be made to this with pediatrics owing to size or to elder patients with significant loss of bone density. A 10 × 12 exposure field may be orientated crosswise or lengthwise according to the part being imaged.

Centering and Collimation

The central ray should be directed to the proper and suggested centering locations. With proper centering, four-sided collimation can be applied to ensure good radiation safety practices as well as the inclusion of all essential anatomy.

Breathing Instructions

With all exposures made with close proximity to the bony thorax, suspended respiration should be implemented to avoid voluntary patient motion. Select exposures such as the transthoracic lateral for the proximal humerus or the AP scapula have the option of suspending respiration or implementing a breathing technique. The breathing technique purposely sets a longer exposure time to as much as 3 or 4 seconds. During the exposure, the patient is instructed to take quick, shallow breaths throughout the entire length of the exposure. The breathing motion of the patient will blur out overlying lung markings and ribs, allowing the stationary anatomy to appear with improved detail.

Identification of Arm Position in Nontrauma Versus Trauma Situations

Patients with potential fracture to a limb should be approached with caution. The technologist may have to deviate from normal protocol to image a part with potential fracture. Certainly, the technologist does not want to worsen an injury or cause the patient additional and unnecessary pain. When the presentation of the patient brings a suspicion of fracture, the technologist should proceed with caution and begin by leaving the arm in the neutral or presenting position while acquiring a minimum of two views 90° apart.

The position of the arm can be determined by identification of the placement position of the greater and lesser tubercles. When the arm is in the anatomic position and the humeral epicondyles are adjusted to align parallel to the imaging plane behind, the greater tubercle is seen laterally in profile, whereas the lesser tubercle is not visualized because it is superimposed upon the proximal humerus due to its anterior location (Figs. 6-23 and 6-24). When the arm is internally rotated and the humeral epicondyles are adjusted to align perpendicular to the imaging plane behind, the lesser tubercle appears in profile medially, toward the glenohumeral joint (Fig. 6-25). With internal rotation, the greater tubercle shifts into an anterior position and superimposes upon the humeral head and is therefore not visualized (Fig. 6-26). When the arm is in the neutral position, the humeral epicondyles are at an approximately 45° angle to the plane behind; therefore, neither the greater nor the lesser tubercle will be seen in profile (Figs. 6-27 and 6-28).

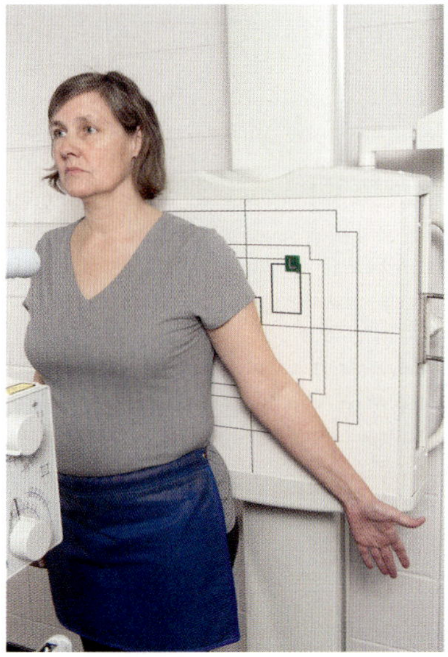

6-23 AP projection of the shoulder with the arm positioned in external rotation.

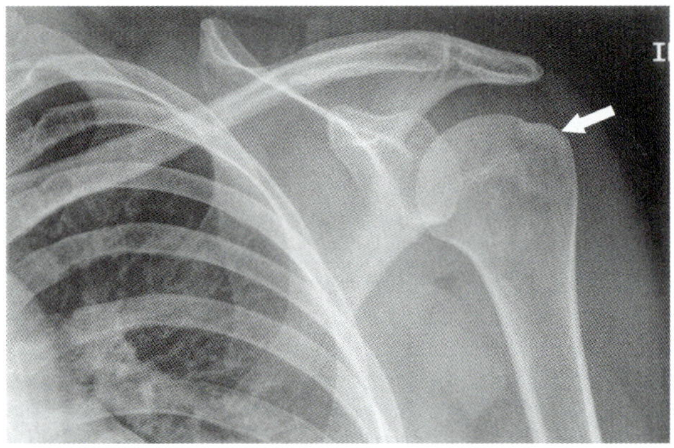

6-24 Greater tubercle in profile laterally.

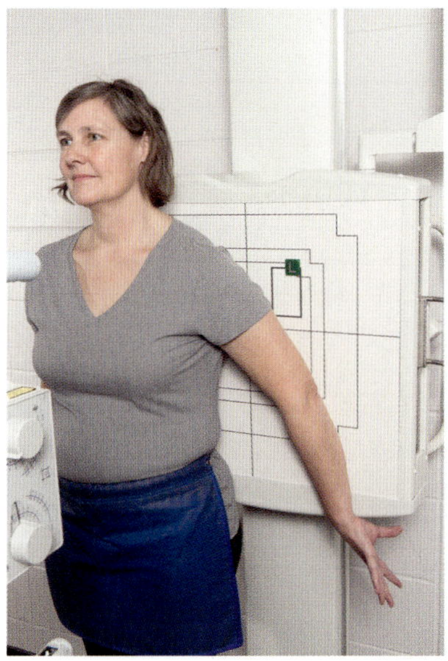

6-25 AP projection of the shoulder with the arm positioned in internal rotation.

TECHNICAL CONSIDERATIONS

Setting a Manual Technique

Manual technique is defined when the radiographer sets the kVp and mAs values independently. A manual technique can be set in the imaging department and on the mobile unit. Tabletop imaging requires the use of manual technique. Kilovoltage is set to penetrate the part thickness and affects the scale of contrast seen on the image. A small focal spot setting is encouraged to improve anatomic resolution. A shortened exposure time when imaging the shoulder girdle to lessen the likelihood of voluntary patient motion during the exposure could be considered.

Setting Technique With Automatic Exposure Control

Automatic Exposure Control (AEC) may be an option when imaging the shoulder. With AEC, the technologist will set the kVp value, will not set an mAs, but rather must select which exposure cell(s) correspond to the anatomy centered and anatomy coverage over the cell(s) according to the projection (Fig. 6-29). The cell(s) will determine when adequate exposure has been reached according to the part thickness and composition, and then the exposure is terminated. After the exposure terminates, the radiographer can briefly examine the mAs value displayed on the control panel. Use of AEC on the shoulder girdle is not recommended for all projections, but when acceptable for use only the center cell is utilized.

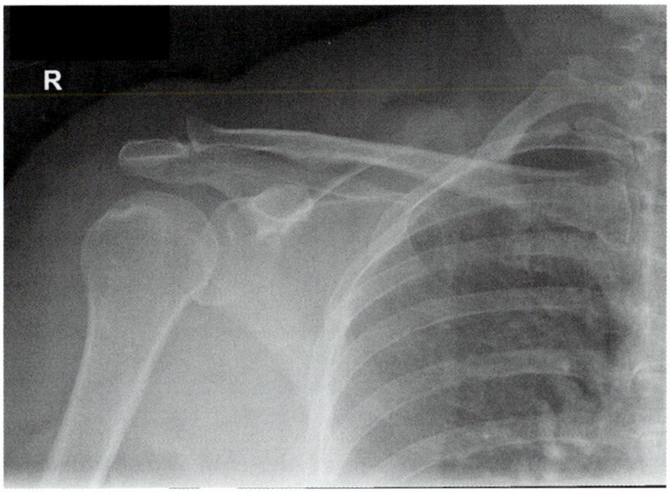

6-26 Lesser tubercle seen in profile medially.

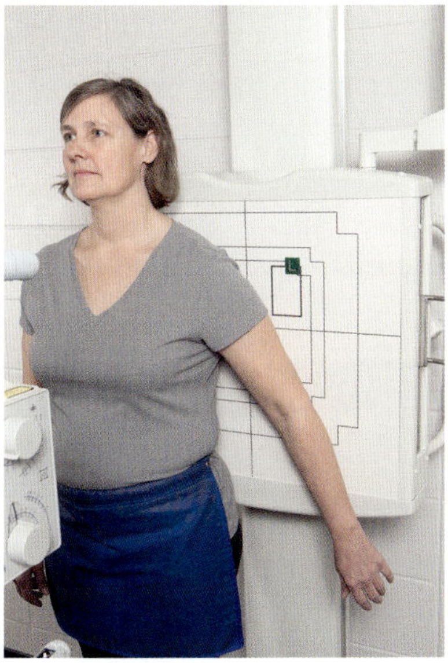

6-27 AP projection of the shoulder with the arm positioned in neutral rotation. Epicondyles are referenced by a 45° angle with the image receptor.

Source-to-Image Distance

40" source to image distance (SID) is employed for most shoulder girdle imaging. A 72" SID is employed to image bilateral AC joints with a single exposure.

Shielding

Acceptable shielding practices include a lap shield. Double shielding around the front and back of the waist should be considered when imaging declared pregnant patients.

Marking the Image

When marking the shoulder girdle when the patient is in a flat or in an oblique position, the anatomic marker should be placed within the collimated exposure field furthest away from the patient's midline or lateral to the part (Figs. 6-30 and 6-31). When marking the lateral position, the anatomic marker is placed along the anterior surface of the part or "in front" of the part and within the collimated exposure field. It is good practice to place the lead marker directly on the image receptor (IR) when the IR is in the table Bucky. When imaging at the upright Bucky, the lead marker can be placed directly in the exposure field on the upright Bucky. Due to the construction design of the upright Bucky, it is sometimes difficult to place the lead marker directly on the image receptor and maintain the position of the lead marker when opening or closing the upright Bucky. When imaging the AC joints, both right and left anatomic markers are placed according to side. Additionally, digital annotations may be added to signify stress or nonstress positions (Fig. 6-32).

Viewing the Image

Assuming the shoulder girdle image was correctly marked, the image is displayed opposite the viewer facing it, as though the part is in the anatomic position (Figs. 6-33 and 6-34).

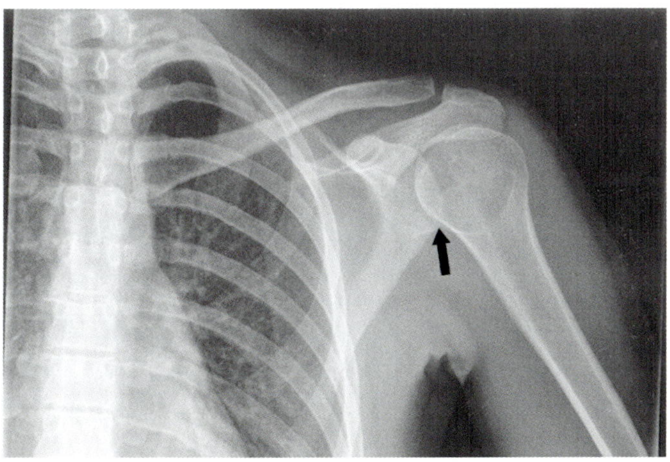

6-28 Neutral arm position—neither greater nor lesser tubercle seen in profile.

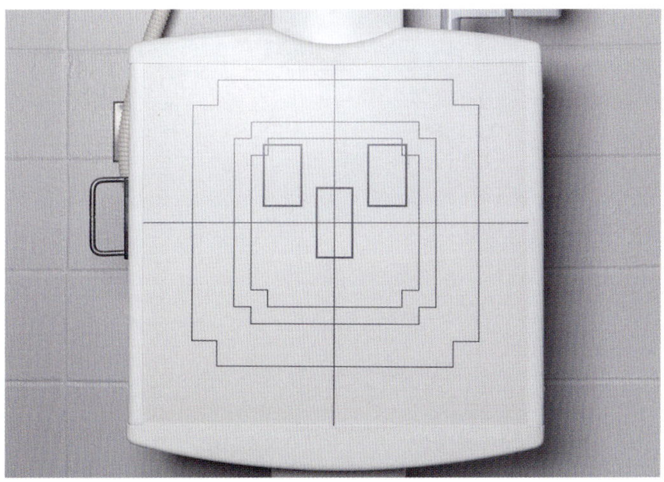

6-29 Upright Bucky showing placement of the three exposure cells.

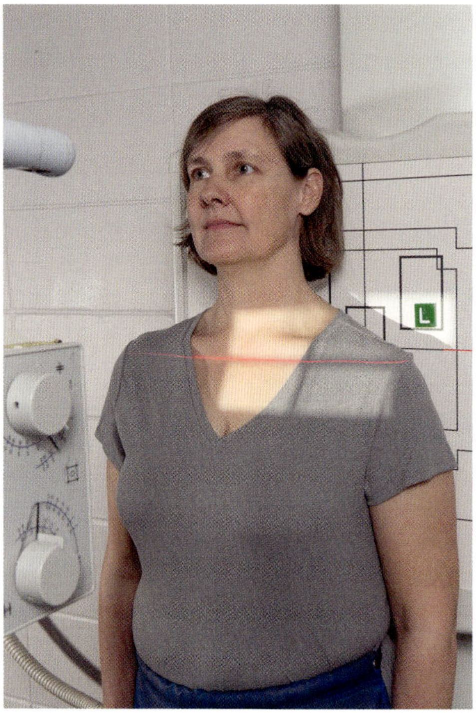

6-30 Correct marker placement for AP projection of the left shoulder.

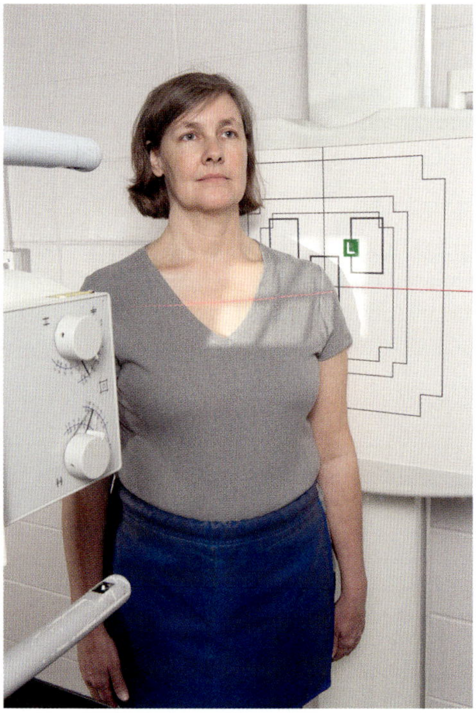

6-31 Correct marker placement for the AP Oblique projection of the left shoulder.

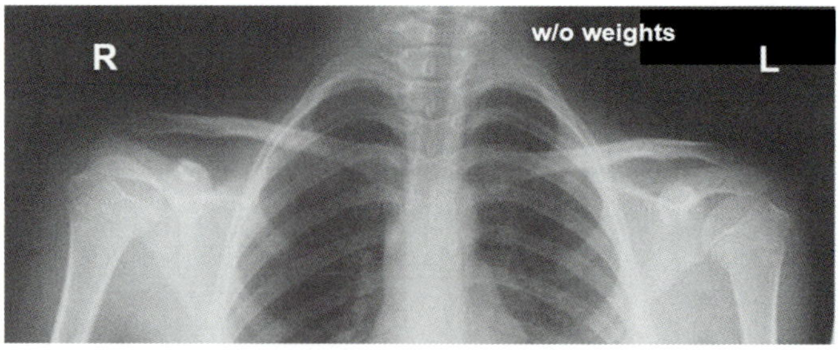

6-32 Correct marker placement and annotations for AC joints.

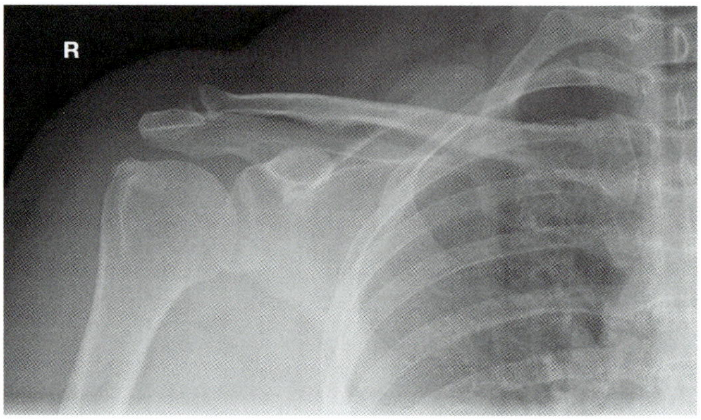

6-33 Correct image display for AP projection of right shoulder.

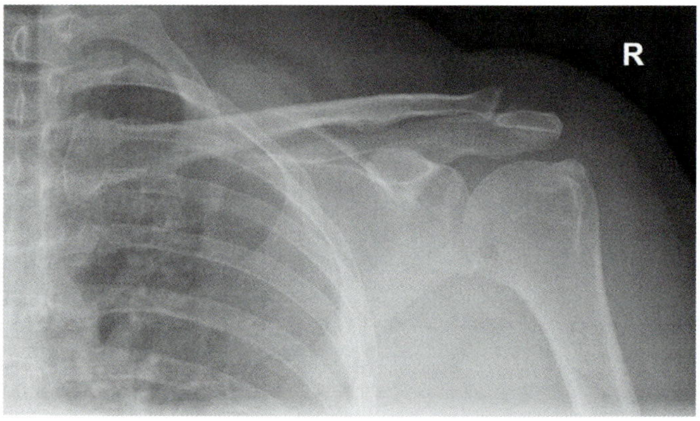

6-34 Incorrect image display for AP projection of right shoulder.

Nontrauma Shoulder

- Projection: AP

Nontrauma Shoulder Protocol
AP (external rotation)
AP (internal rotation)

Technical Considerations

- kVp 70–80
- Center cell AEC or mAs set manually
- 40" SID

Exposure Field Size

- 10 × 12 crosswise to include the entire shoulder girdle

OR

- 10 × 12 lengthwise to include more of the proximal humerus but will fail to include the SC joint

Patient Position (Fig. 6-35)

- Erect or seated on a stool
- Patient may be supine
- Supinate the hand, create anatomic position, and ensure humeral epicondyles are parallel to the imaging plane behind. Palpate the humeral epicondyles to ensure correct position

Centering

- For 10 × 12 crosswise imaging direct the CR 1" inferior to coracoid process and 1" medial to coracoid process. This centering and IR orientation will include the SC joint, entire clavicle, glenohumeral joint, and proximal one-third of the humerus. Inclusion of the SC joint would be verified with the palpation of the jugular notch. Ensure light field to include proximal humerus with proper centering

OR

- For 10 × 12 lengthwise imaging, direct the CR 1" inferior to the coracoid process. This centering and IR orientation will include the proximal humerus, glenohumeral joint, half of the clavicle, and a portion of the scapula

Marking of IR

- Anatomic side marker R or L placed furthest away from midline

Breathing

- Hold breath and instruct the patient to hold still
- Ensure patient holds position while walking away to make the exposure

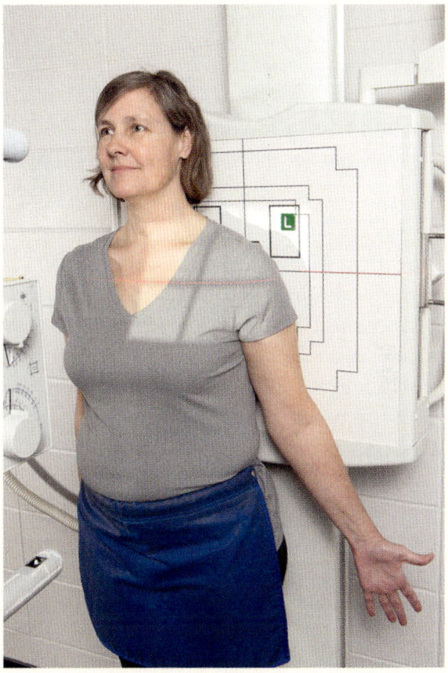

6-35 AP projection with external rotation.

IMAGE CRITIQUE (FIGS. 6-36 and 6-37)

- The relationship of the humeral head to the glenoid fossa is demonstrated
- Proximal humerus included with the greater tubercle seen in profile laterally. The lesser tubercle will not be well visualized as it is superimposed upon the humerus
- Centering and IR orientation will determine how much *or* whether all of the shoulder girdle is visualized
- Properly centered with four-sided collimation

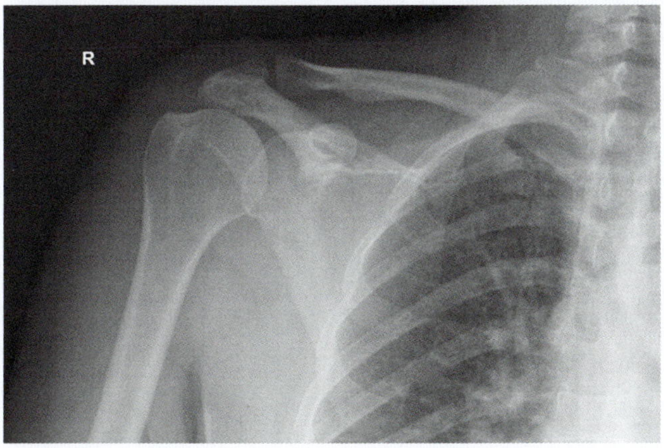

6-36 AP projection with external rotation.

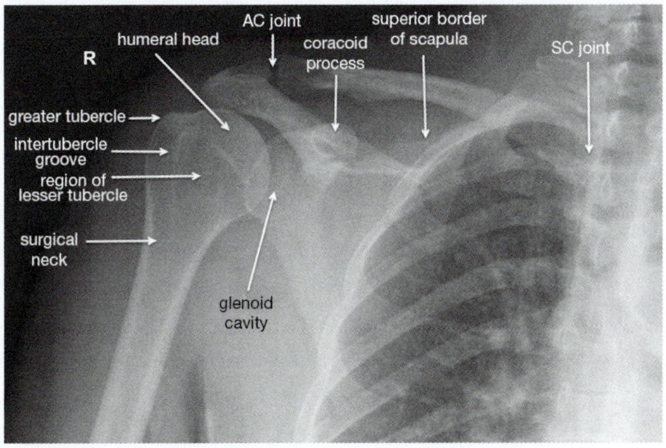

6-37 AP projection with external rotation.

Nontrauma Shoulder

- Projection: AP

Nontrauma Shoulder Protocol
AP (external rotation)
AP (internal rotation)

Technical Considerations

- kVp 70–80
- Center cell AEC or mAs set manually
- 40" SID

Exposure Field Size

- 10 × 12 crosswise to include the entire shoulder girdle
- 10 × 12 lengthwise to include more of the proximal humerus but will fail to include the SC joint

Patient Position (Fig. 6-38)

- Erect or seated on a stool
- Patient may be supine
- Internally rotate hand and arm until the humeral epicondyles are perpendicular to the imaging plane behind. Palpate the humeral epicondyles to ensure proper position

Centering

- For 10 × 12 crosswise imaging, direct the CR 1" inferior to coracoid process and 1" medial to coracoid process. This centering and IR orientation will include the SC joint, entire clavicle, glenohumeral joint, and proximal one-third of the humerus. Inclusion of the SC joint should be verified with the palpation of the jugular notch. Ensure light field appears to include proximal humerus with proper centering
- For 10 × 12 lengthwise imaging, direct the CR 1" inferior to the coracoid process. This centering and IR orientation will include the proximal humerus, glenohumeral joint, half of the clavicle, and a portion of the scapula

Marking of IR

- Anatomic side marker R or L placed furthest away from midline

Breathing

- Hold breath and instruct the patient to hold still
- Ensure patient holds position while walking away to make the exposure

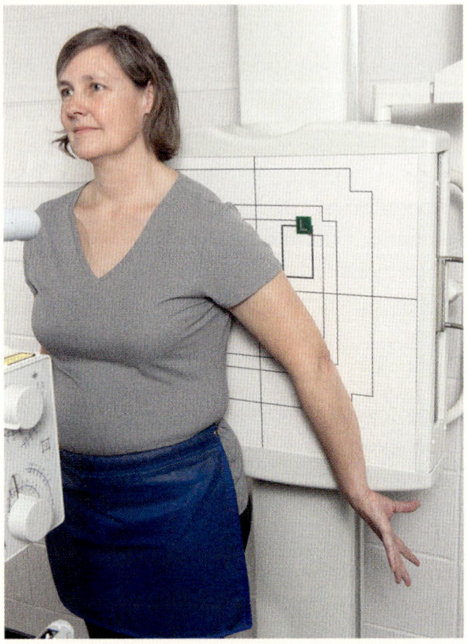

6-38 AP projection with internal rotation.

IMAGE CRITIQUE (FIGS. 6-39 and 6-40)

- The relationship of the humeral head to the glenoid fossa is demonstrated
- Proximal humerus included with the lesser tubercle seen in profile medially (toward the glenoid fossa). The greater tubercle will not be well visualized as the internal rotation of the arm will shift the greater tubercle from its lateral position to be superimposed anteriorly upon the humerus
- Centering and IR orientation will determine how much *or* whether all of the shoulder girdle is visualized
- Properly centered with four-sided collimation

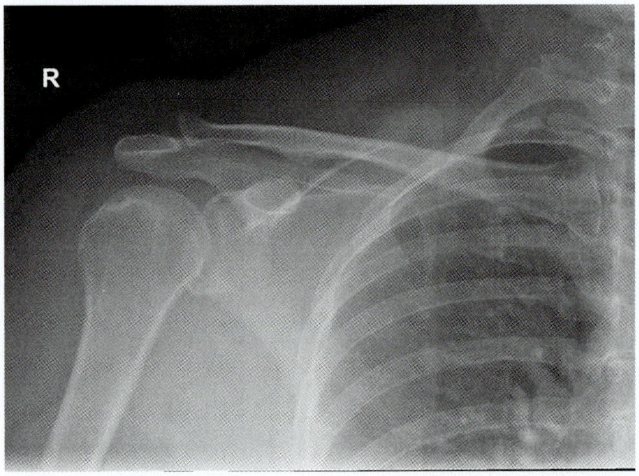

6-39 AP projection with internal rotation.

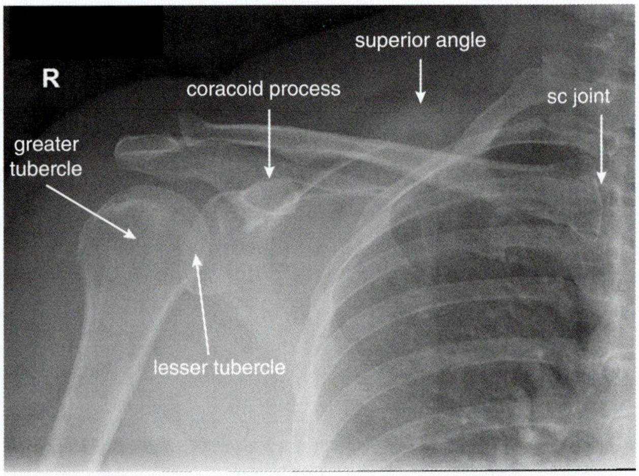

6-40 AP projection with internal rotation.

Nontrauma Shoulder

- Projection: AP Oblique
- Grashey method

Technical Considerations
- kVp 70–80
- Center cell AEC or mAs set manually
- 40" SID

Exposure Field Size
- 8 × 10 or smaller collimated exposure field is encouraged

Patient Position (Fig. 6-41)
- Erect or seated on a stool
- Patient may be supine
- Arm remains in a neutral position (humeral epicondyles are approximately 45° in reference to the IR). (*Ordering physicians may request the arm to be internally or externally rotated*)
- The patient will be rotated into a posterior oblique position with the affected side closest to the IR. The position is trying to achieve visualization of the glenoid fossa in profile and the glenohumeral joint space open
- An average posterior oblique position of about 45°. Rotate the patient toward the affected side

Centering
- Glenohumeral joint space. Move the central ray slightly lateral to the coracoid process

Marking of IR
- Anatomic side marker R or L placed furthest away from midline

Breathing
- Hold breath and instruct the patient to hold still
- Ensure patient holds position while walking away to make the exposure

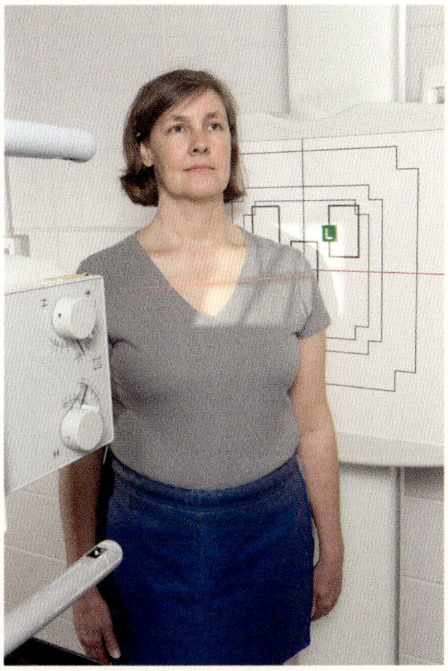

6-41 AP Oblique projection—LPO position.

IMAGE CRITIQUE (FIGS. 6-42 and 6-43)

- Glenoid fossa is seen in profile and the glenohumeral joint space open with proper rotation of the part. With rotation toward the affected side, the distal tip of the coracoid process will shift laterally from anatomic anterior location and towards the joint space
- Over- or underrotation of the patient will result in the glenohumeral joint appearing closed off. The position of the coracoid process could be helpful in determining if the patient was over- or underrotated (Figs. 6-44 and 6-45)
- The clavicle will likely appear distorted owing to the obliquity of the patient's thorax
- Properly centered to the glenohumeral joint with four-sided collimation

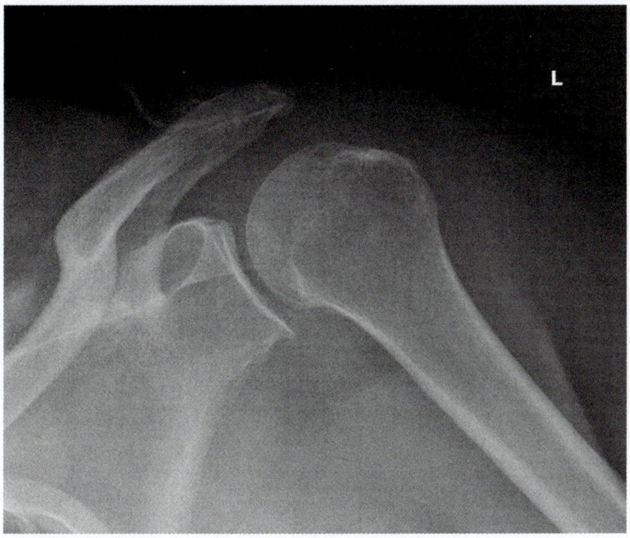

6-42 AP Oblique projection—LPO position.

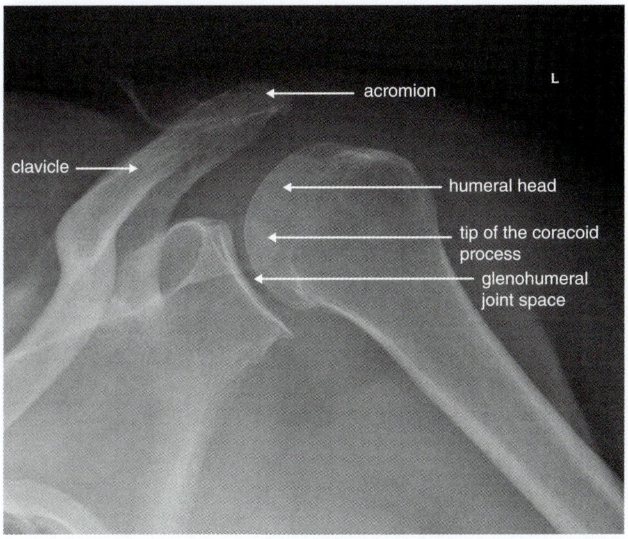

6-43 AP Oblique projection—LPO position.

(continued)

IMAGE CRITIQUE (*Continued*)

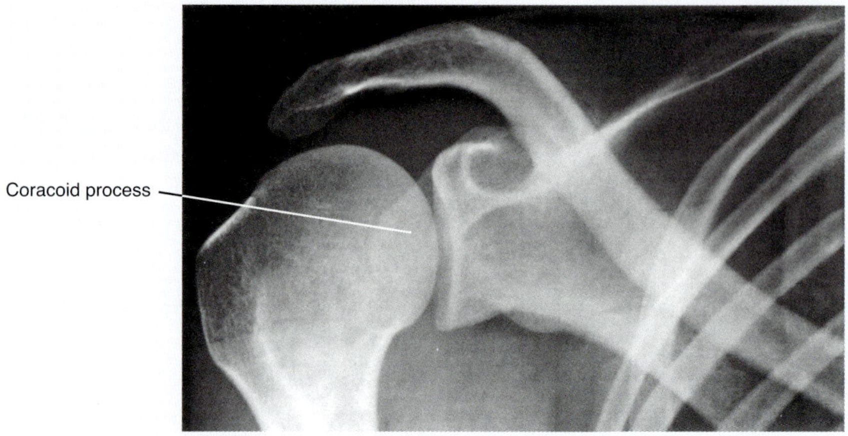

6-44 AP Oblique projection—Overrotated.

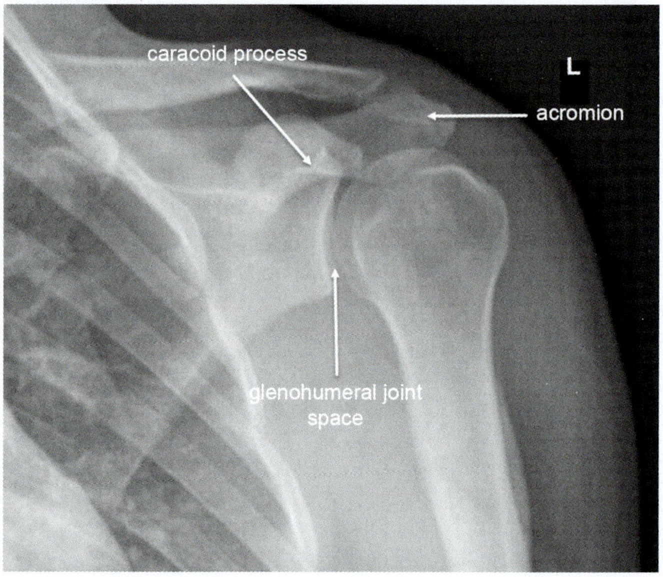

6-45 AP Oblique projection—Underrotated.

Nontrauma Shoulder

- Projection: Inferosuperior axial
- Lawrence method
- *Patient should not undergo this projection if a fracture or dislocation is suspected.*

Technical Considerations

- kVp 70–80
- Manual technique
- Grid versus no grid determined by part thickness
- 40" SID

Exposure Field Size

- 10 × 12 lengthwise with the humerus

Patient Position (Fig. 6-46)

- Patient is supine
- Affected shoulder is built up off the table
- Affected arm abducted 90° from the body. Ensure abducted arm is properly supported
- Palm is supinated, and humeral epicondyles are aligned parallel to the plane behind
- Patient must turn head away from affected side
- Large-breasted females may pull breast tissue up and onto the chest wall to avoid additional tissue superimposition over the shoulder anatomy
- IR is placed superior to the shoulder with the edge of the IR up close to the patient's neck. The IR must drop below the part that has been built up
- The IR is slightly angled out from the neck. The top of the IR should not be flat with the top of the shoulder. The angle of the IR must match the angle of the tube head

Centering (Fig. 6-47)

The tube is rotated 90° to create a horizontal beam. The tube is then angled 20°–30° to the midline of the patient and centered in the midaxilla. If the beam is angled too steep into the midline (for example, 45°), achieving proper collimation with centering to the axilla will be difficult

Marking of IR

- Anatomic side marker R or L placed furthest away from midline and anterior to the part

Breathing

- Hold breath and instruct the patient to hold still
- Ensure patient holds position while walking away to make the exposure

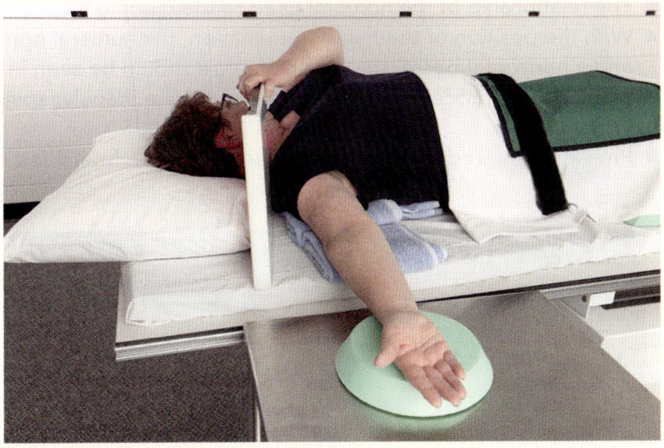

6-46 Inferosuperior axial projection.

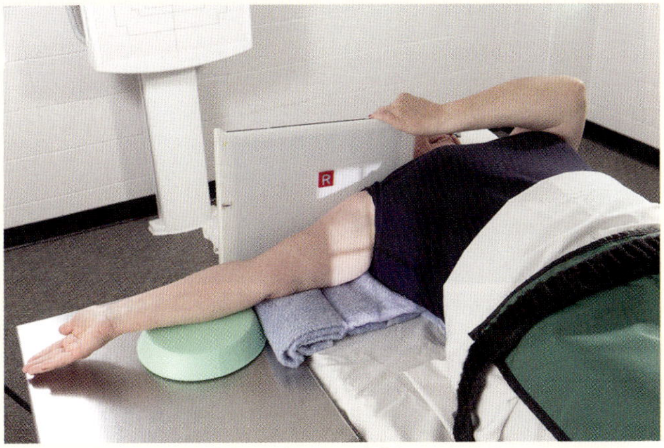

6-47 Inferosuperior axial projection.

IMAGE CRITIQUE (FIG. 6-52)

- Proximal one-third of the humerus included. Neither the greater nor the lesser tubercle will be seen in profile when the arm is in neutral position. Neutral position describes the humeral epicondyles to be positioned in between parallel and perpendicular to the imaging plane behind; likely closer to a 45° reference
- Centering and IR orientation will determine how much *or* whether all of the shoulder girdle is visualized
- Properly centered with four-sided collimation

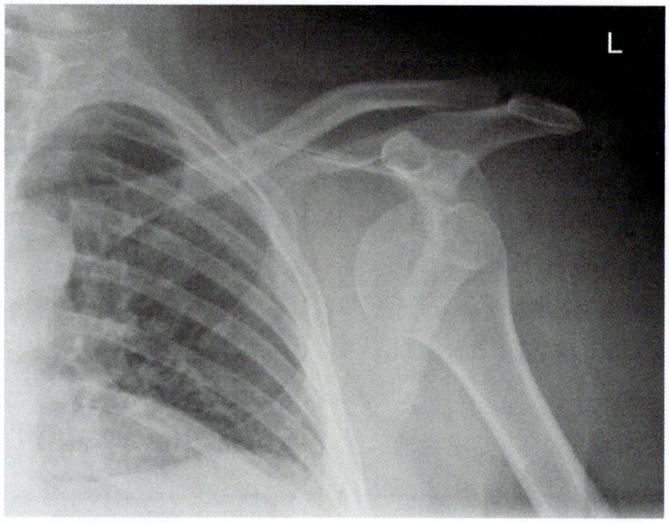

6-52 AP projection—neutral position.

Trauma Shoulder

- Projection: Transthoracic Lateral
- *Do not attempt to reposition the arm if dislocation or fracture is suspected. Affected arm should remain in neutral position*

Trauma Shoulder Protocol
AP (neutral rotation)
Transthoracic Lateral *or* Scapular Y Lateral

Technical Considerations

- kVp 75–80
- Center cell AEC or mAs set manually
- Breathing technique may offer improved image quality
- 40" SID
- Grid

Exposure Field Size

- 10 × 12 lengthwise

Patient Position (Figs. 6-53 and 6-54)

- Erect or seated on a stool
- Patient may be supine
- Patient should be upright in a lateral position or a horizontal beam if patient is supine
- Patient's affected arm should remain in neutral position or presenting position. This will likely cause the humeral epicondyles to be positioned at about a 45° oblique with the plane behind
- Unaffected arm elevated above the patient's head in an attempt to keep the shoulders separated

Centering

- Direct CR to the surgical neck of the affected humerus. The center of the IR should be set to this level
- The beam will enter the midcoronal plane or slightly posterior on the side that is closest to the tube
- The central ray is set to level of the surgical neck of the affected side to allow for proper penetration of the shoulder joint

Marking of IR

- Anatomic side marker R or L indicating affected side closest to the IR. The marker should be placed anterior to the part

Breathing

- Hold breath and instruct the patient to hold still
- Breathing technique is also an option. The breathing technique implements a longer exposure time while the patient purposely breathes through the exposure to blur out lung markings and ribs overlying the stationary humerus. The transthoracic lateral directs the beam through the entire thorax before reaching the affected humerus
- Ensure patient holds position while walking away to make the exposure

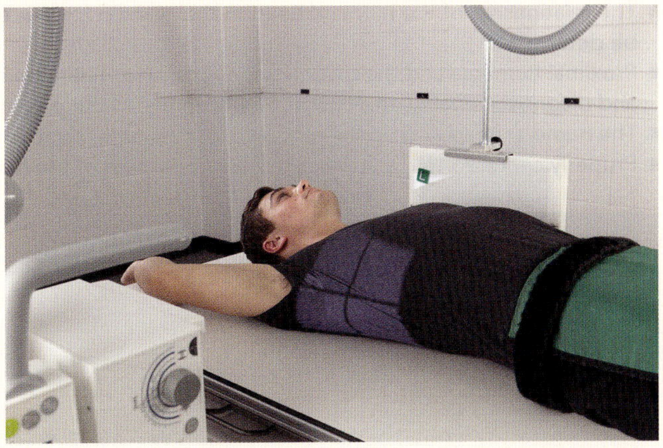

6-53 Transthoracic lateral—patient supine.

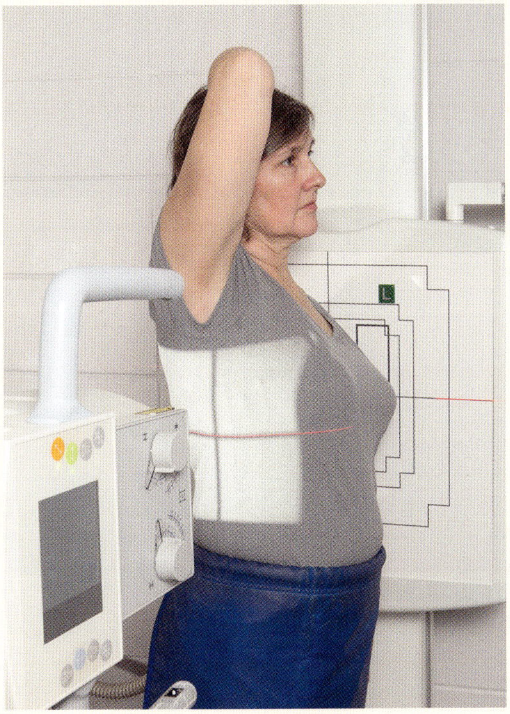

6-54 Transthoracic lateral—patient upright.

Clavicle

Clavicle Protocol
AP
AP Axial

- Projection: AP Axial
- *PA Axial projection would be the best option to place the clavicle closer to the IR (reduced OID), but in the interest of patient comfort and ease of centering, AP Axial projection is most commonly used. If PA Axial is employed, the tube is angled the same degree as the AP Axial; but the direction of tube angle is directed caudal*

Technical Considerations

- kVp 70–80
- mAs set manually
- 40" SID

Exposure Field Size

- 10 × 12 crosswise with collimation down to the clavicle

Patient Position (Figs. 6-67 and 6-68)

- Erect or seated on a stool
- Patient may be supine
- Affect arm remains down at side
- Chin slightly elevated with patient looking straight ahead

Centering

- The tube is angled 15°–30°cephalic. A thinner patient will require more cephalic tube angle (perhaps 30°) than a thicker patient. A thin patient's clavicle is closely situated to the ribs, requiring increased tube angle to create separation between the clavicle and ribs. A thicker, more muscular patient, will have an increased distance in between the clavicle and the ribs; therefore, the degree of angulation may be sufficient when set at 15°–20°
- Midclavicular shaft

Marking of IR

- Anatomic side marker R or L placed furthest away from midline

Breathing

- Hold breath and instruct the patient to hold still
- Ensure patient holds position while walking away to make the exposure

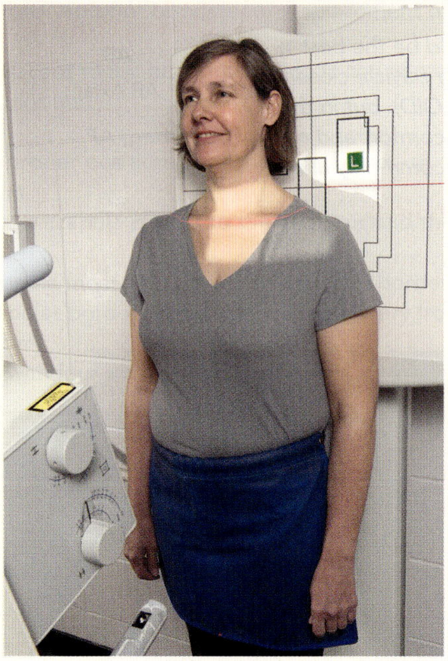

6-67 AP axial—erect.

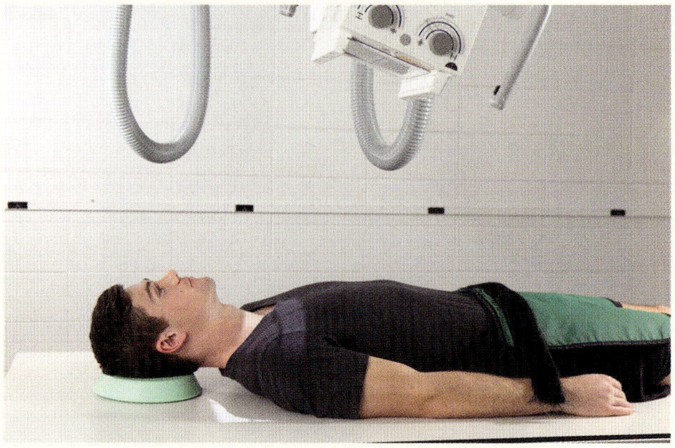

6-68 AP axial—supine.

IMAGE CRITIQUE (FIGS. 6-69 and 6-70)

- Entire clavicle to include the SC joint and the AC joint within the collimated exposure field
- The clavicle will mostly be flattened and projected superiorly to the scapula and the thorax. The SC joint will still remain superimposed upon the ribs
- The SC joint should appear symmetric to the thoracic spine, indicating no rotation of the part
- Properly centered with four-sided collimation. Superior to inferior collimation should be achieved

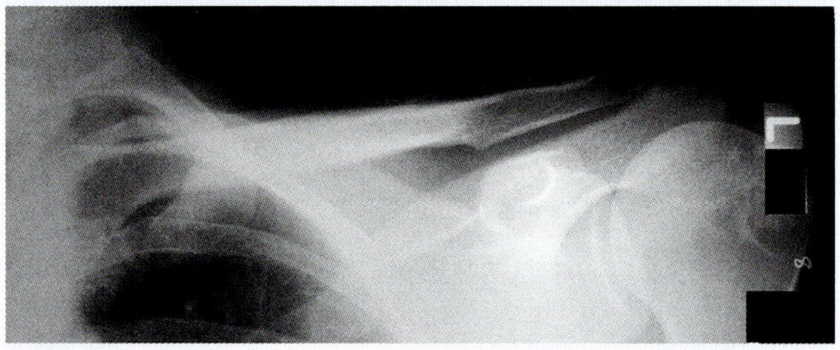

6-69 AP axial clavicle.

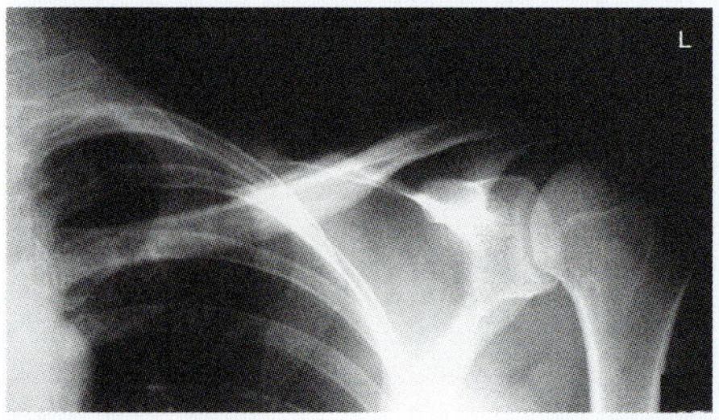

6-70 AP clavicle.

Scapula

- Projection: AP

Scapula Protocol
AP
Lateral

Technical Considerations
- kVp 70–80
- mAs set manually
- Breathing technique may offer improved image quality
- 40" SID

Exposure Field Size
- 10 × 12 lengthwise with collimation down for scapula

Patient Position (Figs. 6-71 and 6-72)
- Erect or seated on a stool
- Patient may be supine
- Elevate patient's chin slightly and have the patient look straight ahead
- Abduct the affected arm 90° from the side of the body. The abduction of the arm will flatten the scapula and align the scapular body parallel to the IR. This abduction also pulls most of the scapula laterally to free it from rib superimposition

Centering
- Midscapular body. 1"–2" below the coracoid process. Palpate the inferior angle of the scapula and adjust accordingly to include the entire scapula. With arm abduction, midscapular body lies near the inferior margin of the axilla

Marking of IR
- Anatomic side marker R or L placed furthest away from midline

Breathing
- Hold breath and instruct the patient to hold still
- Breathing technique is also an option. The breathing technique implements a longer exposure time while the patient purposely breathes throughout the exposure to blur out lung markings and ribs overlying the stationary scapula
- Ensure patient holds position while walking away to make the exposure

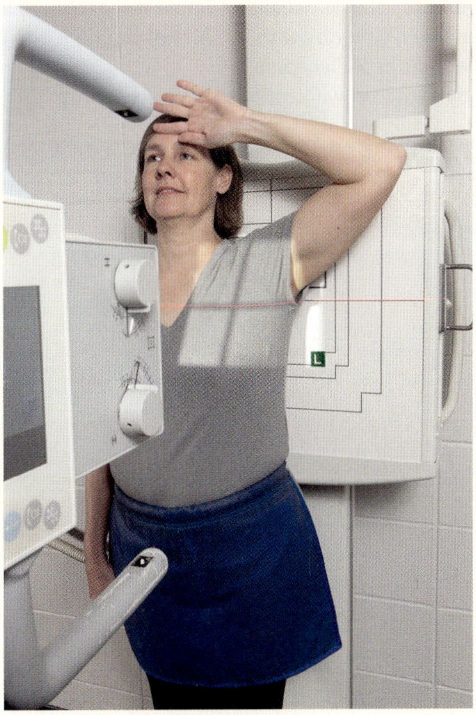

6-71 AP scapula—erect.

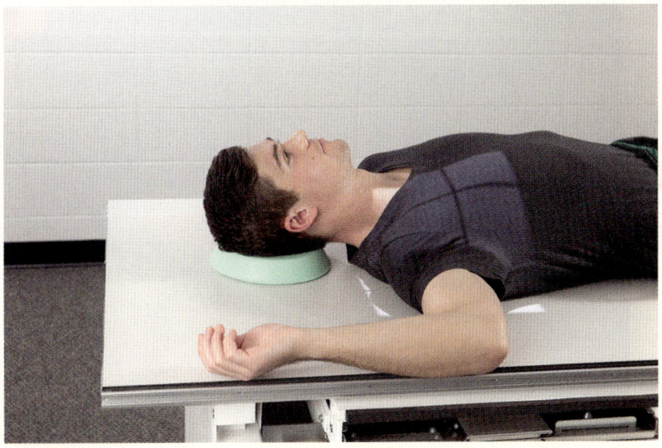

6-72 AP scapula—supine.

IMAGE CRITIQUE (FIGS. 6-77 and 6-78)

- The entire scapula must be demonstrated in the "Y" appearance. The coracoid process should be noted closer to the ribs.
- The humeral shaft will be seen crossing the thorax. This can be a helpful distinguishing identifier of the lateral scapula position (different from the arm position in a Scapular Y lateral when imaged with the trauma arm in neutral position)
- The scapular borders should be directly superimposed, indicating proper positioning of the part. Under- or overrotation can be determined by evaluating the placement of the scapular borders
- Underrotation of the part will display the lateral border of the scapula closest to the humerus and the vertebral border superimposed on the ribs
- Overrotation of the part will display the vertebral border of the scapula most lateral and the axillary border superimposed on or near the ribs. Remember the thickness difference between the scapular borders to help determine the axillary from the vertebral border. The axillary margin has a thick border, whereas the vertebral border is thin (Fig. 6-79)
- Properly centered to display the entire scapula with four-sided collimation

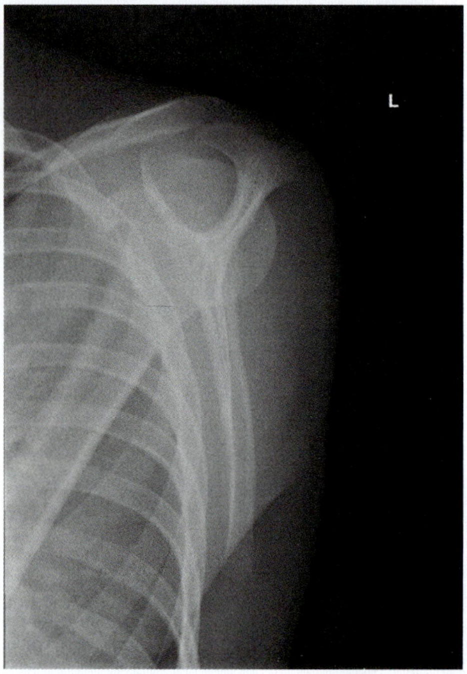

6-77 Lateral scapula.

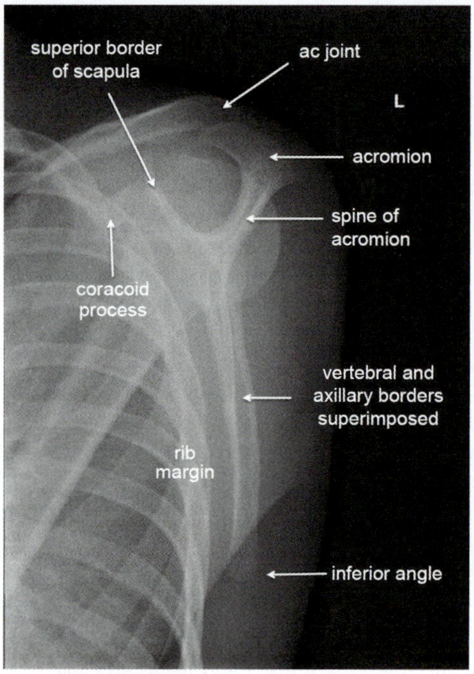

6-78 Lateral scapula.

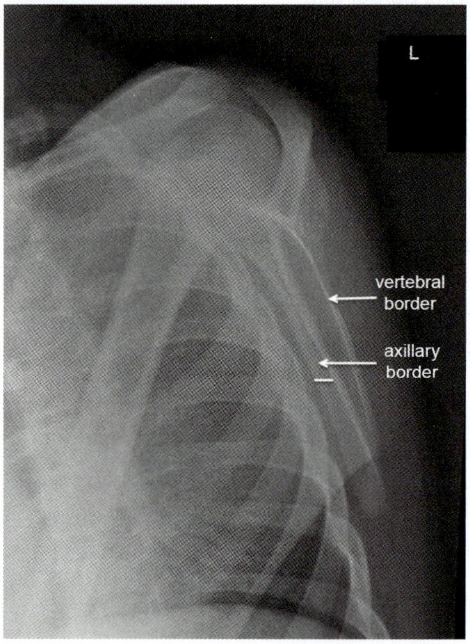

6-79 Lateral scapula—overrotated.

Acromioclavicular Joints

- Projection: AP (potentially 2 projections acquired)
- *AP with neutral position of the arms should be acquired first and checked prior to stressing the patient with wrist weights for the second AP.*

Acromioclavicular Joint Protocol
AP
AP with Stress

Technical Considerations
- kVp 75–80
- mAs set manually
- 72" SID

Exposure Field Size
- 14 × 17 crosswise with collimation down to the clavicles

Patient Position (Figs. 6-80 to 6-83)
- Erect or seated on a stool. This would be preferred for imaging, if possible, because natural effects of gravity may assist with the interpretation of results. Additionally, upright imaging allows for a 72" SID and a bilateral comparison
- Patient may be supine if unable to maintain an erect position. Recumbent imaging will not allow a 72" SID to be achieved
- Both arms remain down at side
- Chin slightly elevated with patient looking straight ahead.
- *The patient will first undergo a neutral image of bilateral joints for comparison and to rule out dislocation or fracture to the clavicles before adding stress or weights to the wrists. This first image should be reviewed and cleared before proceeding to the stress image*
- For stress imaging with the patient standing upright, weights are secured around the patient's wrist prior to exposure to help with depression of the upper limbs. By securing the weights to the wrists, this prevents the patient from resisting the weight. If the patient were to lie recumbent, the two ends of a sheet are put into the patient's hands, and with their own feet the upper limbs are depressed with the sheet by straightening their legs

Centering
- 2" superior to the jugular notch and with midsagittal plane (MSP)

Marking of IR
- Anatomic side marker R and L placed above the corresponding shoulders
- First projection should include additional annotation of "Neutral" or "Without Weights"
- Second projection should include additional annotation of "Stress" or "With Weights"

Breathing
- To increase separation effects of the AC joints, the patient should attempt to achieve maximum relaxation of the shoulder by double breathing, and after the second exhalation the exposure is made
- Ensure patient holds position while walking away to make the exposure
- Immediately after the second exposure, while the patient is stressed with weights, hurry to relieve the patient of the weights from around their wrists

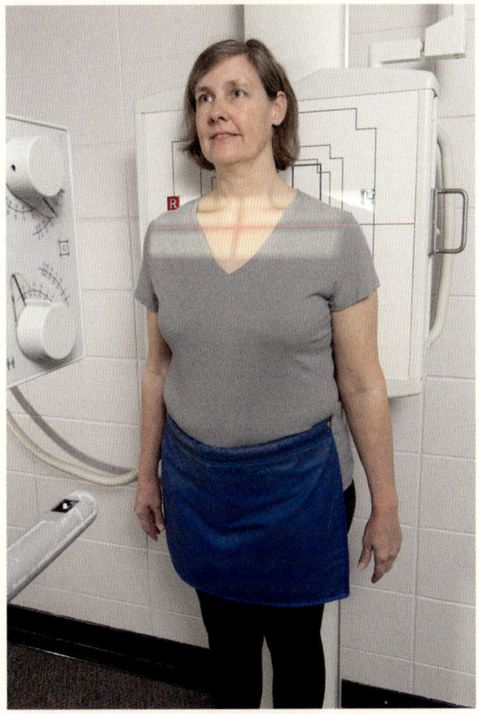

6-80 AC joints—erect.

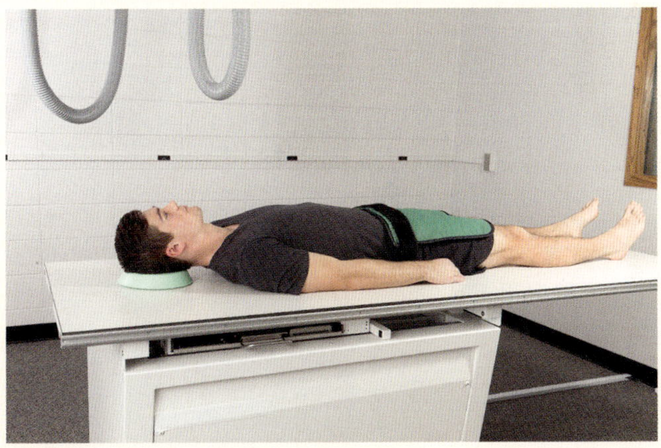

6-81 AC joints—supine.

(continued)

Acromioclavicular Joints (*Continued*)

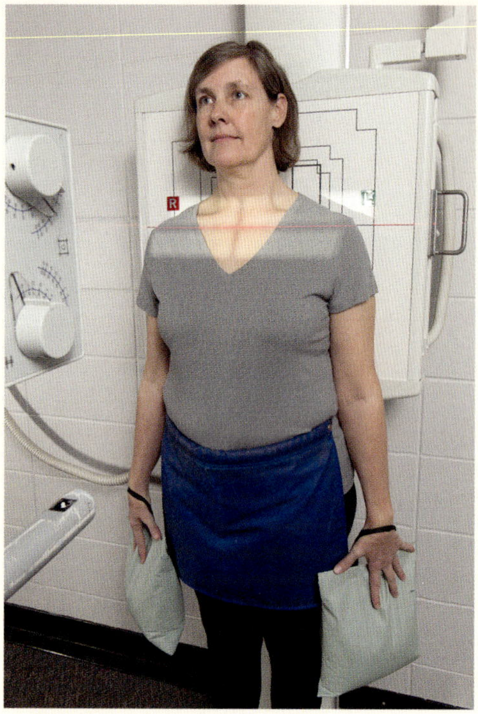

6-82 AC joints—erect with weights.

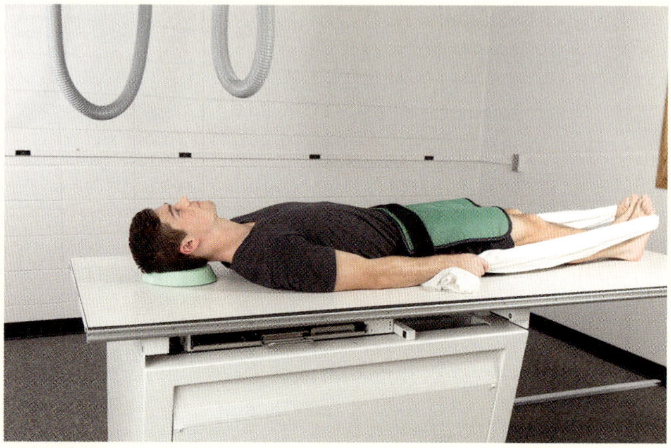

6-83 AC joints—supine with stress.

IMAGE CRITIQUE (FIG. 6-84)

- Bilateral clavicles, including the respective SC joints and the AC joints, are within the collimated exposure field
- This study is acquired bilaterally to allow for comparison of the right to left AC joint and to determine the amount of normal or abnormal AC joint separation
- The SC joints should appear symmetric to the thoracic spine, indicating no rotation of the thorax
- Properly centered with achieved superior to inferior collimation

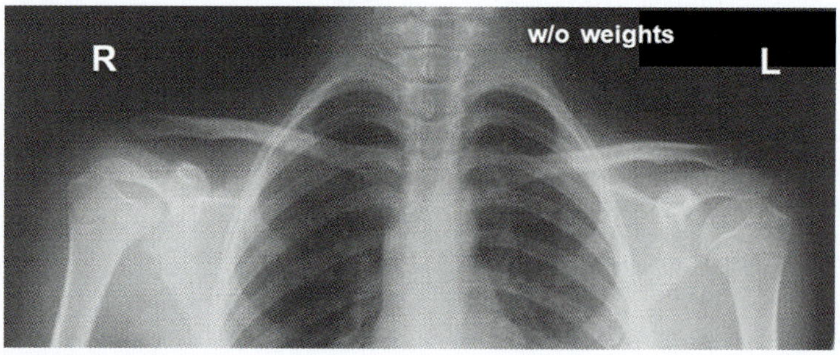

6-84 AC joints.

THE FINAL STEP: IMAGE REVIEW

The technologist must take time to review acquired images to ensure image quality is acceptable. The technologist must have the knowledge proper to their role not only to acquire the images and care for the patient, but also to know how to review the images to ensure diagnostic quality has been attained. In certain instances, a projection may need to be repeated. This is to the discretion of the radiologic technologist. The technologist should review each image for the following.

1. Is all of the necessary anatomy included on the image?
   - Was the central ray (CR) properly directed to the part? An "X" can be drawn to intersect within the collimated exposure field to determine whether the central ray was directed to the correct location.
   - Was essential anatomy in the collimated exposure field?
   - Is the area free of artifact(s)?
2. Is the anatomy well demonstrated?
   - Did the technologist properly position the patient to adequately demonstrate the anatomy?
   - Can the technologist recognize the anatomy best demonstrated with use of different projections?
3. Does the image reflect proper image markings?
   - Did the technologist correctly use a lead marker to identify the right or left side?
   - What additional markings or annotations could be helpful to the radiologist interpreting the exam?
   - Is the image properly displayed?
4. Does the image prove to be technically acceptable?
   - Does the exposure index fall within acceptable range for the operating system? Images that are technically insufficient may appear of good quality if just slightly insufficient or "mottled or pixelated" if severely insufficient. Images that appear "mottled" should be repeated. Images that appear beyond optimal exposure owing to higher technique may display high quality, but the patient has received excessive radiation dose.

CRITICAL THINKING

1. Referring to the Scapular Y view (Fig. 6-85), which of the following correctly characterizes its results?
   a. The image represents good lateral positioning of the part.
   b. The image represents underrotation of the part.
   c. The image represents overrotation of the part.
   d. The image presents proper positioning but incorrect centering.

2. According to the transthoracic lateral acquired for a trauma shoulder (Fig. 6-86), which of the following would characterize its results?
   1. Technically sufficient
   2. Technically insufficient
   3. Centering is directed to inferior on the part.
   4. Centering is directed to superior on the part.
      a. 1 and 3
      b. 2 and 3
      c. 1 and 4
      d. 2 and 4

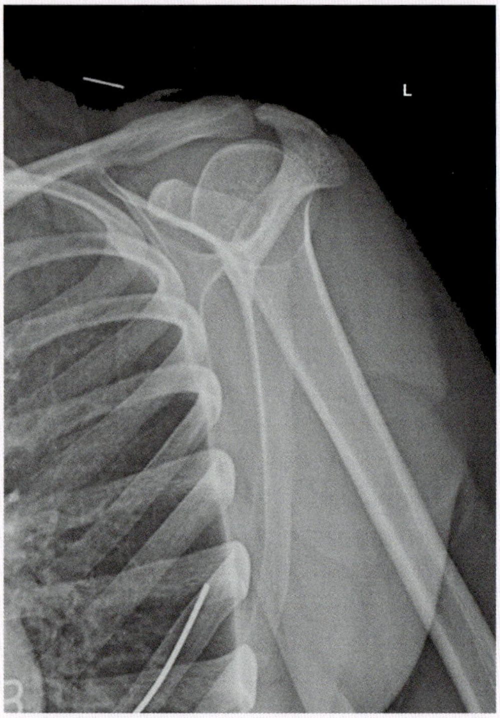

6-85

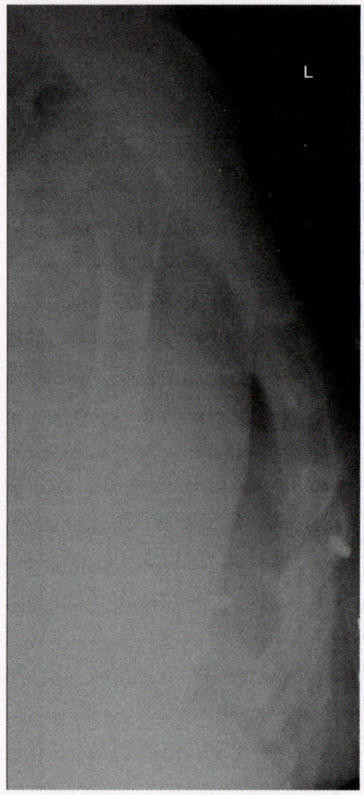

6-86

3. According to the inferosuperior axial shoulder (Fig. 6-87), which of the following adjustments would most improve the quality of the image?
   a. Decrease the kVp.
   b. Increase the kVp.
   c. Direct the central ray more medially on the part.
   d. Direct the central ray more laterally on the part.

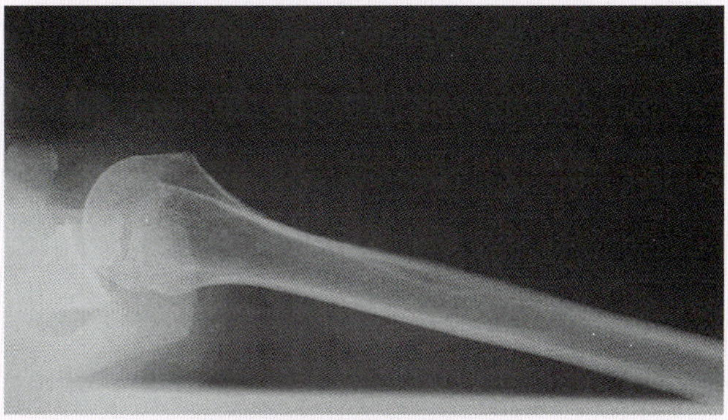

6-87

4. According to the AP Oblique shoulder (Fig. 6-88), which of the following would characterize its results?
   a. Image displays correct centering and proper positioning.
   b. Image displays correct centering and positioning, but too much collimation.
   c. Image displays correct centering, but underrotation.
   d. Image displays correct centering, but overrotation.

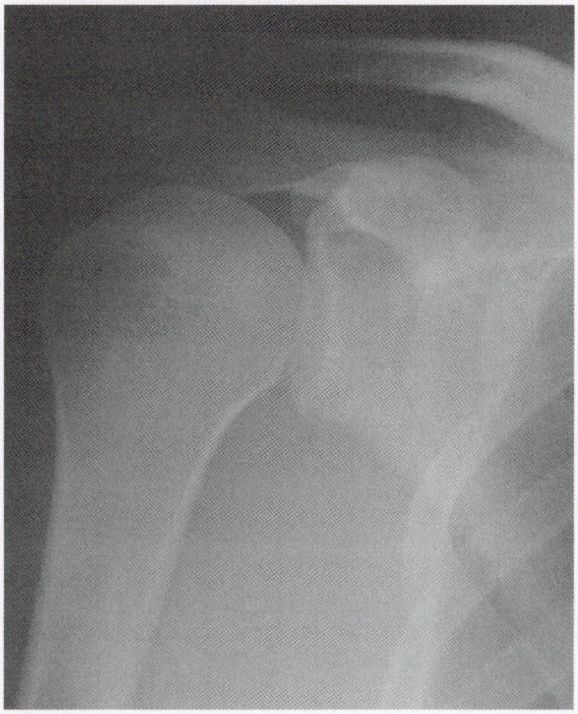

6-88

5. According to the lateral scapula (Fig. 6-89), which of the following characterizes its results?
   1. The central ray is correctly directed to the part.
   2. The central ray is directed to inferiorly on the part.
   3. The central ray is directed to superiorly on the part.
   4. The part represents correct rotation of the part.
   5. The part represents incorrect rotation of the part.
   a. 1 and 4
   b. 1 and 5
   c. 2 and 4
   d. 2 and 5
   e. 3 and 4
   f. 3 and 5

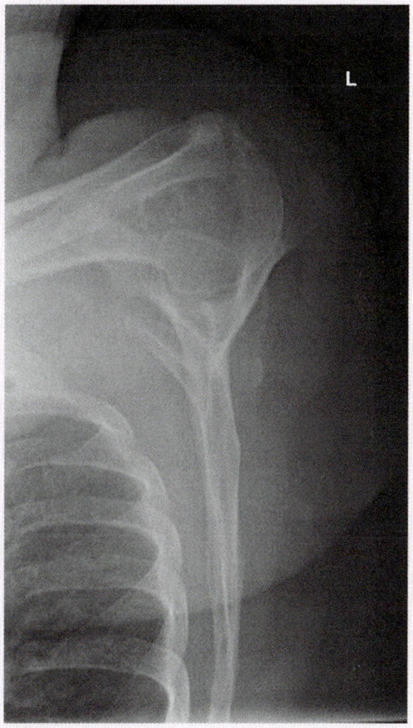

6-89

ANSWERS TO THE CRITICAL THINKING QUESTIONS

1. b
2. b
3. c
4. c
5. e

CHAPTER 7 Lower Extremity

Imaging of the lower extremity will include nontrauma and trauma patient situations. The technologist will need a proficient understanding of nontrauma protocols and be able to critically think and modify protocols in instances of patient trauma. Imaging of the trauma extremity may extend into imaging the patient while in the emergency department, surgical suite, and/or post anesthesia settings.

CLINICAL INDICATIONS

Indications are the symptomatic reasons as to why a particular exam may be ordered by the physician. The technologist should look at the clinical indications before performing a procedure. In certain circumstances, the indication may influence the need to increase or decrease the technical settings. The following briefly introduces common exam indications, but it is not an all-encompassing list.

Gout: A form of hereditary arthritis, more common in men, in which uric acid builds up in the bloodstream and travels to and crystalizes in joints. The most common joint that is first affected is the metatarsophalangeal (MTP) joint. Gout can affect other joints as well. This form of arthritis is not radiographically significant until the condition is chronic (Fig. 7-1).

Osteoarthritis: A form of degenerative disease to the joint resulting in patients experiencing pain and loss of joint mobility. This condition tends to affect patients of increased age and is in joints that are primarily weight bearing such as knees and hips. Advanced disease process will require a reduction in technical settings (Fig. 7-2).

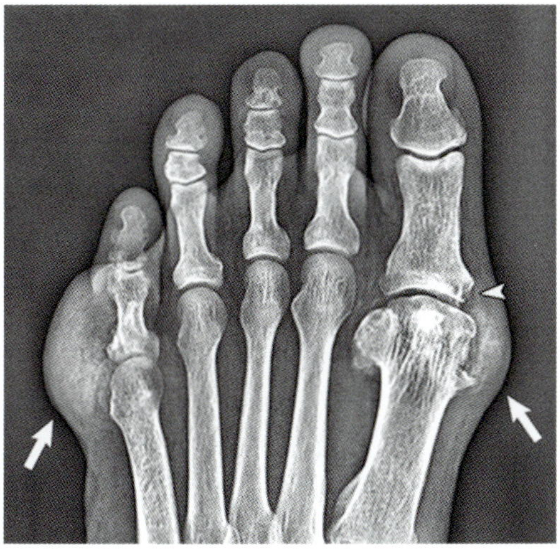

7-1 Gout. *Arrows* depict the accumulation of uric acid.

Jones Fracture: A fracture to the base of the fifth metatarsal. This could be a primary site of injury or a secondary site of injury in some cases. Imaging of the ankle and calcaneus should always include the base of the fifth metatarsal to rule out a secondary injury (Fig. 7-3).

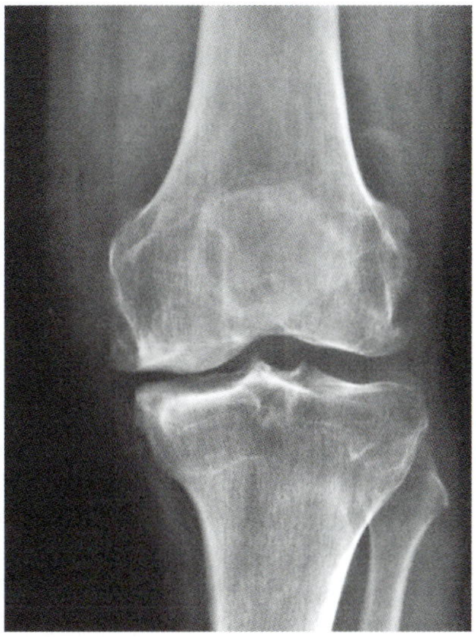

7-2 Osteoarthritis.

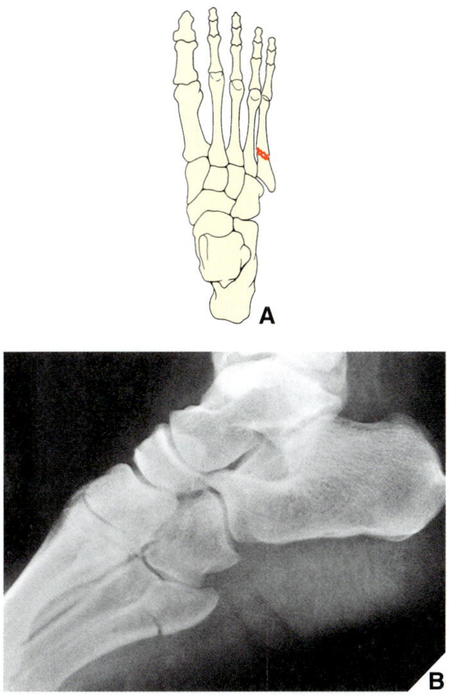

7-3 Jones fracture. **A:** Superior view of foot. **B:** Mediolateral projection.

Bimalleolar Fracture: A fracture to the distal tibia and fibula affecting the medial and lateral malleolus (Fig. 7-4).

Trimalleolar Fracture: A fracture of the ankle to include the medial malleolus, lateral malleolus, and the posterior tip of the tibia. The trimalleolar fracture may not be clearly determined until the ankle is imaged with the lateral projection (Fig. 7-4).

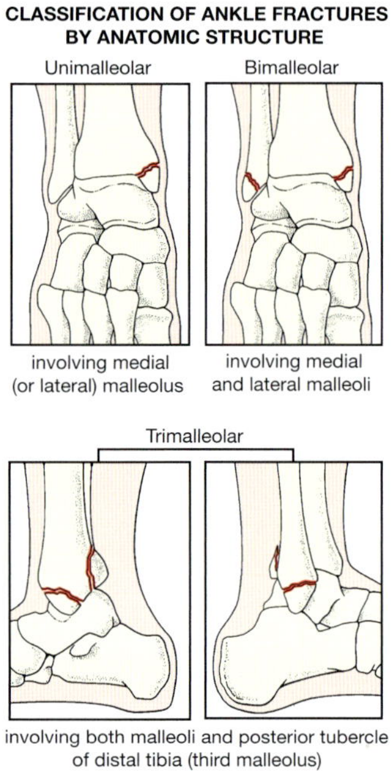

7-4 Bimalleolar versus trimalleolar fracture.

Bone Spur: Calcium deposit at the heel that can cause pain and is often associated with plantar fasciitis (Fig. 7-5).

Ewing's Sarcoma: A primary malignant bone tumor originating from the bone marrow in children and adolescents. This sarcoma commonly presents in long bones (Fig. 7-6).

Osgood–Schlatter Disease: Symptoms and pain to the region of the tibial tuberosity and commonly seen in rapidly growing adolescents. The pain is a result of the long bones growing faster than the attached quadriceps muscle to the tuberosity can stretch. With highly active adolescent boys and their rate of growth, pain is induced with repeated flexion of the knee. An avulsion fracture of the tibial tuberosity may be evident (Fig. 7-7).

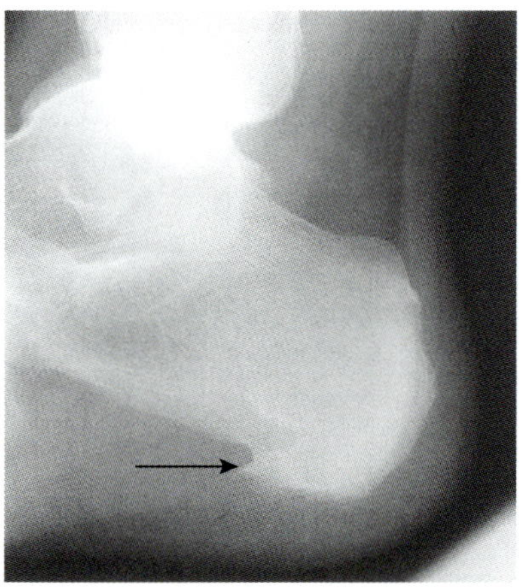

7-5 Bone spur.

Paget's Disease: Disease to the bone that is nonneoplastic and interrupts normal production of new bone. The overproduction of soft, but dense, bone creates a radiographic pattern that resembles "cotton wool." Long bones that are affected and may bow or fracture owing to softening of the bone. Advanced disease process may require an increase in technical settings (Fig. 7-8).

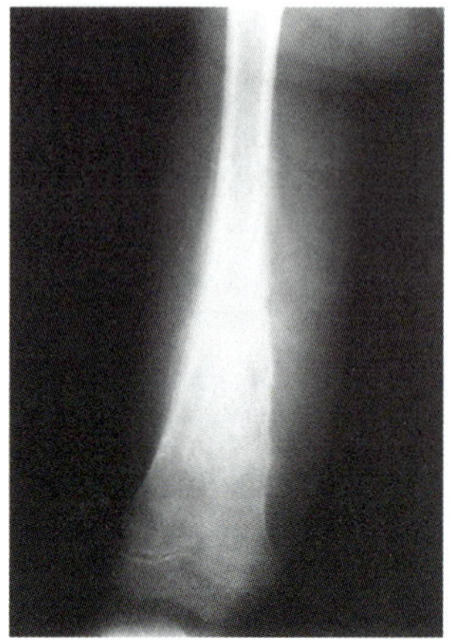

7-6 AP Femur—Ewing sarcoma.

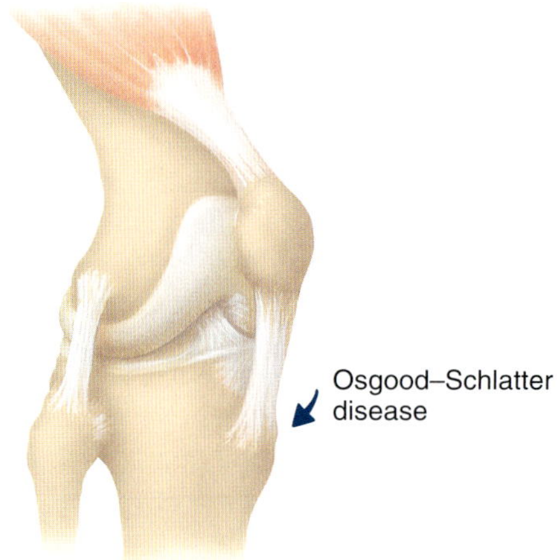

7-7 Osgood–Schlatter disease.

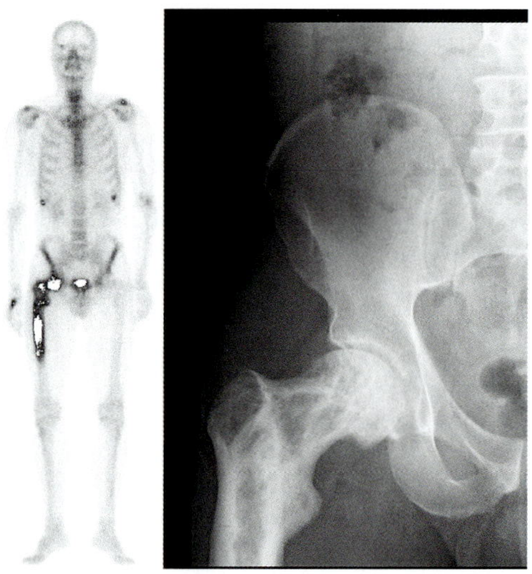

7-8 Paget's Disease. Bone scan reveals increased uptake of the radioisotope in the right femur correlative with the radiograph.

Legg–Calve–Perthes Disease: A necrotic lesion that affects the head of the femur most commonly in young boys, but a small percentage of females could be affected. Most often, the disease is unilateral but can be bilateral (Fig. 7-9).

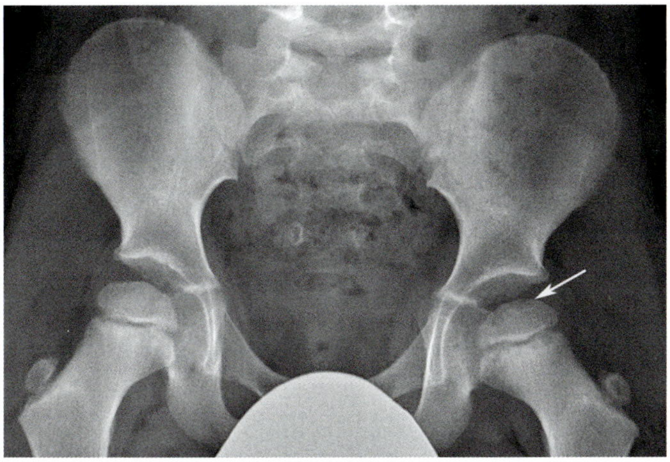

7-9 Legg–Calve–Perthes. Arrow notes change to the left femoral head.

Dislocation: Displacement of a bone from a joint. Pre- and postreduction imaging requires the acquisition of two views 90° apart (Figs. 7-10 to 7-13).

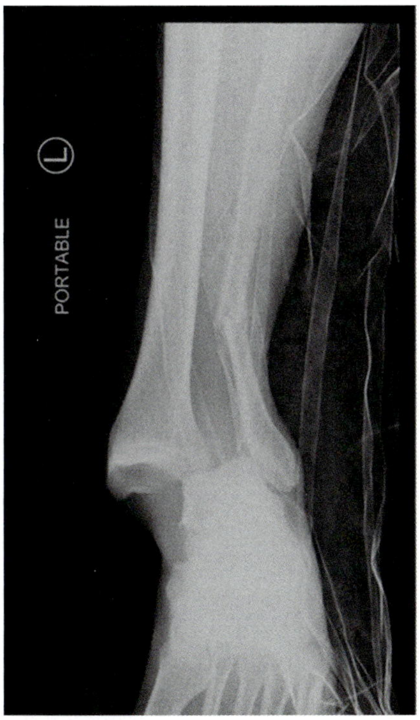

7-10 AP trauma ankle.

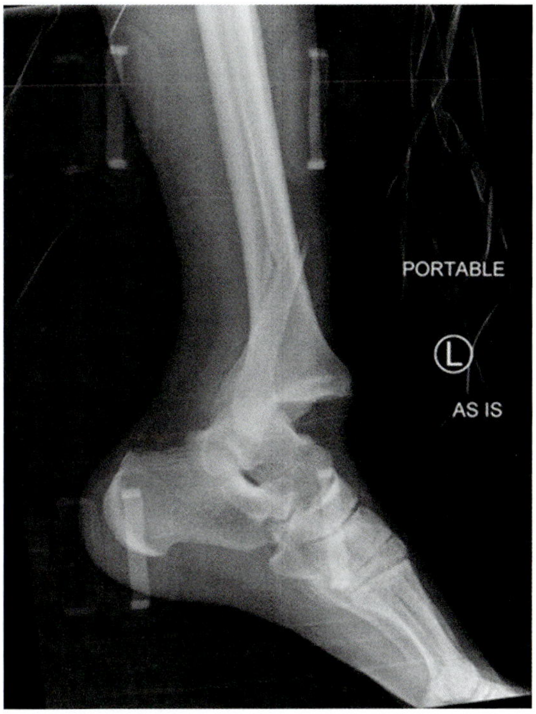

7-11 Lateral trauma ankle.

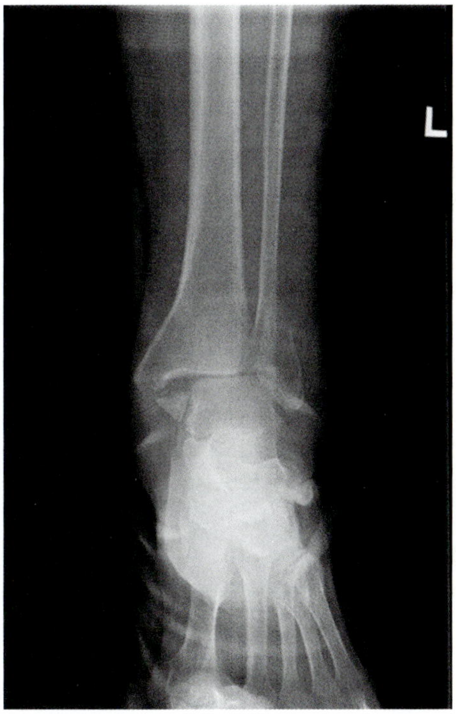

7-12 Postreduction AP ankle.

Foreign Body: Presence of wood, glass, or metal in the extremity. The placement of foreign object must be determined to be within the soft tissue or if it has penetrated the bone. Using a soft tissue technique by decreasing the kilovoltage will be important when trying to locate glass or wood. In some cases, a BB marker can be placed relative to the entrance wound and exit wound if applicable to call attention to the specific area. Two views 90° from one another should be acquired (Fig. 7-14).

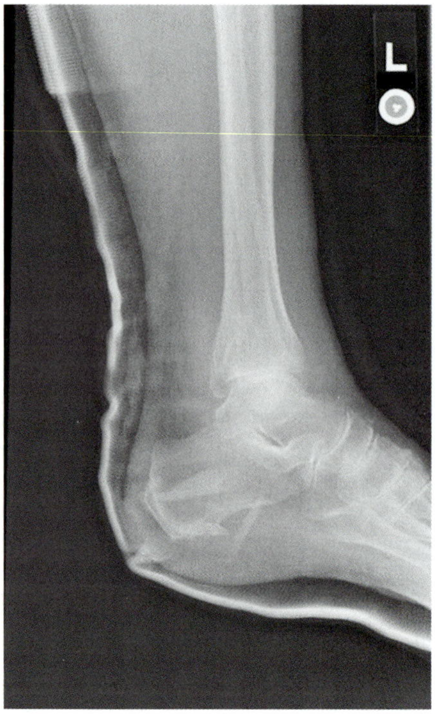

7-13 Postreduction Lateral ankle.

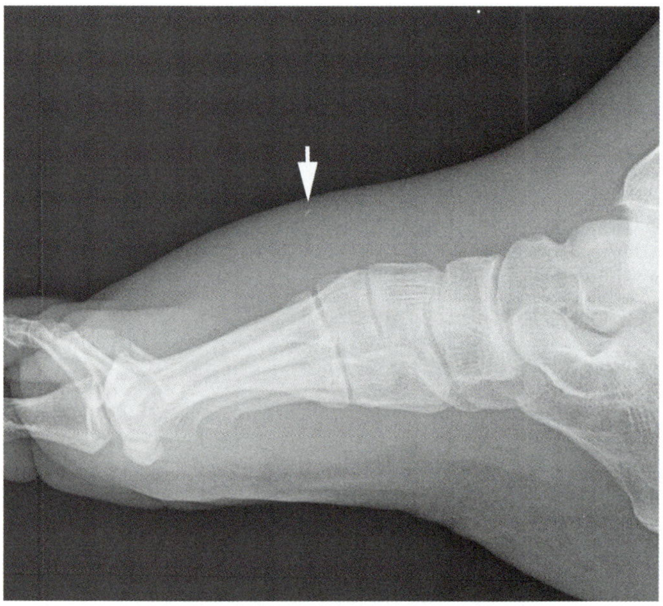

7-14 Foreign body (glass) localized in the dorsum of the foot.

IMAGING CONSIDERATIONS

Patient Dress

The patient may need to remove their pants, socks, and shoes and dress into a patient gown. This will prevent any clothing artifact. Patients need to remove all jewelry from the area of interest.

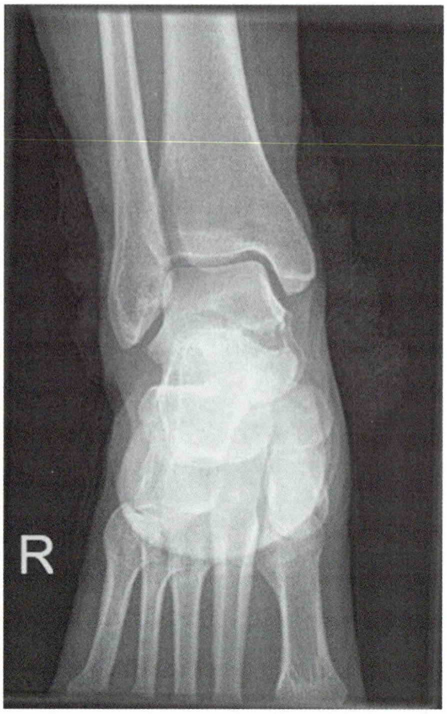

7-15 Artifact from elastic bandage wrap around the ankle.

Artifacts

Artifacts are unwanted objects that appear on the image superimposing pertinent anatomy. Failing to have the patient remove ankle bracelets, toe rings, socks, and certain clothing (containing thick seams or elastic) will cause artifact and potentially obscure essential anatomy. Repeat imaging may be necessary when an artifact obscures the area of interest (Fig. 7-15).

Patient Position

The general position of the patient or part

Seated on imaging table or stretcher—This will allow the patient's extremity to be positioned easily by placing the extremity on the tabletop. Tabletop imaging is common when imaging toes, feet, ankles, and lower leg (Fig. 7-16). When imaging tabletop exams, ensure the table Bucky is moved away from the exposure field to minimize scatter radiation. Patients transported by stretcher may be able to remain on the stretcher for necessary imaging for certain exams—eliminating the need to transfer them over to the imaging table (Fig. 7-17).

Upright—Relative to this chapter, this position could be considered when imaging orders declare the patient to be weight bearing, such as with feet, ankles, or knees.

Recumbent—Routinely used for lower extremity imaging either with the patient laying on the imaging table or stretcher unless the exam is ordered weight bearing.

Ambulatory Patient Imaging

An ambulatory patient is one who can maneuver themselves and bears weight with little to no assistance. Ambulatory patients will be able to walk or may come by wheelchair to the exam room.

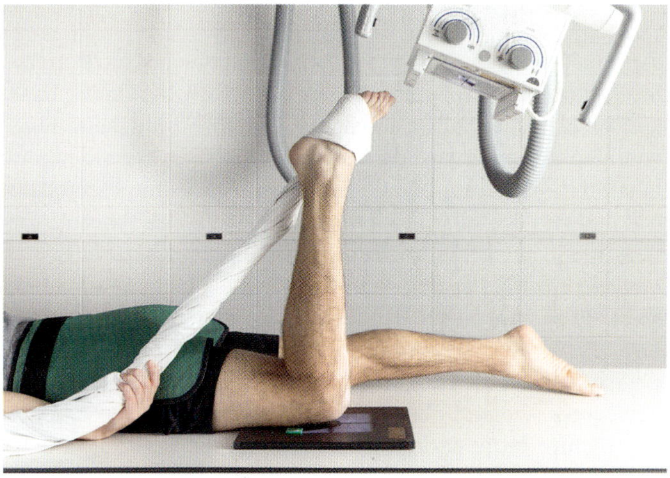

7-16 Tabletop imaging.

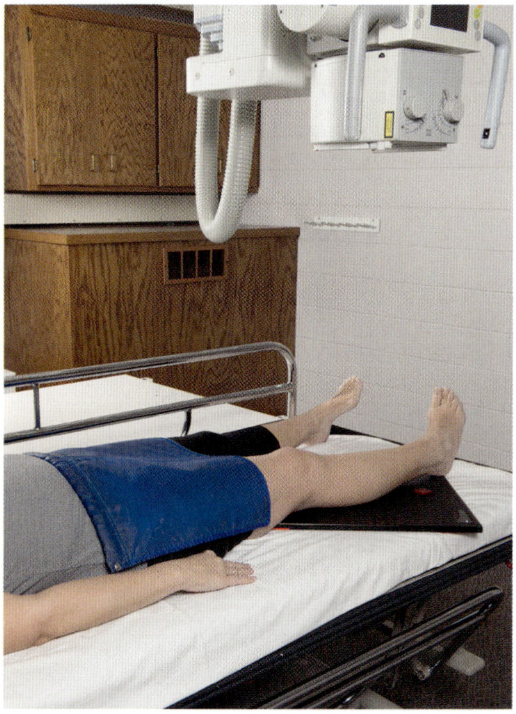

7-17 Imaging the lower extremity with the patient remaining on the stretcher.

Projection(s)

How the x-ray beam passes through the part

- Anteroposterior (AP): The beam is directed to enter through the anterior surface, exit the posterior surface, and strike the image receptor (IR).
- Posteroanterior (PA): The beam is directed to enter the posterior surface, exit the anterior surface, and strike the IR.
- AP Oblique: The beam is directed to enter the anterior surface, exit the posterior surface while the part is positioned into a particular degree of obliquity.
- Mediolateral: The beam will enter the anatomic medial surface and exit the lateral surface, which is closest to the IR.
- Lateromedial: The beam will enter the anatomic lateral surface and exit the medial surface, which is closest to the IR.
- Tangential: The beam skims across a surface.

ANATOMY

Imaging the lower extremity includes the anatomy of the toes, foot, ankle, lower leg, knee, and femur (Fig. 7-18).

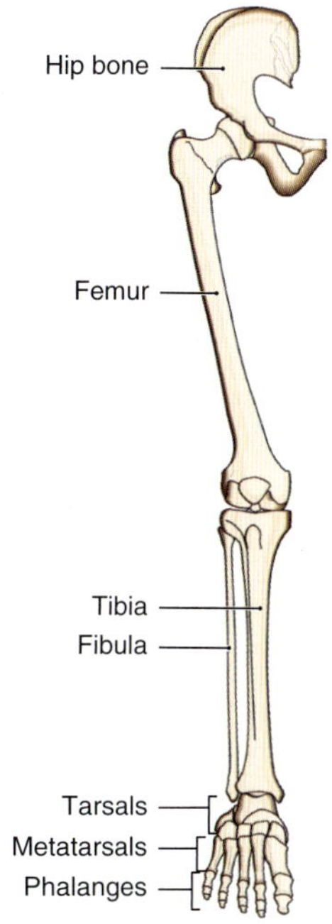

7-18 Lower extremity.

Toes

A toe can also be referred to as a digit. The great (big) toe is digit one. Each digit is comprised of two or three articulated smaller phalanges (phalanx if singular). The great toe only has two phalanges: a proximal and distal. In between the great toe's proximal and distal segments, the articulating joint is the interphalangeal (IP) joint. Digits 2–5 will have three phalanges—a proximal, middle, and distal (Fig. 7-19).

In the digits 2–5, the articulating joint between the distal and middle segment is the distal interphalangeal (DIP) joint. The articulating joint between the middle and proximal

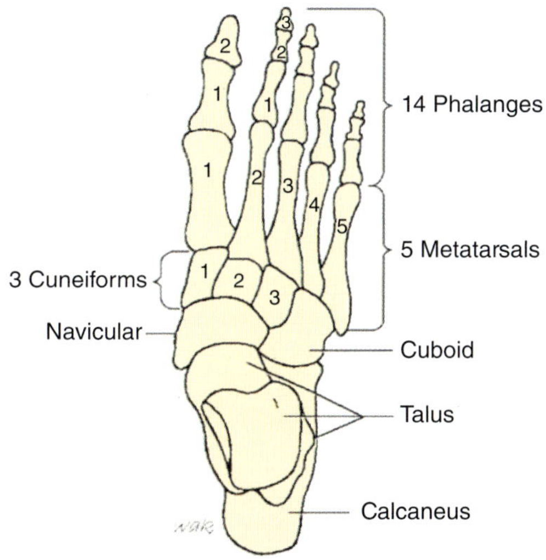

7-19 Digits and foot.

segment is the proximal interphalangeal (PIP) joint (Fig. 7-20). The technologist should attempt to position the digits as parallel to the plane of the image receptor as possible to better ensure these small joint spaces can be evaluated for small avulsion (chip) fractures. However, this is often difficult to impossible to achieve considering the natural curvature of the toes. All IP joints are of synovial and diarthrodial type with ginglymus or hinge-like movement.

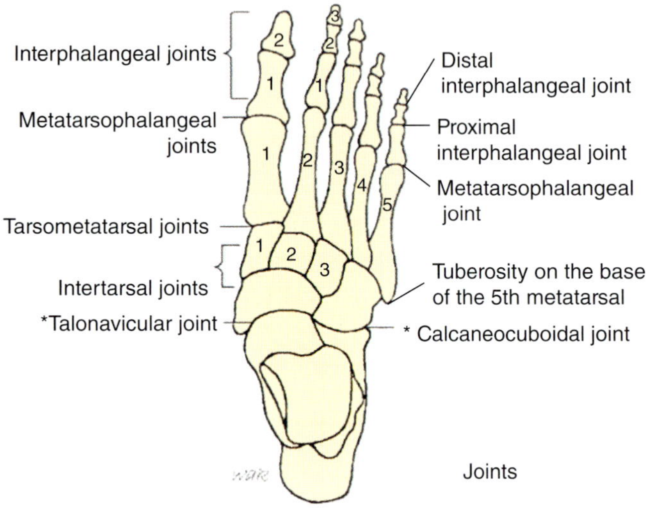

7-20 Joints of the foot.

Foot

The instep of the foot comprises five metatarsals. Each metatarsal is numbered respectably to align with the digits. Each metatarsal, just as each phalangeal segment would, has a head (rounded and most distal), a shaft, and a base (expanded and most proximal) component. The base of the fifth metatarsal is widened and contains a tuberosity (Fig. 7-21). This tuberosity is a common site of fracture known as the Jones fracture.

Distal to the head of each metatarsal, a metatarsophalangeal (MTP) joint exists. Uniquely, at the head of the first metatarsal, two round sesamoid bones are located on the plantar surface of the foot embedded into the tendons. Considering their larger size and plantar surface location, sesamoid bones can fracture more easily compared with the sesamoid bones located at the first metacarpophalangeal joint in the hand (Fig. 7-22). Metatarsophalangeal joints are of synovial and diarthrodial type with condyloid type movement.

Proximal to the base of each metatarsal, a tarsometatarsal (TMT) joint exists. The base of each metatarsal has a respective articulation with the three cuneiforms or the cuboid (Fig. 7-20). The TMT joints are of synovial and diarthrodial type with plane or gliding type movement.

Ankle (Tarsals)

Calcaneus

Of the seven tarsal bones, the calcaneus is the largest. The calcaneal tuberosity is located on the most posterior (heel) and inferior surface of the foot (Figs. 7-23 and 7-24). The Achilles' tendon attaches to the calcaneal tuberosity and can cause symptomatic

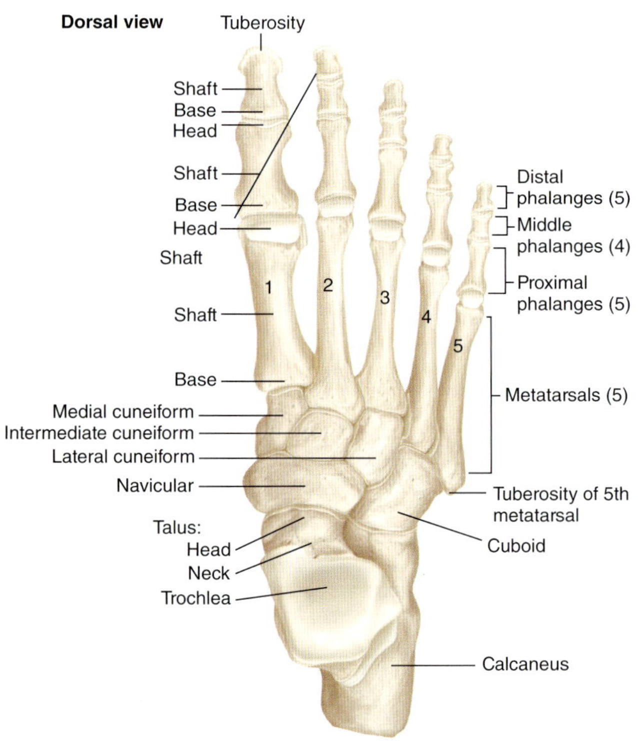

7-21 Dorsal view of the foot.

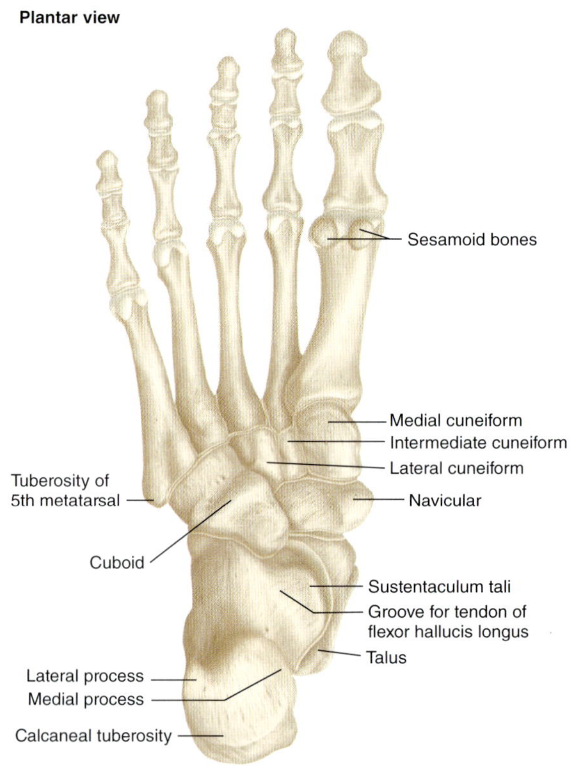

7-22 Plantar view of the foot.

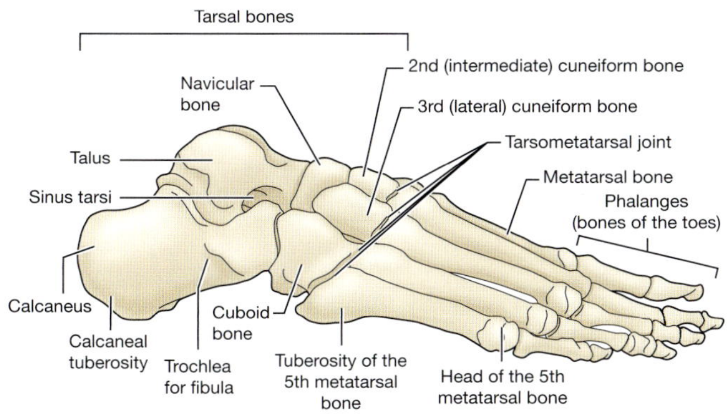

7-23 Lateral view of tarsals.

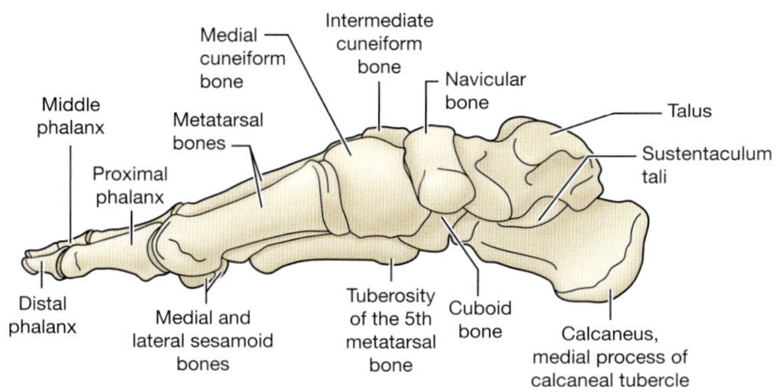

7-24 Medial view of tarsals.

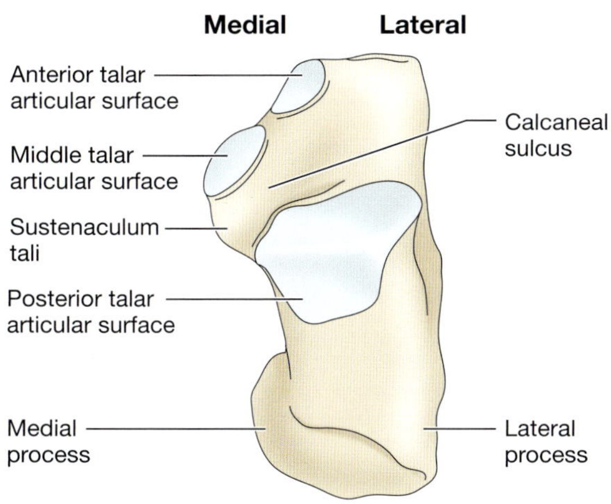

7-25 Superior view of calcaneus.

heel pain. Additionally, bone growths off the tuberosity, such as bone spurs, may also cause heel pain, especially while bearing weight. Upon the medial and lateral surface of the heel, the medial and lateral processes are located (Fig. 7-25).

Moving anteriorly (toward the toes) on the calcaneus, the calcaneus will articulate with the cuboid. On the medial portion of the anterior calcaneus, a prominent bony process, the sustentaculum tali is located. The sustentaculum tali provides additional support for the talus, which sits superior on the calcaneus. On the superior surface of the calcaneus, three articulating facets are present to accept parts of the talus to form the talocalcaneal or subtalar joint (Fig. 7-25). The articulating facets are as follows: anterior, middle, and posterior. The calcaneal sulcus (groove) is located between the middle and posterior facets, which match up with a groove on the inferior talus to form the sinus tarsi (small, round opening) in which ligaments travel through (Fig. 7-23).

Talus

The talus is positioned superior to the calcaneus. The talus helps to distribute the weight of the lower extremity down through the subtalar (talocalcaneal) joint and to the foot. The talus will articulate with the distal tibia and fibula superiorly, the calcaneus inferiorly, and the navicular anteriorly (toward the toes) (Figs. 7-23, 7-24, and 7-26).

Cuneiforms

The cuneiforms are referenced by their location, as they articulate directly with the bases of metatarsals 1–3. The first or medial cuneiform articulates primarily with the base of metatarsal 1. The second or intermediate cuneiform articulates primarily with the base of metatarsal 2 (Fig. 7-26). The third or lateral cuneiform articulates primarily with the base of metatarsal 3. With the close proximity of the cuneiforms with the metatarsal bases, there is slight overlap with each cuneiform to touch more than one metatarsal base. Directly posterior to the cuneiforms (toward the heel) is the navicular (Figs. 7-23 and 7-24).

Cuboid

The cuboid is located laterally on the foot. The cuboid articulates directly with the bases of metatarsals 4 and 5. The cuboid articulates with the third cuneiform. The cuboid also articulates with the calcaneus posteriorly (Figs. 7-23, 7-24, and 7-26).

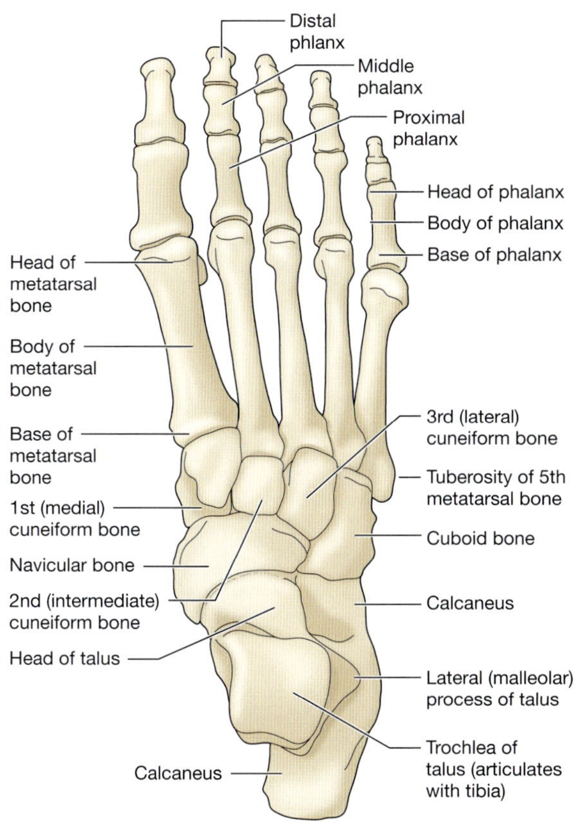

7-26 Superior view of tarsals.

Navicular

The navicular is rectangular in shape and positioned anterior to the talus and posterior the cuneiforms (Figs. 7-23, 7-24, 7-26 to 7-29; Table 7-1).

Arches of the Foot

The foot has two directional arches that run through the foot to aid in absorbing shock and distributing weight. There are two longitudinal arches that run with the instep of the foot formed by the metatarsals and tarsals. The medial longitudinal arch is more pronounced than the lateral longitudinal arch (Fig. 7-30). The foot also has a transverse arch that runs across the foot in the region of the tarsometatarsal joint (TMT) joints and distal row of tarsals (cuneiforms and cuboid) (Fig. 7-31).

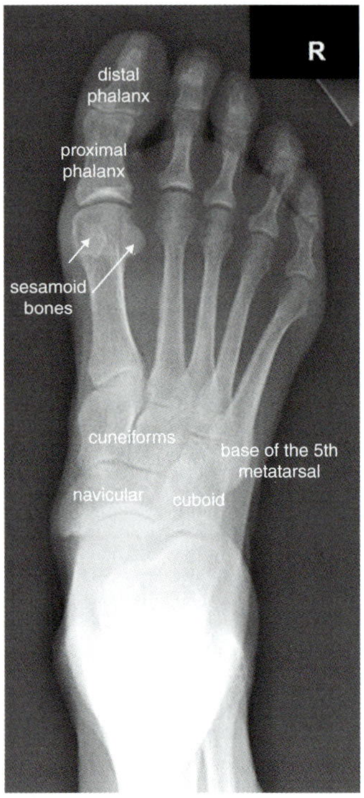

7-27 Dorsoplantar projection of the foot.

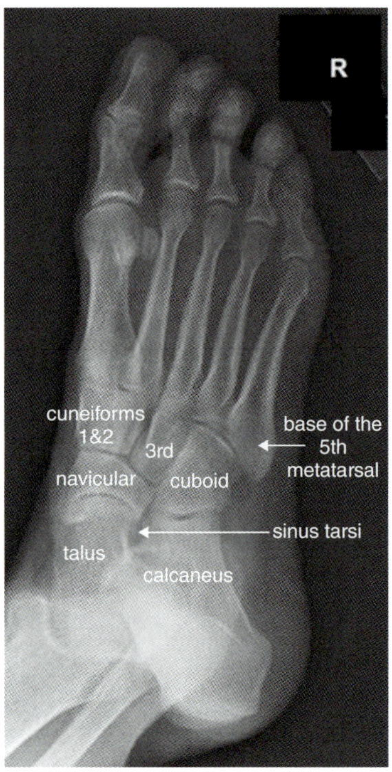

7-28 AP Oblique projection of the foot.

Lower Leg

The lower leg comprises the tibia and fibula, which articulate with one another through the distal and proximal tibiofibular joints. The tibia is located medially on the lower leg and the fibula laterally (Fig. 7-32).

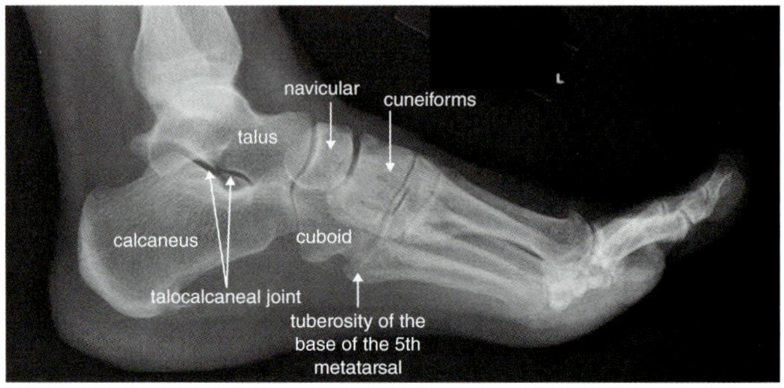

7-29 Mediolateral projection of the foot.

7-1 Tarsal Articulation

Talus	Tibia
	Fibula
	Calcaneus (inferiorly)
	Navicular (anteriorly)
Calcaneus	Talus (superiorly)
	Cuboid (anteriorly)
Navicular	Talus (posteriorly)
	Cuneiforms (anteriorly)
Cuneiforms	Respective metatarsal bases (anteriorly)
	Navicular (posteriorly)
	Medial cuneiform with intermediate cuneiform
	Intermediate cuneiform with medial and lateral cuneiform
	Lateral cuneiform with cuboid
Cuboid	Lateral cuneiform
	Calcaneus (posteriorly)
	Fourth and fifth metatarsals (anteriorly)

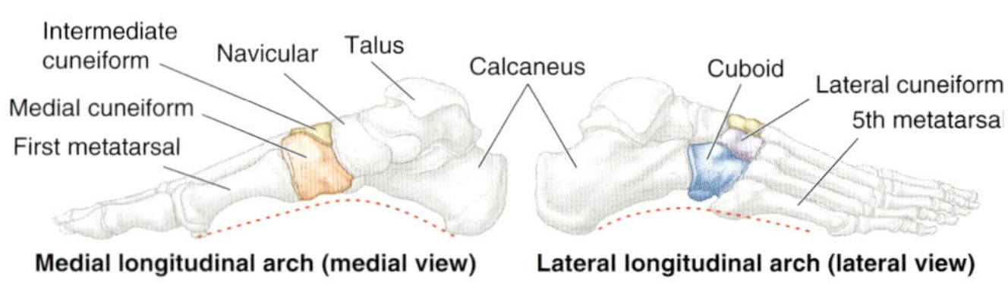

7-30 Medial and lateral longitudinal arches.

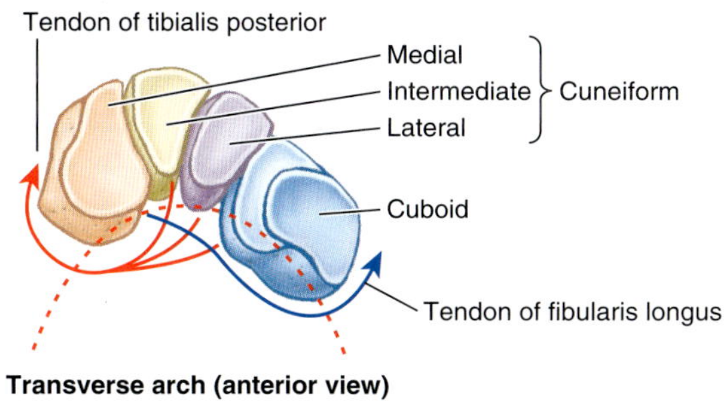

7-31 Transverse arch.

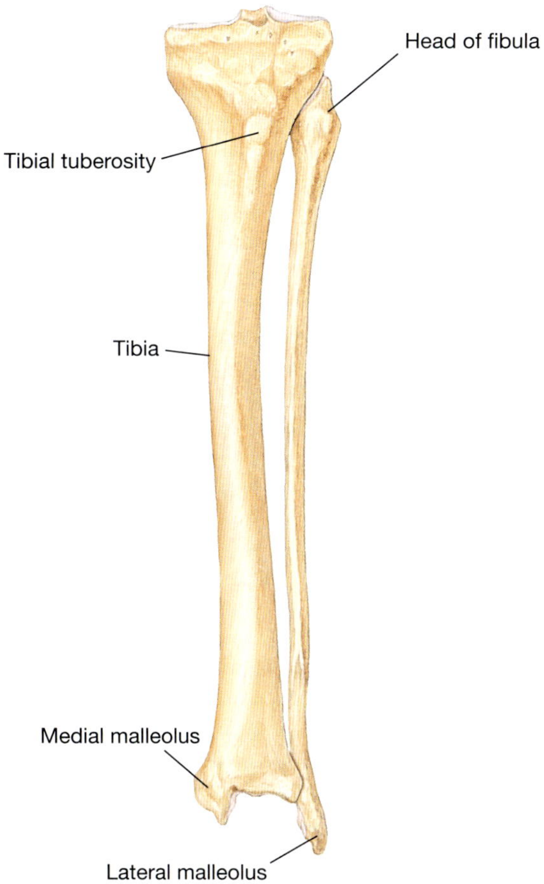

7-32 Anterior view of the right tibia and fibula.

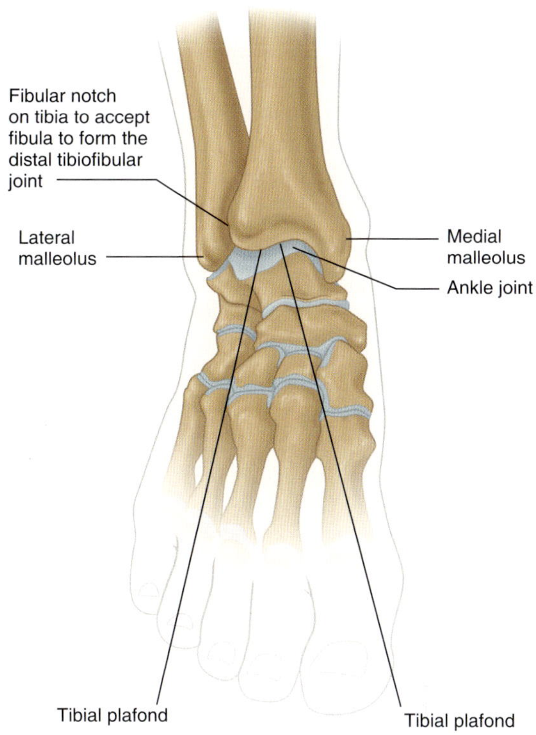

7-33 Anterior view of the distal tibia and fibula.

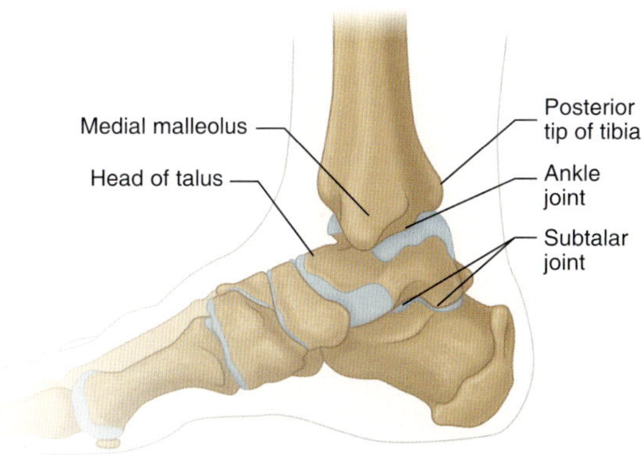

7-34 Lateral view of the distal tibia.

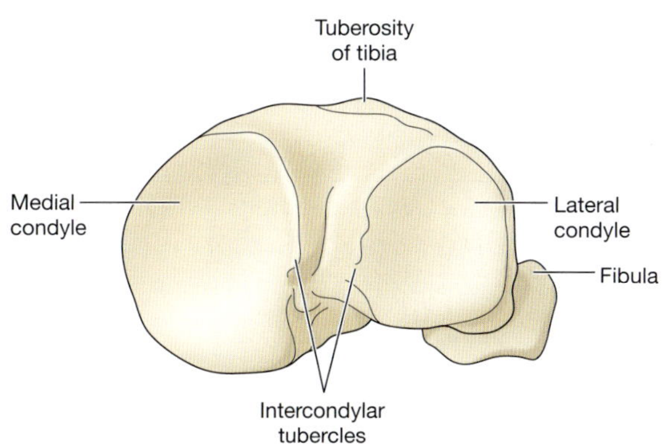

7-35 Superior view of the proximal tibia.

Tibia

The tibia proximally contributes to the knee joint and distally the ankle joint.

Distally, the tibia has a flattened surface, known as the tibial plafond, which articulates with the superior surface of the talus. On the posterior surface of the tibial plafond, the posterior tip of the tibia extends slightly inferior to the level of the tibial plafond. Upon the medial surface of the tibia, the medial malleolus, which is palpable on the ankle, extends inferiorly to the level of the tibial plafond. The tibial plafond and the medial malleolus will contribute to the formation of a socket for the talus to form the ankle joint. On the lateral surface of the tibia, a fibular notch exists to accept the fibula to form the distal tibiofibular joint (Figs. 7-33 and 7-34).

Proximally, two condyles are located on the tibia: the medial and lateral tibial condyles. On the superior surface of the tibia, the intercondylar eminence (tubercles) is located, which divides the articulating surface known as the tibial plateau. The tibial plateau accepts the medial and lateral femoral condyles (Fig. 7-35). The tibial plateau possesses a slight 15°–20°

posterior slope, which is important to consider when imaging the knee. To display an open femorotibial joint space on an AP projection, the central ray must align parallel with the slope of the tibial plateau (Figs. 7-36 and 7-37). The slope of the tibial plateau will directly influence the use of tube angle. Upon the anterior surface of the proximal tibia, a prominent tibial tuberosity provides a site for ligament attachment (Fig. 7-35). This location for ligament attachment is directly affected by rapid growth of adolescents causing pain and potentially an avulsion fracture of the tibial tuberosity.

In between the proximal and distal ends of the tibia is the tibial body or shaft. The anterior crest (ridge) runs from the point of the medial malleolus to the tibial tuberosity (Fig. 7-38).

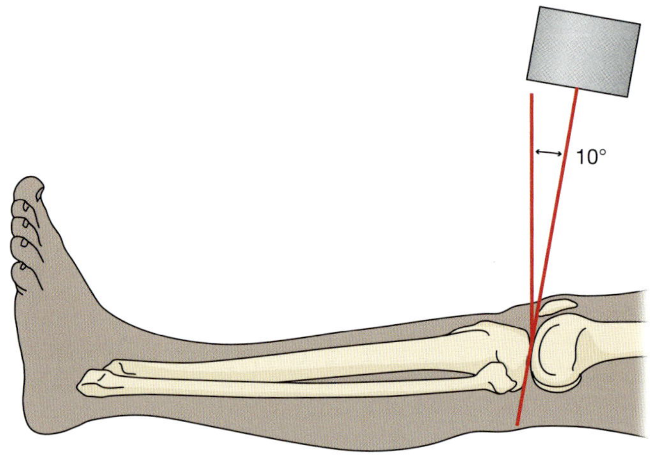

7-36 Posterior slope of the tibial plateau.

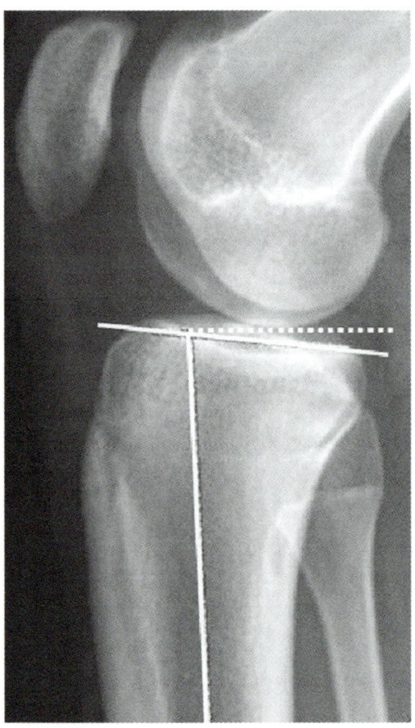

7-37 Posterior slope of the tibial plateau.

Fibula

The fibula, a thin bone, runs parallel with the tibia. It is located lateral to the tibia and sits slightly posterior to the tibia. The tibia and fibula will never entirely and directly superimpose each other when in a lateral position (Fig. 7-39).

Distally, the fibula has a triangular-shaped end and contributes to the socket formation for the ankle joint. The lateral malleolus (distal-most fibula), is palpable on the lateral side of the ankle, and extends down alongside the talus. The lateral malleolus extends slightly inferior to the level of the medial

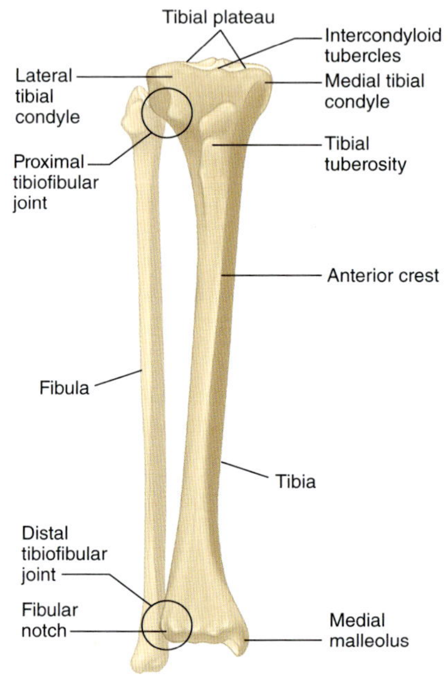

7-38 Anterior view of the right tibia.

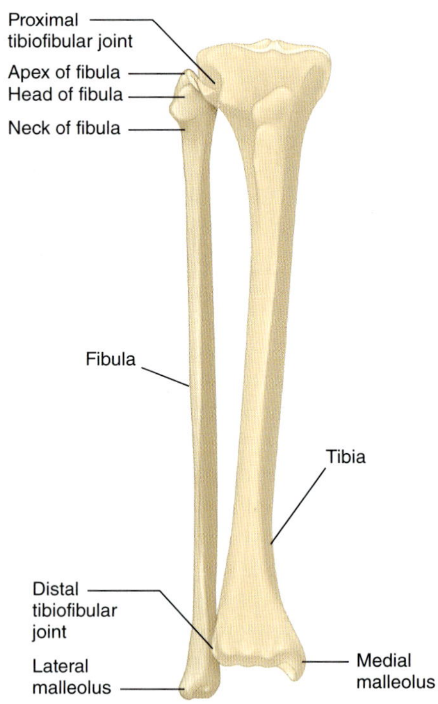

7-39 Anterior view of the right fibula.

malleolus and also sits slightly posterior to the medial malleolus (Fig. 7-40).

Proximally, the fibula has a triangular-shaped end. The most superior point is the apex. Below the apex, the fibula broadens out into the fibular head and then constricts back down into the fibular neck. The fibula articulates with the tibia both proximally and distally at the tibiofibular joints (Figs. 7-39, 7-41, and 7-42).

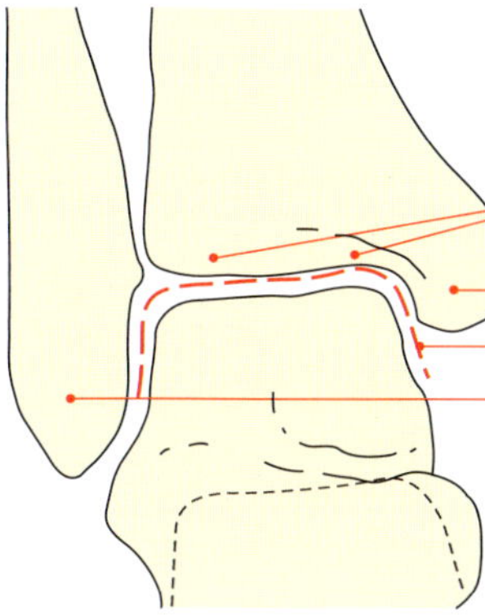

7-40 Relationship of the medial to the lateral malleolus.

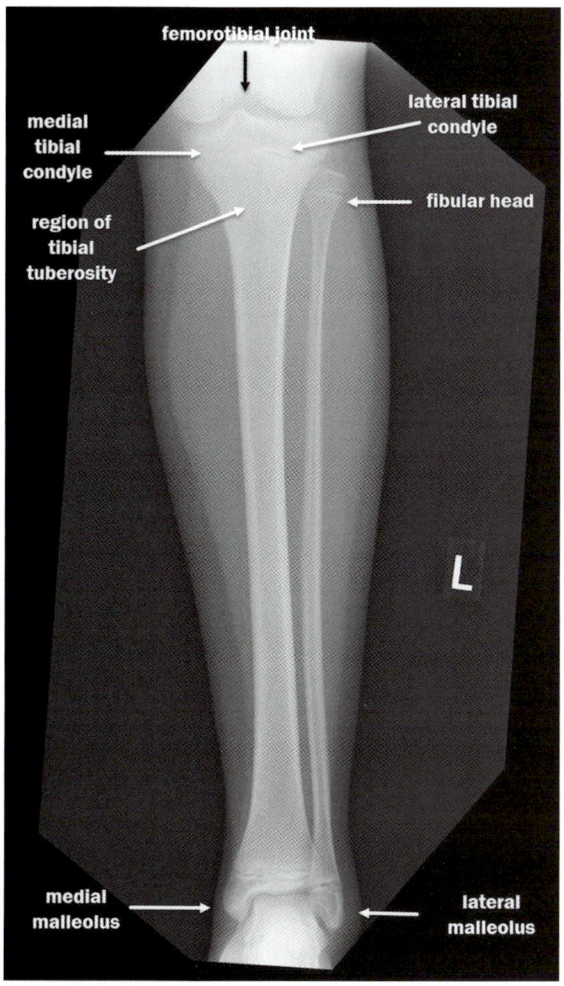

7-41 AP projection of the tibia and fibula.

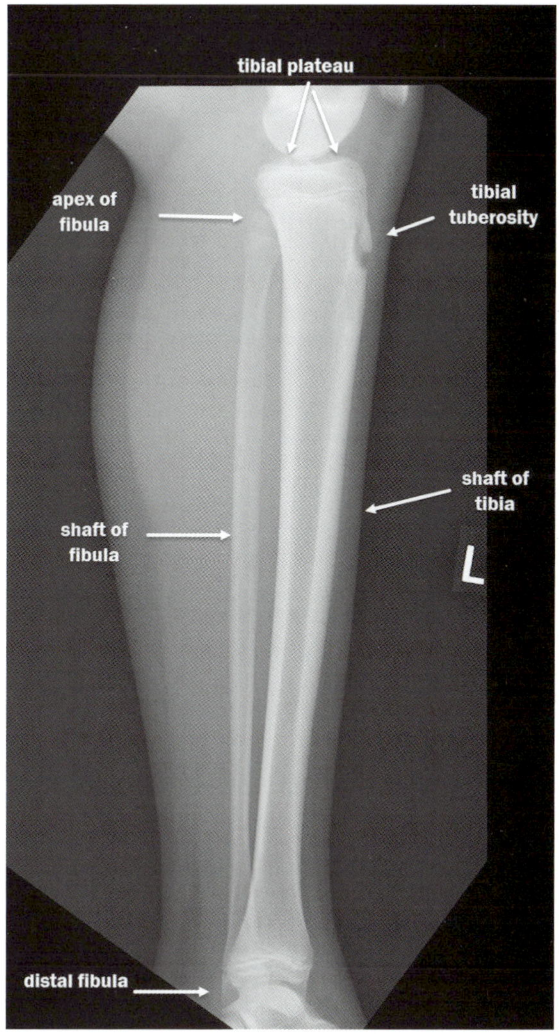

7-42 Mediolateral projection of the tibia and fibula.

Distal Femur

The distal femur has two rounded condyles that articulate with the respective medial and lateral articulating surfaces of the tibial plateau. The medial femoral condyle is round and is characteristically slightly larger in size compared with the lateral femoral condyle and extends slightly more inferiorly than the lateral femoral condyle (Fig. 7-43). In addition, the shaft of the femur deviates 5°–15° off vertical depending on the height stature of a patient to align the hip, knee, and ankle joints (Fig. 7-44). A shorter individual with a wider pelvis will have a greater angle off vertical. These anatomic features paired with natural magnification of the medial condyle must be considered when acquiring the mediolateral projection of the knee. All mediolateral knee projections will need to implement a slight cephalic tube angle to achieve superimposition of the medial and lateral femoral condyles (Figs. 7-45 and 7-46).

Upon the anterior and distal femur, the medial and lateral femoral condyles are separated by a groove—the intercondylar sulcus. The intercondylar sulcus courses inferiorly and on its ascension on the posterior surface of the distal femur, the deep dividing intercondylar fossa presents (Fig. 7-47).

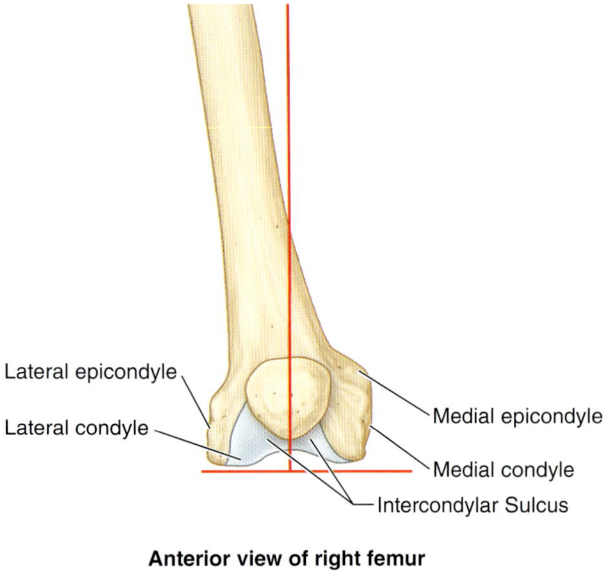

7-43 Anterior view of right distal femur.

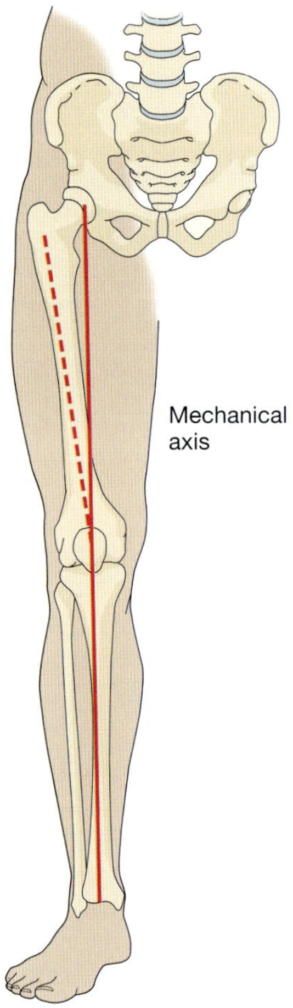

7-44 Angle of the femoral shaft.

Upon the region of the posterior femoral condyles, the lesser prominent epicondyles are present on the medial and lateral condyles. Upon the medial epicondyle, the adductor tubercle is present, which may provide a determinate means for over- and underrotation of the lateral knee position (Figs. 7-47 and 7-48).

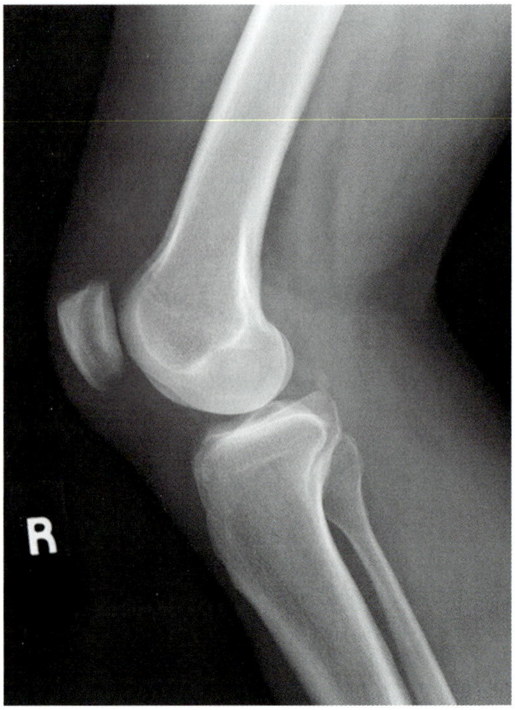

7-45 Mediolateral knee displaying the inferior margins of the femoral condyles superimposed; indicating correct cephalic tube angle was applied.

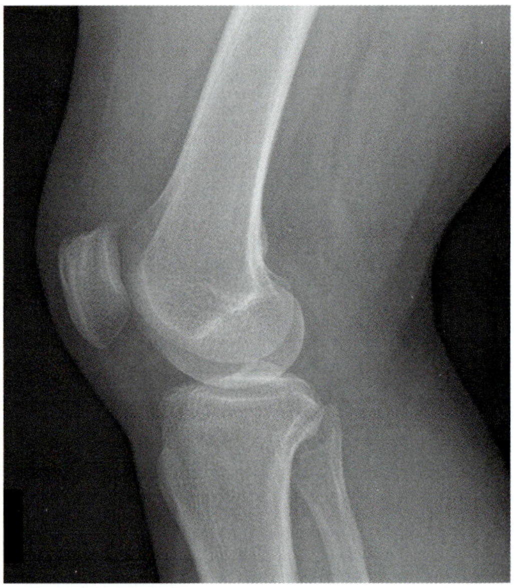

7-46 Mediolateral knee displaying the failure to superimpose the inferior margins of the femoral condyles.

Patella

The patella is the largest sesamoid bone in the body. The patellar base is broad and along the superior border of the patella, while the patellar apex (pointed) is most inferior (Fig. 7-49). The posterior surface of the patella is positioned over the patellar surface on the distal and anterior femur to form the patellofemoral joint (Fig. 7-50). With flexion of the knee, the patella will pull into the intercondylar sulcus on the distal femur and continue to shift inferiorly with increasing flexion.

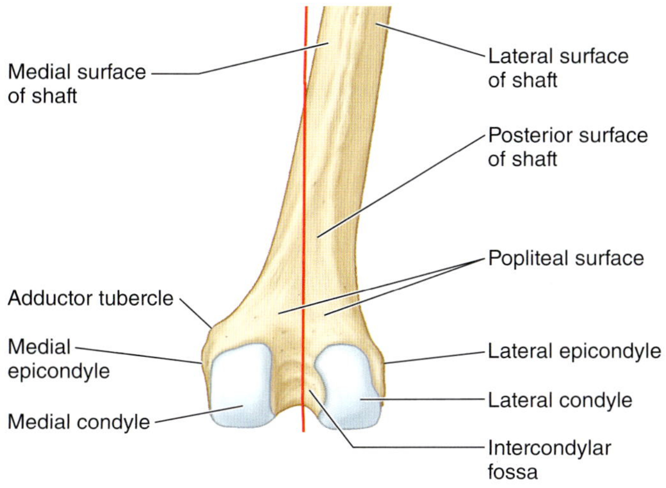

7-47 Posterior distal femur.

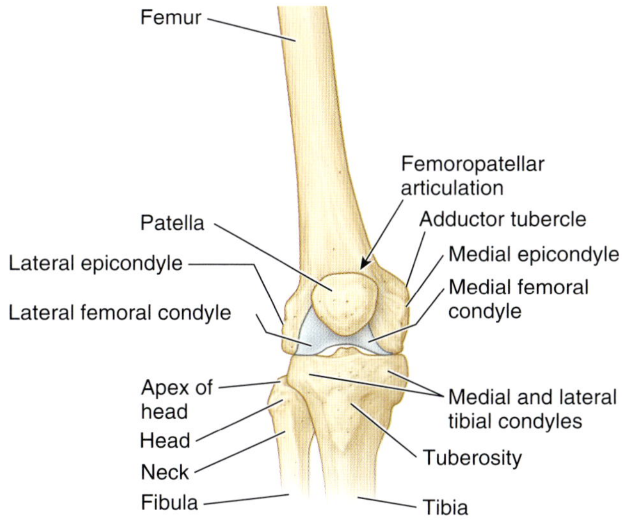

7-50 Anterior view of the femorotibial joint.

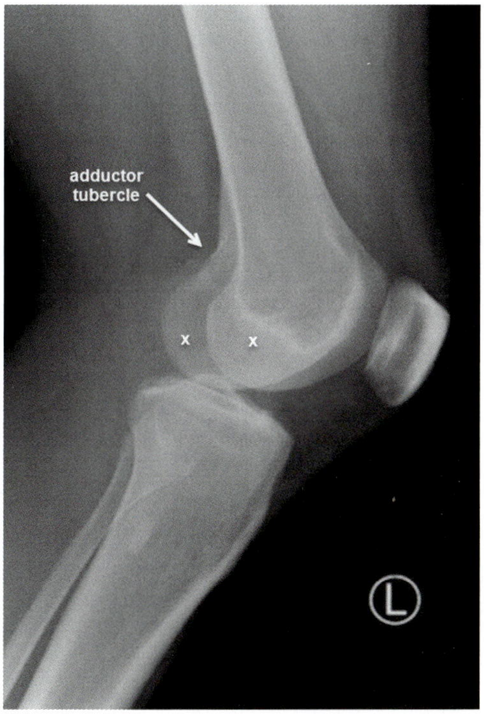

7-48 Mediolateral projection of knee with rotation.

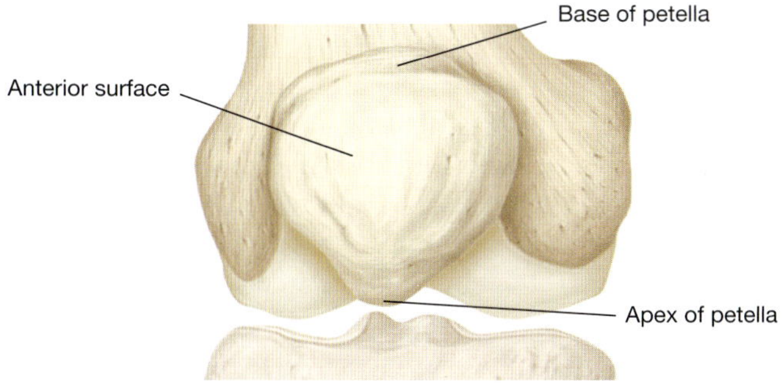

7-49 Anterior view of the patella.

KEY SUMMATION POINTS OF ANATOMY

- The first digit (great toe) contains only an IP joint in between the proximal and distal phalanges. Digits 2–5 contain a DIP joint and a PIP joint.
- The base of the fifth metatarsal is a common site of fracture (Jones fracture), which may be the primary injury or a secondary injury.
- The distal row of tarsals articulates, respectively, with the metatarsal bases. The medial cuneiform articulates primarily with the first metatarsal. The intermediate cuneiform articulates primarily with the second metacarpal. The lateral cuneiform articulates primarily with the third metatarsal. The cuboid articulates with the fourth and fifth metatarsal.
- The inferior surface of the talus articulates directly with the calcaneus through three points of articulation to form the talocalcaneal or subtalar joint.
- The calcaneus is the largest tarsal. It articulates with the talus and the cuboid.
- The tibia and fibula lie parallel to one another. The fibula sits lateral and slightly posterior to the tibia.
- The lateral malleolus sits slightly posterior to the medial malleolus and extends down more inferiorly than the medial malleolus alongside the talus.
- The tibial plateau has a 15°–20° posterior slope. The imaging beam must pass parallel to this slope to image the femorotibial joint open. Therefore, a tube angle may be necessary (influenced by patient habitus) when centering the AP projection of the knee.
- The medial femoral condyle is round and slightly larger than the lateral femoral condyle. In addition, the inferior margin of the medial femoral condyle sits slightly more inferior or distal compared with the lateral femoral condyle. Considering these anatomic features paired with magnification of the medial condyle on the mediolateral projection of the knee; this will require all mediolateral knees to use a slight cephalic tube angle.
- The adductor tubercle (medial condyle) is located on the medial and posterior epicondylar region and can help distinguish the medial femoral condyle from the lateral femoral condyle when under or overrotation of the knee is contemplated.

- The intercondylar fossa is on the posterior distal femur. The deep depression separates and defines the medial and lateral femoral condyles.
- The base of the patella is located superiorly while the pointed apex of the patella is located inferiorly.
- All joints in the lower extremity contain synovial fluid and are diarthrodial (freely movable). Each joint displays a different type of movement (Table 7-2).

7-2 Lower Extremity Joint Classification

Joint	Classification	General Movement	Specific Movement
Interphalangeal joints	Synovial	Diarthrodial	Ginglymus or hinge
Metatarsophalangeal joints	Synovial	Diarthrodial	Ellipsoidal or condyloid
Tarsometatarsal joints	Synovial	Diarthrodial	Plane or gliding
Intertarsal joints	Synovial	Diarthrodial	Plane or gliding
Ankle joint	Synovial	Diarthrodial	Mortise socket forms a saddle joint allowing flexion and extension of the foot
Tibiofibular (distal) joint	Fibrous	Amphiarthrodial	Syndesmosis (ligament bound)
Tibiofibular (proximal) joint	Synovial	Diarthrodial	Plane or gliding
Knee	Synovial	Diarthrodial	Bicondylar (flexion and extension)

POSITIONING CONSIDERATIONS

Patient Part Size and Suggested Image Receptor Orientation

Imaging the lower extremity most commonly includes imaging a part size <10 cm in thickness allowing for tabletop and nongrid imaging. Generally, once a part measures >10 cm, the part should be imaged with a grid. In the lower extremity, the consideration of grid versus nongrid typically occurs at the level of the knee. With digital radiography, one exposure is taken on the digital plate at a time. With one projection per image receptor, the length of the image receptor is orientated with the length of the part. The part should be positioned in the center of the image receptor.

Centering and Collimation

The central ray should be directed to the proper and suggested centering locations. With proper centering, four-sided collimation can be applied to ensure good radiation safety practices and ensure all essential anatomy is included.

Breathing Instructions

Specific breathing instructions are not necessary to be given to the patient because the lower extremities are not affected by the respiratory motions.

Identification Between Nontrauma and Trauma Situations

Patients with potential fracture to a limb should be approached with caution. The technologist may have to deviate from normal protocol and find ways to creatively image a part with a potential fracture. Certainly, the technologist does not want to worsen an injury or cause additional and unnecessary pain to the patient. If the patient presents with a potential fracture, the technologist should proceed with caution leaving the part in its neutral or presenting position while still acquiring a minimum of two views 90° apart (Figs. 7-51 and 7-52).

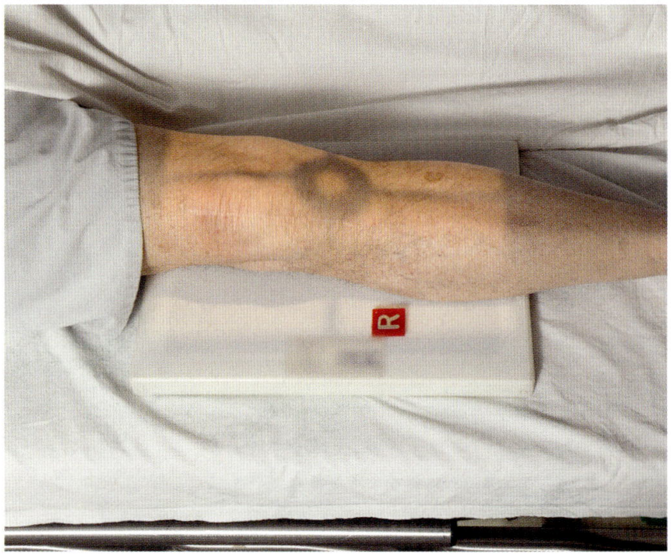

7-51 Trauma AP knee.

TECHNICAL CONSIDERATIONS

Setting a Manual Technique

Manual technique is defined when the radiographer sets the kVp and mAs values. Manual techniques are set for a majority of lower extremity imaging. Tabletop imaging requires the use of manual technique. Kilovoltage is set to penetrate the part thickness and affects the scale of contrast seen on the image. A lower kVp is used for extremity work and set appropriately to penetrate the part thickness. It is desired that a high scale of contrast (less shades with more black-and-white) is achieved

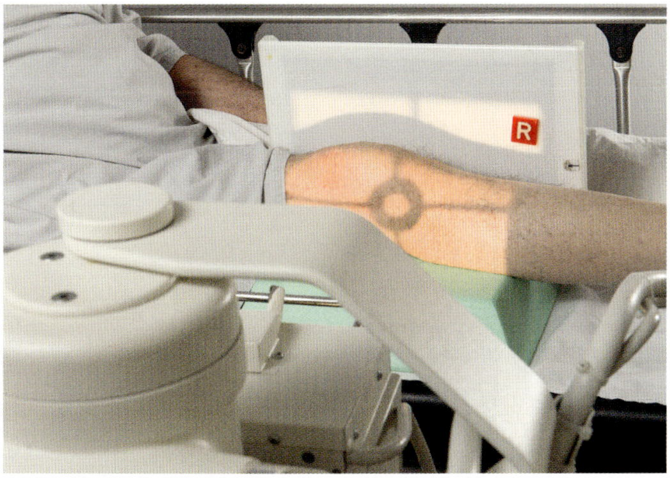

7-52 Lateromedial knee.

for extremity structures. When imaging a patient in a cast, the kVp will increase according to the thickness and the cast material (plaster or fiberglass). A plaster cast may require a 5–10 kVp increase, whereas a fiberglass may only need half the amount increased for a plaster cast. A small focal spot setting is encouraged when imaging extremities in an effort to improve detail, especially for the smallest bones and joints.

Source-to-Image Distance (SID)

40″–44″ SID is used for all extremity imaging.

Exposure Index

With each exposure, the digital system will produce a numeric value taking into account the kVp, mAs, part centering, anatomy, and collimation. The exposure index is typically a range established by the manufacturer and aids the technologist in determining if image was acquired with proper exposure. In instances in which insufficient radiation has reached the IR, indicated by an exposure index, the technologist must repeat the image, as often the image will appear grainy or mottled. The goal of the repeat image is to appropriately increase the exposure to produce a diagnostic quality image when displayed on the radiologist's monitor. In instances in which overexposure is indicated, the image may not need to be reacquired to achieve the image within range, as this will expose the patient to additional and unnecessary radiation. However, the technologist should make note of this to adjust accordingly for future patient exposures. With digital imaging, the wider latitude of systems lessens the exact science of setting kVp and mAs for each exposure. With the flexibility, these wider latitude systems offer, technologists need to learn appropriate combinations of technical settings necessary to acquire diagnostic images within acceptable ranges to avoid unnecessary radiation exposure to patients.

Shielding

Acceptable shielding practices include a lap shield at minimum, but a full lead shield could also be considered. Double shielding around the front and back of the waist and abdomen should be applied when imaging declared pregnant patients.

Marking the Image

When marking an extremity positioned flat or in an oblique position, the anatomic marker should be placed within the collimated exposure field furthest away from the patient's midline or alongside the lateral aspect of the part (Figs. 7-53 and 7-54). When marking the lateral position, the anatomic marker is placed along the anterior surface of the part or "in front" of the part and within the collimated exposure field (Fig. 7-55 and 7-56).

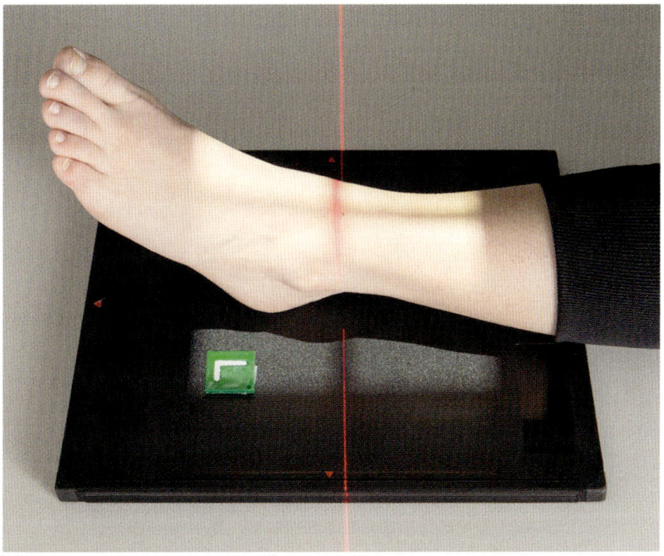

7-53 Correct marker placement for AP projection of left ankle.

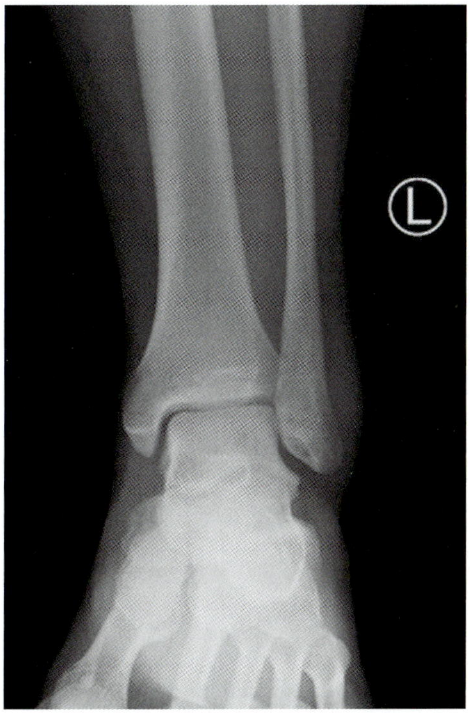

7-54 Correct image display for AP projection of left ankle.

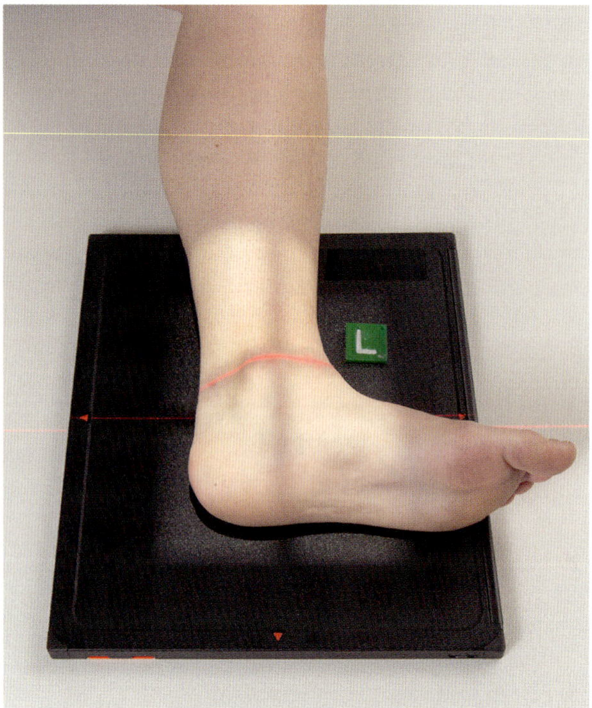

7-55 Correct marker placement for mediolateral projection of left ankle.

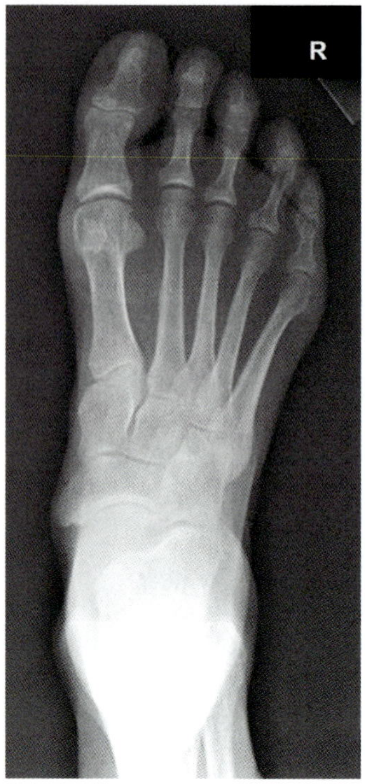

7-57 Correct image display for AP projection of right foot.

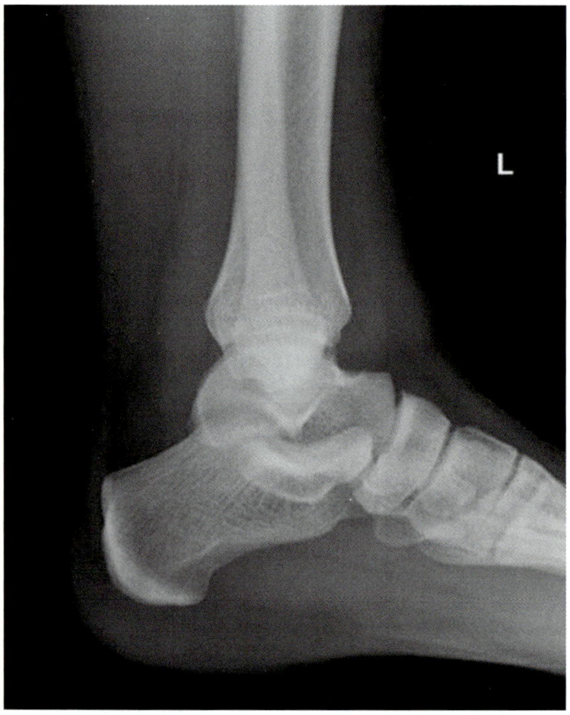

7-56 Correct image display for mediolateral projection of left ankle.

Viewing the Image

When viewing the lower extremities such as toes (all three projections) and feet (AP Axial and AP Oblique), the image is displayed with the toes "up," and as though viewer's part is directly overlaying the image to replicate how the part was positioned (Fig. 7-57).

At the ankle, the image is hung to represent anatomic position, displayed with the hip side, "up." Images of the lateral foot and all ankle, lower leg, knee, and femur images are displayed opposite of the viewer facing it, as though the image is in anatomic position. Therefore, in these cases, the side of the image marked "right" or "left" is opposite of the viewer's right or left side (Fig. 7-58 to 7-60).

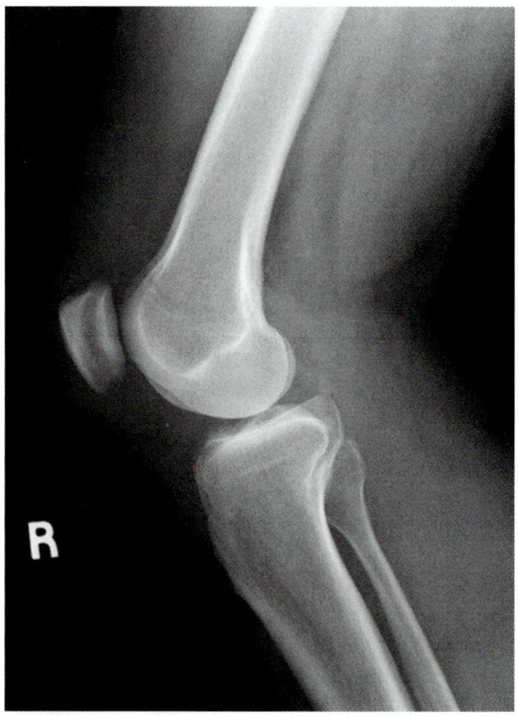

7-58 Correct image display for mediolateral projection of right knee.

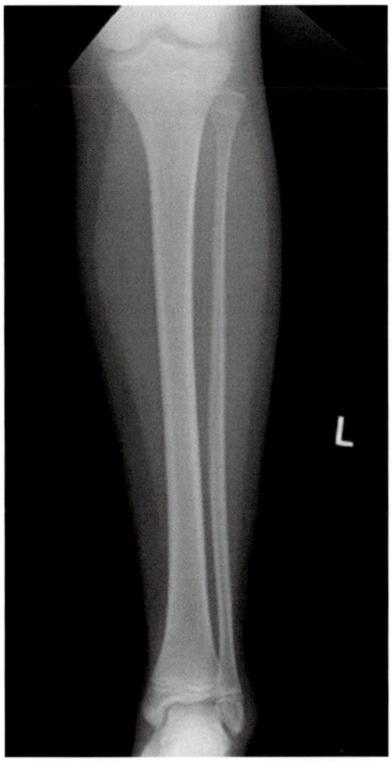

7-59 Correct image display for AP projection of left lower leg.

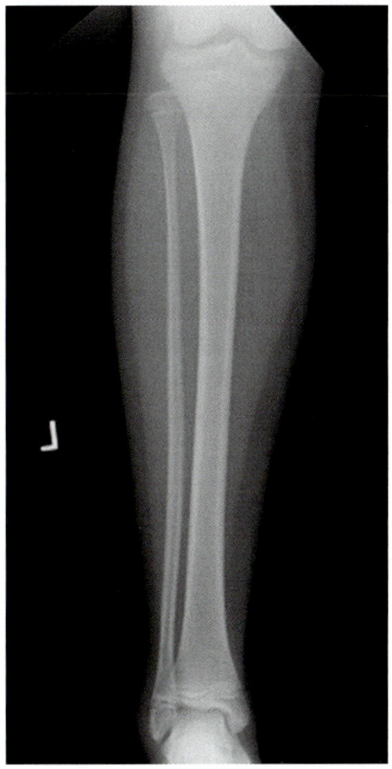

7-60 Incorrect image display for AP projection of left lower leg.

Image Postprocessing

There are a variety of postprocessing options that are available on digital workstations. These options range from windowing, smoothing, subtraction, edge enhancement, black bordering, and annotation. Technologists must realize that the monitor resolution at their workstation will be lower compared with the radiologist's monitor workstation. Additionally, if a technologist postprocesses an image and pushes it over to the department picture archiving and computer system (PACS), this will prevent the radiologist from being able to make any image adjustments for their purpose of interpretation. Therefore, postprocessing by the technologist is not advised. A common postprocessing tool the technologist may utilize is the annotation function. The annotation function should be utilized to add only additional information useful for the purpose of imaging and should not replace the use of standardized minimum right and left markers that should be positioned within the collimated exposure field. Digital annotation of right and left markers cannot replace the need for right and left lead anatomic markers within the original collimated margins. Digital annotations will not uphold in legal litigation cases of malpractice.

Toes

- Projection: AP (Dorsoplantar) Foot

Toes Protocol
AP Foot/AP Toe
AP Oblique
Lateromedial/
Mediolateral

Technical Considerations
- kVp 50–60; nongrid
- mAs set manually
- 40″ SID

Exposure Field Size
- 10 × 12 lengthwise with close collimation down to the foot

Patient Position (Fig. 7-61)
- Seated on the imaging table or stretcher
- Patient's knee flexed 45°
- Position the plantar surface of the foot in contact with the IR

Centering (Fig. 7-62)
- Base of third metatarsal when the entire foot is acquired with a 10°–15° tube angle toward the heel *(a higher longitudinal arch requires the greater angle)* or a 15° wedge sponge is placed under the toes to align the metatarsals parallel to the IR. *(Acquisition of the entire foot will provide an image in which secondary injury can be identified or will provide a comparison of the injured digit to surrounding digits.)*
- If a single digit is protocol for the facility, rather than the entire foot, the central ray is directed to the MTP joint of the digit in question

Marking of IR
- Anatomic side marker R or L placed furthest from the patient's midline or lateral to the part
- Additional marking of the digit in question could be digitally annotated

Breathing
- No specific breathing instructions are given to the patient. Instruct the patient to hold still
- Ensure patient holds position while walking away to make the exposure

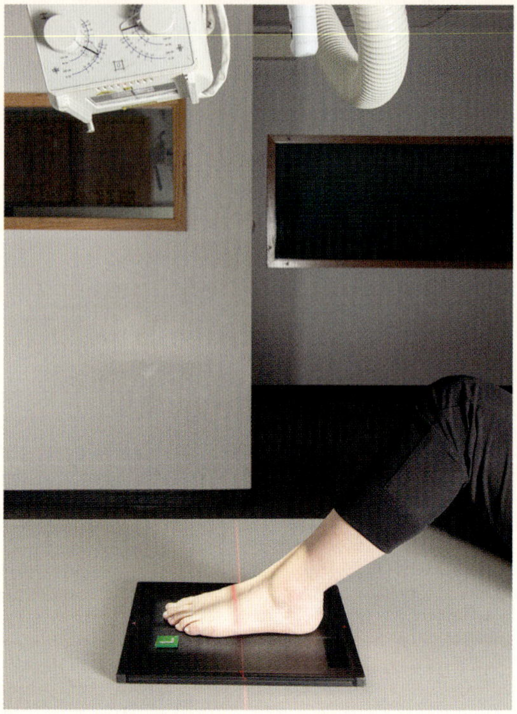

7-61 AP projection of foot.

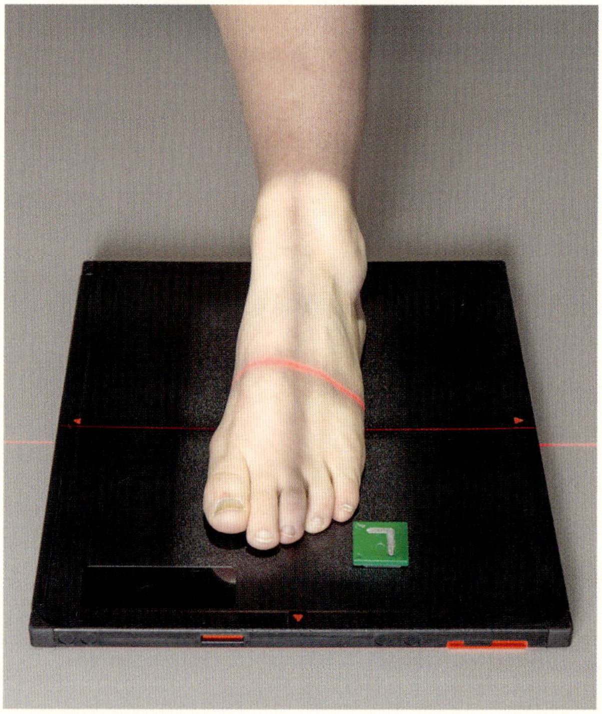

7-62 AP projection of foot.

IMAGE CRITIQUE (FIGS. 7-63 to 7-65)

- If centering for the entire foot, the image must include distal phalanges, metatarsals, tarsals, and calcaneus. When a complete foot is acquired, the other digits provide for comparison to the injured digit. A complete foot will also allow a secondary injury in the foot to be identified
- The bases of metatarsals 2–5 will superimpose
- The distance between metatarsal 1 and 2 shafts will be greater than the distance between metatarsal shafts 2 and 5
- Centering to include the entire foot will not demonstrate the calcaneus and talus clearly owing to the superimposition of the talus and calcaneus
- If centering is for a single digit, the distal phalanx to include the distal one-third of the metatarsal for the digit of interest is needed
- Properly centered with four-sided collimation. Collimation for just the digit will likely include partial or full digit on either side of the one in interest

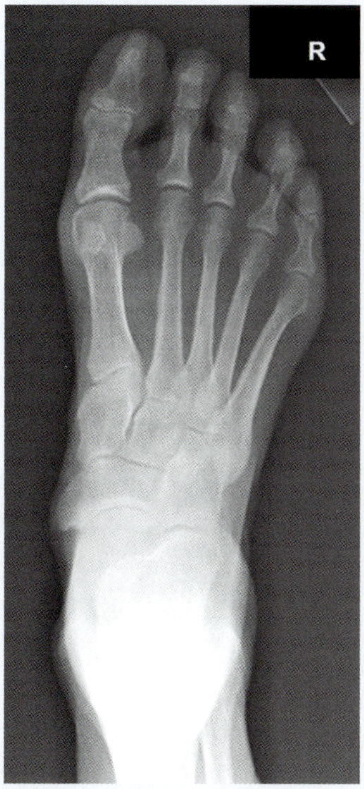

7-63 AP foot.

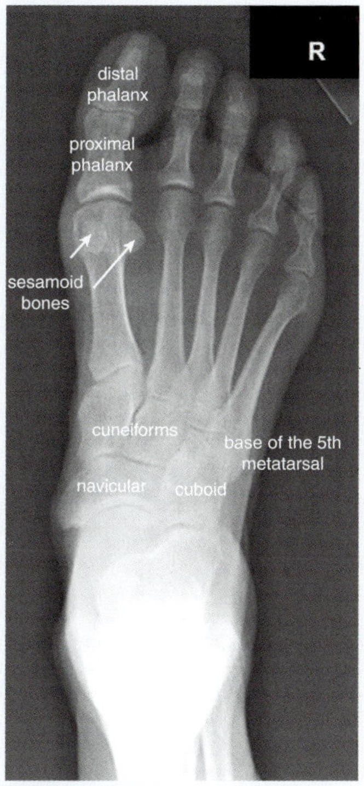

7-64 AP foot.

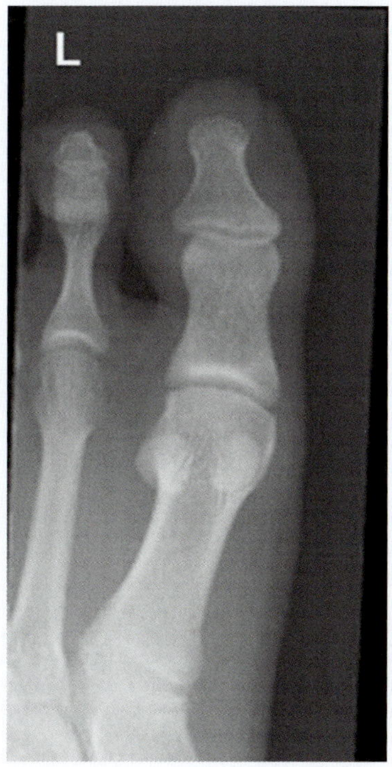

7-65 AP first digit.

Toes

- Projection: AP Oblique of the toe

Toes Protocol
AP Foot/AP Toe
AP Oblique
Lateromedial/
Mediolateral

Technical Considerations
- kVp 50–60; nongrid
- mAs set manually
- 40″ SID

Exposure Field Size
- 10 × 12 with collimation down to the digit of interest.

Patient Position (Figs. 7-66 and 7-67)
- Seated on the imaging table or stretcher
- Patient's knee flexed 45°
- Position the plantar surface of the foot in contact with the IR
- Direction of medial or lateral oblique rotation is determined by rotating the part in the direction that will keep it closest to the IR. Typically, the first and second digit are rotated medially and digits 3–5 are rotated laterally
- Part should be rotated 30°–45°. Stabilization of the foot could be considered
- Digit positioned should remain extended and ideally parallel to the IR

Centering
- MTP joint of the digit in question. Collimate down to the distal phalanx of the toe of interest to include the distal one-third of the metatarsal

Marking of IR
- Anatomic side marker R or L placed furthest from the patient's midline or lateral to the part when possible (Fig. 7-67)

Breathing
- No specific breathing instructions are given to the patient. Instruct the patient to hold still
- Ensure patient holds position while walking away to make the exposure

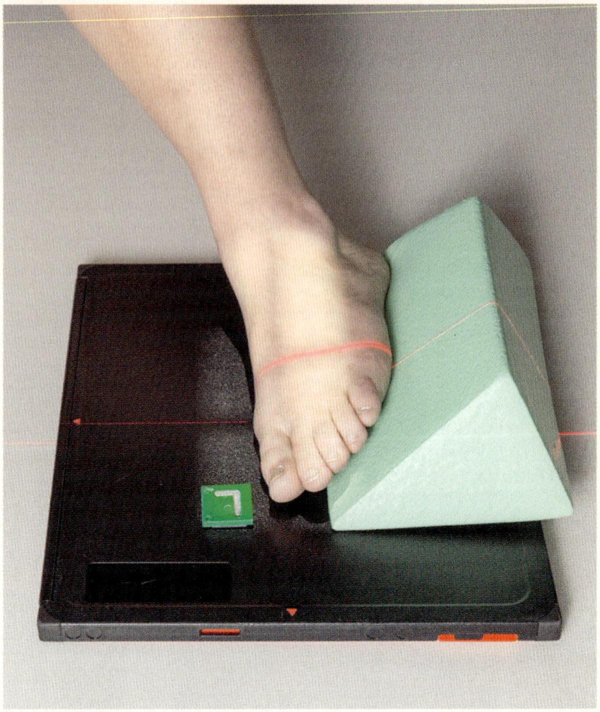

7-66 AP Oblique digit with medial rotation.

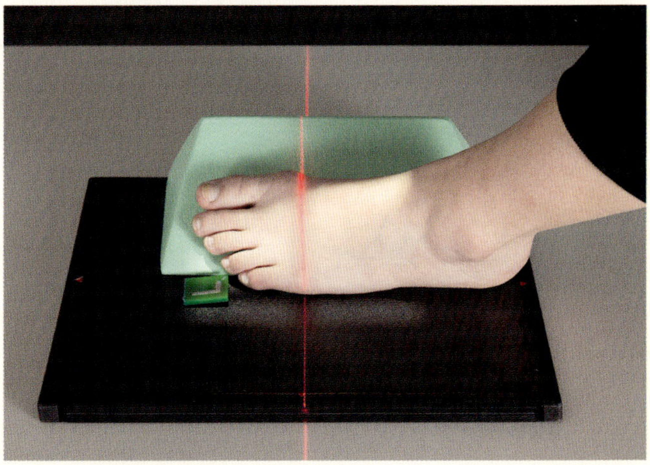

7-67 AP Oblique digit with lateral rotation.

IMAGE CRITIQUE (FIGS. 7-68 and 7-69)

- Distal, middle, and proximal phalanx and the distal one-third of the metatarsal in question are demonstrated for digits 2–5
- Distal and proximal phalanx and the distal one-third of the metatarsal in question for digit 1
- Properly centered with four-sided collimation. Collimation for the digit will likely include partial or full digit on either side of the digit in interest

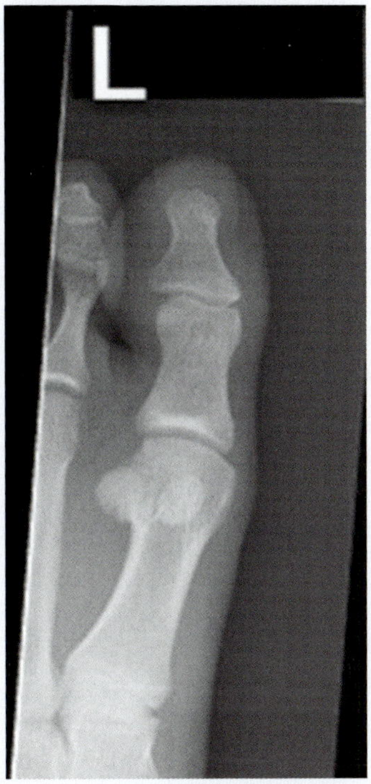

7-68 AP Oblique first digit.

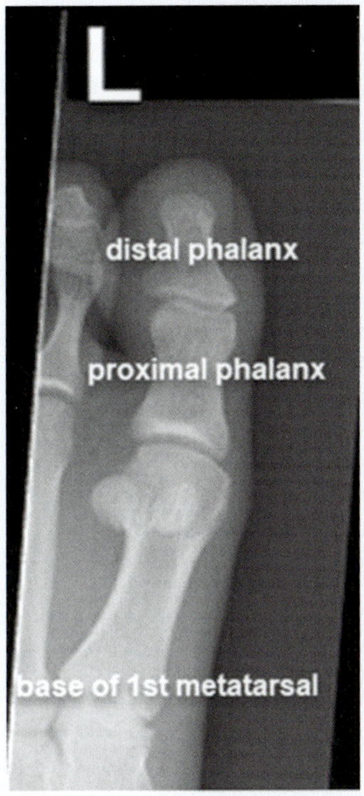

7-69 AP Oblique first digit.

Toes

- Projection: Lateromedial or Mediolateral of affected toe

Toes Protocol
PA
PA Oblique
Lateromedial/ Mediolateral

Technical Considerations
- kVp 50–60; nongrid
- mAs set manually
- 40″ SID

Exposure Field Size
- 10 × 12 with collimation down to the digit of interest

Patient Position (Figs. 7-70 and 7-71)
- Seated on the imaging table or stretcher
- Rotate the leg and foot laterally or medially until the digit of interest is in a true lateral position
- Direction of medial or lateral rotation is determined by rotating the part in the direction that will keep it closest to the IR. Typically, the first and second digits are rotated medially and digits 3–5 are rotated laterally
- Isolating the digit in question is necessary to prevent as much superimposition as possible. Positioning aids, such as gauze, tongue blade, tourniquet, tape, may be considered
- Digit positioned should remain extended as possible and parallel to the IR

Centering
- First digit, the central ray is directed to the IP joint
- Second to fifth digits, the central ray is directed to the PIP joint
- Collimate down to the distal phalanx of the toe of interest to include the distal one-third of the metatarsal

Marking of IR
- Anatomic side marker R or L placed along the anterior surface or "in front" of the part

Breathing
- No specific breathing instructions are given to the patient. Instruct the patient to hold still
- Ensure patient holds position while walking away to make the exposure

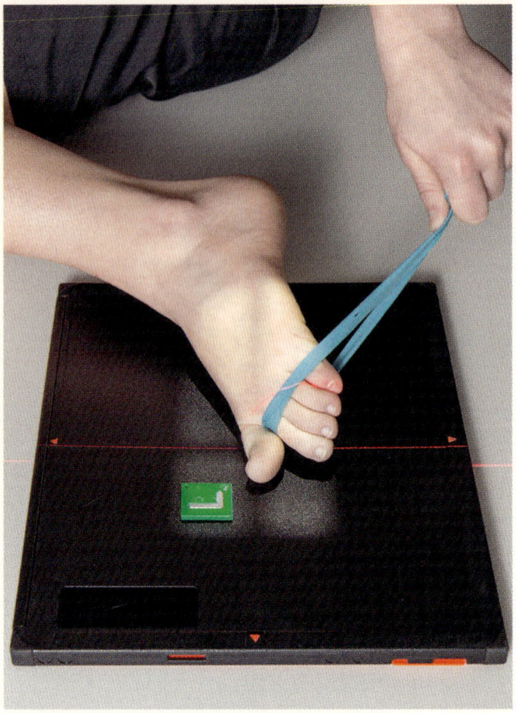

7-70 Lateromedial first digit.

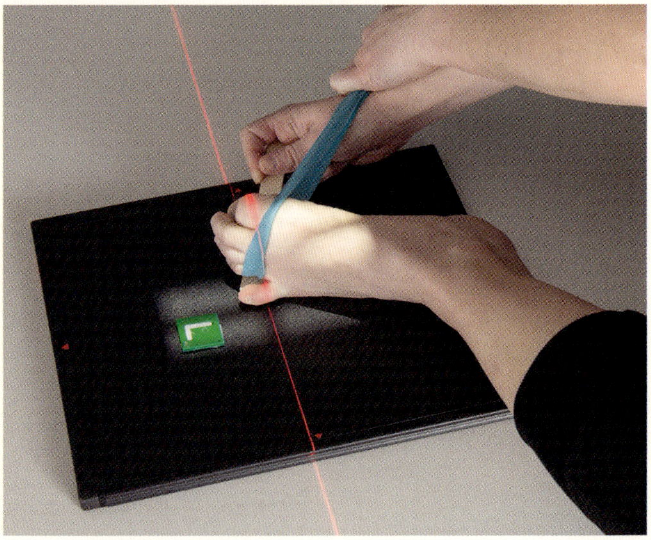

7-71 Mediolateral fifth digit.

IMAGE CRITIQUE (FIGS. 7-72 and 7-73)

- Distal, middle, and proximal phalanx and the distal one-third of the metatarsal in question are demonstrated for digits 2–5
- Distal and proximal phalanx and the distal one-third of the metatarsal in question for digit 1
- Properly centered with four-sided collimation

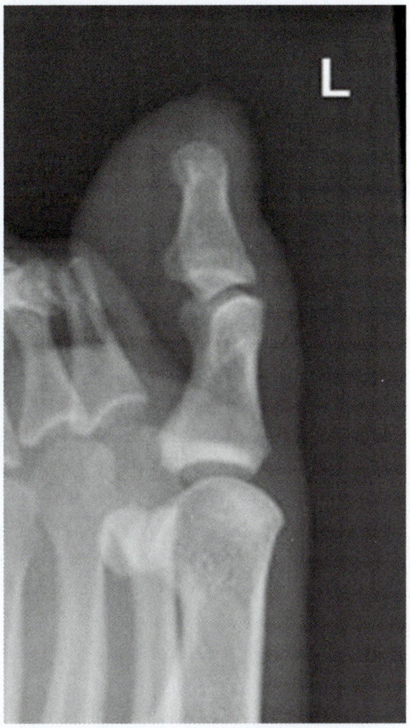

7-72 Lateromedial first digit.

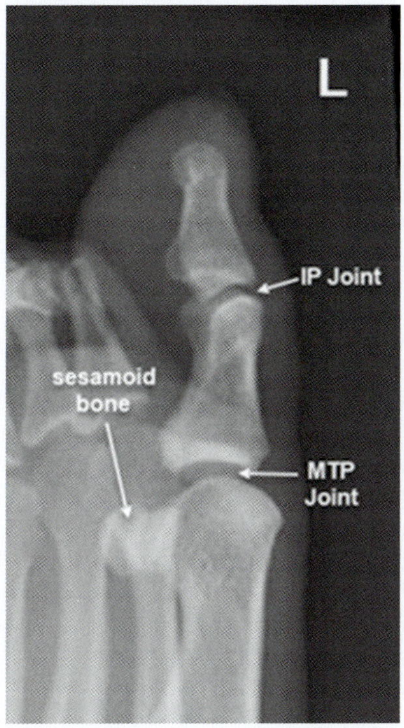

7-73 Lateromedial first digit.

Foot

- Projection: AP (Dorsoplantar) Foot

Foot Protocol
AP
AP Oblique
Mediolateral

Technical Considerations
- kVp 50–60; nongrid
- mAs set manually
- 40″ SID

Exposure Field Size
- 10 × 12 lengthwise with close collimation down to the foot

Patient Position
- Seated on the imaging table or stretcher
- Consider orientating the foot according to the anode heel effect to help attain even exposure density
- Patient's knee flexed 45°
- Position the plantar surface of the foot in contact with the IR

Centering (Figs. 7-74 and 7-75)
- Base of third metatarsal when the entire foot is acquired with a 10°–15° tube angle toward the heel *(a higher longitudinal arch requires the greater angle) or* a 15° wedge sponge is placed under the toes to align the metatarsals parallel to the IR (Acquisition of the entire foot will allow for a secondary injury to be identified or will provide a comparison of the injured digit to surrounding digits)
- Collimate down to include the distal phalanges, calcaneus and distal tibia and fibula

Marking of IR
- Anatomic side marker R or L placed furthest from the patient's midline or lateral to the part

Breathing
- No specific breathing instructions are given to the patient. Instruct the patient to hold still
- Ensure patient holds position while walking away to make the exposure

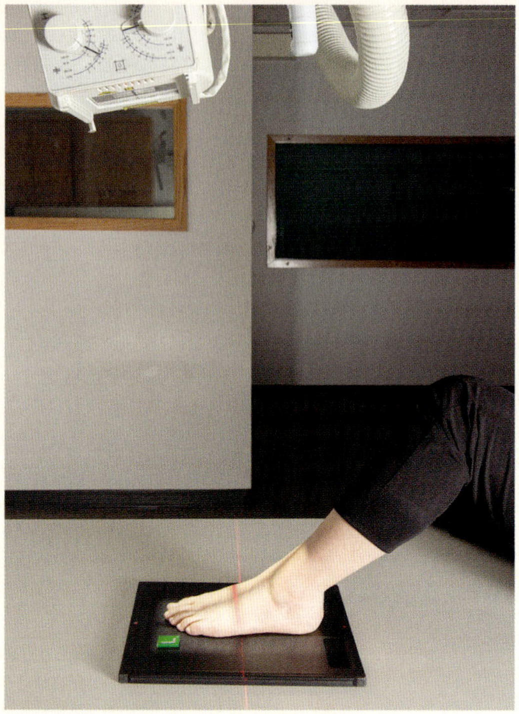

7-74 AP foot.

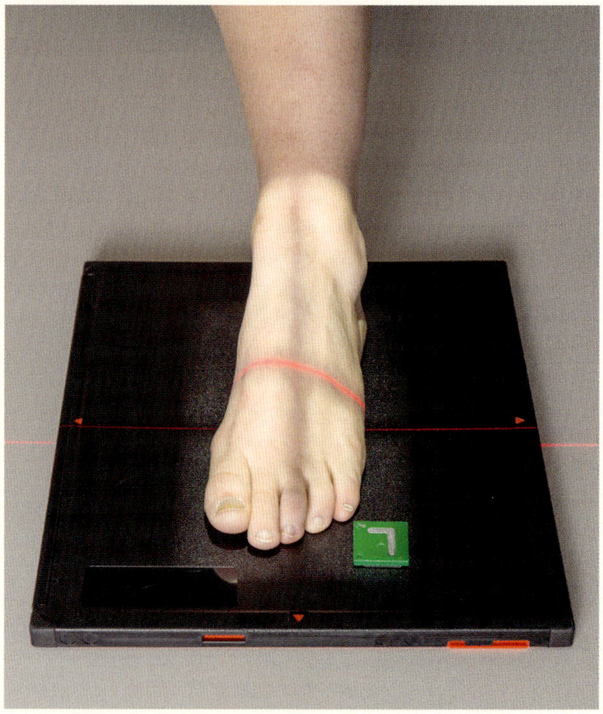

7-75 AP foot.

IMAGE CRITIQUE: (FIGS. 7-76 and 7-77)

- If centering for the entire foot, the image must include distal phalanges, metatarsals, tarsals, and calcaneus. When a complete foot is acquired, the other digits can serve as a comparison to the injured digit. A complete foot will also allow a secondary injury in the foot to be identified
- The bases of metatarsals 2–5 will superimpose
- The distance between metatarsal 1 and 2 shafts will be greater than the distance between metatarsal shafts 2–5
- The calcaneus will be poorly visualized owing to the superimposition of the tibia, fibula, and talus
- Properly centered with four-sided collimation

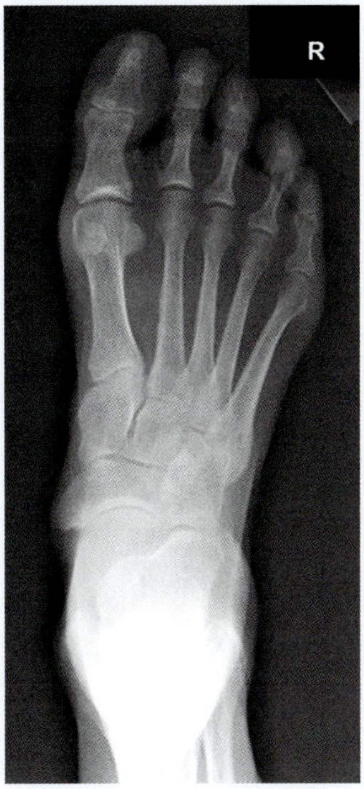

7-76 AP foot.

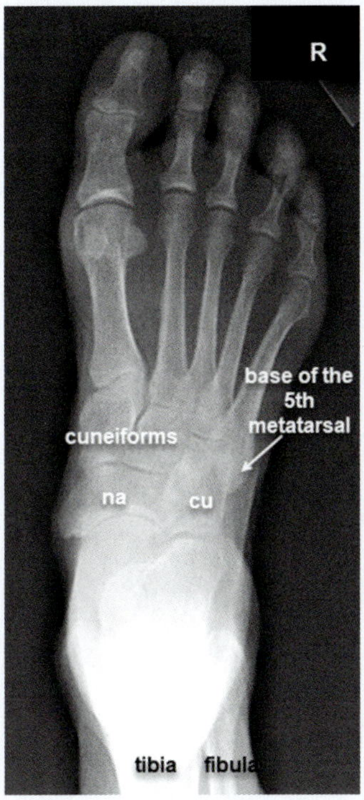

7-77 AP foot.

Foot

- Projection: AP Oblique (medial oblique is routine protocol)

Foot Protocol
PA
AP Oblique
Mediolateral

Technical Considerations
- kVp 50–60; nongrid
- mAs set manually
- 40″ SID

Exposure Field Size
- 10 × 12 lengthwise with close collimation down to the foot

Patient Position (Fig. 7-78)
- Seated on the imaging table or stretcher
- Patient's knee flexed 45°
- Position the plantar surface of the foot in contact with the IR
- Rotate the leg and foot medially 30°–40°

Centering
- Base of the third metatarsal joint with a *perpendicular* beam

Marking of IR
- Anatomic side marker R or L furthest from the patient's midline or lateral to the part when possible

Breathing
- No specific breathing instructions are given to the patient. Instruct the patient to hold still
- Ensure patient holds position while walking away to make the exposure

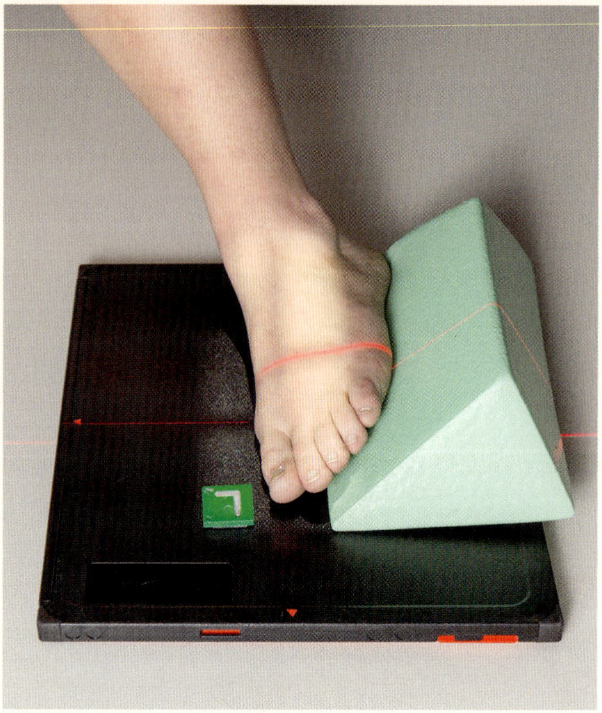

7-78 AP Oblique foot.

IMAGE CRITIQUE: (FIGS. 7-79 and 7-80)

- Entire foot to include distal phalanges, metatarsals, tarsals, and calcaneus within the collimated exposure field
- The bases of metatarsals 1–5 will superimpose
- The distance between all metatarsal shafts will be nearly equal
- The calcaneus and the sinus tarsi will be better visualized
- The base of the fifth metatarsal is of interest and is well visualized
- Properly centered with four-sided collimation

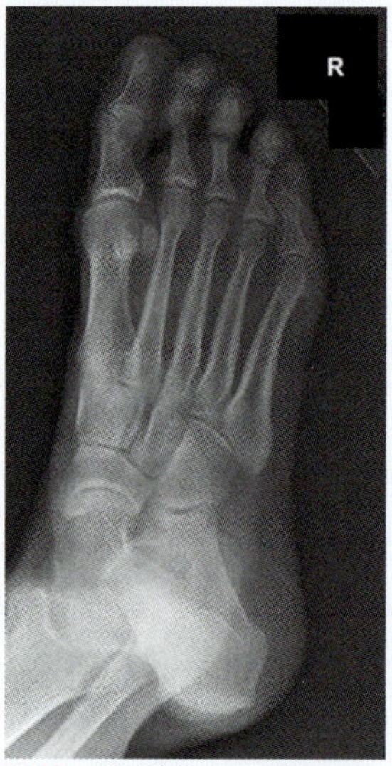

7-79 AP Oblique with medial rotation.

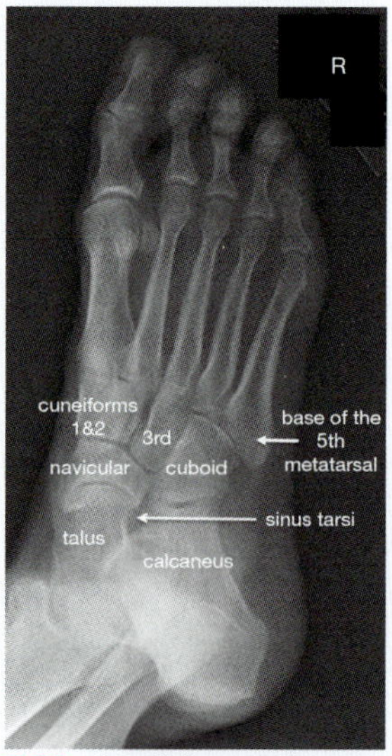

7-80 AP Oblique with medial rotation.

POSITION VARIATION: AP OBLIQUE WITH LATERAL ROTATION (FIGS. 7-81 and 7-82)

The foot is rotated laterally instead of medially approximately 30°. This direction of rotation will better demonstrate the metatarsals 1 and 2, the first and second cuneiforms, and the navicular. The metatarsal shafts of 2–5 will superimpose.

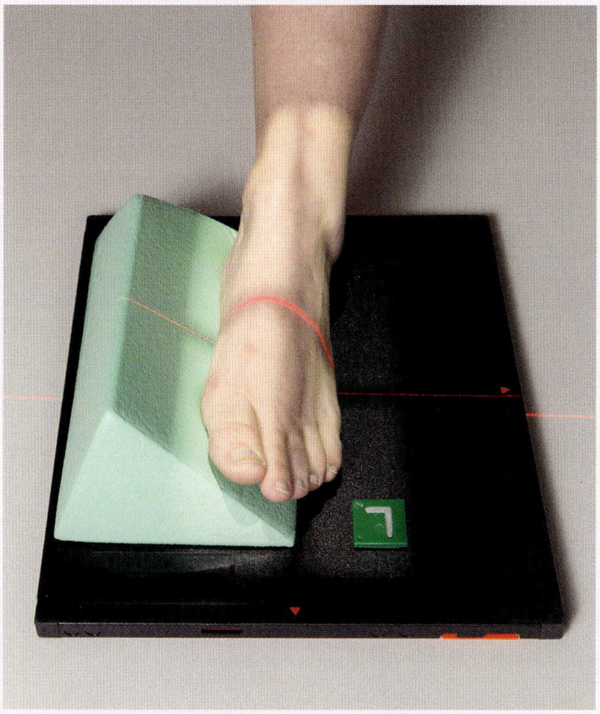

7-81 AP Oblique with lateral rotation.

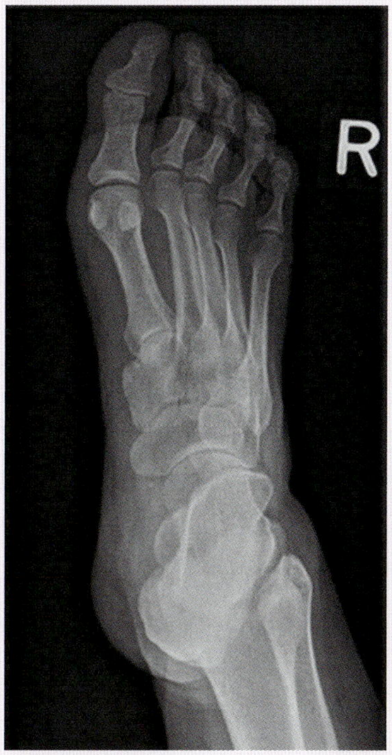

7-82 AP Oblique with lateral rotation.

Foot

- Projection: Mediolateral

Foot Protocol
AP
AP Oblique
Mediolateral

Technical Considerations
- kVp 50–60; nongrid
- mAs set manually
- 40″ SID

Exposure Field Size
- 10 × 12 lengthwise to match the length of the foot

Patient Position (Figs. 7-83 and 7-84)
- Seated on the imaging table or stretcher
- Patient's affected leg is fully extended
- Rotate the leg and foot laterally into a true lateral position
- Dorsiflex the foot until the dorsum of the foot is at a near 90° angle with the lower leg or to the maximum tolerable level for the patient
- Ensure the plantar surface of the foot is perpendicular to the IR. Dorsiflexion of the foot should assist with this. If not, then the patient's knee could be built up off the table until the plantar surface is perpendicular to the IR

Centering
- To the level of the first cuneiform. Collimate down to include the distal phalanges, tarsals, calcaneus and distal tibia and fibula

Marking of IR
- Anatomic side marker R or L placed along the anterior surface of the foot

Breathing
- No specific breathing instructions are given to the patient. Instruct the patient to hold still
- Ensure patient holds position while walking away to make the exposure

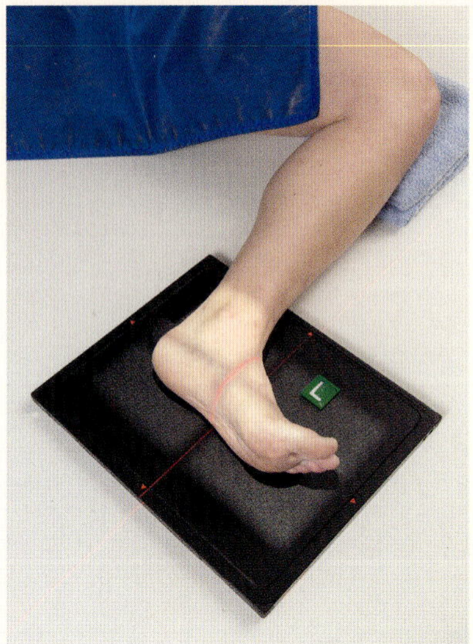

7-83 Knee elevated to help position the plantar surface perpendicular to the IR.

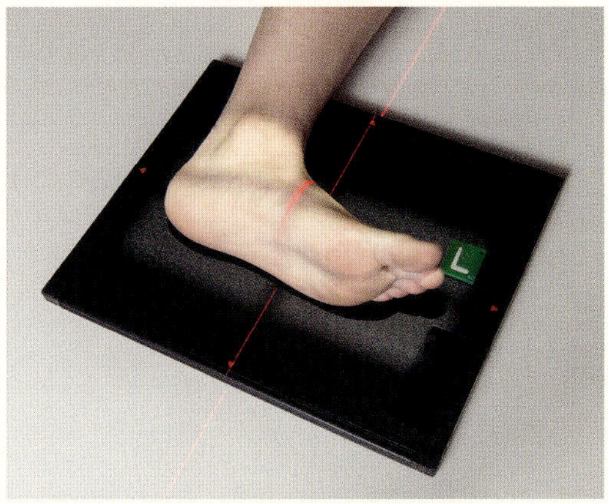

7-84 Mediolateral foot.

IMAGE CRITIQUE (FIGS. 7-85 and 7-86)
- Entire foot to include distal phalanges, metatarsals, tarsals, calcaneus, distal tibia, and fibula are included within the collimated exposure field
- Metatarsals nearly superimposed. Superimposition of the metatarsals improves with dorsiflexion of the foot and the plantar surface aligned perpendicular to the IR
- Base of the fifth metatarsal in profile
- Calcaneus is in profile
- Properly centered with four-sided collimation

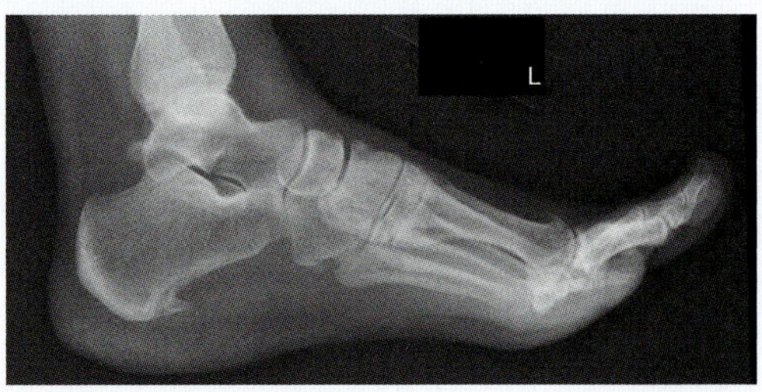

7-85 Mediolateral foot.

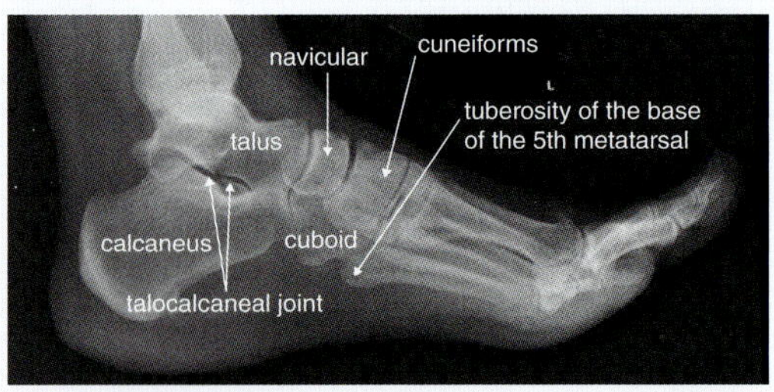

7-86 Mediolateral foot.

Weight Bearing Foot/Feet

- Projection: AP (Dorsoplantar) Foot (Feet)
- *Typically, both feet are imaged to provide comparison. A single projection could center to include both feet or if separate projections are taken of each foot the centering is directed to the foot*

Weight Bearing Foot/Feet Protocol
AP
Mediolateral

Technical Considerations

- kVp 55–60; nongrid
- mAs set manually
- 40″–44″ SID

Exposure Field Size

- 10 × 12 lengthwise (LW) for single projections
- 14 × 17 crosswise (CW) for bilateral projection

Patient Position (Figs. 7-87 and 7-88)

- Erect with weight equally distributed between both feet
- Feet should be parallel to one another
- Patient will stand on the IR

Centering

- Bilateral feet will center the beam with a 15° angle toward the heels midway between both feet at the level of the metatarsal bases
- Each foot could be individually imaged with the 15° angle toward the heel directed to the base of the third metatarsal

Marking of IR

- Anatomic side marker R or L placed furthest from the patient's midline or lateral to the part

Breathing

- No specific breathing instructions are given to the patient. Instruct the patient to hold still
- Ensure patient holds position while walking away to make the exposure

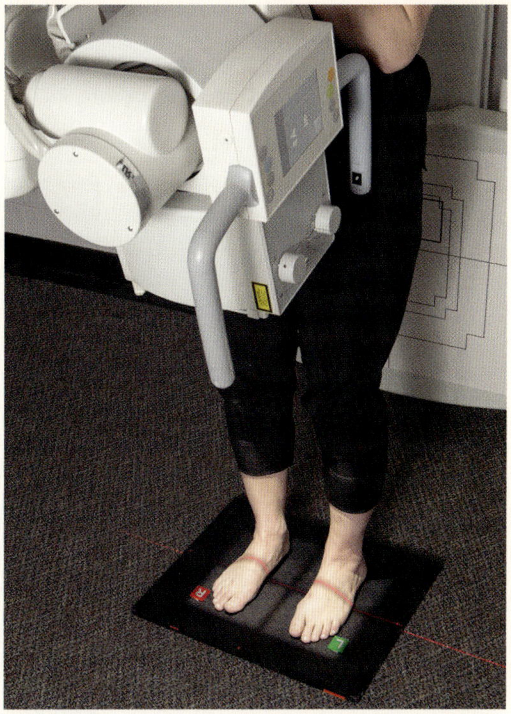

7-87 AP bilateral weight-bearing feet.

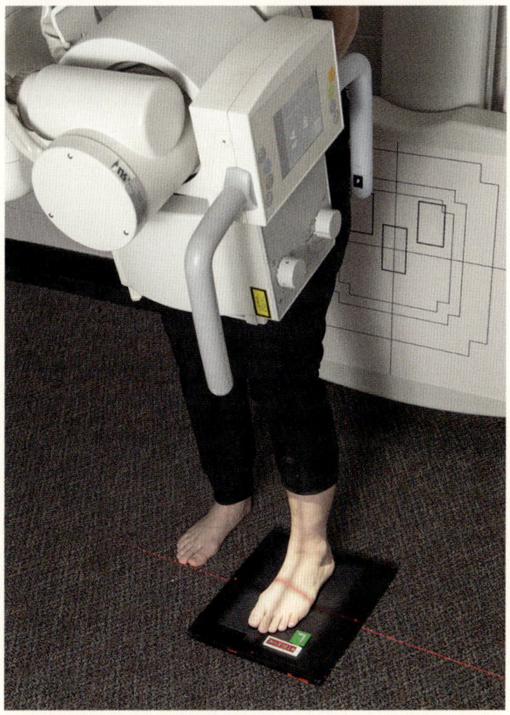

7-88 AP weight-bearing foot.

IMAGE CRITIQUE (FIG. 7-89)

- Image will demonstrate the longitudinal arches of the foot under weight-bearing conditions
- The distal phalanges through the talus must be included. The calcaneus will not be well visualized
- Good penetration of the tarsometatarsal joints
- Properly centered with four-sided collimation

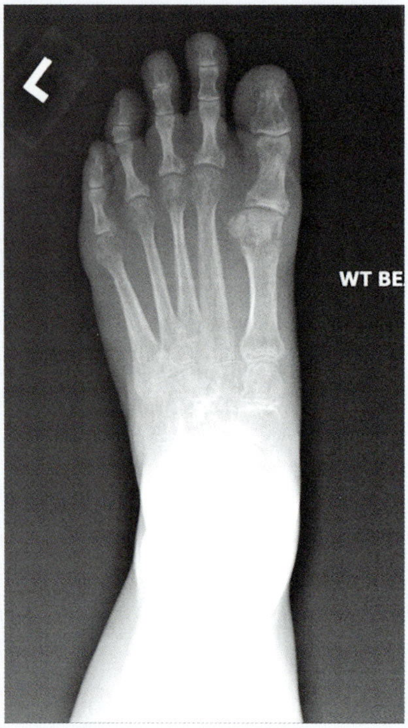

7-89 AP weight-bearing foot.

Weight Bearing Foot/Feet

- Projection: Mediolateral
- *Typically, both feet are imaged to provide comparison. A single projection must be taken of each individual foot while in the standing lateral*

Weight Bearing Foot/Feet Protocol
AP
Mediolateral

Technical Considerations
- kVp 55–60; nongrid
- mAs set manually
- 40″–44″ SID

Exposure Field Size
- 10 × 12 lengthwise with the foot

Patient Position (Fig. 7-90)
- Patient will step up to be elevated up off the floor to allow the horizontal tube head to be dropped down low enough to image the foot
- Ensure the patient is stable while erect and distributing the weight over the affected foot
- Unaffected foot and leg should be positioned behind the affected foot
- A lateromedial projection could be a substitute projection for a patient not stable enough to stand for the preferred mediolateral projection. With the lateromedial approach, the patient would stand with weight distributed between both feet. The IR is positioned between the feet. The central ray is directed to enter on the lateral surface of the foot at the level of the base of the third metatarsal

Centering
- To the level of the first cuneiform. Collimate down to include the distal phalanges, tarsals, calcaneus and distal tibia and fibula

Marking of IR
- Anatomic side marker R or L placed along the anterior surface of the foot

Breathing
- No specific breathing instructions are given to the patient. Ensure patient is stable
- Ensure patient holds position while walking away to make the exposure

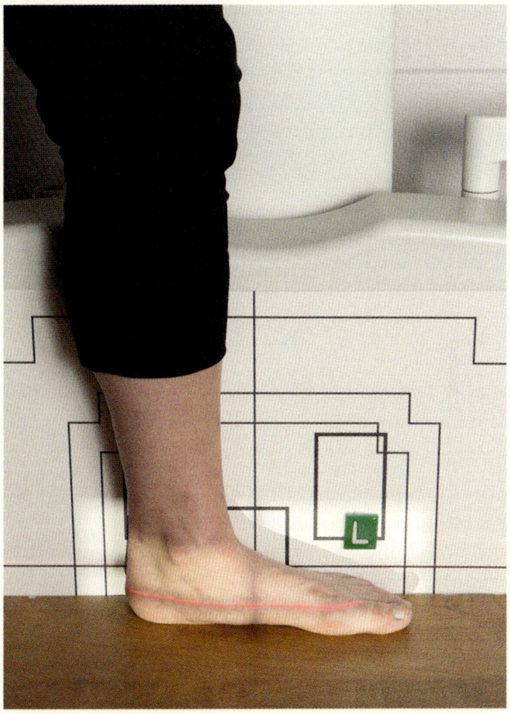

7-90 Mediolateral weight-bearing foot.

IMAGE CRITIQUE (FIG. 7-91)

- Entire foot to include distal phalanges, metatarsals, tarsals, calcaneus, distal tibia, and fibula included within the collimated exposure field
- Longitudinal arch seen under weight-bearing conditions
- Metatarsals nearly superimposed. Base of the fifth metatarsal in profile. Calcaneus is in profile
- Properly centered with four-sided collimation

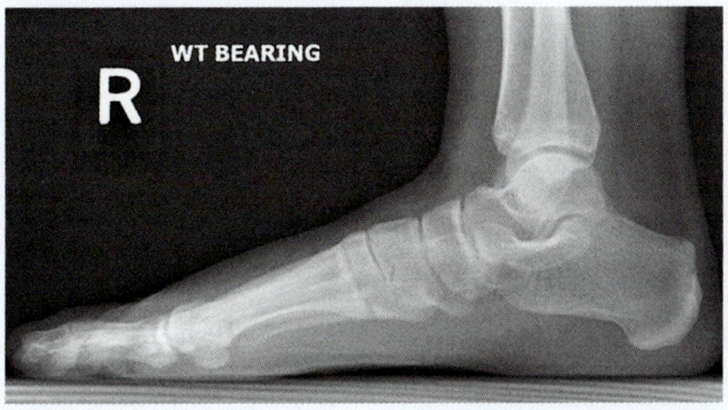

7-91 Mediolateral weight-bearing foot.

Calcaneus

- Projection: Plantodorsal Axial

Calcaneus Protocol
Plantodorsal Axial
Mediolateral

Technical Considerations
- kVp 60–65; nongrid
- mAs set manually
- 40″ SID

Exposure Field Size
- 10 × 12 lengthwise with the lower leg with collimation down to the calcaneus

Patient Position (Fig. 7-92)
- Seated on the imaging table or stretcher
- Patient's affected leg is fully extended
- Affected foot is dorsiflexed to align the plantar surface of the foot perpendicular to the IR

Centering (Fig. 7-93)
- 40° cephalic (toward the heel) tube angle directed to enter on the plantar surface of the foot at the base of the third metatarsal (beam should appear to exit the level of the lateral malleolus or slightly below). Collimate to include the entire calcaneus and the talocalcaneal joint

Marking of IR
- Anatomic side marker R or L placed furthest from the patient's midline or lateral to the part

Breathing
- No specific breathing instructions are given to the patient. Instruct the patient to hold still
- Ensure patient holds position while walking away to make the exposure

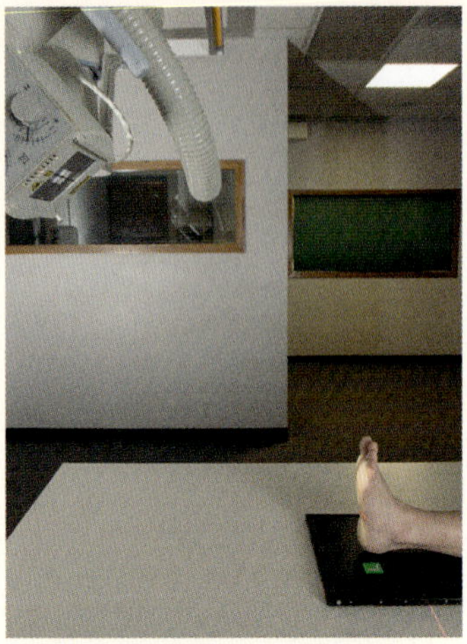

7-92 Plantodorsal axial calcaneus.

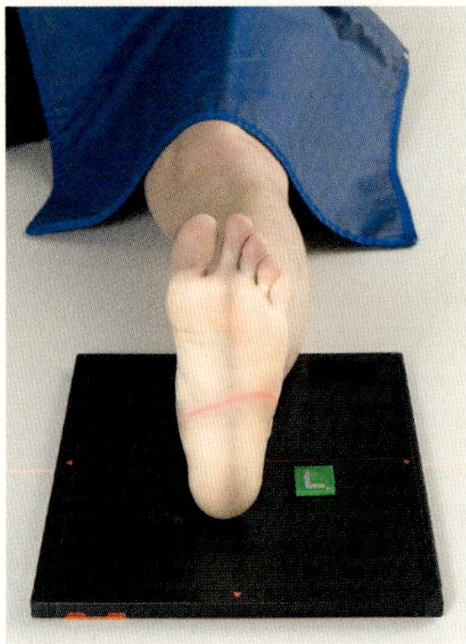

7-93 Plantodorsal axial calcaneus.

IMAGE CRITIQUE (FIGS. 7-94 and 7-95)

- The talocalcaneal joint visualized anteriorly on the image with the joint adequately penetrated
- Calcaneal tuberosity visualized posteriorly. The sustentaculum tali (anterior and medial on the calcaneus) visualized
- Properly centered with four-sided collimation

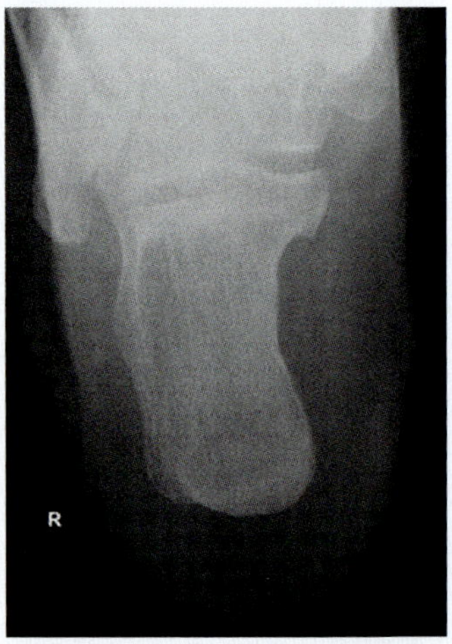

7-94 Plantodorsal axial calcaneus.

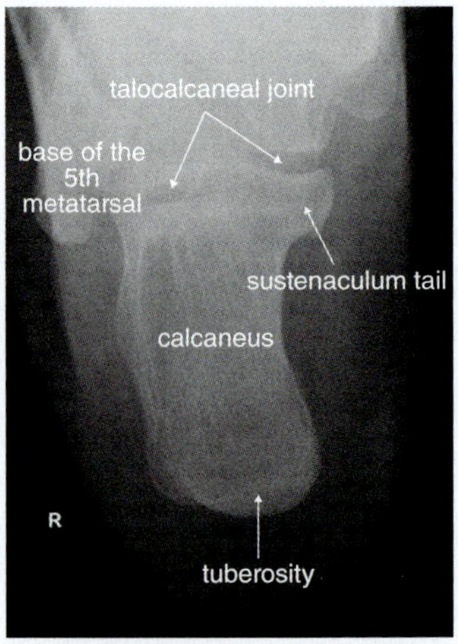

7-95 Plantodorsal axial calcaneus.

Calcaneus

- Projection: Mediolateral

Calcaneus Protocol
Plantodorsal Axial
Mediolateral

Technical Considerations
- kVp 60; nongrid
- mAs set manually
- 40″ SID

Exposure Field Size
- 10 × 12 lengthwise with the length of the lower leg

Patient Position (Fig. 7-96)
- Seated on the imaging table or stretcher
- Patient's affected leg is fully extended
- Rotate the leg and foot laterally into a true lateral position
- Dorsiflex the foot until the dorsum of the foot is at a near 90° angle with the lower leg
- Ensure the plantar surface of the foot is perpendicular to the IR. Dorsiflexion of the foot should assist with this. If not, then the patient's knee could be built up off the table until the plantar surface is perpendicular to the IR

Centering
- 1″ inferior to the medial malleolus. Collimate down to include the base of the 5th metatarsal, entire calcaneus and distal tibia and fibula

Marking of IR
- Anatomic side marker R or L placed along the anterior surface of the foot

Breathing
- No specific breathing instructions are given to the patient. Instruct the patient to hold still
- Ensure patient holds position while walking away to make the exposure

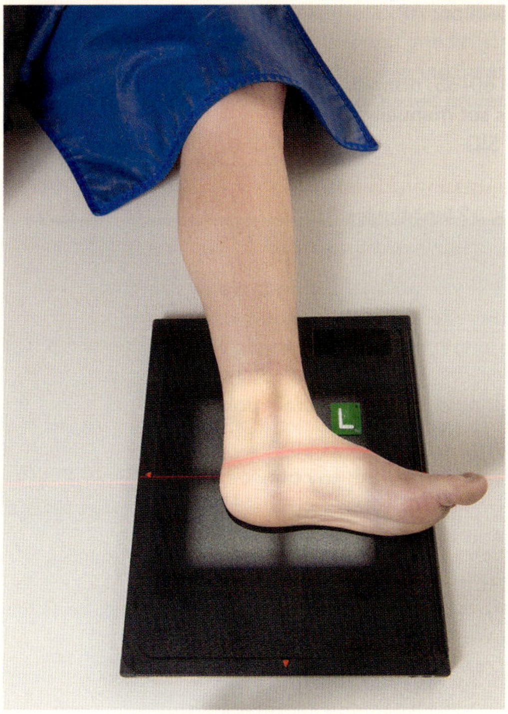

7-96 Mediolateral calcaneus.

IMAGE CRITIQUE (FIGS. 7-97 and 7-98)

- Calcaneus is in profile to include the talus, distal tibia, and fibula along with the base of the fifth metatarsal within the collimated exposure field
- The talocalcaneal joint may include visualization of the sinus tarsi
- Properly centered with four-sided collimation

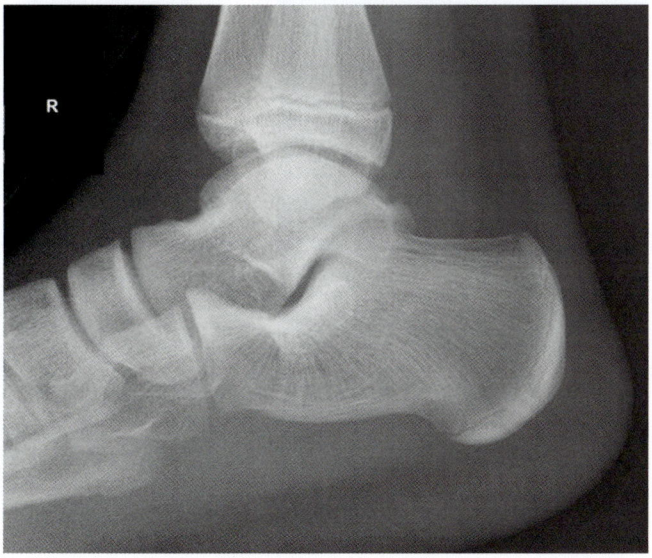

7-97 Mediolateral calcaneus.

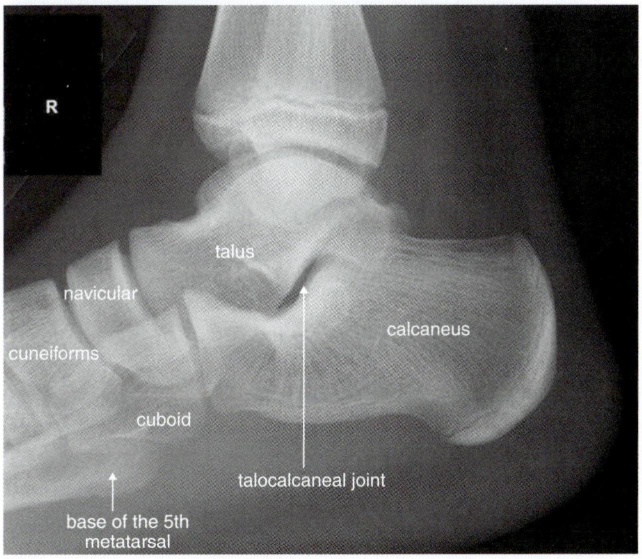

7-98 Mediolateral calcaneus.

Ankle

- Projection: AP Oblique with 45° medial rotation
- *Oblique position (45° or mortise) determined by physician/radiologist preference.*

Ankle Protocol
AP
AP Oblique 45° *or*
AP Oblique Mortise
Mediolateral

Technical Considerations
- kVp 60–65; nongrid
- mAs set manually
- 40″ SID

Exposure Field Size
- 10 × 12 lengthwise

Patient Position (Fig. 7-106)
- Patient seated on imaging table or stretcher
- Patient's leg is fully extended.
- The patient's leg and ankle are medially rotated 45°
- Dorsiflex the foot. This is critical to prevent superimposition of the distal fibula upon the calcaneus

Centering
- Midankle joint (midway between the malleoli). Collimate down to include the proximal metatarsals, tarsals and distal tibia and fibula

Marking of IR
- Anatomic side marker R or L placed furthest away from midline

Breathing
- No specific breathing instructions are given to the patient. Instruct the patient to hold still
- Ensure patient holds position while walking away to make the exposure

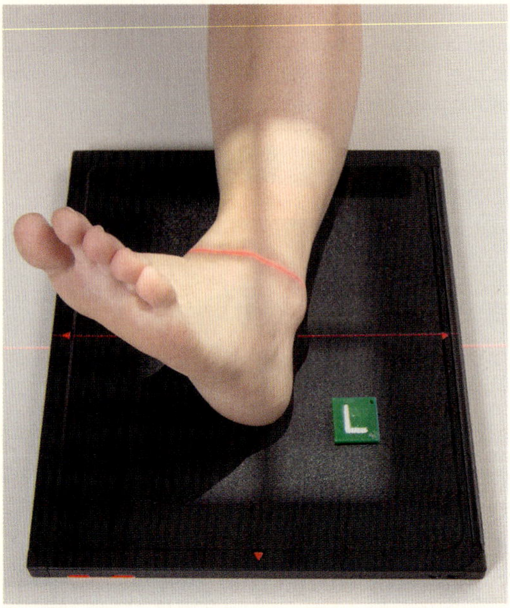

7-106 AP Oblique ankle with 45° medial rotation.

IMAGE CRITIQUE (FIGS. 7-107 and 7-108)

- Distal tibia and fibula, talus, and the proximal-most ends of the metatarsals included in the collimated exposure field. Specific attention given to the base of the fifth metatarsal
- The distal tibiofibular joint is of interest. The joint may entirely open or may show only minimal superimposition of the tibia and fibula, but a visible change at this joint between the AP and the 45° medial AP Oblique should be noticed
- The medial side of the mortise joint will be closed, and the lateral side of the mortise joint will be open
- The distal fibula (lateral malleolus) is free of superimposition from the calcaneus with foot dorsiflexion
- Properly centered with four-sided collimation

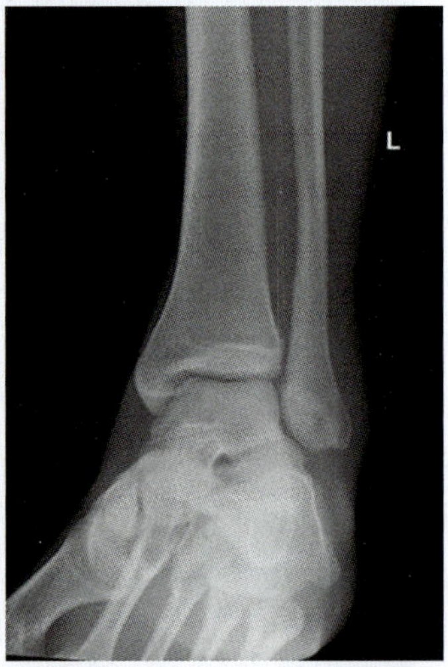

7-107 AP Oblique ankle with 45° medial rotation.

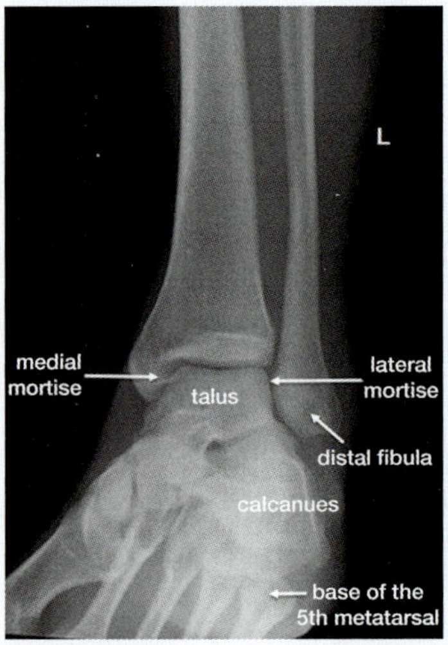

7-108 AP Oblique ankle with 45° medial rotation.

Ankle

- Projection: AP Oblique with 15°–20° medial rotation (Mortise)
- *Oblique position (45° or mortise) determined by physician/ radiologist preference*

Ankle Protocol
AP
AP Oblique 45° *or*
AP Oblique Mortise
Mediolateral

Technical Considerations
- kVp 60–65; Tabletop
- mAs set manually
- 40″ SID

Exposure Field Size
- 10 × 12 lengthwise

Patient Position (Fig. 7-109)
- Patient seated on imaging table or stretcher
- Patient's leg is fully extended
- The patient's foot should remain in a natural position
- The patient's leg and ankle are medially rotated 15°–20° until the intermalleolar line is parallel to the imaging plane

Centering
- Midankle joint (midway between the malleoli). Collimate down to include the proximal metatarsals, tarsals and distal tibia and fibula

Marking of IR
- Anatomic side marker R or L placed furthest away from midline

Breathing
- No specific breathing instructions were given to the patient. Instruct the patient to hold still
- Ensure patient holds position while walking away to make the exposure

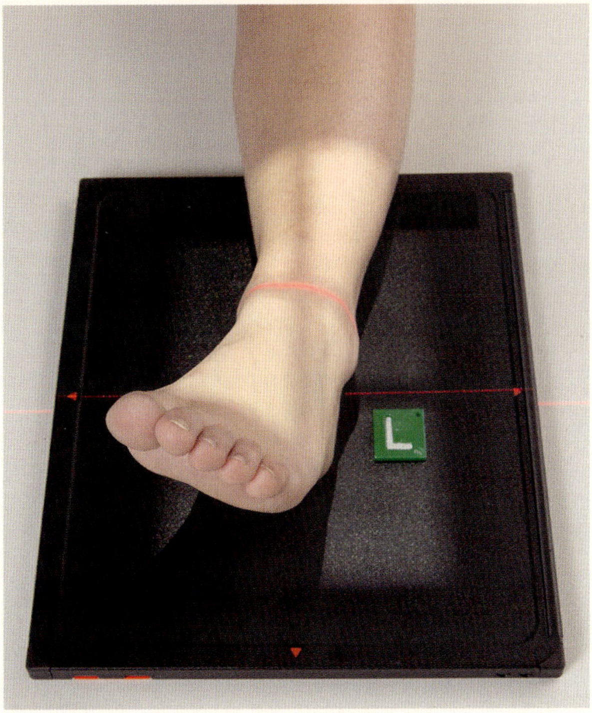

7-109 AP Oblique ankle with 15°–20° medial rotation.

IMAGE CRITIQUE (FIGS. 7-110 and 7-111)

- Distal tibia and fibula, talus, and the proximal-most ends of the metatarsals are included within the collimated exposure field. Specific attention given to the base of the fifth metatarsal
- The entire mortise joint is of interest. Proper obliquity will display the medial and lateral sides of the mortise joint open
- Properly centered with four-sided collimation

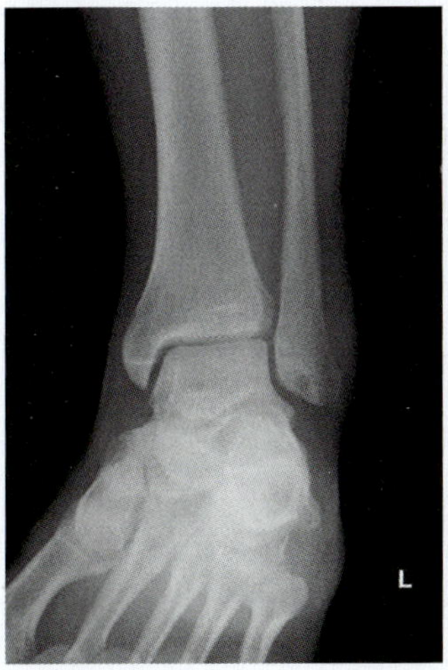

7-110 AP Oblique ankle with 15°–20° medial rotation.

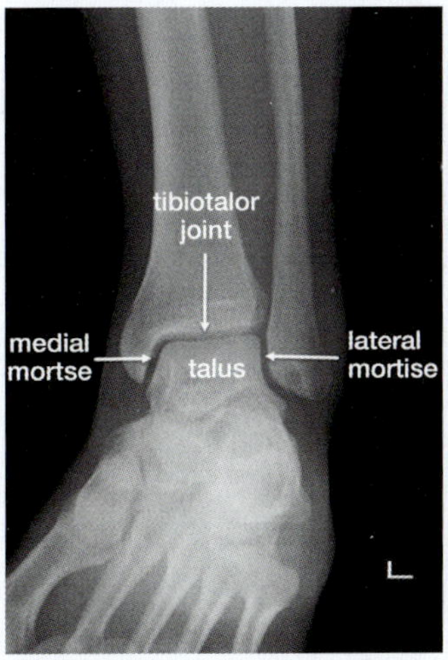

7-111 AP Oblique ankle with 15°–20° medial rotation.

Ankle

- Projection: Mediolateral

Ankle Protocol
AP
AP Oblique 45° *or* AP Oblique Mortise
Mediolateral

Technical Considerations

- kVp 60–65; nongrid
- mAs set manually
- 40″ SID

Exposure Field Size

- 10 × 12 lengthwise

Patient Position (Fig. 7-112)

- Seated on the imaging table or stretcher
- Patient's affected leg is fully extended
- Rotate the leg and foot laterally into a true lateral position
- Dorsiflex the foot until the dorsum of the foot is at a near 90° angle with the lower leg
- Ensure the plantar surface of the foot is perpendicular to the IR. Dorsiflexion of the foot should assist with this. If not, then the patient's knee could be built up off the table until the plantar surface is perpendicular to the IR

Centering

- To the level of the medial malleolus. Collimate down to include the proximal metatarsals, tarsals and distal tibia and fibula

Marking of IR

- Anatomic side marker R or L placed along the anterior surface of the foot

Breathing

- No specific breathing instructions are given to the patient. Instruct the patient to hold still
- Ensure patient holds position while walking away to make the exposure

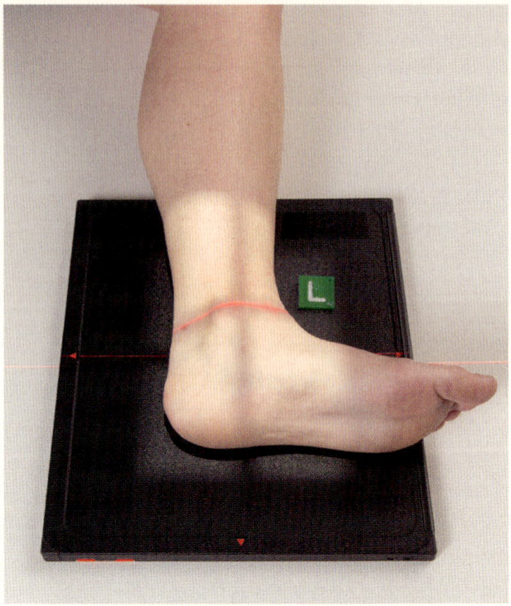

7-112 Mediolateral ankle.

IMAGE CRITIQUE (FIGS. 7-113 and 7-114)

- Distal tibia and fibula, talus, and the proximal-most ends of the metatarsals are included within the collimated exposure field
- The distal fibula will superimpose the posterior ½ of the tibia
- Base of the fifth metatarsal in profile. Calcaneus is in profile
- Anterior to posterior displacement of the part can be determined if a fracture is noted or dislocation is present
- Properly centered with four-sided collimation

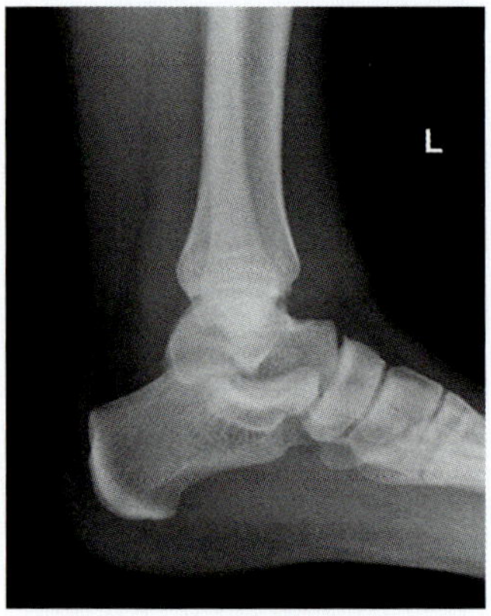

7-113 Mediolateral ankle.

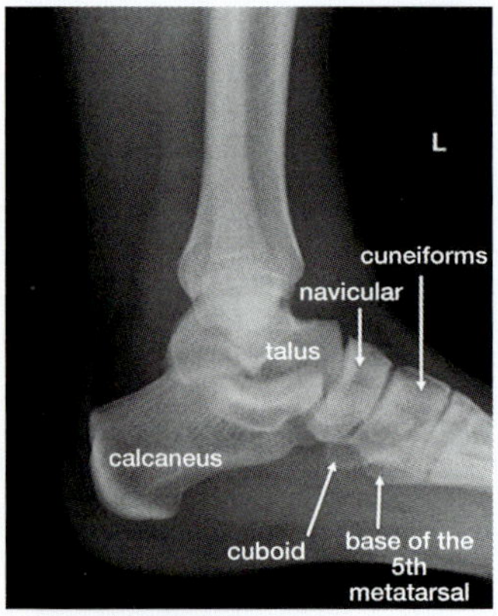

7-114 Mediolateral ankle.

Trauma Ankle

- Projection: AP
- A minimum of two views 90° apart are required.
- *Trauma extremity routine described here is an example that can be applied similarly to other lower extremities. Trauma protocol may be elected for pre- and postsurgical patients*

Trauma Ankle Protocol
AP
Mediolateral or Lateromedial

Technical Considerations
- kVp 60–65; nongrid
- mAs set manually
- Technical changes in consideration of a cast. A 3–10 increase in kVp can be considered
- 40″ SID

Exposure Field Size
- 10 × 12 lengthwise with collimation down to the ankle

Patient Position (Fig. 7-115)
- Patient condition may be variable. Imaging may include patients in the emergency department, recovery room, or operating room. Mobile imaging is possible
- Erect and seated on a stretcher
- Patient may be supine
- The technologist will have to adapt to the patient's ability and creatively find an approach to best image the patient
- If the patient is in the operating room, the IR(s) will be given to the nurse to drop into a sterile covering. The operating room surgeon or scrub nurse will touch the sterile IR and place it under the patient's part. The technologist while being very aware of the sterile field will center to the part and keep the collimation open to include all the anatomy. Center where designated by the surgeon

Centering
- Midankle joint—midway between the medial and lateral malleolus unless designated differently by the surgeon

Marking of IR
- Anatomic side marker R or L placed furthest from the patient's midline or lateral to the part
- Marking the IR when imaging in a sterile field (operating room) is not possible

Breathing
- No specific breathing instructions are given to the patient. Instruct the patient to hold still
- Ensure patient holds position while walking away to make the exposure

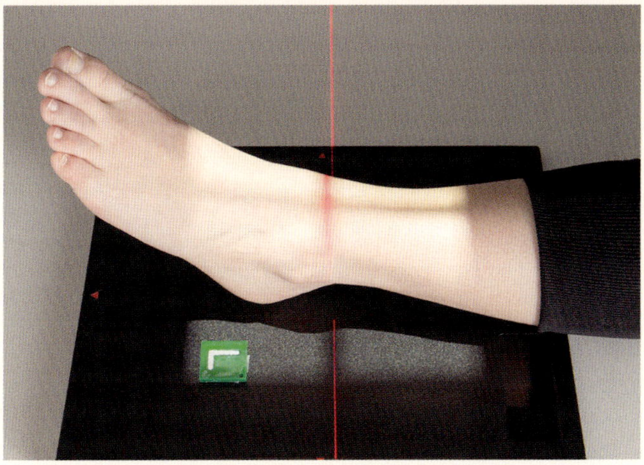

7-115 AP trauma ankle. Neutral or presenting position.

IMAGE CRITIQUE (FIGS. 7-116 and 7-117)

- Distal tibia and fibula, talus, and the proximal-most ends of the metatarsals included within the collimated exposure field. Specific attention was given to the base of the fifth metatarsal
- Tibia and fibula should appear parallel to one another and articulate at the distal tibiofibular joint
- Imaging joint spaces to appear open may not be achievable due to the patient limitations
- Images acquired in the OR suite or postoperatively must set the collimated exposure field to include surgical metal implants in their entirety (Fig. 7-118)
- Patients that are post open reduction internal fixation (ORIF) will require that all metal plates, wires, pins, and screws be included on the image

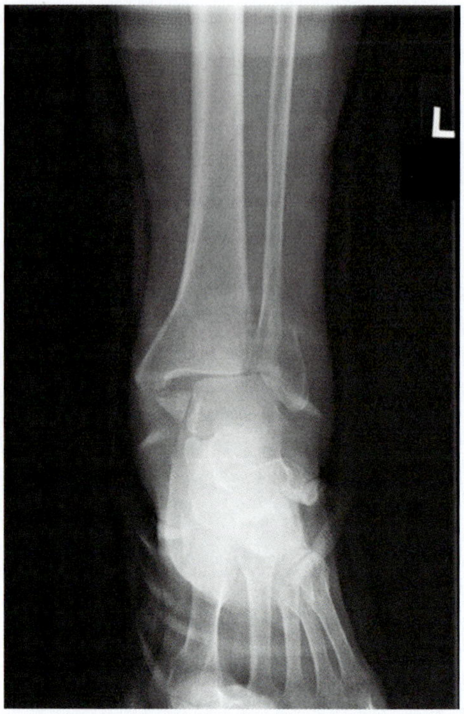

7-117 AP trauma ankle. Postreduction.

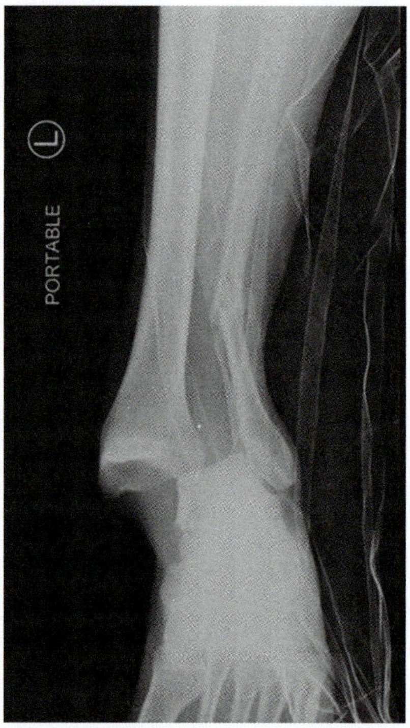

7-116 AP trauma ankle. Neutral or presenting position.

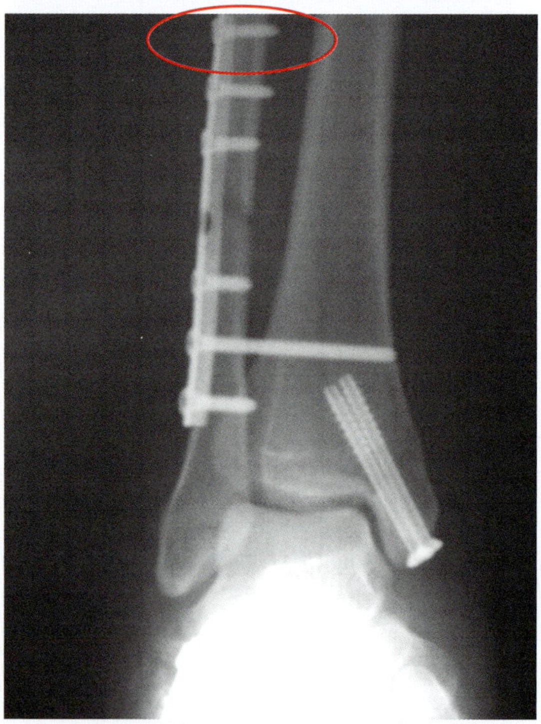

7-118 Failure to include the entirety of the surgical implant.

Trauma Ankle

- Projection: Mediolateral or Lateromedial (depends on the patient situation)
- A minimum of two views 90° apart are required
- *Trauma extremity routine described here is an example that can be applied similarly to other lower extremities. Trauma protocol may be elected for pre- and postsurgical patients*

Trauma Ankle Protocol
AP
Mediolateral *or* Lateromedial

Technical Considerations

- kVp 60–65; nongrid
- mAs set manually
- Technical changes in consideration of a cast. A 3–10 increase in kVp can be considered
- 40″ SID

Exposure Field Size

- 10 × 12 lengthwise

Patient Position (Fig. 7-119)

- Patient able to moderately ambulate.
  - Seated on the imaging table or could remain on stretcher
  - Patient's affected leg is fully extended
  - Rotate the leg and foot laterally into a true lateral position. This will allow a mediolateral projection of the part to be attained
  - Dorsiflex the foot only if tolerated by the patient to their maximum point. If unable to dorsiflex, leave the foot in natural position
- Patient unable to ambulate
  - Patient remains supine and a horizontal beam will be utilized
  - Patient's lower leg and ankle are elevated slightly up off the table allowing the IR to drop below the anatomy. Typically, due to the condition of the patient, the IR is positioned along the medial side of the lower leg and ankle. Due to this IR placement, a lateromedial projection of the part is attained (Fig. 7-120)

Centering

- To the level of the medial malleolus or lateral malleolus depending on projection utilized
- If in the surgical suite, center where designated by the surgeon

Marking of IR

- Anatomic side marker R or L placed along the anterior surface of the foot
- Marking the IR when imaging in a sterile field (operating room) is not possible

Breathing

- No specific breathing instructions are given to the patient. Instruct the patient to hold still
- Ensure patient holds position while walking away to make the exposure

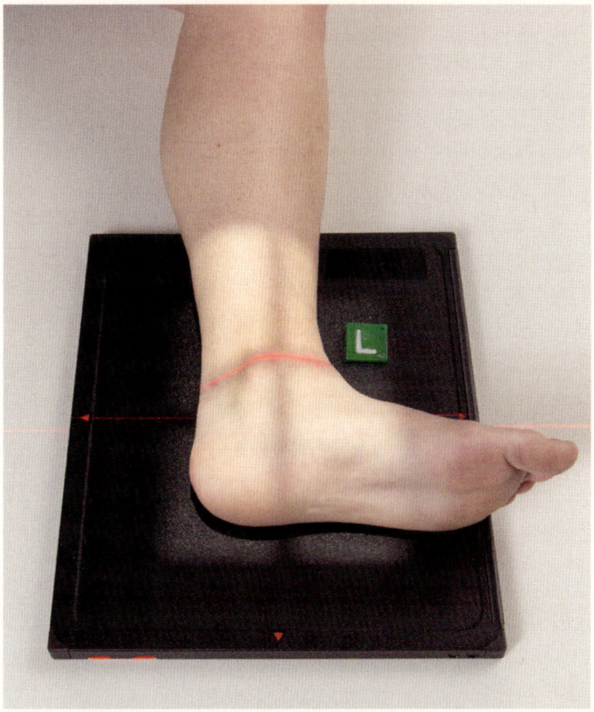

7-119 Mediolateral trauma ankle.

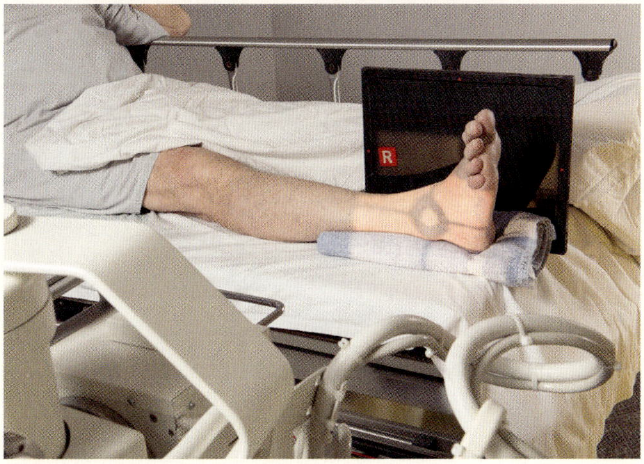

7-120 Lateromedial trauma ankle.

IMAGE CRITIQUE (FIGS. 7-121 and 7-122)

- Distal tibia and fibula, talus, and the proximal-most ends of the metatarsals within the collimated exposure field
- The distal fibula will superimpose the posterior ½ of the tibia
- Base of the fifth metatarsal in profile
- Calcaneus is in profile and included entirely
- Anterior to posterior displacement of the part can be determined if a fracture or dislocation is present
- Images acquired in the OR suite or postoperative, the collimated exposure field must include surgical metal implants in their entirety
- Patient's that are post ORIF (open reduction internal fixation) will require all the metal plates, wires, pins, and screws to be included on the image

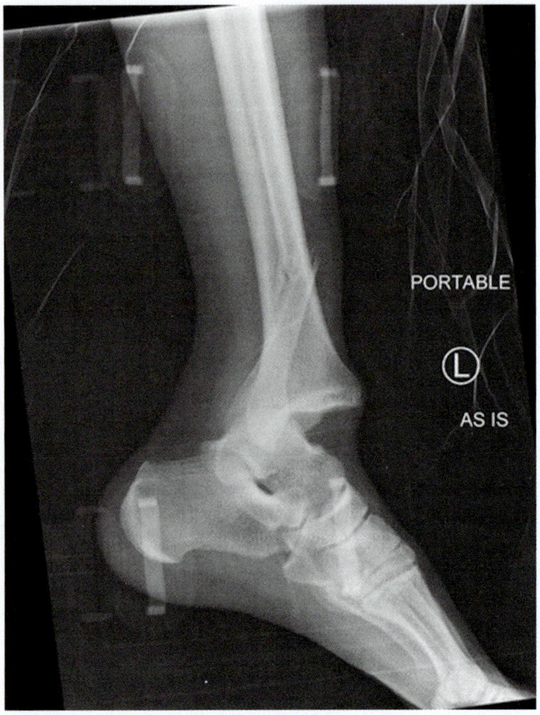

7-121 Lateromedial trauma ankle.

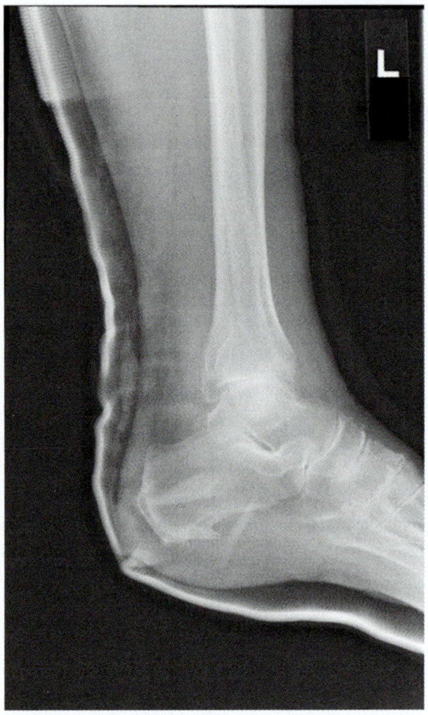

7-122 Lateromedial trauma ankle.

Lower Leg

- Projection: AP

Lower Leg Protocol
AP
Mediolateral

Technical Considerations
- kVp 65; nongrid
- mAs set manually
- 40″–44″ SID (44″ SID may be necessary to attain entire lower leg and both joints with a single projection)

Exposure Field Size
- 14 × 17 diagonal with collimation down to lower leg
- A combination of a 10 × 12 lengthwise and a 14 × 17 lengthwise exposure field sizes may be needed to acquire the entire length of the lower leg with two separate exposures. The two images must display a point of anatomic overlap

Patient Position
- Patient seated on imaging table or stretcher
- Patient's leg is fully extended
- Foot moderately dorsiflexed
- Slight medial rotation (3°–5°) of the leg to align the tibial condyles parallel with the image receptor

Centering (Figs. 7-123 to 7-125)
- Single 14 × 17 diagonal: Midshaft of the lower leg
- Overlapping exposure fields: With the bottom of the 10 x 12 exposure field placed just below the calcaneus, center to the IR to image ankle joint and up towards mid-shaft. The second AP takes the 14 x 17 exposure field placed just above the knee joint and then is centered on the IR on image knee joint down

Marking of IR
- Anatomic side marker R or L placed furthest away from midline

Breathing
- No specific breathing instructions are given to the patient. Instruct the patient to hold still
- Ensure patient holds position while walking away to make the exposure

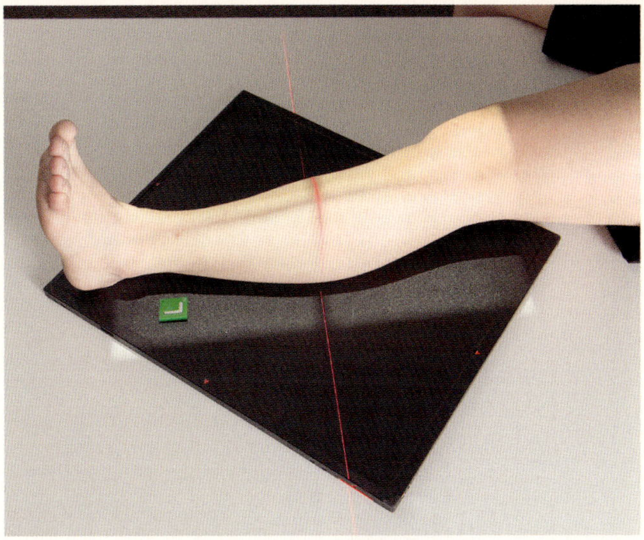

7-123 AP tibia and fibula.

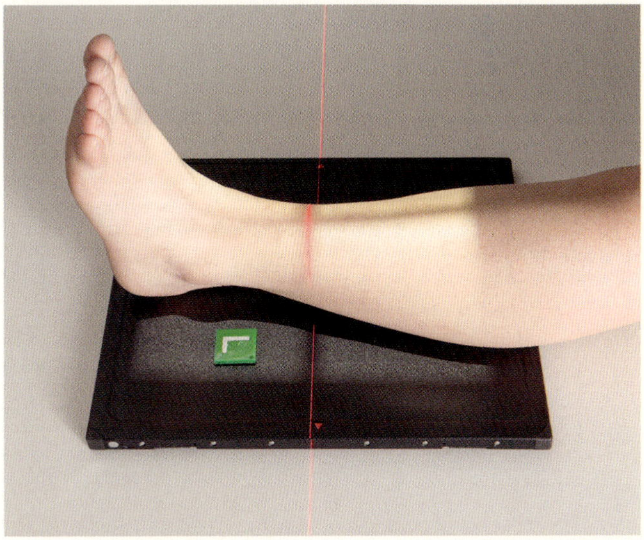

7-124 AP tibia and fibula distal.

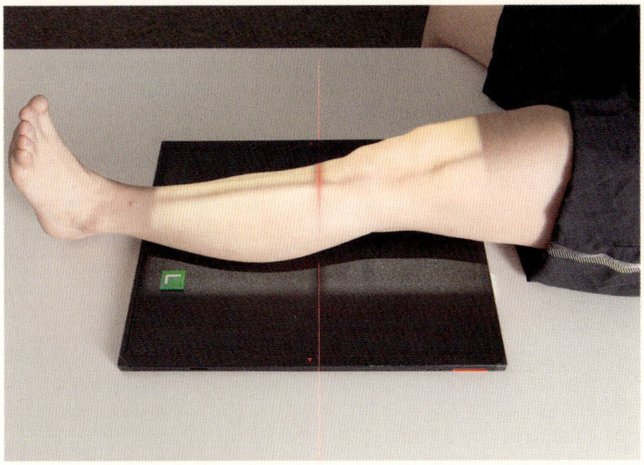

7-125 AP tibia and fibula proximal.

IMAGE CRITIQUE (FIGS. 7-126 to 7-128)

- Entire tibia and fibula are included along with visualization of both the ankle and knee joints within the collimated exposure field
- Tibia and fibular should appear parallel to one another
- Properly centered with four-sided collimation

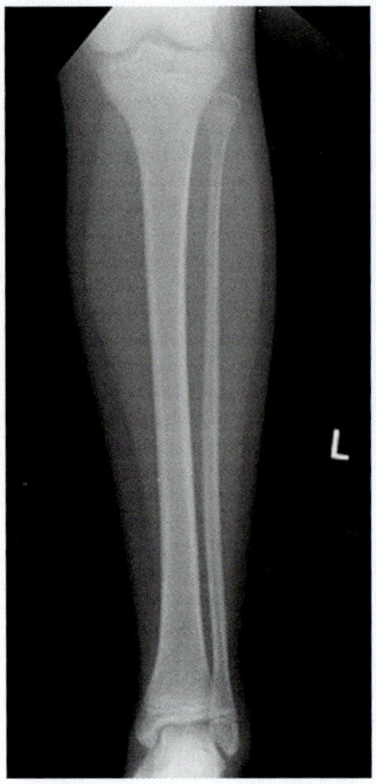

7-126 AP tibia and fibula.

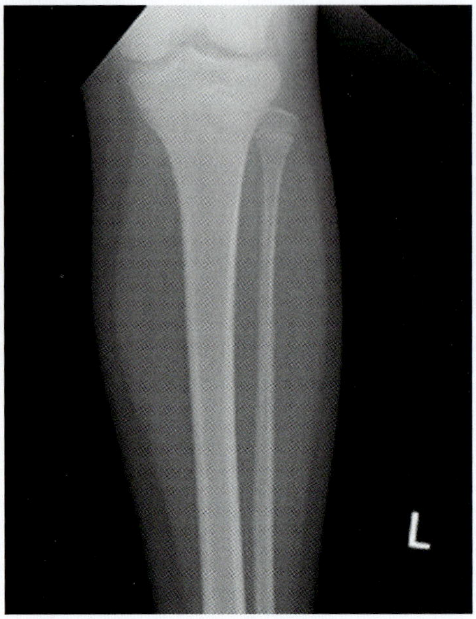

7-127 AP tibia and fibula proximal.

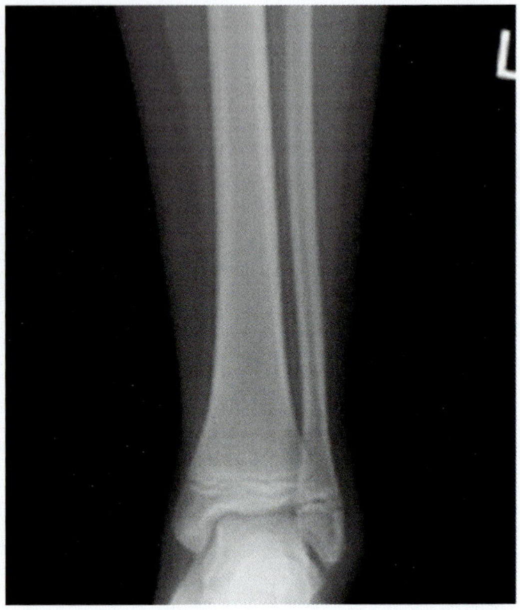

7-128 AP tibia and fibula distal.

Lower Leg

- Projection: Mediolateral

Lower Leg Protocol
AP
Mediolateral

Technical Considerations

- kVp 65; nongrid
- mAs set manually
- 40″–44″ SID (44″ SID may be necessary to attain entire lower leg and both joints with a single projection)

Exposure Field Size

- 14 × 17 diagonal with collimation down to lower leg.
- A combination of a 10 × 12 lengthwise and a 14 × 17 lengthwise exposure field sizes may be needed to acquire the entire length of the lower leg with two separate exposures. The two images must display a point of anatomic overlap. If overlap method is used, switch the placement location of the IRs from the AP to avoid the images showing the anatomy overlapping near the same point on both projections

Patient Position

- Patient seated on imaging table or stretcher
- Patient's leg is fully extended
- Flex the knee 45° and rotate the leg and foot laterally
- Ensure the lower leg is parallel to the plane of the IR. If the ankle is substantially smaller than the knee, the ankle could be supported slightly
- Adjust the knee into a true lateral by palpating the medial and lateral borders of the patella and adjust until perpendicular to the IR
- Slightly dorsiflex the foot

Centering (Figs. 7-129 to 7-131)

- Single 14 × 17 LW: Midshaft of the lower leg
- Overlapping exposure fields: With the top of the 10 x 12 exposure field placed just above the knee joint, center to the IR. The second AP takes 14 x 17 exposure field placed just below the calcaneus and then is centered on the IR to image ankle joint up

Marking of IR

- Anatomic side marker R or L placed along the anterior surface or "in front" of the part

Breathing

- No specific breathing instructions are given to the patient. Instruct the patient to hold still
- Ensure patient holds position while walking away to make the exposure

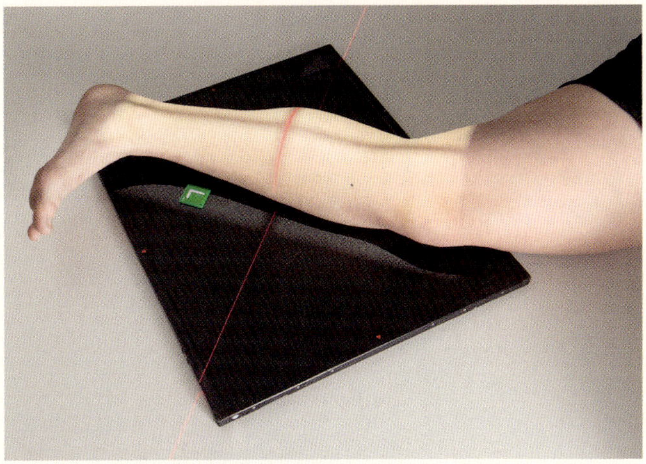

7-129 Mediolateral tibia and fibula.

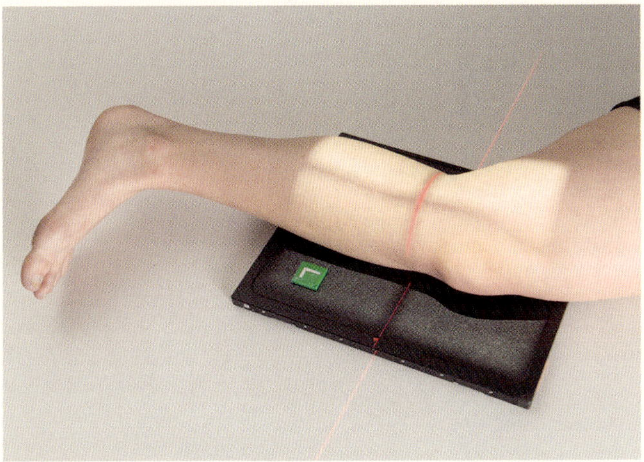

7-130 Mediolateral tibia and fibula proximal.

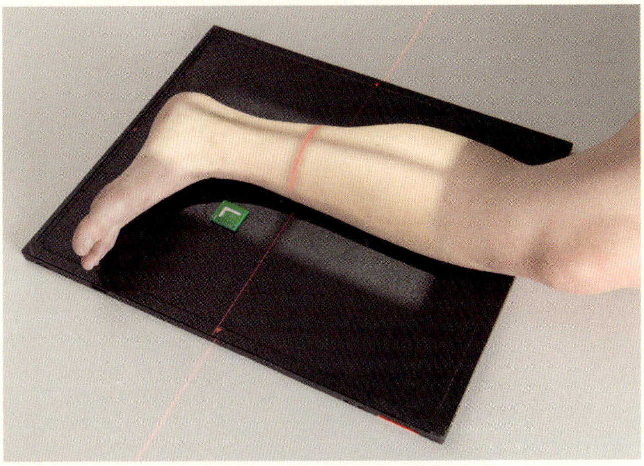

7-131 Mediolateral tibia and fibula distal.

IMAGE CRITIQUE (FIGS. 7-132 to 7-134)

- Entire tibia and fibula are included along with visualization of both the ankle and knee joints within the collimated exposure field
- The fibula sits posterior to the tibia
- Anterior to posterior displacement of the part can be determined
- Properly centered with four-sided collimation

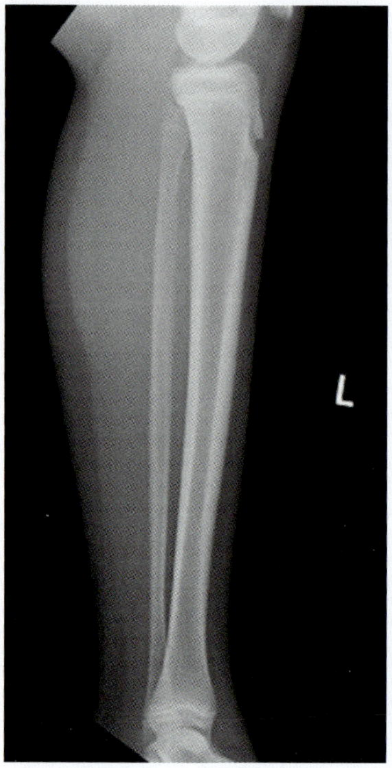

7-132 Mediolateral tibia and fibula.

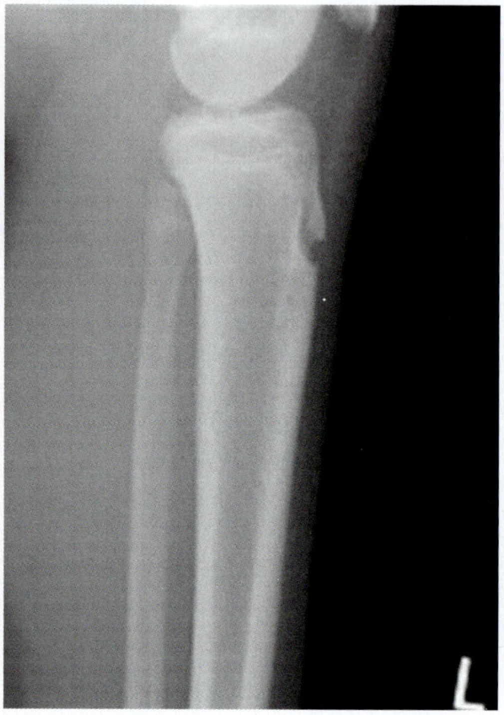

7-133 Mediolateral tibia and fibula proximal.

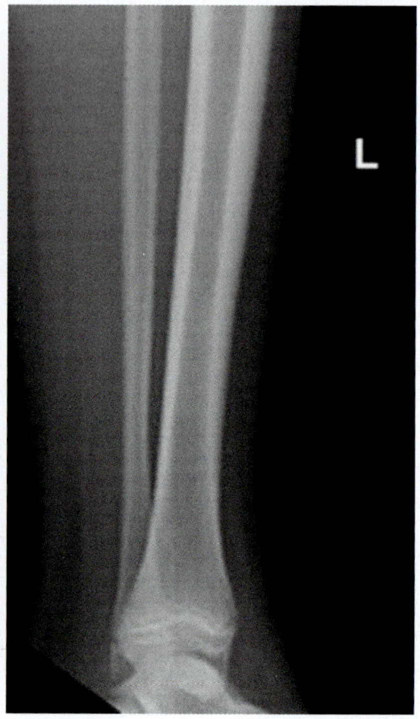

7-134 Mediolateral tibia and fibula distal.

Pediatric Lower Leg

- Projection: AP

Pediatric Lower Leg Protocol
AP
Mediolateral

Technical Considerations
- kVp 55–60; nongrid
- mAs set manually
- 40″ SID

Exposure Field Size
- 14 × 17 lengthwise or smaller with collimation down to lower leg

Patient Position (Fig. 7-135)

AP Lower Leg
- Patient seated on imaging table or stretcher
- Patient's leg is fully extended
- Foot slightly dorsiflexed
- Slight medial rotation (3°–5°) of the leg may be necessary to align the tibial condyles parallel with the IR
- Immobilize as necessary considering the age of the patient

Mediolateral Lower Leg
- Patient seated on imaging table or stretcher
- Flex the knee 45° and rotate the leg and foot laterally
- Adjust the knee into a true lateral by palpating the medial and lateral borders of the patella and adjust until perpendicular to the IR
- Slightly dorsiflex the foot
- Immobilize as necessary considering the age of the patient (Fig. 7-136)

Centering
- Single exposure: Midshaft of the lower leg. Adjust collimation to include the entire tibia, fibular, ankle joint, and femorotibial joint

Marking of IR
- Anatomic side marker R or L placed furthest away from midline

Breathing
- No specific breathing instructions are given to the patient. Ensure the safety of the patient on the table
- Ensure patient holds position while walking away to make the exposure

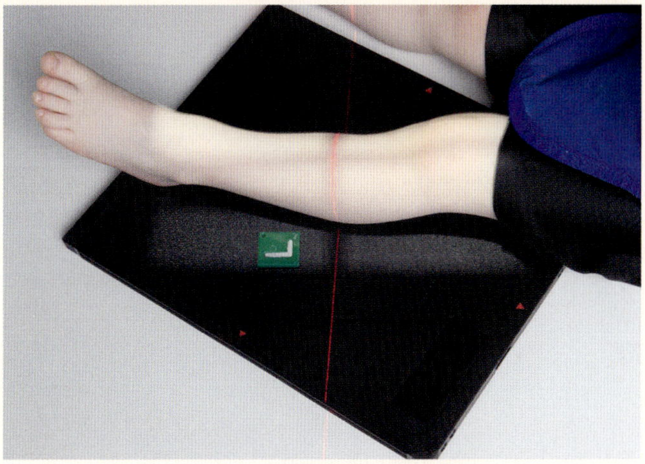

7-135 Pediatric AP tibia and fibula.

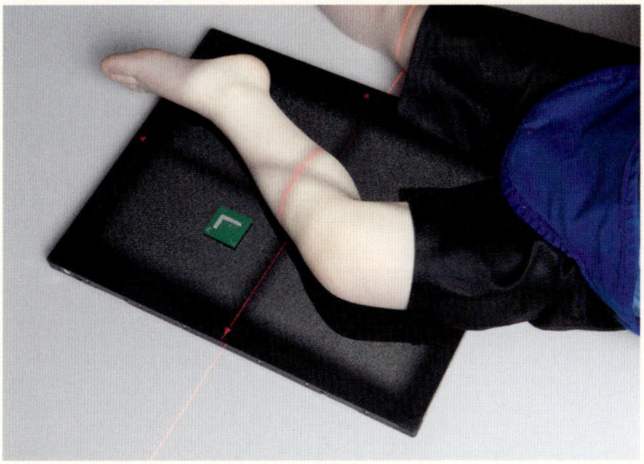

7-136 Pediatric mediolateral tibial and fibula.

IMAGE CRITIQUE (FIGS. 7-137 and 7-138)

AP

- Entire tibia and fibula are included along with visualization of both the ankle and knee joints within the collimated exposure field
- Tibia and fibular should appear parallel to one another
- Properly centered with four-sided collimation

Mediolateral

- Entire tibia and fibula are included along with visualization of both the ankle and knee joints
- The fibula sits posterior to the tibia
- Anterior to posterior displacement of the part can be determined
- Properly centered with four-sided collimation

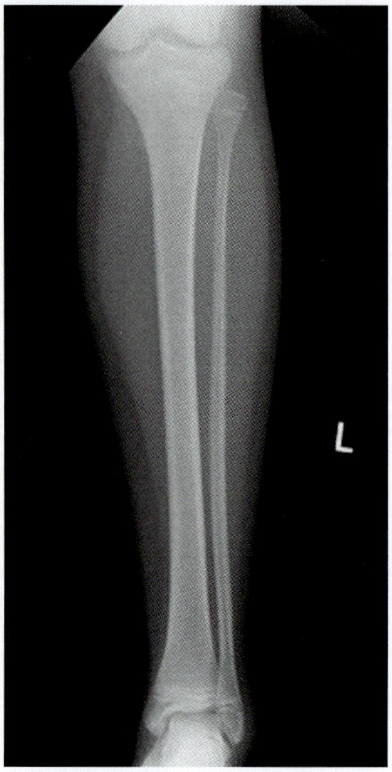

7-137 Pediatric AP tibia and fibula.

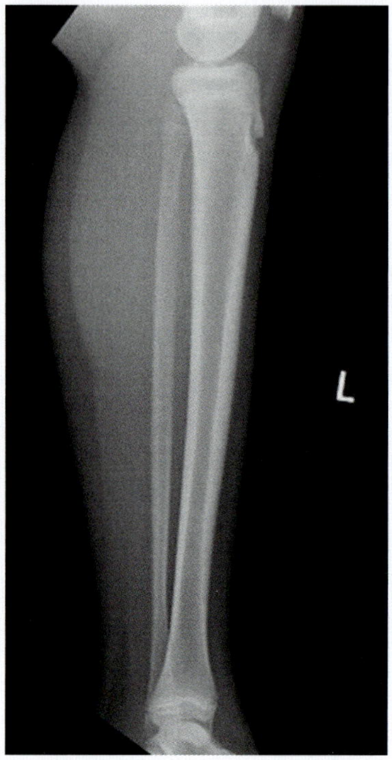

7-138 Pediatric mediolateral tibial and fibula.

Knee

- Projection: AP

Knee Protocol
AP
AP Oblique
Mediolateral

Technical Considerations
- kVp 65; nongrid
- kVp 70-75; grid
- mAs set manually
- 40″ SID

Exposure Field Size
- 10 × 12 lengthwise

Patient Position
- Patient supine or seated on the imaging table
- Leg fully extended
- Slight medial rotation (3°–5°) until the femoral condyles are parallel to the IR

Centering (Figs. 7-139 and 7-140)
- Femorotibial joint—1/2″ (1 finger) inferior to the apex of the patella
- To assist with displaying an open femorotibial joint, the technologist may need to consider the application of a tube angle. The central ray is directed to match the slope of the tibial plateau, which is influenced by the patient's body habitus
- The central ray may be directed perpendicular, slightly cephalic or slightly caudal as needed through the femorotibial joint

Marking of IR
- Anatomic side marker R or L placed furthest away from midline

Breathing
- No specific breathing instructions are given to the patient. Instruct the patient to hold still
- Ensure patient holds position while walking away to make the exposure

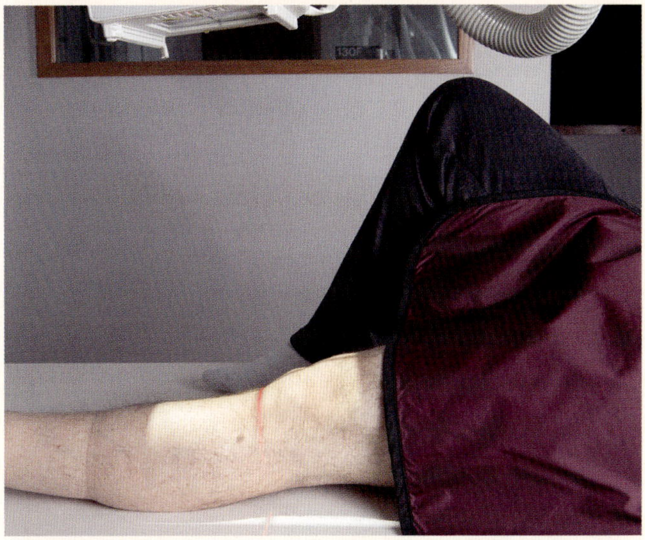

7-139 AP knee hypersthenic patient.

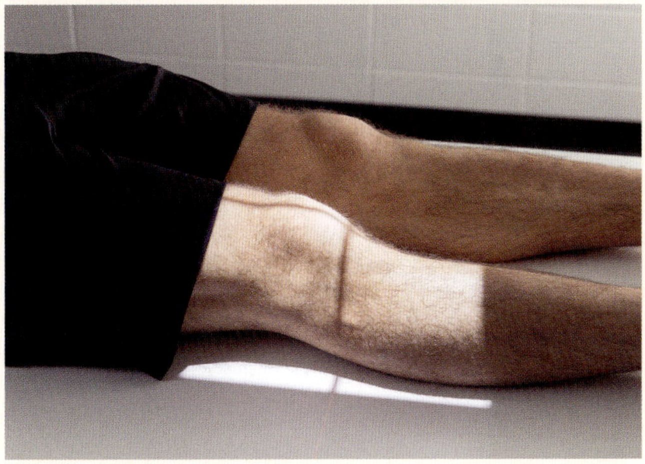

7-140 AP knee sthenic patient.

IMAGE CRITIQUE (FIGS. 7-141 and 7-142)

- Distal femur and proximal tibia and fibula are included within the collimated exposure field
- Femorotibial joint open
- Fibular apex and head superimposed on the proximal and lateral tibia
- The patella is centered over the distal femur
- Properly centered with medial to lateral-sided collimation

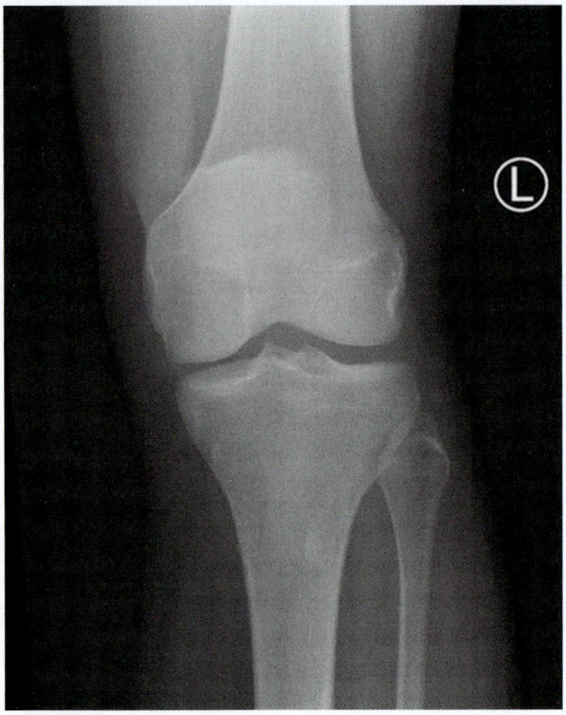

7-141 AP knee.

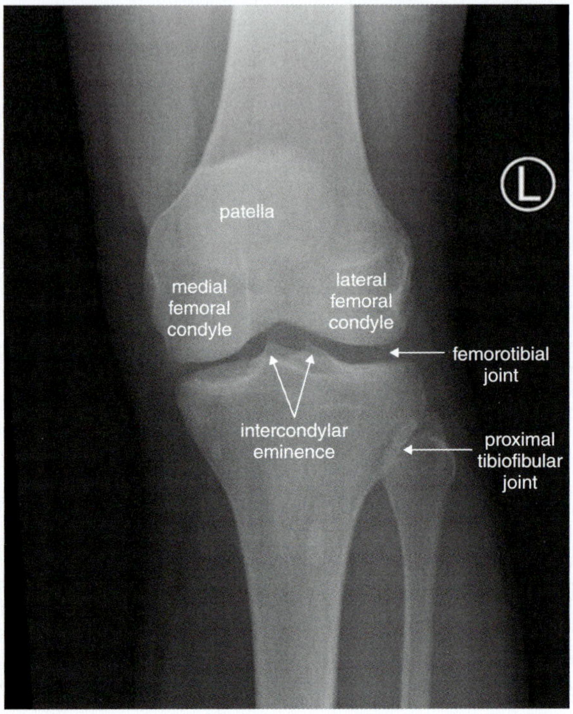

7-142 AP knee.

POSITION VARIATION AP OR PA BILATERAL WEIGHT-BEARING KNEES (FIGS. 7-143 to 7-145)

- Weight-bearing knees are often acquired to evaluate and compare the femorotibial joints for joint degenerative disease and to determine candidacy for a knee joint replacement. Both right and left knees are acquired side-by-side on a 14 × 17 crosswise IR with the center directed to the level of the femorotibial joints and midway between both knees to provide comparison of both knees. A unilateral knee could also be acquired. If AP projection is required, the central ray should include a 5°–10° caudal tube angle in attempt to match the slope of the tibial plateau to better demonstrate the femorotibial joint. If PA Axial projection or Rosenberg method is acquired at the site, the knees are flexed 45° and the central ray is angled 10° caudal in attempt to match the slope of the tibial plateau.

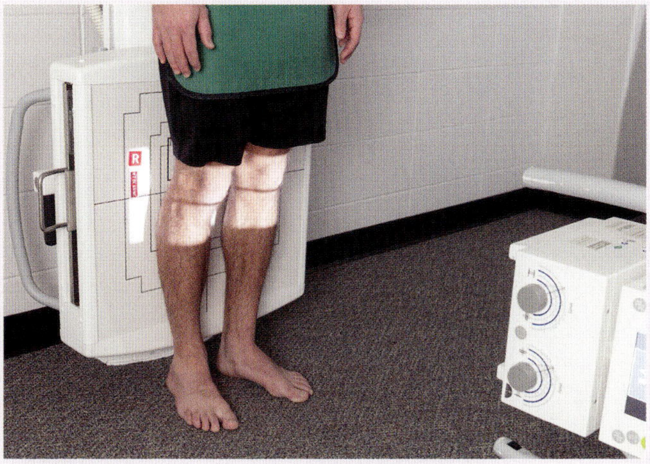

7-143 AP weight-bearing knees.

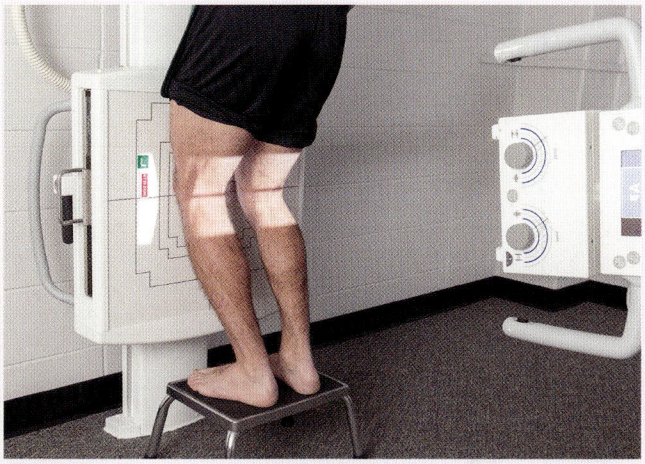

7-144 PA Axial—Rosenberg method.

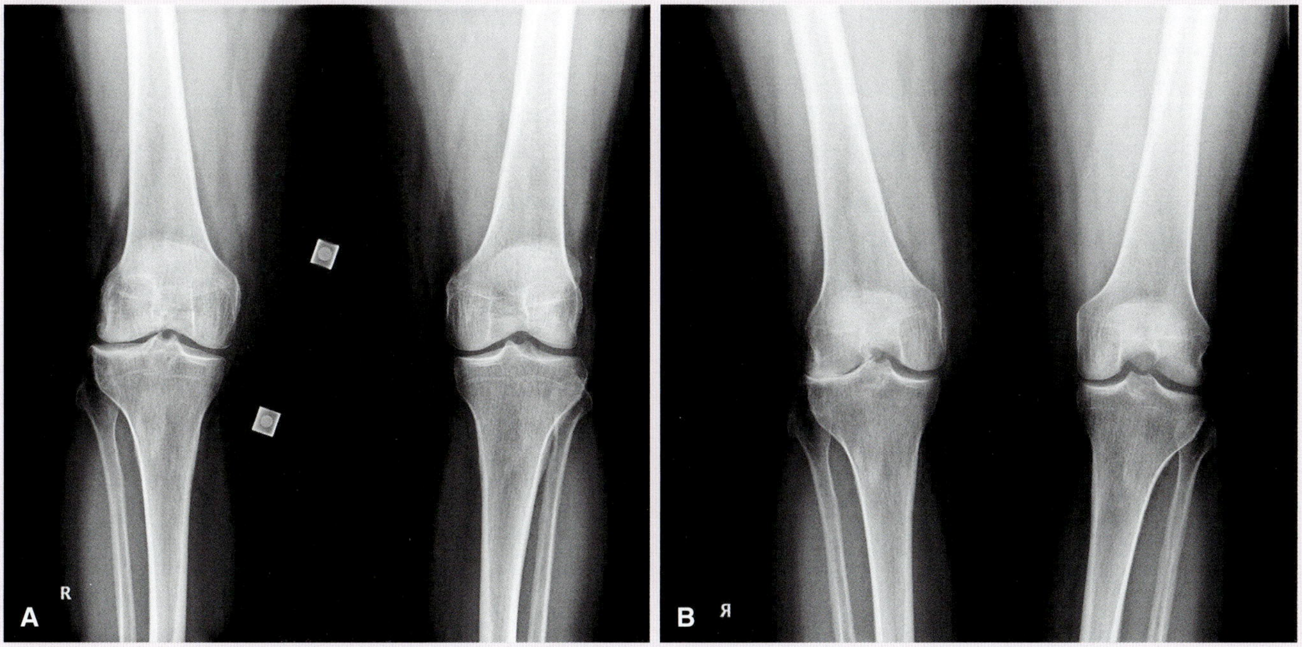

7-145 Weight-bearing knees. **A:** AP weight-bearing knees. **B:** PA axial knees.

Knee

- Projection: AP Oblique with 45° medial rotation

Knee Protocol
AP
AP Oblique
Lateromedial

Technical Considerations

- kVp 65; nongrid
- kVp 70–75; grid
- mAs set manually
- 40″ SID

Exposure Field Size

- 10 × 12 lengthwise

Patient Position (Fig. 7-146)

- Patient supine or seated on the imaging table
- Leg fully extended
- Entire leg rotated 45° into a medial oblique

Centering

- Femorotibial joint—1/2″ (1 finger) inferior to the apex of the patella with a *perpendicular beam*

Marking of IR

- Anatomic side marker R or L placed furthest away from midline

Breathing

- No specific breathing instructions are given to the patient. Instruct the patient to hold still
- Ensure patient holds position while walking away to make the exposure

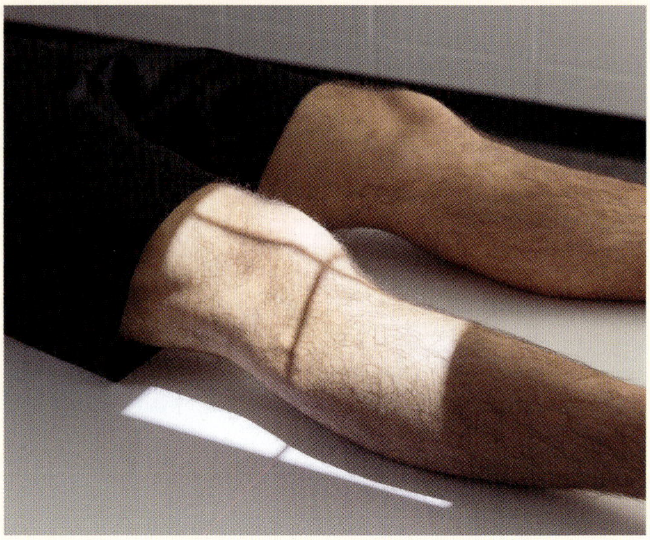

7-146 AP Oblique knee with medial rotation.

IMAGE CRITIQUE (FIGS. 7-147 and 7-148)

- Distal femur and proximal tibia and fibula are included within the collimated exposure field
- Lateral femoral and tibial condyles are in profile (the first time the lateral femoral condyle is free of bony superimposition)
- Approximately, ½ of the patella will superimpose the medial femoral condyle. The remaining patella will shift off the femur and be free of superimposition. Underrotation will present the patella still superimposed on the medial femoral condyle
- Fibular apex and head will shift laterally from the tibia. The proximal tibiofibular joint is of interest
- Properly centered with lateral-sided collimation

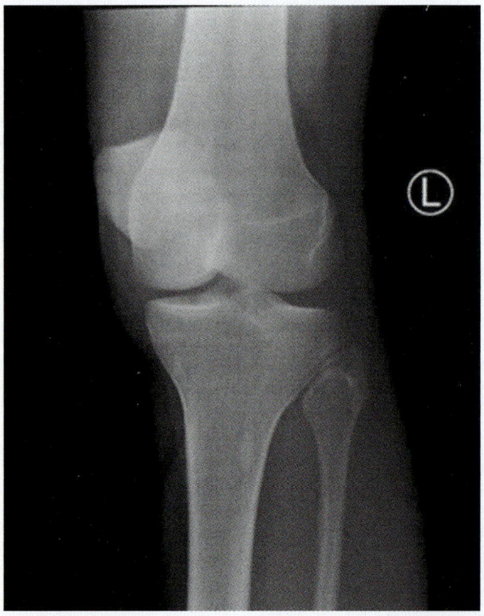

7-147 AP Oblique knee with medial rotation.

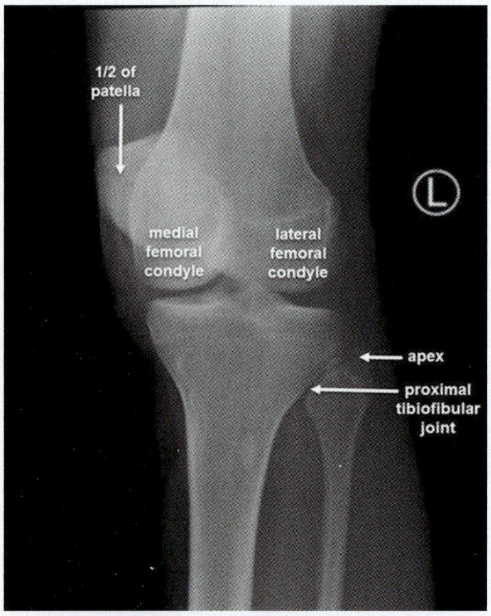

7-148 AP Oblique knee with medial rotation.

POSITION VARIATION AP OBLIQUE WITH 45° LATERAL ROTATION (FIGS. 7-149 to 7-151)

The 45° lateral rotation will shift half of the patella over the lateral femoral condyle and the other half free of femoral superimposition. The medial femoral and tibial condyles are viewed in profile. The lateral oblique position will superimpose the proximal tibia and fibula.

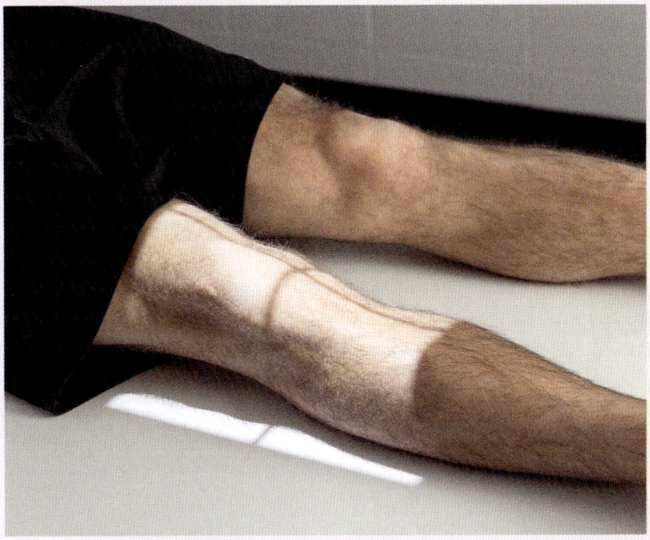

7-149 AP Oblique knee with lateral rotation.

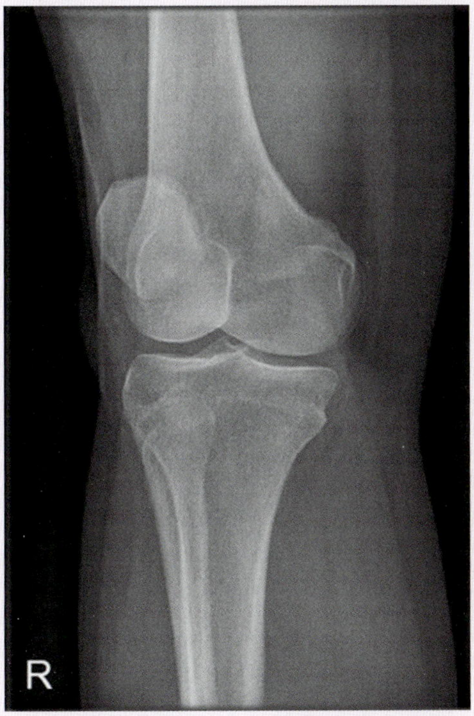

7-150 AP Oblique knee with lateral rotation.

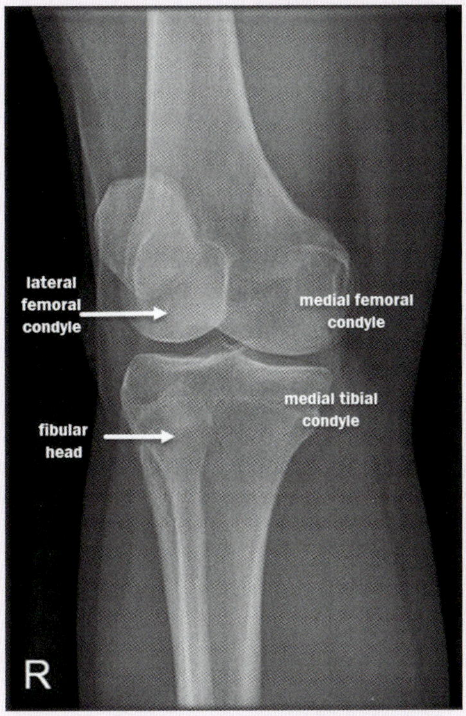

7-151 AP Oblique knee with lateral rotation.

Knee

- Projection: Mediolateral

Knee Protocol
AP
AP Oblique
Mediolateral

Technical Considerations

- kVp 65; nongrid
- kVp 70–75; grid
- mAs set manually
- 40″ SID

Exposure Field Size

- 10 × 12 lengthwise

Patient Position (Figs. 7-152 and 7-153)

- Start with patient supine
- Roll the patient up onto their affected side
- The unaffected leg could stay behind the affected leg or cross over in front of the affected leg. Determine what is best for the patient position
- Flex the knee 20°–30°. Overflexion of the part will result in the patella drawing in too close to the distal femur resulting in a closed patellofemoral joint
- Rotate the part into a true lateral by palpating the medial and lateral patellar borders and aligning perpendicular to the IR

Centering

- Femorotibial joint—From the medial femoral condyle, move 1/2″ inferior
- A 5°–7° cephalic tube angle is applied to every nontrauma lateral knee. The greater angle for a shorter patient and the lesser angle for a taller patient. The cephalic tube angle will aid in projecting the magnified medial femoral condyle *(remember the medial condyle lies slightly inferior to the lateral condyle)* upon the lateral femoral condyle to aid in opening up the femorotibial joint

Marking of IR

- Anatomic side marker R or L placed along the anterior surface or "in front" of the part

Breathing

- No specific breathing instructions are given to the patient. Instruct the patient to hold still
- Ensure patient holds position while walking away to make the exposure

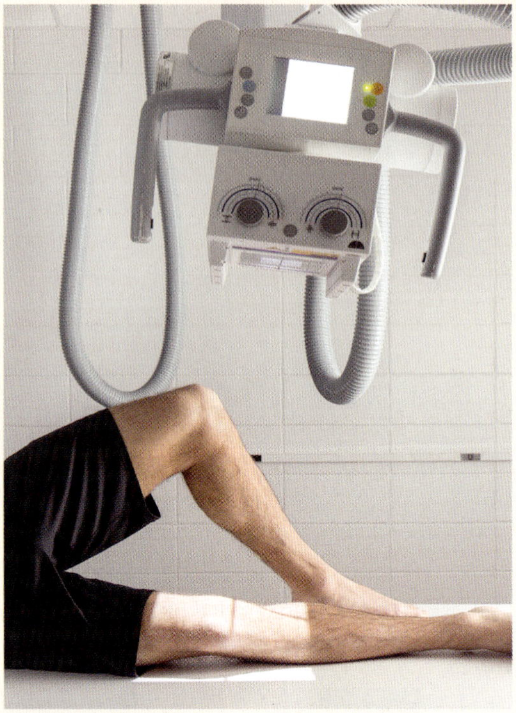

7-152 Mediolateral knee.

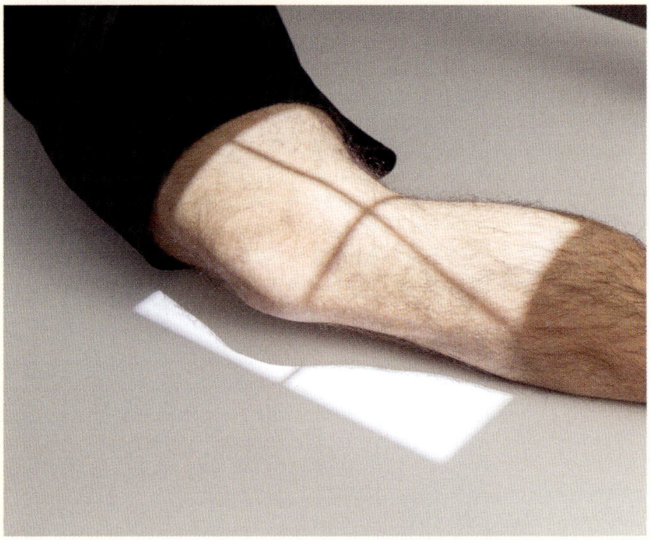

7-153 Mediolateral knee.

IMAGE CRITIQUE (FIGS. 7-154 and 7-155)

- Distal femur and proximal tibia and fibula are included within the collimated exposure field
- The patella in profile and the patellofemoral joint space open
- Creating an open patellofemoral joint is influenced by two positioning criteria:
  - Proper flexion of the knee. Overflexion will close the patellofemoral joint (Fig. 7-156)
  - Rotation. Under- or overrotation of the part will shift the medial or lateral femoral condyle into the patellofemoral joint space. Identification of the adductor tubercle on the superior and posterior border of the medial condyle will help identify under- or overrotation of the part (Fig. 7-157). Underrotation will display the medial femoral condyle posterior to lateral femoral condyle. Overrotation will display the medial femoral condyle anterior to the lateral femoral condyle
- The inferior margins of the medial and lateral femoral condyles are superimposed indicating the correct 5°–7° cephalic tube angle has been applied (Fig. 7-158). Figs. 7-154 and 7-158 reveal a mediolateral knee lacking the appropriate tube angle
- The proximal fibula will sit posterior to the tibia
- Properly centered with anterior and posterior-sided collimation

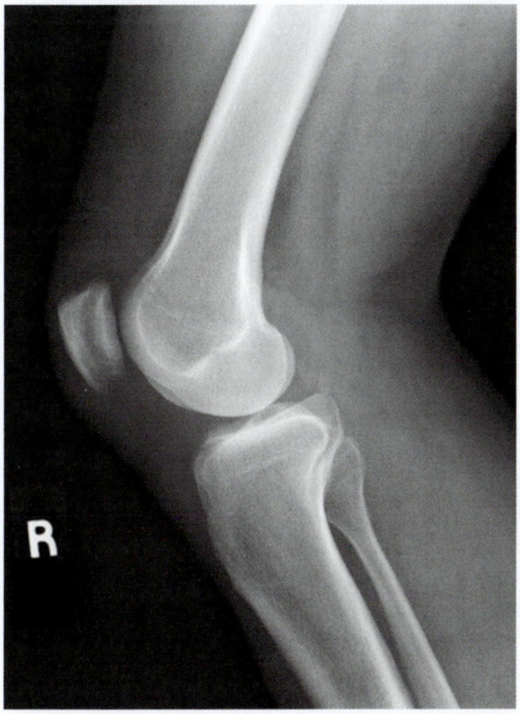

7-154 Mediolateral knee.

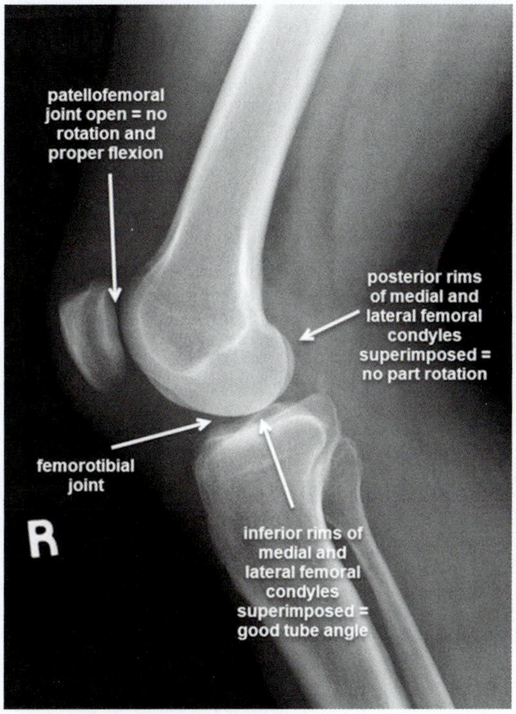

7-155 Mediolateral knee.

(continued)

IMAGE CRITIQUE (*Continued*)

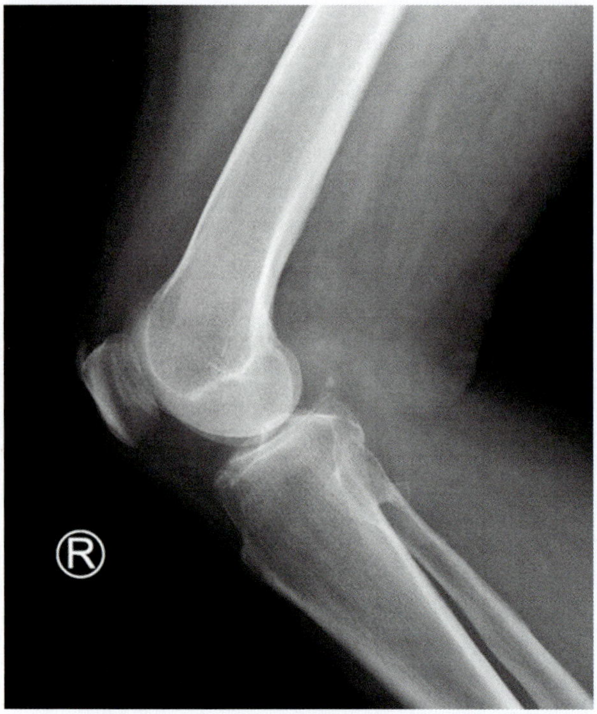

7-156 Overflexed lateral knee. Patellofemoral space closed up.

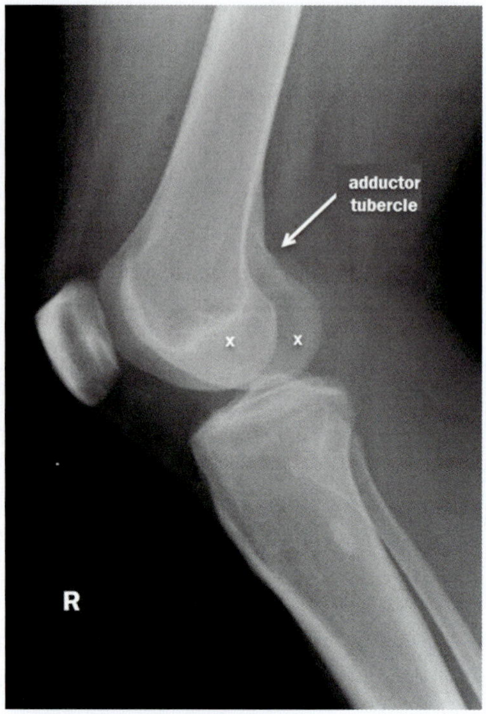

7-157 Rotated lateral knee.

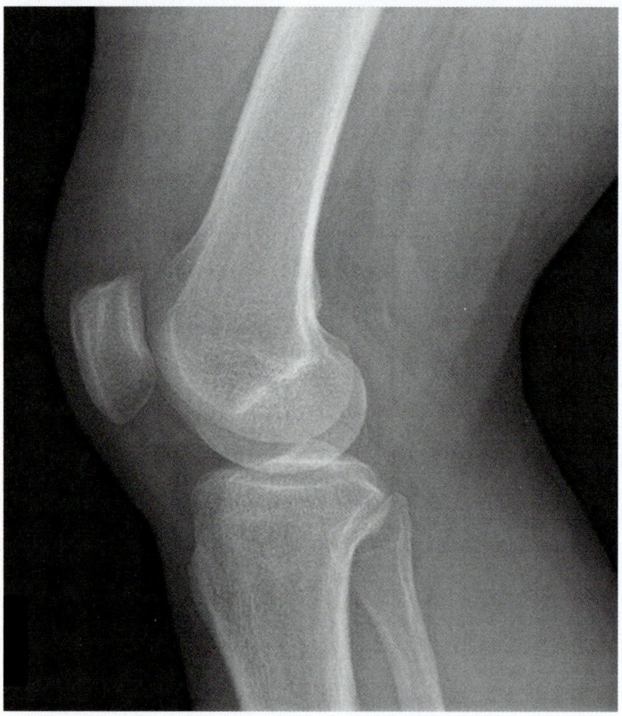

7-158 Insufficient cephalic tube angle. Femorotibial joint space obscured.

Trauma Knee

- Projection: AP
  - A minimum of two views 90° apart are required
  - *Trauma extremity routine described here is an example that can be applied similarly to other lower extremities. Trauma protocol may be elected for pre- and postsurgical patients*

Trauma Knee Protocol
AP
Lateromedial

Technical Considerations
- kVp 65; nongrid
- kVp 70–75; grid
- mAs set manually
- 40″ SID

Exposure Field Size
- 10 × 12 lengthwise

Patient Position
- Supine on the imaging table or stretcher
- Leave the patient's part in its presenting position

Centering (Fig. 7-159)
- Femorotibial joint. (Could move 1/2″ inferior to the apex of the patella OR in cases in which the patella is not palpable the technologist could consider using the level of the midpopliteal crease to mark the approximate joint space)

Marking of IR
- Anatomic side marker R or L placed furthest away from midline
- Marking the IR when imaging in a sterile field (operating room) is not possible

Breathing
- No specific breathing instructions are given to the patient. Instruct the patient to hold still
- Ensure patient holds position while walking away to make the exposure

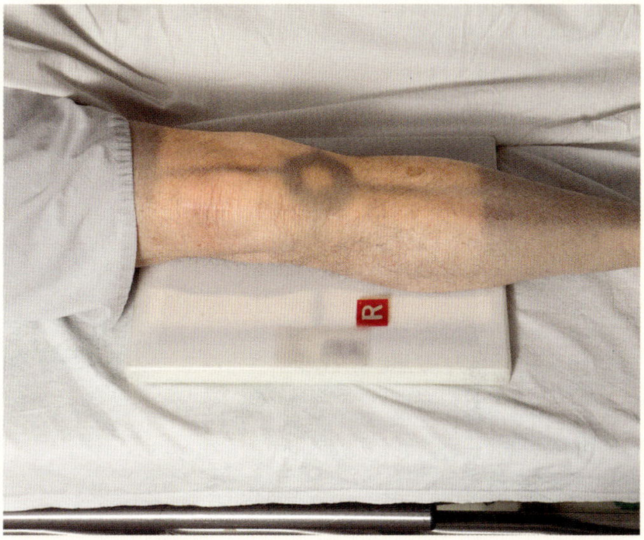

7-159 AP Trauma knee.

IMAGE CRITIQUE (FIG. 7-160)

- Distal femur, proximal tibia, and fibula included within the collimated exposure field
- Femorotibial joint centered on the image. The femorotibial joint space may not appear open and will not if a tube angle was not directed toward it correctly
- Images acquired in the OR suite or postoperatively, the collimated exposure field must include surgical metal implants in their entirety
- Patients that are postsurgical for knee replacement will require that the entire metal prosthesis is included on the image

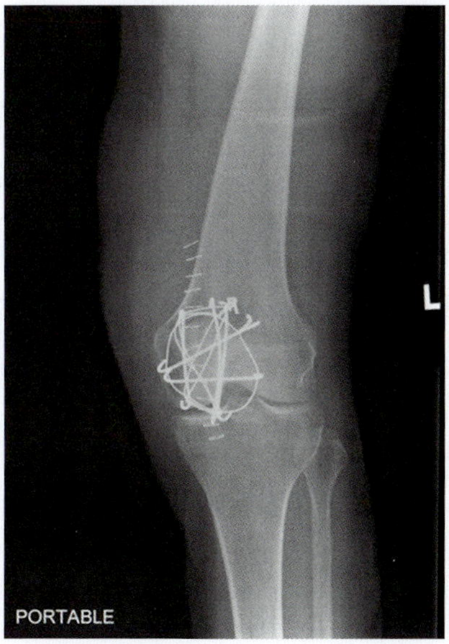

7-160 AP Trauma knee.

Trauma Knee

- Projection: Lateromedial
  - A minimum of two views 90° apart are required
  - *Trauma extremity routine described here is an example that can be applied similarly to other lower extremities. Trauma protocol may be elected for pre- and postsurgical patients*

Trauma Knee Protocol
AP
Lateromedial

Technical Considerations

- kVp 65; nongrid
- kVp 70–75; grid
- mAs set manually
- 40″ SID

Exposure Field Size

- 10 × 12 lengthwise

Patient Position (Fig. 7-161)

- Roll patient into a lateral position if able
- Patient who remains supine is imaged 90° from the AP projection with the use of a horizontal beam. Patient's knee is elevated slightly up off the table allowing the IR to drop below the anatomy. Typically, due to the condition of the patient, the IR is positioned along the medial side of the knee. Due to this IR placement, a lateromedial projection of the part is attained

Centering

- Femorotibial joint entering on the lateral surface (the level of the midpopliteal region)

Marking of IR

- Anatomic side marker R or L placed along the anterior surface or "in front" of the part

Breathing

- No specific breathing instructions are given to the patient. Instruct the patient to hold still
- Ensure patient holds position while walking away to make the exposure

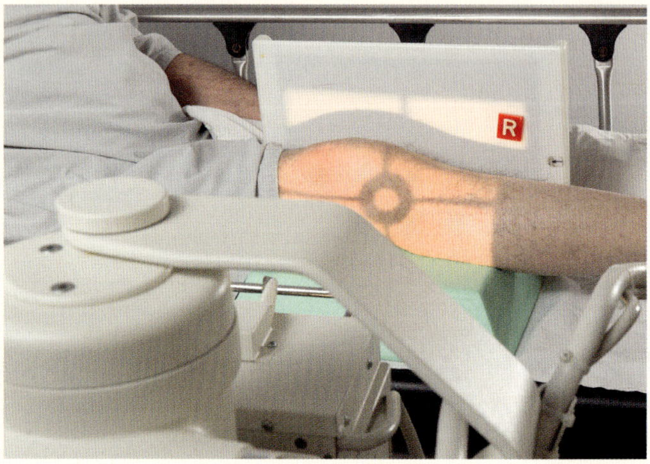

7-161 Horizontal beam—Lateromedial projection.

IMAGE CRITIQUE (FIG. 7-162)

- The distal femur, proximal tibia, and fibula within the collimated exposure field
- Anterior to posterior displacement evaluation of anatomy can be determined
- Femorotibial joint is centered within the exposure field
- Images acquired in the OR suite or postoperatively, the collimated exposure field must include surgical metal implants in their entirety
- Patients that are postsurgical for a knee replacement will require that the entire metal prosthesis is included on the image

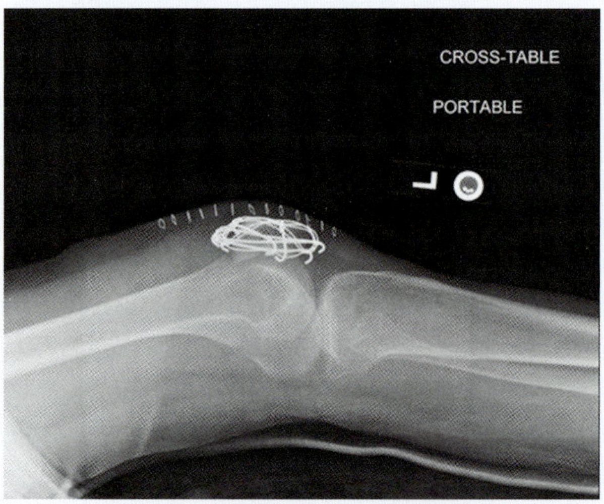

7-162 Horizontal beam lateral knee.

Patella

- Projection: PA
  - *PA projection is preferred as the patella is positioned closer to the image receptor for improved spatial resolution*

Patella Protocol
PA
Mediolateral
Tangential

Technical Considerations
- kVp 65–70; grid
- mAs set manually
- 40″ SID

Exposure Field Size
- 10 × 12 lengthwise

Patient Position (Fig. 7-163)
- Start with patient supine and then have the patient roll into a prone position. If the patient is unable to roll prone, acquire the patella with an AP projection, realizing the patella will magnify
- If the patient has pain due to pressure of the patella being in direct contact with the imaging surface, the technologist could consider building the part up off the table slightly with support added beneath the distal femur and beneath the proximal lower leg
- Ensure the femoral condyles are aligned parallel with the plane of the IR

Centering
- Perpendicular beam to the midpopliteal crease

Marking of IR
- Anatomic side marker R or L placed along the lateral of the part

Breathing
- No specific breathing instructions were given to the patient. Instruct the patient to hold still
- Ensure patient holds position while walking away to make the exposure

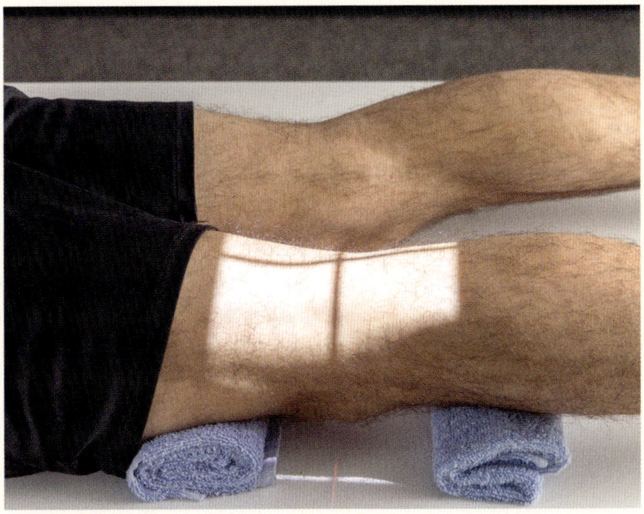

7-163 PA patella.

IMAGE CRITIQUE (FIG. 7-164)
- The patella is imaged with the least amount of magnification when a PA projection is utilized
- Patella should be centered over the distal femur
- Inclusion of the femorotibial joint
- Properly centered with four-sided collimation

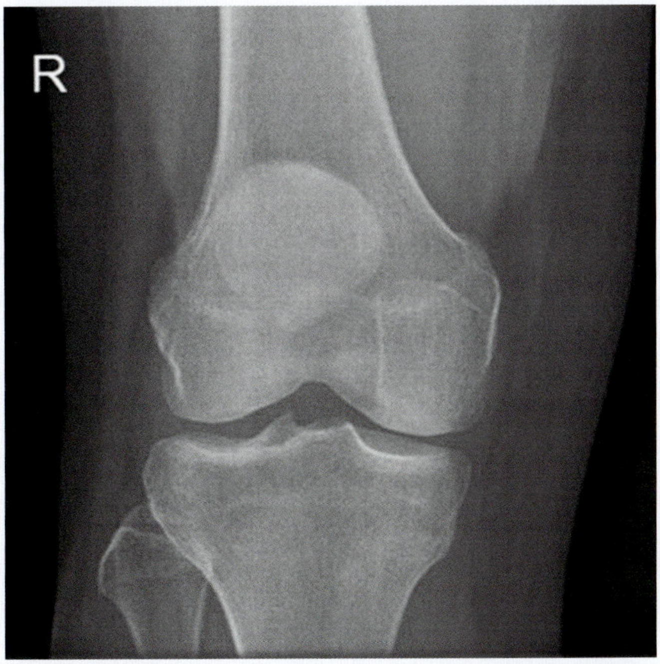

7-164 PA patella.

Patella

- Projection: Mediolateral
  - *Minimal flexion is applied for the lateral patella to avoid patellar fracture displacement if there is concern for fracture*

Patella Protocol
PA
Mediolateral
Tangential

Technical Considerations
- kVp 65–70; grid
- mAs set manually
- 40″ SID

Exposure Field Size
- 10 × 12 lengthwise

Patient Position (Fig. 7-165)
- Roll the patient up onto their affected side
- The unaffected leg could stay behind the affected leg or cross over in front of the affected leg
- Flex the knee 5°–10°. Overflexion of the part will result in the patella drawing in too close to the distal femur closing off the patellofemoral joint. Overflexion of the part may displace fractured segments. If fracture is suspected, flexion of the knee should not be applied
- Rotate the part into a true lateral by palpating the medial and lateral patellar borders or femoral condyles and aligning perpendicular to the IR

Centering
- Perpendicular beam to the patellofemoral joint

Marking of IR
- Anatomic side marker R or L placed along the anterior surface or "in front" of the part

Breathing
- No specific breathing instructions are given to the patient. Instruct the patient to hold still
- Ensure patient holds position while walking away to make the exposure

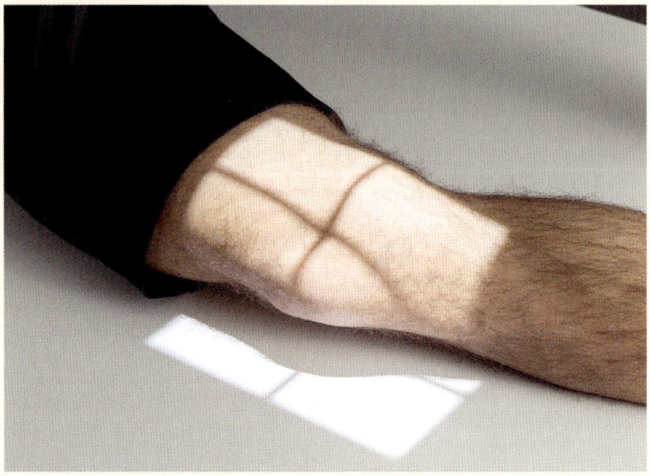

7-165 Mediolateral patella.

IMAGE CRITIQUE (FIG. 7-166)

- Distal femur and proximal tibia and fibula are included within the collimated exposure field
- The patella is in profile and the patellofemoral joint space open
- Creating an open patellofemoral joint is influenced by two positioning criteria:
  - Proper flexion (5°–10°) of the knee. Overflexion will close the patellofemoral joint
  - Rotation. Under- or over-rotation of the part will shift the medial or lateral femoral condyle into the patellofemoral joint space. Identification of the adductor tubercle on the superior and posterior border of the medial condyle will help identify under or overrotation of the part
- Properly centered with four-sided collimation

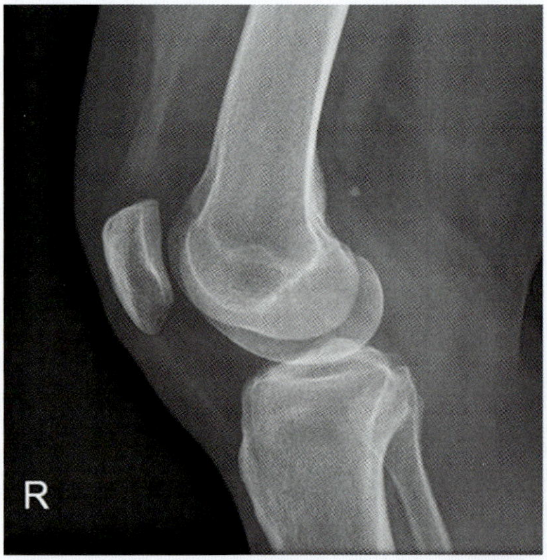

7-166 Mediolateral patella.

Patella

- Projection: Tangential (variety of methods exist)
    - *Fracture of the patella must be ruled out before flexing the patient's knee to the required amount*
    - *A variety of projections exist to demonstrate the patellofemoral joint. The technologist must consider the best and safest approach for a patient on a case-by-case basis*

Patella Protocol
PA
Mediolateral
Tangential

Technical Considerations

- kVp 65–70; nongrid
- mAs set manually
- 40″ SID (or 72″ SID necessary only for the Merchant method)

Exposure Field Size

- Size will depend on if the image is acquired unilateral or bilateral. Collimation down to the part is important

Inferosuperior Axial (Figs. 7-167 and 7-168)

- Patient lays supine with the knee(s) flexed 45°. The technologist should consider the proper wedge angle under the knees to ensure proper flexion and femoral quadriceps relaxation
- The IR rests on midthighs at an angle that will match the tube head. Stabilize the IR position. This may present a challenge with certain patients trying to remain supine while stabilizing the IR; therefore, an alternative may be better to prevent unnecessary exposure to the neck and face if the patient were to sit up
- With a minimum of 40″ SID, the central ray is angled 10°–20° cephalic beyond the 90° horizontal beam
- Direct the CR to the patellofemoral joint. This projection could also provide a bilateral assessment if requested or is protocol. The CR would directed midway between the patellae

Inferosuperior Axial—Hughston Method (Fig. 7-169)

- Patient lays prone with the knee flexed up off the IR 50°–60° from full extension. Ensure patient's leg flexion is stable
- The IR is placed under the distal femur
- With a minimum of 40″ SID, the central ray is angled 45° cephalic
- Direct the CR to the patellofemoral joint

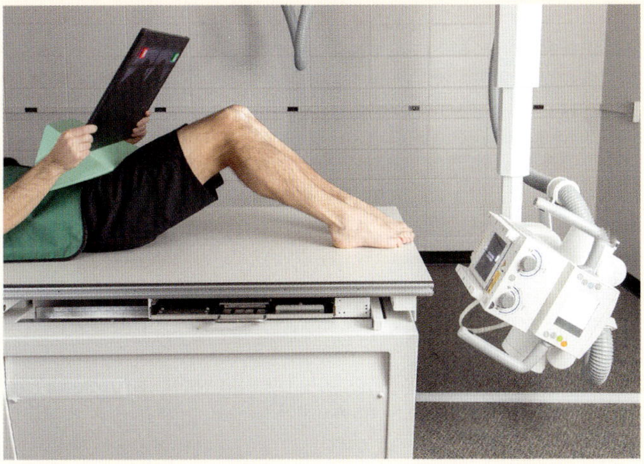

7-167 Inferosuperior axial.

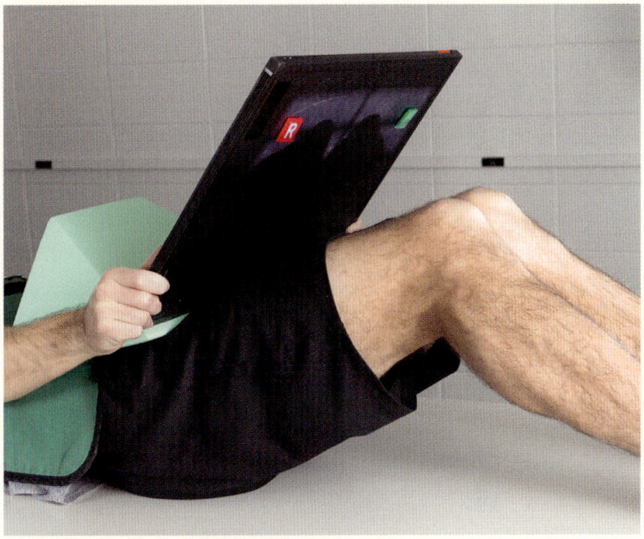

7-168 Inferosuperior axial.

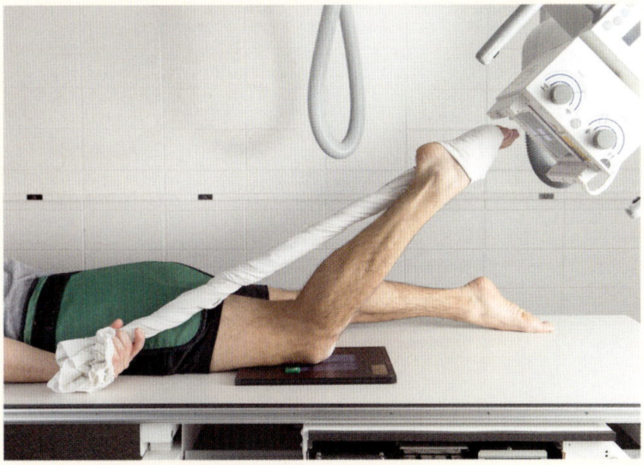

7-169 Inferosuperior axial—Hughston method.

(continued)

Patella (*Continued*)

Inferosuperior Axial—Settegast Method (Fig. 7-170)

- Patient lays prone with the affected knee flexed 90°. Ensure patient's leg flexion is stable
- The IR is placed under the distal femur
- With a minimum of 40″ SID, the central ray is angled 15°–20° cephalic
- Direct the CR to the patellofemoral joint

Superoinferior Axial—Merchant Method (Fig. 7-171)

- Bilateral assessment for comparison requires a 60″–72″ SID
- Patient is supine with knees flexed 40° and supported off end of the table
- Secure lower legs together side-by-side without rotation and ensure the legs are relaxed. Relaxation of the femoral quadriceps will ensure an accurate representation of the patellar placement to the intercondylar sulcus
- The 14 × 17 IR is placed about 3″ above the ankles. The IR and tube head must be aligned parallel to one another to ensure the CR intersects the IR perpendicularly
- The tube is angled 30° caudal off horizontal
- CR is directed between the two patellae

Marking of IR

- Anatomic side markers R and L were placed furthest away from midline. Bilateral knee imaging for comparison should mark both the right and left anatomic sides

Breathing

- No specific breathing instructions are given to the patient. Instruct the patient to hold still
- Ensure patient holds position while walking away to make the exposure

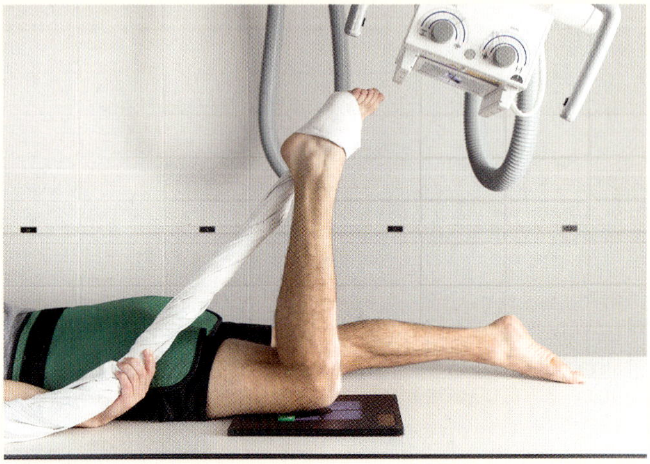

7-170 Inferosuperior axial—Settegast method.

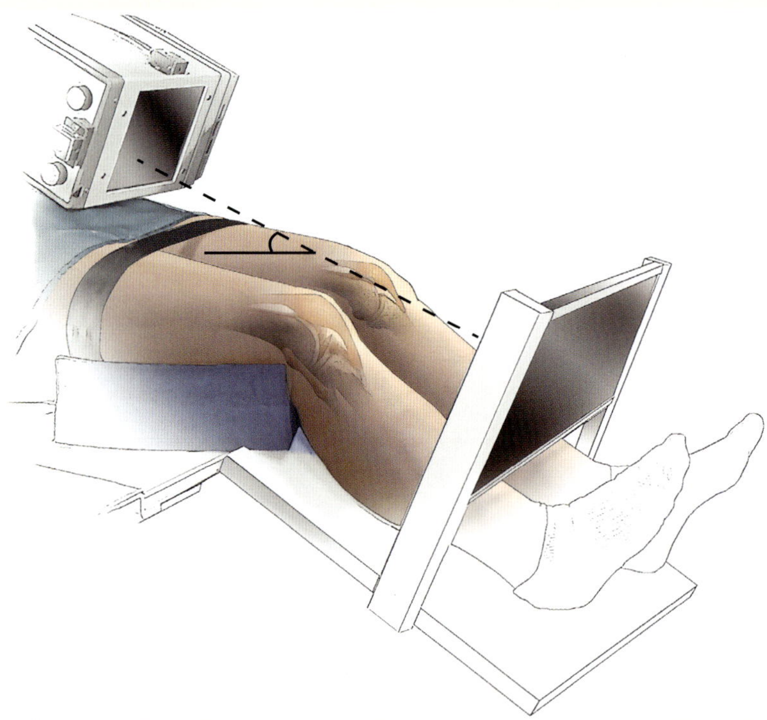

7-171 Superoinferior axial—Merchant method. Note the parallel relationship of the tube and the image receptor.

IMAGE CRITIQUE (FIGS. 7-172 to 7-174)

**Regardless of the method utilized to image the patient, the radiographic result will all appear similar*

- Patellofemoral joint(s) is best visualized and ideally visualized open within the collimated exposure field
- Patella visualized in profile
- Distal femur and patella properly centered within four-sided collimation

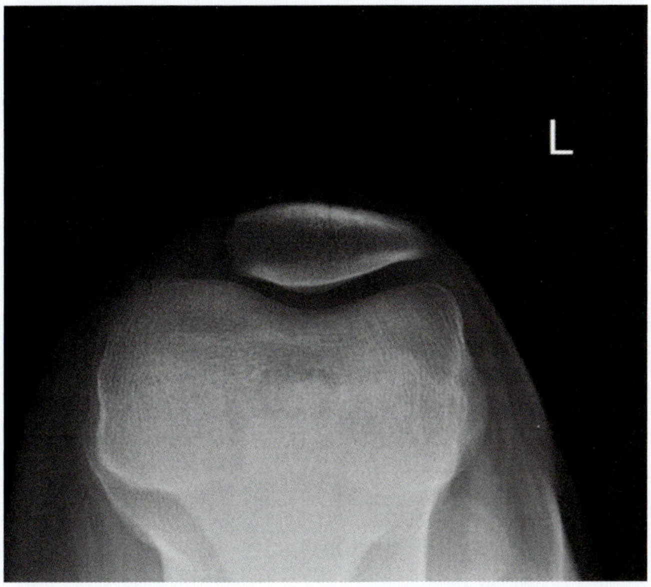

7-172 Patellofemoral joint.

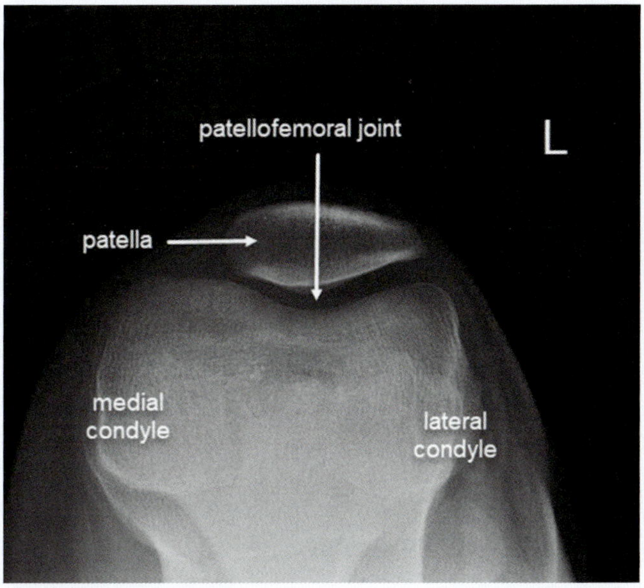

7-173 Patellofemoral joint.

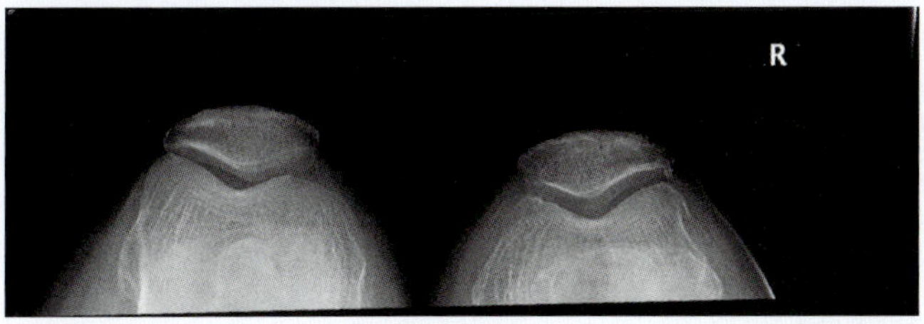

7-174 Bilateral patellofemoral joints.

Intercondylar Fossa of the Knee

- Projection: PA, PA Axial, or AP Axial
  - *A variety of projections exist to demonstrate the intercondylar fossa. The technologist must consider the best and safest approach for a patient on a case-by-case basis*

Technical Considerations

- kVp 70–75
- mAs set manually
- 40″ SID

Holmblad Method (Figs. 7-175 and 7-176)

- Patient is in a kneeling position on x-ray table or patient standing on unaffected leg with affected leg supported on a chair
- From a 90° flexion lean forward about 30° creating a 60°–70° knee flexion
- The IR is placed parallel to the lower leg
- With a minimum of 40″ SID, the central ray is directed perpendicularly to the lower leg into the midpopliteal space

Camp–Coventry (Fig. 7-177)

- Patient is prone with the knee flexed 40°–50° from full extension with support provided under the ankle
- The IR is placed under the distal femur
- With a minimum of 40″ SID, the central ray is angled 40°–50° caudal to intersect perpendicular with the lower leg
- Direct the CR to the midpopliteal space

Béclere Method (Fig. 7-178)

- Patient is supine with the knee flexed 40°–45° with support provided under the knee
- A small IR is placed directly beneath the knee and supported on top of the knee support. There will be object to image distance (OID) present
- With a 40″ SID, the central ray is angled 40°–50° cephalic, so it is perpendicular to the lower leg
- Direct the CR just distal to the apex of the patella

Marking of IR

- Anatomic side marker R or L placed furthest away from midline

Breathing

- No specific breathing instructions are given to the patient. Instruct the patient to hold still
- Ensure patient holds position while walking away to make the exposure

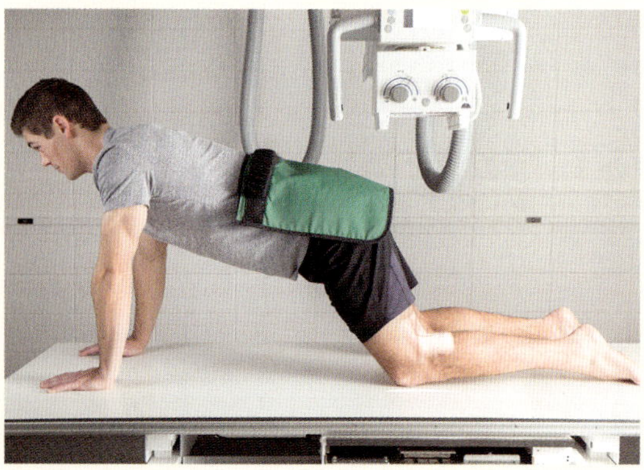

7-175 Intercondylar fossa—Holmblad method.

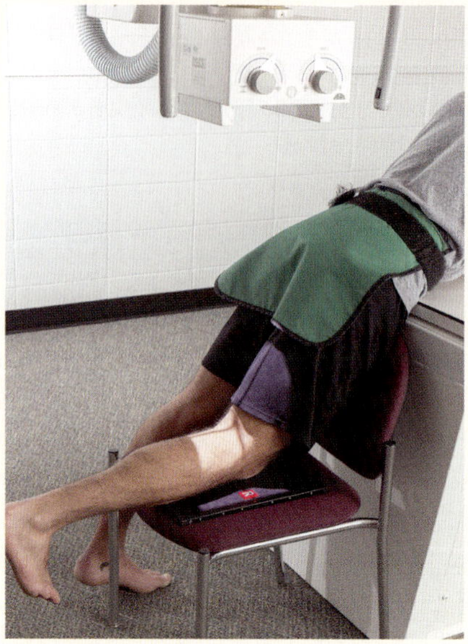

7-176 Intercondylar fossa—Holmblad method.

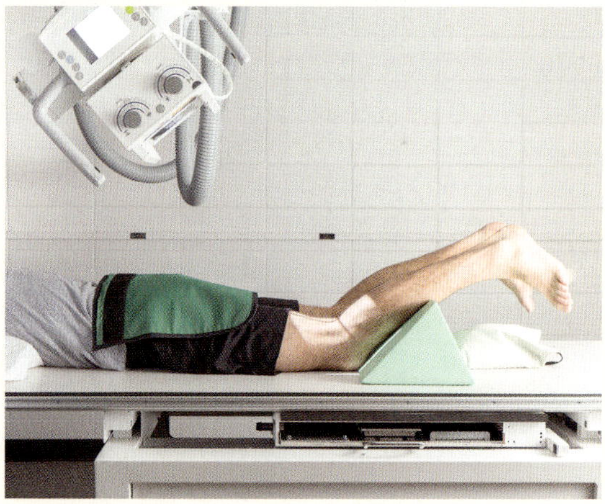

7-177 Intercondylar fossa—Camp–Coventry method.

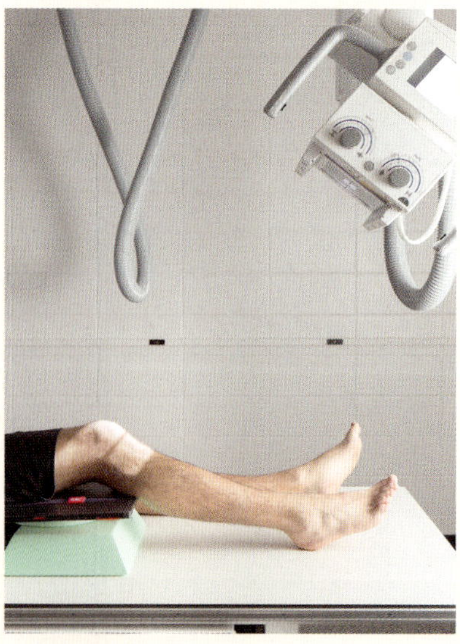

7-178 Intercondylar fossa—Béclere method.

IMAGE CRITIQUE (FIGS. 7-179 to 7-181)

**Regardless of the method utilized to image the patient, the radiographic results will all appear similar*

- Intercondylar fossa is best visualized within the collimated exposure field
- Femoral condyles symmetrical ensuring no rotation of the part
- Distal femur and proximal tibia and fibula properly centered within the four-sided collimation

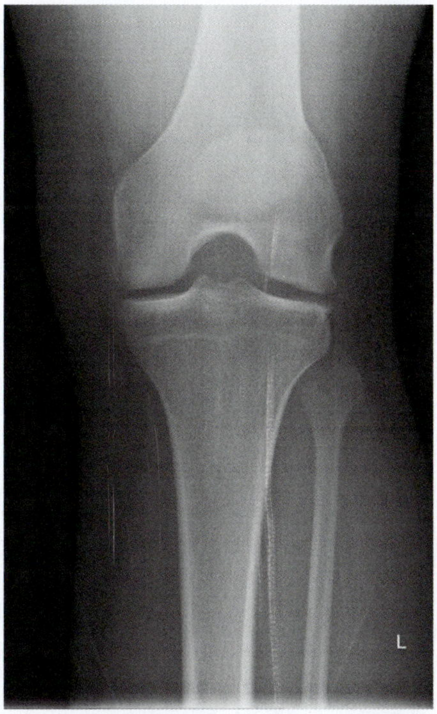

7-179 Intercondylar fossa.

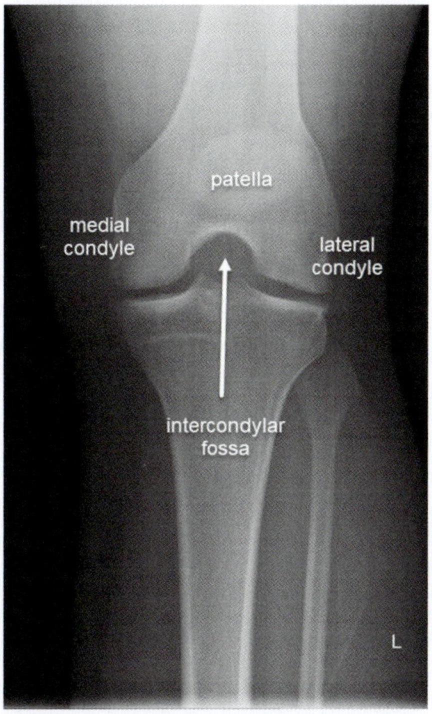

7-180 Intercondylar fossa.

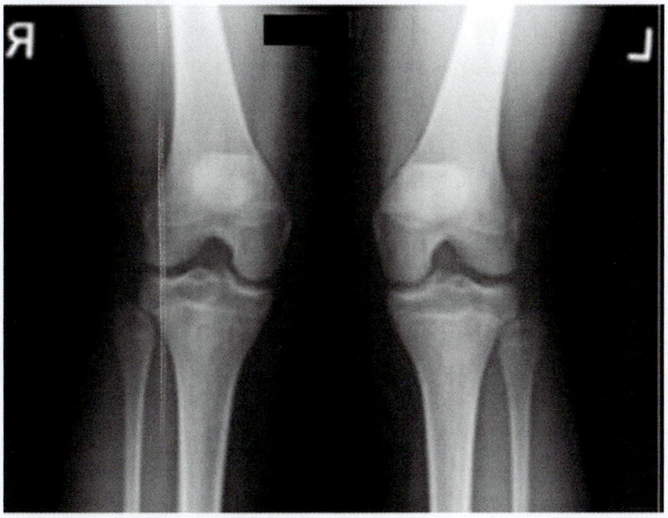

7-181 Intercondylar fossae.

Nontrauma Femur (Trauma Femur Covered in Chapter 8)

- Projection: AP

Femur Protocol
AP
Mediolateral

Technical Considerations

- kVp 70–75; part thickness will require a grid
- mAs set manually
- 40″ SID

Exposure Field Size

- 2-AP projections will be necessary due to the length of the adult femur
- 14 × 17 lengthwise for distal femur with collimation to reduce the width of the field size
- 10 × 12 lengthwise for proximal femur (acquire the AP hip)

Patient Position (Fig. 7-182)

- Patient supine
- Leg fully extended
- Imaging of Distal Femur
  - The distal femur will need a slight medial rotation (3°–5°) until the femoral condyles are parallel to the IR
- Imaging of Proximal Femur
  - The proximal femur will need internal rotation of the entire leg, knee, and ankle 15°–20° medially (Fig. 7-183)

Centering (Ensure Tube and Bucky Are Aligned) (Fig. 7-184)

- Distal femur: The bottom of the 14 × 17 LW positioned just below the femorotibial joint and the central ray directed to the femur. Collimate in to the medial and lateral sides of the femur
- Proximal femur: The central ray is directed to the femoral neck, as it is for the AP hip with a 10 × 12 LW exposure field size

Marking of IR

- Anatomic side marker R or L placed furthest away from midline

Breathing

- Breathing should be suspended with exposures in the region of the pelvis. Instruct the patient to hold still
- Ensure patient holds position while walking away to make the exposure

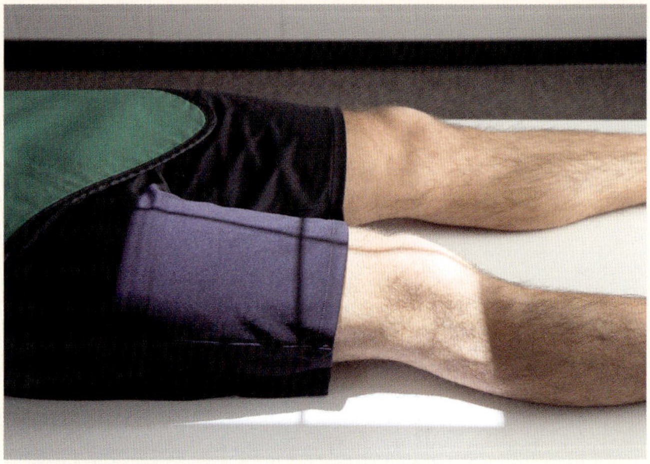

7-182 AP distal femur.

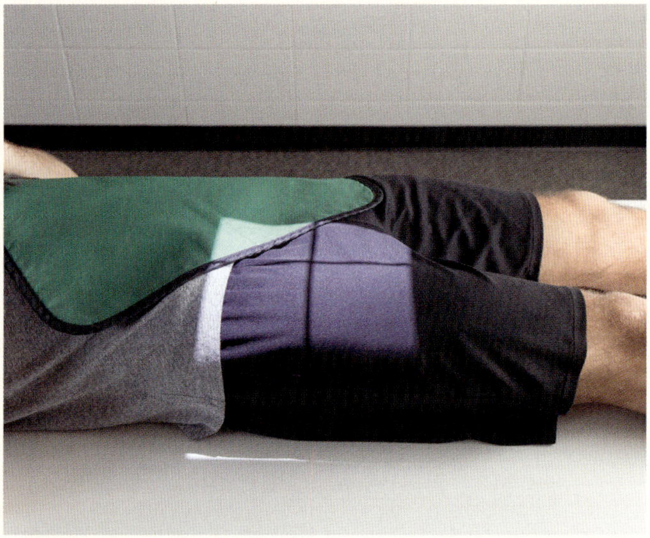

7-183 AP proximal femur.

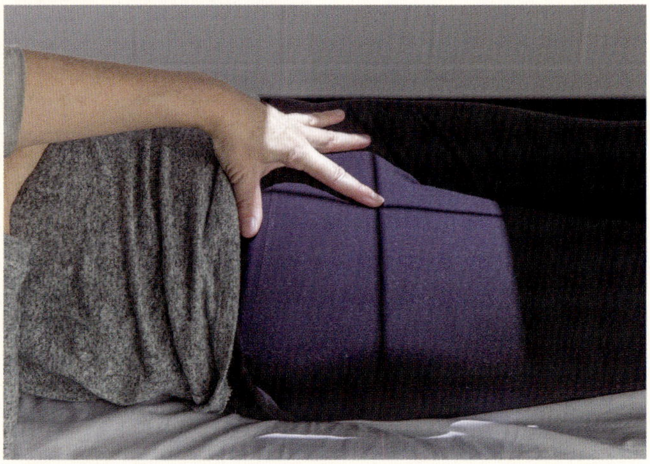

7-184 AP hip centering.

IMAGE CRITIQUE (FIGS. 7-185 and 7-186)

- Entire femur, proximal to distal, to include the knee and the hip joint visualized within the collimated exposure field
- The proximal femur must include the hip joint, the greater trochanter in profile laterally. The lesser trochanter will be nonvisible when superimposed on the posterior surface of the femur
- The distal femur must include the knee joint. The patella will center over the distal femur
- Properly centered with anterior to posterior-sided collimation

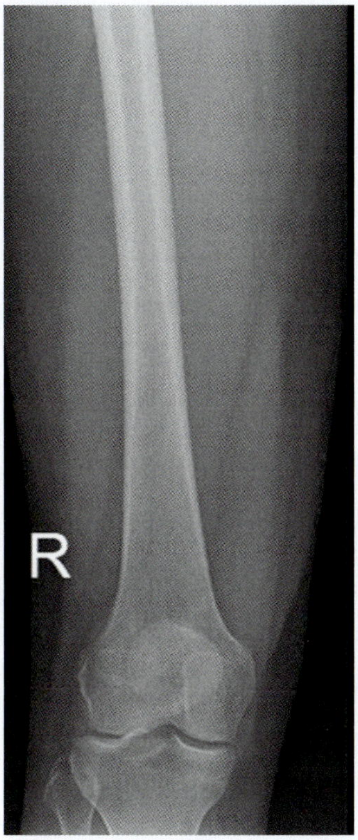

7-185 AP distal femur.

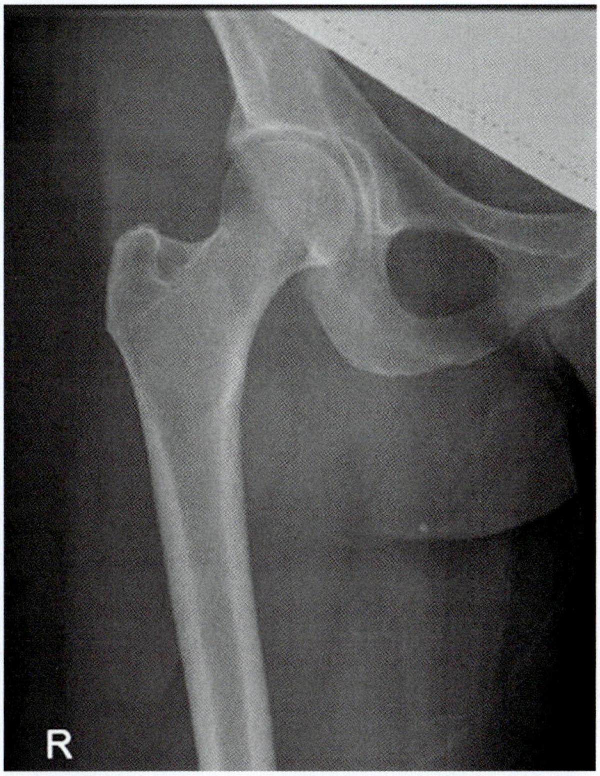

7-186 AP proximal femur.

Nontrauma Femur (Trauma Femur Covered in Chapter 8)

- Projection: Mediolateral

Femur Protocol
AP
Mediolateral

Technical Considerations
- kVp 75; part thickness will require a grid
- mAs set manually
- 40″ SID

Exposure Field Size
- Two Mediolateral projections will be necessary due to the length of the femur
- 14 × 17 lengthwise for proximal femur
- 10 × 12 lengthwise for distal femur

Patient Position (Fig. 7-187)
- Patient begins supine
- Patient rolls up onto the affected side. Unaffected leg is positioned behind (posterior) to the affected leg
- The technologist should align the patient's hip joint with the knee joint in efforts to try to align the femur to run straight up and down on the table
- The affected knee flexed 45°
- Palpate the medial and lateral patellar borders and adjust the patella until perpendicular to the IR

Centering *(ensure tube and Bucky are aligned)* (Figs. 7-187 and 7-188)
- Proximal femur: The top of the 14 × 17 LW aligned with the level of the ASIS and centered on the femur
- Distal femur: The bottom of the 10 × 12 LW is positioned below the level of the knee joint and centered on the femur

Marking of IR
- Anatomic side marker R or L placed anterior to the part

Breathing
- Breathing should be suspended as imaging approaches the region of the pelvis. Instruct
- Ensure patient holds position while walking away to make the exposure

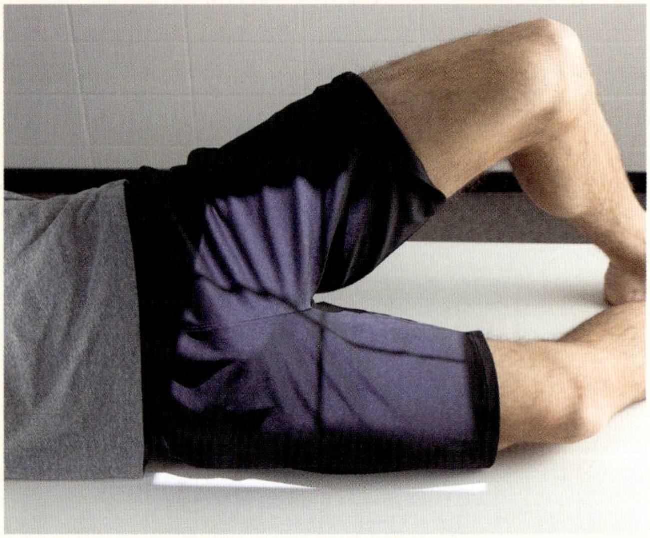

7-187 Mediolateral proximal femur.

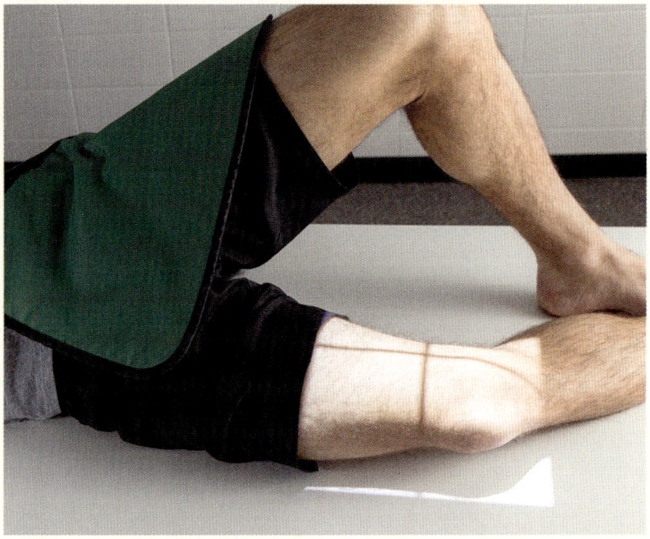

7-188 Mediolateral distal femur.

IMAGE CRITIQUE (FIGS. 7-189 and 7-190)

- Entire femur, proximal to distal, to include the knee and the hip joint visualized within the collimated exposure field
- The proximal femur must include the hip joint. The greater and lesser trochanters will superimpose on the femoral neck
- The distal femur must include the knee joint. The patella in profile. The inferior margins of the femoral condyles will not appear directly superimposed since the distal lateral femur is not acquired with a cephalic tube angle (as done for the mediolateral knee) to assist with femoral condyle superimposition
- Properly centered with anterior to posterior-sided collimation

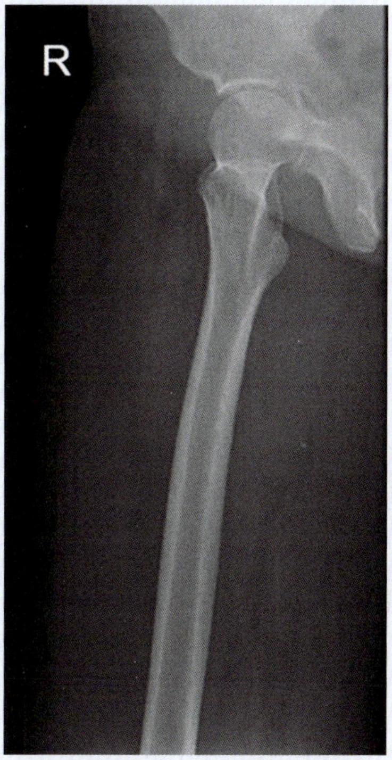

7-189 Mediolateral proximal femur.

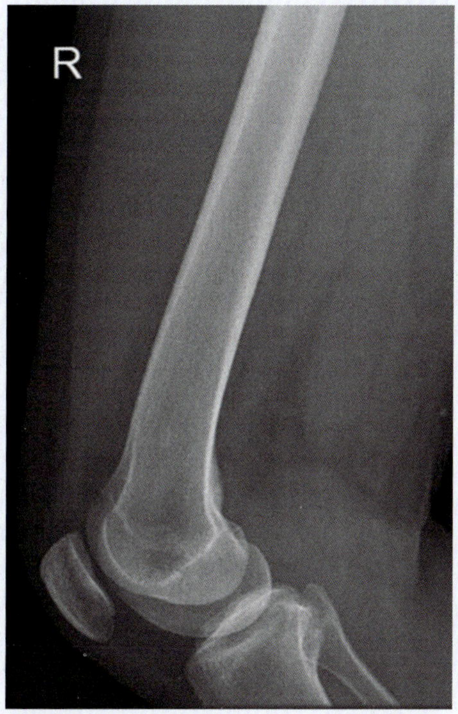

7-190 Mediolateral distal femur.

THE FINAL STEP IMAGE REVIEW

The technologist must take time to review acquired images to ensure image quality is acceptable. The technologist must have the knowledge within their role to not only acquire the images and care for the patient but also know how to review the images to ensure diagnostic quality has been attained. In certain instances, a projection may need to be repeated. This is to the discretion of the radiologic technologist. The technologist should review each image for the following.

1. Is all of the necessary anatomy included on the image?
   - Was the central ray (CR) properly directed to the part? An "X" can be drawn to intersect within the collimated exposure field to determine if the CR was directed to the correct location.
   - Was essential anatomy in the collimated exposure field?
   - Is the area free of artifact(s)?
2. Is the anatomy well demonstrated?
   - Did the technologist properly position the patient to adequately demonstrate the anatomy?
   - Can the technologist recognize the anatomy best demonstrated with use of different projections?
3. Does the image reflect proper image markings?
   - Did the technologist correctly use a lead marker to identify the right or left side?
   - What additional markings or annotations could be helpful to the radiologist interpreting the exam?
   - Is the image properly displayed?
4. Does the image prove to be technically acceptable?
   - Does the exposure index fall within acceptable range for the operating system? Images that are technically insufficient may appear of good quality if just slightly insufficient or "mottled or pixelated" if severely insufficient. Images that appear "mottled" should be repeated. Images that appear beyond optimal exposure due to higher technique may display high quality, but the patient has received excessive radiation dose.

CRITICAL THINKING

1. In review of the nontrauma lateral foot (Fig. 7-191), how well was the part positioned?
   a. The part appears properly positioned.
   b. The part does not represent a true lateral.
   c. The part would have been imaged better if the foot was dorsiflexed.
   d. The part would have been better imaged if the foot was plantarflexed.

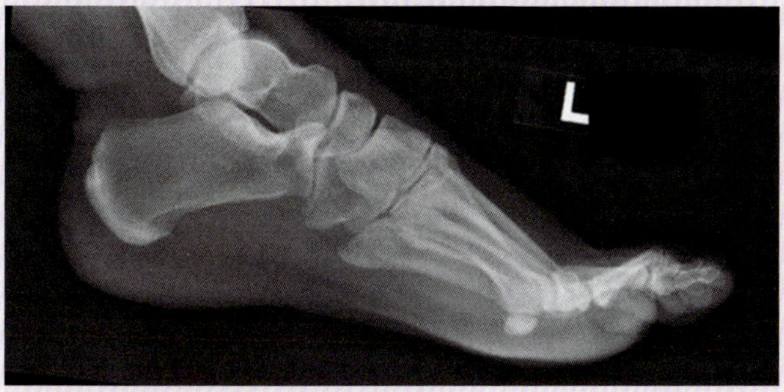

7-191

2. In review of the AP Oblique ankle with 45° medial rotation (Fig. 7-192), characterize the results.
   a. Image passes; all criteria met.
   b. Image fails; image is technically insufficient.
   c. Image fails; central ray directed to high clipping essential anatomy.
   d. Image fails; part is improperly positioned.

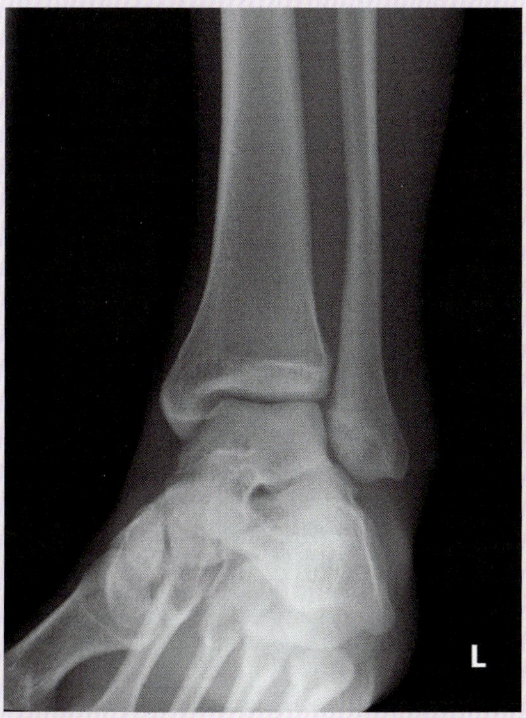

7-192

3. In review of the plantodorsal axial (Fig. 7-193), characterize the results.
   a. Image passes; all image criteria met.
   b. Image fails; image is technically insufficient.
   c. Image fails; central ray is directed to low clipping essential anatomy.
   d. Image fails; central ray is directed to high clipping essential anatomy.

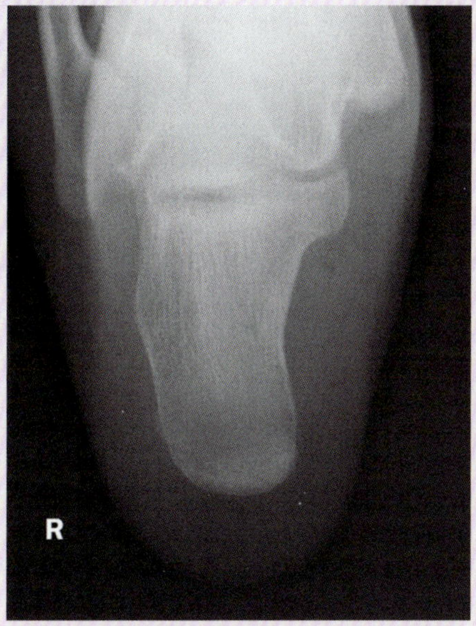

7-193

4. In review of the AP Oblique knee (Fig. 7-194), characterize the results.
   a. Image passes; all image criteria met.
   b. Image fails; image is technically insufficient.
   c. Image fails; femur appears to be underrotated.
   d. Image fails; part appears to be overrotated.

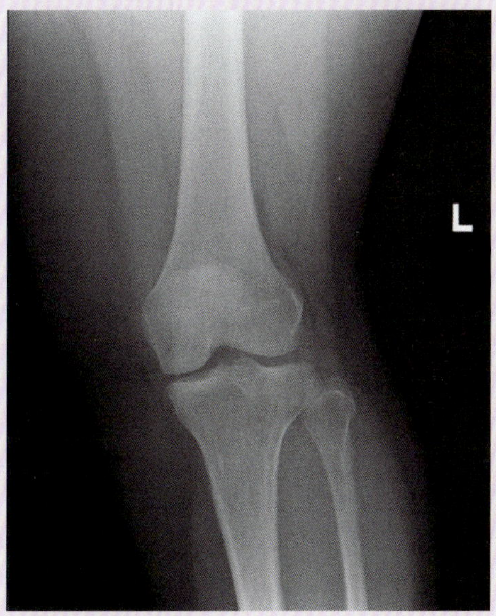

7-194

5. In review of the postoperative mediolateral knee (Fig. 7-195), characterize the results.
   a. Image passes; all image criteria met.
   b. Image fails; image is technically insufficient.
   c. Image fails; tibiotalar joint space is closed
   d. Image fails; surgical hardware not entirely included.

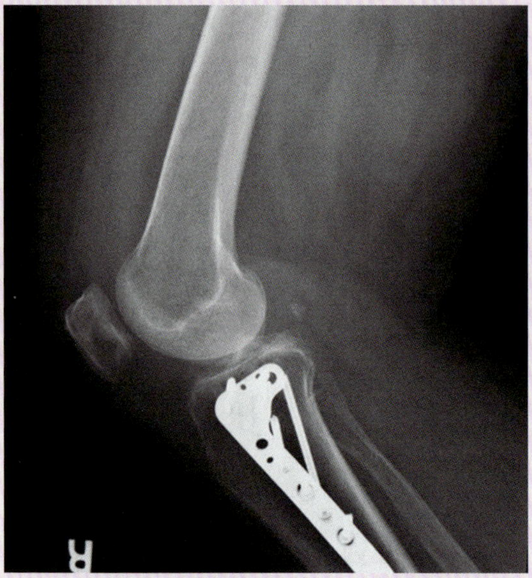

7-195

6. In review of the AP Oblique foot (Fig. 7-196), characterize the positioning results.
   a. Image passes; all positioning criteria is met.
   b. Image passes; distal fibula is superimposing the calcaneus.
   c. Image fails; the part appears overrotated.
   d. Image fails; the part appears underrotated.

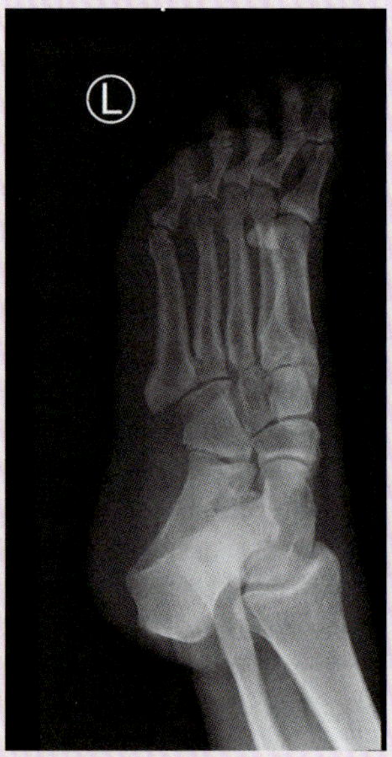

7-196

7. In review of the mediolateral knee (Fig. 7-197), characterize the positioning results.
   a. Image represents no rotation of the part.
   b. Image represents overflexion of the part.
   c. Image represents overrotation of the part.

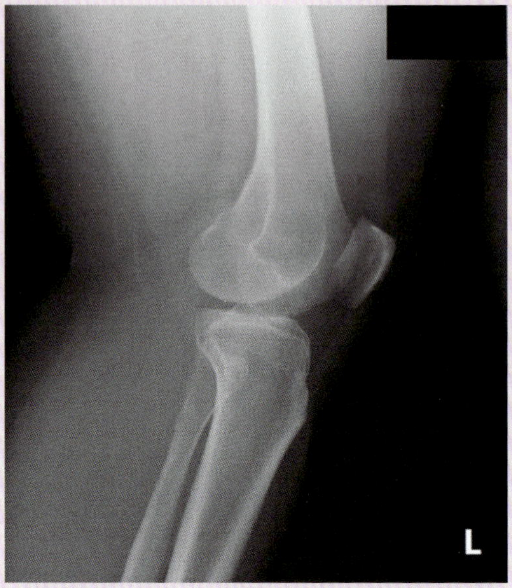

7-197

8. In review of the mediolateral knee (Fig. 7-198), the primary positioning error of concern is:
   a. Rotation
   b. Insufficient tube angle
   c. Underflexion of the part
   d. Overflexion of the part

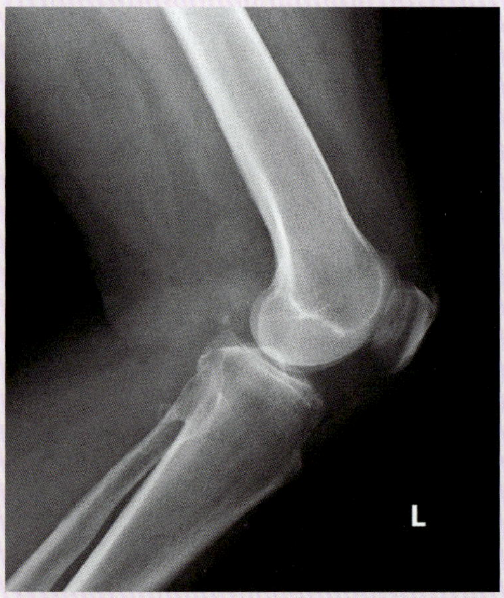

7-198

9. In review of the AP distal trauma femur (Fig. 7-199), the primary concern is:
   a. Rotation
   b. Failure to include the entire prosthetic implant
   c. Failure to include the knee joint
   d. Failure to include the entire length of the femur

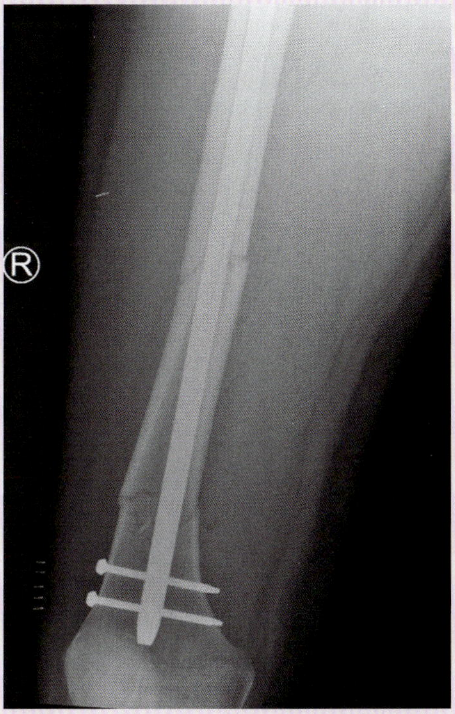

7-199

10. In review of the mediolateral lower leg (Fig. 7-200), characterize the results.
   a. Image fails to include all essential anatomy.
   b. Image passes as it includes all essential anatomy.
   c. Image demonstrates rotation of the part.
   d. Image demonstrates insufficient technique.

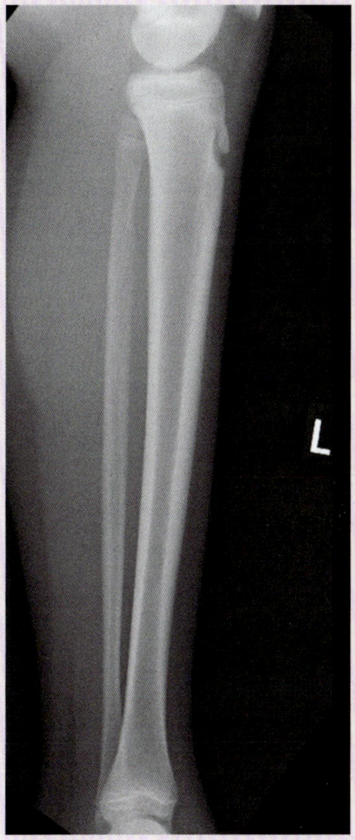

7-200

ANSWERS TO THE CRITICAL THINKING QUESTIONS

1. c
2. a
3. a
4. c
5. d
6. c
7. c
8. d
9. c
10. a

CHAPTER 8 Pelvis and Hip

Imaging of the pelvis and hip will include nontrauma and trauma case situations on patients that may be very young and span to the elderly. Traumatic injuries can commonly result in fractures in the elder population owing to a loss of bone density. Exams may have to be modified to accommodate the patient's condition or implement specialty views with altered positioning and/or tube angles to image necessary anatomy. The technologist must take into consideration patient variables such as size, age, ability, and pathology, which can all pose challenges to attaining the highest quality images.

CLINICAL INDICATIONS

Indications are the symptomatic reasons as to why a particular exam may be ordered by the physician. The technologist should look at the clinical indications before performing a procedure. The following briefly introduces common exam indications, but it is not an all-encompassing list. In certain circumstances, the indication may influence the need to increase or decrease the technical settings.

Osteoarthritis: A form of degenerative disease to the joint resulting in patients experiencing pain and reduced joint mobility. This condition tends to affect patients of increased age and in joints that are primarily weight-bearing such as knees and hips (Fig. 8-1).

Osteoporosis: A loss of bone density caused by a deficiency of calcium needed for bone formation. The condition affects primarily aging females and can result in fractures to the hip (Fig. 8-2).

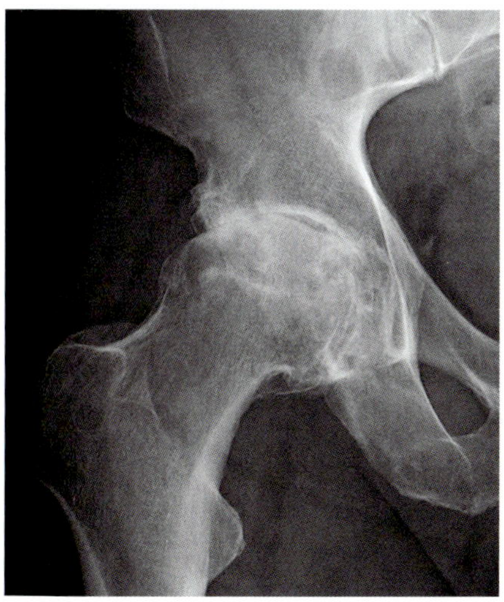

8-1 Osteoarthritis.

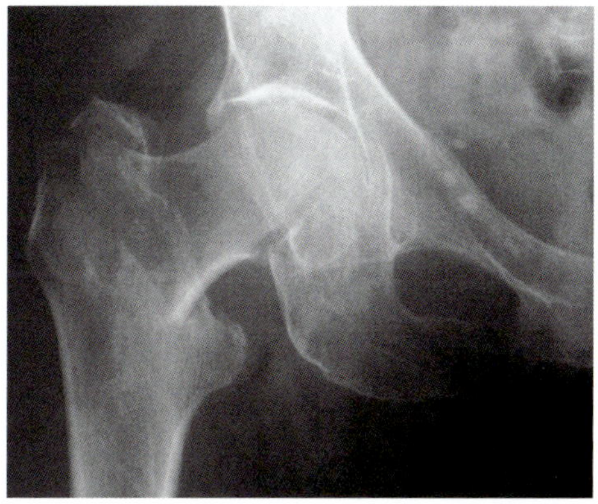

8-2 Osteoporosis.

Hip Fracture: A result of trauma or osteoporotic condition paired with traumatic injury. Most commonly, the proximal femur will fracture at the femoral neck, a thinner and less stable portion of bone, particularly with the weakend and brittle bones in older female patients. The classic presenting sign of a femoral neck fracture is the patient's affected leg and foot will appear externally rotated. The proximal femur may also incur an intertrochanteric fracture, a fracture that is located on the intertrochanteric crest that lies between the greater and lesser trochanter on the posterior aspect of the proximal femur. Hip fracture typically results in a prosthetic hip replacement (Fig. 8-3).

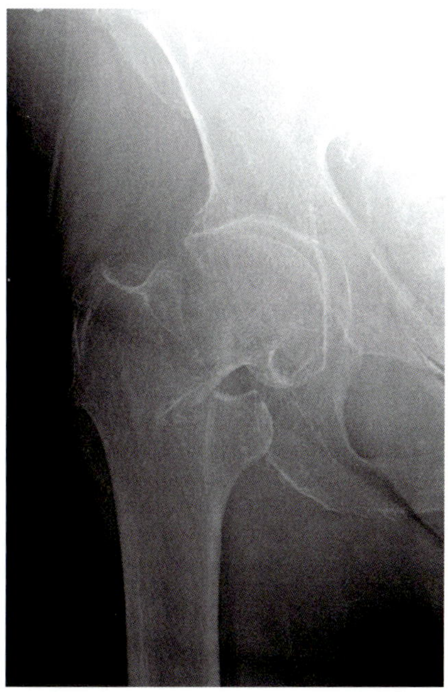

8-3 Hip Fracture.

Postreduction: A fracture or dislocation is reduced back into correct anatomic placement with or without internal fixation with surgical implants. Postreduction imaging is common (Fig. 8-4).

Congenital Hip Dysplasia or Developmental Dysplasia of the Hip: A condition that affects neonates, causing the hips to dislocate owing to a lax joint capsule. This condition occurs more commonly in females. Bilateral hip radiographic imaging may assist with diagnosis, but the use of ultrasound is increasingly sought. Undiagnosed cases can result in necrosis caused by lack of blood supply (Figs. 8-5 and 8-6).

Legg–Calve–Perthes Disease: A condition found more often in young boys with a lesion commonly seen in the head of the femur. The patient will present with pain and a limp. This lesion will over time cause a flattened appearance to the femoral head and may show signs of necrosis (cellular death) (Fig. 8-7).

Trochanteric Bursitis: Inflammation to the bursa sac that covers the trochanter, often as a result of repetitive activity, causing the bursa sacs of the gluteus maximus and the trochanter to build friction. The patient will present with point tenderness at the greater trochanter (Fig. 8-8).

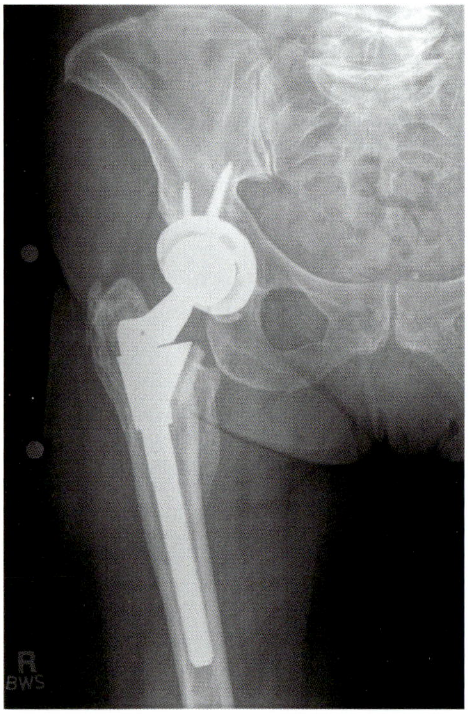

8-4 Postreduction hip to document prosthetic placement.

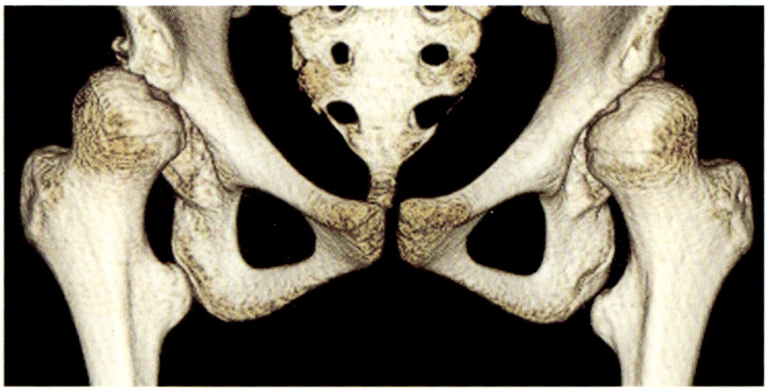

8-5 3D reconstructed CT displaying bilateral congenital hip dysplasia.

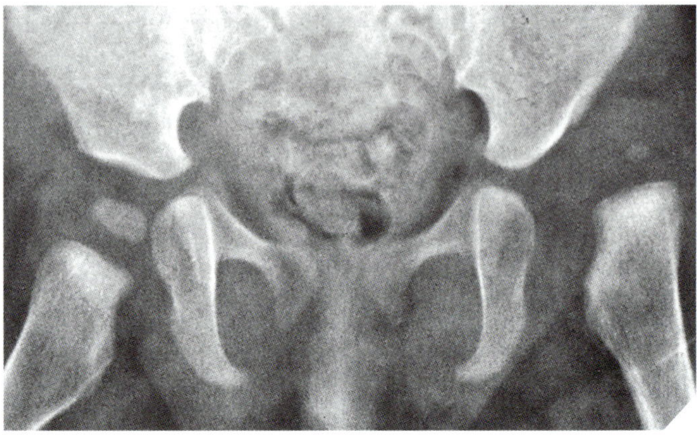

8-6 Congenital hip dysplasia.

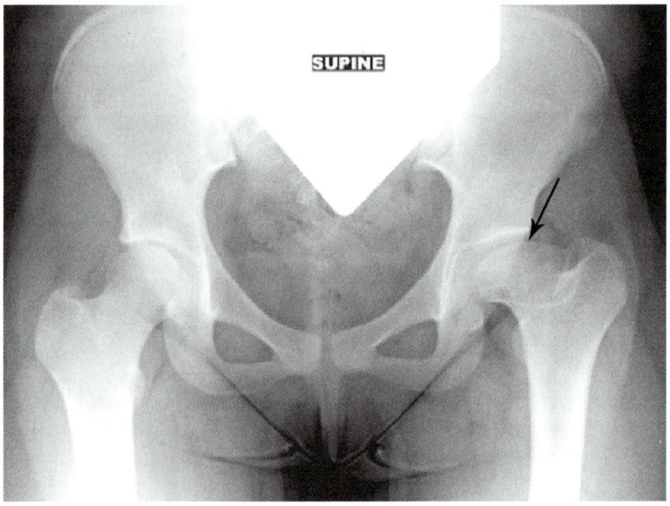

8-7 Legg–Calve–Perthes disease.

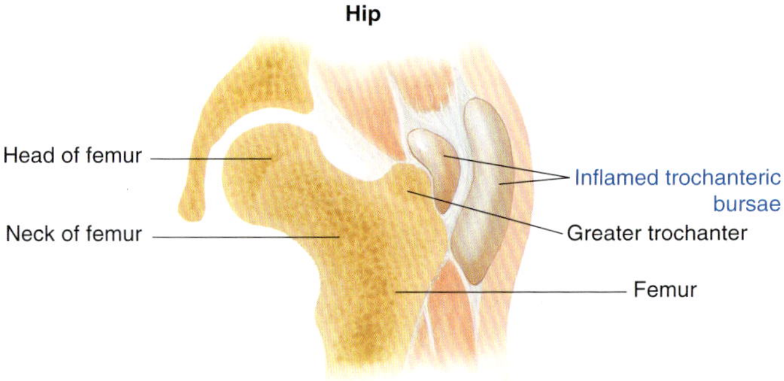

8-8 Trochanteric bursitis.

IMAGING CONSIDERATIONS

Patient Dress

Patient will need to change from the waist area down, removing all metal/plastic objects from clothing and/or jewelry that might present as artifact on the image. The patient should be dressed into a gown. For patients already dressed into a hospital gown, the radiographer should check the area of interest to ensure the area is free of artifact before imaging. When imaging toddlers and infants wearing diapers, diapers should be clean and dry or removed before imaging.

Artifacts

Artifacts are unwanted objects that appear on the image superimposing pertinent anatomy. This includes snaps, buttons, safety pins, jewelry, and waistbands. Considering the higher detail acquired with digital imaging, components such as waistbands, pockets, soiled diapers, and embroidering stitching are easily identified on images and are considered artifacts that will constitute a repeat image (Fig. 8-9).

Patient Position

The general position of the patient or part

Supine—Most common position for both trauma and nontrauma situations.

Posterior Oblique—The beam is directed to enter the anterior surface and exit the posterior surface while the body is positioned into a particular degree of obliquity. The patient will be rotated into a right or left posterior oblique (Fig. 8-10).

Ambulatory Patient Imaging

An ambulatory patient is one who can maneuver themselves and bear weight with little to no assistance. However, it should be considered that elderly patients may still need assistance on and off the imaging table to ensure their safety. When exams are completed recumbent, technologists could improve the patient care experience by placing a pad on the hard tabletop surface and providing the patient a blanket during imaging. Patients are often chilled in the exam rooms while dressed in a hospital gown. Ambulatory patients may also be imaged upright while bearing weight.

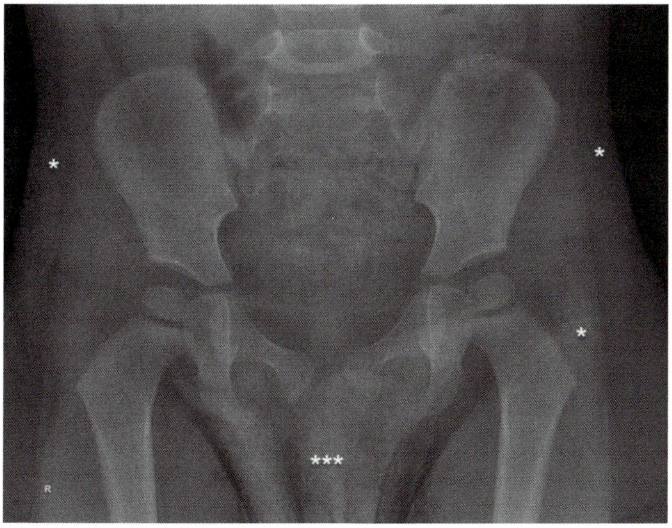

8-9 Diaper artifact.

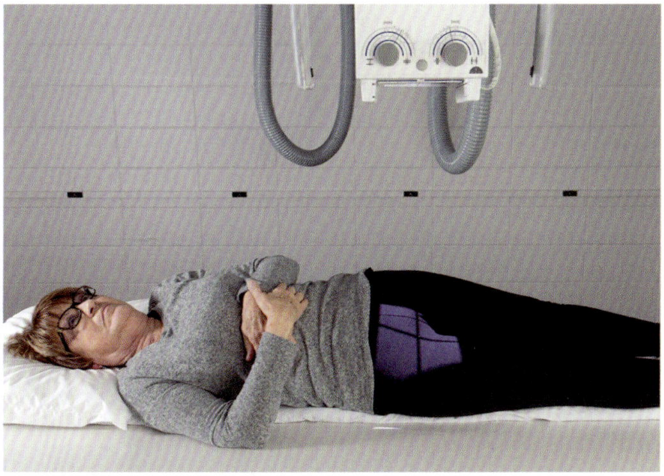

8-10 Right posterior oblique position and utilizing an AP Oblique projection.

Nonambulatory Patient Imaging

Patients transported by stretcher to the department for a study will require the assistance of at least a second radiographer to help carefully transfer the patient from the stretcher to the imaging table. Exams may be modified to adapt to the patient condition or include specialty views to better image anatomy.

Mobile Patient Imaging

Mobile imaging is reserved for the patient unable to ambulate owing to their condition. Mobile exams can be performed in the emergency department, intensive care unit, PACU, surgery, and inpatient rooms. When imaging the pelvis, a single anteroposterior (AP) projection is acquired. If imaging the hip, a minimum of two views are attained with a trauma protocol approach. Patients who are postsurgical for open reduction internal fixation (ORIF) will require a minimum of two views of the part to include the entire prosthetic device implanted.

Projection(s)

How the x-ray beam passes through the part

- AP (Anteroposterior): The beam is directed to enter through the anterior surface, exit the posterior surface, and strike the image receptor (IR).
- AP Oblique: The beam is directed to enter the anterior surface and exit the posterior surface while the body is positioned into a particular degree of obliquity (Fig. 8-10).
- Mediolateral: The beam will enter the lateral positioned part on the anatomic medial surface and exit the lateral surface that is closest to the IR.
- AP or PA Axial: The beam directs anterior to posterior (AP) or posterior to anterior (PA), with an added specified tube (axial) angle directed to the part.
- Inferosuperior Axial: The beam is directed inferiorly to superiorly on a part with an angle applied to the beam.

ANATOMY

The pelvis is comprised of the right and left hip bones that articulate with the sacrum and coccyx posteriorly and at the symphysis pubis anteriorly (Fig. 8-11). Each hip bone is comprised of three bones: ilium, ischium, and pubis (Fig. 8-12). These three bones form the acetabulum and begin to fuse together during the adolescent years. The pelvis serves to distribute weight from the vertebral column down to the lower extremities.

Ilium

The ilium, the largest division of the hip bone, comprises the superior portion of the hip bone and contributes to the upper region of the acetabulum. The body of the ilium is just superior to the acetabulum (Fig. 8-13). Moving superiorly from the body, the ilium thins out into the wing or ala. Continuing to the most superior point of the ilium is the iliac crest. The iliac crest runs in between two bony points, the anterior superior iliac spine (ASIS) and the posterior superior iliac spine (PSIS). Respectively below the ASIS and PSIS, a lesser prominence is located. The anterior inferior iliac spine (AIIS) is located just inferior to the palpable ASIS, and the posterior inferior iliac spine (PIIS) is just inferior to the posterior PSIS (Fig. 8-14).

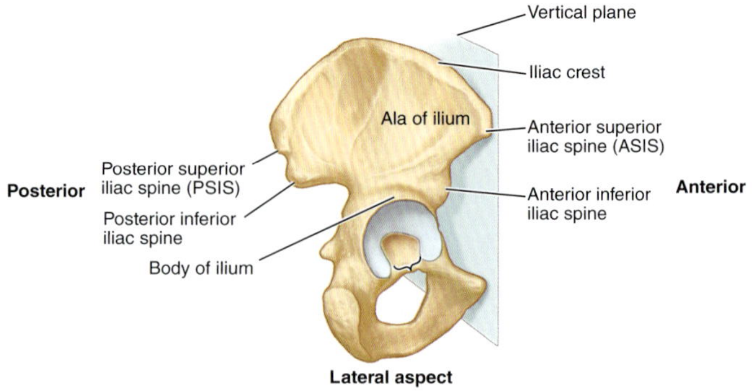

8-13 Lateral view of ilium.

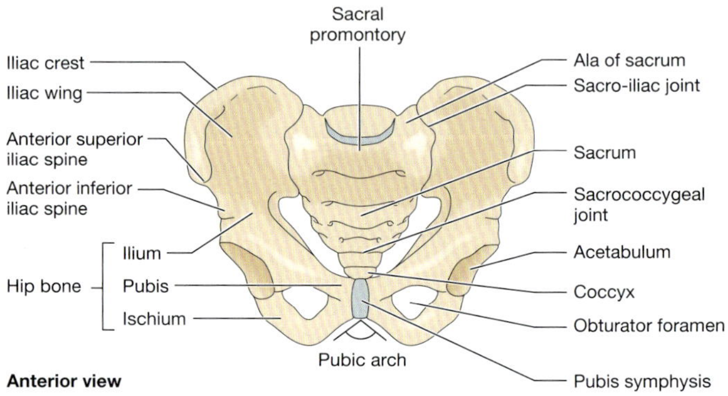

8-14 Frontal view of pelvis.

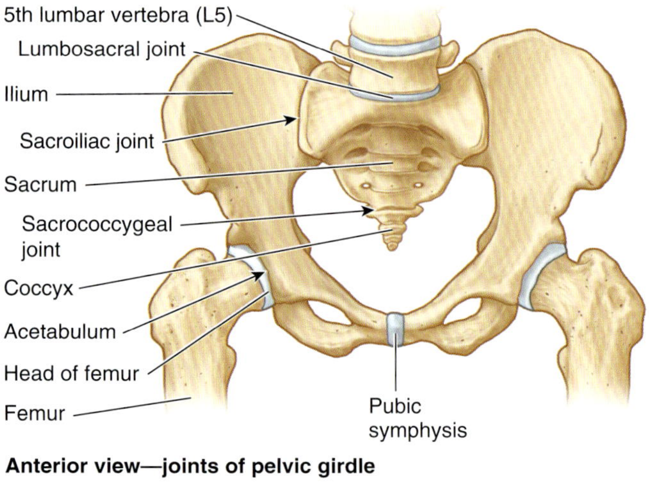

8-11 Pelvis.

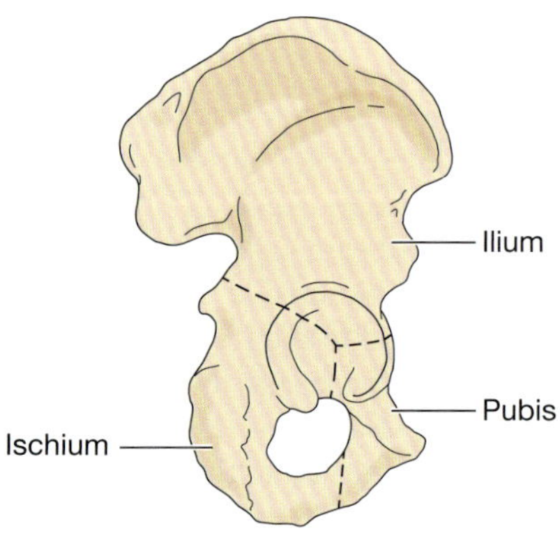

8-12 Lateral view of hip bone.

Ischium

The ischium contributes to the formation of the posterior inferior region of the acetabulum. The body of the ischium is closest to the acetabulum. Directly posterior to the acetabulum, a small prominence, the ischial spine is noted. When imaging the pelvis in a true AP, the right and left ischial spines should barely be visible along the pelvic brim, just medial to the acetabulum (Fig. 8-14). Superiorly to the ischial spine sits a large pronounced notch, the greater sciatic notch. Inferiorly to the ischial spine sits a smaller, less pronounced notch, the lesser sciatic notch. Again, referencing the ischial body with its proximity adjacent to the acetabulum, the body travels inferiorly and terminates at the ischial tuberosity (Fig. 8-15). The ischial tuberosities support the weight of the body when in the seated position. From the ischial tuberosity a ramus extends anteriorly toward the inferior ramus of the pubic bone.

Pubis

The pubis comprises the anterior and inferior region of the acetabulum. The body of the pubis extends anteriorly from the proximity of the acetabulum. The body gives rise to the superior ramus (Fig. 8-16). The superior ramus of the right pubis and the superior ramus of the left pubis unite at midline and form the articulation of the symphysis pubis. The right and left pubic bones are separated by a cartilage pad at midline (Figs. 8-14 and 8-16). This cartilage pad allows for limited movement of the pelvis. The symphysis pubis is classified as

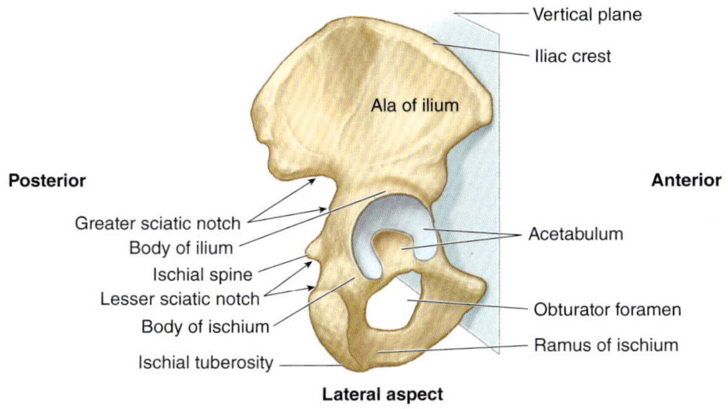

8-15 Lateral view of ischium.

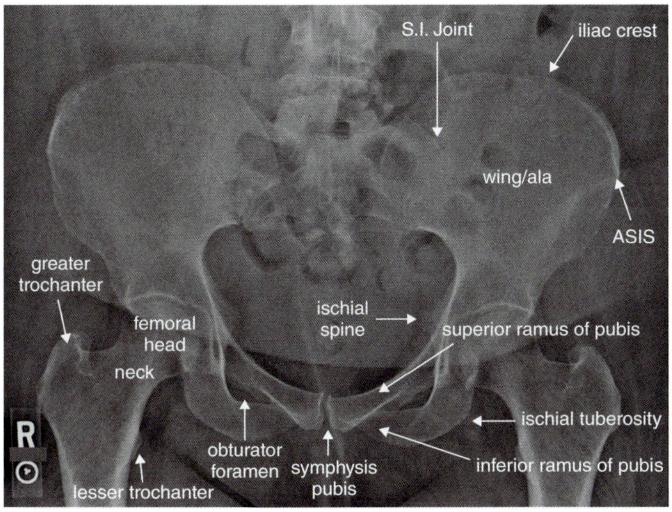

8-16 AP pelvis.

a cartilaginous type with amphiarthrodial movement. From the symphysis pubis, an inferior ramus extends inferiorly and runs laterally toward the ischial tuberosity to connect with the ramus of the ischium. Between the superior and the inferior ramus of the pubis, the largest opening, or foramen, in the body is formed and is referred to as the obturator foramen (Fig. 8-17). The shape of the obturator foramen can be observed for symmetry during pelvic imaging to help identify potential rotation of the positioned pelvis.

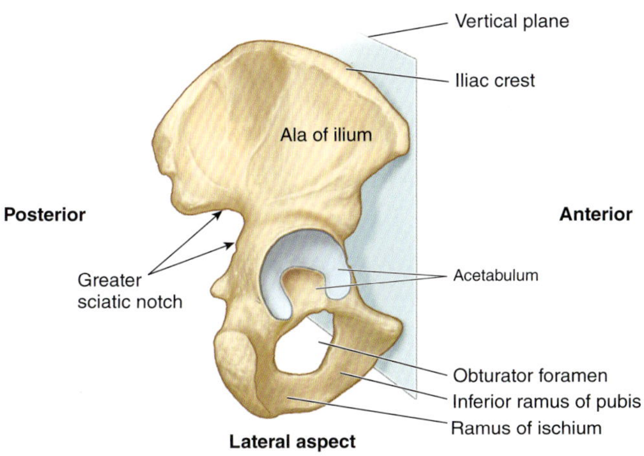

8-17 Lateral view of pubis.

Proximal Femur

The proximal femur consists of the rounded femoral head, which fits into the acetabulum of the pelvis. The hip articulation is a diarthrodial joint with ball and socket movement. The ball and socket joint of the hip provides a greater stability of the hip joint compared to the ball and socket joint of the shoulder owing to the depth of the socket (Fig. 8-18).

A small depression located in the center of the femoral head, which is sometimes visible on a radiograph, is the fovea capitis. The fovea capitis serves as a site for ligament attachment. The femoral neck tapers from the head and connects to the femoral shaft. The femoral neck is a common location for a hip fracture to occur (Fig. 8-19).

The femoral head and neck sit at a 15°–20° anterior angle to the acetabulum compared to the shaft of the femur. This anatomic angle requires the femurs and lower legs to be internally

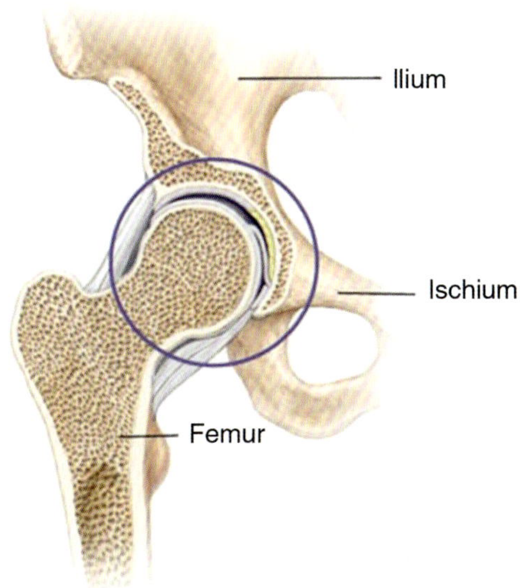

8-18 Hip joint.

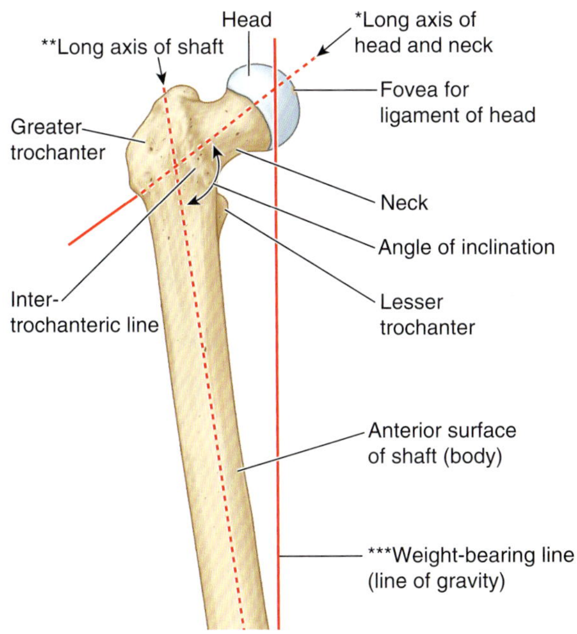

8-19 Proximal femur—anterior view.

rotated 15°–20° to achieve a true AP view of the femoral neck(s) (Fig. 8-19).

Lastly, on the proximal femur are two prominences. On the superior and lateral aspect of the proximal femoral shaft, the prominent and palpable greater trochanter is located. The greater trochanter sits in close reference to the plane of the symphysis pubis. The lesser trochanter is located on the medial and posterior portion of the proximal shaft. The greater and lesser trochanters are connected posteriorly by a ridge of bone known as the intertrochanteric crest (Figs. 8-20 and 8-21).

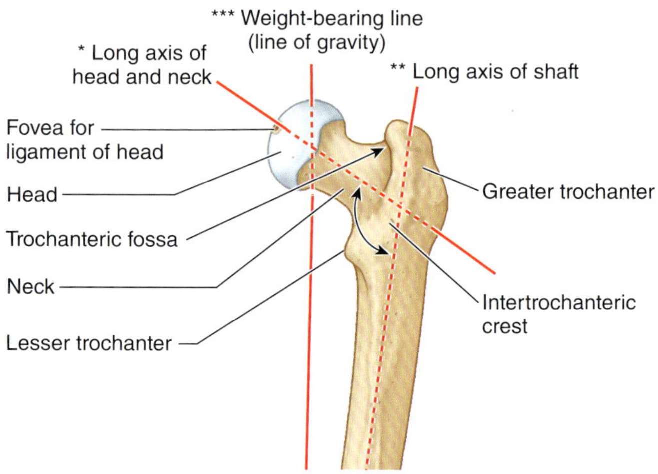

8-20 Proximal femur—posterior view.

Characteristics of the Male and Female Pelvis

Radiographically, the male pelvis can be distinguished from the female pelvis. Distinguishable factors are:

1. The overall shape appearance of the pelvis. The female pelvis will display iliac wings with more lateral flare, contributing to a wider appearance. The male pelvis will display a narrower pelvis as the iliac wings are less flared. The appearance of the female pelvic brim will be more rounded compared to the male pelvic brim (Figs. 8-22 and 8-23).
2. The angle of the pubic arch. The angle of the pubic arch on a female may appear flattened because the angle is >90°. The male patient will have the appearance of an acute angle at the pubic arch (Figs. 8-22 to 8-25).

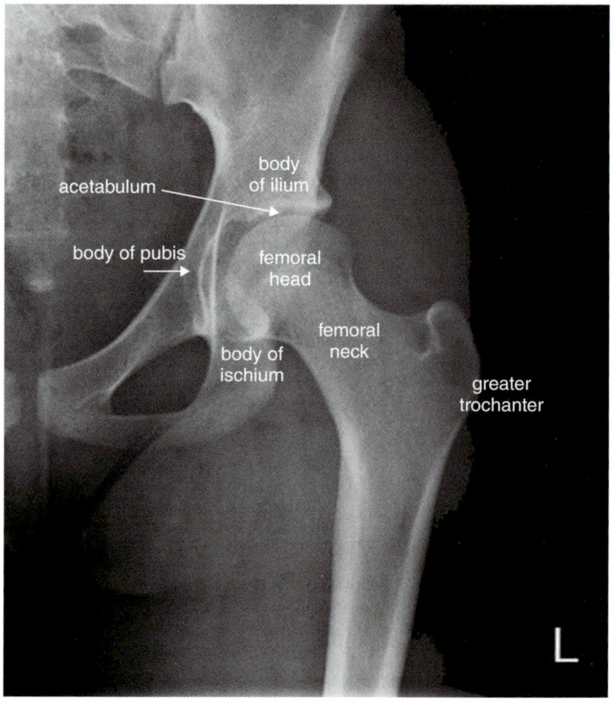

8-21 AP hip.

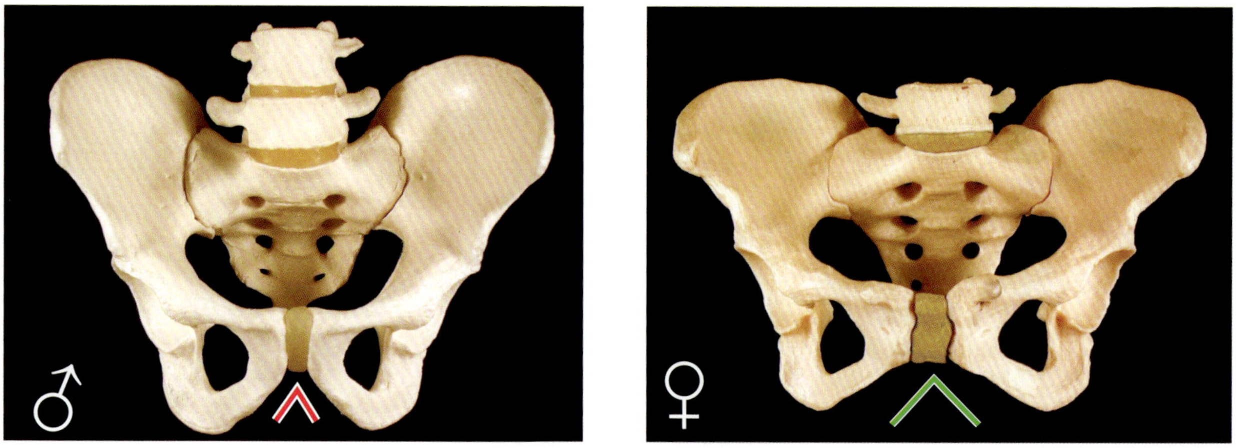

8-22 Characteristics of the male and female pelvis.

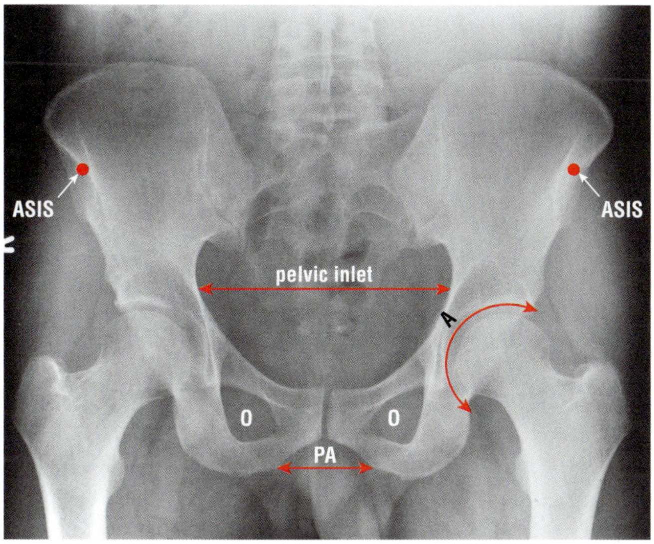

A

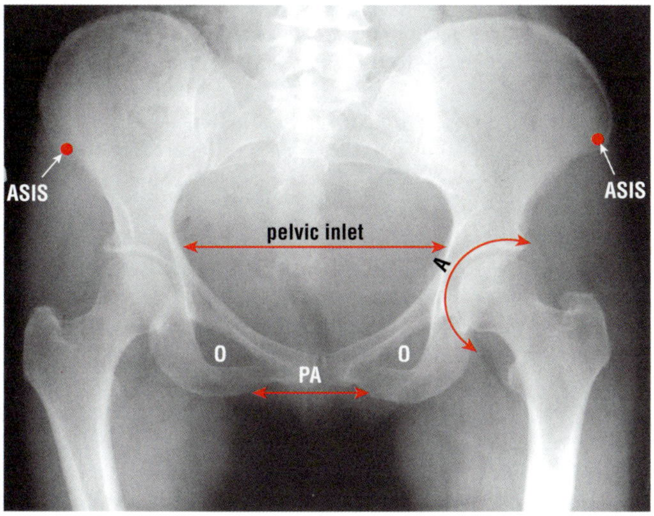

B

8-23 Radiographic comparison of male and female pelvis. **A**: Anteroposterior radiograph, male pelvis. **B**: Anteroposterior radiograph, female pelvis.

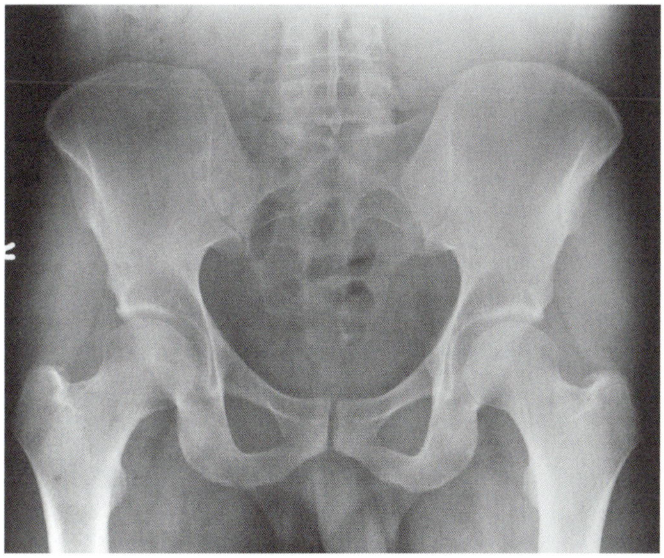

8-24 Male pelvis.

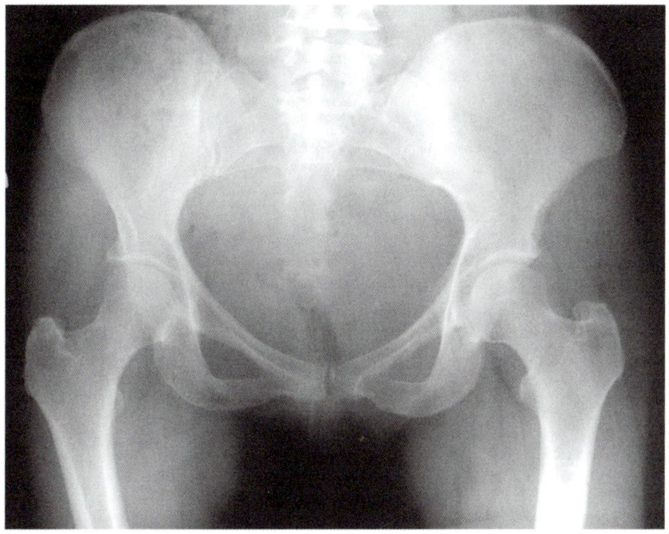

8-25 Female pelvis.

True and False Pelvis

The pelvic brim or linea terminalis divides the pelvis into true and false divisions. The pelvic brim or linea terminalis is the bony circular opening that runs from the point of the sacral promontory down to the symphysis pubis and back up around to the sacral promontory. The area directly superior to the pelvic brim is the false pelvis. The false pelvis supports the lower abdominal organs. The area directly inferior to the pelvic brim is the true pelvis (Fig. 8-26). The true pelvis forms the birth canal. With reference to the birthing process, the female pelvic brim is also the pelvic inlet, which the fetal head passes through first. The pelvic outlet is delineated by the two ischial tuberosities and the tip of the coccyx. The space in between the pelvic inlet and the outlet is the pelvic cavity (Fig. 8-27).

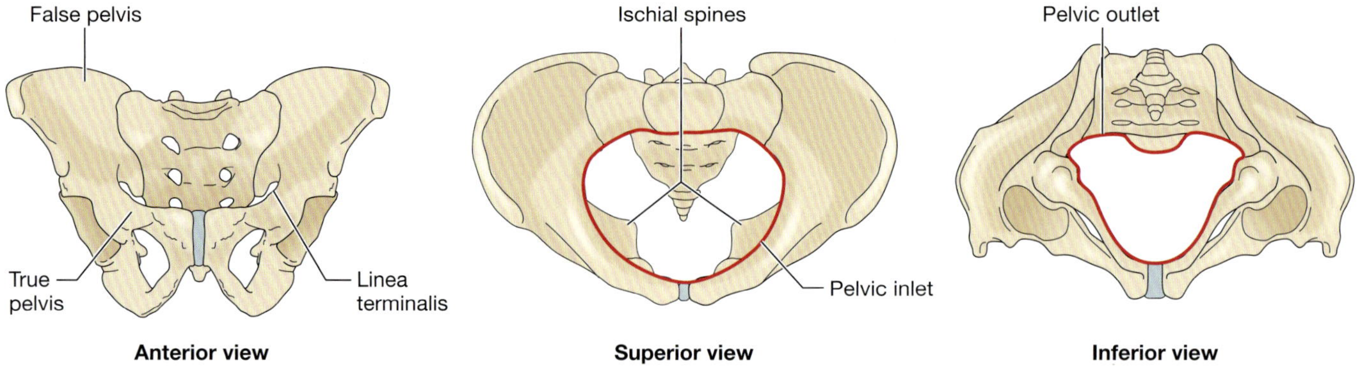

8-26 True and false pelvis divisions.

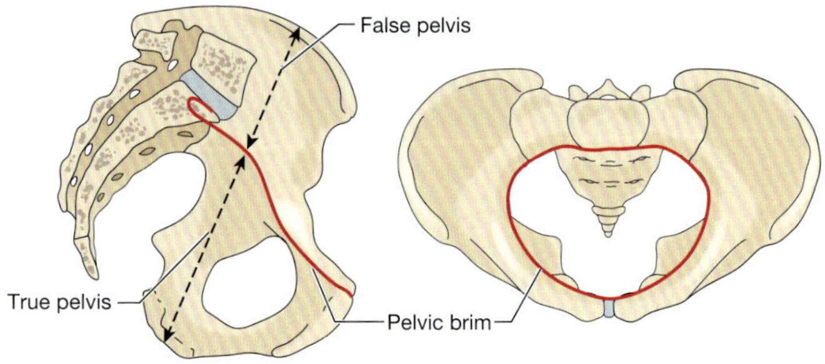

8-27 Lateral view of true and false pelvis divisions.

Joints of the Pelvis (Fig. 8-28 and Table 8-1)

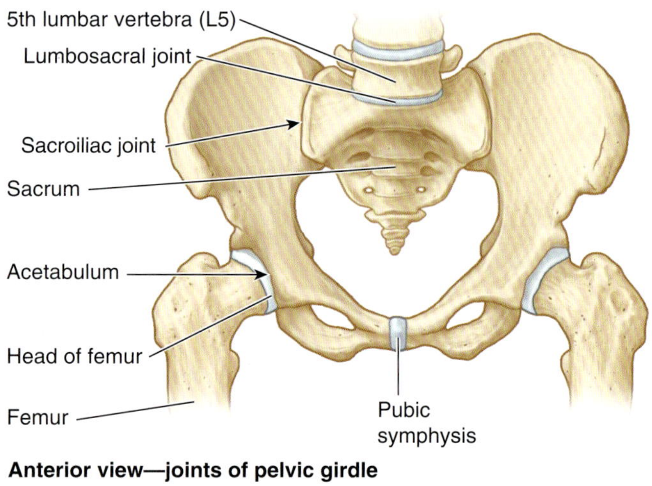

8-28 Joints of the pelvis.

8-1 Joints of the Pelvis

Joint	Classification	General Movement	Specific Movement
Hip joint	Synovial	Diarthrodial	Spheroidal or ball and socket
Sacroiliac joint	Synovial	Amphiarthrodial	–
Symphysis pubis	Cartilaginous	Amphiarthrodial	–

KEY SUMMATION POINTS OF ANATOMY

- The hip bone is comprised of three separate bones that fuse together at adulthood. The three bones are the ilium, ischium, and pubis. All three bones contribute to the formation of the acetabulum.
- The iliac crest is the most superior landmark on the pelvis. The true location of the iliac crest at its most superior location should be palpated on the side of the patient. The level of the iliac crest corresponds to lumbar vertebral levels 4–5.
- The iliac crest runs between two bony landmarks: The ASIS and the PSIS. The ASIS is a palpable landmark on the anterior pelvis.
- The ischial spine is located on the posterior border of the ischium. Superior to the ischial spine is the greater sciatic notch. Inferior to the ischial spine is the lesser sciatic notch. Bilateral ischial spines may be barely visible on an AP pelvis radiograph when the positioning is free of body rotation. Ischial spines will appear just medial to the acetabulum.
- The ischial tuberosities represent the most inferior point on the pelvis. The ischial tuberosities support the weight of the body when in a seated position.
- The femoral head and neck sit with a slight anterior angulation compared to the femoral shaft in order to articulate with the acetabulum. It is for this reason that internal rotation of the femurs and lower limbs will position the femoral necks parallel to the IR.
- The characteristics of the male pelvis are: narrower across, less flare of the iliac wings, and has a pubic arch <90°.
- The characteristics of the female pelvis are: wider across, more flare of the iliac wings, a round pelvic brim, and a pubic arch >90°.
- The pelvis is divided into true and false divisions. The false pelvis sits superior to the pelvic brim and supports the lower abdominal structures. The true pelvis sits inferior to the pelvic brim and allows for the formation of the birthing canal.
- The female pelvis is characterized as also having a pelvic inlet and outlet that allow for birthing. The pelvic inlet is anatomically the same as the pelvic brim. The pelvic outlet is delineated by both the ischial tuberosities and the tip of the coccyx.
- There are three primary joints of the pelvis: hip joint, sacroiliac joint, and the symphysis pubis (Fig. 8-28 and Table 8-1).

POSITIONING AND TECHNICAL CONSIDERATIONS

Body Habitus and Suggested Image Receptor Orientation

In consideration of different body types among the population, all imaging of the adult pelvis will use a 14 × 17 IR orientated crosswise. When imaging the hip, typically a 10 × 12 is utilized or collimated to this size owing to the length and orientation of the part dependent on the projection.

Centering

Proper centering to the pelvis and hip may be better accomplished with the use of topographic landmarks such as the iliac crest, xiphoid process, ASIS, and the symphysis pubis (Fig. 8-29).

KEY ANATOMIC LANDMARKS (FIG. 8-29)

- Iliac crest corresponds to lumbar vertebral levels L4–L5
- ASIS corresponds to the first sacral segment
- Symphysis pubis
- Greater trochanter serves as an alternate landmark for the superior margin of the symphysis pubis
- Jugular notch, xiphoid process, and spine would all be landmarks for midsagittal plane (MSP)

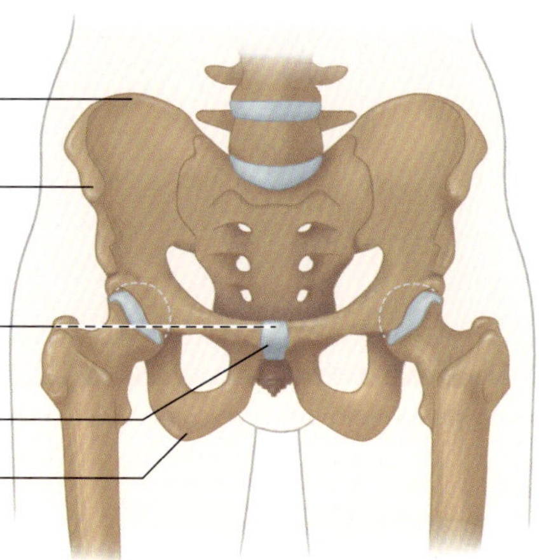

8-29 Topographic landmarks.

Measuring from landmarks will assist in centering on the proximal femur. To locate the femoral neck for centering, the technologist can:

1. Measure 1″–2″ (2–3 fingers) medial to the ASIS and then inferiorly 4″ (one hand width) (Figs. 8-30).
1. Create a line that runs in between the ASIS and symphysis pubis. From this line, the technologist can extend the index finger (approximately 2″) to the femoral neck from the midpoint of this line (Figs. 8-31 and 8-32).

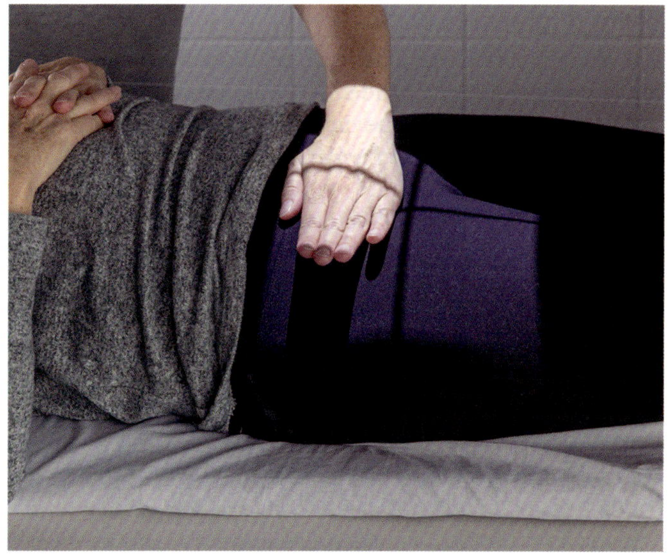

8-30 A 1″–2″ medial to the ASIS and then 4″ inferior to locate the femoral neck.

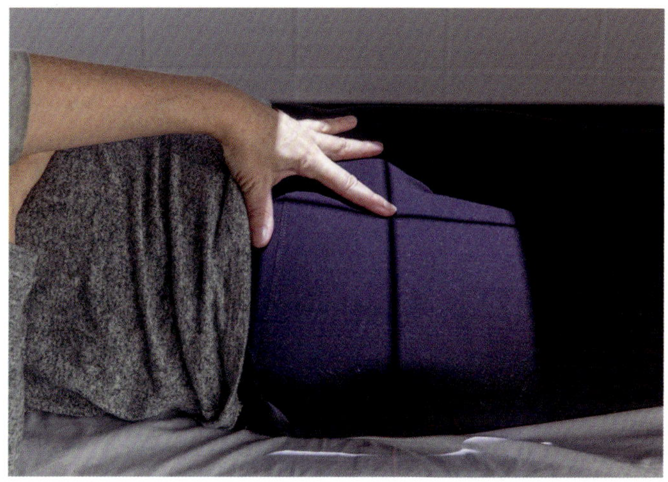

8-31 Three-finger technique to locate the femoral neck on the right hip.

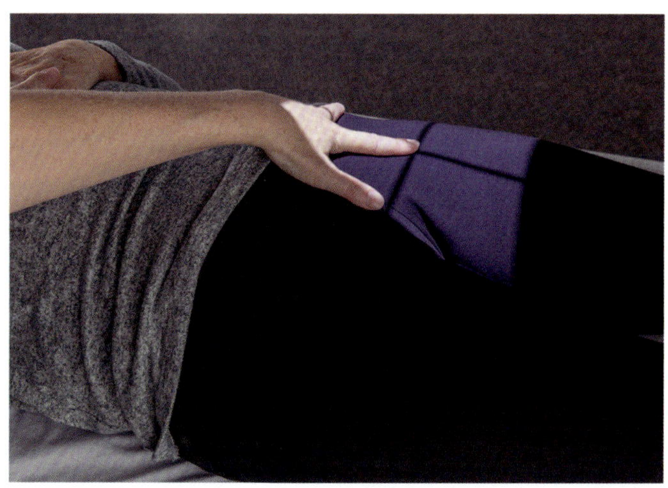

8-32 Three-finger technique to locate the femoral neck on the left hip.

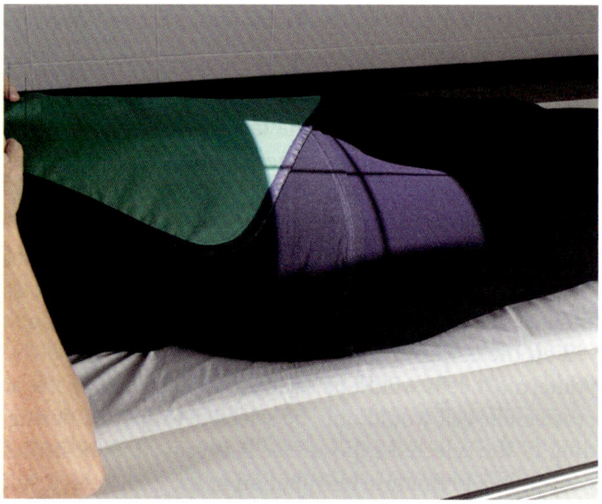

8-40 Placement of lap shield for female patient.

lap apron shielding may be carefully applied to minimize exposure to the reproductive organs (Fig. 8-40). Ultimately, the technologist should take proper care with centering and collimation to ensure the image may be successfully acquired on the first attempt to avoid the need for a repeat exposure.

Marking the Image

All images must be accurately marked with a right or left lead marker to avoid superimposition with bony anatomy. Markers should be placed lateral to the part with frontal projections (Figs. 8-41 and 8-42).

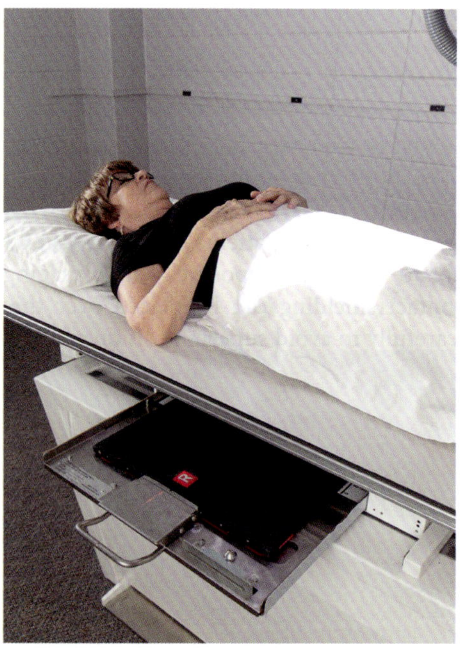

8-41 Suggested marker placement for AP pelvis.

Markers should be placed anterior to the part with lateral projections (Fig. 8-43).

Viewing the Image

Assuming the pelvis or hip image was correctly marked, the image is displayed opposite the viewer facing it, as though the image is in anatomic position (Figs. 8-44 to 8-46).

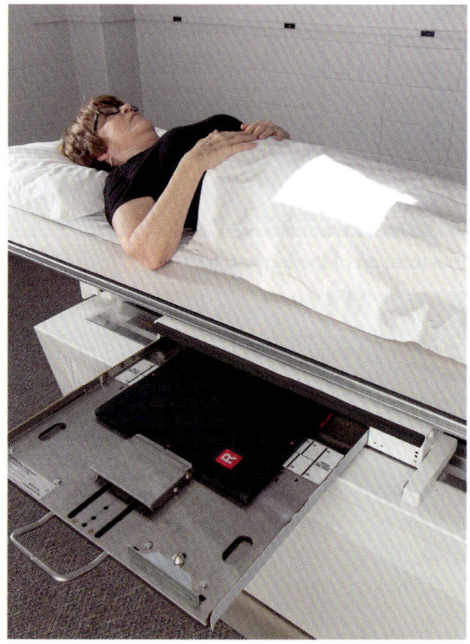

8-42 Suggested marker placement for AP hip.

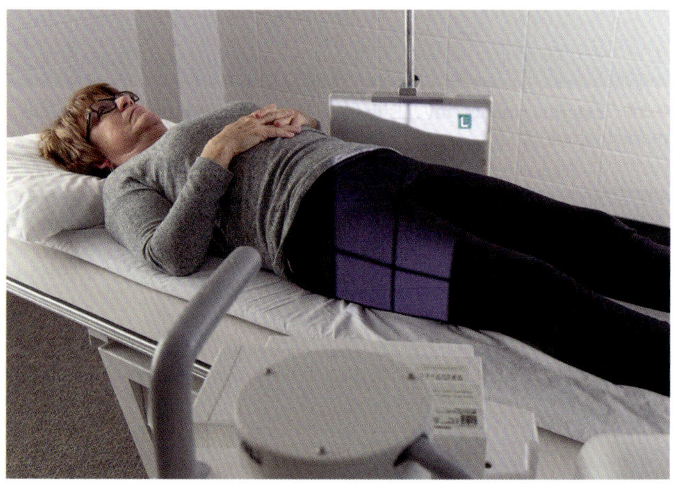

8-43 Suggested marker placement for the inferosuperior axiolateral hip.

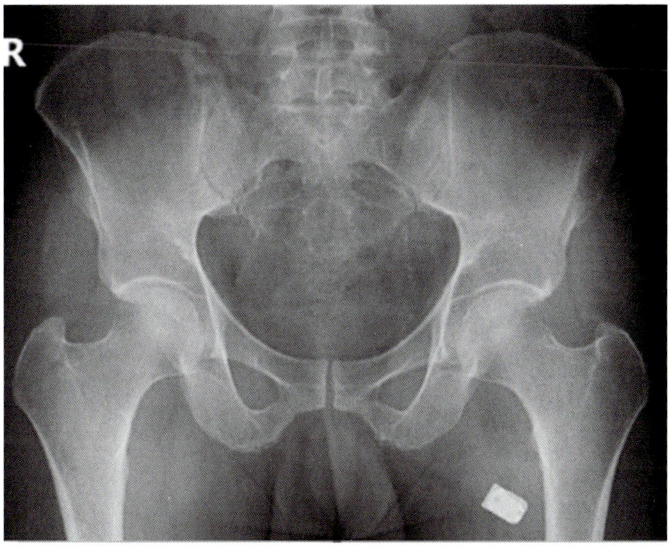

8-44 Correct display of AP pelvis.

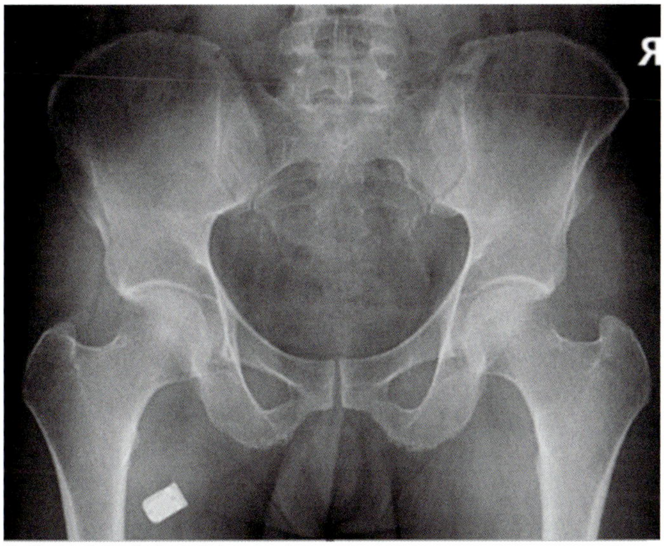

8-46 Incorrect display of AP pelvis.

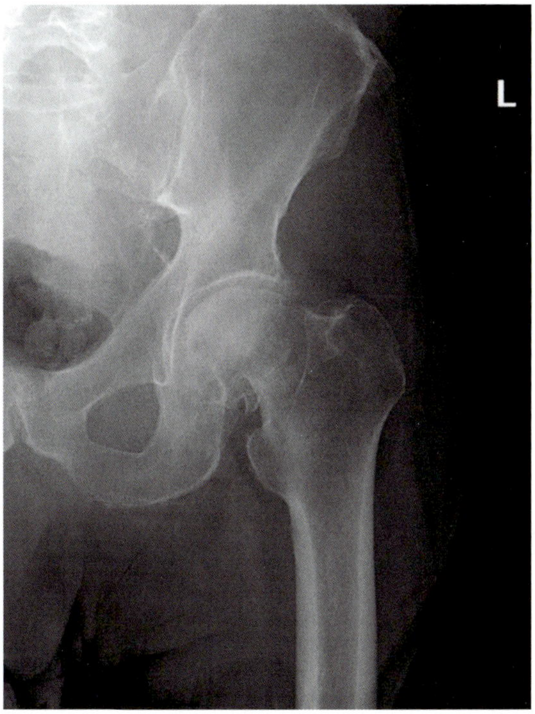

8-45 Correct display of AP left hip.

Pelvis

- Projection: AP

Pelvis Protocol
AP

Technical Considerations
- kVp 70–85
- Two outermost AEC cells selected for table Bucky or upright Bucky if weight bearing
- 40″ SID

Exposure Field Size
- 14 × 17 crosswise for all adult sized patients
- 10 × 12 crosswise for younger pediatric patients

Patient Position (Fig. 8-47)
- Supine with no rotation of the torso
- Arms removed from the imaging field
- **Nontrauma** patients should have legs slightly separated and then internal rotation may be performed of the entire both lower limbs 15°–20°. The technologist should have everything set for exposure before internally rotating the limbs to avoid the patient having to hold this position of the legs. With patients that do have difficulty holding position of the legs, sandbags could be placed to secure outside the legs and feet, or a band around the feet could stabilize the part position. These assistive measures are only possible with a supine patient
- **Trauma** patients are in the same general position as nontrauma patients, but should not have any internal rotation of the legs applied. The patient's legs should remain in their presenting position until a fracture has been ruled out

Centering
- MSP and midway between the levels of the symphysis pubis and ASIS. With proper centering, approximately 1″ of light will appear superior to the iliac crest

Marking of IR
- Right or left marker according to correct side

Breathing
- Suspend respiration
- Ensure patient holds position while walking away to make the exposure

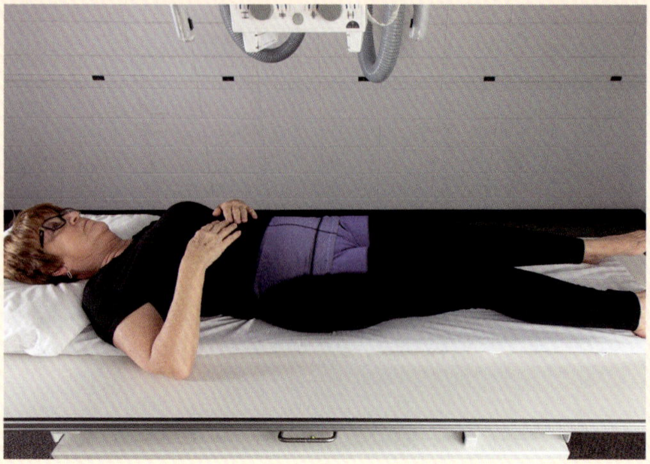

8-47 AP pelvis.

IMAGE CRITIQUE (FIGS. 8-48 and 8-49)

- Entire pelvis and proximal one-third of the femurs visualized
- IR properly orientated, properly centered, and collimated
- Symmetry of the iliac wings, ischial spines, and the obturator foramen ensure minimal to no rotation of the part. With nonsymmetry, the smaller obturator foramen indicates the rotation to that side (Fig. 8-50)
- **Nontrauma** patients with proper internal rotation of the legs will display the greater trochanters in profile laterally and femoral necks positioned parallel to the IR. The lesser trochanters should be rotated posterior to the proximal femur and be nonvisible to only slightly visible
- **Trauma** patients will display foreshortening of the femoral neck(s) and the lesser trochanter in profile medially owing to lack of internal leg rotation (Fig. 8-51)

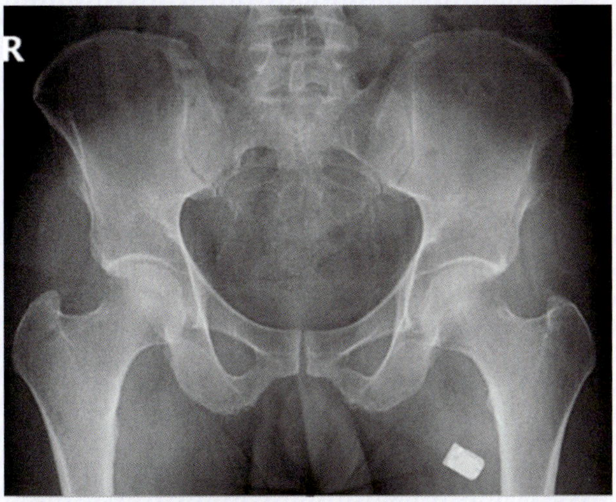

8-48 Nontrauma AP pelvis.

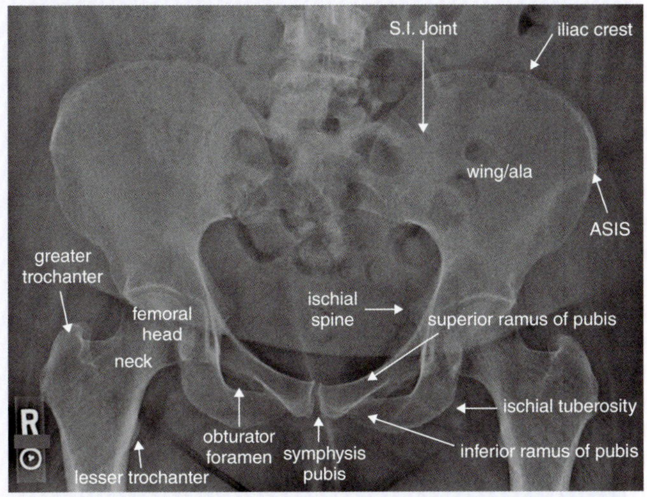

8-49 Nontrauma AP pelvis.

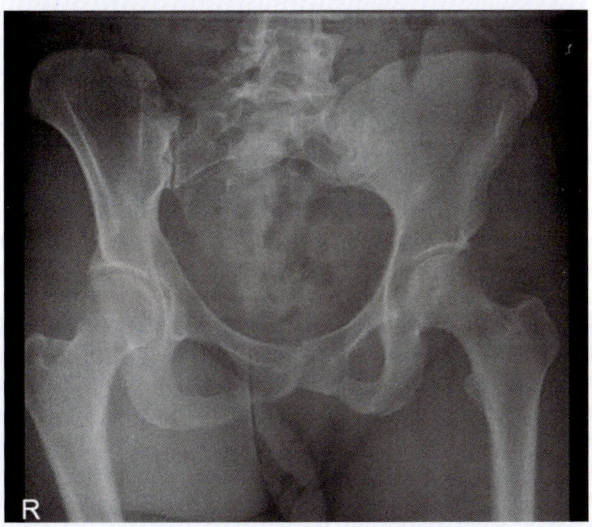

8-50 AP pelvis with rotation.

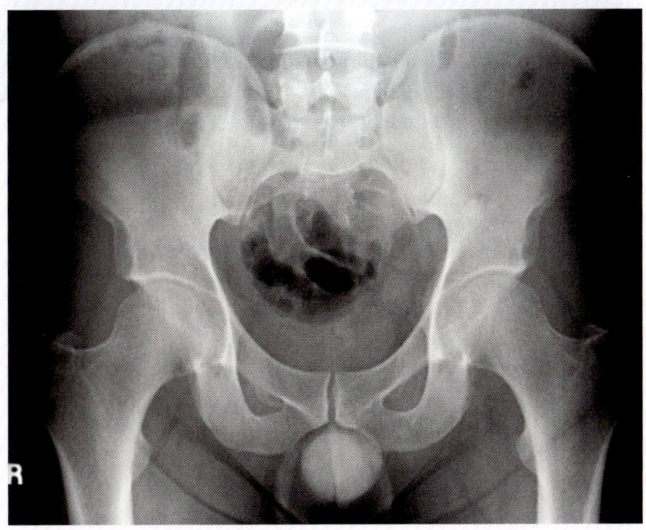

8-51 Trauma AP pelvis.

Trauma Hip

- Projection: AP
- *Do not attempt to move or reposition the leg if dislocation or fracture is suspected*

Trauma Hip Protocol
AP
Inferosuperior Axiolateral

Technical Considerations
- kVp 70–85
- Center AEC cell selected for table Bucky
- 40″ SID

Exposure Field Size
- 10 × 12 lengthwise

Patient Position (Fig. 8-63)
- Supine with no rotation of the torso
- Arms removed from the imaging field
- Trauma patients should not have any internal rotation to the leg applied. The patient's leg should remain in its presenting position

Centering
- Femoral neck. Location of the femoral neck is found by measuring 1″–2″ medial to the ASIS on the side of interest and then 4″ or one hand width or 2″ inferiorly from the midpoint on the imaginary line between the ASIS and the symphysis pubis. When utilizing a 10 × 12 LW and proper centering is established, the top of the exposure field should correspond to the level of the ASIS

Marking of IR
- Right or left marker according to correct side and lateral to the part

Breathing
- Suspend respiration
- Ensure patient holds position while walking away to make the exposure

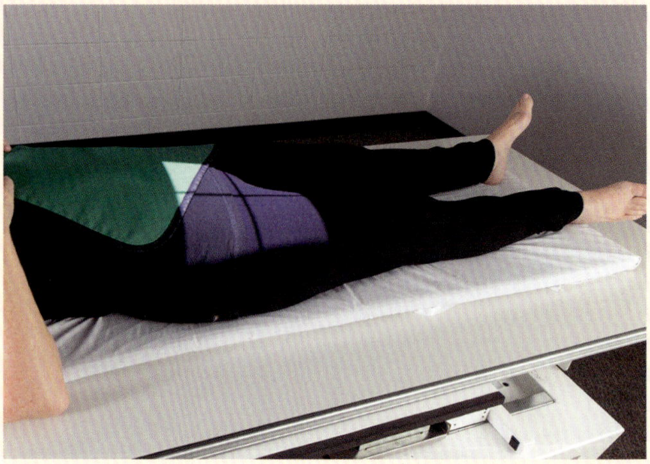

8-63 Trauma AP hip.

IMAGE CRITIQUE (FIGS. 8-64 and 8-65)

- Proximal one-third of the femur, acetabulum, and the symphysis pubis are included within the collimated exposure field
- Trauma patients will display foreshortening to the femoral neck and the lesser trochanter in profile medially

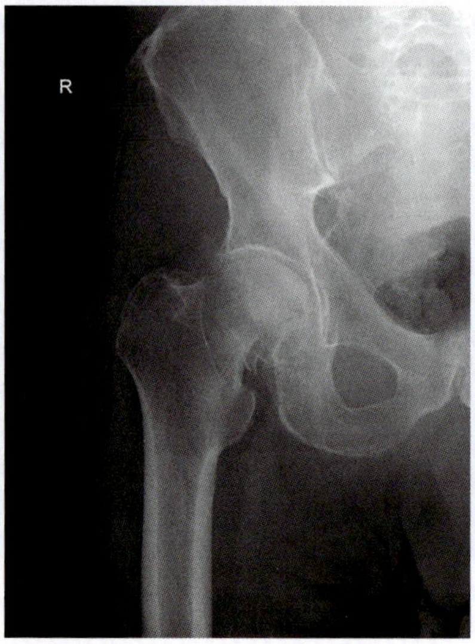

8-64 Trauma AP hip.

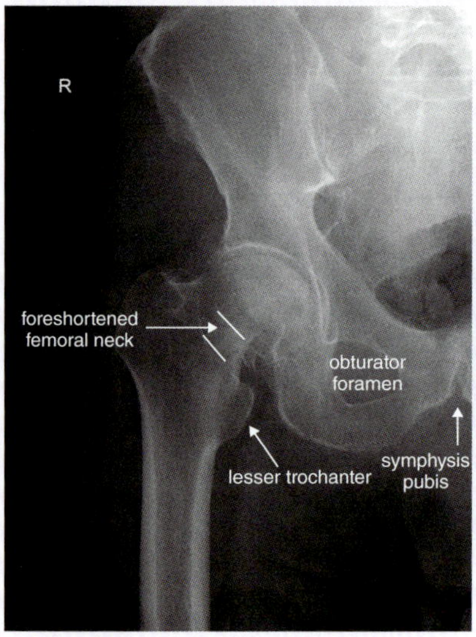

8-65 Trauma AP hip.

Trauma Hip

- Projection: Inferosuperior Axiolateral
- Danelius–Miller method
- *Do not attempt to move or reposition the leg if dislocation or fracture is suspected*

Trauma Hip Protocol
AP
Inferosuperior Axiolateral

Technical Considerations

- kVp 75–85
- mAs set manually
- Grid
- 40″ SID

Exposure Field Size

- 10 × 12 lengthwise orientation of grid to run with the length of the femur

Patient Position

- Supine with no rotation of the torso
- Arms removed from the imaging field
- Trauma patients should not have any internal rotation to the leg applied. The patient's affected leg should remain in its presenting position
- Maximum flexion (toward the patient's head) of the *unaffected* knee and leg to remove overlying bone and soft tissue over the affected proximal femur is necessary

Centering (Figs. 8-66 to 8-68)

- Place the top of the 10 × 12 LW exposure field with grid at or slightly above the iliac crest. Rotate the "foot" end of the grid out from the lateral side of the thigh to align the IR parallel to the femoral neck. If using a 14 × 17 digital IR plate, collimation of the exposure field to a 10 × 12 is encouraged
- The tube must be dropped to create a horizontal beam. The tube head is angled while in the horizontal position toward the patient's head until it lines up and is parallel to the plane of the IR. The beam must exit the tube and intersect the plane of the IR perpendicularly
- Align the CR with the center of the grid
- Correctly position the unaffected leg as described previously with maximum flexion and abduction
- Stabilize the unaffected leg with a stool or box propped up on the x-ray table. Only if necessary, should the technologist can dress in lead attire and hold the patient's unaffected leg up in the proper position
- Drop the central ray down after aligning with the grid to enter the patient's femoral neck (about the crease of the leg). Ensure the collimation is set to the length of the IR, and ensure the exposure field to include anterior and posterior sides of the part

Marking of IR

- Right or left marker according to correct side and anterior to the proximal femur

Breathing

- Suspend respiration
- Ensure patient holds position while walking away to make the exposure

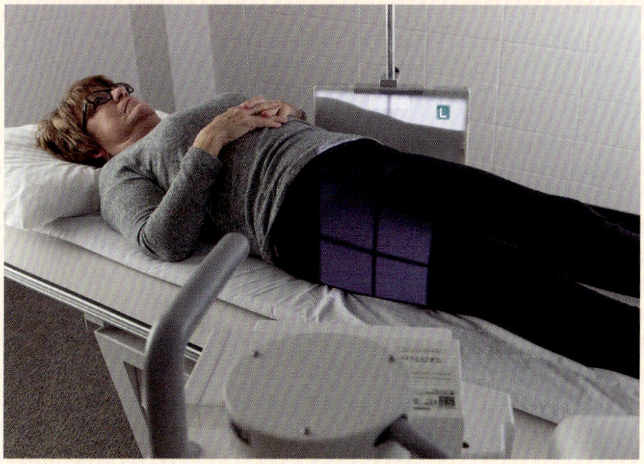

8-66 10 × 12 grid and horizontal beam setup.

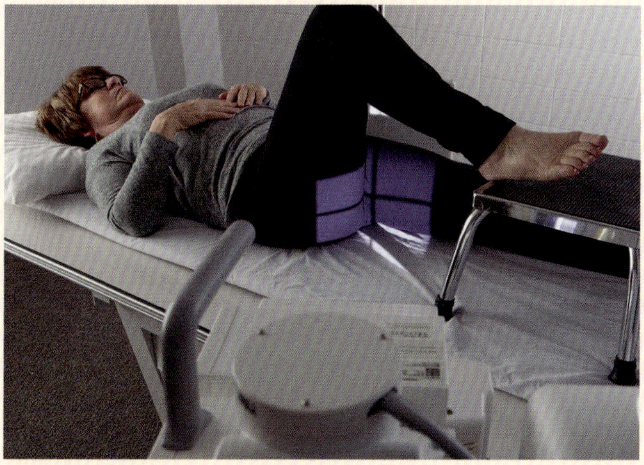

8-67 Flexion of the nonaffected leg with CR to femoral neck.

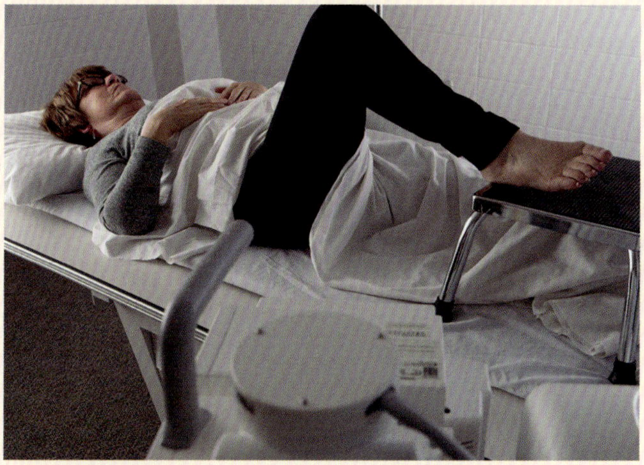

8-68 Example of draping the patient to maintain modesty.

IMAGE CRITIQUE (FIGS. 8-69 and 8-70)

- Proximal one-third of the femur, acetabulum, and the ischial tuberosity are visualized within the collimated exposure field size
- The femoral neck should be well visualized with greater trochanter superimposing upon the femoral neck
- If the patient is postoperative with a prosthesis, the image must include the entire prosthetic device, which, in some cases, may require the use of a longer collimated exposure field with a 14 × 17 IR to accommodate the length of the prosthesis

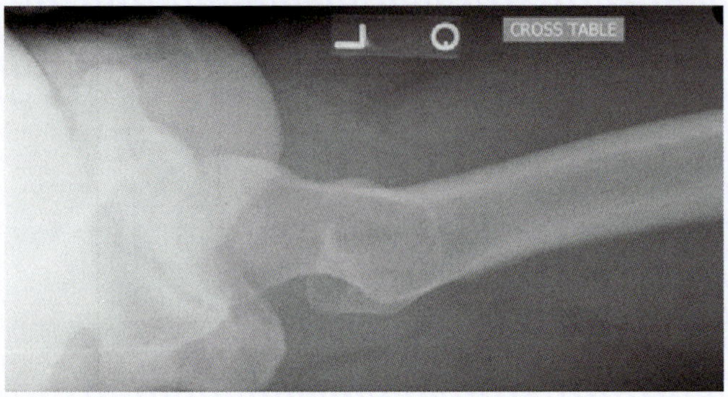

8-69 Inferosuperior axiolateral.

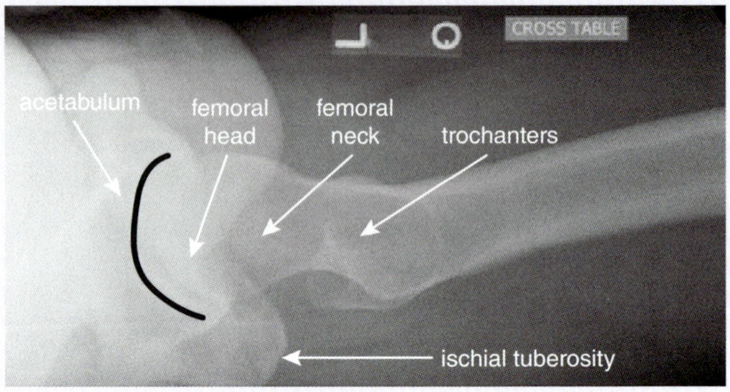

8-70 Inferosuperior axiolateral.

POSITION VARIATION MODIFIED AXIOLATERAL PROJECTION/CLEMENTS–NAKAYAMA METHOD (FIGS. 8-71 and 8-72)

For patients with potential trauma and/or the inability to move either lower limb, this projection could be modified by eliminating the need for the patient to elevate the unaffected leg. The 10 × 12 lengthwise grid positioned with the top at about the iliac crest and angled out to align parallel to the femoral neck is then tilted back about 15°–20° from the vertical. The tube is then angled 15°–20° from the horizontal toward the floor until the tube head and the IR are parallel to one another. Direct the CR to enter the anterior and medial side of the femoral neck.

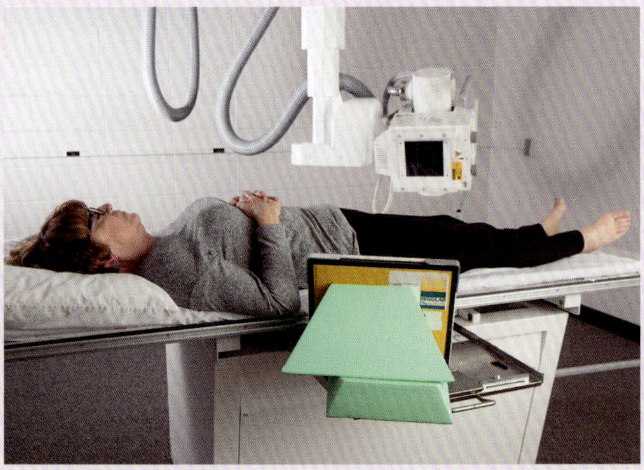

8-71 Modified Axiolateral projection—Clements–Nakayama method.

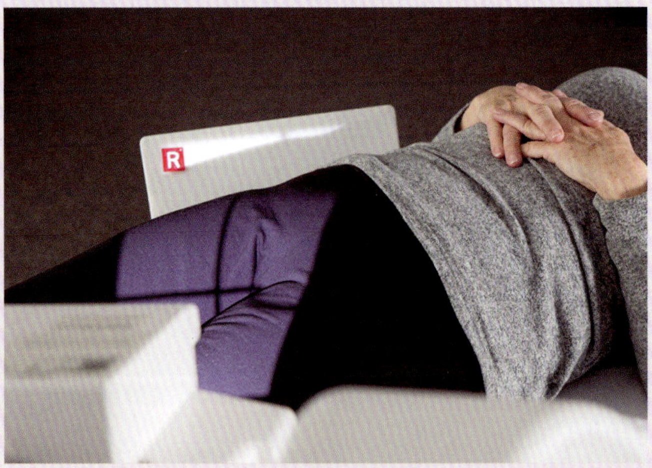

8-72 Modified Axiolateral projection—Clements–Nakayama method.

Trauma Femur (Nontrauma Femur Covered in Chapter 7)

- Projections: 2 AP's and 2 Laterals

Technical Considerations

- kVp 70–80
- mAs set manually
- 40″ SID

Exposure Field Size

- 10 × 12 lengthwise
- 14 × 17 lengthwise

Patient Position

- Patient supine
- Patient's leg remains in a neutral position

Centering (Figs. 8-73 to 8-76)

- AP Femur
  - Proximal femur: 10 × 12 LW centered to the femoral neck
  - Distal femur: 14 × 17 LW with the bottom of the IR positioned below the level of the knee joint and centered on the femur
- Lateral Femur
  - Proximal Femur: Acquire a Danelius–Miller method for the lateral hip
  - Distal Femur: With a horizontal beam, image the patient with a lateromedial or a mediolateral projection, depending on the situation, with the bottom of the IR positioned below the level of the knee joint and centered on the femur

Marking of IR

- Anatomic side marker R or L placed lateral to the part for the AP and anterior to the part for the lateral

Breathing

- Breathing should be suspended as imaging approaches the region of the pelvis. Instruct the patient to hold still
- Ensure patient holds position while walking away to make the exposure

Trauma Femur Protocol

AP Femur Proximal and Distal

Inferosuperior Axiolateral Proximal and

Lateromedial Distal

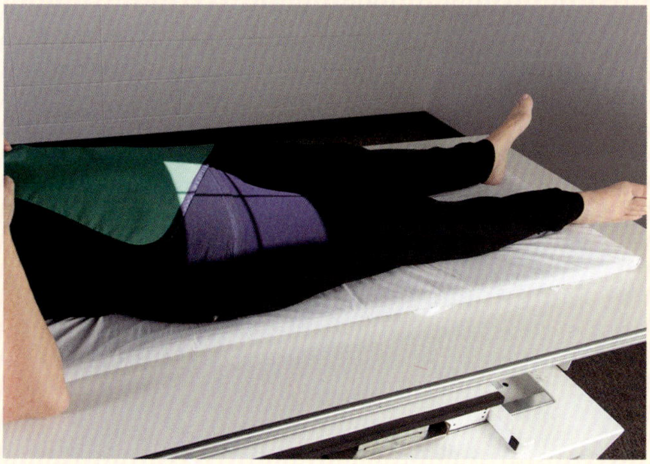

8-73 Trauma AP Proximal femur.

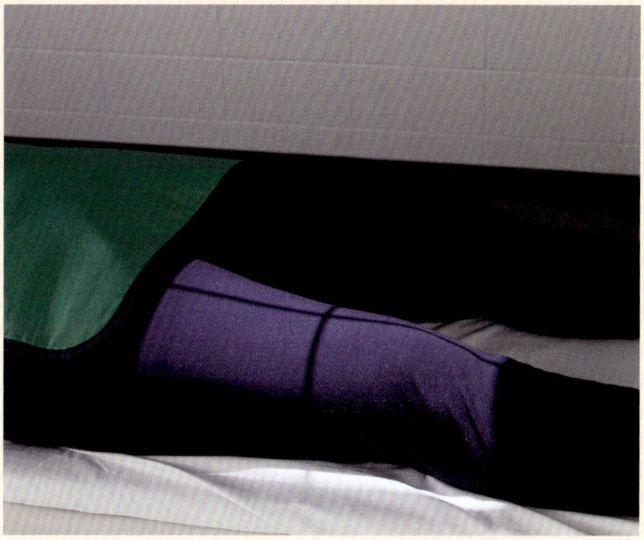

8-74 Trauma AP Distal femur.

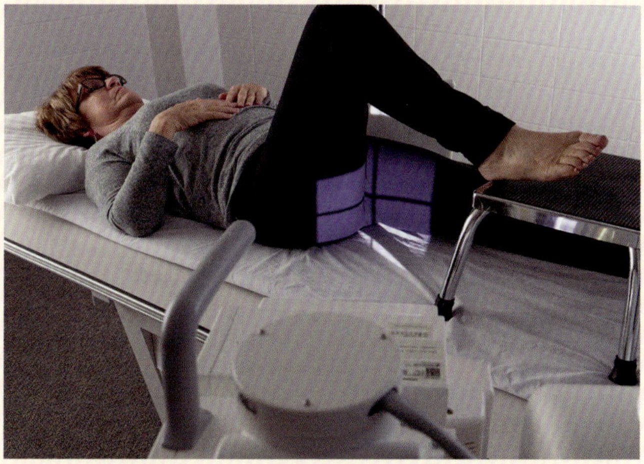

8-75 Inferosuperior axiolateral hip for proximal trauma femur.

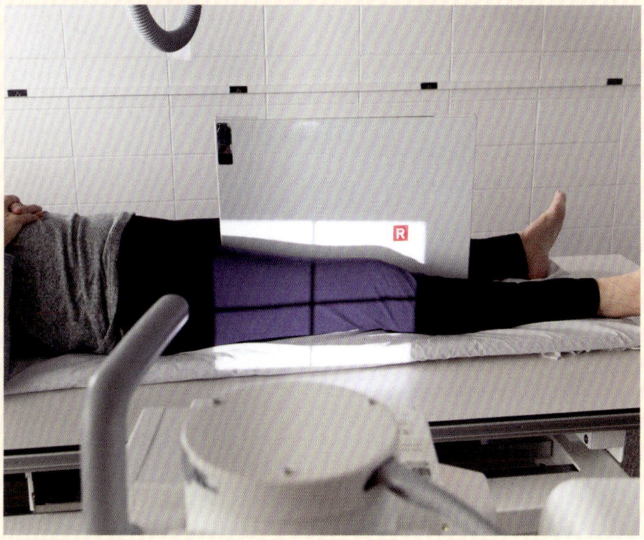

8-76 Lateromedial projection for distal trauma femur.

IMAGE CRITIQUE (FIGS. 8-77 to 8-80)

- Entire femur proximal to distal to include the knee and the hip joint within the collimated exposure field
- The AP proximal femur must include the hip joint. The greater and lesser trochanters will likely be visible with the patient's leg in a trauma leg position. The AP distal femur must include the knee joint and the majority of the femoral shaft
- The proximal lateral femur must include the hip joint with acceptable technical exposure. The greater and lesser trochanters will likely be visible with a trauma leg position. The distal lateral femur must include the knee joint. The femoral condyles will not directly superimpose because the trauma distal lateral femur is acquired with a perpendicular beam directed to the part

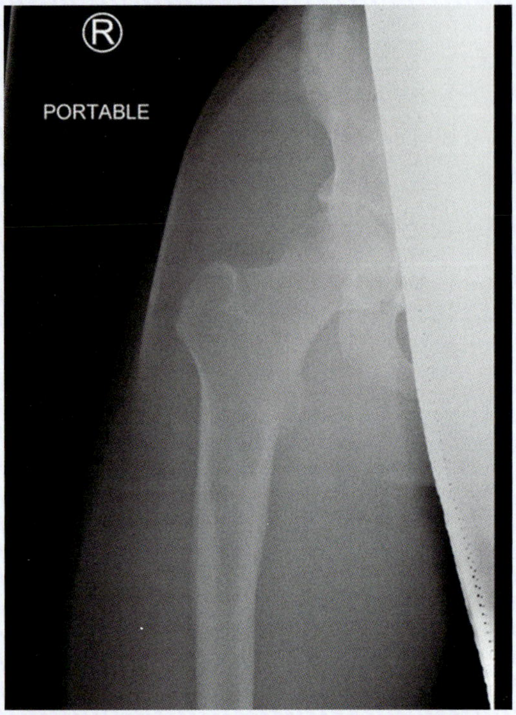

8-77 Trauma AP Proximal femur.

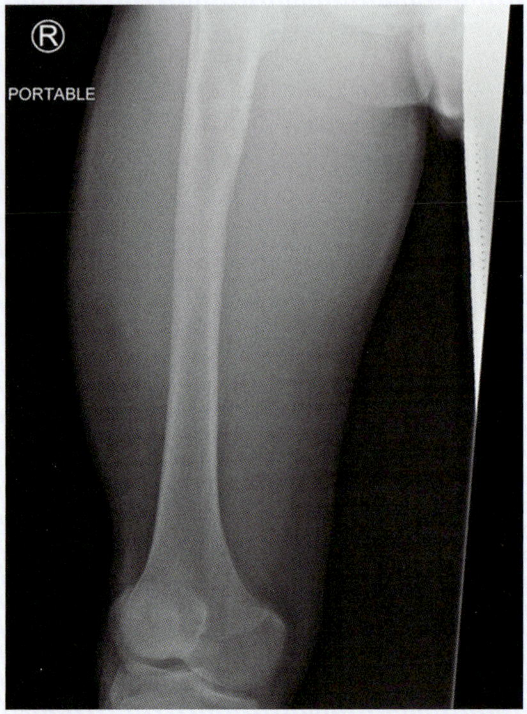

8-78 Trauma AP Distal femur.

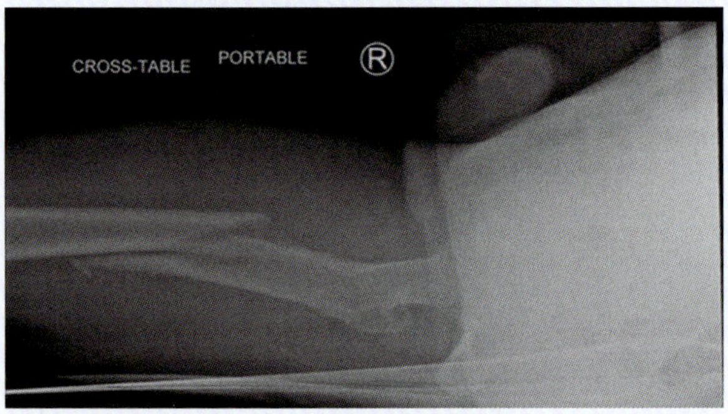

8-79 Inferosuperior axiolateral proximal femur.

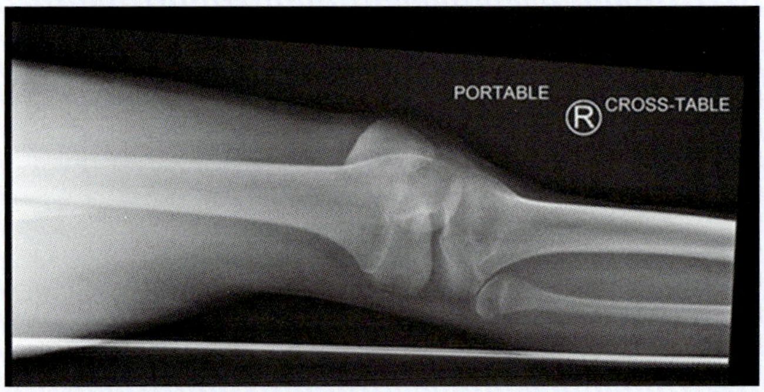

8-80 Lateromedial distal femur.

Pelvis

- Projection: AP Oblique
- Judet method

Technical Considerations
- kVp 75–85
- Center AEC cell selected for table Bucky
- 40″ SID

Exposure Field Size
- 10 × 12 lengthwise

Patient Position
- Supine with a 45° posterior oblique position of the torso and pelvis
- Both posterior obliques (RPO and LPO) are often acquired to provide a means of comparison

Centering
- The centering can be directed to the upside or downside hip. Centering on the upside or downside hip joint will better demonstrate either the anterior or the posterior rim of the acetabulum
  - *To demonstrate the anterior rim of the acetabulum*, the CR is directed 2″ medial and 2″ inferior to the ASIS closest to the IR (Fig. 8-81)
  - *To demonstrate the posterior rim of the acetabulum*, the CR is directed 2″ inferior to the ASIS furthest from the IR (Fig. 8-82)

Marking of IR
- Mark the side down or side closest to the IR

Breathing
- Suspend respiration
- Ensure patient holds position while walking away to make the exposure

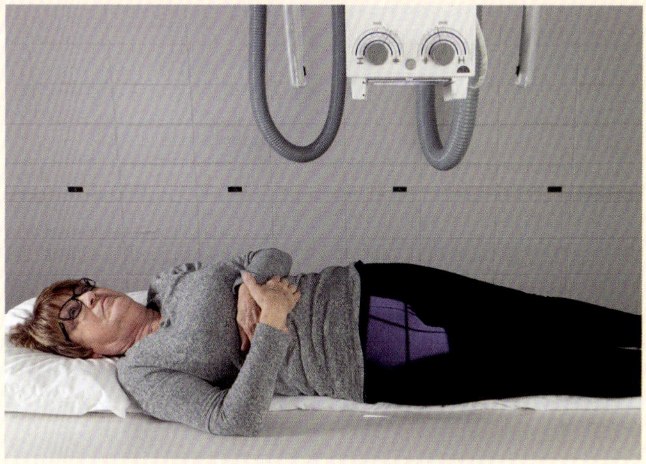

8-81 Judet method to demonstrate the anterior rim of the acetabulum.

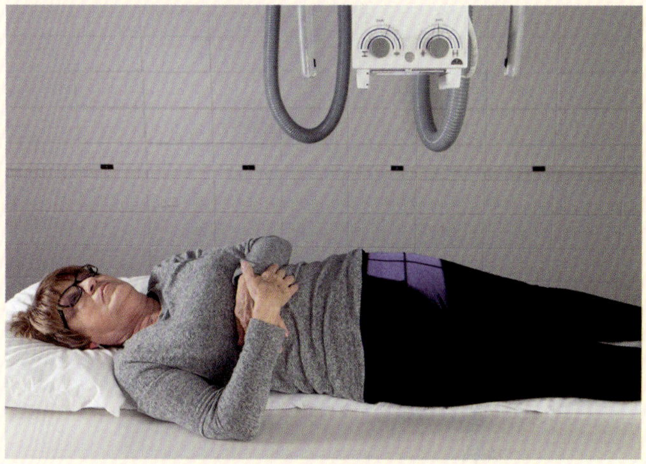

8-82 Judet method to demonstrate the posterior rim of the acetabulum.

IMAGE CRITIQUE (FIGS. 8-83 and 8-84)

- Correct obliquity of the patient is evidenced by an open joint space in between the femoral head and the anterior or posterior rim of the acetabulum
- When centering on the downside acetabulum, the iliac crest will appear flared open (Fig. 8-83)
- When centering on the upside acetabulum, the ASIS and the PSIS will superimpose on each other (Fig. 8-84)

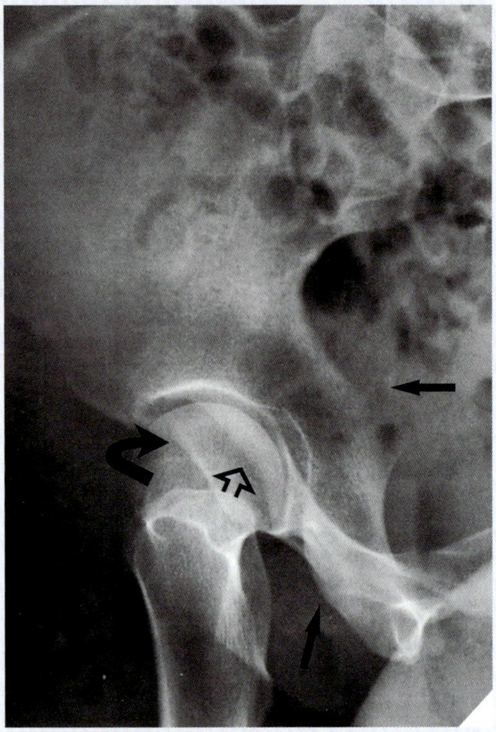

8-83 Centered on the downside ASIS to demonstrate the anterior acetabular rim (*curved arrow*). The open arrow represents the posterior acetabular rim. The solid arrows represent the iliopubic region.

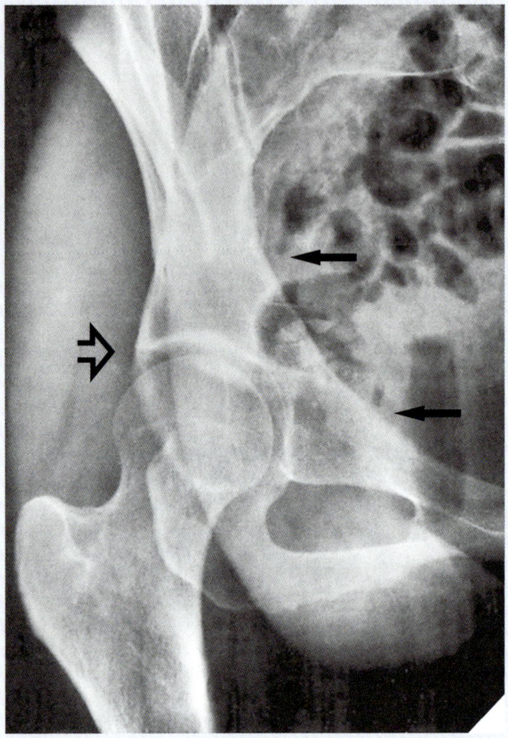

8-84 Centered on the upside ASIS to demonstrate the posterior acetabular rim (*open arrow*). The solid arrows represent the iliopubic region.

Pelvis

- Projection: AP Axial for Pelvic Outlet
- Taylor method to demonstrate the pelvic outlet demonstrating fracture or displacement of the pubic and ischial bones

Technical Considerations
- kVp 75–85
- Center AEC cell selected for table Bucky
- 40″ SID

Exposure Field Size
- 14 × 17 crosswise

Patient Position
- Supine with torso flat and free of rotation

Centering (Fig. 8-85)
- Angle the CR cephalic toward the pelvic outlet
  - For males 20°–35° cephalic
  - For females 30°–45° cephalic
- MSP with the central ray directed to enter 1″–2″ inferior to the symphysis pubis
- Collimation to include the inferior pelvis and proximal-most femoral heads and acetabulum is encouraged

Marking of IR
- Mark the right or left side

Breathing
- Suspend respiration
- Ensure patient holds position while walking away to make the exposure

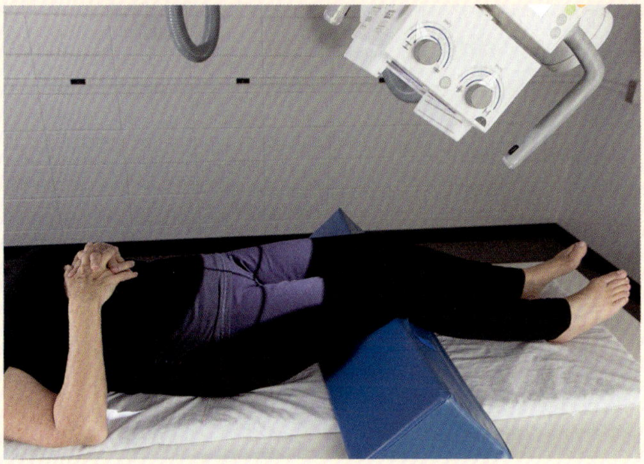

8-85 AP Axial for pelvic outlet.

IMAGE CRITIQUE (FIG. 8-86)

- Superior and inferior rami, ischial body, and ischial tuberosities are of interest
- The cephalic tube angle will elongate of the anatomy of interest

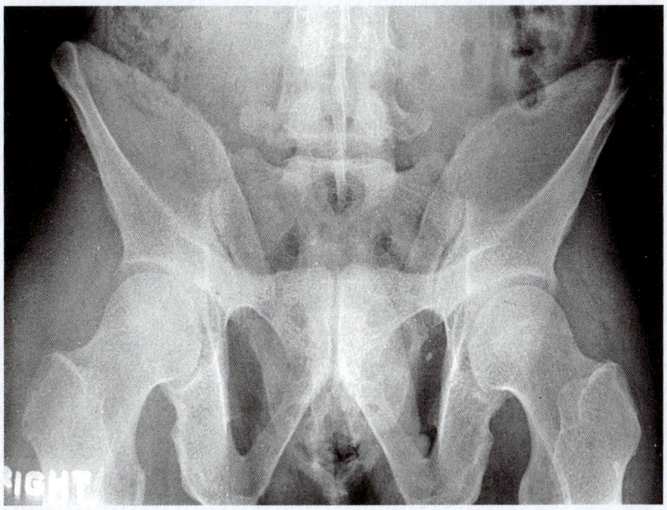

8-86 Pelvic outlet.

Pelvis

- Projection: AP Axial for Pelvic Inlet
- Bridgman method

Technical Considerations

- kVp 75–85
- Two outer cells AEC selected for table Bucky
- 40″ SID

Exposure Field Size

- 14 × 17 crosswise

Patient Position

- Supine with torso flat and free of rotation

Centering (Fig. 8-87)

- Angle the CR 40° caudal toward the pelvic inlet
- The CR is directed to MSP at the level of the ASIS

Marking of IR

- Mark the right or left side

Breathing

- Suspend respiration
- Ensure patient holds position while walking away to make the exposure

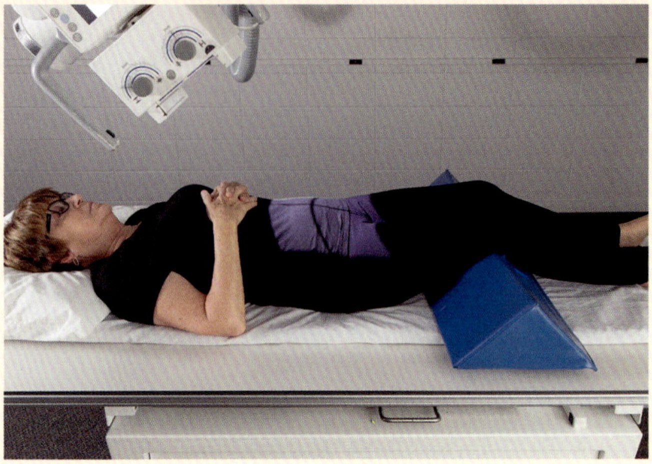

8-87 AP Axial for pelvic inlet.

IMAGE CRITIQUE (FIG. 8-88)

- The pelvic inlet from the sacral promontory to the symphysis pubis is demonstrated
- The ischial spines are visible and equally visible, indicating no rotation of the pelvis
- The caudal tube angle will create elongation of the anatomy of interest

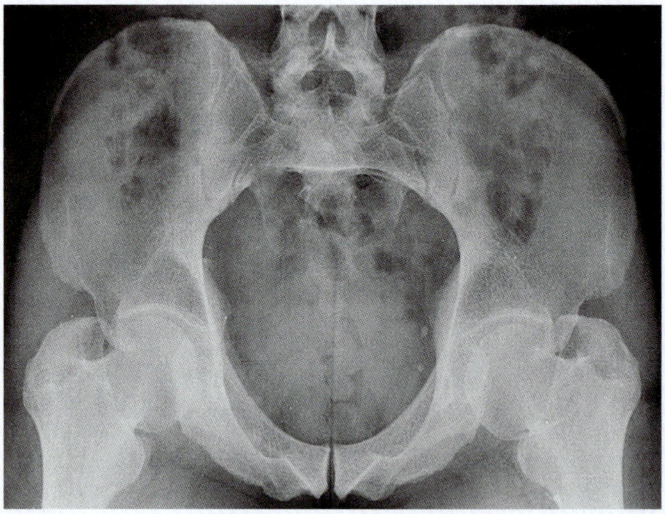

8-88 Pelvic inlet.

THE FINAL STEP: IMAGE REVIEW

The technologist must take time to review acquired images to ensure image quality is acceptable. The technologist must have the knowledge proper their role not only to acquire the images and care for the patient, but also to know how to review the images to ensure diagnostic quality has been attained. In certain instances, a projection may need to be repeated. This is left to the discretion of the radiologic technologist. The technologist should review each image for the following.

1. Is all of the necessary anatomy included on the image?
   - Was the central ray (CR) properly directed to the part? An "X" can be drawn to intersect within the collimated exposure field to determine whether the CR was directed to the correct location.
   - Was essential anatomy in the collimated exposure field?
   - Is the area free of artifact(s)?
2. Is the anatomy well demonstrated?
   - Did the technologist properly position the patient to adequately demonstrate the anatomy?
   - Can the technologist recognize the anatomy best demonstrated with use of different projections?
3. Does the image reflect proper image markings?
   - Did the technologist correctly use a lead marker to identify the right or left side?
   - What additional markings or annotations could be helpful to the radiologist interpreting the exam?
   - Is the image properly displayed?
4. Does the image prove to be technically acceptable?
   - Does the exposure index fall within acceptable range for the operating system? Images that are technically insufficient may appear of good quality if just slightly insufficient or "mottled or pixelated" if severely insufficient. Images that appear "mottled" should be repeated. Images that appear beyond optimal exposure owing to higher technique may display high quality, but the patient has received excessive radiation dose.

CRITICAL THINKING

1. In reference to the nontrauma AP pelvis (Fig. 8-89), which of the following correctly characterizes its results?
   1. The image appears correctly centered.
   2. The image appears with the CR directed slightly to superior.
   3. The image appears with the CR directed slightly to inferior.
   4. The image should pass.
   5. The image should fail.
      a. 1 and 4
      b. 1 and 5
      c. 2 and 4
      d. 2 and 5
      e. 3 and 4
      f. 3 and 5

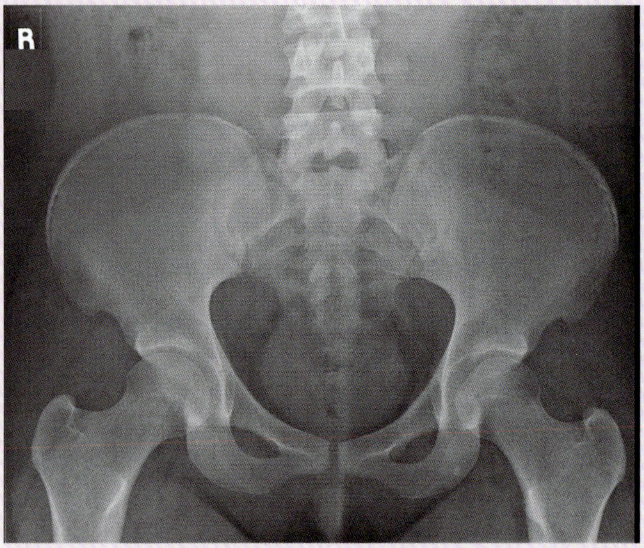

8-89

2. Referring to the nontrauma AP pelvis (Fig. 8-90), which of the following should the technologist consider?
   a. The technologist should pass the image because all criteria appear to be met.
   b. The technologist should repeat the image with lowered centering to include the entire right hip prosthesis.
   c. The technologist should repeat the image with higher centering to include the entire right hip prosthesis.
   d. The technologist should complement this AP pelvis with an AP hip image with centering potentially adjusted to ensure the entire prosthesis is included.

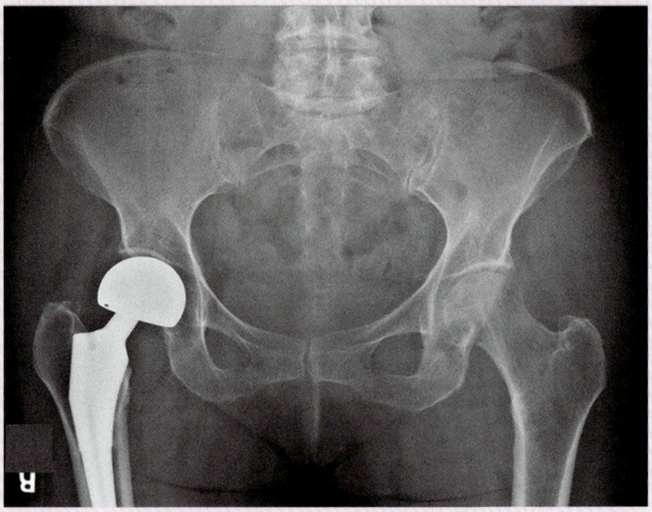

8-90

3. Referring to the nontrauma AP pelvis (Fig. 8-91), which of the following could the technologist consider in an effort to improve the overall technical quality of the image?
   a. The image is sufficient, nothing to consider.
   b. The technologist could decrease the technical factors.
   c. The technologist could have the patient pull lower abdominal tissue up toward their head.
   d. The technologist could have the patient lie prone to decrease the tissue thickness.

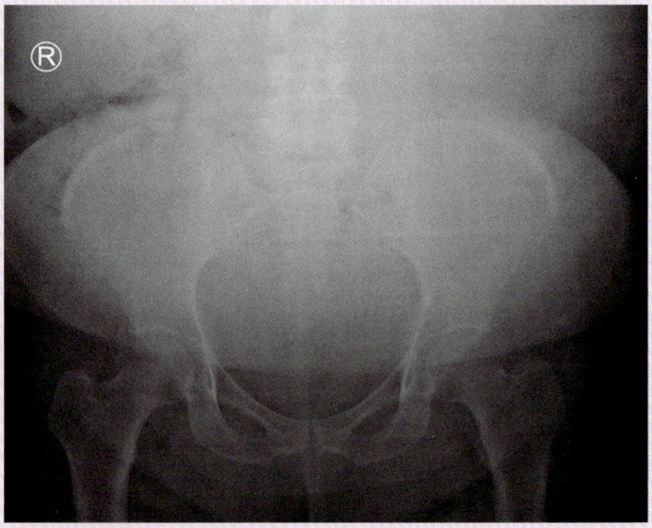

8-91

4. In reference to the inferosuperior axiolateral hip (Fig. 8-92), which of the following could the technologist consider in an effort to improve the overall technical quality of the image?
  a. The image is sufficient, nothing to consider.
  b. Ensure the central ray is directed to the femoral neck.
  c. Ensure the tube and the grid are aligned.
  d. Increase collimation.

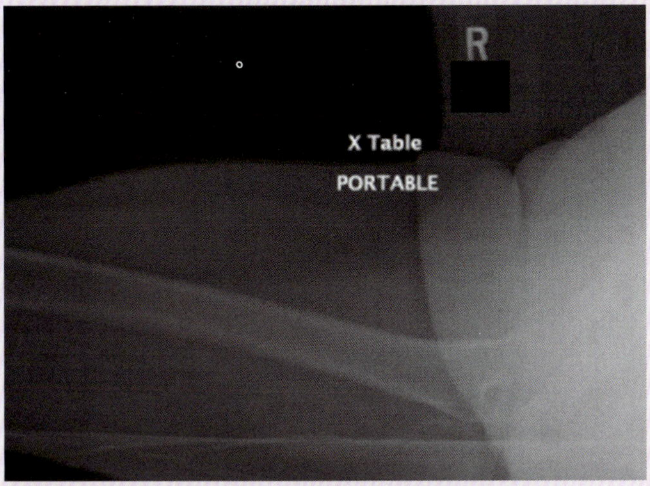

8-92

5. In reference to the nontrauma AP hip (Fig. 8-93), which of the following should the technologist consider?
  a. The technologist should pass the image because all image criteria are met.
  b. The technologist should repeat the image because the leg was not internally rotated.
  c. The technologist should repeat the image ensuring rotation of the pelvis has been eliminated.
  d. The technologist should repeat the image because the centering is incorrectly directed to the level of the femoral neck.

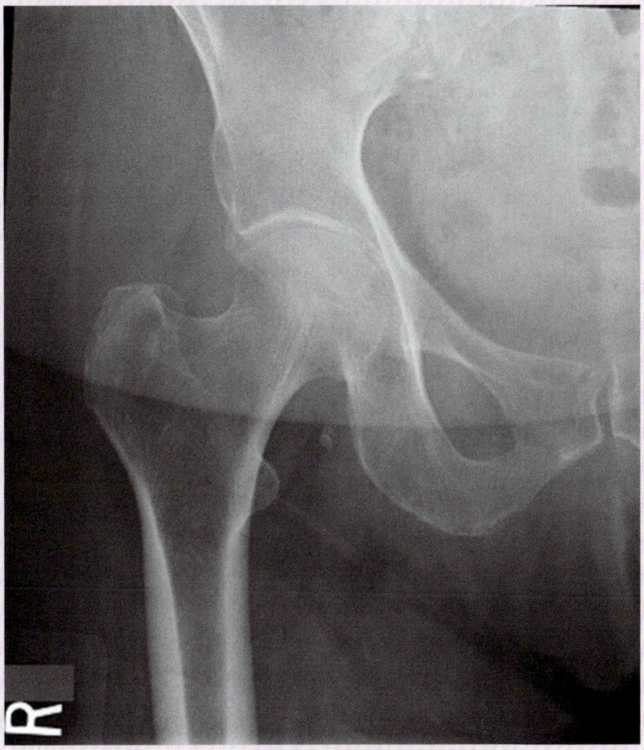

8-93

ANSWERS TO THE CRITICAL THINKING QUESTIONS

1. d
2. d
3. c
4. b
5. b

CHAPTER 9 Vertebral Column

Imaging of the vertebral column will include nontrauma and trauma patient situations. The technologist needs a proficient understanding of nontrauma protocols and the ability to critically think to modify protocols in instances of patient limitations and trauma. Imaging of the spine will extend beyond outpatient imaging. Patients will be encountered in the emergency department, the operating room, and/or PACU.

CLINICAL INDICATIONS

Indications are the symptomatic reasons as to why a particular exam may be ordered by the physician. The technologist should look at the clinical indications before performing a procedure. The following briefly introduces common exam indications, but it is not an all-encompassing list. In certain circumstances, the indication may influence the need to increase or decrease the technical settings.

Jefferson's Fracture: Fracture to both the anterior and the posterior arches of C1. Stability of this fracture will determine the treatment of the patient (Fig. 9-1).

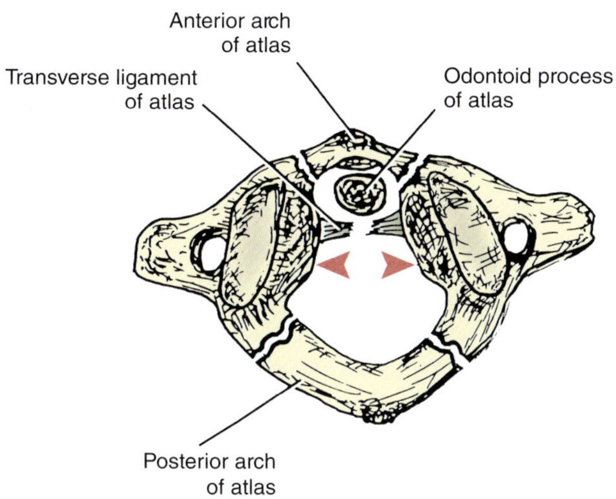

9-1 Jefferson fracture. Arrowheads represent lateral masses of C1.

Hangman Fracture: Extreme hyperextension of the neck as implied with the term *hangman* causing fracture through the C2 pedicles. This hyperextension may result in anterior subluxation of C2–C3, injuring the cord (Fig. 9-2).

Subluxation: The shift (dislocation) of a vertebra out of its normal alignment in the succession of the vertebral column. Subluxation is identified on a lateral projection (Fig. 9-3).

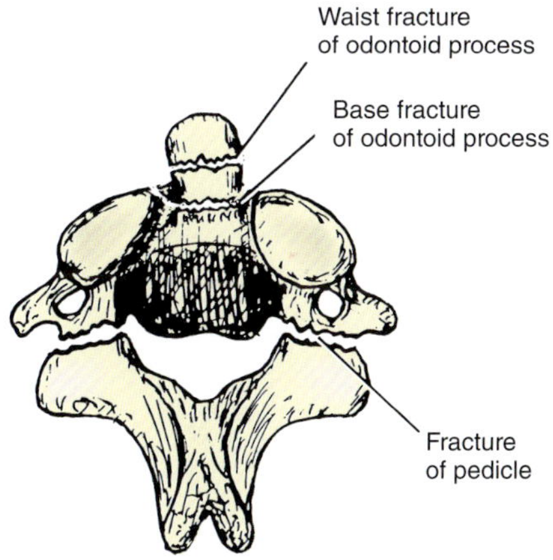

9-2 Hangman's fracture.

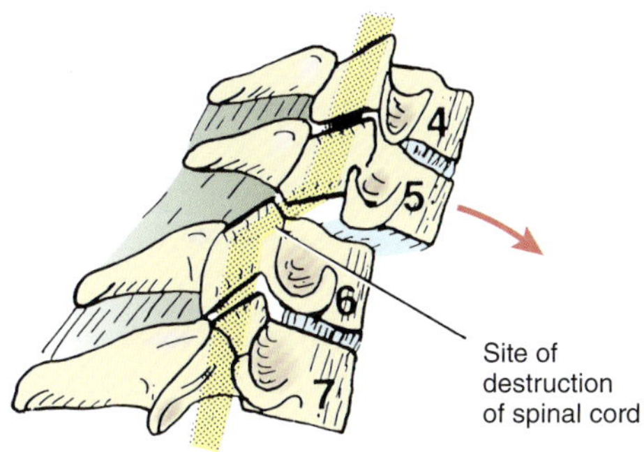

9-3 Subluxation.

Compression Fracture: The vertebral body loses its normal height and appears wedge-shaped or compacted. This is most easily noticed in a lateral view of the vertebral column. The thoracic and lumbar bodies are most commonly affected (Fig. 9-4).

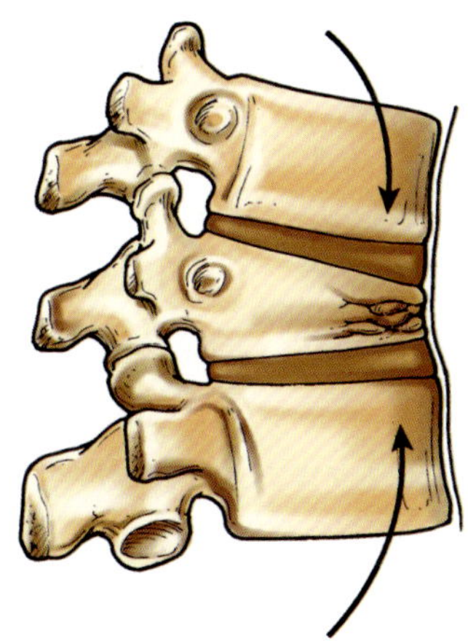

9-4 Compression fracture.

Osteoporosis: A loss of bone density over time typically associated with age, loss of estrogen (postmenopausal women), lifestyle considerations, and, possibly, with long-term use of certain medications. Patients with advanced osteoporosis will require a decrease in technical factors (Fig. 9-5).

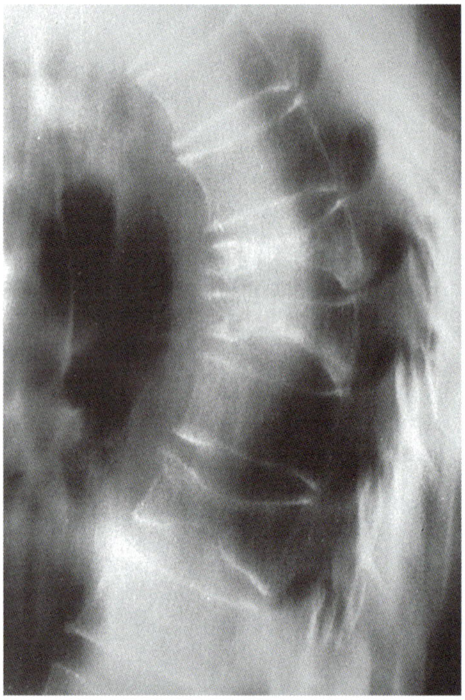

9-5 Compression fracture secondary to osteoporosis.

Osteoarthritis: A form of degenerative disease of the joint(s) resulting in patients experiencing pain and reduced joint mobility. This condition may reveal the presence of osteophytes on the vertebral bodies (Fig. 9-6).

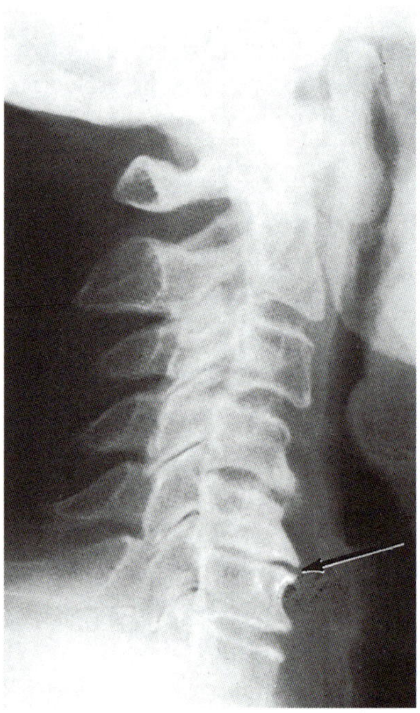

9-6 Osteophytes (arrow) of vertebral bodies reveals osteoarthritis.

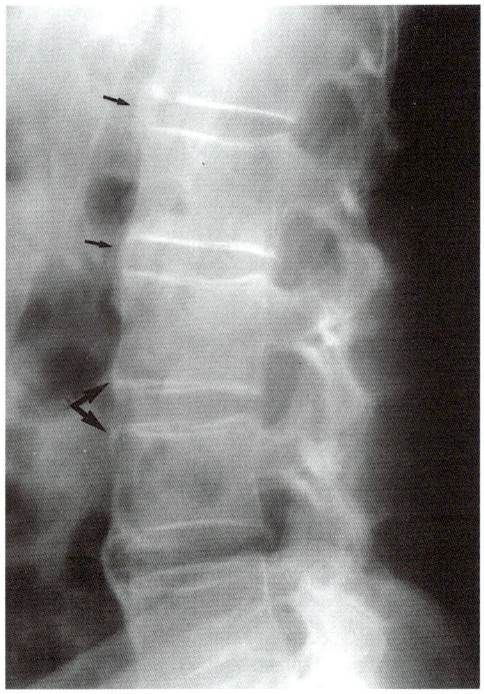

9-7 Spondylitis reveals bone erosion present at the margins of the vertebral bodies (large arrows). Small arrows represent hardening of the anterior intervertebral disks.

Spondylitis: Vertebral inflammation (Fig. 9-7).

Spondylolysis: A fracture to one or both pars interarticularis on a lumbar vertebra (Fig. 9-8).

Spondylolisthesis: Develops as a result of a defect in the pars interarticularis or from degenerative bone conditions, causing an anterior subluxation (shift) of a vertebra. This commonly affects the L5–S1 or L4–L5 location. This condition may be asymptomatic or may cause symptoms in the lower back, buttocks, and legs if more severe. Surgical fusion may be necessary in severe cases (Fig. 9-9).

Sciatica: Inflammation of the sciatic nerve that causes lower back pain and often pain down a buttock and leg. This condition may be associated with a herniated disk (Fig. 9-10).

Spinal Fusion: Added stability between vertebral bodies by connecting them surgically and permanently.

Spina Bifida: A congenital condition that results when the laminar portions of the lumbar fail to fuse and close off the posterior vertebral arch. The spinal meninges may herniate outside of the vertebral column of variable severity. This condition is most commonly seen at the L5 location (Fig. 9-11).

Herniated Disk: A condition in which the jellylike center of a disk herniates out of its protective outer shell (annulus fibrosis) and is most commonly seen in the lower lumbar division. This condition may cause symptomatic pain such as sciatica (Fig. 9-12).

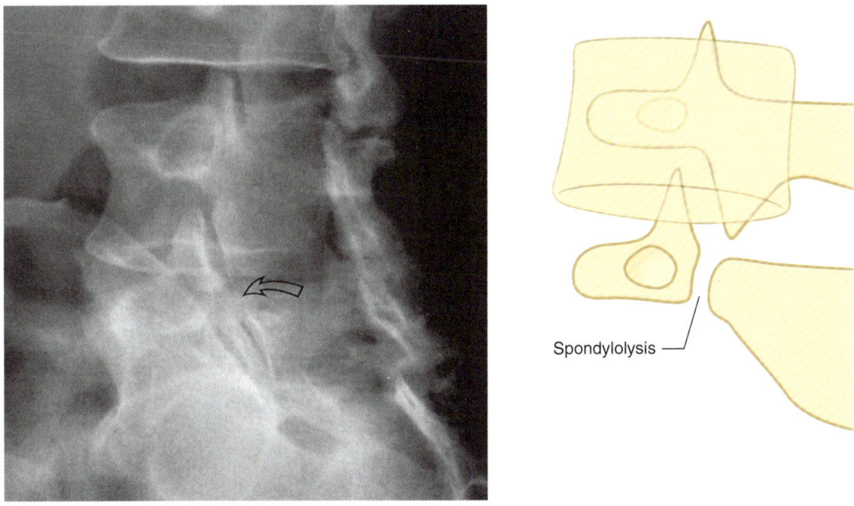

9-8 Spondylolysis presents as a defect within the pars interarticularis. Arrow represents the defect within the pars interarticularis.

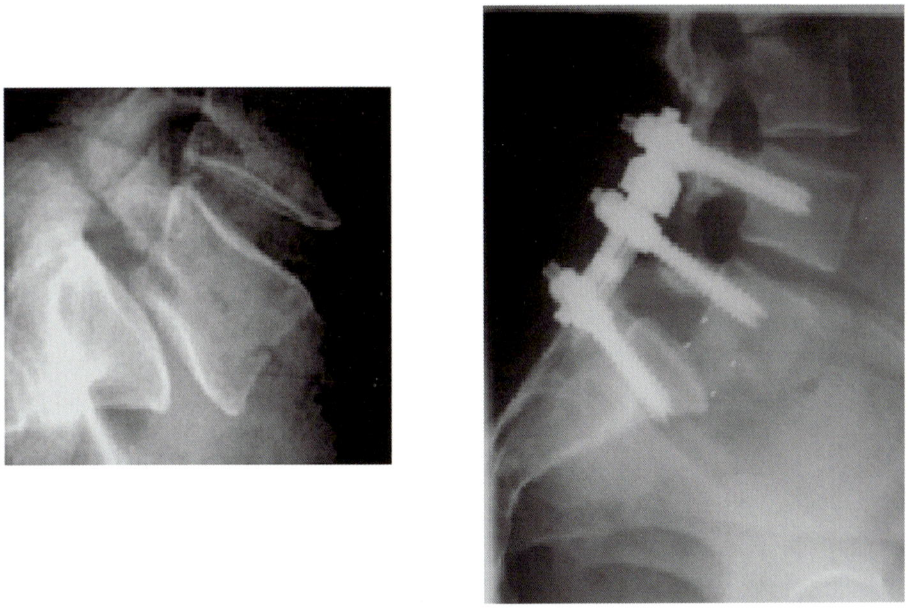

9-9 Spondylolisthesis reveals a point of vertebral subluxation that may require surgical fusion for vertebral stability.

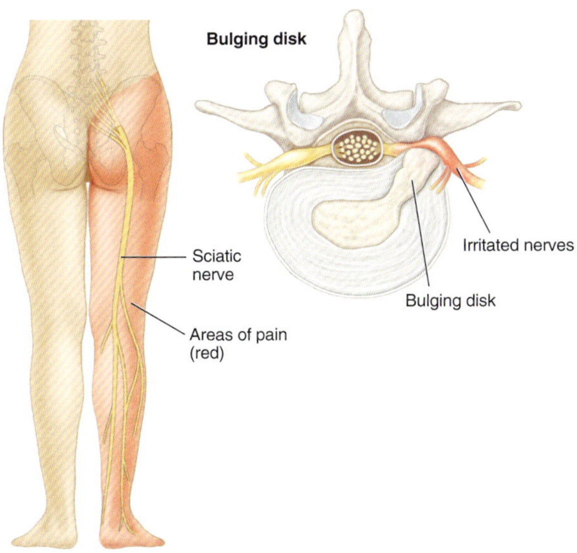

9-10 Sciatica.

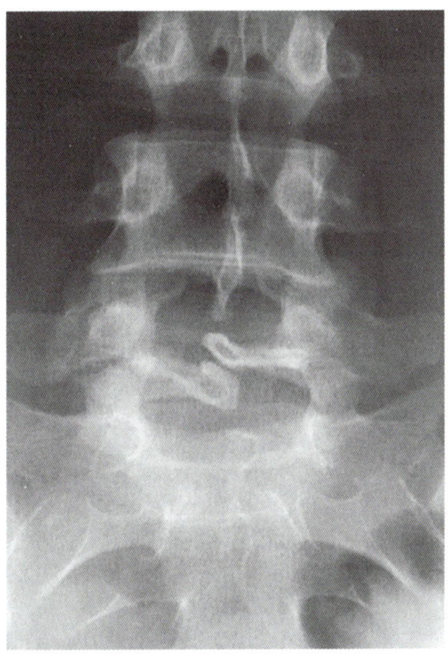

9-11 Spina bifida.

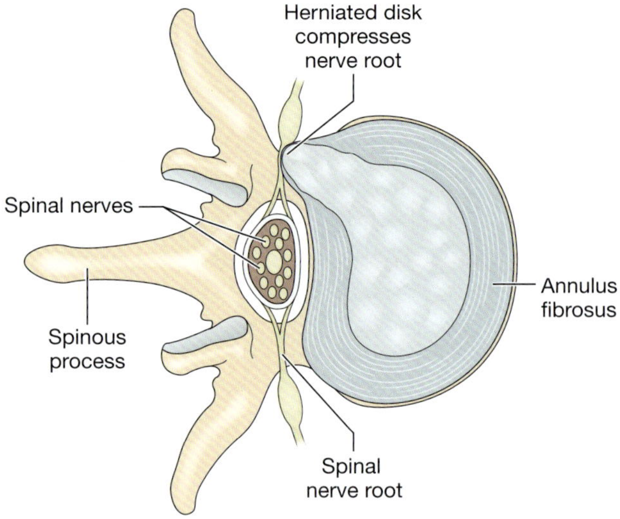

9-12 Herniated disk.

Laminectomy: The surgical removal of the laminar portions of the vertebral arch performed to potentially relieve pressure on the cord caused by vertebral stenosis, herniated intervertebral disk, or abnormal growths (Fig. 9-13).

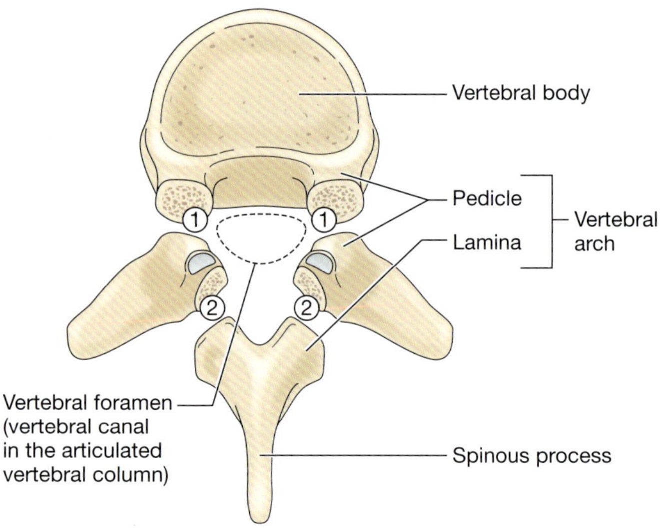

9-13 Laminectomy.

Kyphosis: An abnormal exaggerated convex curvature that affects the thoracic spine. This condition is typically a result of osteoporosis and is seen more commonly in postmenopausal women. Compression fractures may accompany this kyphotic condition. Patients with kyphosis will exhibit a degree of "hunchback" stature, which in some individuals is more pronounced than in others (Fig. 9-14).

Lordosis: An abnormal exaggerated concave curvature that affects the lumbar spine. This condition is typically a result of poor posture, pregnancy, or excess abdominal weight (Fig. 9-14).

Scoliosis: Severe lateral curvature that can affect the thoracic and lumbar spine, which may affect the position of the pelvis as well. This condition is most associated with adolescents and females (Fig. 9-14).

IMAGING CONSIDERATIONS

Patient Dress

Patient will need to remove all clothing from the region of the spine being imaged and remove jewelry from the area of interest (Fig. 9-15). Elastic bands in pants, underwear, and sports bras can create distracting lines and creases on the image that may overlie vertebral anatomy. Female patients should be instructed to remove their bras if it will interfere with the field of interest. The patient should dress into a gown when imaging the thoracic or lumbar region of the spine. For patients already dressed in a hospital gown, the radiographer should still check the area of interest to ensure it is free of artifact before imaging. When imaging in the region of the cervical spine, patients wearing assistive aids such as eyeglasses or hearing aids, will have to remove them prior to making the exposure. Assistive aids should be the very last thing removed after the technologist explains the exam to the patient and answers any questions they may have.

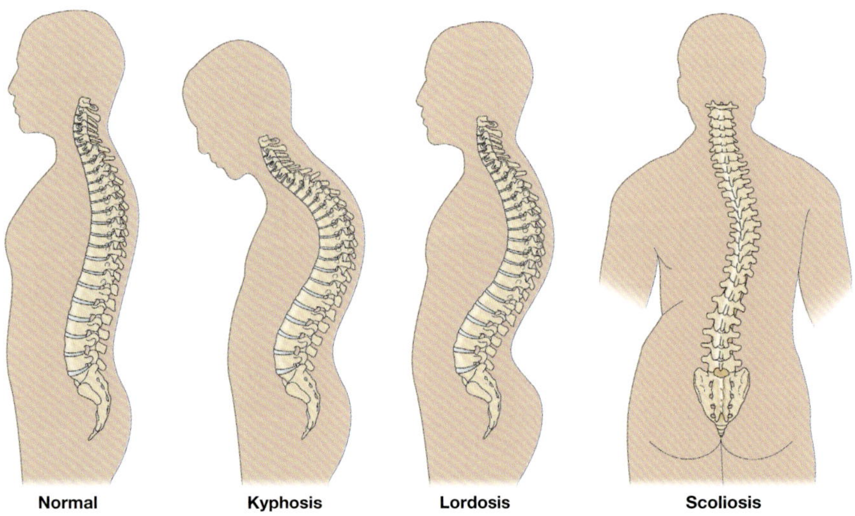

9-14 Abnormal curvatures of the spine.

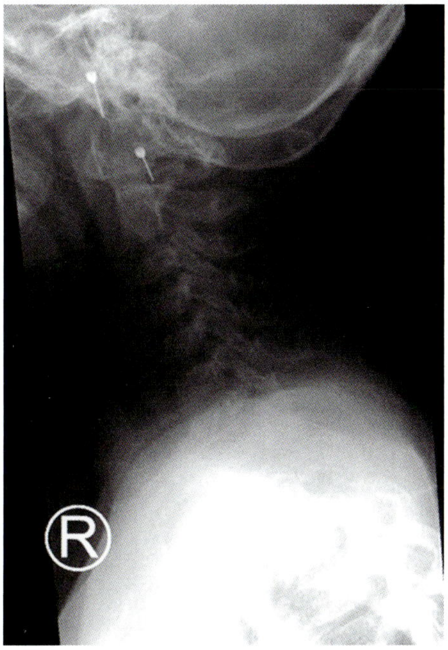

9-15 Earring(s) artifact.

Artifacts

Artifacts are unwanted objects that appear on the image superimposing pertinent anatomy. This includes snaps, buttons, bras, and jewelry. Other artifacts that may appear could be intravenous (IV) lines, electrocardiogram (ECG) patches, oxygen tubing, or safety pins that may secure a line to the patient's gown. The radiographer should assess the patient's lines and tubing, pins, snaps, etc., and try to reposition to avoid obscuring the spine anatomy (Figs. 9-16 and 9-17). This could be encountered with trauma patients and postsurgical patients. Considering the higher detail attained with digital imaging, clothing components such as waist bands, pockets, thick seams, and embroidery stitching may constitute a repeat image.

Patient Position

The general position of the patient or part.

Upright—Relative to this chapter, this position is implemented when imaging orders declare the patient to be weight-bearing such as for lumbar spine and scoliosis. Nontrauma cervical spine is typically imaged upright because it will allow for the longer source-to-image distance (SID) necessary to compensate for the object-to-image distance (OID) created between the neck and the image receptor (IR).

Recumbent—Applicable to imaging certain divisions of the spine or in instances in which the patient is not stable enough to stand erect.

Ambulatory Patient Imaging

An ambulatory patient is one who can maneuver themselves and bear weight with little to no assistance. Ambulatory patients will be able to walk or may come by wheelchair to the exam room. Patients transported by stretcher will be transferred over to the imaging table.

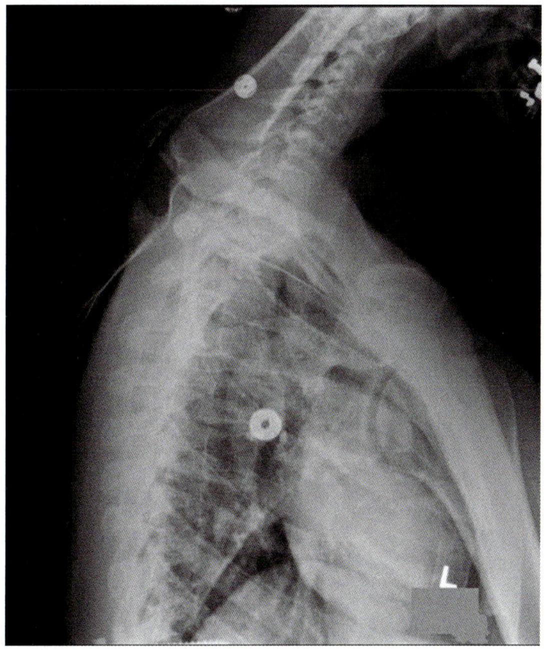

9-16 Gown snaps.

Projection(s)

How the x-ray beam passes through the part.

- Anteroposterior (AP): The beam is directed to enter through the anterior surface, exit the posterior surface, and strike the IR.
- AP Axial: The beam is directed to enter through the anterior surface and exit the posterior surface with the use of a tube angle.
- Posteroanterior (PA): The beam is directed to enter the posterior surface, exit the anterior surface, and strike the IR.
- AP Axial Oblique: The beam is directed to enter the anterior surface and exit the posterior surface while the part is positioned into a particular degree of obliquity with the use of an applied tube angle.

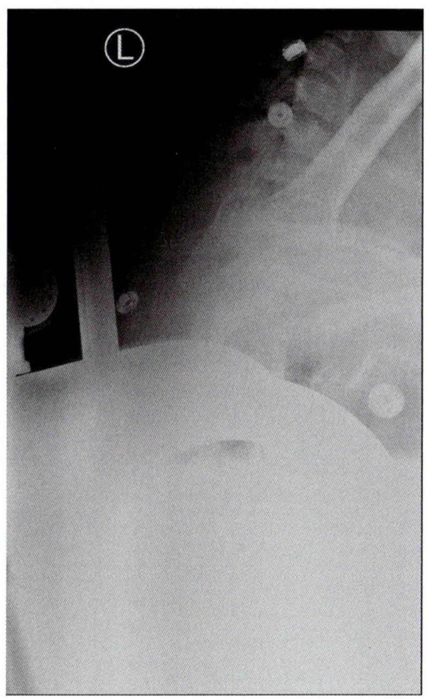

9-17 Artifact from patient gown. Wheelchair also noted within image exposure field.

- PA Axial Oblique: The beam is directed to enter the posterior surface and exit the anterior surface while the part is positioned into a particular degree of obliquity with the use of an applied tube angle.
- Lateral: The beam will enter the lateral surface and exit the lateral surface of the torso.

ANATOMY

Imaging the vertebral column includes cervical, thoracic, lumbar, and sacral and coccyx divisions of the vertebral column. There are 7 cervical vertebrae, 12 thoracic vertebrae, 5 lumbar vertebrae, 1 sacrum, and 1 coccyx in the adult vertebral column (Fig. 9-18). There are a total of 26 bones within the adult vertebral column. The column consists of concave and convex curvatures to increase the strength and support of the column (Fig. 9-19). The concave curvatures are the cervical and lumbar divisions, whereas the convex curvatures are the thoracic and sacral divisions. Formation of these curvatures begins in infancy and transform as the infant develops to hold their head up, sit up, crawl, and eventually walk (Fig. 9-20).

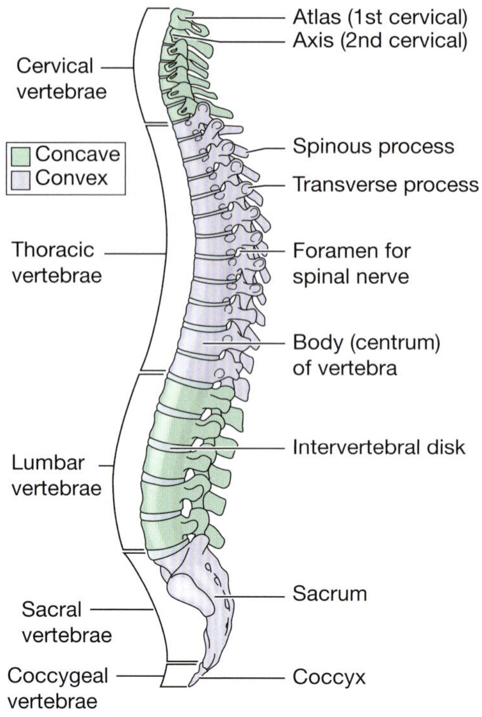

9-19 Concave and convex curvatures of the spine.

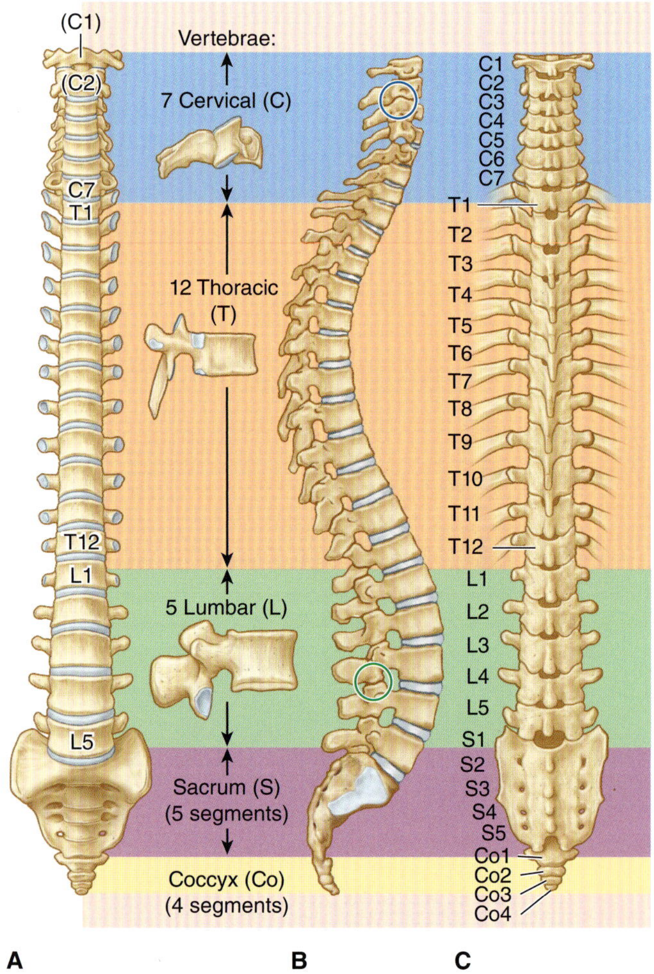

9-18 Divisions of the vertebral column. **A:** Anterior view. **B:** Lateral view. **C:** Posterior view with vertebral ends of ribs.

Typical Vertebral Anatomy

The vertebrae within the thoracic and lumbar divisions resemble each other, with similar anatomy and the formation of significant anatomic structures.

Vertebral Body

The vertebral body is the weight-bearing portion of the vertebra. The vertebral bodies increase in size as they progress down the column from the cervical division. Above and

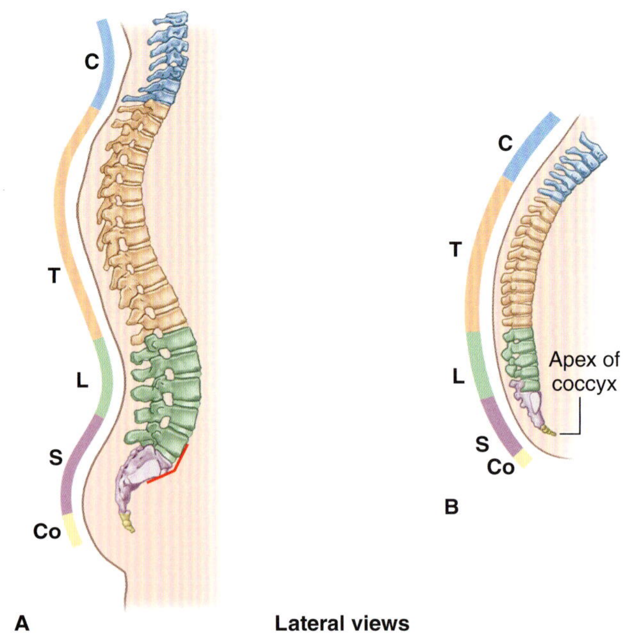

9-20 Curvature development from infancy. **A:** Adult. **B:** Fetus.

below each vertebral body an intervertebral disk is found to act as a cushion and shock absorber in between the vertebrae (Fig. 9-21).

Intervertebral Disks

Intervertebral disks have two main components. The center of the disk is the nucleus pulposis. Its soft center is contained by the protective outer shell referred to as the annulus fibrosis. Herniation of the nucleus pulposis through the annulus fibrosis is more common in the lumbar division, given its weight-bearing responsibilities (Fig. 9-21). Patients suffering from a herniated disk experience lower back pain that may also cause pain down the buttock and leg. Diagnosis of the condition may start with radiographic imaging of the lumbar spine, but magnetic resonance imaging (MRI) is often a better alternative.

Vertebral Arch

The vertebral arch extends off the posterior aspect of the vertebral body. The lateral sides of the arch are framed in by the right and left pedicles. The posterior portion of the arch is framed by the right and left laminae. The formation of the bony vertebral arch creates the opening or vertebral foramen, which allows for the passage of the spinal cord (Fig. 9-22).

Pedicles

The pedicles are the first bony structures to extend posteriorly off each lateral-most edge of the posterior vertebral body. There is a right and a left pedicle. On the superior border of the pedicle, a superior vertebral notch is noted, whereas on the inferior border of the pedicle an inferior vertebral arch is noted. The inferior vertebral arch is more pronounced than the superior vertebral notch (Fig. 9-23). The significance of the superior and inferior vertebral notches is that when the vertebral bodies are stacked together in succession, the notches align to form an intervertebral (in between the vertebrae) foramen (Fig. 9-23). There is a right intervertebral and a left intervertebral foramen between each vertebra. Intervertebral foramina serve as a route for nerves and vessels to travel.

Lamina

The lamina closes off the back side of the vertebra arch. Fusion of the right and left laminae will form the midline posterior bony extension known as the spinous process (Fig. 9-24). Failure of the laminae to fuse together can result in a pathologic condition known as spina bifida.

Transverse Process

With the union of a pedicle and a lamina, the bony lateral extension, known as the transverse process, projects off each side of the vertebra. The transverse processes serve as a site for muscles to attach (Fig. 9-24).

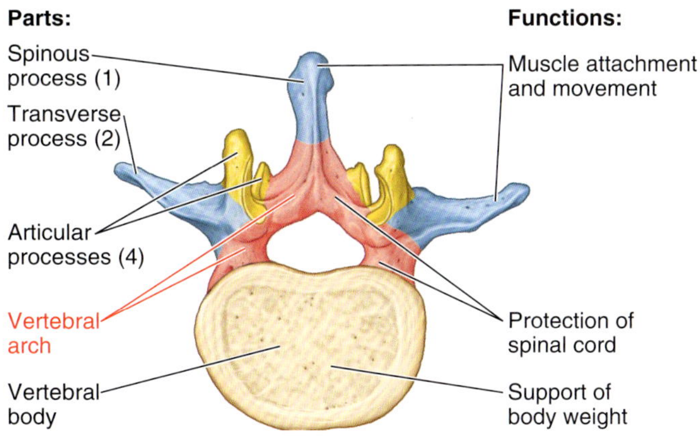

9-22 Vertebral body and vertebral arch.

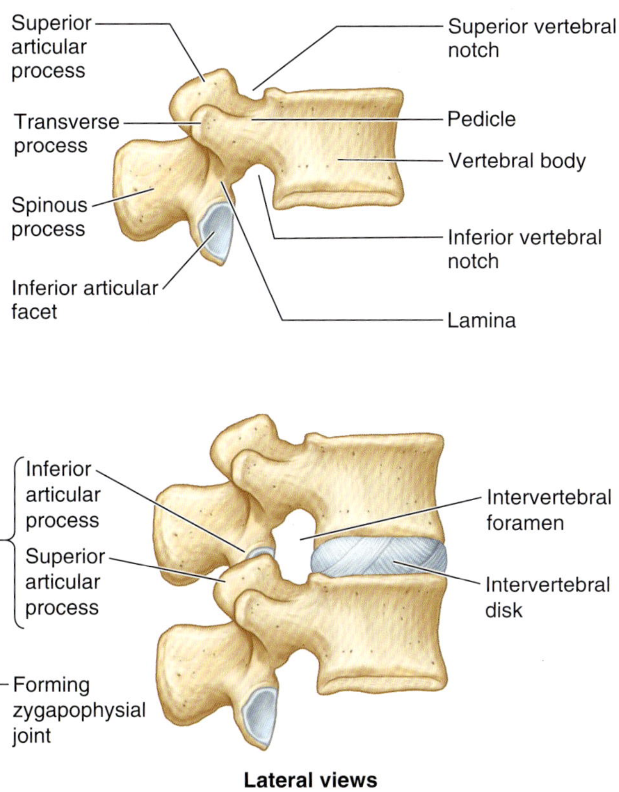

9-23 Pedicles contribute to the formation of the intervertebral foramen (*foramina*).

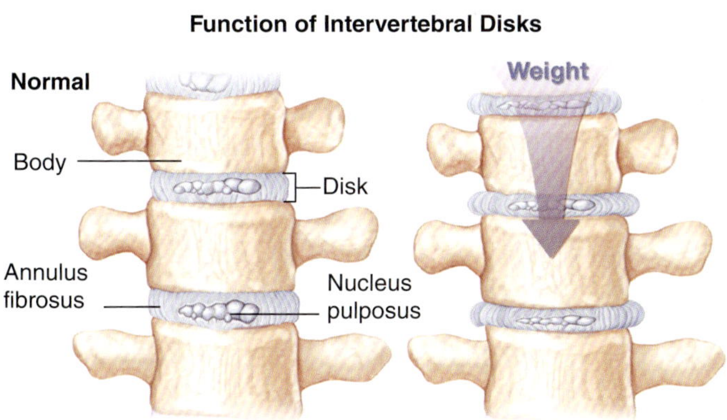

9-21 Intervertebral disks.

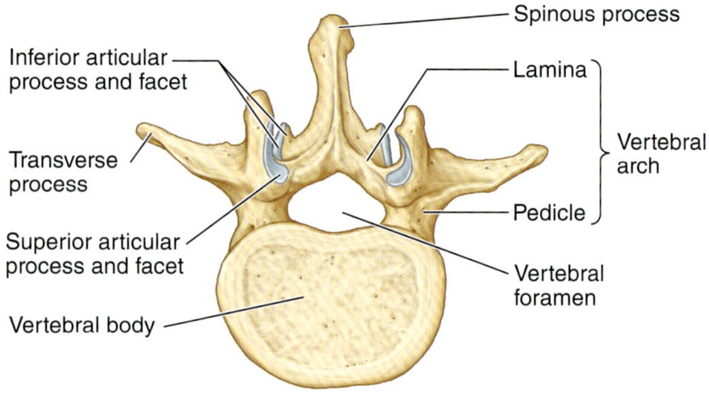

9-24 Superior view of the vertebra.

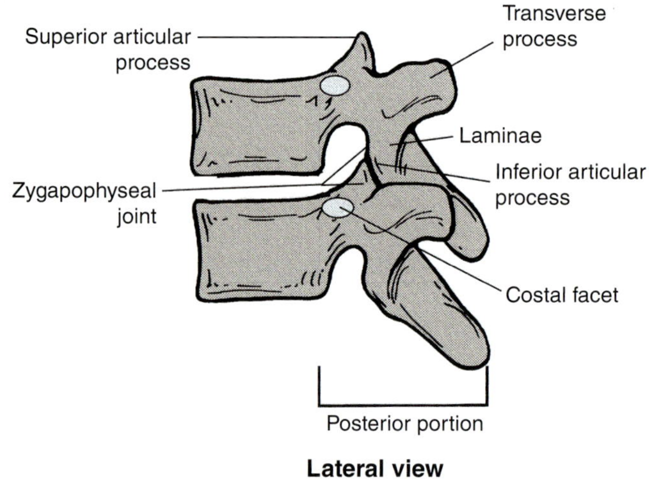

9-26 Stacking of the vertebral bodies allows superior and inferior articular processes to form the zygapophyseal joints.

Superior and Inferior Articular Processes

A superior articular process and an inferior articular process extend, respectively, at the junction point of the pedicle and lamina. Each vertebra has two superior articular processes and two inferior articular processes (Fig. 9-25). When a superior articular process meets an inferior articular process, a zygapophyseal joint is formed. A right and a left zygapophyseal joint exist between each vertebra (Fig. 9-26).

Cervical Vertebral Anatomy

The cervical vertebrae are the smallest and most atypical in shape. The articulation of these atypical characteristics allows for range of movement, including flexion, extension, and rotation of the neck. C1 and C2 are very different from one another. Cervical vertebrae three through six are similar to one another, and the seventh cervical vertebra begins to resemble the first thoracic vertebra (Fig. 9-18).

C1-Atlas

The first cervical vertebra lacks the typical vertebral structures such as the body, pedicles, and laminae. C1 is comprised of an anterior arch and a posterior arch, each with a tubercle. The lateral-most sides are referred to as the lateral masses. The lateral masses are thick and supportive to accommodate the weight of the skull. Extending laterally off each lateral mass is the transverse process. The transverse process contains a transverse foramen that allows for passage of the vertebral arteries, veins, and nerves (Fig. 9-27). On the superior aspect of the lateral masses, the superior articular facets accept the occipital condyles to form the atlantooccipital joints. On the inferior aspect of the lateral masses, the inferior articular processes will articulate with the superior articular processes of C2 to form a right and a left zygapophyseal joint (Fig. 9-28).

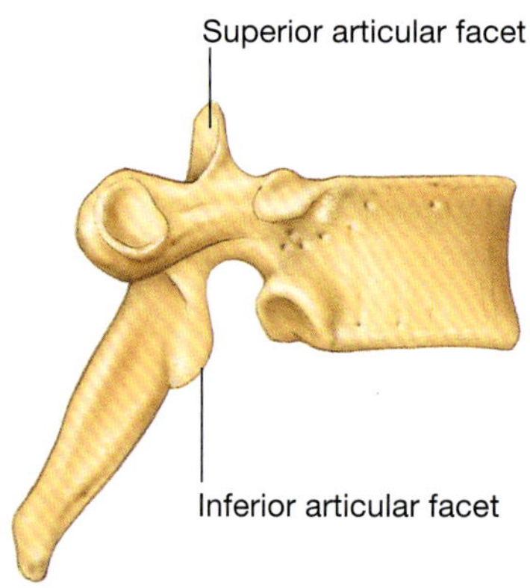

9-25 Lateral view of the vertebra.

C2-Axis

The second cervical vertebra has the largest body of all cervical vertebrae because it contains its original body along with the odontoid process or dens fused superior to its body. The odontoid process fits behind the anterior arch of C1 and is secured by the transverse ligament, which passes behind it to help stabilize it into place (Fig. 9-29). C2 possesses pedicles and laminae. At the junction of the pedicle with each side of the body, a transverse process originates that contains a transverse foramen. The right and left laminae close off the posterior portion of the vertebral arch. The spinous processes on C2–C6 have a bifid (split) tip (Fig. 9-30). The superior articular processes sit slightly more anterior than the inferior articular processes (Fig. 9-31). Considering the anatomic differences and articulation of C1 and C2, the zygapophyseal joints are seen only through the AP open mouth projection (Fig. 9-32).

C3–C7

The third through the seventh cervical vertebrae all have similar characteristics to one another. As with C2, the transverse processes arise from the junction of each pedicle to the body. The transverse processes all contain transverse foramina. The transverse foramen allows for the passage of the vertebral artery, vein, and nerves (Fig. 9-33). The laminae close off the posterior vertebral arch and give rise to the spinous process, which terminates in a bifid tip, with the exception of C7 (Fig. 9-34). The spinous process of C7 resembles the spinous

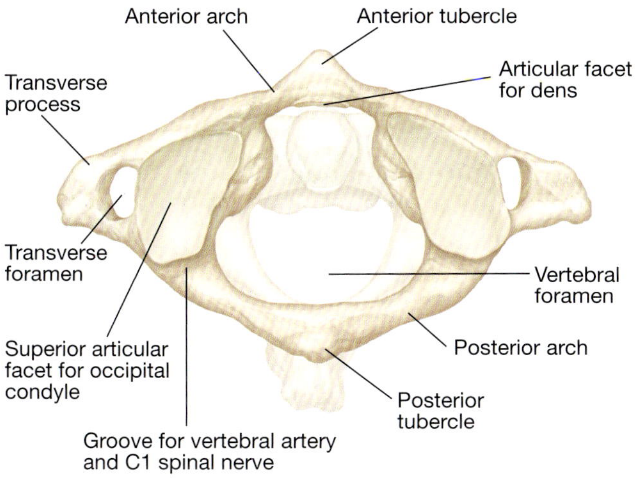

9-27 Superior view of C1.

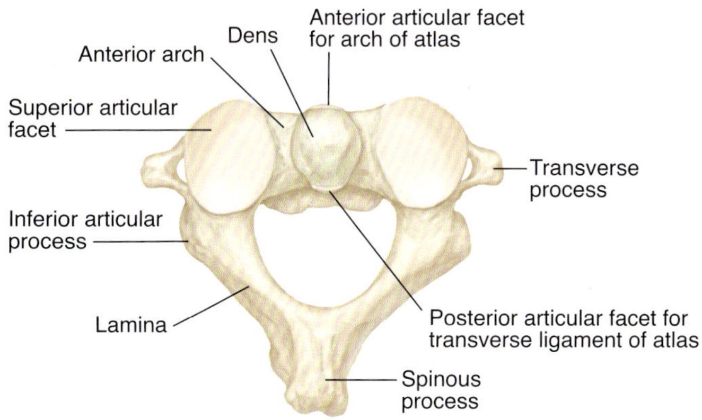

9-30 Superior view of C2.

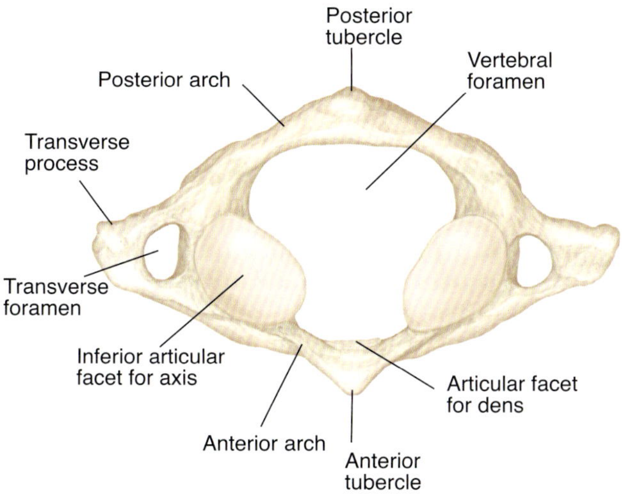

9-28 Inferior view of C1.

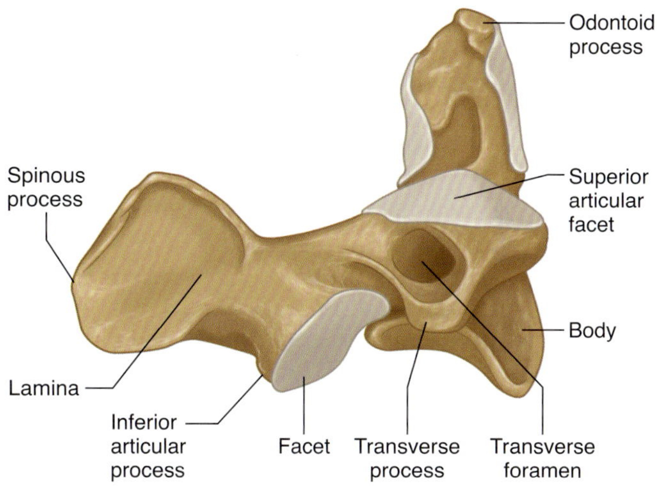

9-31 Lateral view of C2.

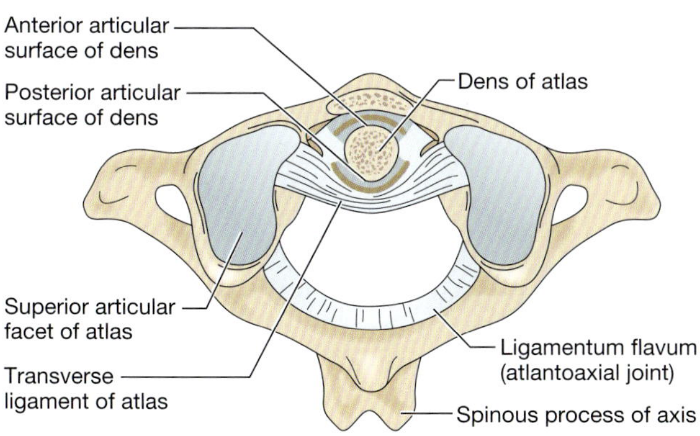

9-29 C1–C2 articulation.

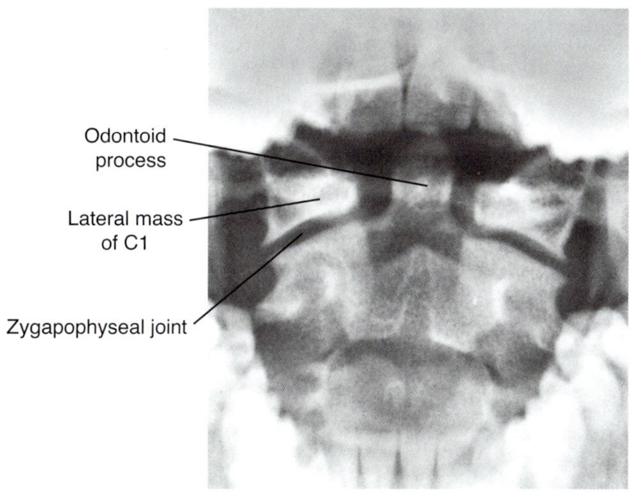

9-32 C1–C2 zygapophyseal joints.

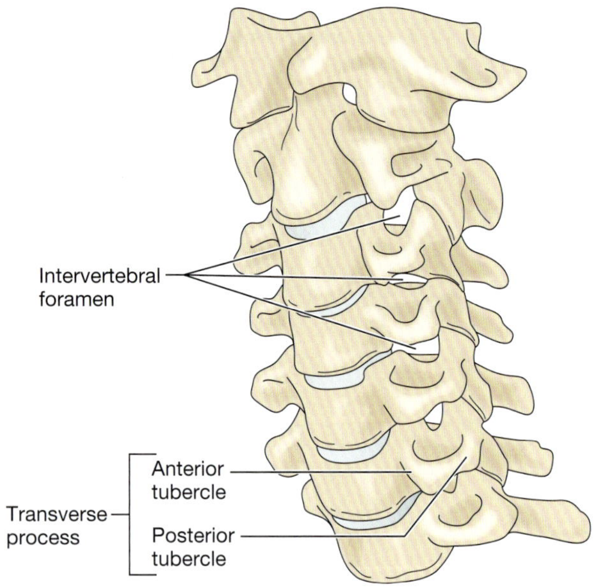

9-33 Succession of intervertebral foramina.

process of the thoracic vertebrae (Fig. 9-35). This prominent, palpable spinous process at the base of the neck is referred to as the vertebra prominens. Right- and left-sided zygapophyseal joints are best visualized with a true lateral position for C3-7 and are formed with articulation of the superior and inferior articular processes. In between these processes, the articular pillar is present and provides additional strength to the cervical division (Figs. 9-36 to 9-38). Right- and left-sided intervertebral foramina are present between C2 and C7 when the superior and inferior vertebral notches above and below each pedicle align and are visualized with an oblique patient position. (Fig. 9-39).

Distinguishing Features of Thoracic and Lumbar Vertebrae

Although the thoracic and lumbar vertebrae have similar basic structural anatomy, they also have distinct characteristics that set them apart.

Thoracic Vertebrae

The thoracic vertebrae models many of the features of a traditional vertebra previously described (Fig. 9-40). However, additionally, the thoracic vertebrae provide the site for rib articulation. Each head of a rib articulates with a facet (full depression) or demi-facet (half depression) on the lateral, posterior edge of the vertebral body (Fig. 9-41). This articulation creates the costovertebral joint. All 12 ribs have a right and left costovertebral joint. Each tubercle of the rib articulates with the transverse process of the vertebra (Figs. 9-41 to 9-43). This

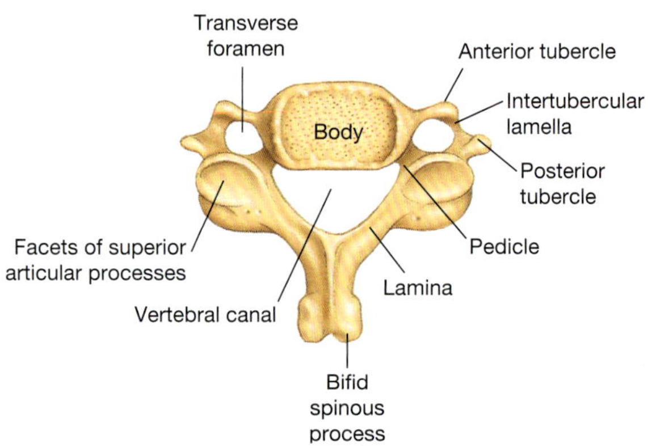

9-34 Superior view of C3–C6.

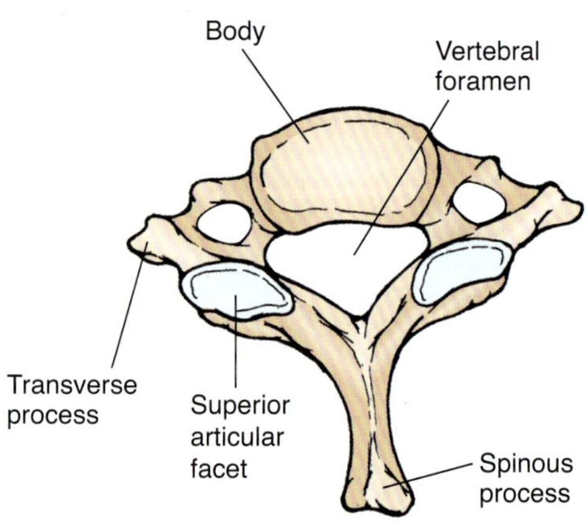

9-35 Superior view of C7.

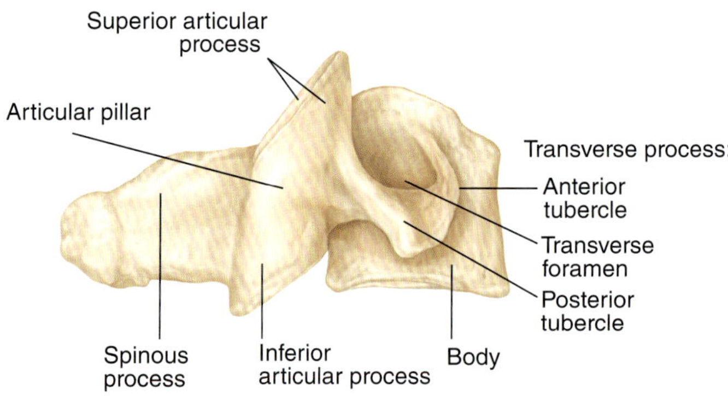

9-36 Lateral view of cervical vertebra C3–C7.

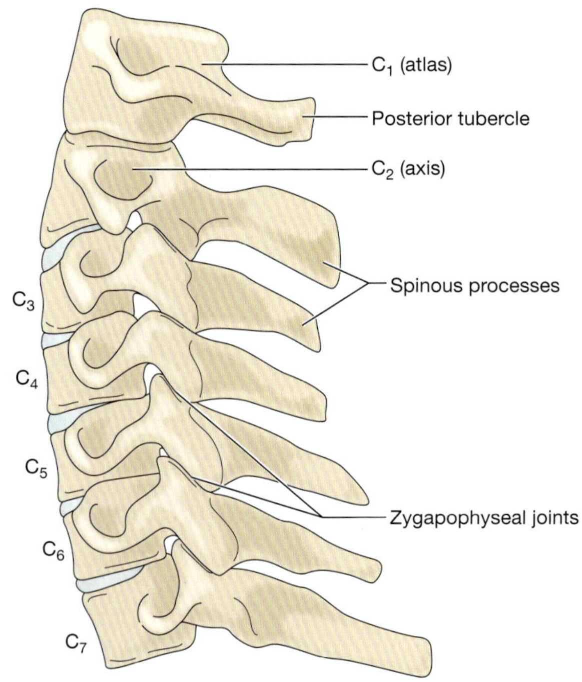

9-37 Zygapophyseal joints of C3–C7.

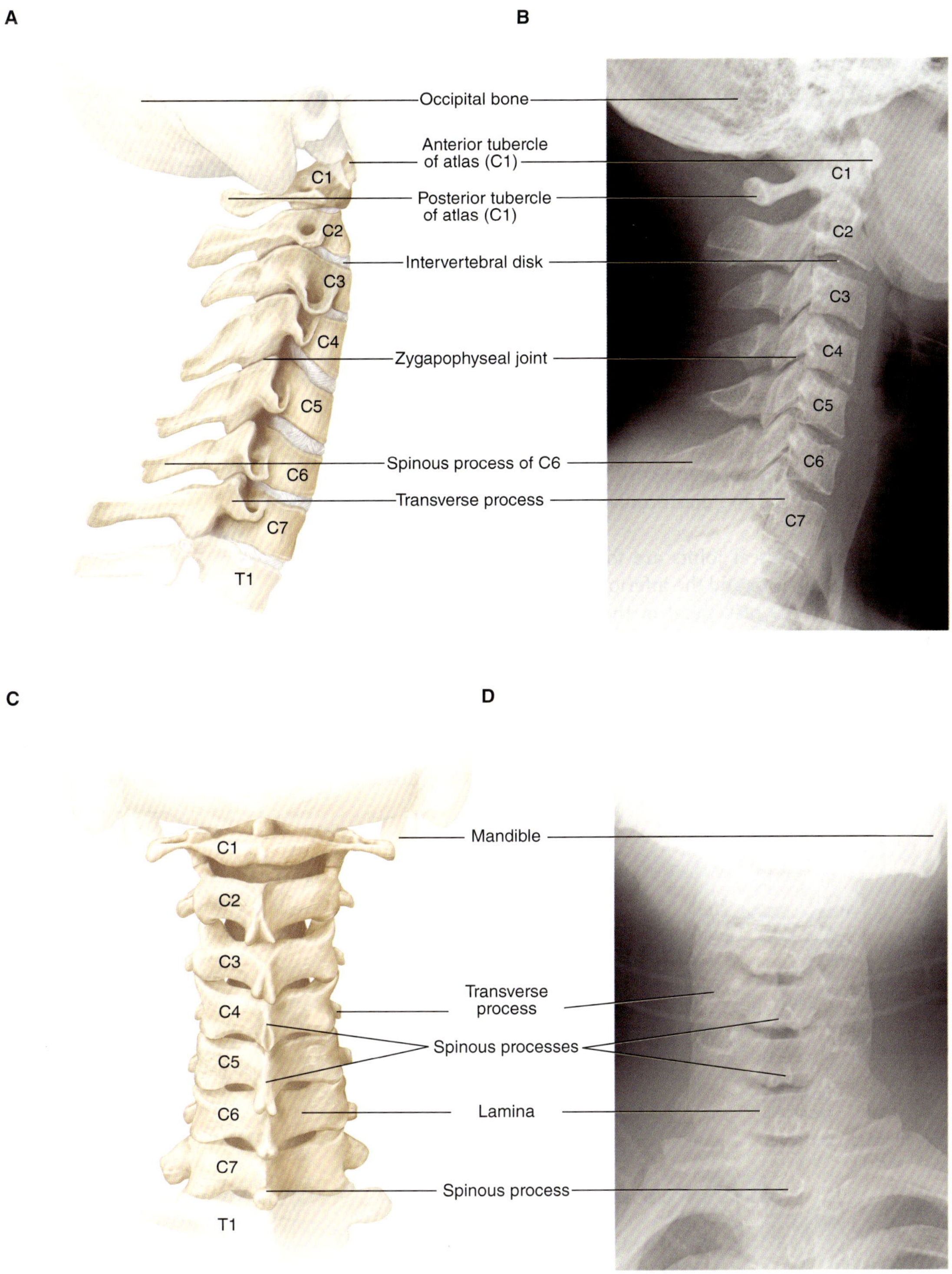

9-38 Cervical spine. **A:** Lateral view. **B:** Radiograph of cervical vertebrae, lateral view. **C:** Posterior view. **D:** Radiograph of cervical vertebrae, AP view.

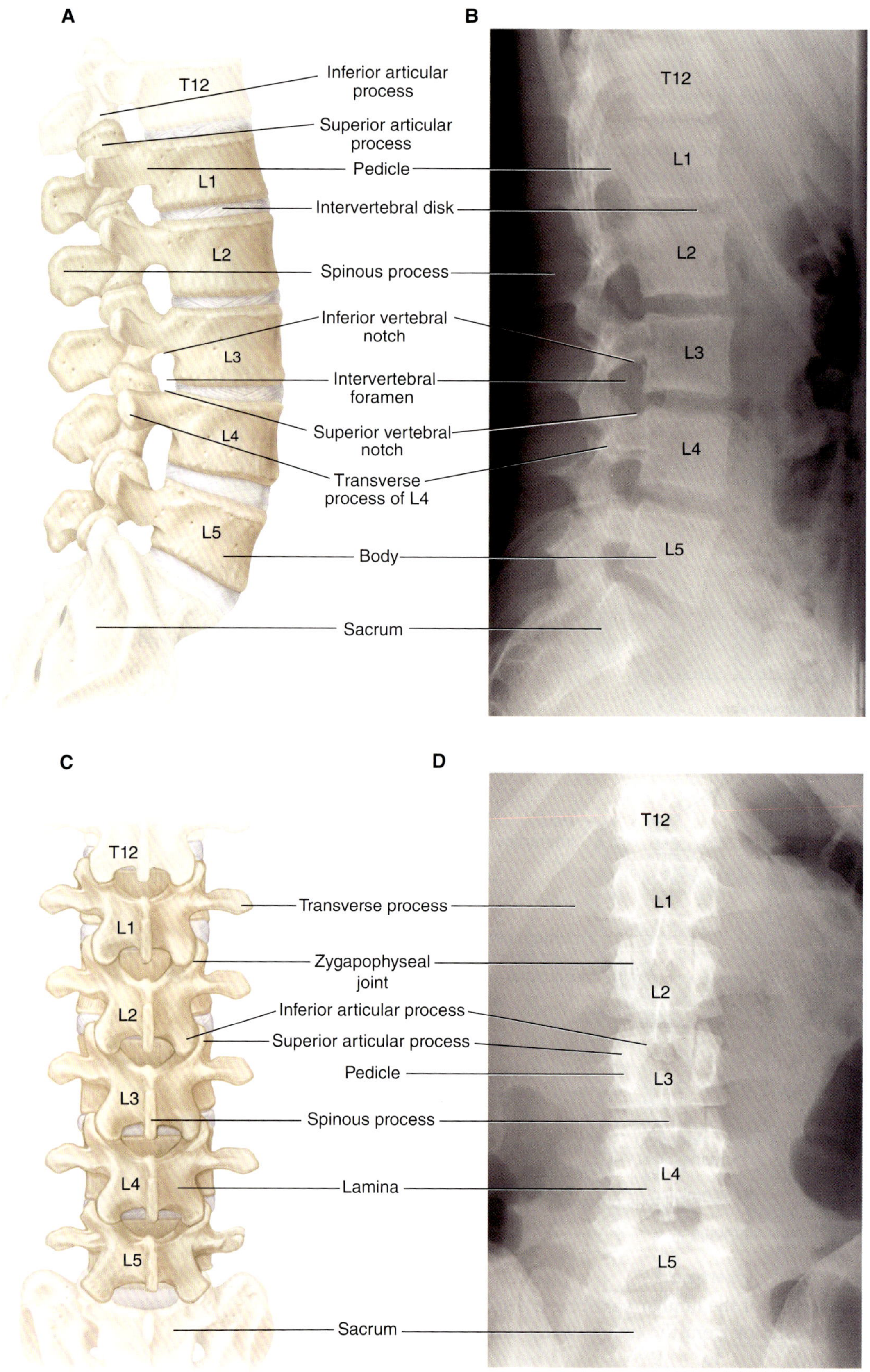

9-48 AP and lateral views of the lumbar spine. **A:** Lateral view. **B:** Radiograph of lumbar vertebrae, lateral view. **C:** Posterior view. **D:** Radiograph of lumbar vertebrae, AP view.

This obliquity will best demonstrate the zygapophyseal joints in the midlumbar column. If the zygapophyseal joints of T12–L1 or L1–L2 are of interest, an increased obliquity (slightly greater than 45°) will better demonstrate them. Recall that the zygapophyseal joints in the thoracic division are demonstrated with a 70° oblique. If the zygapophyseal joints at L5–S1 are of interest, a decreased obliquity (slightly less than 45°) would better demonstrate. Despite the noted differences in degrees of body obliquity necessary to demonstrate the zygapophyseal joints, the average 45° oblique is practiced. Visualization of the radiographic "Scottie Dog" in the lumbar spine reveals proper rotation of the patient. The significant components of the "Scottie Dog" and the anatomic part representation are as follows: eye (pedicle), ear (superior articular process), front leg (inferior articular process), nose (transverse process), neck (pars interarticularis), body (lamina), and tail (superior articular process of opposite side) (Figs. 9-49 and 9-50).

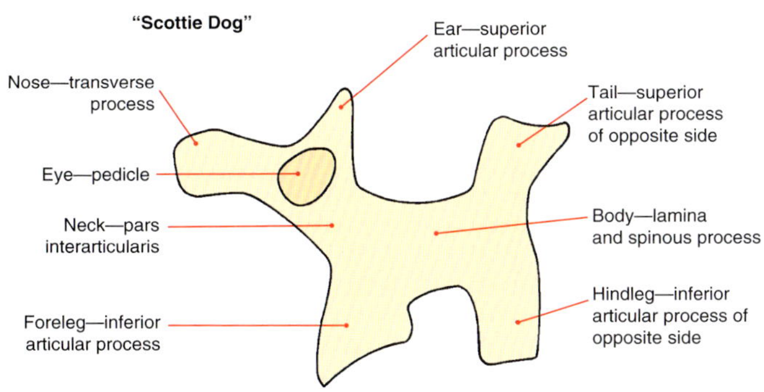

9-49 Lumbar "Scottie Dog."

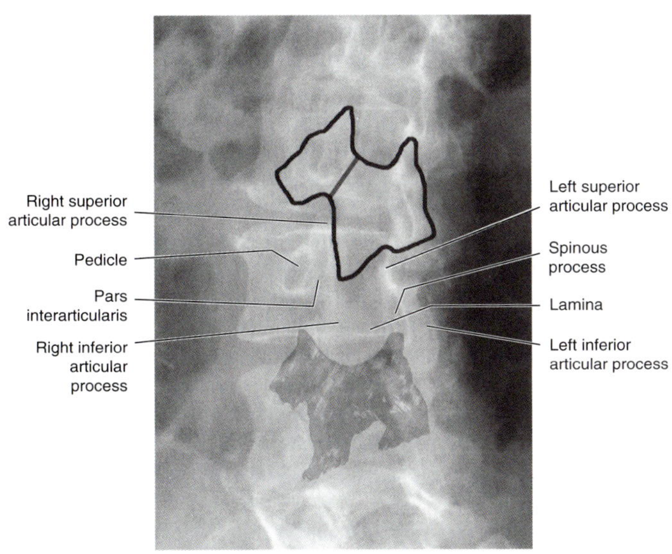

9-50 Oblique view of the lumbar spine.

Sacrum

The sacrum is comprised of a base and an apex. The base is located superiorly. The apex will articulate with the coccyx. The sacrum is comprised initially of five sacral segments that fuse into one at adulthood (Fig. 9-51). The sacrum has concave curvature. Considering this curvature, it requires the use of a 15° cephalic tube angle to direct the central ray perpendicular to the sacrum. Along the superior border of the sacral base are two superior articular processes. These superior articular processes articulate with the inferior articular processes of L5, creating the last zygapophyseal joints within the vertebral column (Fig. 9-51). On the body of the sacrum and the first sacral segment lies the sacral promontory. Lateral to the sacral promontory are the sacral wings or alae. On the lateral sides of the sacrum, the auricular (ear-shaped) processes are present to articulate with the right and left ilia to form the sacroiliac (SI) joints (Fig. 9-52). Within the sacral segments continuing down toward the apex of the sacrum, right and left sacral foramina are present. Sacral foramina represent the continuation of the intervertebral foramina, which allow for the continued passage of nerves and vessels (Fig. 9-53).

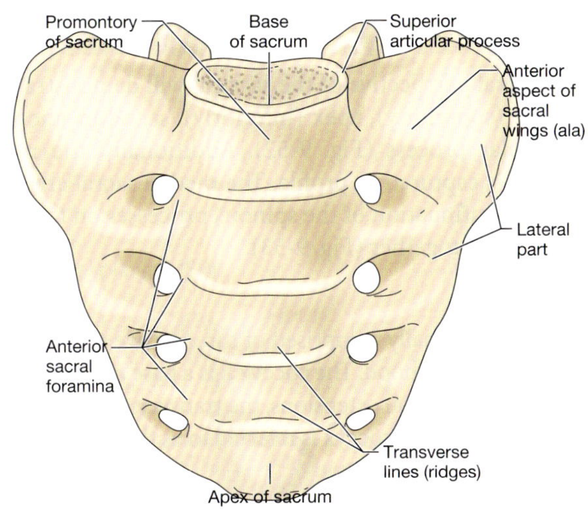

9-51 Frontal view of sacrum.

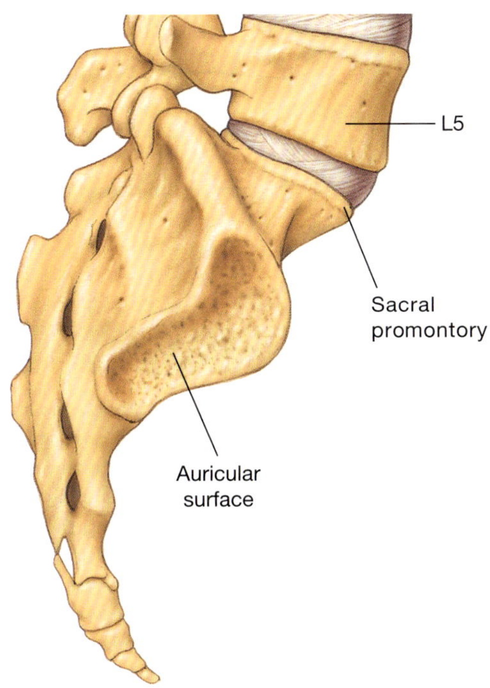

9-52 Lateral view of sacrum.

POSITIONING CONSIDERATIONS

Patient Part Size and Suggested Image Receptor Orientation

Imaging the spine always includes imaging a part size greater than 10 cm in thickness requiring grid imaging. Image receptor orientation regardless of size will be lengthwise.

Centering and Collimation

The central ray should be directed to the proper and suggested centering locations to ensure the best technical results and collimation. Topographical landmarks can be assistive to proper centering. With proper centering, four-sided collimation can be applied to ensure good radiation safety practices as well as the inclusion of all essential anatomy. Close collimation is essential when considering the increased technical settings and part thickness to reduce as much scatter from reaching image receptor.

Extremely obese or bariatric patients often present the challenge of palpating key anatomic landmarks to assist with centering. Consider the following:

- Pulling the lower abdominal tissue or pannicular tissue upward to allow closer palpation to bony landmarks. This may be helpful with the anterior superior iliac spine (ASIS) and the symphysis pubis.
- The greater trochanter can also serve as an alternative means to locate the level of the symphysis pubis.
- The jugular notch may be the best landmark to determine the MSP if the xiphoid tip is difficult to palpate. The umbilicus is not a reliable midline reference.

Breathing Instructions

Breathing instructions to the patient could be suspended breathing to prevent motion on the image. When imaging in the thoracic region, it is recommended that the patient suspend breath after expiration to remove air volume from the lungs. A breathing technique could also be implemented on the lateral thoracic spine or Swimmer's lateral (Figs. 9-56 and 9-57). When imaging in the lumbar region, it is recommended that the patient suspend breath after expiration in order to move the diaphragm to its most superior level to prevent lung superimposition on the first lumbar vertebra.

Identification Between Nontrauma Versus Trauma Situations

Patients with potential trauma to the vertebral column or who are postsurgical should be approached with extra care. The technologist may have to deviate from normal protocol to image the patient unable to roll or move. This may require the implementation of a horizontal beam. Trauma imaging requires a minimum of two views 90° apart.

Weight-Bearing

It is becoming more commonplace for the spine to be imaged in its natural state while bearing weight. Upright imaging may be part of standard protocol at facilities based on physician preferences.

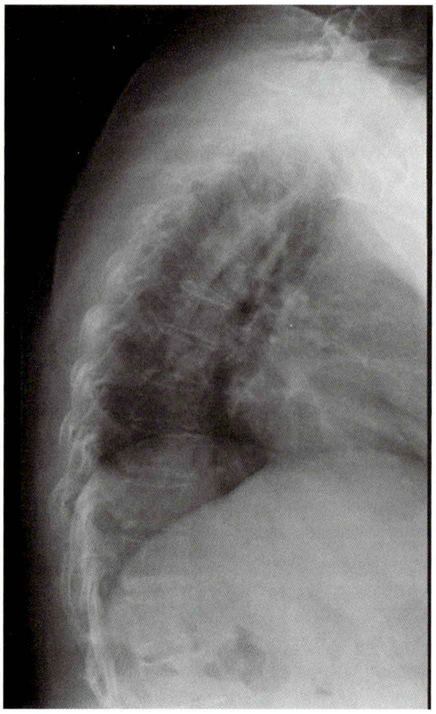

9-56 Lateral thoracic spine acquired with a manual technique.

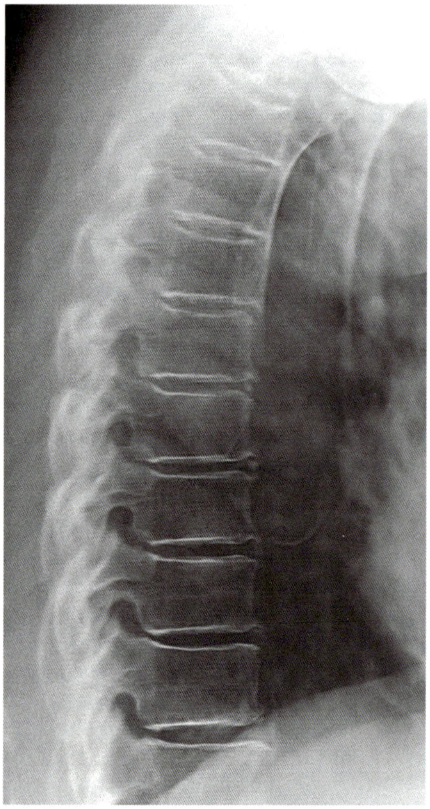

9-57 Lateral thoracic spine acquired with a breathing technique.

TECHNICAL CONSIDERATIONS

Setting a Manual Technique

Manual technique is defined when the radiographer sets the kVp and mAs values (Fig. 9-56). A manual technique can be set in the department and on a mobile imaging unit.

Kilovoltage is set to penetrate the part thickness and affects the scale of contrast seen on the image. A midlevel kVp, 70–85 is used for different regions of the vertebral column. The determination of mAs would be influenced by part size, considering the amount of soft tissue in the region. In situations of known potential destructive pathologies, such as osteoporosis, a manual technique will allow appropriate decreased modifications of kVp and mAs levels.

Setting Technique With Automatic Exposure Control

Automatic exposure control (AEC) may be an option in the imaging department. With AEC, the technologist will set the kVp value, will not set a mAs but rather must select which exposure cell(s) correspond to the anatomy centered and the anatomic coverage over the cell(s) according to the projection. The cell(s) will determine when adequate exposure has been reached according to the part thickness and tissue composition, and then the exposure is terminated. After the exposure terminates, the radiographer can then see the mAs value displayed on the control panel. When imaging the vertebral column, only the center cell must be selected. A pitfall to using AEC during spine imaging is failing to achieve proper centering of the spine over the designated exposure cell. An upright patient who is unbalanced may result in a small shift in their position away from the selected exposure cell, resulting in early exposure termination resulting in image underexposure.

Source-to-Image Distance

Forty to seventy-two–inch SID is employed for the vertebral column. Certain regions of the column will institute different distances. Increased distances are necessary when patient positioning results in increased object to image distance (OID) between the patient's part and the image receptor to compensate for structure magnification.

Shielding

Acceptable shielding practices include a lap shield when imaging the cervical and thoracic regions. Application of gonadal shielding when imaging the lumbar and sacral regions is not possible for females, and therefore proper centering, positioning, good collimation, and proper selection of technical settings are crucial in efforts to minimize repeat exposures.

Shadow shields may be employed to protect the breasts and gonads when imaging patients with scoliosis. Patients with scoliosis require imaging throughout the course of their diagnosis and treatment. Keep in mind that these patients are usually within their adolescent and teenage years. Shadow shields are secured on the glass window in between the tube and the patient. Shadow shields can be adjusted in their position to correctly cast a "shadow" over the reproductive anatomy.

In addition to efforts on shielding, the technologist must question all patients of reproductive age regarding the possibility of pregnancy. It is important to rule out pregnancy with any direct exposure to the abdominal and pelvic area.

Marking the Image

When marking the spine with the patient positioned flat, the anatomic marker should be placed within the collimated exposure field furthest away from the patient's midline to identify correctly the right or left side of the patient. When marking the lateral position, the anatomic marker is placed along the anterior surface of the part or "in front" of the part and within the collimated exposure field (Fig. 9-58). When marking an oblique position, the lead marker should be placed within the collimated exposure field, indicating the anatomic side closest to the IR (Fig. 9-59). For example, with a left posterior oblique position, the left marker is placed lateral to the patient's left side (Fig. 9-60).

Viewing the Image

Assuming the spine image was correctly marked, the image is displayed opposite of the viewer facing it, as though the image is in the anatomic position. Therefore, the side of the image marked "Right" or "Left" is opposite of the viewer's right or left side (Figs. 9-61 and 9-62).

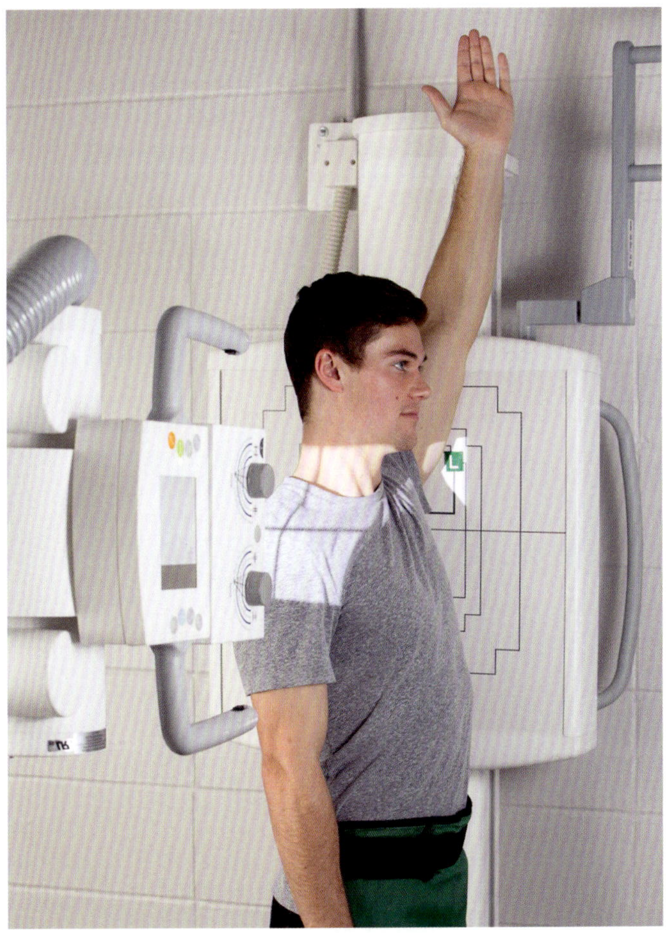

9-58 Marker placement for the lateral thoracic spine.

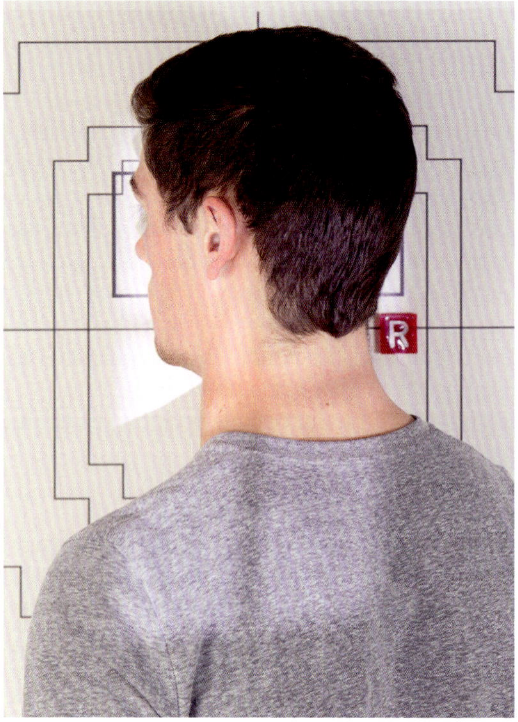

9-59 Marker placement for the RAO upright spine position.

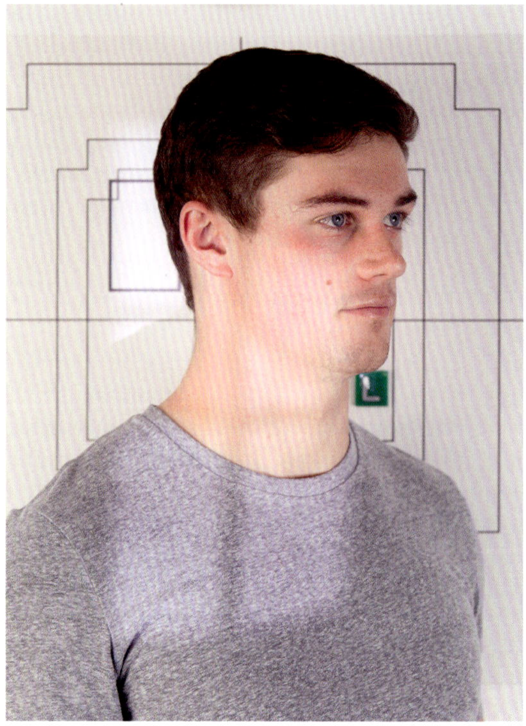

9-60 Marker placement for the LPO upright spine position.

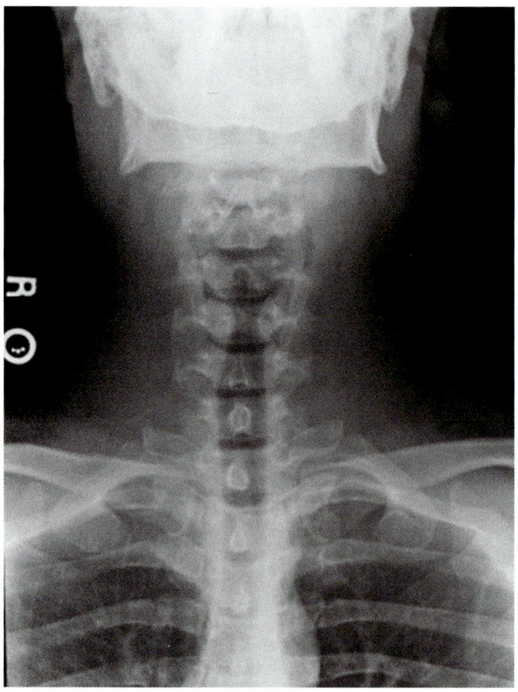

9-61 Correct image display for AP axial cervical spine.

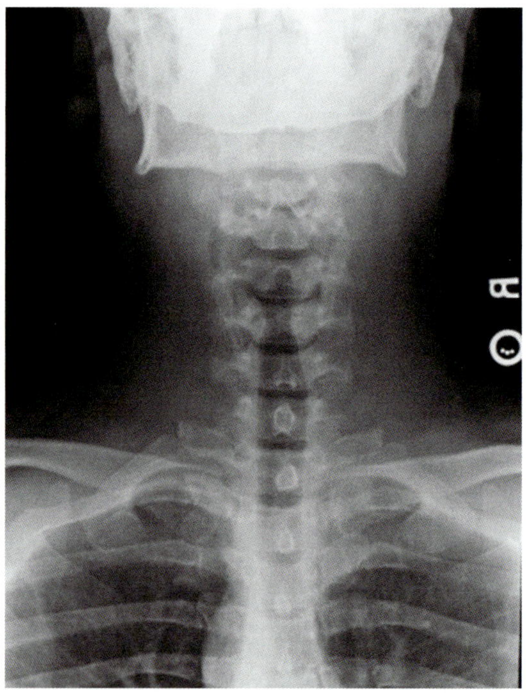

9-62 Incorrect image display for AP axial cervical spine.

Nontrauma Cervical Spine

- Projection: Lateral
- Summation of entire cervical spine protocol is found in Table 9-2

Cervical Spine Protocol

Lateral

AP Obliques or PA Obliques

AP Axial

AP Open Mouth

Technical Considerations

- kVp 75–85
- mAs set manually or center AEC cell
- 72″ SID (increased SID compensates for the OID created between neck and IR)

Exposure Field Size

- 10 × 12 lengthwise

Patient Position (Fig. 9-64)

- Erect
- Ensure patient is in a true left lateral and is looking straight ahead
- If patient is free of upper extremity injury, neck pain, and is not postsurgical, clinical facilities *may* use sandbags applied around each wrist of the patient to aid in shoulder depression to assist with the demonstration of all seven cervical vertebrae. If weights are applied, this should happen just prior to the exposure

Centering (Fig. 9-63)

- C5 (Adam's apple) and MCP (mid-coronal plane)

Marking of IR

- Anatomic L side marker placed along the anterior surface of the patient

Breathing

- Suspend respiration after the second expiration. Instruct the patient to "take a deep breath in, blow it out and hold it out, and relax your shoulders down"
- The control panel should have already been set before administering the weights to the patient's wrists, allowing an immediate exposure after breathing is suspended on exhalation
- Ensure patient holds position while walking away to make the exposure

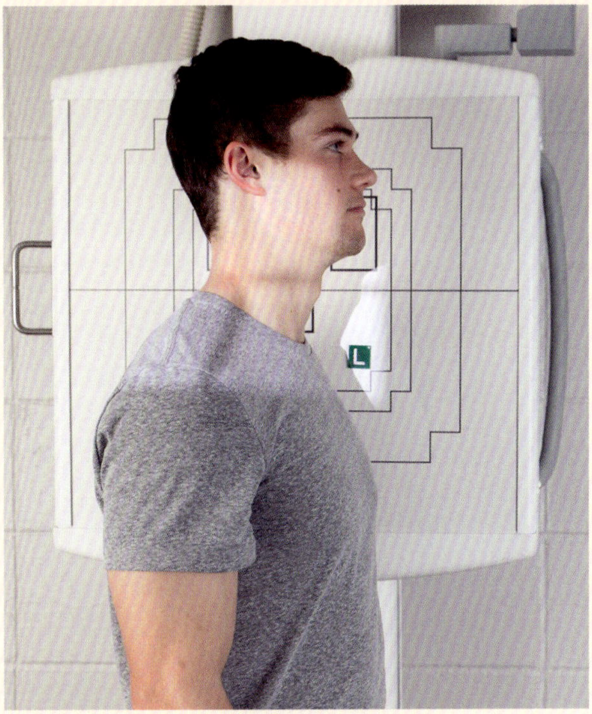

9-63 Ambulatory lateral C-spine.

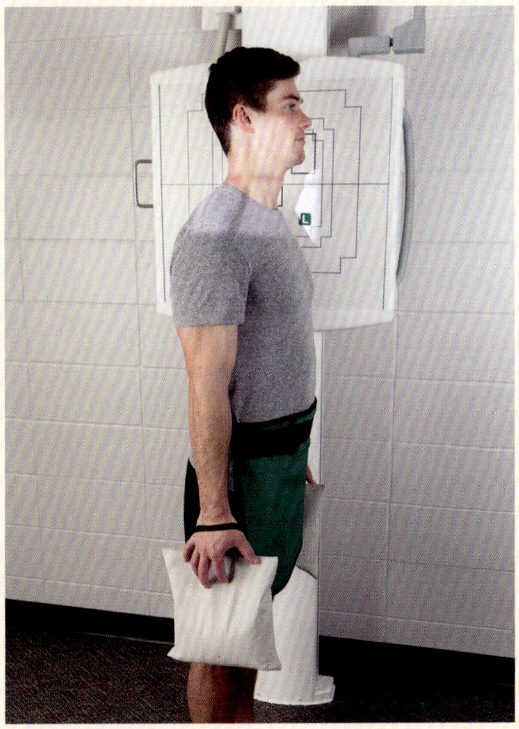

9-64 Lateral C-spine with weights.

IMAGE CRITIQUE (FIGS. 9-65 and 9-66)

- Cervical vertebral C1–C7 bodies and spinous processes should be seen in profile
- Anterior to posterior alignment of the cervical vertebrae
- Height of vertebral bodies and intervertebral disk spaces observed
- Zygapophyseal joints of C3–C7 visualized (Table 9-7)
- C1 and C2 should be free of superimposition from the base of the skull and mandibular rami. Excessive extension of the chin will cause the base of the skull to drop down on C1. Excessive flexion of the chin will cause the mandibular rami to superimpose on C1 and C2 (Figs. 9-67 and 9-68)
- Demonstrating the transition of C7–T1 is ideal if possible to achieve
- Properly centered with four-sided collimation

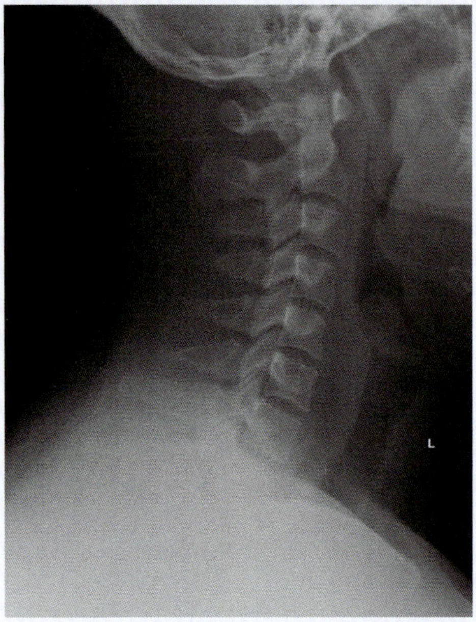

9-65 Lateral C-spine.

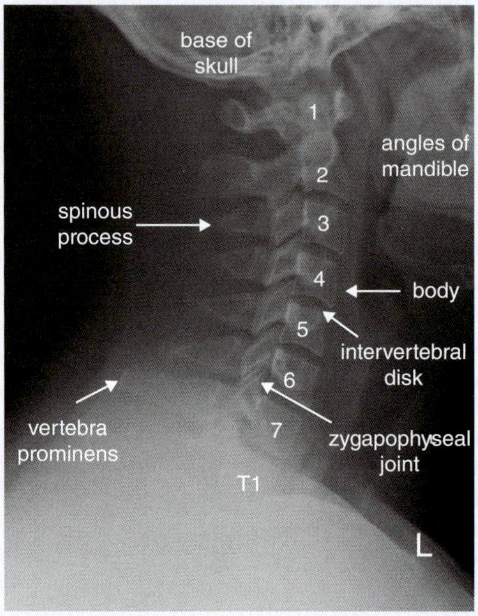

9-66 Lateral C-spine.

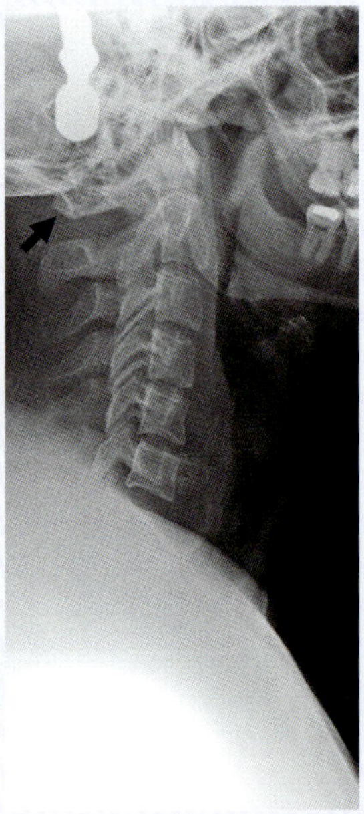

9-67 Lateral C-spine with overextension.

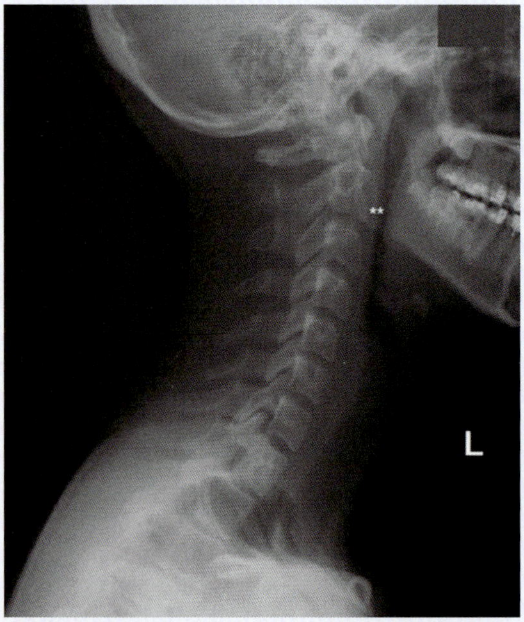

9-68 Lateral C-spine with flexion. Asterisks denote mandibular angle.

POSITION VARIATION: HYPEREXTENSION AND HYPERFLEXION LATERALS

Flexion and extension laterals may be ordered as an additional two views to a complete C-spine order or perhaps only as two view flexion and extension cervical views. Flexion and extension laterals are ordered to assess the range of movement with presurgical, postsurgical recovery (such as a cervical fusion), or after a whiplash type injury. These comparative laterals are set up similarly to the lateral cervical spine projection, but with added maximum flexion and extension positions achieved to the tolerance of the patient (Figs. 9-69 to 9-72).

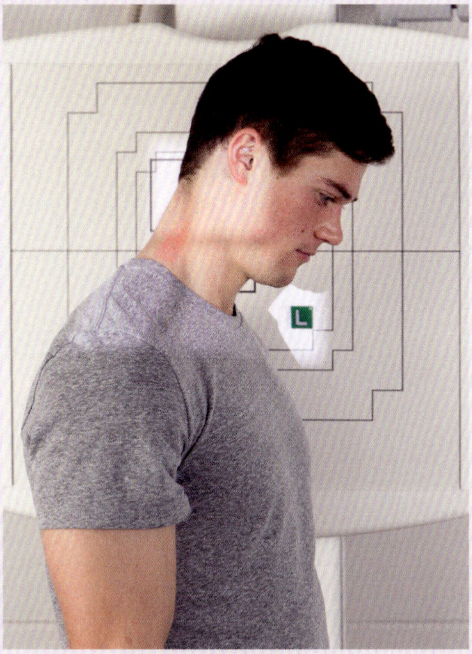

9-69 Lateral C-spine with hyperflexion.

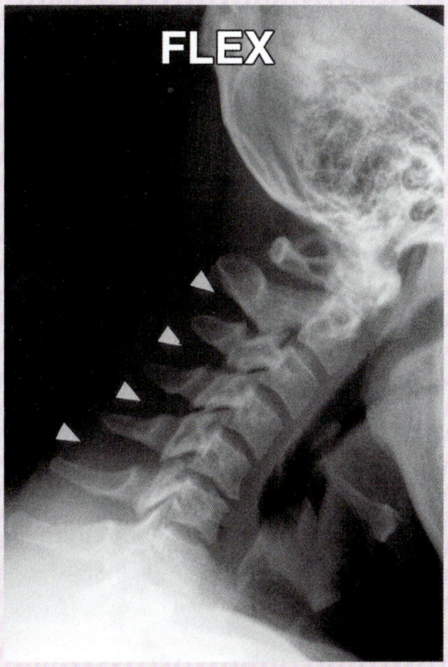

9-70 Lateral C-spine with hyperflexion. Arrowheads reveal increased space between spinous processes.

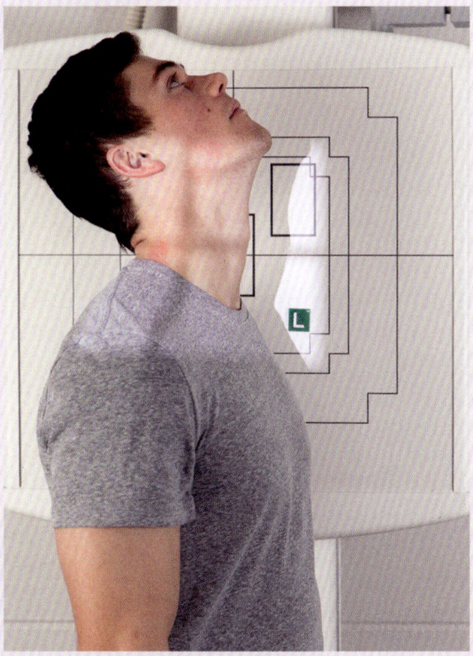

9-71 Lateral C-spine with hyperextension.

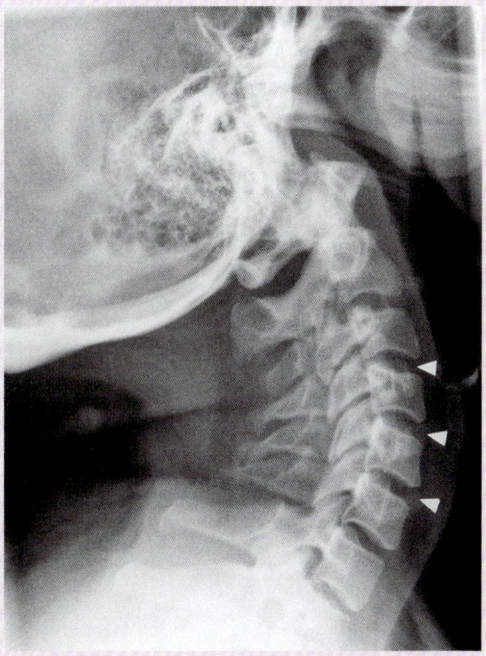

9-72 Lateral C-spine with hyperextension.

Nontrauma Cervical Spine

- Projection: AP Axial Oblique or PA Axial Oblique
- Summation of entire cervical spine protocol is found in Table 9-2

Cervical Spine Protocol

Lateral

AP Axial Obliques or PA Axial Obliques

AP Axial

AP Open Mouth

Technical Considerations

- kVp 70–85
- mAs set manually or center AEC cell
- 60″–72″ SID is recommended to compensate for the OID between the cervical spine and IR

Exposure Field Size

- 10 × 12 lengthwise

Patient Position

- Erect with patient looking straight ahead
- Patient is rotated into a 45° posterior oblique or anterior oblique. Only one complete set of posterior oblique(s) (right posterior oblique/left posterior oblique [RPO/LPO]) or anterior oblique(s) (right anterior oblique/left anterior oblique [RAO/LAO]) are acquired. Using the anterior oblique positions (RAO and LAO) with the PA oblique projection would deliver the least amount of entrance dose to the thyroid (Figs. 9-73, 9-74, and 9-75)

Centering

- C5 (Adam's apple) and midway between the borders of the neck
  - 15°–20° cephalic tube angle is applied to the AP axial oblique projections (Fig. 9-74)
  - 15°–20° caudal tube angle is applied to the PA axial oblique projections (Fig. 9-76)

Marking of IR

- Anatomic side marker R or L placed to indicate the patient's anatomic side closest to the IR

Breathing

- Suspend respiration. Instruct the patient to "hold their breath"
- Ensure patient holds position while walking away to make the exposure

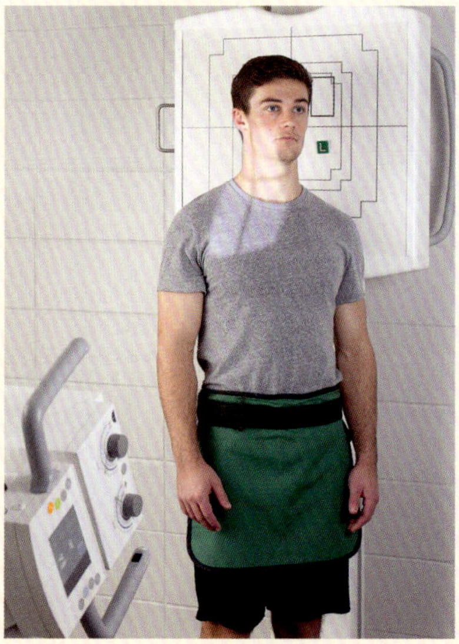

9-73 AP Oblique projection.

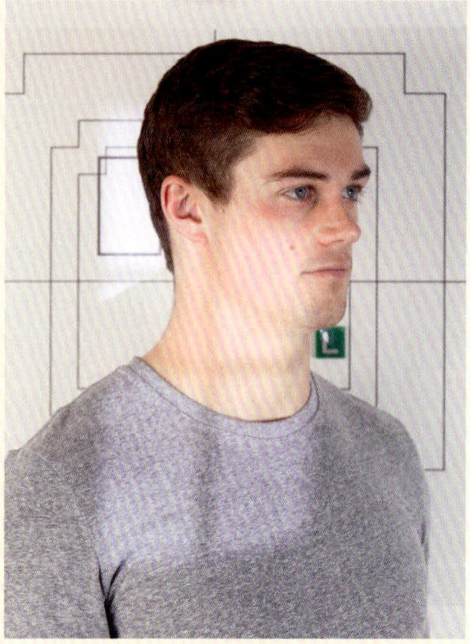

9-74 LPO cervical spine position.

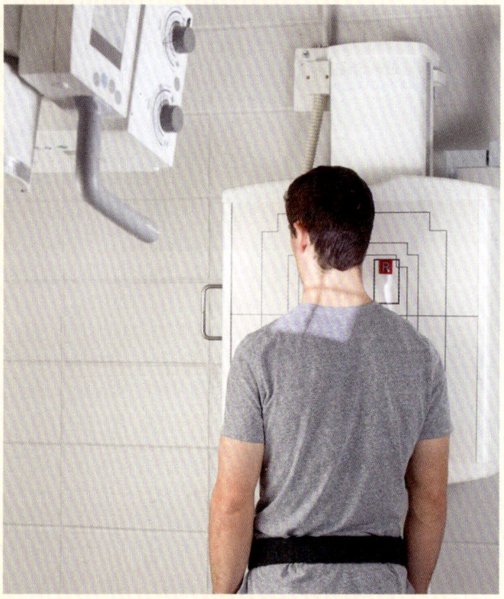

9-75 PA Oblique projection.

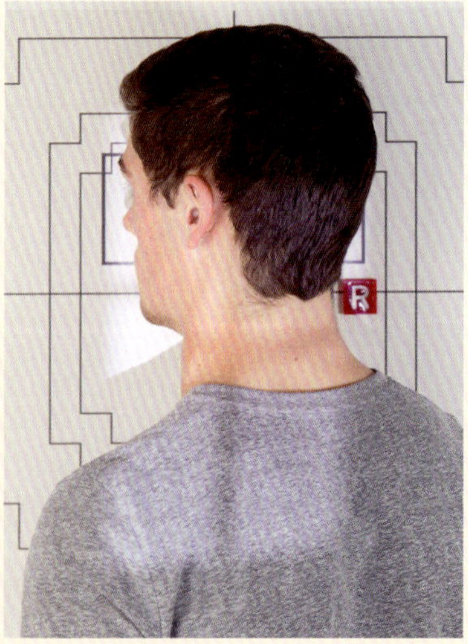

9-76 RAO cervical spine position.

IMAGE CRITIQUE (FIGS. 9-77 and 9-78)

- Intervertebral foramina of C2–C7 are open, indicating the patient was rotated into the correct degree of obliquity
  - Posterior oblique positions (RPO/LPO) demonstrate the foramina furthest from the IR. The RPO position demonstrates the left-sided intervertebral foramina (Table 9-7)
  - Anterior oblique positions (RAO/LAO) demonstrate the foramina closest to the IR. The RAO position demonstrates the right-sided intervertebral foramina (Table 9-7)
- Under-rotation of the patient will fail to display an open intervertebral foramina. Both pedicles may be visible on the lateral-most edges of the vertebral body, similar to a frontal view of the spine (Fig. 9-79)
- Over-rotation of the patient is evident when the spinous process becomes visible (Fig. 9-80)
- The tube angle applied will help create separation between the vertebral bodies and open up the intervertebral foramina
- Properly centered with four-sided collimation

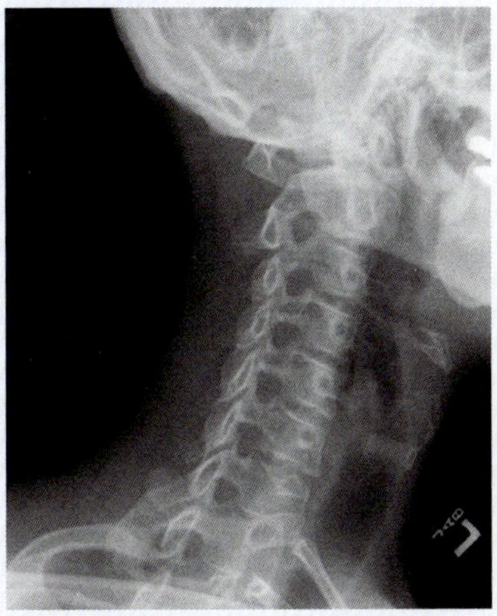

9-77 Oblique cervical spine.

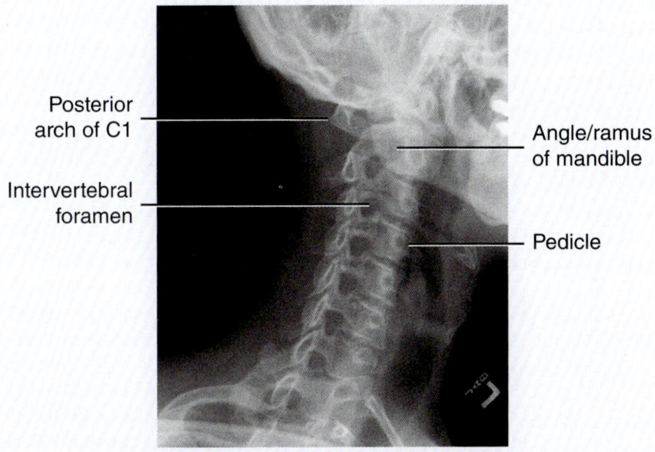

9-78 Oblique cervical spine.

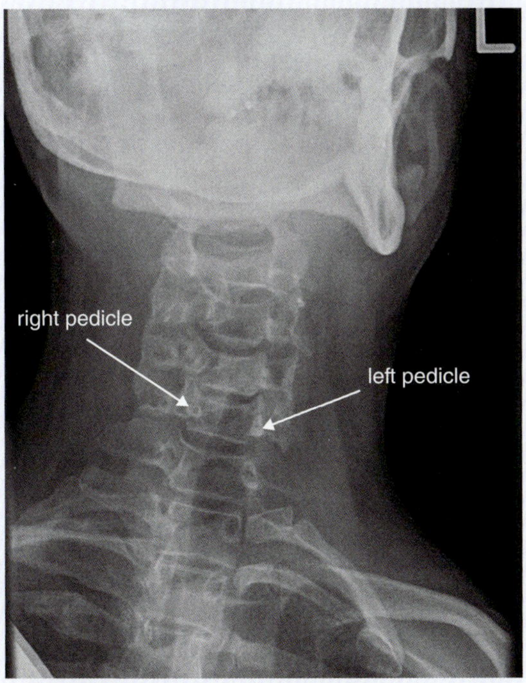

9-79 Underrotated oblique cervical spine.

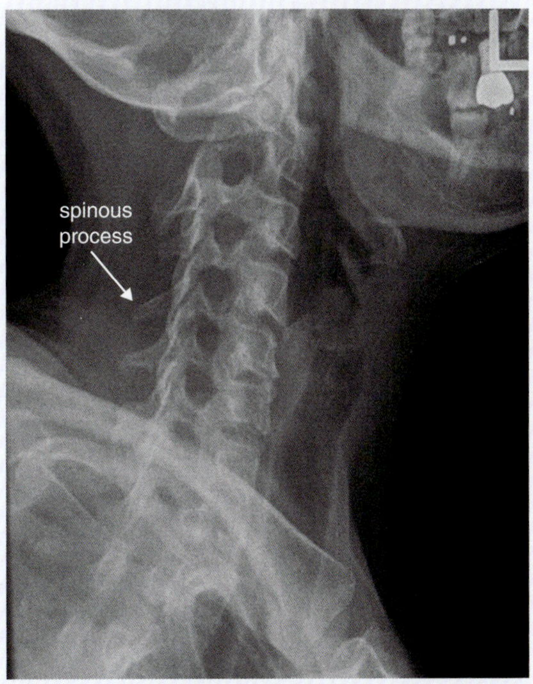

9-80 Overrotated oblique cervical spine.

Nontrauma Cervical Spine

- Projection: AP Axial
- Summation of entire cervical spine protocol is found in Table 9-2

Cervical Spine Protocol

Lateral

AP Axial Obliques OR PA Axial Obliques

AP Axial

AP Open Mouth

Technical Considerations

- kVp 70–80
- mAs set manually or center AEC cell
- 40″ SID

Exposure Field Size

- 10 × 12 lengthwise

Patient Position

- Supine or erect
- Ensure patient is flat with no rotation and is looking straight ahead

Centering

- C5 (Adam's apple) and MSP
- 15° cephalic tube angle is applied to the supine patient (Fig. 9-81)
- 20° cephalic tube angle is applied to the erect patient to account for increased curvature of the cervical spine (Fig. 9-82)

Marking of IR

- Anatomic side marker R or L placed furthest from the patient's midline

Breathing

- Suspend respiration. Instruct the patient to "hold their breath"
- Ensure patient holds position while walking away to make the exposure

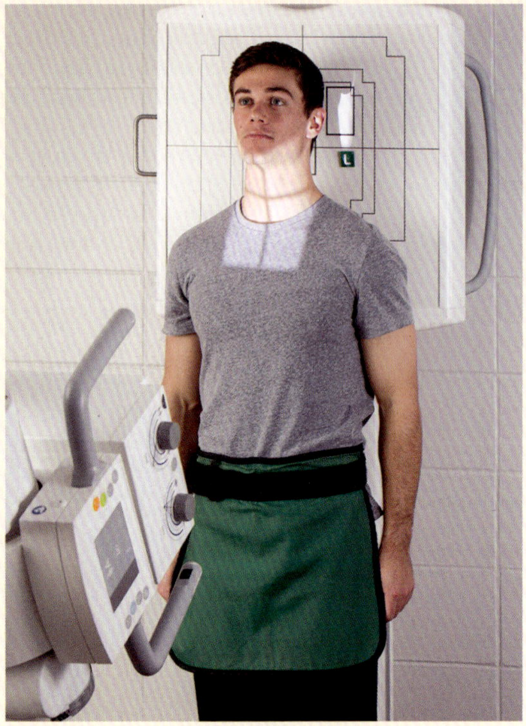

9-81 AP axial cervical spine.

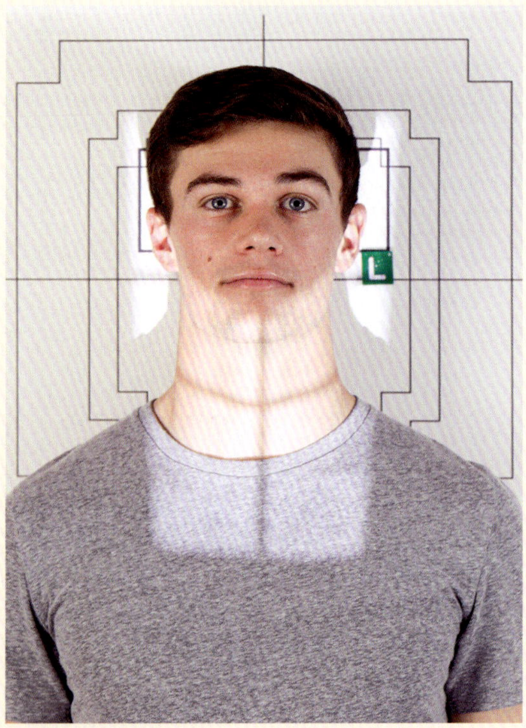

9-82 AP axial cervical spine.

IMAGE CRITIQUE (FIGS. 9-83 and 9-84)

- Cervical vertebrae C3–C7 should be seen free of rotation. Symmetry of the vertebral pedicles can aid in ruling out rotation. Sternoclavicular (SC) joints can also reveal rotation
- C1 and C2 will be superimposed by the base of the skull and mandible. Ensure that the mandible or base of the skull is not superimposing C3 (Figs. 9-85 and 9-86)
- Demonstrating the transition of C7–T1 is recommended
- Intervertebral disk spaces may appear open if the tube angle has been correctly applied if and the patient's cervical region still possesses healthy intervertebral disks
- Properly centered with four-sided collimation

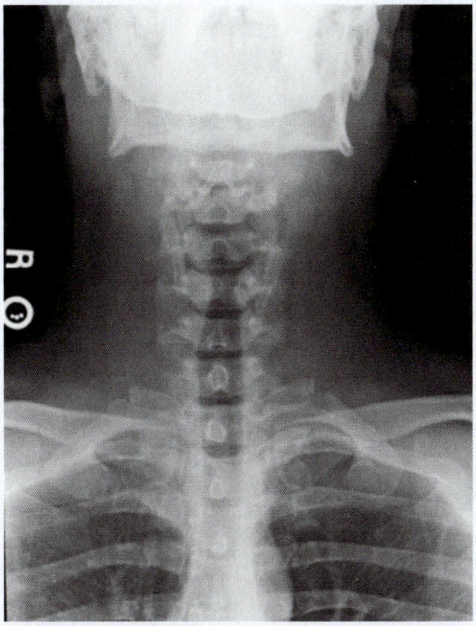

9-83 AP axial cervical spine.

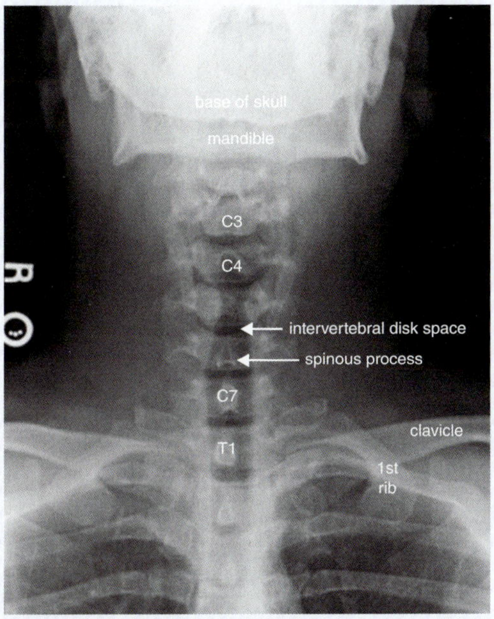

9-84 AP axial cervical spine.

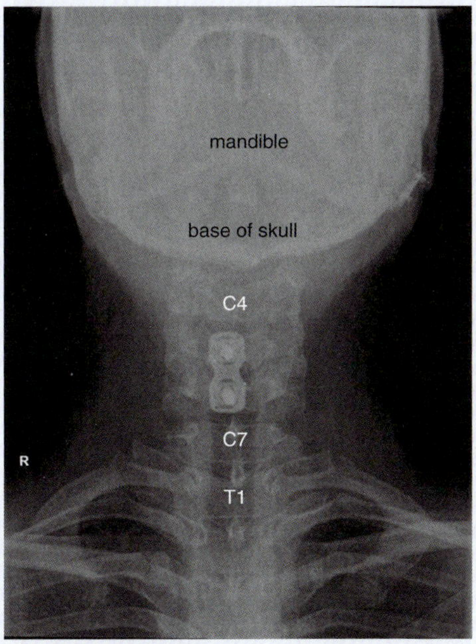

9-85 AP axial cervical spine with chin too elevated.

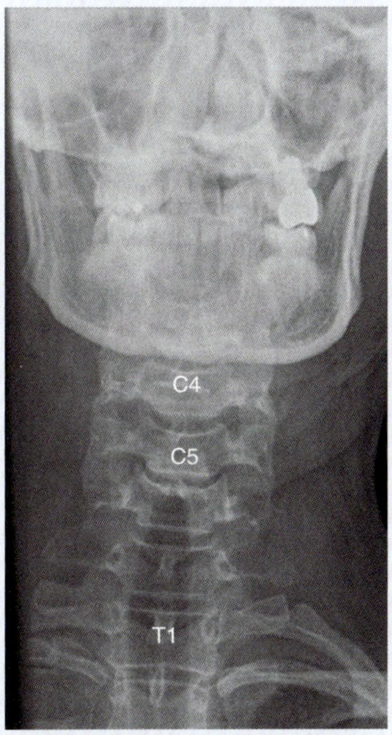

9-86 AP axial cervical spine with chin depressed.

Nontrauma Cervical Spine

- Projection: AP Open Mouth
- Summation of entire cervical spine protocol is found in Table 9-2

Cervical Spine Protocol

Lateral

AP Axial Obliques

OR PA Axial Obliques

AP Axial

AP Open Mouth

Technical Considerations

- kVp 75–80
- mAs set manually; center AEC cell
- 40″ SID

Exposure Field Size

- 8 × 8 or smaller

Patient Position

- Supine or erect. Supine may provide better stabilization of the part
- Ensure patient is flat with no rotation or tilt of the skull
- Have patient open their mouth wide. Slightly depress or extend the chin until the lower margin of the upper teeth aligns with the base of the skull. Base of the skull can be located by the mastoid tip (Fig. 9-87)

Centering

- Center of the open mouth (Figs. 9-88 and 9-89)

Marking of IR

- Anatomic side marker R or L placed furthest from the patient's midline

Breathing

- With the patient's mouth wide open, have them suspend respiration. Instruct the patient to "hold their breath"
- Ensure you watch the patient the entire time while walking away to make the exposure

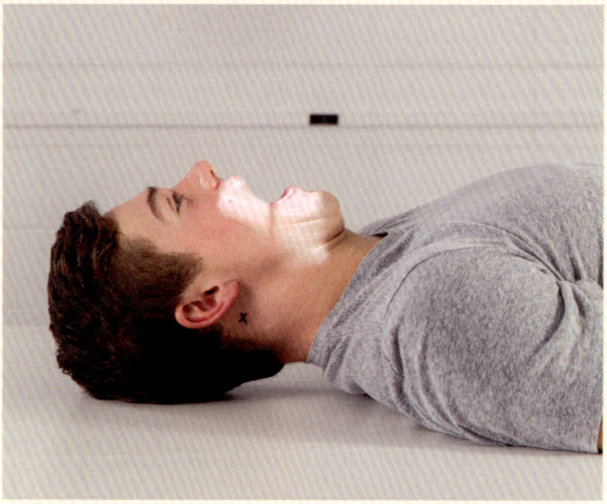

9-87 AP open mouth.

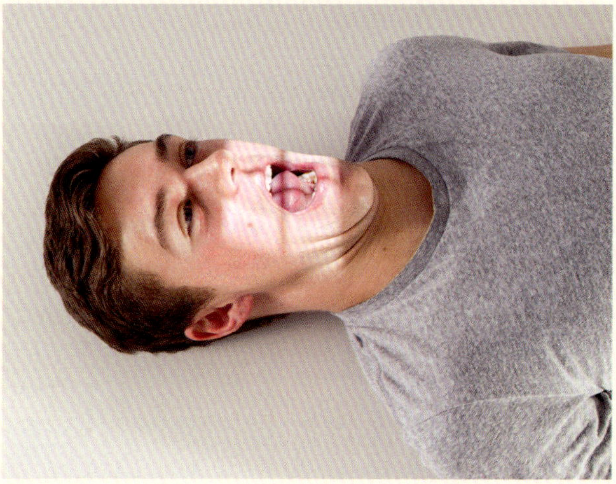

9-88 AP open mouth.

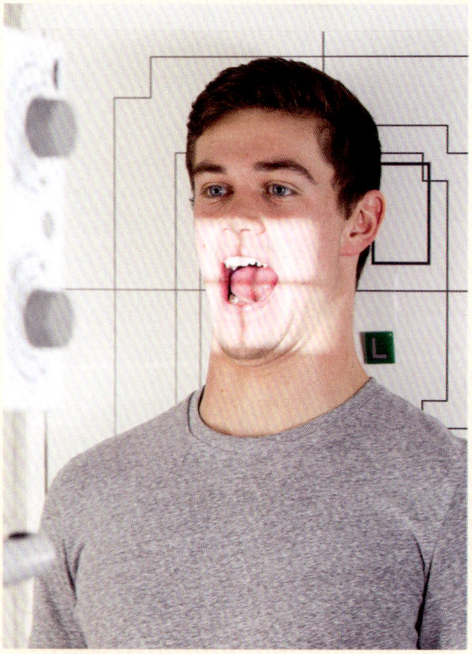

9-89 AP open mouth.

IMAGE CRITIQUE (FIGS. 9-90 to 9-92)

- C1 and C2 should be seen centered within the open mouth. With rotation of the head, C1 and C2 will shift closer toward a mandibular ramus (Fig. 9-93). As a result of the rotation, the transverse process will shift and may become superimposed by the ramus
- The symmetry and height of the zygapophyseal joints between C1 and C2 are visualized (Table 9-7)
- The odontoid process should be visualized free of superimposition from the base of the skull or teeth
    - When the base of the skull is visualized superimposed on the odontoid process, the chin is too extended (Fig. 9-94)
    - When the teeth are visualized superimposed on the odontoid process, the chin is too depressed (Fig. 9-95)
- Properly centered with four-sided collimation

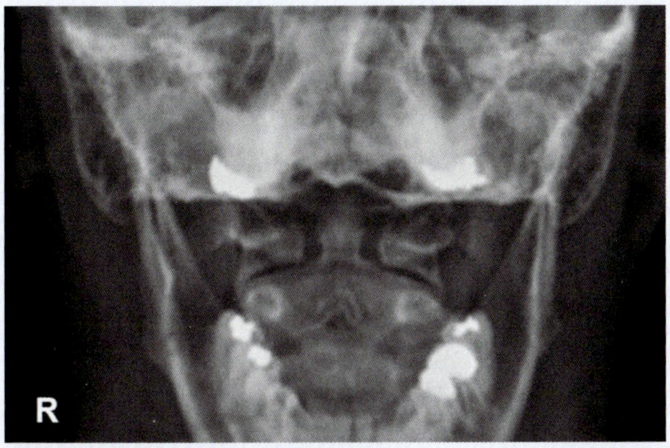

9-90 AP open mouth.

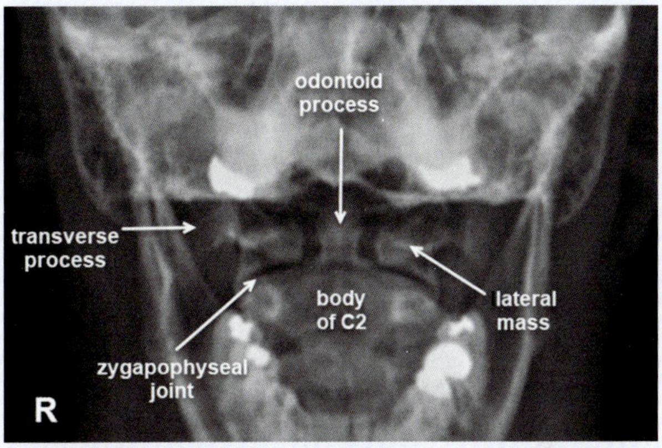

9-91 AP open mouth.

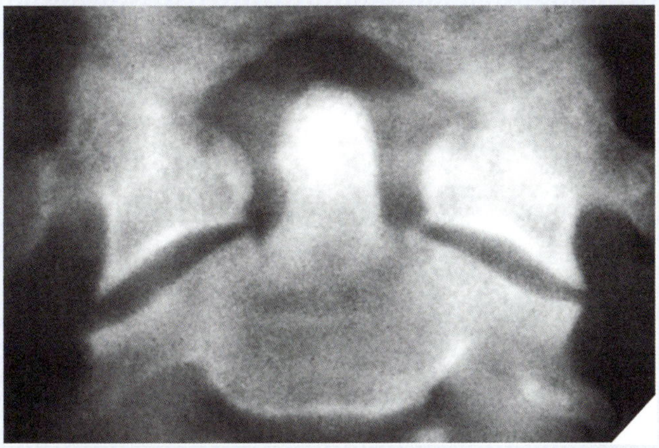

9-92 Tomogram of C1–C2.

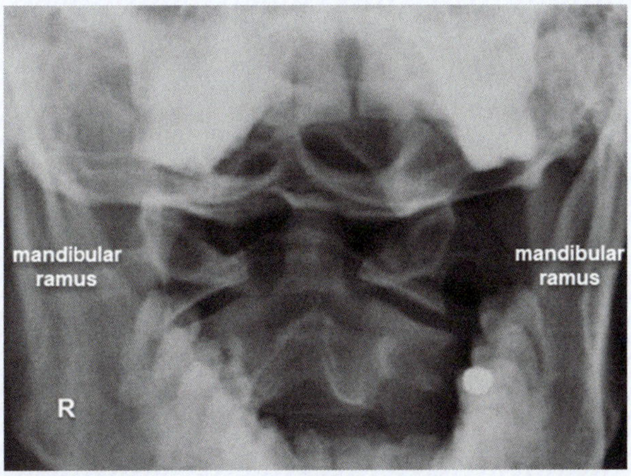

9-93 AP open mouth with rotation.

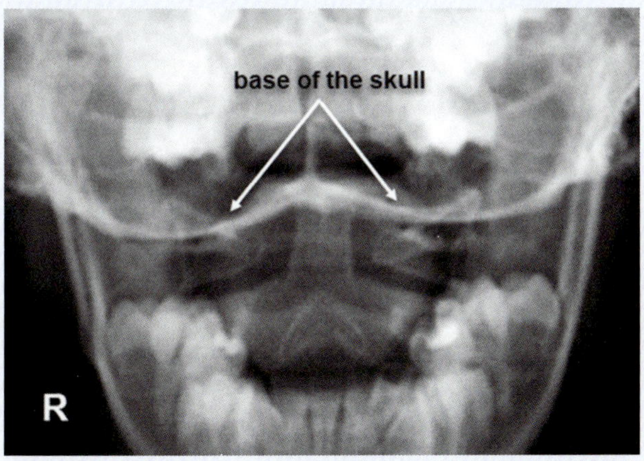

9-94 AP open mouth with the base of the skull over C1.

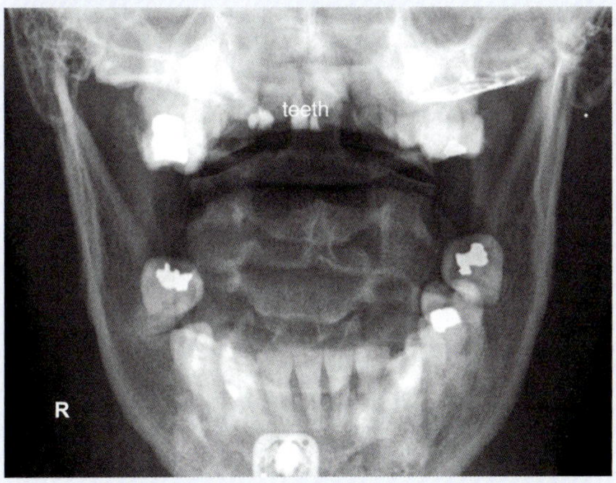

9-95 AP open mouth with teeth over C1.

POSITION VARIATION: FUCHS METHOD (A.K.A. REVERSE WATERS PROJECTION)

A Fuchs method could be attempted to supplement the AP open mouth projection in instances when the odontoid process cannot be successfully cleared. For the Fuchs method, the patient should extend their chin up until the mentomeatal line (MML) is perpendicular to the image receptor. If the patient is unable to extend the chin, the central ray can be angled slightly cephalic until parallel to the MML. The central ray is directed to enter just below the chin. When properly positioned, the odontoid process should appear within the foramen magnum (Figs. 9-96 to 9-99).

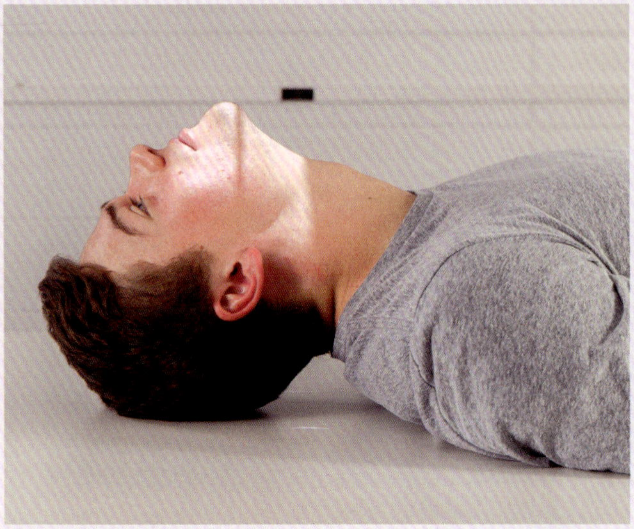

9-96 Fuchs method.

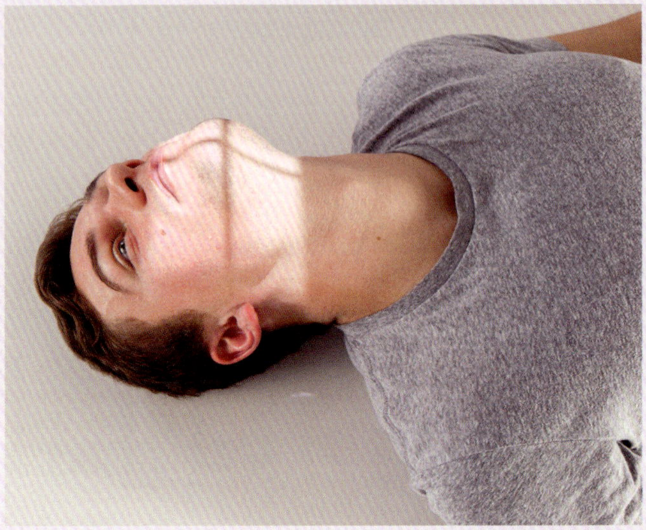

9-97 Centering for Fuchs method.

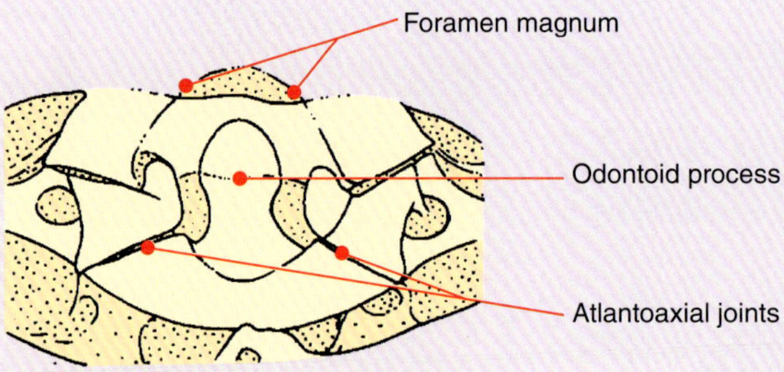

9-98 Fuchs method.

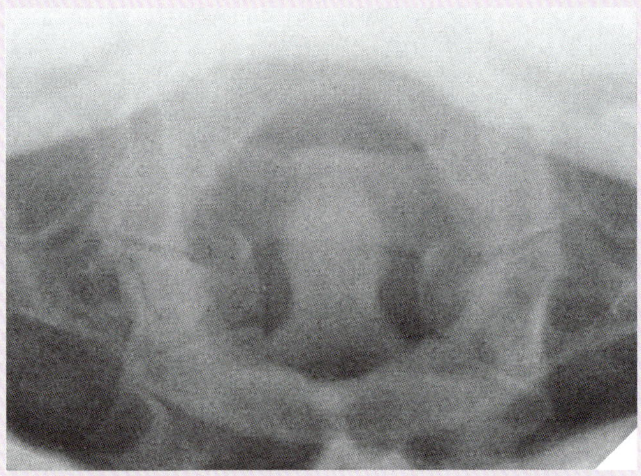

9-99 Fuchs method.

Nontrauma Cervical Spine or Thoracic Spine

- Projection: Swimmer's Lateral
- *Swimmer's Lateral may be used to complement a non-trauma cervical or thoracic spine protocol series or trauma cervical or thoracic spine protocol series*

Technical Considerations

- kVp 70–85
- mAs set manually or center AEC cell
- 40″–72″ SID

Exposure Field Size

- 10 × 12 lengthwise

Patient Position

- Left lateral recumbent (Figs. 9-100 and 9-101)
    - Roll patient into a left lateral position. The left arm should be extended straight up. The right arm should reach down toward the toes. This will help separate the thickness of the shoulders. Ensure the patient raises chin to look straight ahead to help align the cervical spine with the thoracic spine
    - The alternate right lateral recumbent could be used if arm position needs to be reversed for a patient's upper extremity injury
- Erect (Fig. 9-102)
    - Position the patient into an erect left lateral. The left arm (arm closest to the Bucky) reaches straight up. The right arm should relax down toward toes. SID may be determined by site preference but can be increased to as much as 72″
- If there is ever an instance in which the left arm is injured and the arm cannot move or reach straight up, the right lateral position could be considered to reverse the arm positions

Centering

- C7–T1 and MCP

Marking of IR

- Anatomic L side marker placed along the anterior surface of the patient

Breathing

- Suspend respiration or a breathing technique could be implemented
- Ensure patient holds position while walking away to make the exposure

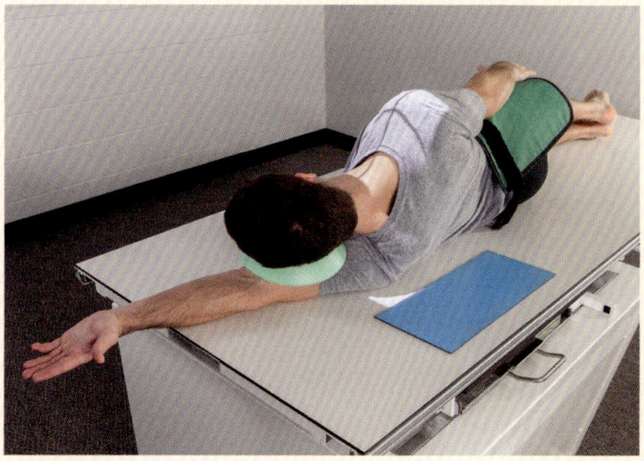

9-100 Recumbent Swimmer's left lateral.

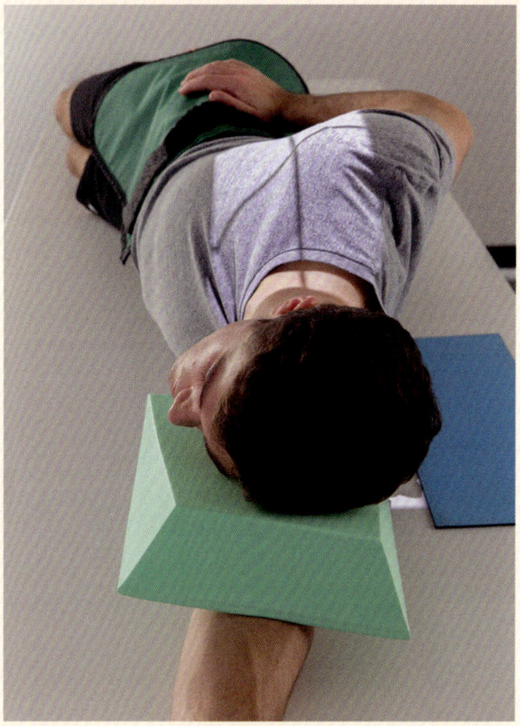

9-101 Recumbent Swimmer's left lateral. Arm position is slightly variated with the hand on the hip and the shoulder dropped back to bring the humeral head more posterior aiming to avoid rotation of the thorax.

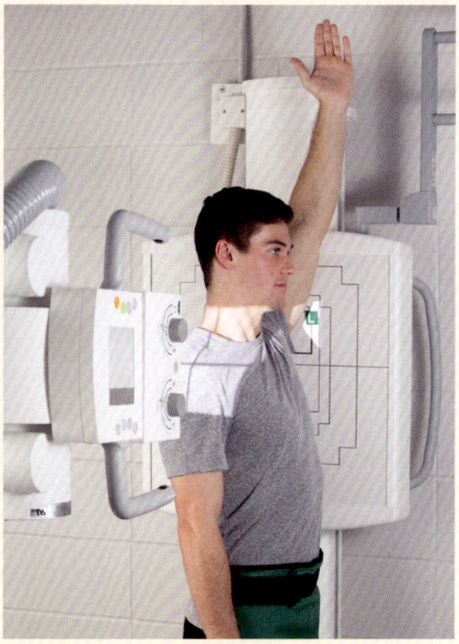

9-102 Erect Swimmer's left lateral.

IMAGE CRITIQUE (FIGS. 9-103 and 9-104)

- The lower cervical and upper thoracic vertebrae are imaged (cervicothoracic region)
- The alignment of C7–T1 bodies is of interest as are intact spinous processes
- The Swimmer's lateral can complement a C-spine or T-spine series
  - Swimmer's lateral for C-spine will demonstrate the lower cervical vertebrae that may technically be nonvisible owing to the thickness of the shoulders
  - Swimmer's lateral for a T-spine will demonstrate the upper thoracic vertebrae when they are technically nonvisible owing to the thickness of the shoulders
- Height of vertebral bodies and intervertebral disk spaces observed
- Zygapophyseal joints of C5–C7 are visualized
- Demonstrating the region free of part rotation (Fig. 9-105)
- Properly centered with four-sided collimation

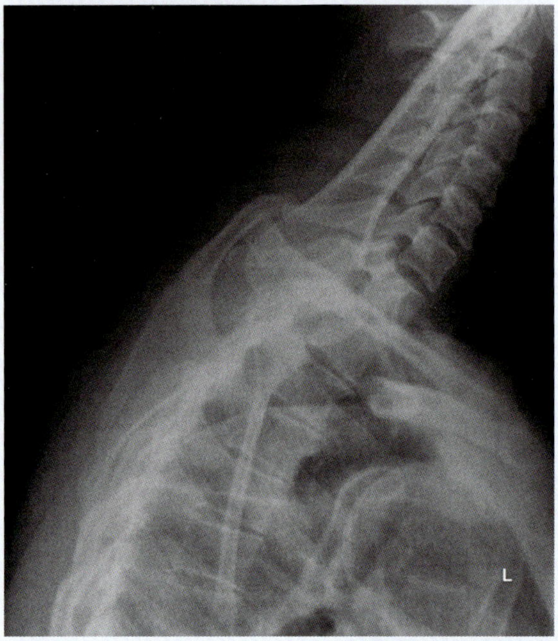

9-103 Swimmer's lateral.

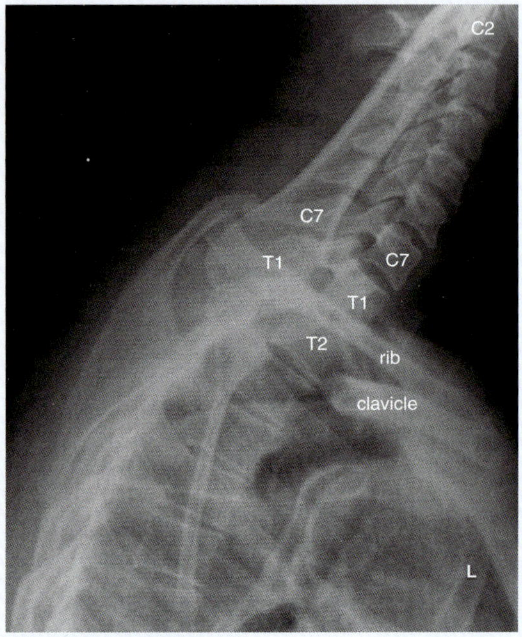

9-104 Swimmer's lateral.

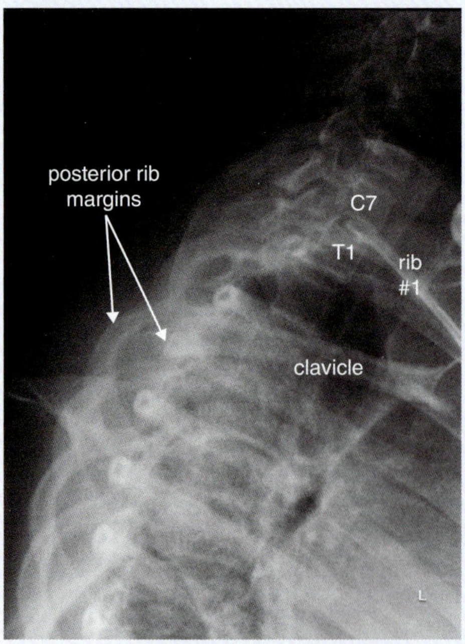

9-105 Swimmer's lateral with rotation.

POSITION VARIATION: HORIZONTAL BEAM SWIMMER'S LATERAL PROJECTION

A horizontal beam Swimmer's lateral could be attempted to supplement a horizontal beam cervical or thoracic lateral in trauma situations in which lower cervical and/or upper thoracic vertebrae need visualization. With the patient recumbent, a horizontal beam is set at a 40″–72″ SID. With a grid placed, an exposure field size is set at 10 × 12 lengthwise. The patient's arm closest to the IR is positioned to extend above their head. The patient's opposite arm is allowed to remain at their side. The central ray is set to enter just above the level of the shoulder at approximately C7–T1 and with MCP. A right horizontal beam lateral can be switched for a left lateral if the patient has arm injury that prevents the aforementioned positioning (Figs. 9-106 and 9-107).

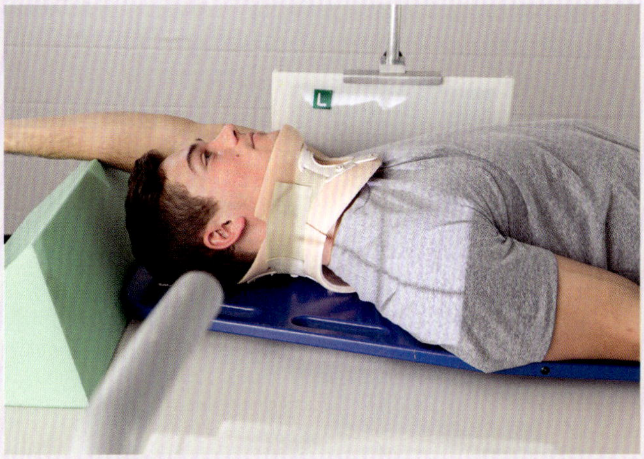

9-106 Horizontal beam Swimmer's lateral.

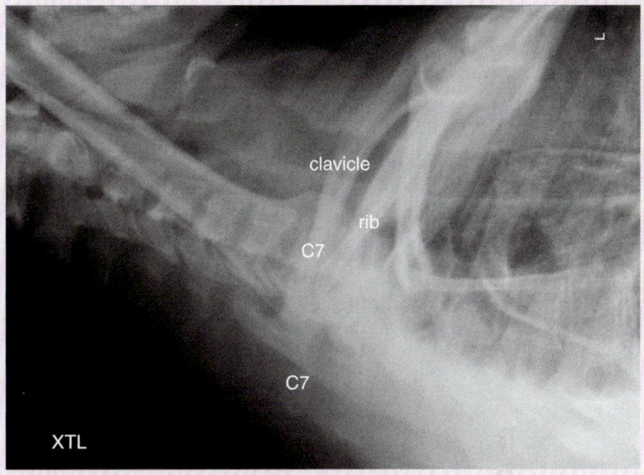

9-107 Horizontal beam Swimmer's lateral.

9-2 Nontrauma Cervical Spine Protocol

Projection	SID	Positioning	Central Ray	Best Visualizes
Lateral 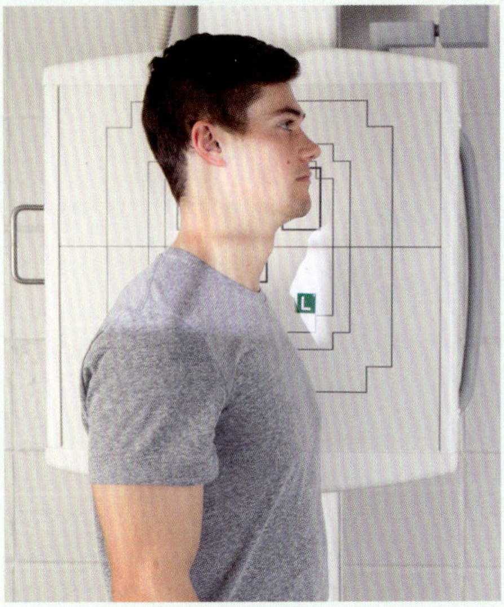	72″	Erect left lateral. Patient looks straight ahead. Shoulders may be further depressed with use of weights.	C5 and MCP	C1–C7 Zygapophyseal joints C2–C7 Spinous processes in profile Anterior to posterior alignment of the vertebral bodies
PA Axial Oblique(s)[a] 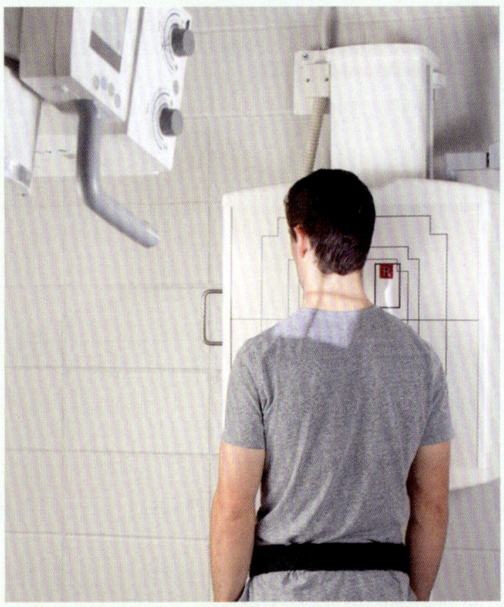	40″–72″	Erect 45° RAO and LAO positions. Patient looks straight ahead.	15°–20° caudal tube angle to C5 and midway between neck borders.	Intervertebral foramina of C2–C7 closest to the IR. Example: RAO demonstrates the right intervertebral foramina.
AP Axial Oblique(s)[a] 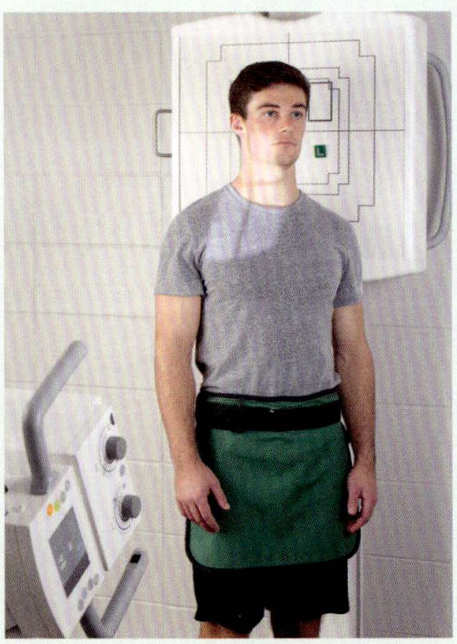	40″–72″	Erect 45° RPO and LPO positions. Patient looks straight ahead.	15°–20° cephalic tube angle to C5 and midway between neck borders	Intervertebral foramina of C2–C7 furthest from the IR. Example: RPO demonstrates the left intervertebral foramina.

Projection	SID	Positioning	Central Ray	Best Visualizes
AP Axial 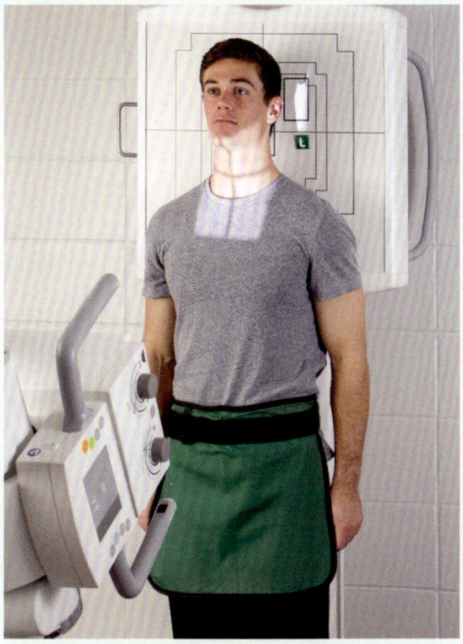	40″	Erect or supine	If erect, 20° cephalic angle If recumbent, 15° cephalic angle C5 and MSP	C3–C7 must be visualized. C1 and C2 will be superimposed by the base of the skull. Inclusion of C7–T1 articulation is ideal. Intervertebral disk spaces open Symmetry of the spine displayed with symmetric pedicles and centered spinous processes.
AP open mouth 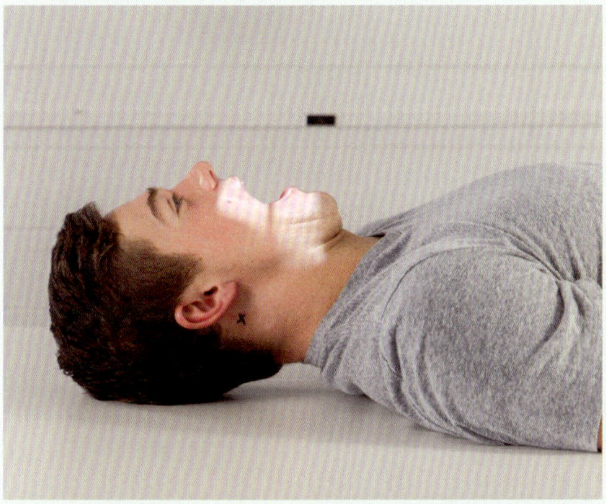	40″	Erect or supine Open mouth wide Tuck or extend the chin until the lower margin of the upper teeth aligns with the base of the skull.	Center of open mouth	C1 and C2 centered within the open mouth, indicating no rotation. Zygapophyseal joints between C1 and C2 are visualized. The odontoid process is free of superimposition from the teeth or base of the skull.
Swimmer's lateral 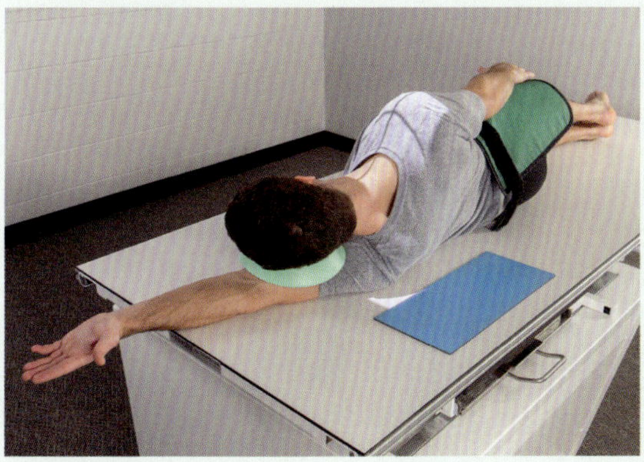	40″ recumbent	Erect left lateral or left lateral recumbent Left arm is elevated above head up toward the left ear. Right arm is left at side and relaxed down toward the feet. Make sure patient lifts chin to ensure a true lateral C-spine.	Just above the humeral head and MCP to the level of C7–T1	Relationship of C7–T1 evaluating disk space and anterior to posterior alignment True lateral upper T-spine should display the intervertebral foramina.

[a]Indicates that only the PA Axial Obliques *OR* AP Axial Obliques are obtained, not both.

Trauma Cervical Spine

- Projection: Horizontal Beam Lateral
- Summation of entire trauma spine protocol is found in Table 9-8

Trauma Cervical Spine Protocol

Horizontal Beam Lateral

AP Axial

AP Open Mouth

Technical Considerations

- kVp 75–85
- mAs set manually
- 72″ SID (compensates for the OID created between neck and IR)

Exposure Field Size

- 10 × 12 lengthwise

Patient Position

- Supine
- Owing to trauma and spinal precautions, the patient position should not be altered
- If patient is free of upper extremity injury, neck pain, and paralysis, clinical facilities may have the technologist put on personnel protective garments and manually depress the patient's shoulders. *Manual depression of the shoulders may not be allowed at facilities or allowed only when physician consent is given*
- Manual depression of the shoulders is applied by gently pulling down on the patient's wrists during delivery of patient breathing. Manual depression could assist with the demonstration of all seven cervical vertebrae

Centering

- C5 (Adam's apple) and MCP (Fig. 9-108)

Marking of IR

- Anatomic L side marker placed along the anterior surface of the patient

Breathing

- Suspend respiration after the second expiration. Instruct the patient to "take a deep breath in, blow it out and hold it out, and relax your shoulders down"
- Ensure you watch the patient the entire time while walking away to make the exposure
- In cases where manual depression of the shoulders is utilized, the technologist depressing the patient's shoulders will signal to the technologist at the control panel when to make the exposure

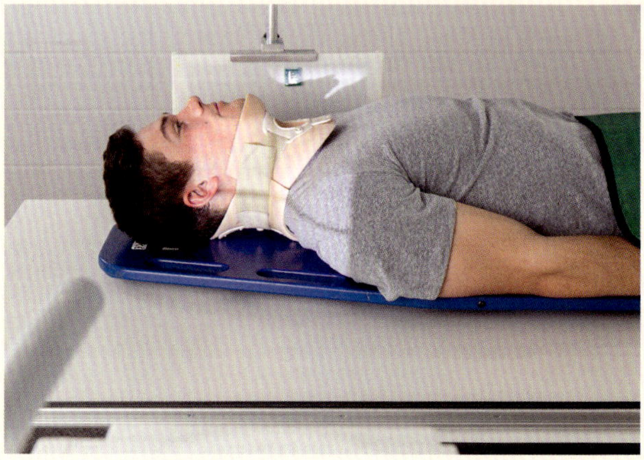

9-108 Horizontal beam trauma lateral C-spine.

IMAGE CRITIQUE (FIGS. 9-109 and 9-110)

- Cervical vertebral C1–C7 bodies and spinous processes should be seen in profile. In cases where not all seven cervical vertebrae are visualized, a horizontal beam Swimmer's lateral projection may complement the horizontal beam cervical lateral
- Anterior to posterior alignment of the cervical vertebrae
- Height of vertebral bodies and intervertebral disk spaces observed
- Zygapophyseal joints of C3–C7 visualized
- C1 and C2 should be free of superimposition from the base of the skull and mandibular rami but may not be, considering the trauma position of the patient that cannot be altered
- Demonstrating the transition of C7–T1 is ideal if possible to achieve
- Properly centered with four-sided collimation

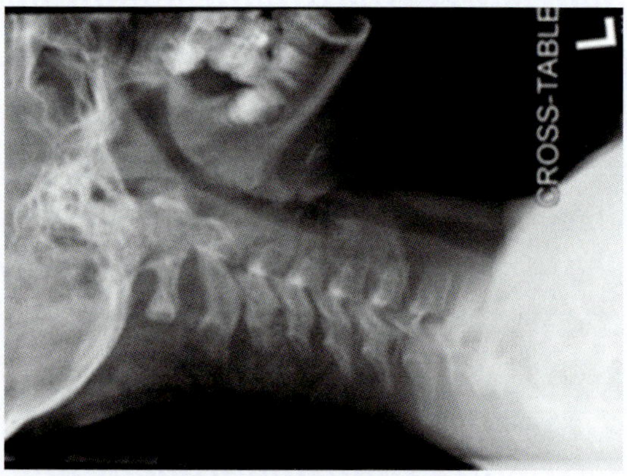

9-109 Horizontal beam trauma lateral C-spine.

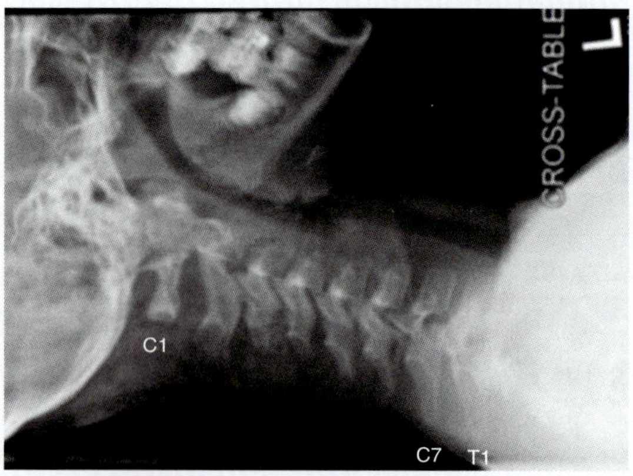

9-110 Horizontal beam trauma lateral C-spine.

Trauma Cervical Spine

- Projection: AP Axial

Trauma Cervical Spine Protocol
Horizontal Beam Lateral
AP Axial
AP Open Mouth

Technical Considerations
- kVp 70–80
- mAs set manually or center AEC cell
- 40″ SID

Exposure Field Size
- 10 × 12 lengthwise

Patient Position
- Supine
- Owing to trauma and spinal precautions, the patient position should not be altered

Centering
- C5 (Adam's apple) and MSP
- 15° cephalic tube angle is applied to the supine patient (Fig. 9-111)

Marking of IR
- Anatomic side marker R or L placed lateral to the patient's side

Breathing
- Suspend respiration. Instruct the patient to "hold their breath"
- Ensure patient holds position while walking away to make the exposure

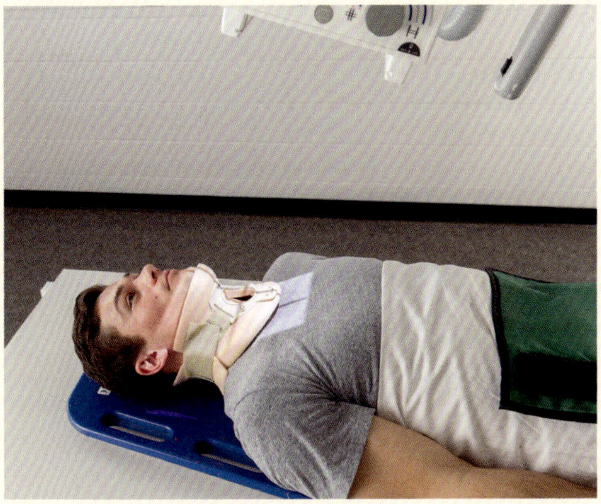

9-111 Trauma AP axial C-spine.

IMAGE CRITIQUE (FIGS. 9-112 and 9-113)

- Cervical vertebrae C3–C7, ideally, are seen free of rotation; however, this may be difficult to avoid. Symmetry of the vertebral pedicles can aid in ruling out rotation
- C1 and C2 will likely be superimposed by the base of the skull and mandible. The mandible or base of the skull may superimpose C3, considering the trauma position of the patient confined to a cervical collar, that cannot be altered
- Demonstrating the transition of C7–T1 is recommended
- Intervertebral disk spaces may appear open if the tube angle has been applied
- Properly centered with four-sided collimation

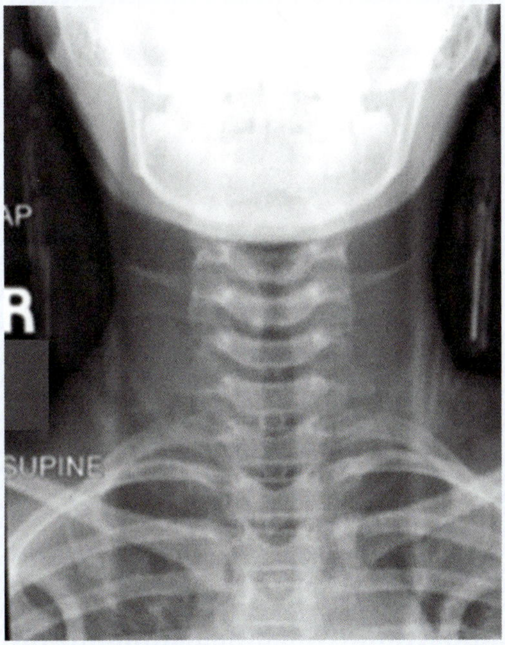

9-112 Trauma AP axial C-spine.

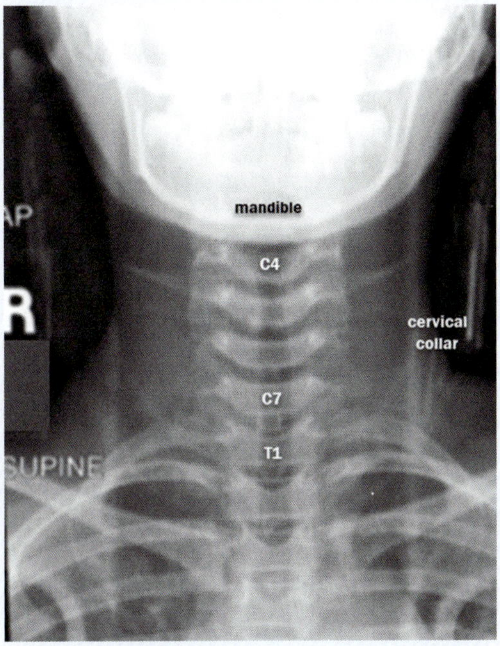

9-113 Trauma AP axial C-spine.

Trauma Cervical Spine

- Projection: AP Open Mouth

Trauma Cervical Spine Protocol
Lateral
AP Axial
AP Open Mouth

Technical Considerations
- kVp 75–80
- mAs set manually
- 40″ SID

Exposure Field Size
- 8 × 8 or smaller

Patient Position
- Supine
- Owing to trauma and spinal precautions, the patient's head and neck position should not be altered
- Have patient open their mouth wide; the cervical collar will be restrictive (Fig. 9-114)

Centering
- Center of the open mouth

Marking of IR
- Anatomic side marker R or L placed furthest from the patient's midline

Breathing
- With the patient's mouth wide open, have them suspend respiration. Instruct the patient to "hold their breath"
- Ensure patient holds position while walking away to make the exposure

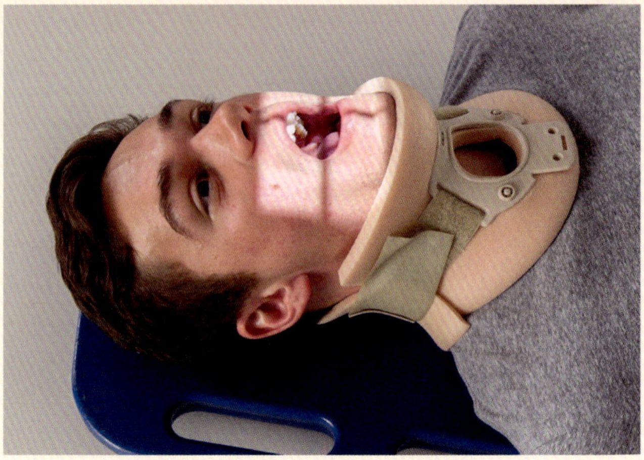

9-114 Trauma AP open mouth.

IMAGE CRITIQUE (FIG. 9-115)

- Ideally, C1 and C2 should be seen centered within the open mouth, although the inability to align the lower margin of the upper teeth with the base of the skull may prevent this from being achieved
- The height of the zygapophyseal joints of C1 and C2 are visualized and evaluated
- The odontoid process should be visualized free of superimposition from the base of the skull or teeth. In cases in which this is not achieved in the trauma circumstance, a Fuchs method (Reverse Waters) could be attempted. Rather than extending the chin to align MML perpendicular to the IR, the central ray is angled cephalic until it is parallel to the MML (Figs. 9-116 and 9-117)
- Properly centered with four-sided collimation

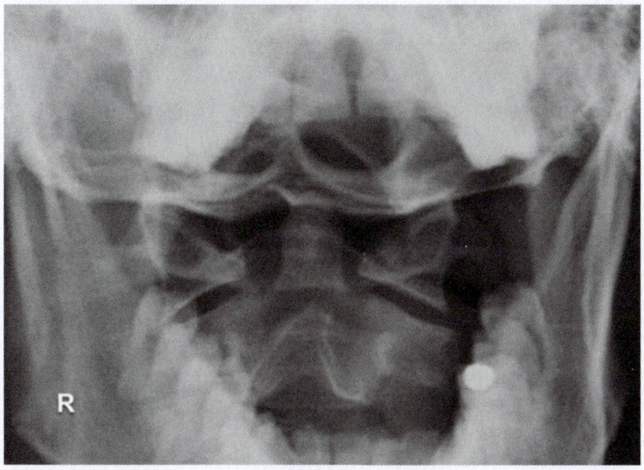

9-115 Trauma AP open mouth prevents the R.T. from adjusting the head and neck owing to the cervical collar.

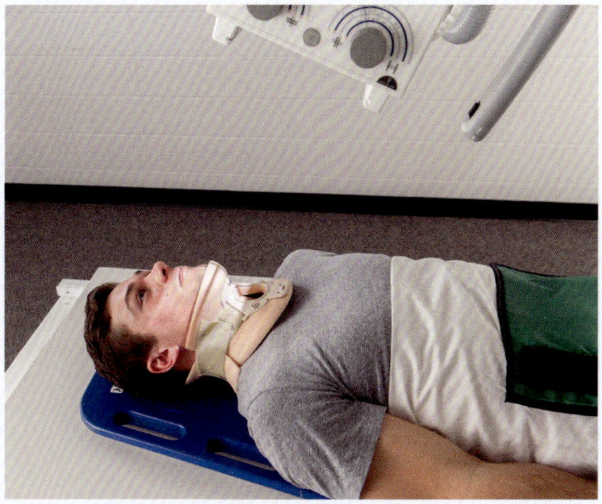

9-116 Reverse Waters method.

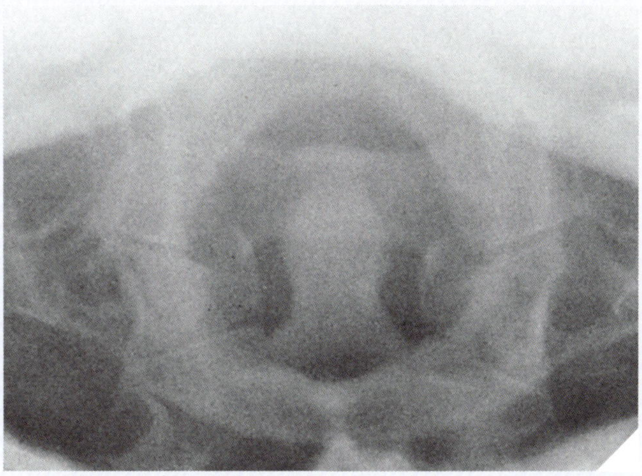

9-117 Odontoid seen within the foramen magnum.

Nontrauma Thoracic Spine

- Projection: AP
- Summation of entire thoracic spine protocol is found in Table 9-3

Thoracic Spine Protocol

AP

Left Lateral

Technical Considerations

- kVp 75–80
- mAs set manually or center AEC cell
- 40″ SID
- Consider positioning the patient according to the anode heel effect or implement a compensating filter

Exposure Field Size

- 14 × 17 lengthwise (restrict the beam side to side)

Patient Position

- Supine (Fig. 9-118)
- Erect if ordered weight-bearing (Fig. 9-119)
- Arms slightly abducted from patient's sides
- Orientate the patient's neck with the anode side of the tube and the abdomen with the cathode side of the tube to achieve a more even density between the thickness differences of the patient. Consider using the anode heel effect and/or apply a compensating filter

Centering

- Level of T7/8 (Locate by measuring approximately 3″–4″ inferior to jugular notch)
- Align to the MSP

Marking of IR

- R or L marker placed above the correct side in the shoulder region within the collimated exposure field

Breathing

- Instruct patient to hold their breath after expiration
- Ensure patient holds position while walking away to make the exposure

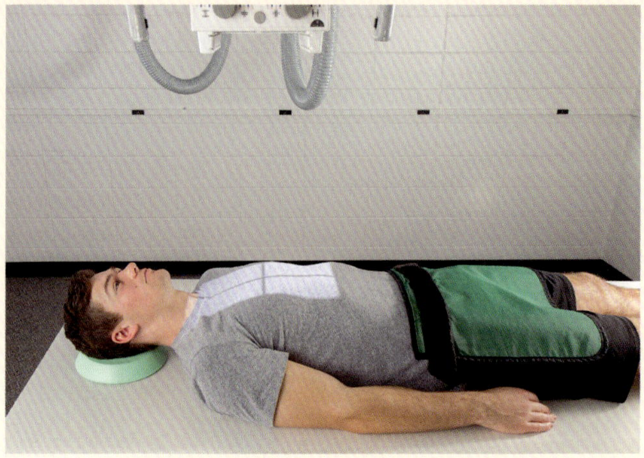

9-118 AP T-spine recumbent.

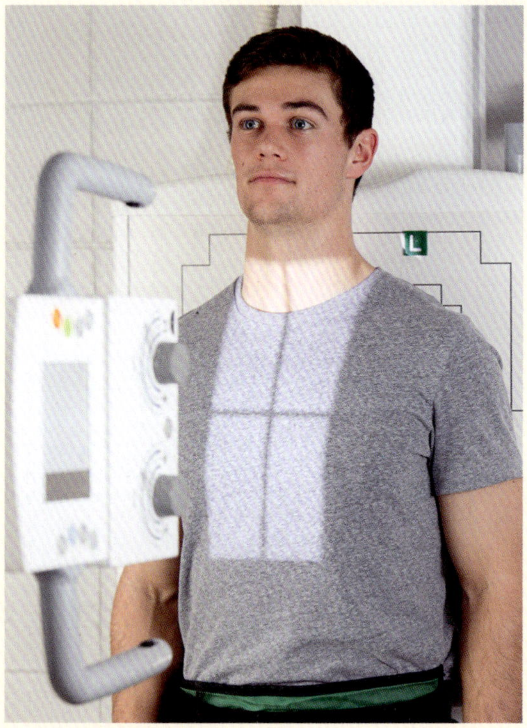

9-119 AP T-spine erect.

IMAGE CRITIQUE (FIGS. 9-120 and 9-121)

- C7–T1 junction, all 12 thoracic vertebrae, and T12–L1 junction visualized
- No rotation of the thoracic vertebrae evidenced when the spinous processes are centered upon the vertebral bodies and pedicles are symmetric on the lateral and superior edges of the bodies
- Clavicles near horizontal. This indicates that the shoulders were relaxed
- Sternoclavicular (SC) joints symmetric. This indicates that the patient was not rotated toward the right or the left shoulder (Fig. 9-122)
- Even density achieved between the upper and the lower portions of the thoracic column (Fig. 9-123)
- Properly centered and collimated

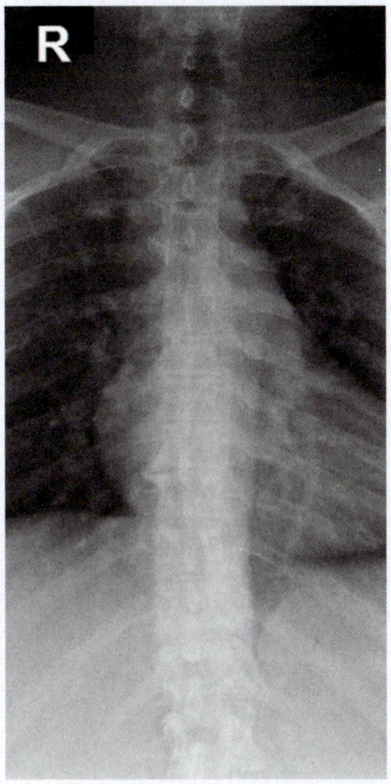

9-120 AP T-spine.

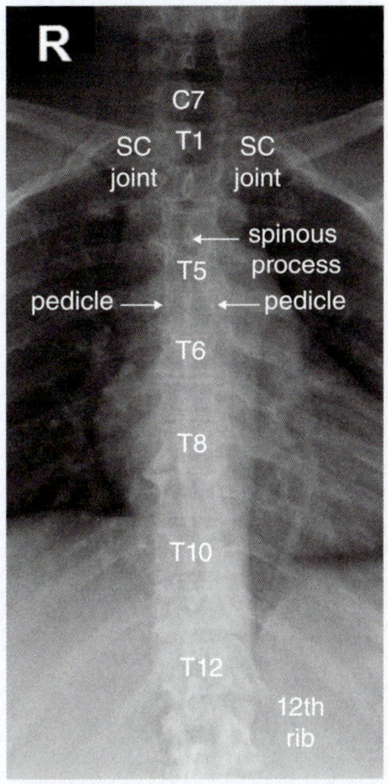

9-121 AP T-spine.

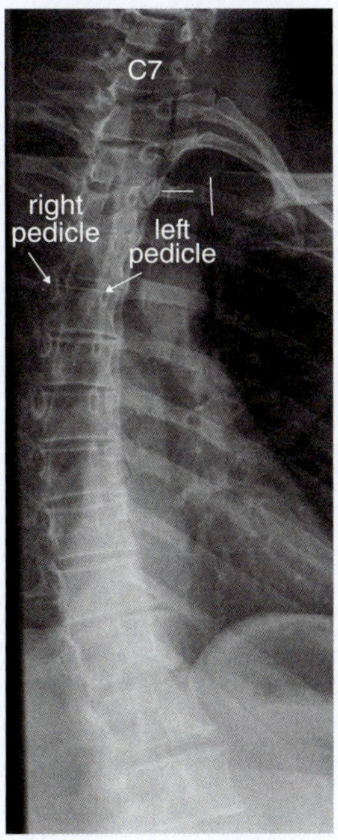

9-122 AP T-spine with rotation.

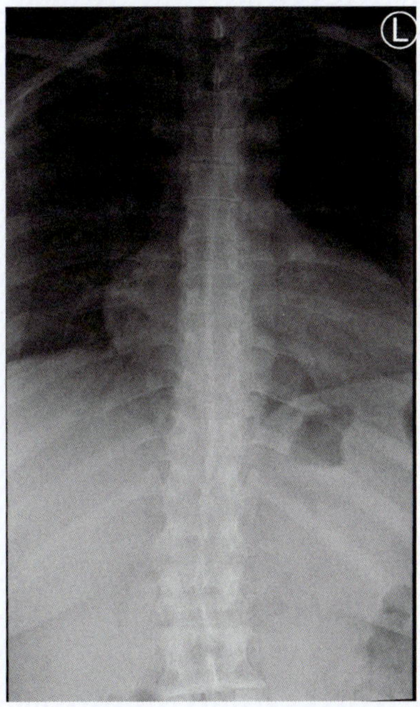

9-123 Example of uneven density achieved throughout the thoracic spine.

Nontrauma Thoracic Spine

- Projection: Left Lateral
- Summation of entire thoracic spine protocol is found in Table 9-3

Thoracic Spine Protocol
AP
Left Lateral

Technical Considerations

- kVp 75–85
- mAs set manually
- 40″ SID

Exposure Field Size

- 14 × 17 lengthwise for all patients (restrict the beam anterior to posterior)

Patient Position

- Recumbent left lateral
  - Ensure true lateral position of thorax. The shoulders directly superimposed and aligned with the hips. Bend knees slightly for patient stability and pull knees up slightly toward chest. Bend the elbows and raise 90° from the chest. Elevate chin to align cervical spine with thoracic spine (Fig. 9-124)
- Erect left lateral position if ordered weight-bearing
  - Ensure true lateral position of thorax by aligning hips and shoulders. Step feet apart for stability. Arms elevated to hold onto chest positioning bar. Elevate chin to align cervical spine with thoracic spine (Fig. 9-125)

Centering

- Level of T7/8 (inferior angle of scapula) and slightly posterior to MCP. Collimate the beam as tight as possible anterior to posterior on the patient to minimize scatter radiation. Skimming light should be seen only on the posterior surface of the patient

Marking of the IR

- L marker placed on the anterior surface within the collimated exposure field

Breathing

- *Two options:*
  - The patient is instructed to take in a breath, exhale, and hold their breath out. The image is acquired after expiration
  - The patient breathes continuously throughout a 3–4 second exposure by taking shallow, quick breaths
- Ensure patient holds position while walking away to make the exposure

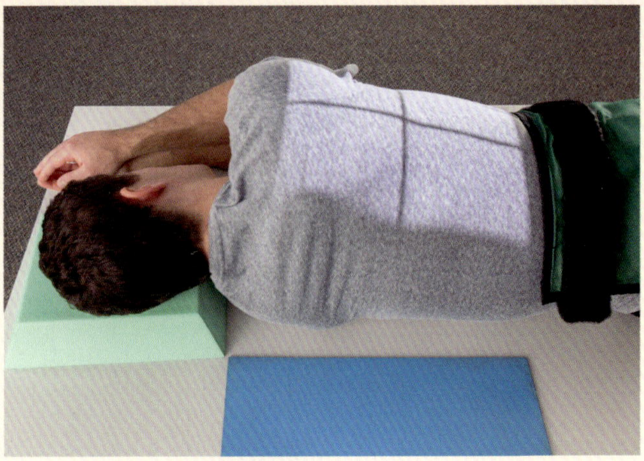

9-124 Lateral T-spine recumbent.

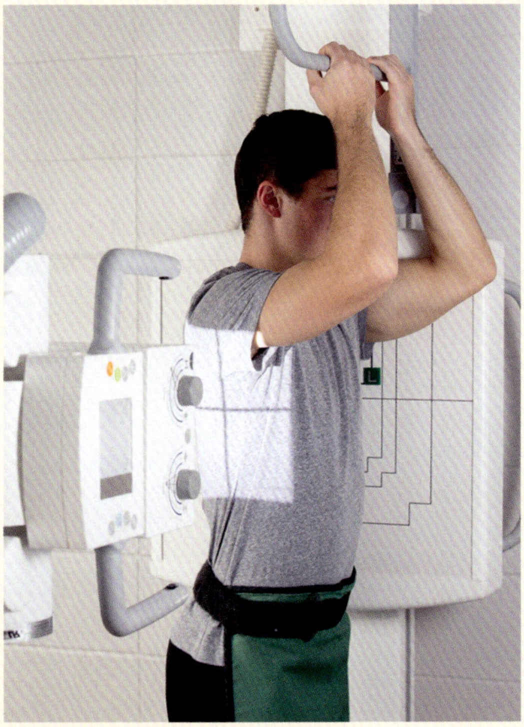

9-125 Lateral T-spine erect.

IMAGE CRITIQUE (FIGS. 9-126 and 9-127)

- T1–T3/4 may be difficult to visualize technically owing to the thickness of both shoulders being superimposed. A Swimmer's lateral projection may be needed to complement this lateral projection to demonstrate the upper thoracic vertebrae
- Anterior to posterior alignment of the thoracic vertebrae
- Height of vertebral bodies and intervertebral disk spaces observed
- Intervertebral foramina are open, indicating minimal to no rotation of the thorax (Table 9-7). Superimposition of the posterior rib margins indicates the thorax is not rotated. Rotation evidenced as posterior rib margins separate apart (Fig. 9-128)
- Spinous processes may be noted in profile
- Properly centered and collimated

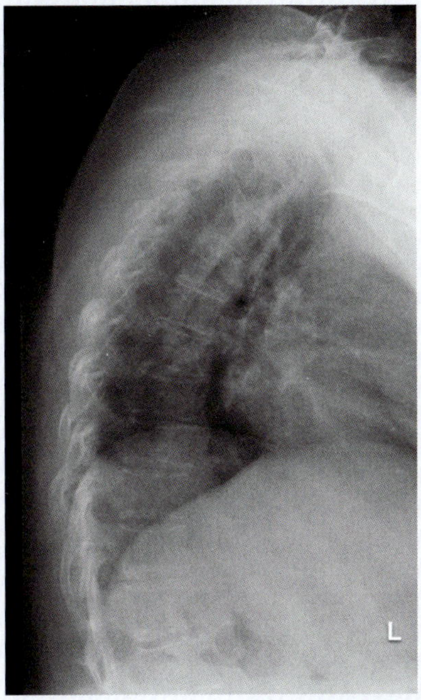

9-126 Lateral T-spine.

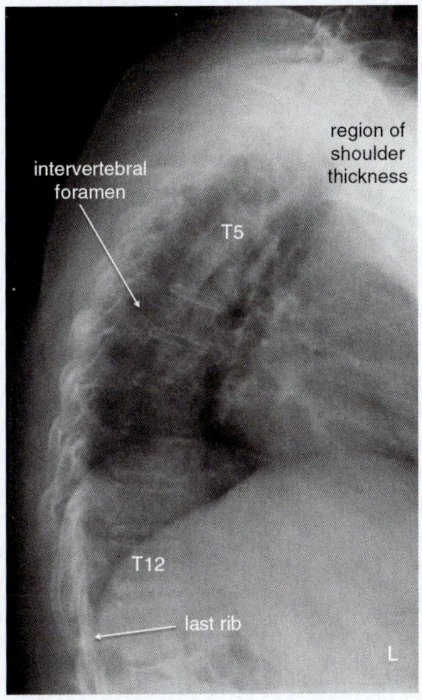

9-127 Lateral T-spine.

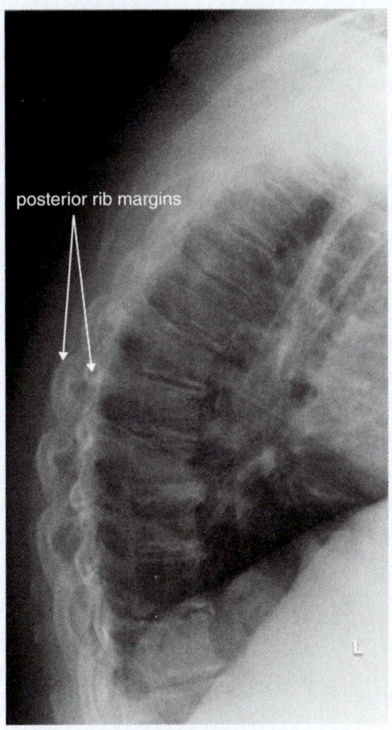

9-128 Lateral T-spine with rotation.

9-3 Nontrauma Thoracic Spine Protocol

Projection	SID	Positioning	Central ray	Best Visualizes
AP 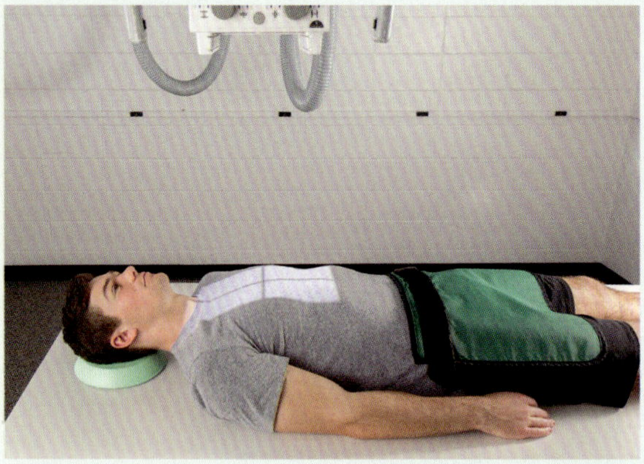	40″	Supine Arms at side and no rotation of the shoulders, spine, or pelvis.	T7–T8 and MSP (CR resembles AP chest centering)	T1–T12 visualized. Inclusion of C7–T1 and T12–L1 transitions is ideal. Intervertebral disk spaces open. Symmetry of the spine displayed with symmetric pedicles and centered spinous processes.
Lateral 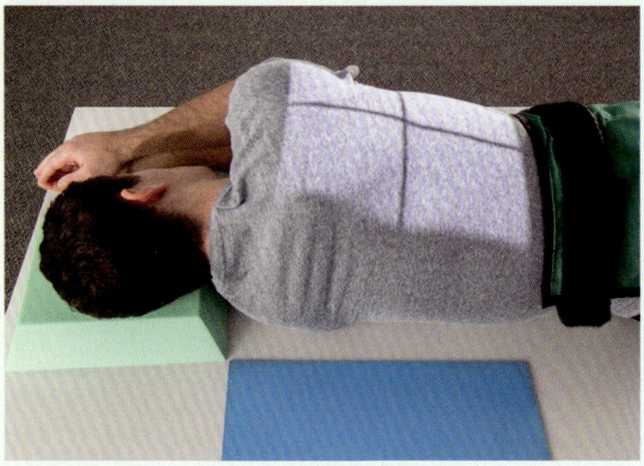	40″	Recumbent left lateral Ensure true lateral with shoulder and hips stacked and aligned.	T7–T8 and MCP or slightly posterior (CR resembles Lateral chest centering)	T1–T4 may be difficult to visualize owing to the thickness of the shoulders. Swimmer's lateral may need to accompany. True lateral evidenced by superimposed posterior rib margins and intervertebral foramina open. Anterior to posterior alignment of the vertebral bodies. Intervertebral disk spaces and vertebral body height.
Swimmer's lateral 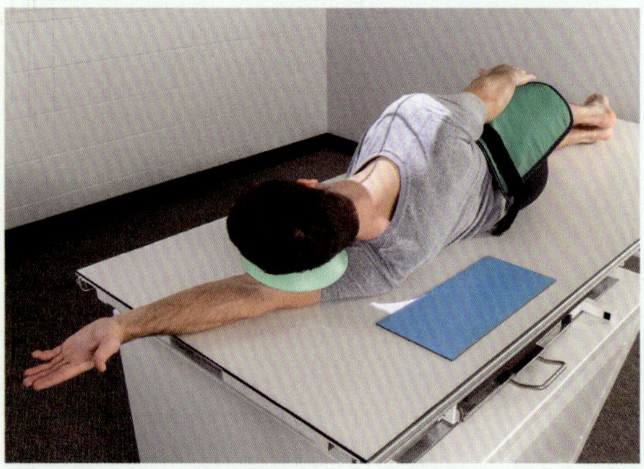	40″	Recumbent left lateral Left arm is elevated above head up toward the left ear. Right arm is left at side and relaxed down toward the feet. Make sure patient lifts chin to ensure a true lateral C-spine.	Just above the humeral head and MCP to the level of C7–T1.	Cervicothoracic region demonstrating the lower C-spine and upper T-spine. Relationship of C7–T1 evaluating disk space and anterior to posterior alignment of the vertebral bodies. True lateral upper T-spine should display the intervertebral foramina.
AP oblique or PA oblique[a] (not shown)	40″	70° anterior or posterior oblique		Zygapophyseal joints

[a]Indicates that oblique T-spine projections are not typically acquired.

Nontrauma Lumbar Spine

- Projection: AP
- *PA projection is not typically practiced owing to the increased OID created between the spine and the IR caused by the abdominal tissue*
- Summation of entire lumbar spine protocol is found in Table 9-4

Lumbar Spine Protocol

AP

AP Obliques

Lateral

Technical Considerations

- kVp 75–85
- mAs set manually or center AEC cell
- 40″ SID

Exposure Field Size

- 14 × 17 lengthwise (restrict the beam side to side)

Patient Position

- Supine with patient lying comfortably on the table Support provided under the patient's knees will reduce the lordotic lumbar curvature and position the lumbar spine parallel to the plane of the IR. A parallel spine will allow the natural beam divergence to pass through intervertebral disk spaces, allowing them to appear open if no pathology is present (Figs. 9-129 to 9-132)
- Erect if ordered weight-bearing (Fig. 9-133)
- Arms slightly abducted from patient's sides or resting on chest

Centering

- Level of the iliac crest and to MSP. Centering resembles the supine abdomen with added collimation

Marking of IR

- Anatomic side marker R or L down in the lowest corner margin of the IR (down in the area of the greater trochanter) within the collimate exposure field

Breathing

- The patient is instructed to take in a breath, exhale, and hold their breath out
- The image is acquired after expiration. This respiratory phase will move the diaphragm superiorly and prevent lung superimposition upon L1
- Ensure patient holds position while walking away to make the exposure

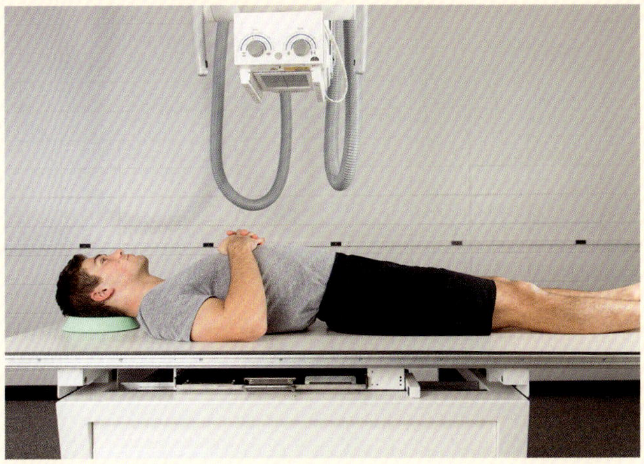

9-129 Full leg extension creating lordotic curvature of spine.

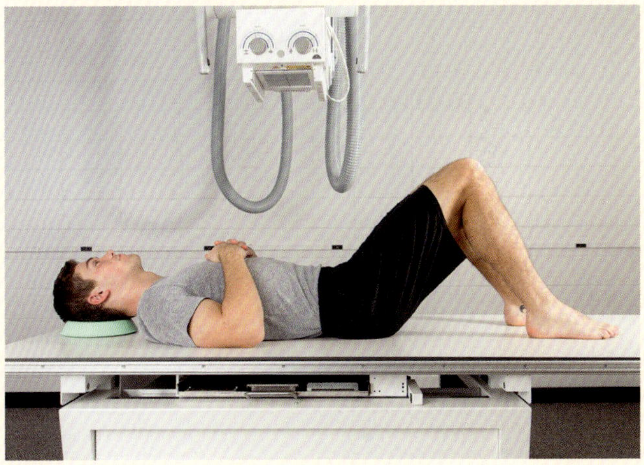

9-130 Full leg flexion flattens the lumbar spine.

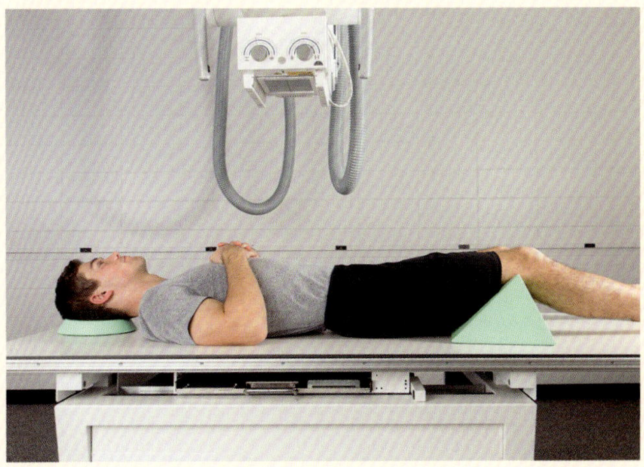

9-131 Ideal position for AP lumbar spine.

(continued)

Nontrauma Lumbar Spine (*Continued*)

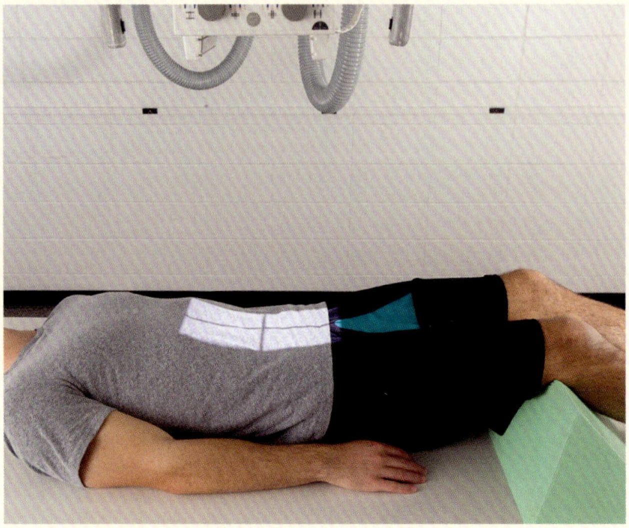

9-132 AP L-spine recumbent.

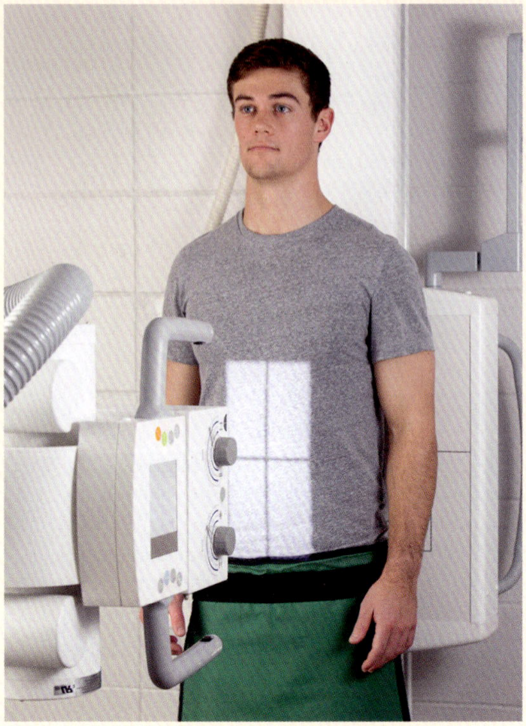

9-133 AP L-spine erect.

IMAGE CRITIQUE (FIGS. 9-134 and 9-135)

- T12–L1 junction, all five lumbar vertebrae, and L5–S1 junction and sacroiliac joints visualized
- No rotation of the lumbar vertebrae evidenced when the pedicles are symmetrically displayed on the lateral edges of the bodies (Fig. 9-136). In addition, the iliac wings should appear symmetric and the ribs extending laterally from the low thoracic vertebral bodies
- Properly centered and collimated for inclusion of necessary anatomy

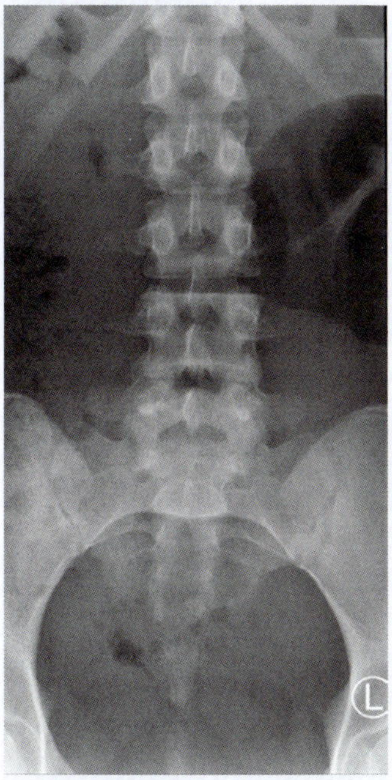

9-134 AP L-spine.

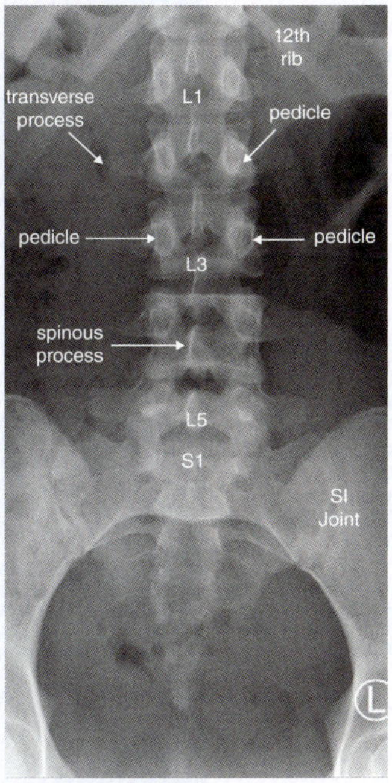

9-135 AP L-spine.

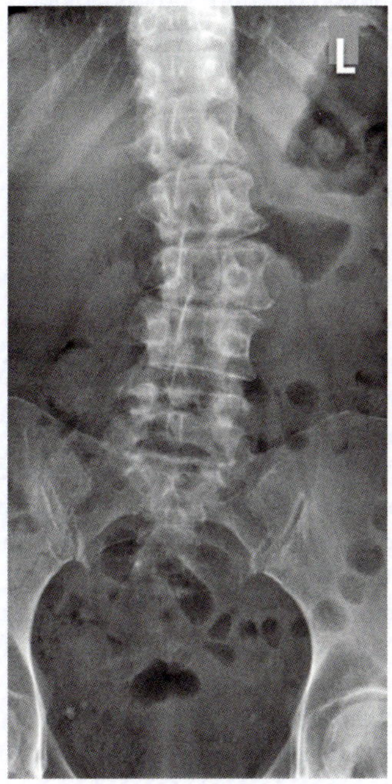

9-136 AP L-spine with rotation.

IMAGE CRITIQUE (*Continued*)

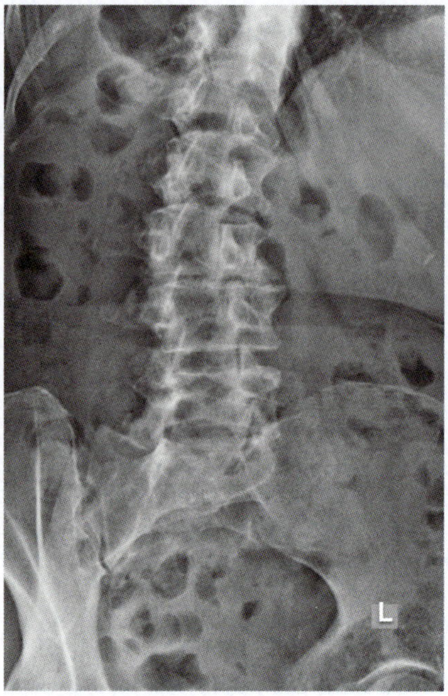

9-141 AP Oblique L-spine—underrotated.

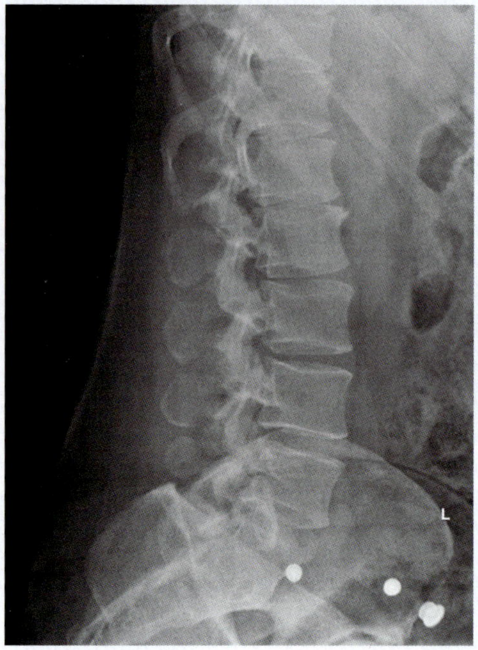

9-142 AP Oblique L-spine—overrotated.

Nontrauma Lumbar Spine

- Projection: Lateral
- Summation of entire lumbar spine protocol is found in Table 9-4

Lumbar Spine Protocol
AP
AP Obliques
Lateral

Technical Considerations

- kVp 80–85
- mAs set manually or center AEC cell
- 40″ SID

Exposure Field Size

- 14 × 17 lengthwise for all patients (restrict the beam anterior to posterior)

Patient Position

- Recumbent left lateral
  - Ensure true lateral position of thorax and abdomen. The shoulders directly superimposed and by aligning hips. Bend knees slightly for patient stability and pull knees up slightly toward chest (Fig. 9-143)
  - Bend the elbows and raise 90° from the chest
  - Consider providing a supportive wedge to the waist area just above the iliac crest in cases of an extremely small-waisted patient when comparing their shoulders to their hips. A supportive wedge will attempt to keep the spine parallel to the IR to assist with visualization of open intervertebral disk spaces. Ideally, the divergence of the beam will align with the disk spaces to demonstrate them open
- Erect left lateral position if ordered weight-bearing
  - Ensure true lateral position of thorax by aligning hips and shoulders. Step feet apart for stability. Arms elevated to hold onto chest positioning bar. Elevate chin to align cervical spine with thoracic spine (Fig. 9-144)

Centering

- Level of L4/5 (iliac crest) and with MCP
- Collimate the beam as tight as possible anterior to posterior on the patient to minimize scatter radiation. Skimming light should be seen only on the posterior surface of the patient and may not be seen on all patients

Marking of the IR

- L marker placed on the anterior surface within the collimated exposure field

Breathing

- The patient is instructed to take in a breath, exhale, and hold their breath out
- The image is acquired after expiration
- Ensure patient holds position while walking away to make the exposure

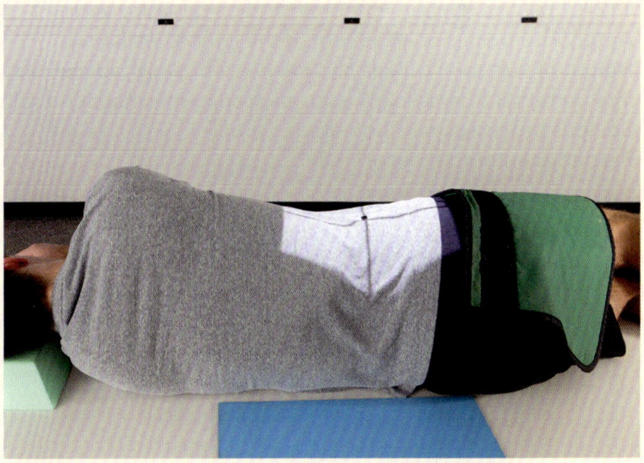

9-143 Lateral L-spine recumbent.

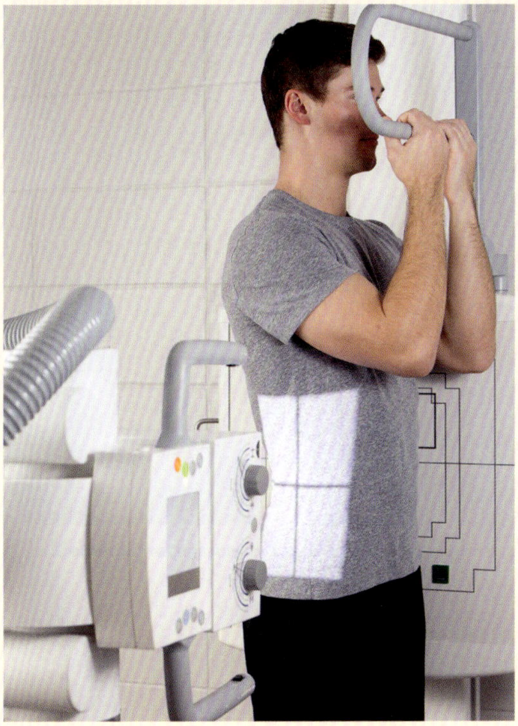

9-144 Lateral L-spine erect.

IMAGE CRITIQUE (FIGS. 9-149 and 9-150)

- L4–L5 and L5–S1 is visualized
- Anterior to posterior alignment of the lumbar vertebrae to the first sacral segment
- Height of vertebral bodies and intervertebral disk spaces observed
- Intervertebral foramina are open, indicating minimal to no rotation of the spine
- Spinous processes may be noted in profile
- Properly centered with four-sided collimation

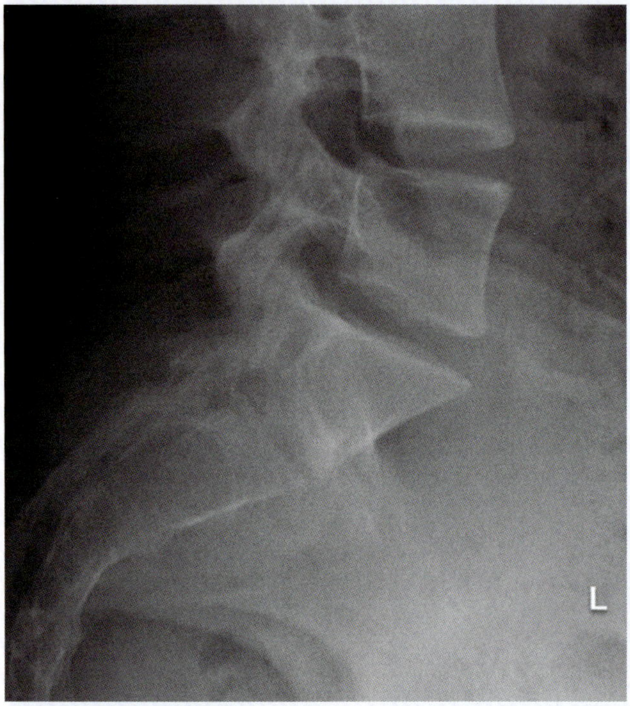

9-149 Lateral L5–S1 spot.

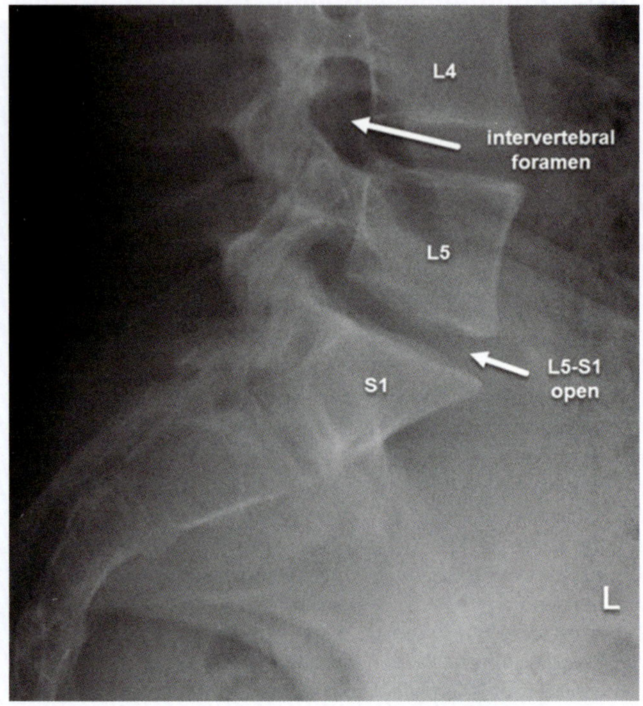

9-150 Lateral L5–S1 spot.

9-4 Nontrauma Lumbar Spine Protocol

Projection	SID	Positioning	Central Ray	Best Visualizes
AP 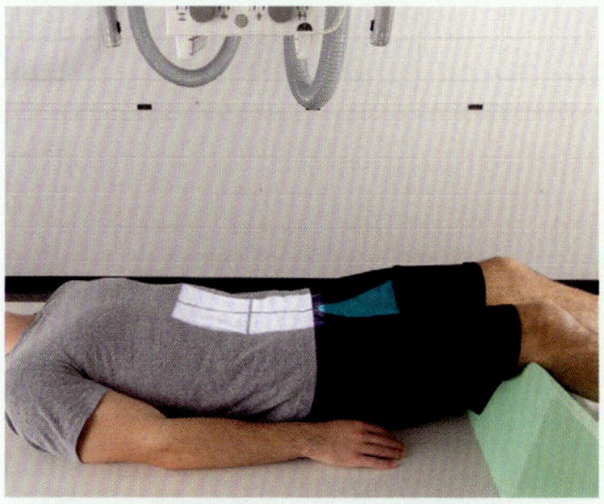	40″	Supine or upright Arms at side and no rotation of the shoulders, spine, or pelvis. Flex knees slightly to align lumbar spine more parallel to the IR.	L4–L5 and MSP (CR resembles supine abdomen centering)	L1–L5 visualized. Inclusion of T12–L1 and L5–S1 transitions is ideal. Intervertebral disk spaces open. Symmetry of the spine displayed with symmetric pedicles and centered spinous processes.
AP oblique(s)[a] (preferred) 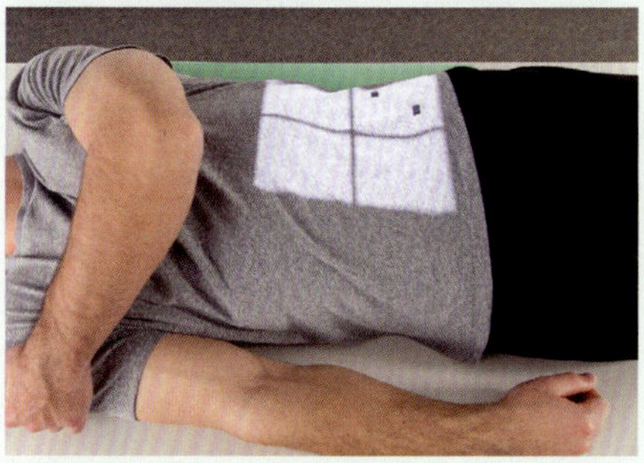	40″	From supine roll into a supine oblique(s). 45° RPO and LPO Ensure shoulders through hips are evenly rotated and supported to hold the position. May also be acquired upright	1″ superior to the iliac crest and 1″ medial to upside ASIS	L1–L5 zygapophyseal joints on the downside are best demonstrated. For example, RPO demonstrates the right zygapophyseal joint. T12–L1 and L5–S1 articulations are included.
PA oblique(s)[a] (not shown)	40″	From prone roll into prone oblique(s). 45° RAO and LAO		L1–L5 zygapophyseal joints on the upside are best demonstrated. For example, RAO demonstrates the left zygapophyseal joint. T12–L1 and L5–S1 articulations are included.
Lateral 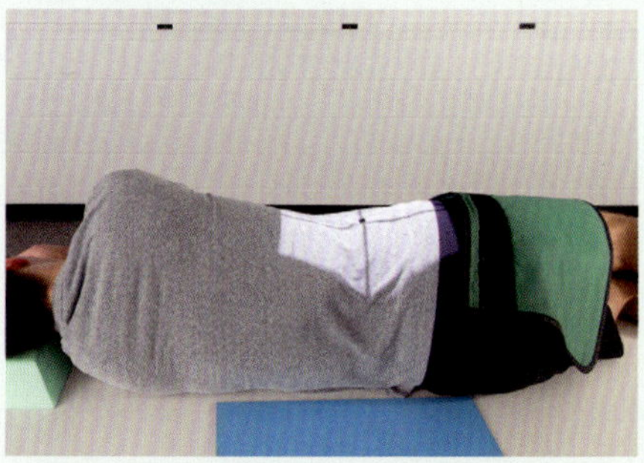	40″	Left lateral recumbent or upright Ensure true lateral with shoulder and hips stacked and aligned. Consider support under the waist to eliminate exaggerated spinal sag when recumbent.	L4–L5 and MSP	L1–L5 visualized. T12–L1 and L5–S1 articulations are included. True lateral evidenced by superimposed posterior rib margins and intervertebral foramina open. Anterior to posterior alignment of the vertebral bodies. Intervertebral disk spaces and vertebral body height.
Lateral L5–S1 spot[b] 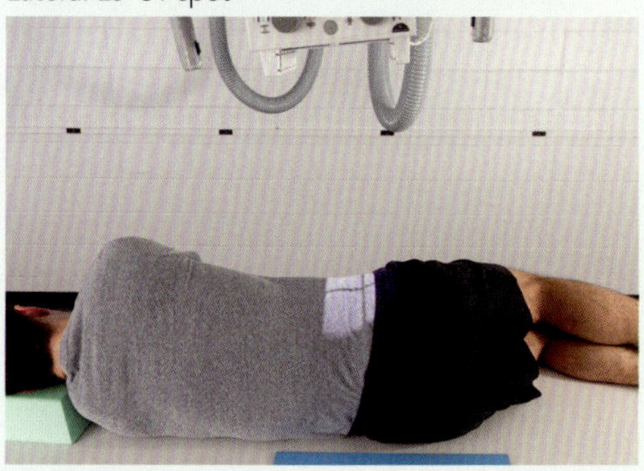	40″	Left lateral recumbent or upright Ensure true lateral with shoulder and hips stacked and aligned.	1½″ inferior to iliac crest and 1″ posterior to MCP 5°–8° caudal tube angle typically applied	L5–S1 disk space open and centered to the collimated field. L4–L5 may also be included. True lateral position will evidence the intervertebral foramina open at L4–L5 and L5–S1.

[a]Indicates that only the AP Obliques (RPO/LPO) *OR* PA Obliques (RAO/LAO) are obtained, not both. AP Obliques are preferred.
[b]Indicates that the L5–S1 may be standard protocol for every exam at your facility or only a complementary image when needed.

Nontrauma Lumbar Spine - Hyperextension & Hyperflexion Laterals

- Projection: Lateral
- *Assessment of range of motion at the spinal fusion is observed through the comparative flexion and extension positions*

Technical Considerations

- kVp 80–85
- mAs set manually or center AEC cell
- 40″ SID

Exposure Field Size

- 14 × 17 lengthwise for all patients

Patient Position

- Recumbent left lateral
  - Ensure true lateral position of thorax and abdomen
  - Hyperflexion (Fig. 9-151)
    - Leaving the pelvis stationary, have the patient curl up, pulling the knees toward their elbows
  - Hyperextension (Fig. 9-152)
    - Leaving the pelvis stationary, have the patient pull shoulders and legs back behind them until the position is intolerable
- Erect left lateral position
  - Hyperflexion (Fig. 9-153)
    - Leaving the pelvis stationary, have the patient bend forward as much as possible. Ensure the patient is stable for length of exposure. Positioning the patient from sitting on a stool could also be considered
  - Hyperextension (Fig. 9-154)
    - Leaving the pelvis stationary, have the patient lean backward until the position is intolerable. Ensure the patient is stable for length of exposure. Positioning the patient from sitting on a stool could also be considered

Centering

- 1″–2″ superior to the level of the iliac crest or to the level of known spinal fusion
- Collimate the beam as tight as possible anterior to posterior on the patient to minimize scatter radiation. Collimation may be limited as the entire spine is included in this special position

Marking of the IR

- L marker placed on the anterior surface within the collimated exposure field

Breathing

- The patient is instructed to take in a breath, exhale, and hold their breath out
- The image is acquired after expiration
- Ensure patient holds position while walking away to make the exposure

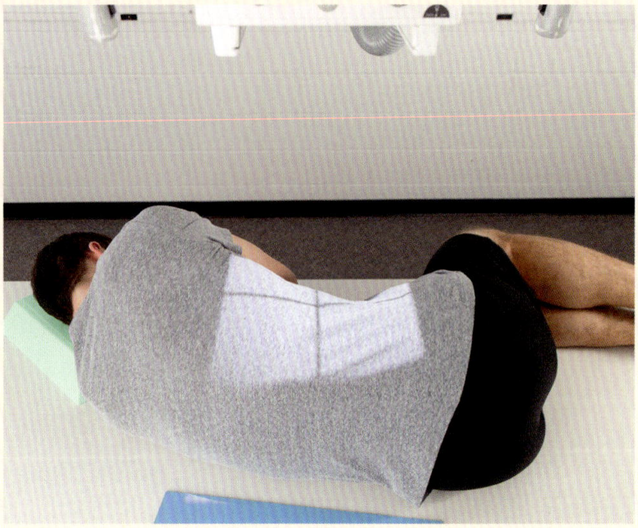

9-151 Hyperflexion L-spine lateral recumbent.

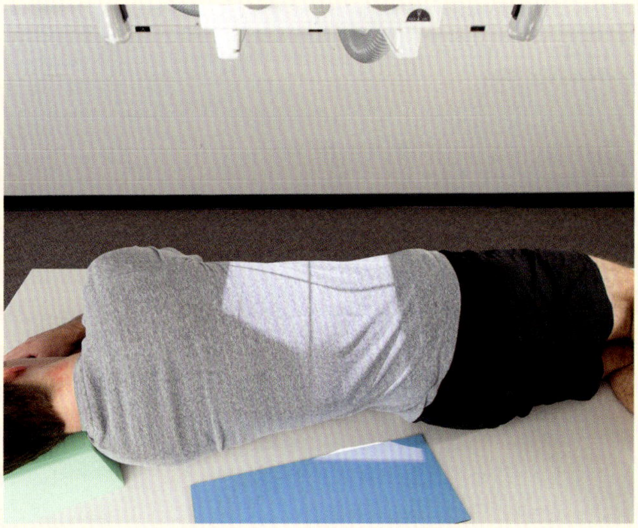

9-152 Hyperextension L-spine lateral recumbent.

(continued)

Nontrauma Lumbar Spine (*Continued*)

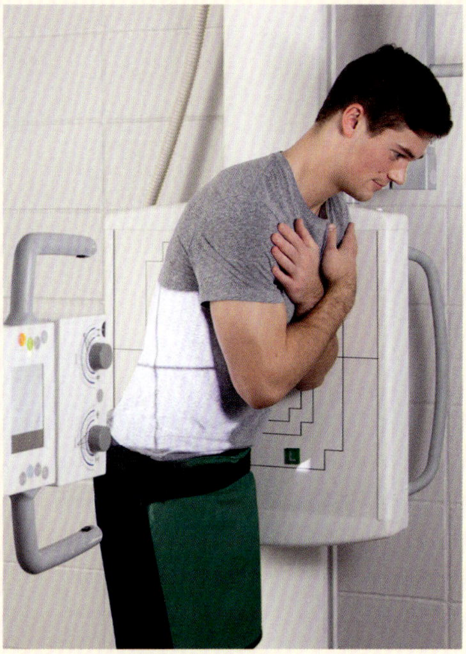

9-153 Hyperflexion L-spine lateral erect.

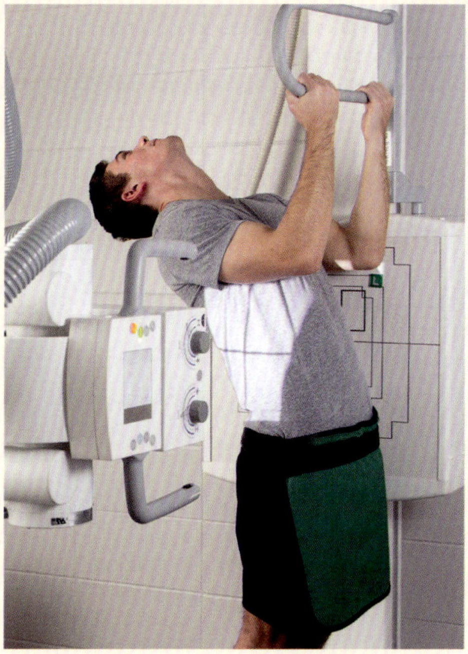

9-154 Hyperextension L-spine lateral erect.

IMAGE CRITIQUE (FIGS. 9-155 and 9-156)

- Thoracic and lumbar vertebrae demonstrated in a true lateral position evidenced with open intervertebral foramina
- Height of vertebral bodies and intervertebral disk spaces observed
- Spinous processes may be noted in profile
- Properly centered and collimated

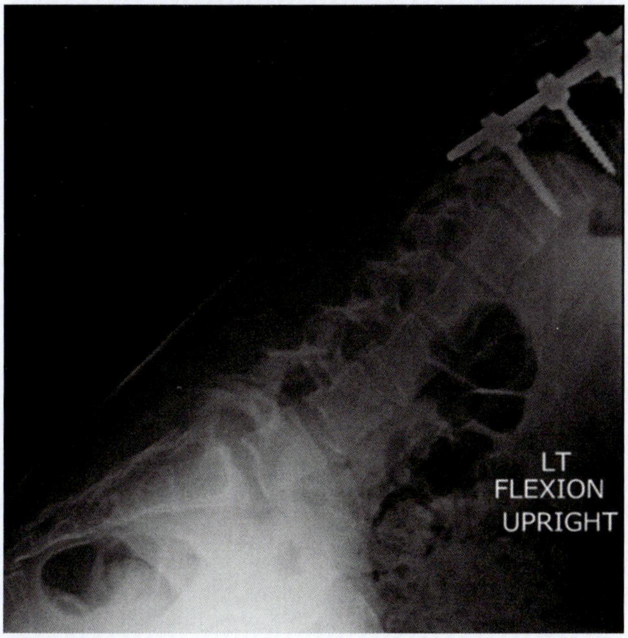

9-155 Hyperflexion L-spine.

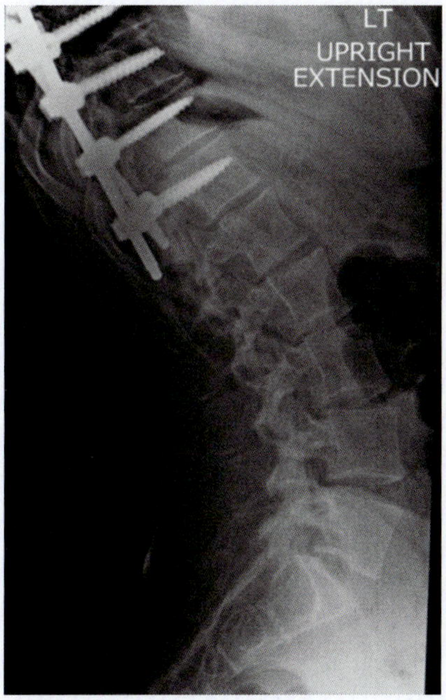

9-156 Hyperextension L-spine.

Nontrauma Spine - Right and Left Bending Laterals

- Projection: PA or AP
- *PA projection preferred to reduce entrance dose to radiosensitive tissues such as breast and thyroid*
  - *These positions may be used to assess range of motion for a scoliosis patient or a spinal fusion patient*

Technical Considerations

- kVp 75–85
- mAs set manually
- Compensating filter could be considered to achieve a more uniform density
- 40″–60″ SID dependent on IR size used for amount of spine inclusion

Exposure Field Size

- 14 × 17 or 14 × 36 (if an option) lengthwise

Patient Position

- Erect facing the upright Bucky (Fig. 9-157)
  - Patient stands with equal weight distribution through the lower limbs. Arms are placed down at their side
  - Keeping the pelvis as the center of gravity, the patient must bend laterally at the waist until intolerable. Have the patient reach with their right hand/arm down toward their right foot. Both a right and a left bending lateral position will be acquired
- Recumbent with supine (Fig. 9-158)
  - Ensure patient is flat with avoidable rotation if possible. Oftentimes, owing to their condition, this cannot be prevented. Arms are placed down at their side
  - The patient's pelvis must remain in a stationary position, whereas the upper body is bent laterally until intolerable. Have the patient reach with their right hand/arm down toward their right foot. Both a right and a left bending lateral position will be acquired (Figs. 9-157 and 9-158)

Centering

- 14 × 17—CR is directed to the level of the iliac crest and MSP
- 14 × 36—CR is directed 2″ superior to the iliac crest and MSP

Marking of IR

- Anatomic side marker R or L placed furthest from the patient's midline or lateral to the part
- If erect, annotate this position

Breathing

- The patient is instructed to take in a breath, exhale, and hold their breath out
- The image is acquired after expiration
- Ensure patient holds position while walking away to make the exposure

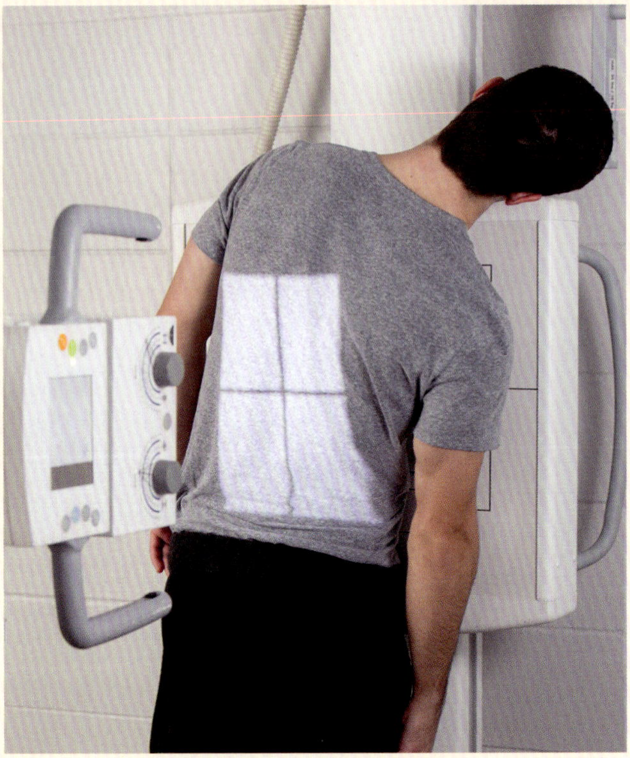

9-157 Bending lateral erect.

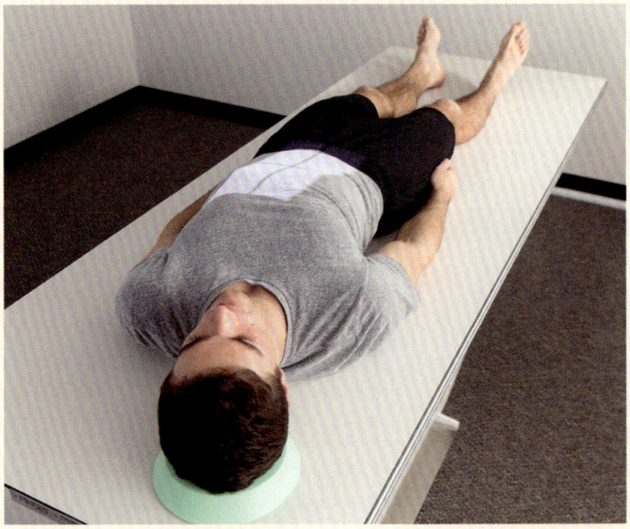

9-158 Bending lateral recumbent.

IMAGE CRITIQUE (FIG. 9-159)

- The thoracic and lumbar portions of the vertebral column are assessed for range of motion
- Symmetry of the spine may not be obtainable owing to the varying degrees of deformity
- Properly centered with side-to-side collimation to minimize tissue exposure

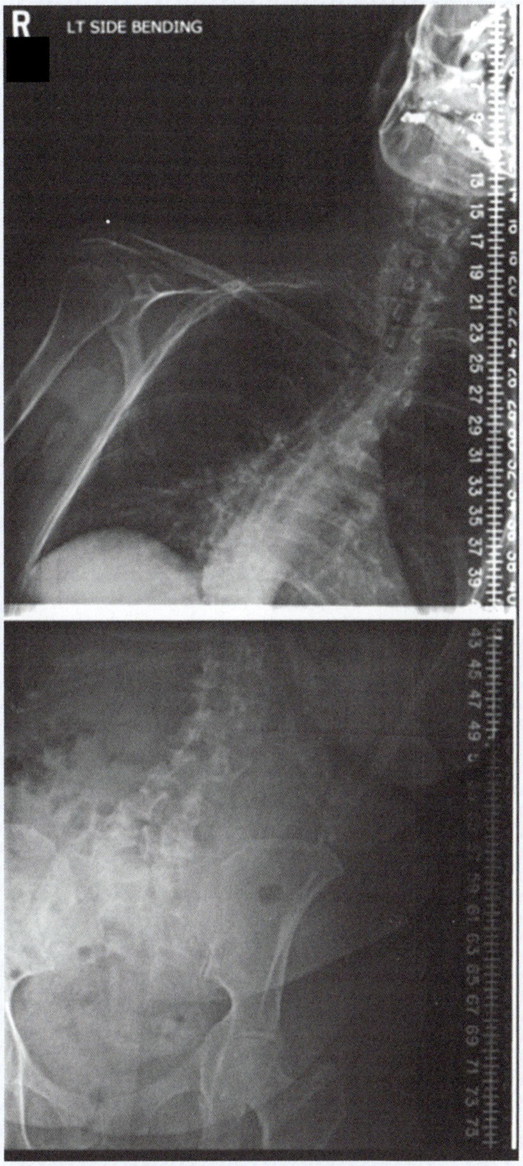

9-159 Bending lateral.

Sacrum and Coccyx

- Projection: AP Axial
- *An AP Axial will be acquired for the sacrum and a separate AP Axial for the coccyx*
- Summation of entire sacrum and coccyx protocol is found in Table 9-5

Sacrum and Coccyx Protocol

AP Axial

Lateral

Technical Considerations

- kVp 70–80
- mAs set manually or center AEC cell
- 40″ SID

Exposure Field Size

- 10 × 12 lengthwise

Patient Position

- Supine
- Ensure patient is flat with no rotation. Support could be provided under the patient's knees to reduce the lordotic lumbar curvature and position the lumbar spine parallel to the plane of the IR

Centering

- Midway between the ASIS and symphysis pubis and MSP
- AP Axial Sacrum
    - 15° cephalic tube angle is applied to the supine patient. The cephalic tube angle will intersect the sacrum perpendicularly. This aids in flattening the concave curvature of the sacrum to better visualize the sacral foramina (Fig. 9-160)
- AP Axial Coccyx
    - 10° caudal tube angle is applied to the supine patient. The caudal tube angle will aid in pushing the symphysis pubis down to prevent superimposition upon the coccyx (Fig. 9-161)

Marking of IR

- Anatomic side marker R or L placed furthest from the patient's midline

Breathing

- Suspend respiration. Instruct the patient to "hold their breath"
- Ensure patient holds position while walking away to make the exposure

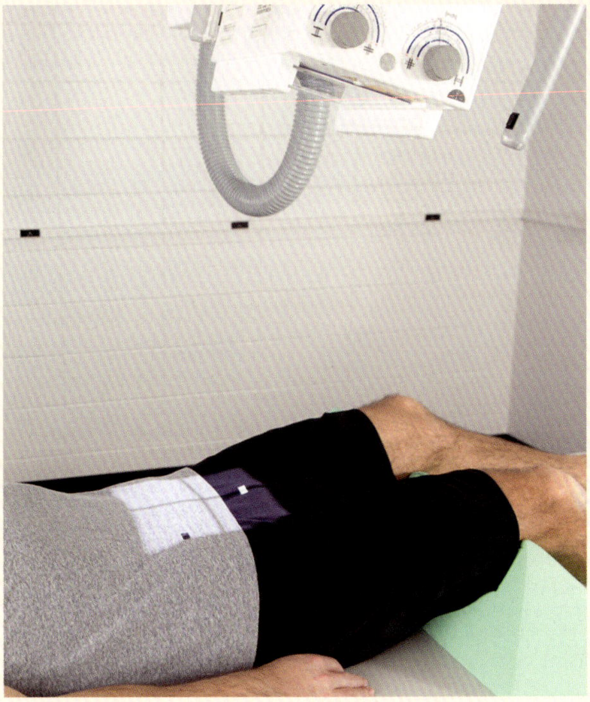

9-160 AP axial sacrum.

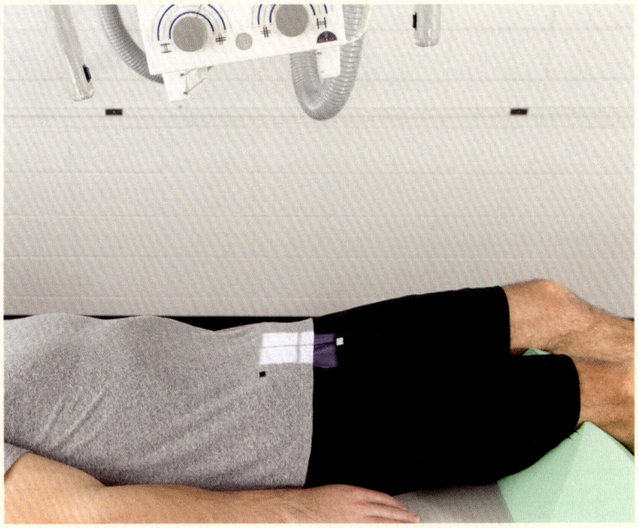

9-161 AP axial coccyx.

IMAGE CRITIQUE (FIGS. 9-162 to 9-165)

- Sacrum
  - L5–S1 joint space must be included along with both right and left SI joints
  - Open sacral foramina (which represent the continuation of the intervertebral foramina down the vertebral column)
  - Coccyx is not necessarily of interest and will likely be superimposed by the symphysis pubis
  - No rotation of the part is determined when the sacrum is centered within the pelvic brim
  - Properly centered with four-sided collimation
- Coccyx
  - Coccyx must be free of superimposition from the symphysis pubis
  - No rotation of the part is determined when the coccyx is centered within the pelvic brim. Tightly collimated borders may make it difficult to judge centering within the pelvic brim
  - Properly centered with four-sided collimation

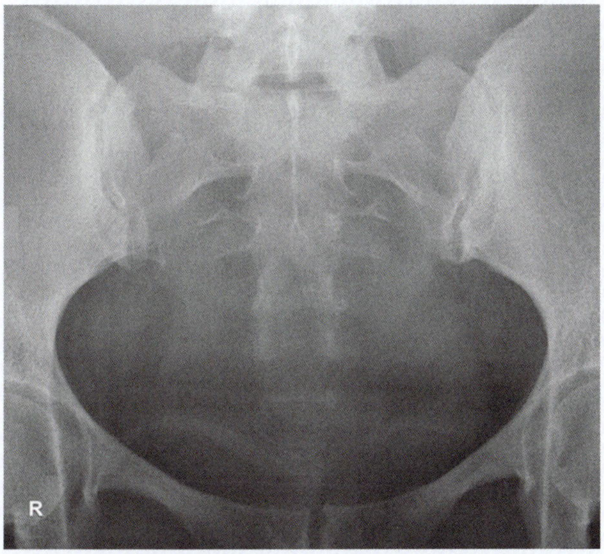

9-162 AP axial sacrum.

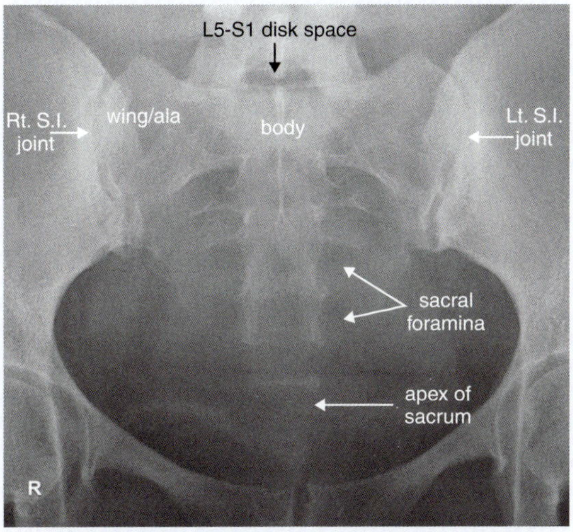

9-163 AP axial sacrum.

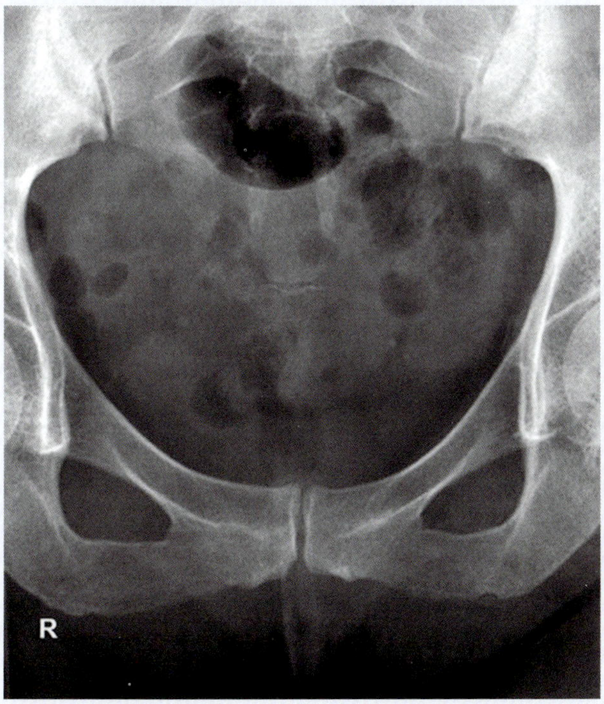

9-164 AP axial coccyx.

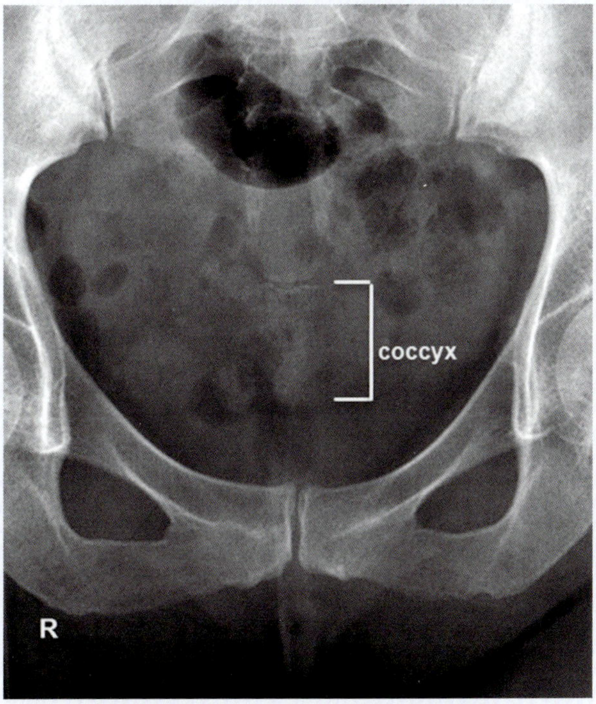

9-165 AP axial coccyx.

Sacrum and Coccyx

- Projection: Lateral
- Summation of entire sacrum and coccyx protocol is found in Table 9-5

Sacrum and Coccyx Protocol
AP Axial
Lateral

Technical Considerations

- kVp 75–85
- mAs set manually or center AEC cell
- 40″ SID

Exposure Field Size

- 10 × 12 lengthwise

Patient Position

- Recumbent left lateral
- Ensure true lateral position of thorax and abdomen. The shoulders should be directly superimposed and aligned with the hips
- Bend knees slightly for patient stability and pull knees up slightly toward chest. Bend the elbows and raise 90° from the chest
- If using a supportive wedge positioned just above the iliac crest, necessary in cases of an extremely small-waisted patient comparing to their shoulders and hips, this supports the spine to be parallel to the IR. This will assist with visualization of open L5–S1 intervertebral disk space (Fig. 9-166)

Centering

- To the level of the ASIS and 2″ posterior to the MCP. Collimate the beam as tight as possible on the patient to minimize scatter radiation. Skimming light may be seen only on the posterior surface of the patient, but not necessarily all patients

Marking of the IR

- L marker placed on the anterior surface within the collimated exposure field

Breathing

- The patient is instructed to hold their breath
- Ensure patient holds position while walking away to make the exposure

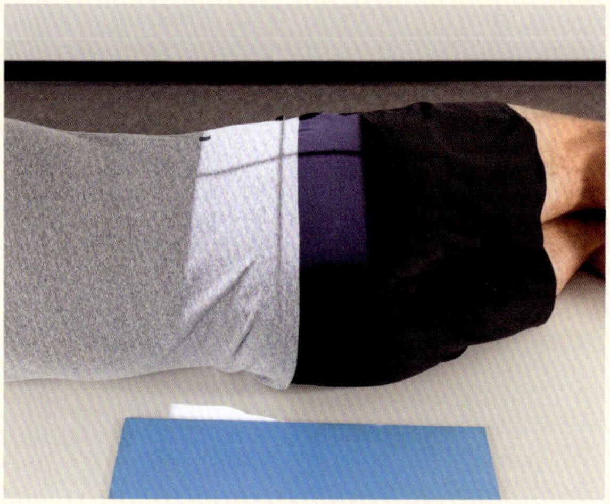

9-166 Lateral sacrum and coccyx.

IMAGE CRITIQUE (FIGS. 9-167 and 9-168)

- L5–S1 is visualized with the sacrum and coccyx in profile
- The medial sacral crest (which represents the continuation of fused spinous processes) may be noted in profile
- Near superimposition of the greater sciatic notches, indicating minimal to no rotation of the pelvis
- Properly centered with four-sided collimation

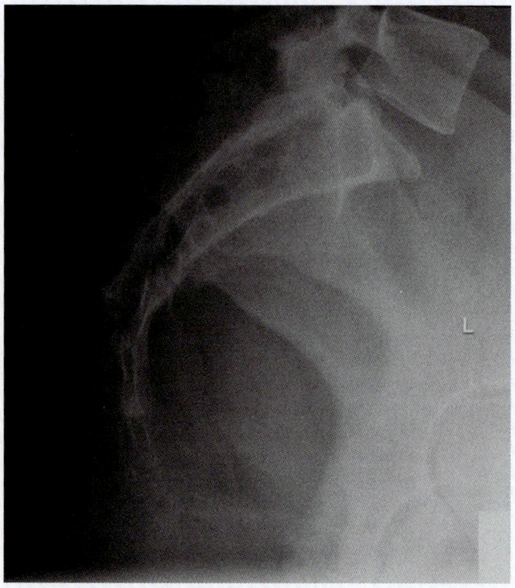

9-167 Lateral sacrum and coccyx.

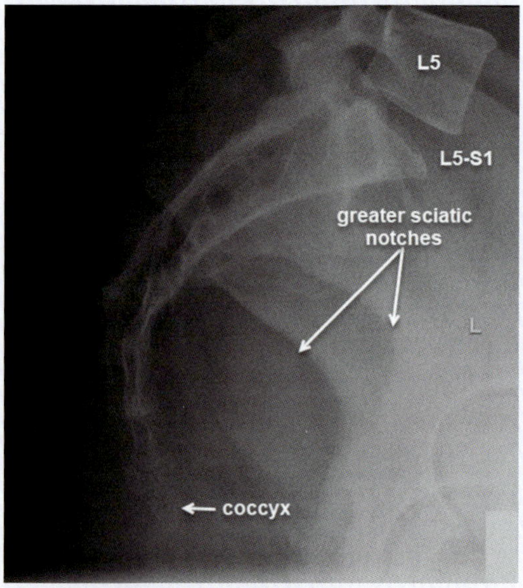

9-168 Lateral sacrum and coccyx.

9-5 Sacrum and Coccyx Protocol

Projection	SID	Positioning	Central Ray	Best Visualizes
AP axial sacrum 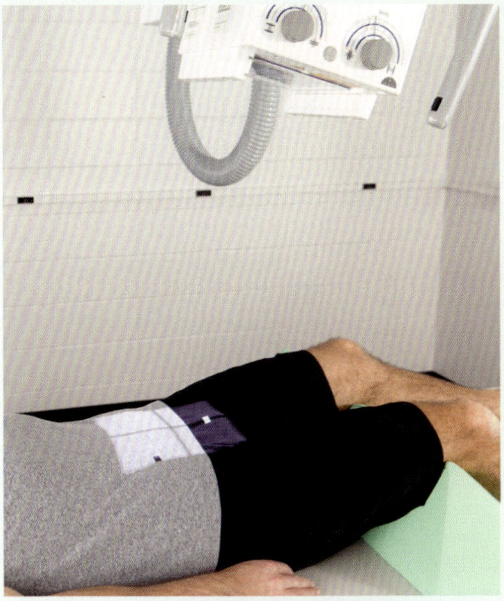	40″	Supine Arms at side and no rotation of the shoulders, spine, or pelvis. Flex knees slightly to align lumbar spine parallel with the IR.	Midway between ASIS and symphysis pubis and MSP 15° cephalic tube angle	L5–S1 visualized. Sacrum centered within the pelvic brim. Apex of the sacrum free of symphysis pubis superimposition.
AP axial coccyx 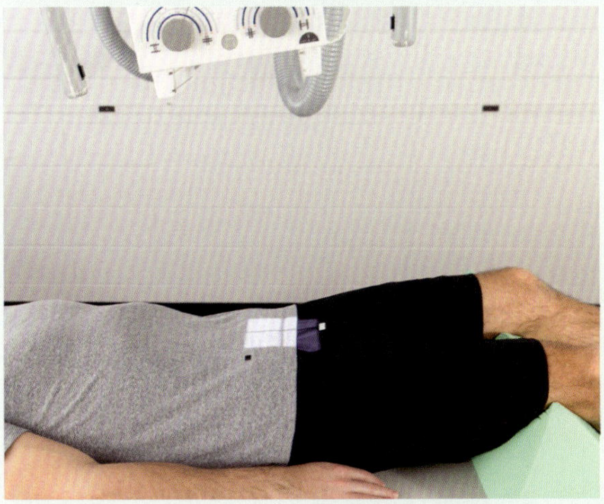	40″	Supine Arms at side and no rotation of the shoulders, spine, or pelvis. Flex knees slightly to align lumbar spine parallel to the IR.	Midway between ASIS and symphysis pubis and MSP 10° caudal tube angle	Sacrum/Coccyx centered within the pelvic brim. Coccyx free of symphysis pubis superimposition.
Lateral sacrum and coccyx 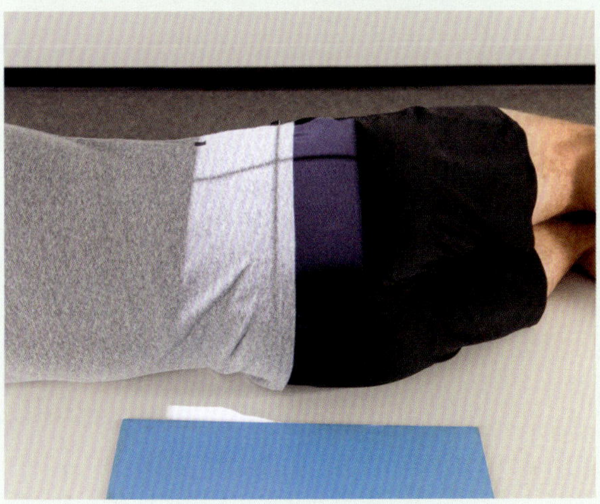	40″	Left lateral position Ensure shoulders and hips are truly lateral and in alignment with one another.	At the level of the ASIS and posterior to MCP	Profile perspective of the sacrum and coccyx. L5–S1 visualized. Near superimposition of the greater sciatic notches, indicating minimal to no rotation of the part.

Scoliosis

- Projection: PA
- *PA projection preferred to reduce entrance dose to radiosensitive tissues such as breast and thyroid*

Scoliosis Protocol

PA

Lateral

Technical Considerations

- kVp 75–85
- mAs set manually
- Compensating filter could be considered to achieve a more uniform density
- 40″–60″ SID dependent on IR size

Exposure Field Size

- (2)14 × 17's lengthwise to overlap or 14 × 36 if available

Patient Position

- Erect facing the upright Bucky (Fig. 9-169)
  - Patient stands with equal weight distribution through the lower limbs. Arms are placed down at their side
- Recumbent in supine position (this may be a requested to accompany the erect)
  - Ensure patient is flat and avoiding rotation if possible. Oftentimes, owing to their condition, this cannot be prevented. Arms are placed down at their side

Centering

- 14 × 36
  - To the level of T10 and with MSP
- (2)14 × 17's to overlap
  - The bottom of the first 14 × 17 set to the ASIS and MSP. The bottom of the second 14 × 17 set to overlap, so approximately at the level of the xiphoid process to allow light to center up and include C1

Marking of IR

- Anatomic side marker R or L placed furthest from the patient's midline or lateral to the part
- If erect, annotate this position

Breathing

- The patient is instructed to take in a breath, exhale, and hold their breath out
- The image is acquired after expiration
- Ensure patient holds position while walking away to make the exposure

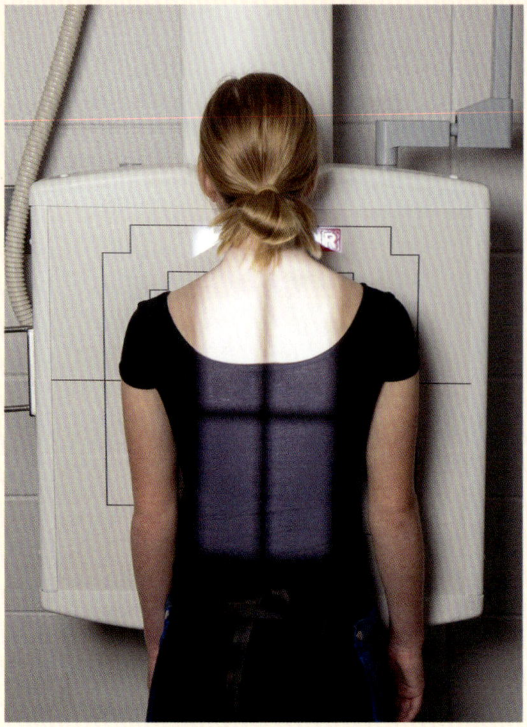

9-169 PA scoliosis.

IMAGE CRITIQUE (FIG. 9-170)

- Cervical, thoracic, lumbar vertebrae are included along with the upper portion of the sacrum
- Symmetry of the spine may be unobtainable owing to the varying degrees of deformity
- Properly centered with side-to-side collimation to minimize tissue exposure. Shadow shields are encouraged

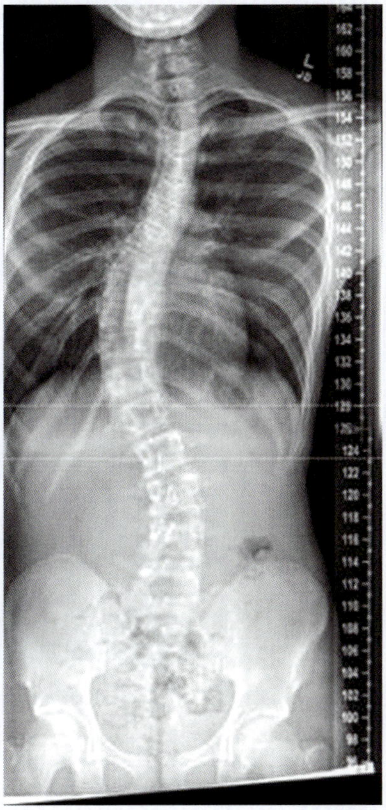

9-170 PA scoliosis.

Scoliosis

- Projection: Lateral

Scoliosis Protocol
PA
Lateral

Technical Considerations

- kVp 75–85
- mAs set manually
- 40″–60″ SID dependent on IR size

Exposure Field Size

- (2)14 × 17's lengthwise to overlap or 14 × 36 if available

Patient Position (Fig. 9-171)

- Erect and lateral position
- Patient stands with equal weight distribution through the lower limbs. Arms are elevated similar to their position for a lateral chest

Centering

- 14 × 36
  - To the level of T10 and with MCP
- (2)14 × 17's to overlap
  - The bottom of the first 14 × 17 set to the ASIS and MCP. The bottom of the second 14 × 17 set to overlap, so approximately at the level of the xiphoid process to allow light to center up and include C1

Marking of IR

- Anatomic side marker R or L placed along the anterior surface of the patient, indicating which side of the patient is closest to the IR
- If erect, annotate this position

Breathing

- The patient is instructed to take in a breath, exhale, and hold their breath out
- The image is acquired after expiration
- Ensure patient holds position while walking away to make the exposure

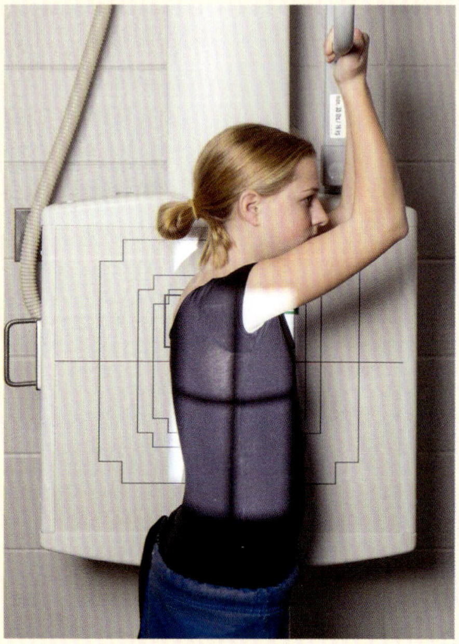

9-171 Lateral scoliosis.

IMAGE CRITIQUE (FIG. 9-172)

- Lateral perspective of the cervical, thoracic, lumbar vertebrae is included along with the upper portion of the sacrum
- Symmetry of the spine may be unobtainable owing to the varying degrees of deformity
- Properly centered with anterior to posterior collimation to minimize tissue exposure. Shadow shields are encouraged

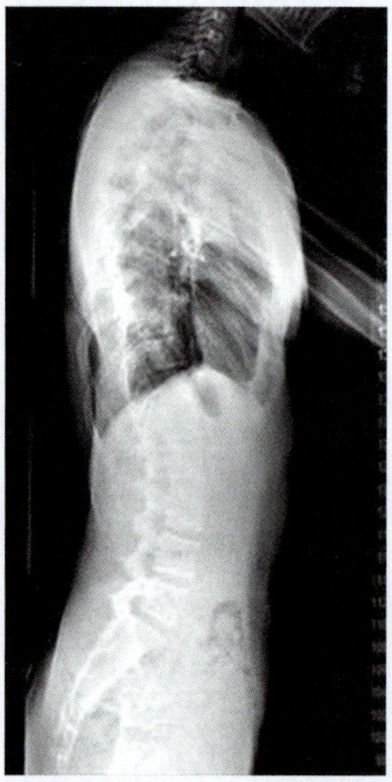

9-172 Lateral scoliosis.

Sacroiliac Joints

- Projection: AP Axial
- Summation of entire sacroiliac joint protocol is found in Table 9-6

Sacroiliac Joints Protocol
AP Axial
AP Obliques

Technical Considerations
- kVp 75–85
- mAs set manually or center cell AEC
- 40″ SID

Exposure Field Size
- 10 × 12 crosswise

Patient Position (Fig. 9-173)
- Supine
- Ensure patient is flat with no rotation. Support could be provided under the patient's knees to reduce the lordotic lumbar curvature and position the lumbar spine parallel to the plane of the IR

Centering
- Midway between the ASIS and symphysis pubis and MSP
- 30°–35° cephalic tube angle is applied

Marking of IR
- Anatomic side marker R or L placed furthest from the patient's midline. It is suggested that both right and left sides be marked on this bilateral study

Breathing
- Suspend respiration. Instruct the patient to "hold their breath."
- Ensure patient holds position while walking away to make the exposure

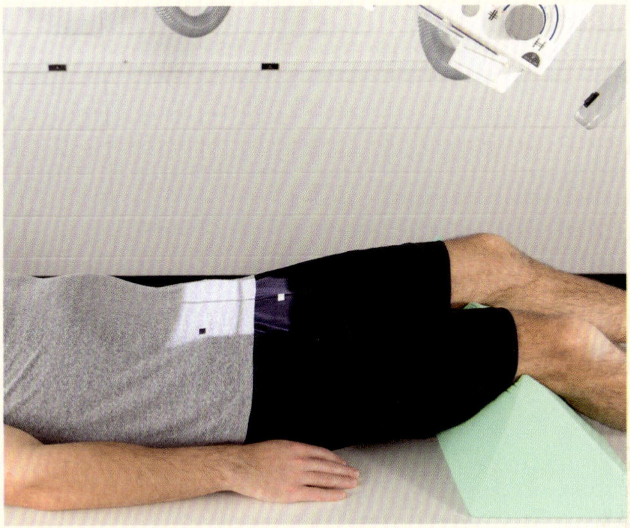

9-173 AP axial SI joints.

IMAGE CRITIQUE (FIGS. 9-174 and 9-175)

- L5–S1 joint space must be visualized along with both right and left SI joints
- No rotation of the part is determined when the sacrum is centered within the pelvic brim
- Properly centered with four-sided collimation

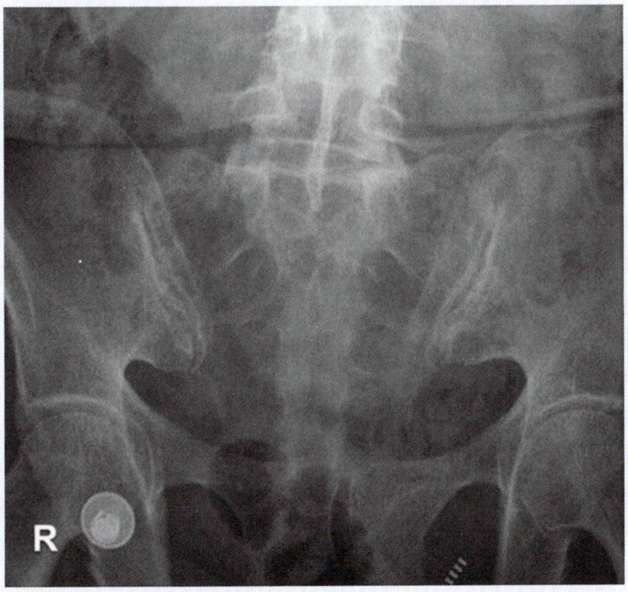

9-174 AP axial SI joints.

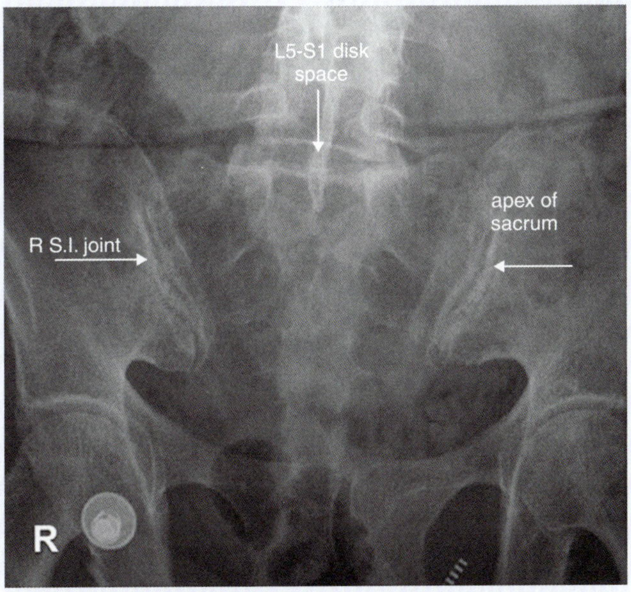

9-175 AP axial SI joints.

Sacroiliac Joints

- Projection: AP Oblique
- *Both right and left SI joints are imaged for purpose of comparison*
- Summation of entire sacroiliac joint protocol is found in Table 9-6

Sacroiliac Joint Protocol
AP Axial
AP Obliques

Technical Considerations

- kVp 75–85
- mAs set manually
- 40″ SID

Exposure Field Size

- 10 × 12 crosswise or lengthwise

Patient Position

- Recumbent posterior oblique is sought in order to keep the SI joints closer to the IR (Figs. 9-176 and 9-177)
- Patient is rotated into a 25°–30° posterior oblique. Ensure the shoulders are rotated evenly with the hips. A complete set of posterior oblique positions (RPO/LPO) are acquired for comparison. A support wedge should be placed beneath the patient to support their shoulders and hips. *Using the anterior oblique positions (RAO and LAO) with the PA Oblique projection will result in magnification of structures and a loss of detail owing to part magnification and is therefore not typically implemented*

Centering

- 1″ medial to the upside ASIS. The centering is directed over the upside SI joint

Marking of IR

- Anatomic side marker R or L placed to indicate the patient's anatomic side closest to the IR

Breathing

- The patient is instructed to hold their breath
- Ensure patient holds position while walking away to make the exposure

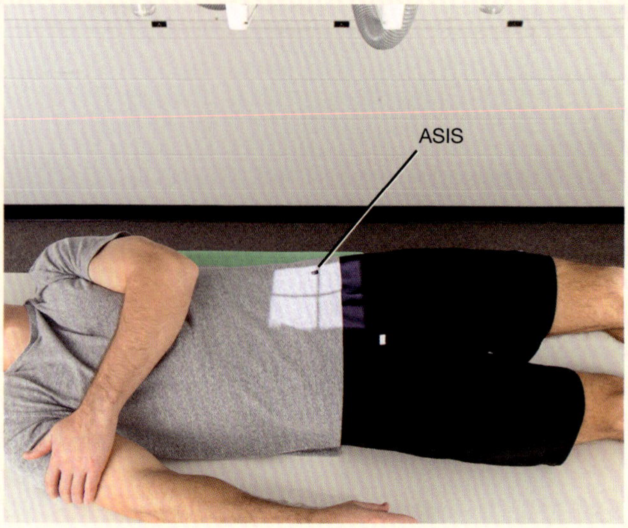

9-176 AP oblique SI joint—RPO position.

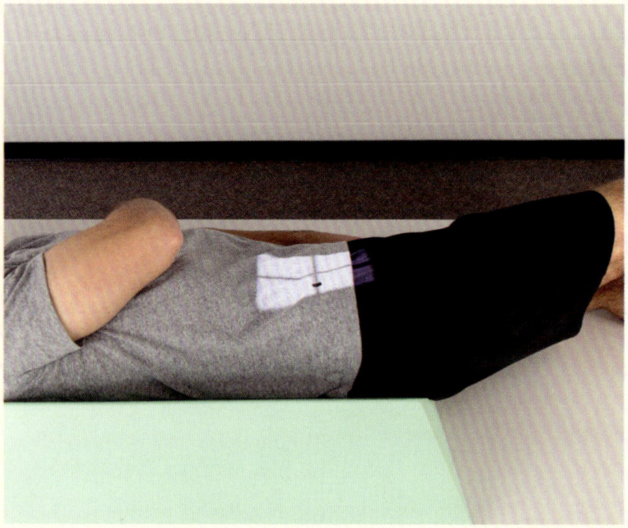

9-177 AP oblique SI joint—LPO position.

IMAGE CRITIQUE (FIGS. 9-178 and 9-179)

- Visualization of the SI joint of interest open
  - Posterior oblique positions (RPO/LPO) demonstrate the SI joint furthest from the IR open. The RPO position demonstrates the left SI joint. The LPO position demonstrates the right SI joint
  - Anterior oblique positions (RAO/LAO) demonstrate the SI joint closest to the IR. The RAO position demonstrates the right SI joint. The LAO position demonstrates the left SI joint. Again, owing to magnification of the spine and the comfort and ability of the patient, anterior oblique positions are not typically protocol
- Over-rotation of the patient will be evidenced when the ilium shifts to superimpose the SI joint of interest
- Properly centered with four-sided collimation

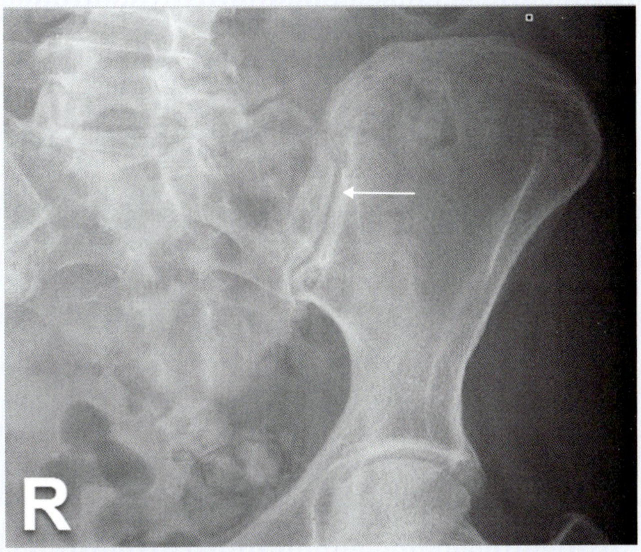

9-178 AP oblique SI joint. Arrow depicts an open left S.I. joint.

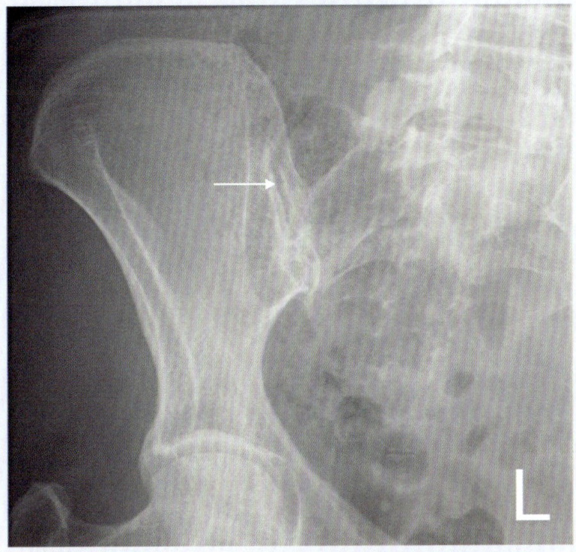

9-179 AP oblique SI joint. Arrow depicts and open right S.I. joint.

9-6 Sacroiliac Joint Protocol

Projection	SID	Positioning	Central Ray	Best Visualizes
AP Axial 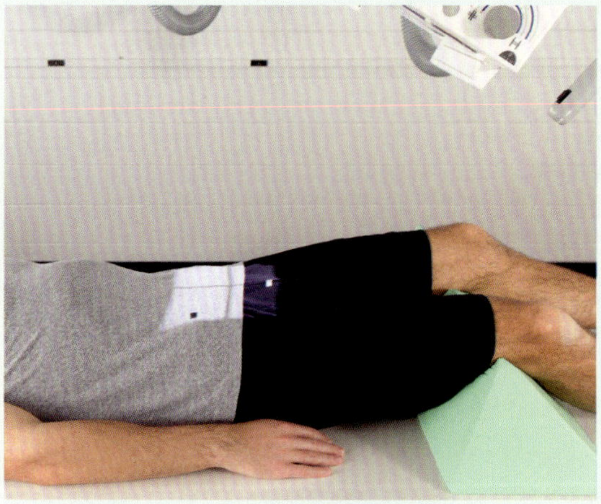	40″	Supine Arms at side and no rotation of the shoulders, spine, or pelvis. Flex knees slightly to align lumbar spine parallel to the IR.	Midway between ASIS and symphysis pubis and MSP. 30°–35° cephalic tube angle	L5–S1 visualized and open. Symmetry of the spine displayed with symmetric pedicles and centered spinous processes.
AP Oblique[a] 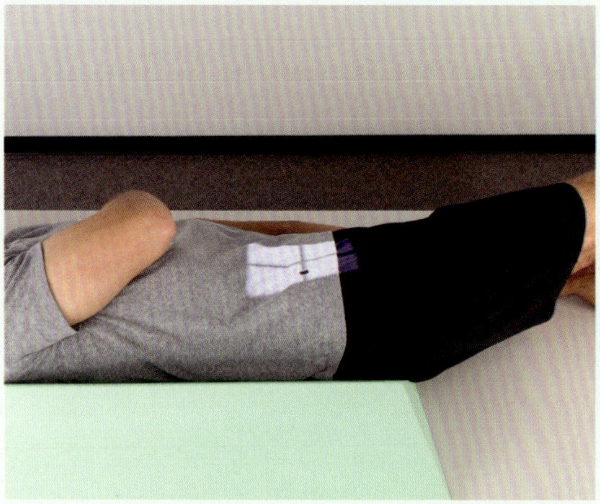 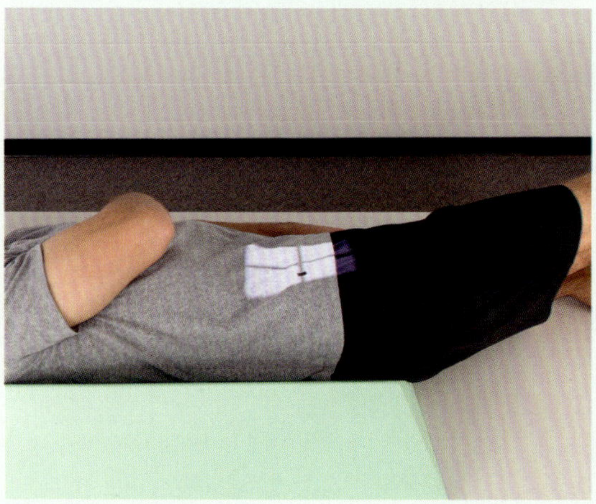	40″	25°–30° RPO and LPO Ensure shoulders through hips are evenly rotated.	1″ medial to upside ASIS	SI joint on the upside is demonstrated open, indicating the patient was in the proper degree of rotation. For example, RPO demonstrates the left SI joint.
PA oblique[a] (not shown)	40″	25°–30° RAO and LAO		SI joint on the downside is demonstrated open, indicating the patient was in the proper degree of rotation. For example, RAO demonstrates the right SI joint.

[a]Indicates that the AP Oblique are preferred as the S.I. joints are positioned closer to the image receptor.

9-7 Anatomy Best Demonstrated in the Vertebral Column

	Intervertebral Foramina	Zygapophyseal Joints
Cervical spine	45° oblique(s) Posterior oblique positions (RPO/LPO) demonstrate upside Anterior oblique positions (RAO/LAO) demonstrate downside	AP open mouth for C1–C2 Lateral demonstrates C2–C7
Thoracic spine	90° lateral	70° anterior or posterior oblique
Lumbar spine	90° lateral	45° oblique(s) Posterior oblique positions (RPO/LPO) demonstrate downside Anterior oblique positions (RAO/LAO) demonstrate upside

9-8 Trauma Spine Protocol

Projection	SID	Positioning	Central Ray	Best Visualizes
Horizontal beam lateral C-spine 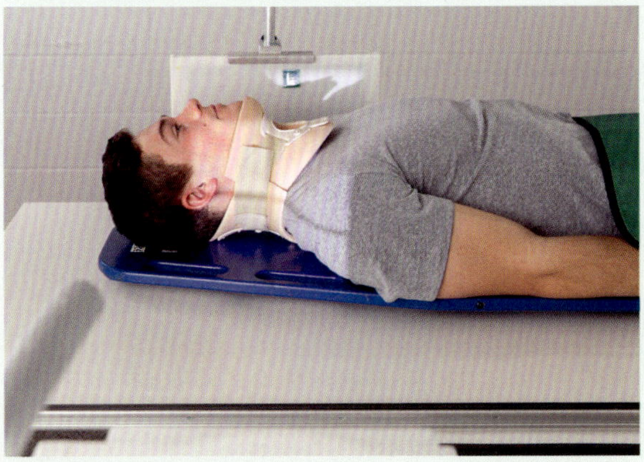 9-180 Horizontal beam lateral C-spine.	72"	Supine Arms at side Do not reposition of the body, head, or neck.	Horizontal beam C5 and MCP	C1–C7 and C7–T1 vertebral bodies and spinous processes are visualized in profile. Rule out subluxation, compression fracture, or other vertebral fracture.
Swimmer's lateral 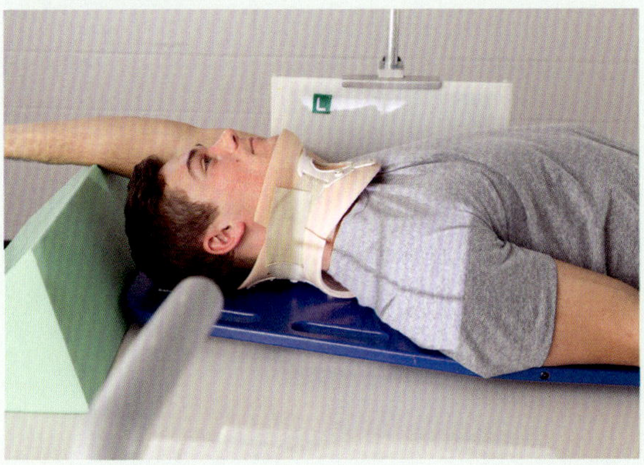 9-181 Horizontal beam lateral Swimmers.	40"–72"	Supine Left arm lifted and directed above head. Right arm and shoulder remain in position.	Horizontal beam C7–T1 disk space. CR enters just above the right shoulder and MCP	C5–T3 region with specific focus on C7–T1

Projection	SID	Positioning	Central Ray	Best Visualizes
AP axial C-spine 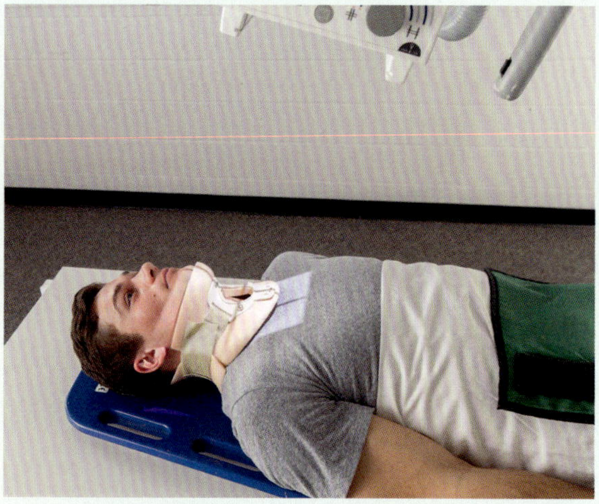 **9-182** Trauma AP axial C-spine.	40″	Supine	C5 and MSP 15° cephalic angle	C3–T1 vertebral bodies and disk spaces.
AP open mouth 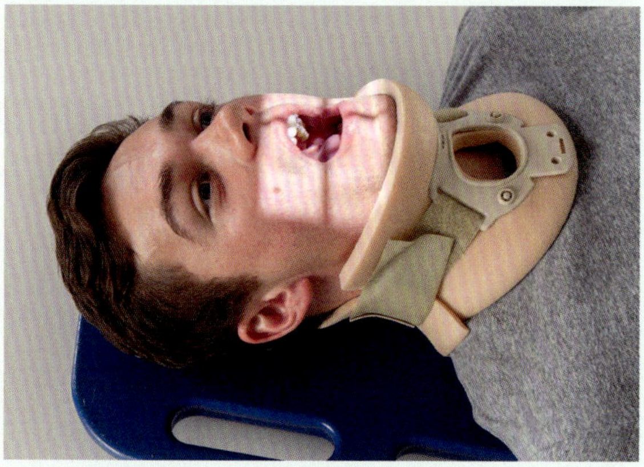 **9-183** Trauma AP open mouth.	40″	Supine Open mouth as much as possible without movement of the neck.	Center of open mouth	Zygapophyseal joints of C1–C2 are evaluated for height and symmetry. Odontoid would ideally be visualized, but may obscured by the base of the skull or teeth as the neck position may not be adjusted.
Fuchs method (a.k.a. Reverse Waters) 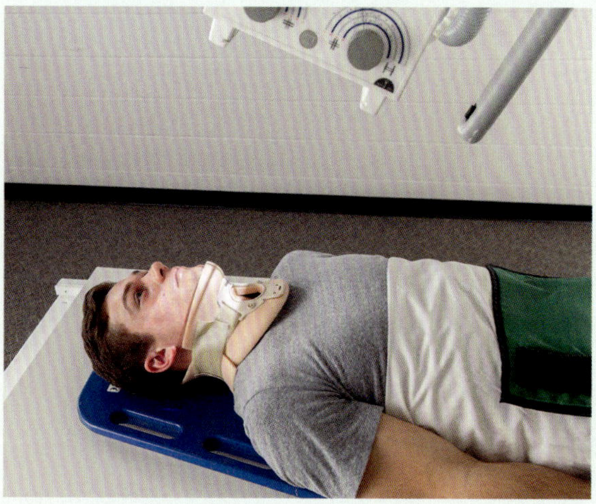 **9-184** Fuchs method.	40″	Supine	Angle the tube cephalic until parallel to MML since the patient is unable to alter position Center beneath the mentum and MSP.	Odontoid visualized through the foramen magnum. This image may complement the AP open mouth to visualize the odontoid process.

Projection	SID	Positioning	Central Ray	Best Visualizes
AP T-spine 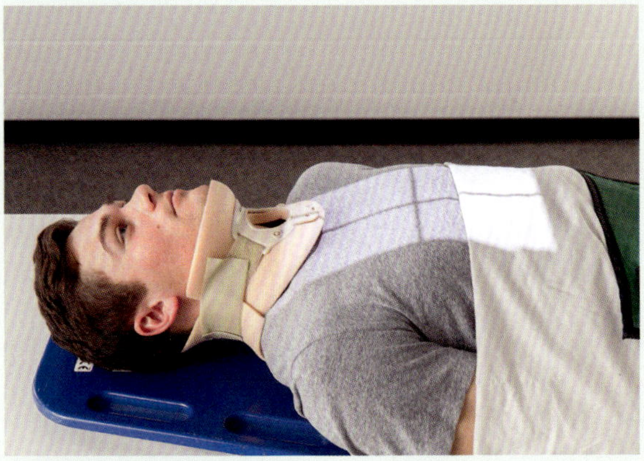 9-185 Trauma AP T-spine.	40″	Supine	T7–T8 and MSP	C7–T1; T1–T12; T12–L1 Vertebral bodies and intervertebral disk spaces are visualized.
AP L-spine 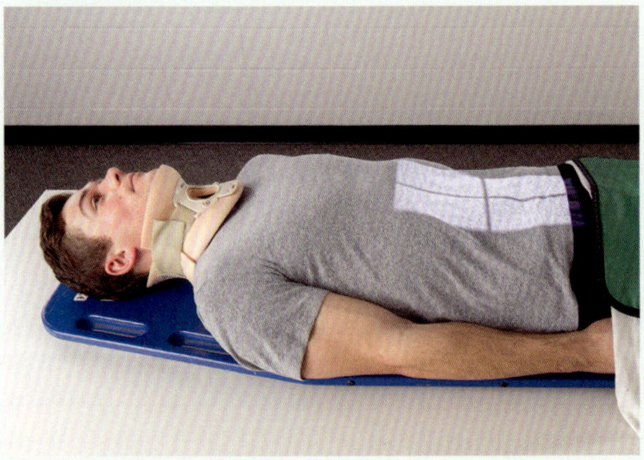 9-186 Trauma AP L-spine.	40″	Supine	L4–L5 and MSP	T12–L1; L1–L5; L5–S1 Vertebral bodies and intervertebral disk spaces are visualized.
Horizontal beam lateral T-spine 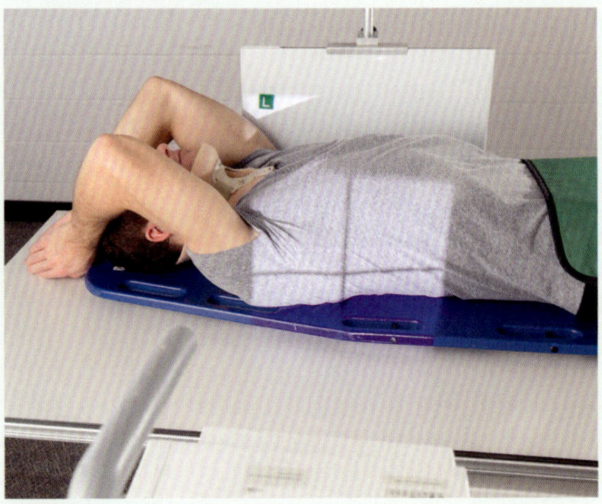 9-187 Horizontal beam lateral T-spine.	40″	Supine Both arms elevated above head as long as there is no fracture to upper extremity.	T7/8 and MCP	T1–T12 although upper T-spine may be poorly visualized owing to the thickness of the shoulders. Swimmer's will better demonstrate this region. Rule out subluxation, compression fracture or other vertebral fracture. Vertebral bodies and spinous processes are visualized in profile.

Projection	SID	Positioning	Central Ray	Best Visualizes
Horizontal beam lateral L-spine 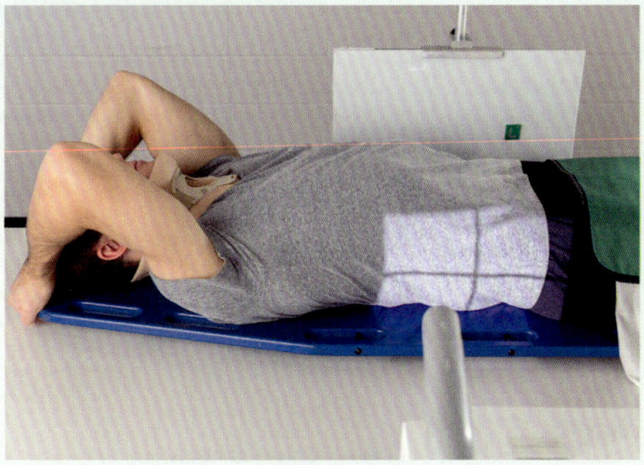 9-188 Horizontal beam lateral L-spine.	40″	Supine Both arms elevated above head as long as there is no fracture to upper extremity.	L4/5 and MCP	L1–L5; T12-L1 transition; L5-S1 transition. Rule out subluxation, compression fracture, or other vertebral fracture. Vertebral bodies and spinous processes are visualized in profile.

THE FINAL STEP: IMAGE REVIEW

The technologist must take the time to review acquired images to ensure image quality is acceptable. The technologist must have the knowledge within their role not only to acquire the images and care for the patient, but also to know how to review the images to ensure diagnostic quality has been attained. In certain instances, a projection may need to be repeated. This is to the discretion of the radiologic technologist. The technologist should review each image for the following.

1. Is all of the necessary anatomy included on the image?
   - Was the central ray (CR) properly directed to the part? An "X" can be drawn to intersect within the collimated exposure field to determine whether the CR was directed to the correct location.
   - Was essential anatomy in the collimated exposure field?
   - Is the area free of artifact(s)?
2. Is the anatomy well demonstrated?
   - Did the technologist properly position the patient to adequately demonstrate the anatomy?
   - Can the technologist recognize the anatomy best demonstrated with use of different projections?
3. Does the image reflect proper image markings?
   - Did the technologist correctly use a lead marker to identify the right or left side?
   - What additional markings or annotations could be helpful to the radiologist interpreting the exam?
   - Is the image properly displayed?
4. Does the image prove to be technically acceptable?
   - Does the exposure index fall within an acceptable range for the operating system? Images that are technically insufficient may appear of good quality if just slightly insufficient or "mottled or pixelated" if severely insufficient. Images that appear "mottled" should be repeated. Images that appear beyond optimal exposure owing to higher technique may display high quality, although the patient has received an excessive radiation dose.

CRITICAL THINKING

1. In review of the AP open mouth (Fig. 9-189), the primary positioning error is as follows:
   a. Odontoid process is entirely superimposed by the base of the skull.
   b. Odontoid process is superimposed by the teeth.
   c. Zygapophyseal joints are asymmetric because of tilt.
   d. C1 and C2 are not centered within the open mouth because of rotation.

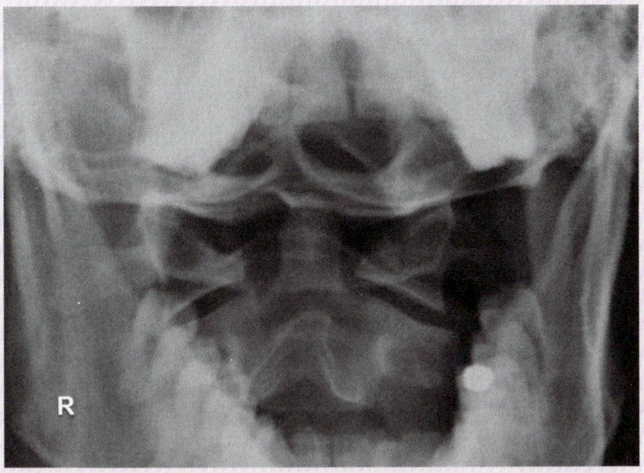

9-189

2. In review of the AP Axial Oblique C-spine (Fig. 9-190), what is the anatomy of interest?
   a. Right zygapophyseal joint
   b. Left zygapophyseal joint
   c. Right intervertebral foramina
   d. Left intervertebral foramina

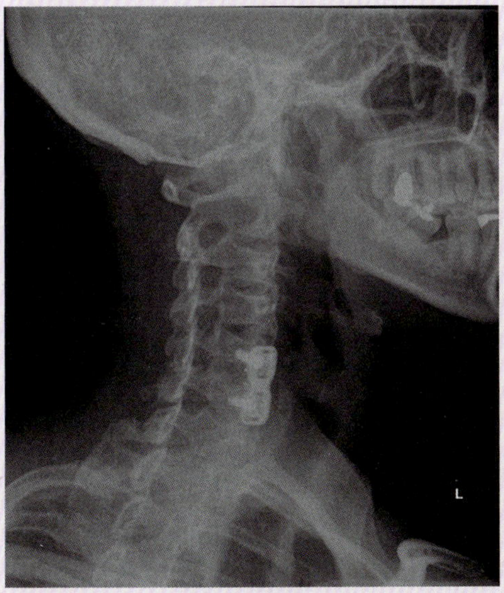

9-190

3. In review of the Swimmer's lateral (Fig. 9-191), which letter identifies C7?
   a. A
   b. B
   c. C
   d. D

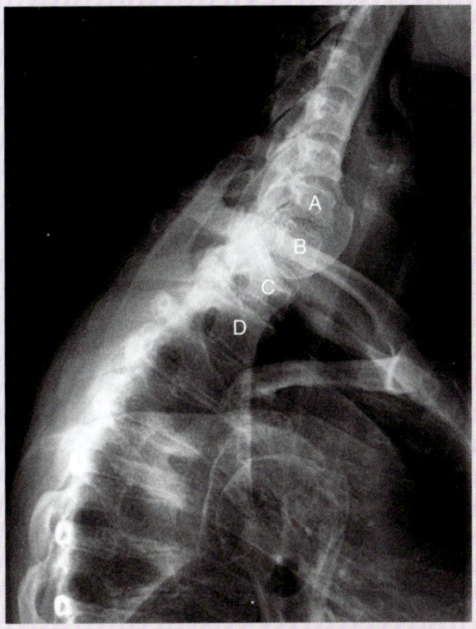

9-191

4. Review of the lateral L-spine (Fig. 9-192). In order to better evaluate the L5–S1 relationship, how should the technologist proceed?
   a. Repeat the lateral with increased technical settings.
   b. Acquire an L5–S1 spot with a perpendicular beam.
   c. Acquire an L5–S1 spot with a 5°–8° cephalic angle.
   d. Acquire an L5–S1 spot with a 5°–8° caudal angle.

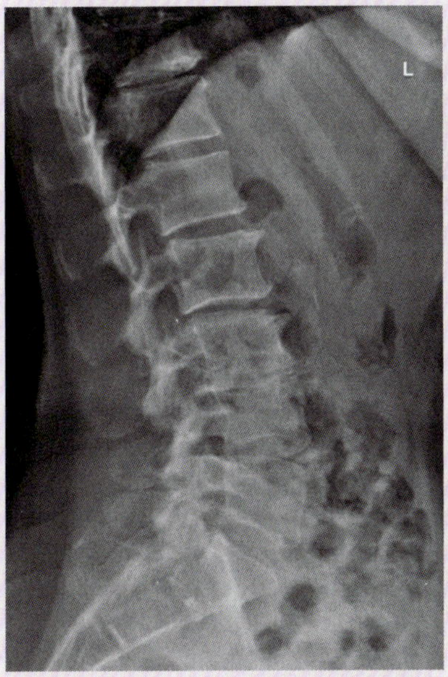

9-192

5. In review of the AP oblique L-spine (Fig. 9-193), what is the anatomy of interest?
   a. Right zygapophyseal joint
   b. Left zygapophyseal joint
   c. Right intervertebral foramina
   d. Left intervertebral foramina

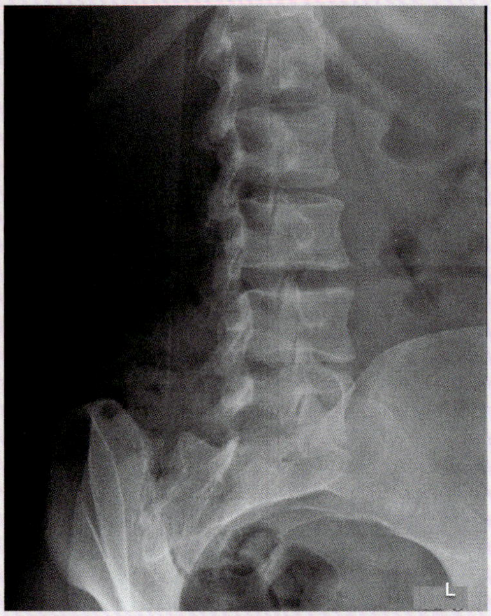

9-193

6. In review of the AP T-spine (Fig. 9-194), characterize the image results.
   a. Image may be improved with use of the anode heel affect when positioning.
   b. Image satisfactorily represents all 12 thoracic vertebrae.
   c. Image represents centering to high on the thoracic vertebral column.
   d. Image represents centering to low, which fails to include T1.

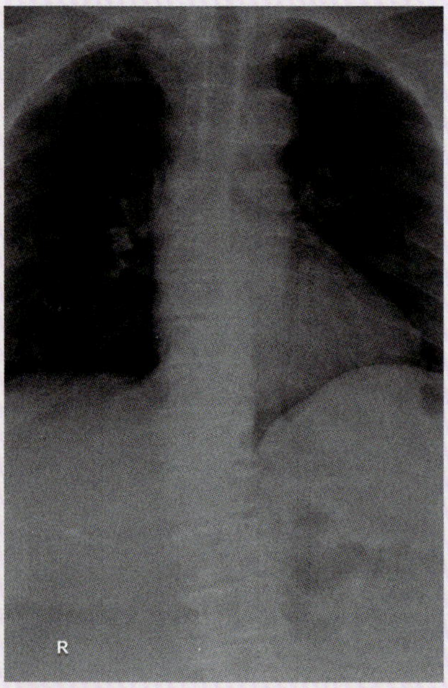

9-194

7. In review of the lateral T-spine (Fig. 9-195), identify the thoracic vertebra number indicated by the letter "A."
   a. T9
   b. T10
   c. T11
   d. T12

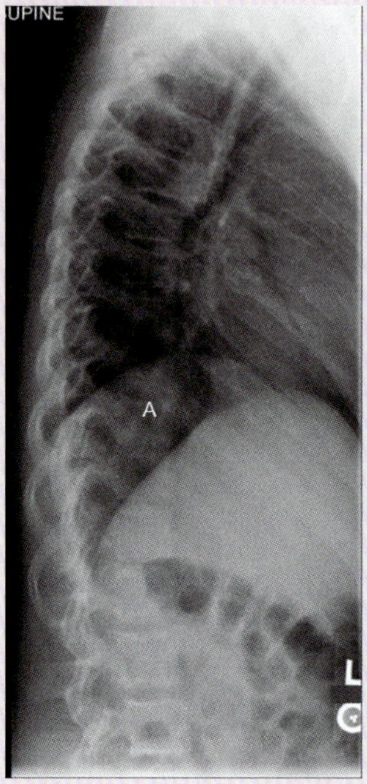

9-195

8. In review of the Swimmer's lateral (Fig. 9-196), characterize the positioning results.
   a. Image correctly represents correct positioning.
   b. Increased flexion of the neck would improve the outcome.
   c. Increased extension of the neck would improve the outcome.
   d. The addition of a tube angle would improve inclusion of C7.

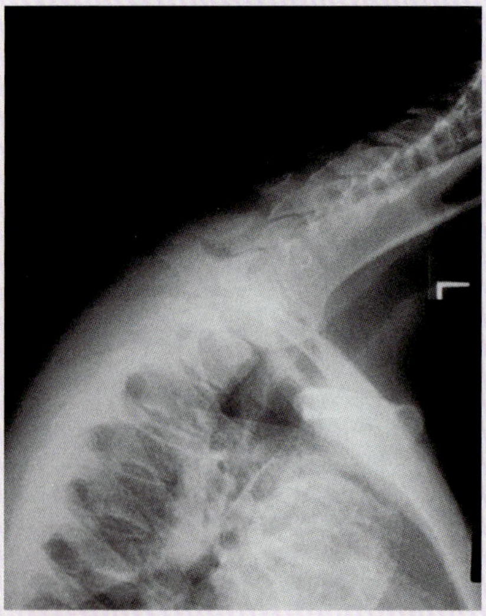

9-196

9. In review of the AP Oblique SI joint (Fig. 9-197), what is the position of the patient and the anatomy of interest?
   a. RAO position to demonstrate the right SI joint
   b. LAO position to demonstrate the left SI joint
   c. RPO to demonstrate the left SI joint
   d. LPO to demonstrate the right SI joint

10. In review of the AP Axial C-spine (Fig. 9-198), which vertebrae are adequately demonstrated?
    a. C3–T1
    b. C4–T1
    c. C5–C7
    d. C5–T1

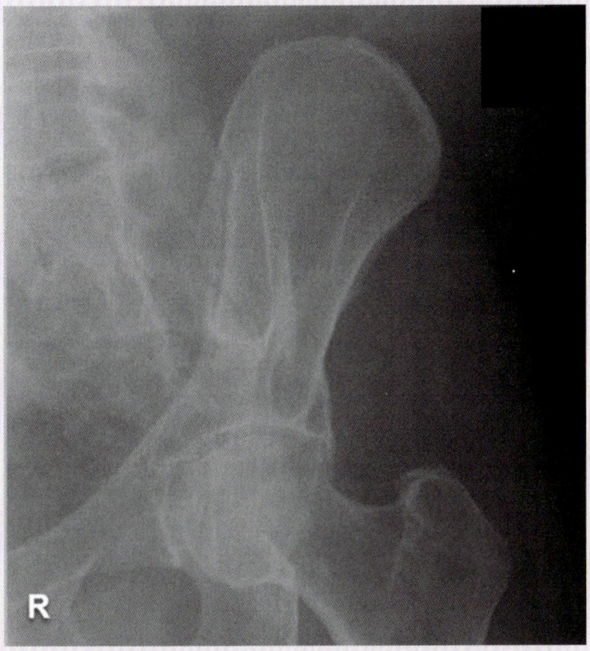

9-197

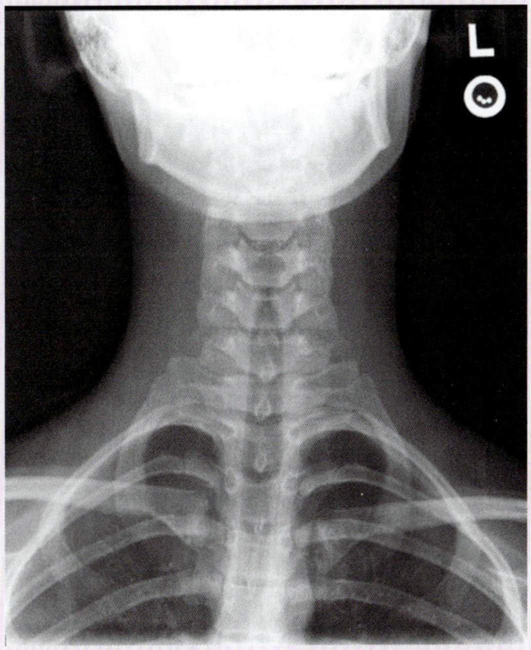

9-198

ANSWERS TO THE CRITICAL THINKING QUESTIONS

1. d
2. c
3. b
4. d
5. b
6. d
7. b
8. c
9. c
10. b

CHAPTER 10 Headwork

Imaging of the skull, facial bones, and sinuses have been largely replaced with the modality of computed tomography (CT). While diagnostic imaging offers lower radiation exposure and less expense for the patient, the determination of whether CT or diagnostic imaging will be ordered may depend on what the imaging facility has to offer and/or what the physician preference may be. Since the number and variety of cranial diagnostic imaging exams have decreased, many facilities have streamlined their image protocols.

CLINICAL INDICATIONS

Indications are the symptomatic reasons as to why a particular exam may be ordered by the physician. The technologist should look at the clinical indications before performing a procedure. The following briefly introduces common exam indications, but it is not an all-encompassing list.

Blowout Fracture: The floor of the orbit "blows out" into the maxillary sinus cavity when a direct force impacts the base of the orbit (Fig. 10-1).

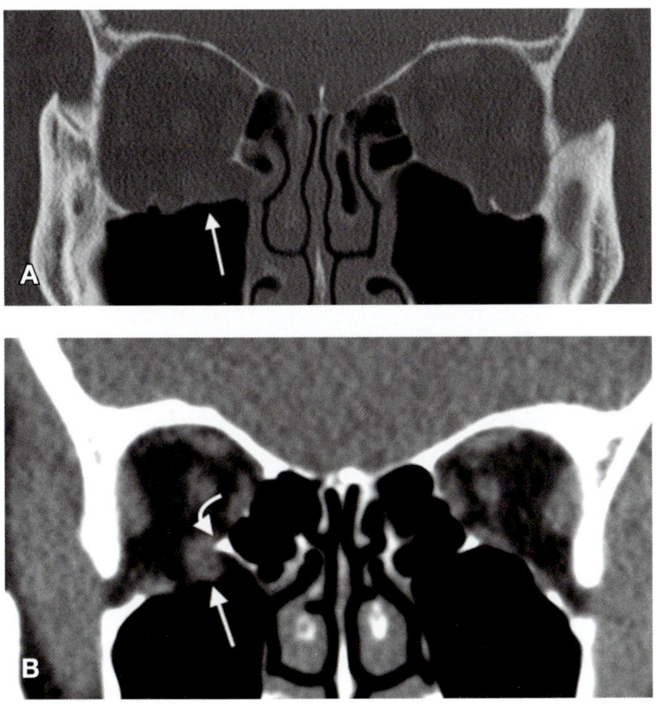

10-1 **A:** Blowout fracture to the right orbit. **B:** Defect to the floor of the right orbit is confirmed with CT.

Tripod Fracture: An impact to the cheekbone could result in the zygoma separating away from its three points of connection: the maxilla, the frontal bone, and the zygomatic arch (Figs. 10-2 and 10-3).

Le Fort Fracture: Trauma to the maxilla resulting in horizontal fractures leading to an instable segment of bone (Fig. 10-4).

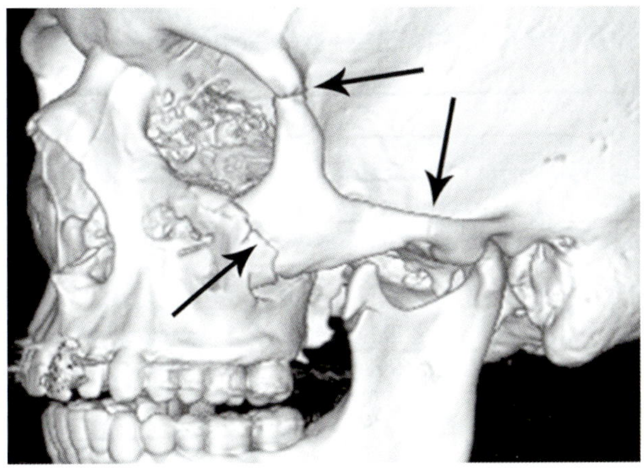

10-2 Tripod fracture. Arrows signify the points of fracture from the frontal bone, maxilla, and the zygomatic arch.

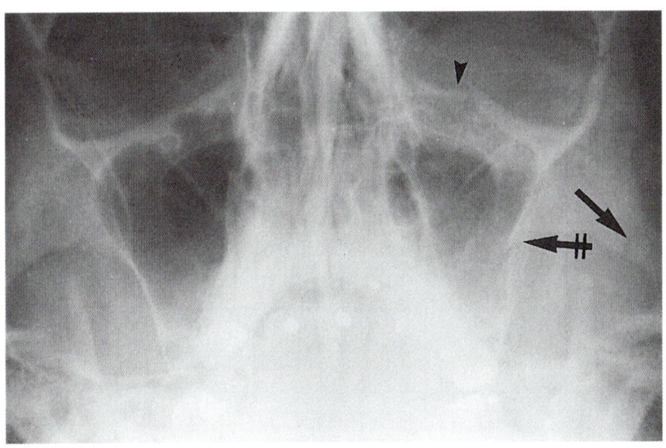

10-3 Tripod fracture. Arrow reveals fracture to the zygmatic arch. Crossed arrow reveals fracture to the maxilla. Arrow head reveals fracture to the orbit.

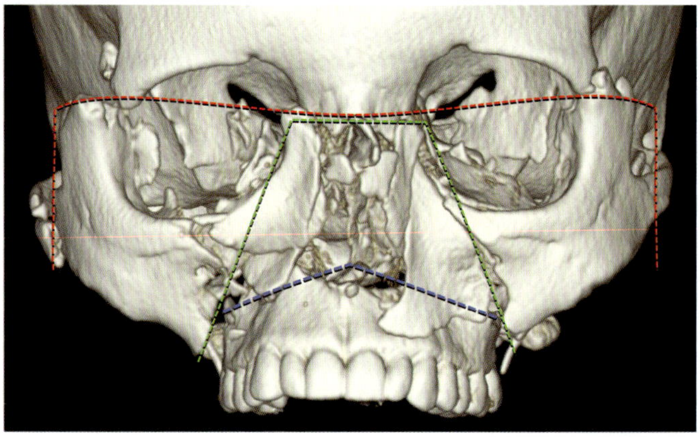

10-4 Le Fort fracture. Each color dotted line represents a different type of Le Fort fracture.

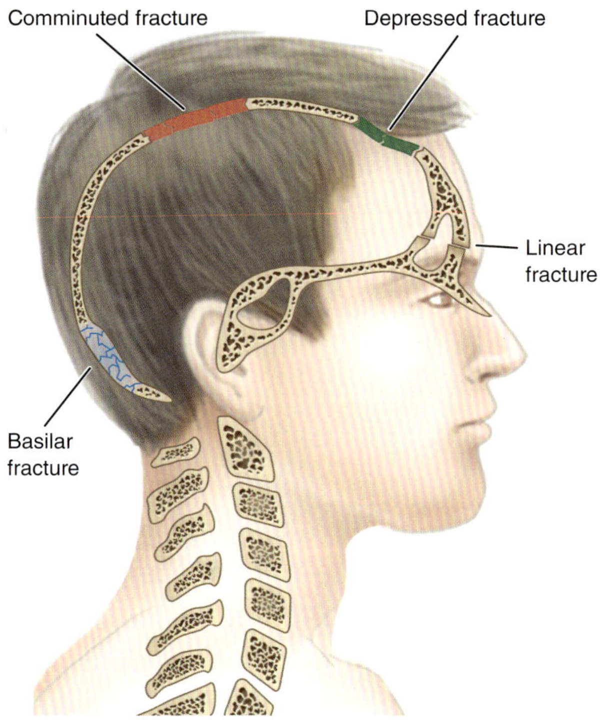

10-5 Basilar fracture.

Basilar Fracture: A fracture that occurs at the suture line of the sphenoid bone and occipital bone in the base of the skull. Radiography may not be able to detect this type of fracture unless a sphenoid effusion is present. Sphenoidal effusion is a result of cerebrospinal fluid pooling within the sphenoid sinus. A horizontal beam would be necessary to demonstrate the fluid level in this trauma instance. CT would be the preferred diagnostic modality to detect a basilar fracture (Fig. 10-5).

Depression Fracture: A depressed fragment that appears like a "dent" in the calvarium in result to a direct blow to the cranium (Fig. 10-6).

Gunshot Wound: Localization of the bullet in trauma or postmortem instances (Fig. 10-7).

Sinusitis: Acute or chronic infection of the sinus.

Foreign Body in the Eye: Presence of wood, glass, or metal fragments within the eye. Patients with job-specific concerns of potential foreign bodies within the eye often undergo preliminary imaging of the orbits to rule out metal fragments within the eye as the magnetic field with magnetic resonance image (MRI) would cause the metal fragment to shift. A shift that could potentially sever the optic nerve.

TMJ Syndrome: Dysfunction of the temporomandibular joint (TMJ) may be present with pain or popping of the joint. Imaging of the TMJs should provide a right to left comparison and include the joint displayed with the mouth closed and open as long as a mandibular fracture is of no concern (Fig. 10-8).

IMAGING CONSIDERATIONS

Patient Dress

The patient will need to remove their jewelry, glasses, hairpins, hair ties, hairpieces, wigs, hearing aids, dentures, and partials. Preventing artifacts from obscuring the anatomy of interest must be considered.

Artifacts

Artifacts are unwanted objects that appear on the image superimposing pertinent anatomy. Failing to have the patient remove earrings, facial piercing, hairpieces, glasses, and hearing aids will cause artifact and potentially obscure essential anatomy (Fig. 10-9). Repeat imaging may be necessary when artifact obscures the area of interest.

Patient Position

The general position of the patient or part

Upright—Relative to this chapter, this position would be most desired because it is easier for the patient to assume necessary positions. Additionally, upright imaging will allow for the evaluation of air–fluid levels.

Supine—Generally only reserved for trauma imaging

Topographical Landmarks

Landmarks that assist with centering and adjusting positioning lines

Ear (Fig. 10-10)

- External Auditory Meatus (EAM)—Center of the external ear canal
- Top of the Ear Attachment (TEA)—Where the top of the auricle attaches to the head; the TEA corresponds to the internal level of the petrous ridge.

Eye (Fig. 10-11)

- Superior Orbital Margin (SOM)—Superior bony orbit
- Inferior Orbital Margin (IOM)—Inferior bony orbit
- Inner Canthus—Where the eyelids junction medially
- Outer Canthus—Where the eyelids junction laterally

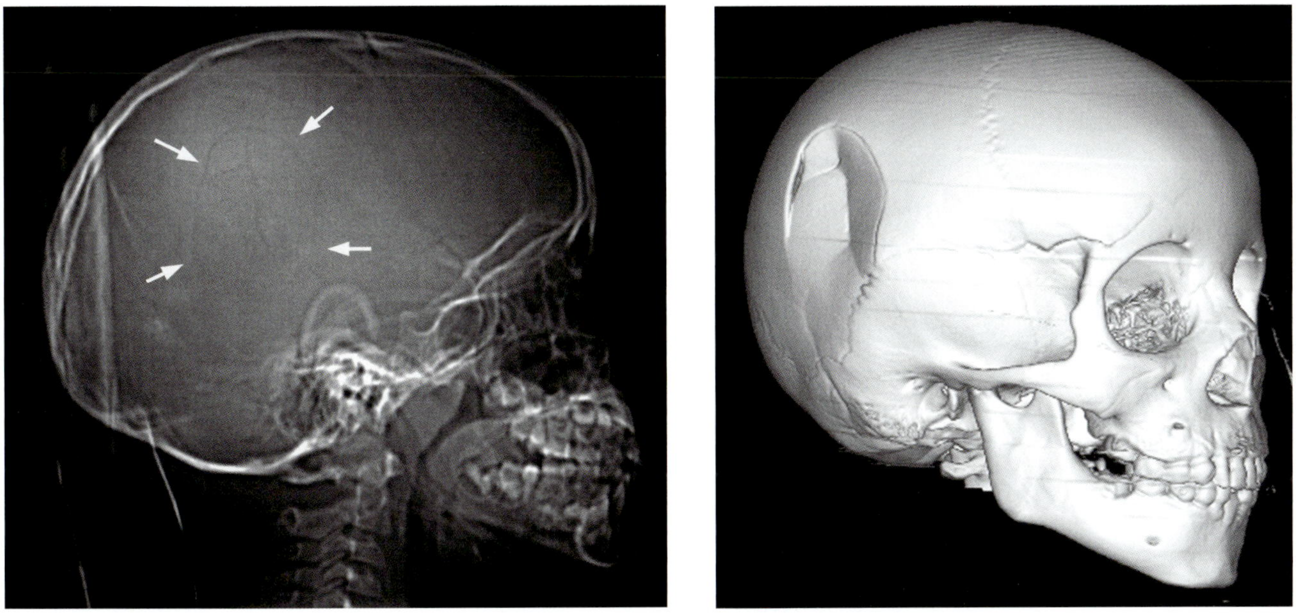

10-6 Depression fracture denoted by arrows on the image to correlate with the 3D CT reconstruction.

Face (Figs. 10-10 and 10-12)

- Glabella—Lies just superior to the nasion; on the frontal bone between the eyebrows
- Nasion—The bridge of the nose where the nasal bones articulate with the frontal bone

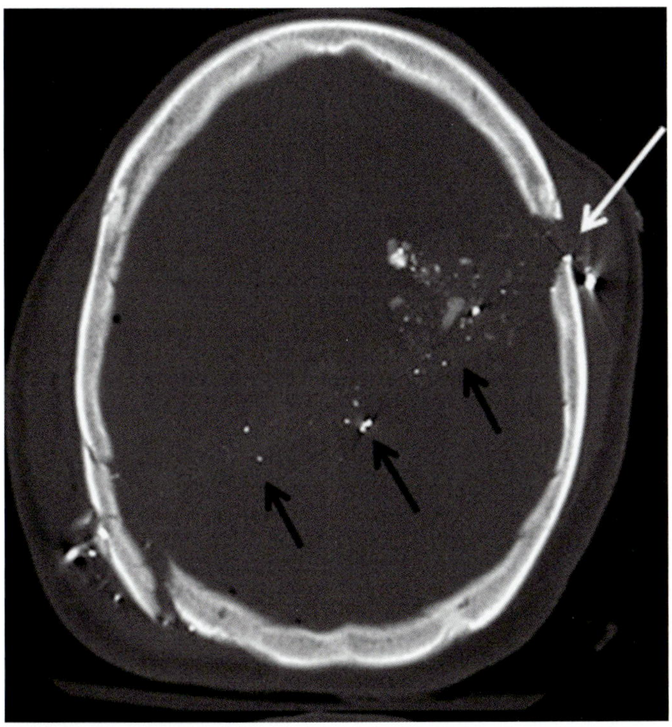

10-7 Axial CT reveals gunshot wound to right temple with metal fragments and bone denoted by the black arrows.

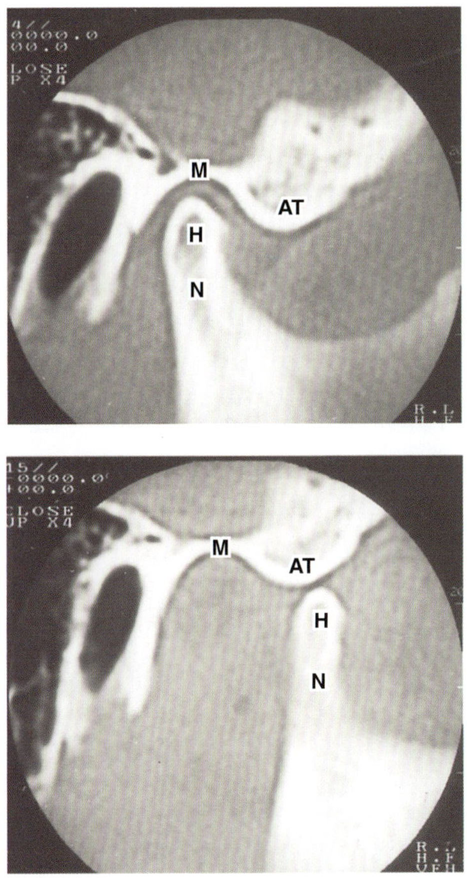

10-8 Sagittal CT of TMJ with mouth closed and opened. (H) Mandibular head (N) Neck (M) Temporomandibular fossa (AT) Articular tubercle on the temporal bone.

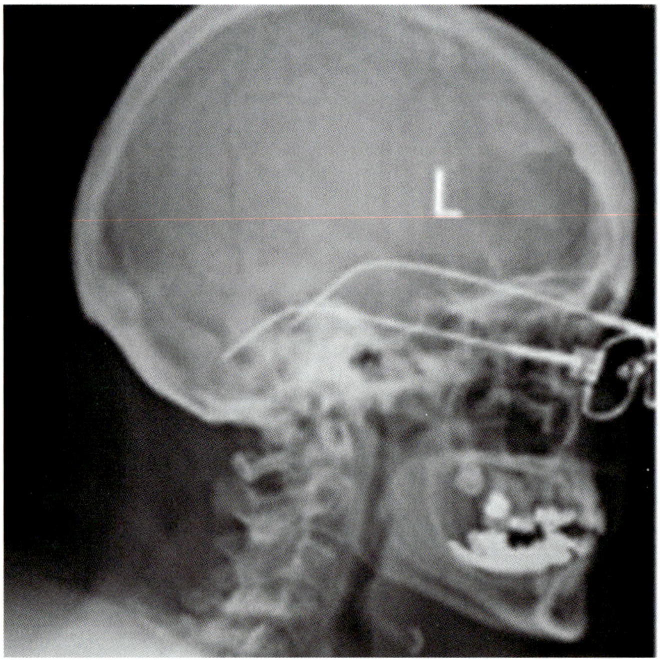

10-9 Patient artifact.

- Acanthion—At the base of the nasal septum
- Mentum—The center of the chin
- Ramus/Angle of the mandible—The palpable posterior-most point of the mandible. This curve separates the body from the ramus (Fig. 10-10).

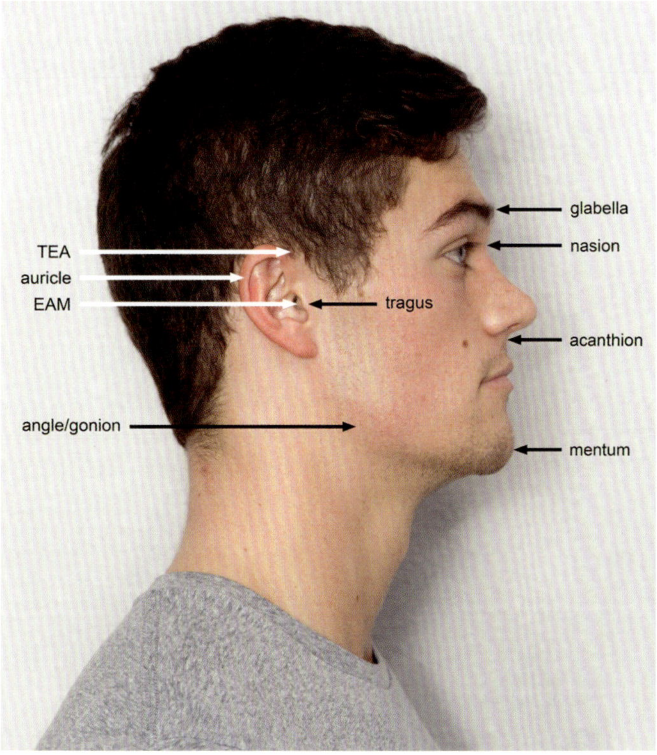

10-10 Landmarks of the ear.

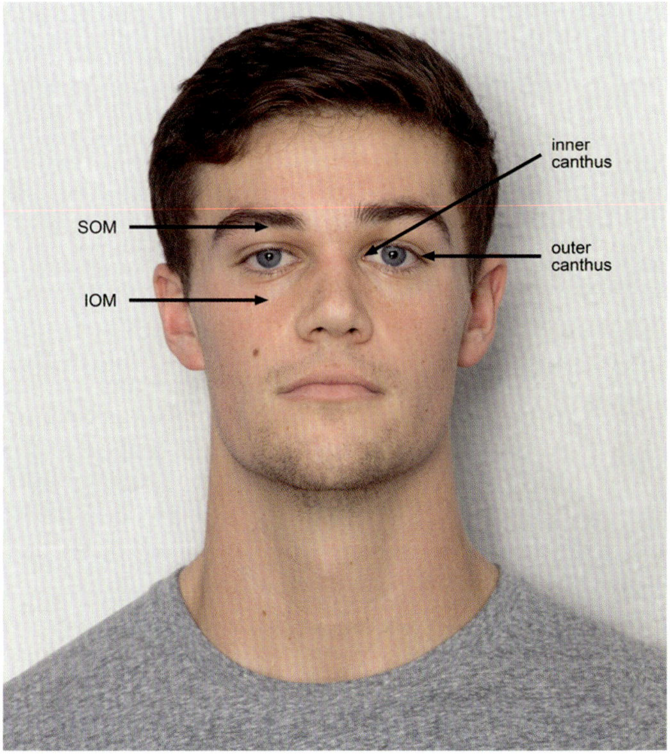

10-11 Landmarks of the eye.

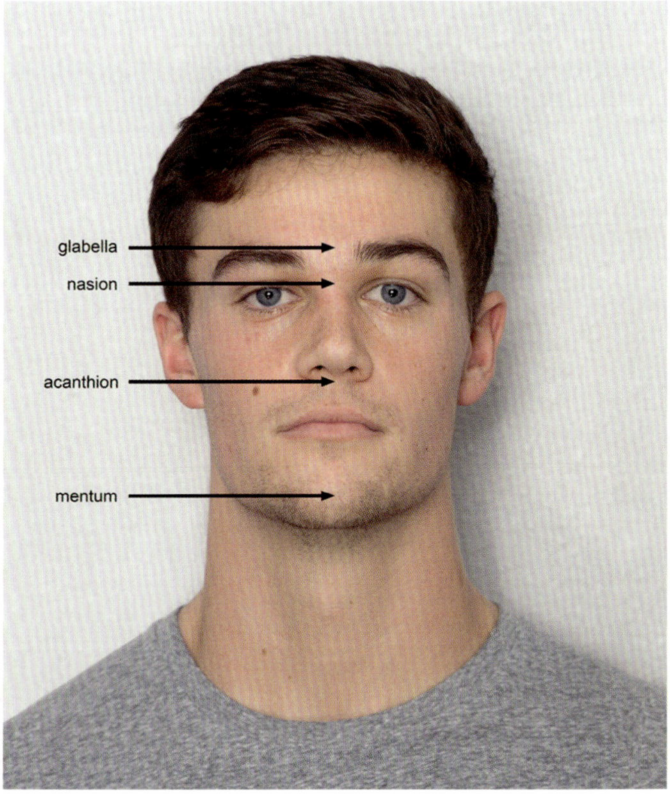

10-12 Landmarks of the face.

Positioning Lines

To attempt to achieve proper positioning of the skull, facial bones, or sinuses, the technologist must identify the positioning lines that connect landmarks. Positioning lines are adjusted to intersect parallel or perpendicular with the image receptor (IR) by depressing or extending the chin. Two landmark points could be connected with a straight edge to help visualize the positioning line (Figs. 10-13 and 10-14).

Orbitomeatal Line (OML)—A line that connects the outer canthus of the orbit to the middle of the EAM

Infraorbitomeatal Line (IOML)—A line that connects the inferior orbital margin to the middle of the EAM. An older reference to the IOML was Reid's baseline. There is a 7° difference between the OML and IOML

Acanthiomeatal Line (AML)—A line that connects the acanthion to the middle of the EAM

Lip Meatal Line (LML)—A line that connects the lip junction to the middle of the EAM

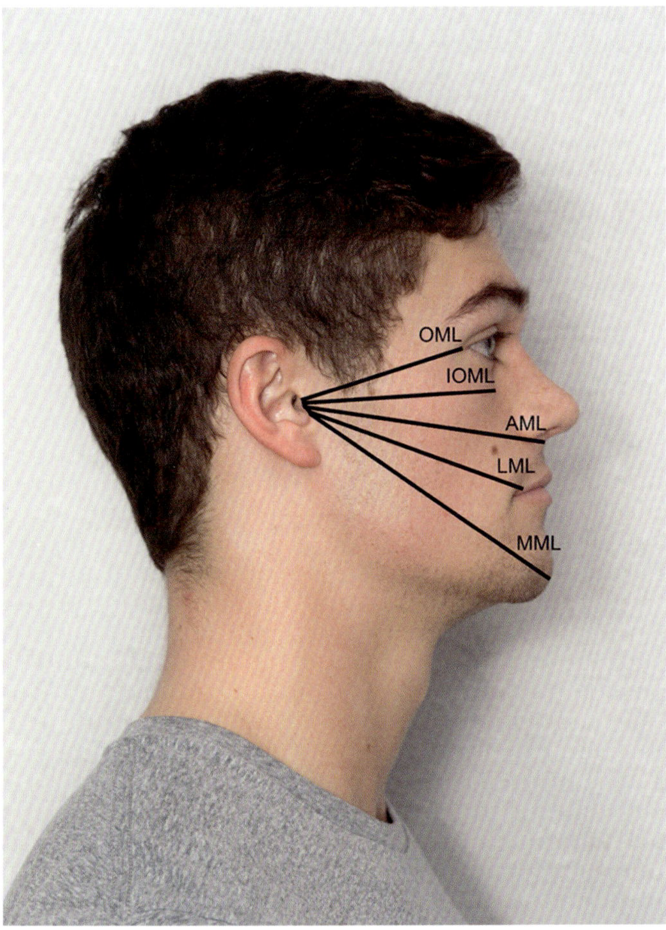

10-13 Lateral positioning lines.

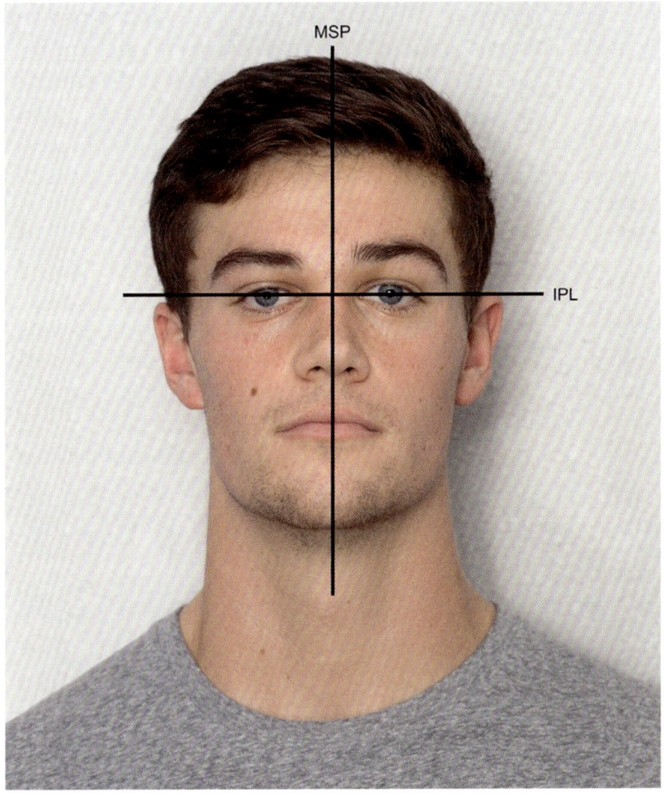

10-14 Frontal positioning lines.

Mentomeatal Line (MML)—A line that connects the mentum to the middle of the EAM

Interpupillary Line (IPL)—A line that intersects both pupils

Midsagittal Line (MSP)—A line that divides the face into equal right and left halves

Ambulatory Patient Imaging

Ambulatory patients will be able to tolerate the imaging projections, while seated on a stool or chair, which is ideal for headwork imaging to display an air–fluid level if present. Ambulatory patients will be able to walk or may come by wheelchair to the exam room (Fig. 10-15). Patients transported by stretcher will be transferred to the imaging table. If an air–fluid level is of concern with this type of patient, it would have to be determined with the use of a horizontal beam (Fig. 10-16).

Projection(s)

How the x-ray beam passes through the part

- Anteroposterior (AP): The beam is directed to enter through the anterior surface, exit the posterior surface, and strike the IR.
- Posteroanterior (PA): The beam is directed to enter the posterior surface, exit the anterior surface, and strike the IR.

- Lateral: The beam will enter the lateral positioned part on the lateral surface and exit the opposite lateral surface.
- AP Axial: An angled beam is directed through the anterior surface and exits the posterior surface before striking the IR.
- PA Axial: An angled beam is directed through the posterior surface and exits the anterior surface before striking the IR.

ANATOMY

Imaging of the head can provide an overall survey of the anatomic area. Exams could also be ordered to image a very specific part, such as skull, nasal bones, orbits, mandible, sinuses, or facial bones. When a specific part is ordered (i.e., nasal bones), this allows for specific centering and improved collimation for the anatomy of interest.

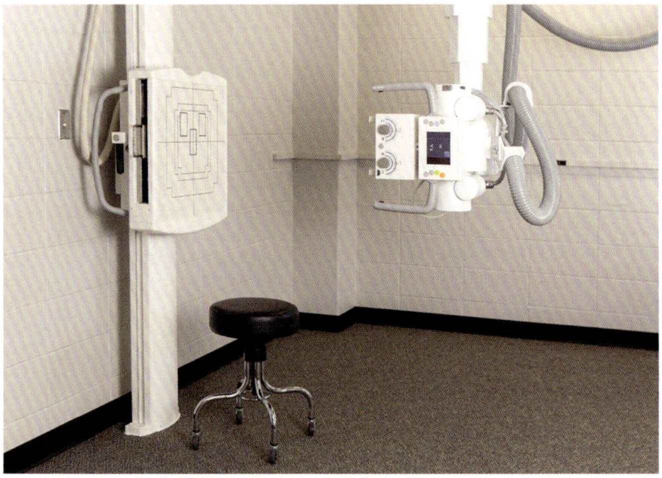

10-15 Room set-up for ambulatory patient.

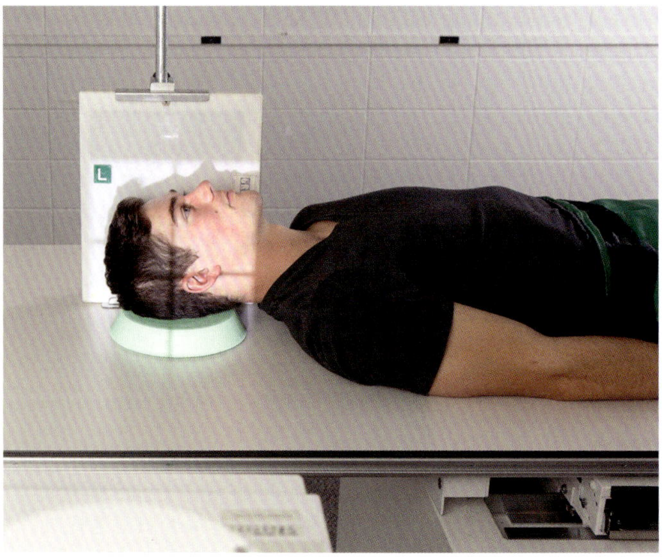

10-16 Horizontal beam imaging.

Skull

The skull is divided into the calvarium (cap) and the skull base. The calvarium consists of a portion of the frontal bone, occipital bone, and both parietal bones (Fig. 10-17). The skull base is composed of the sphenoid bone, ethmoid bone, and paired temporal bones (Fig. 10-18).

Skull bones articulate by the way of serrated sutures that ossify in the adult patient forming a synarthrodial articulation. Intersecting sutures create points of interest.

Sutures (Figs. 10-19 and 10-20)

Sagittal suture—Midline suture that divides the right and left parietal bones

Coronal suture—Suture that divides the frontal bone from the two parietal bones

Lambdoidal suture—Suture that divides the occipital bone from the two parietal bones

Squamosal suture—Suture that divides the temporal bone from the parietal bone

Suture Points of Intersection (Figs. 10-21 to 10-23)

Bregma—Intersection of the frontal suture with the sagittal suture (Figs. 10-21 and 10-22)

Lambda—Intersection of the lambdoidal suture with the sagittal suture (Fig. 10-22)

Pterion—Intersection of the squamosal suture with the frontal suture (Fig. 10-23)

Asterion—Intersection of the squamosal suture with the lambdoidal suture (Fig. 10-23)

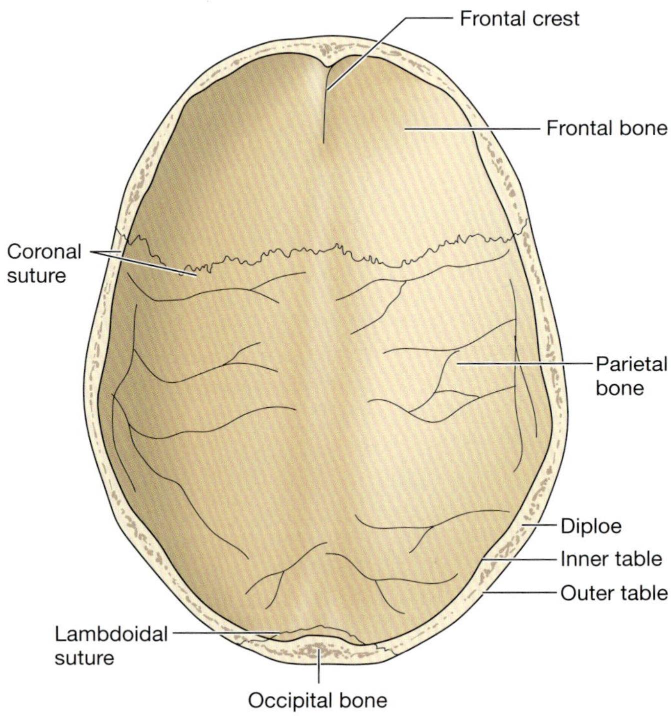

10-17 Calvarium.

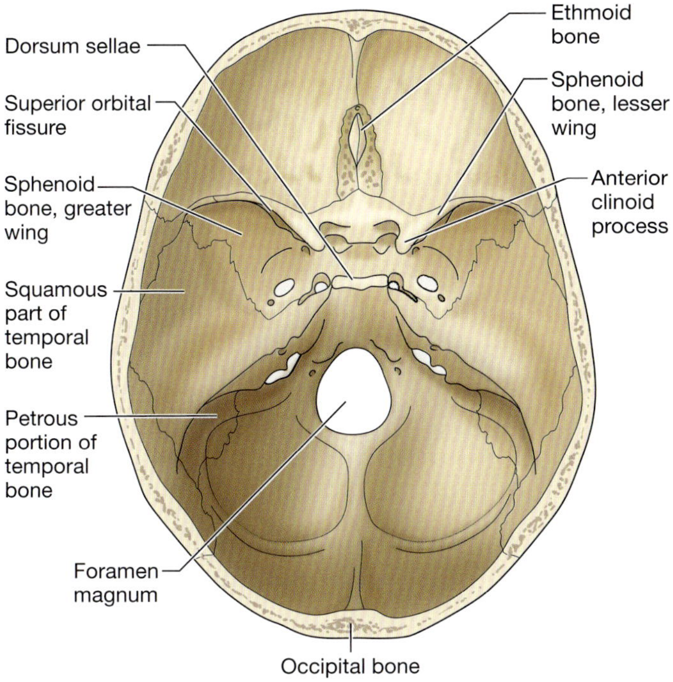

10-18 Skull base.

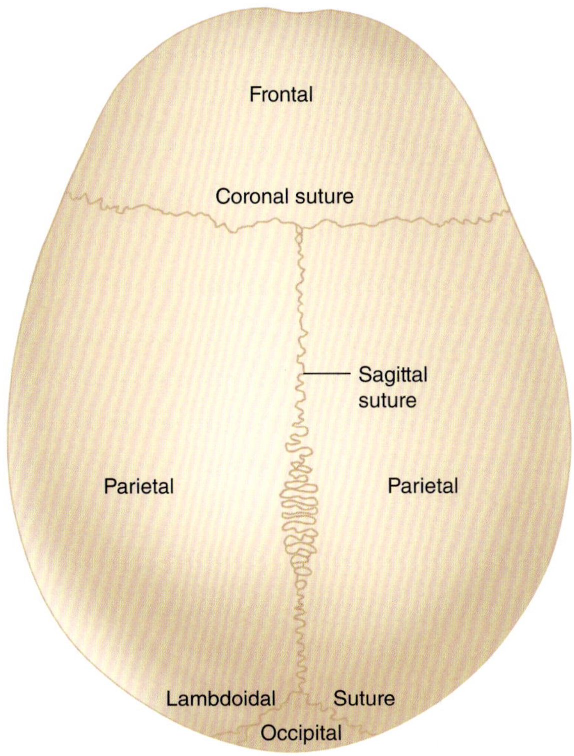

10-19 Superior view of skull sutures.

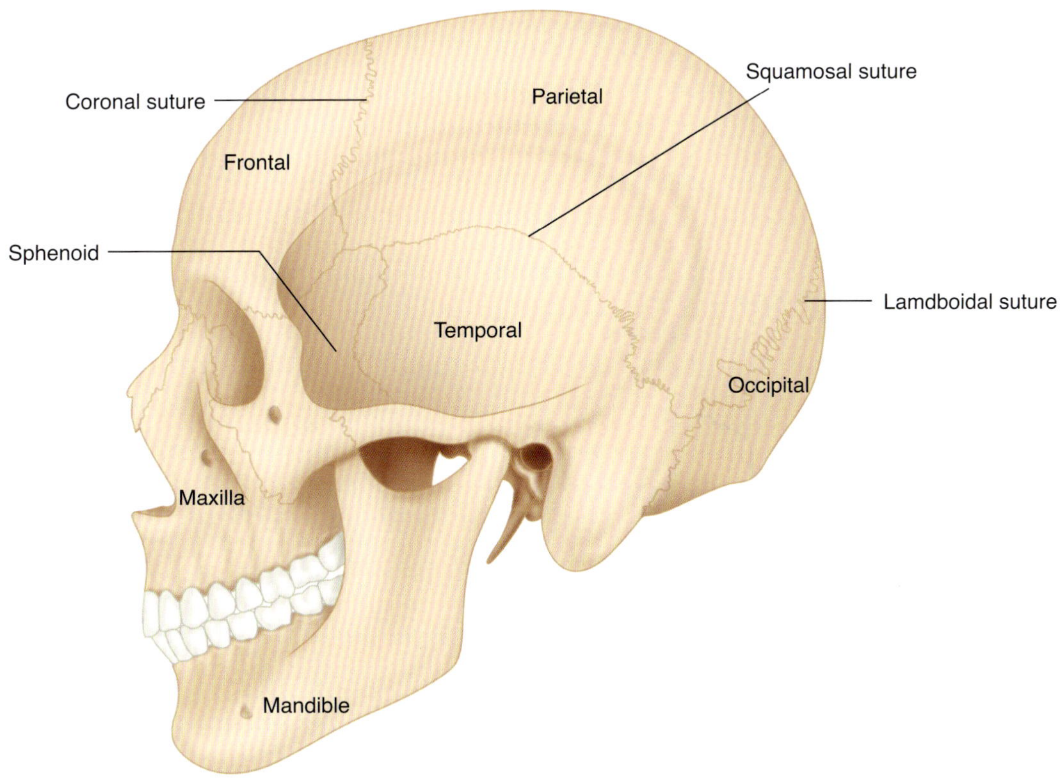

10-20 Lateral view of skull sutures.

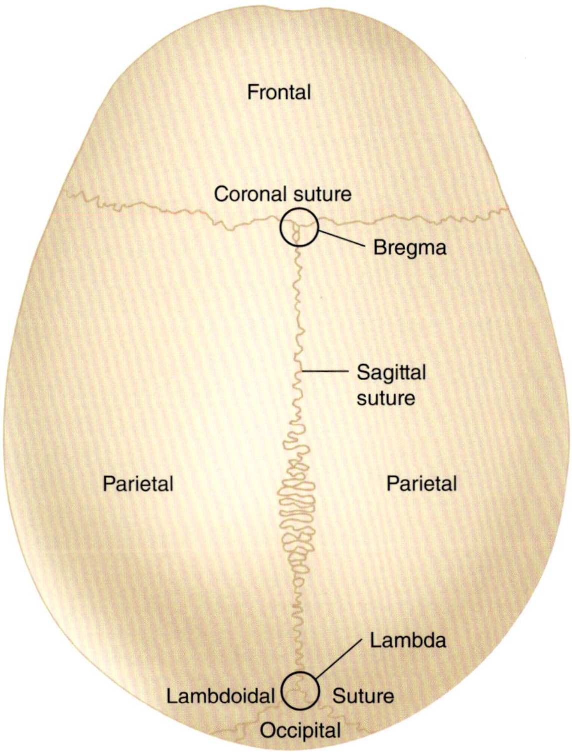

10-21 Superior view of suture points of intersection.

Frontal Bone

The horizontal portion of the frontal bone forms the roofs of the orbits. The vertical, squamous portion creates the forehead. On the forehead, just above the superior orbital margins (SOMs), the superciliary ridges or arches (bony arch beneath the eyebrows) lie. Just superior to the superciliary ridge, a depression marks the supraorbital groove. The flattened, smooth area located between the eyebrows is the glabella. Posterior to the glabella and between the inner and outer skull tables, the frontal sinus cavity exists (Figs. 10-24 and 10-25).

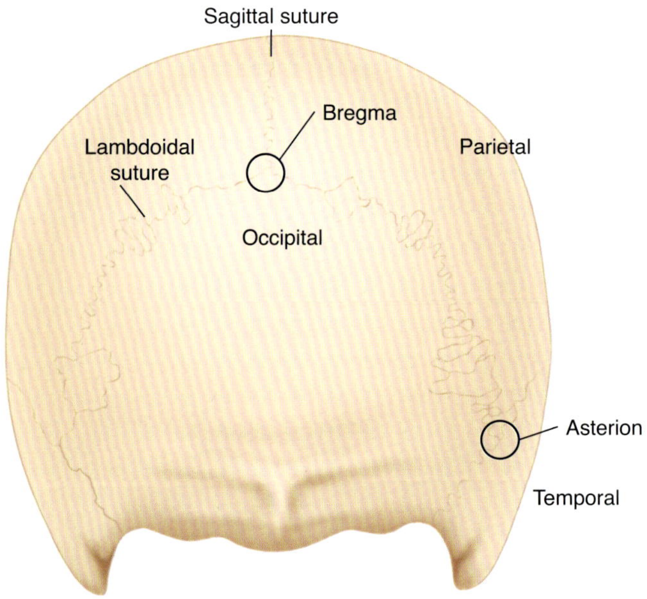

10-22 Posterior view of suture points of intersection.

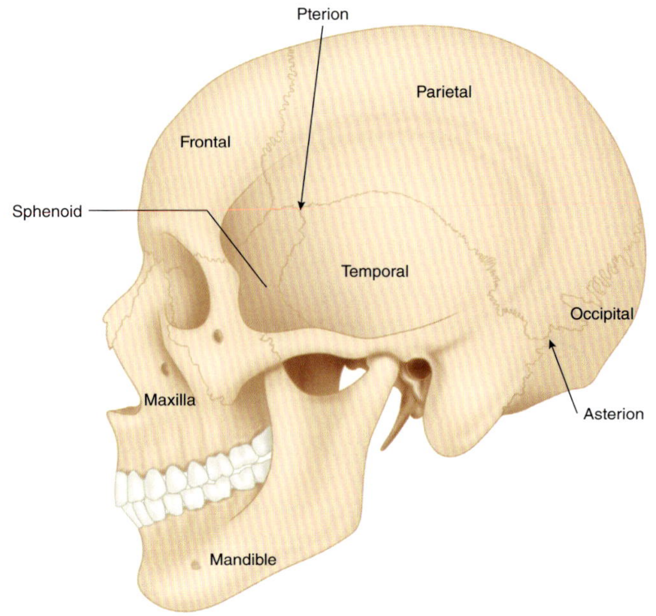

10-23 Lateral view of suture points of intersection.

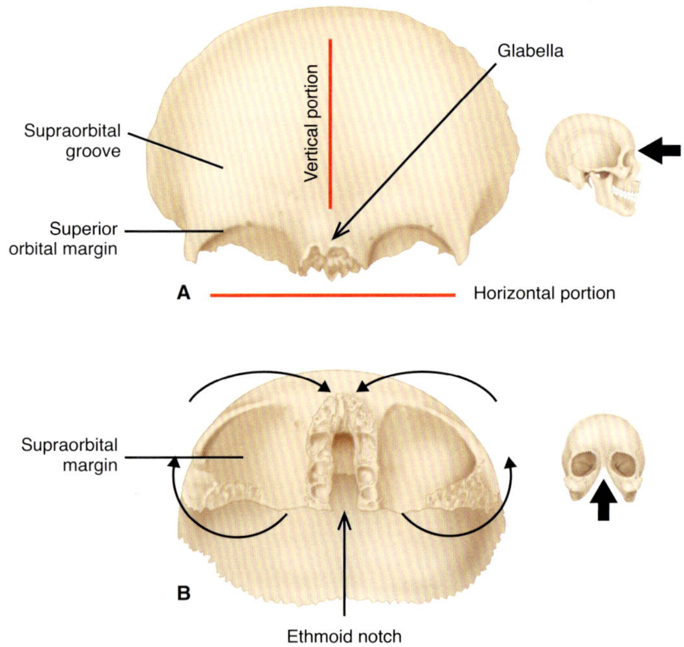

10-24 Frontal view (A) and inferior view (B) of the frontal bone.

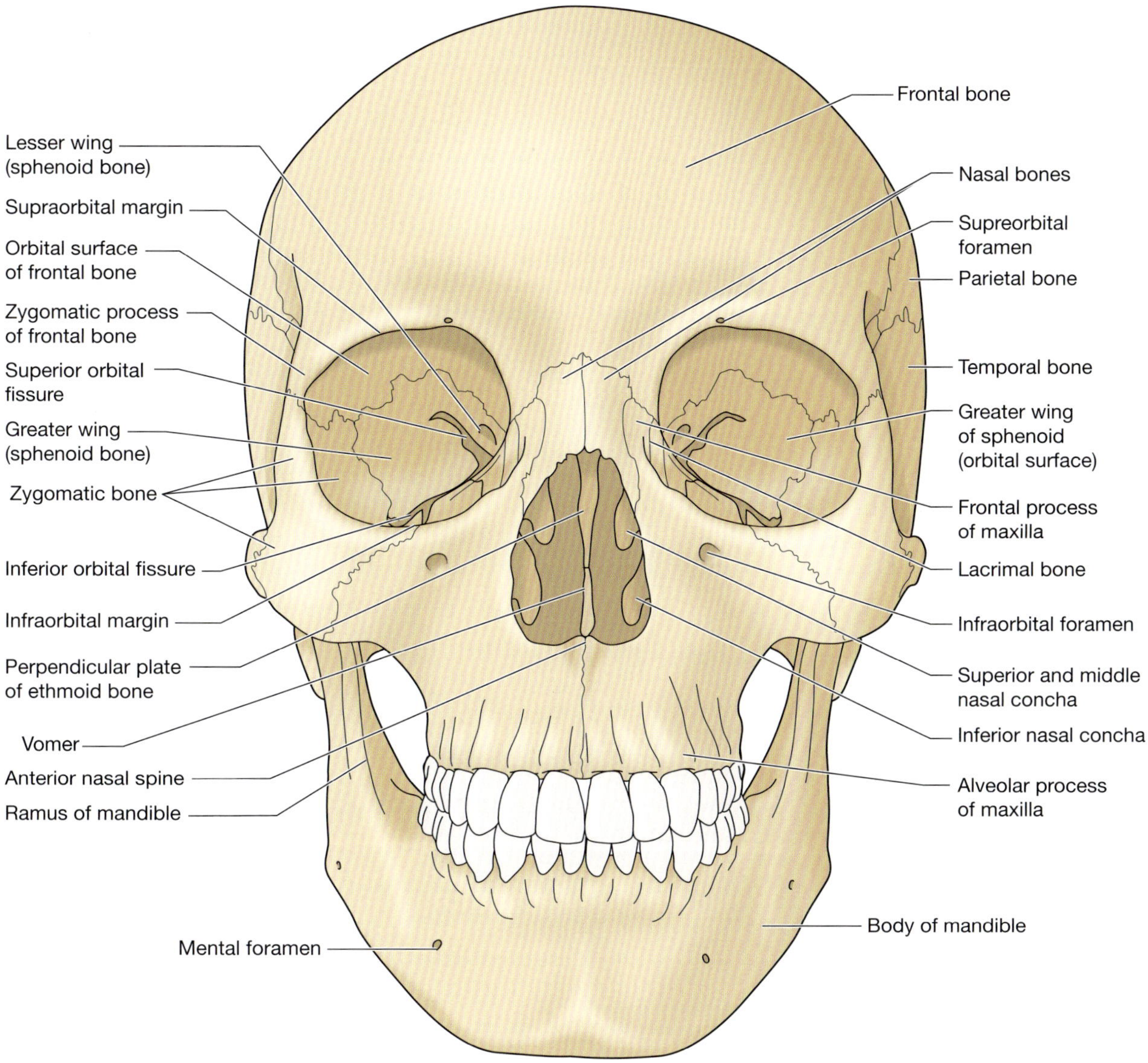

10-25 Frontal view of skull.

Parietal Bones

The parietal bones form the superior and lateral portions of the skull. The superior most point of the skull is termed the vertex. The widest dimension of the skull lies between the two parietal eminences (Figs. 10-26 and 10-27).

Occipital Bone

The occipital bone forms the posterior and inferior portion of the skull. Most inferiorly on the occipital bone, the foramen magnum is located to allow for the continued inferior travel of the spinal cord. On each lateral side of the foramen magnum, an occipital condyle exists and will articulate with the superior facets on the atlas (C1) to form the atlanto-occipital joints (Fig. 10-28).

The posterior occipital bone has an extremely pronounced convex curvature. On this portion, the external occipital protuberance (small elevated bony prominence) or inion is located. When imaging the skull to visualize the occipital bone, a tube angle is necessary to elongate this portion of the bone to lengthen its extreme curvature. Superior to the external occipital protuberance and up to the point of the lambdoidal suture, the flattened portion, known as the squamous portion of the occipital bone is identified (Fig. 10-29).

Temporal Bone

The temporal bone contains and protects the organs of hearing and balance. Aside from the external anatomic features, the internal portion of the temporal bone is the densest portion

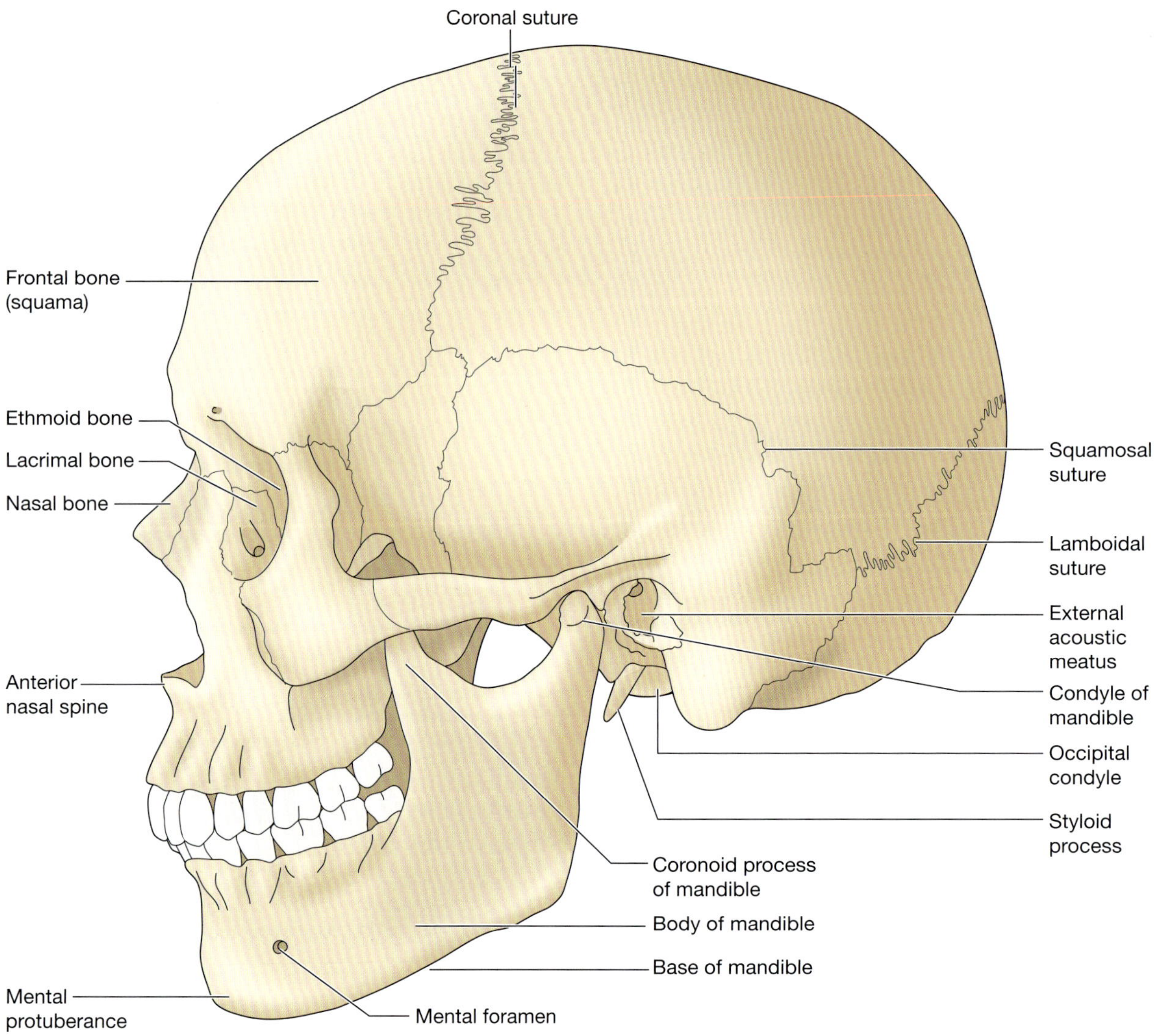

10-26 Lateral view of skull.

of the skull and is known as the petrous pyramid. Petrous pyramids are visible on all head images and provide a means to evaluate for proper positioning (Figs. 10-30 and 10-31).

The EAM is easily identifiable on the external temporal bone. Superior to the EAM, the squamous portion of the temporal bone extends up to the squamosal suture line. Posterior to the EAM is the mastoid portion. The mastoid portion contains the mastoid air cells. The most inferior point of the mastoid portion is the mastoid tip. Slightly anterior and inferior from the EAM, a slender styloid process projects inferiorly from the temporal bone (Fig. 10-32). The styloid process provides a site for facial muscle attachment. Anterior to the EAM, a slender process projects anteriorly toward the face to contribute to the formation of the zygomatic arch. Just inferior to the zygomatic process, the temporomandibular fossa is located to accept the condyle of the mandible (Fig. 10-32).

The petrous pyramids or the petrous portions are located interiorly on the temporal bone. The petrous pyramids are each triangular in shape. Each right and left petrous pyramids run from the EAM at an anterior angle toward the midline. The most superior point of the petrous pyramids is referred to as the petrous ridge. Located posteriorly on each petrous pyramid, a small opening can be found; the internal auditory meatus. The petrous pyramids protect all the inner ear organs of hearing (Fig. 10-30).

Sphenoid Bone

The sphenoid bone is the anchor for all cranial bones to articulate with. Centrally on the sphenoid, the sella turcica is located. The sella turcica has the appearance of a depressed saddle. The sella turcica will support the pituitary gland (Fig. 10-33). Directly inferior to the sella turcica is the body of the sphenoid bone, which will contain the sphenoid sinus cavity. The anterior clinoid

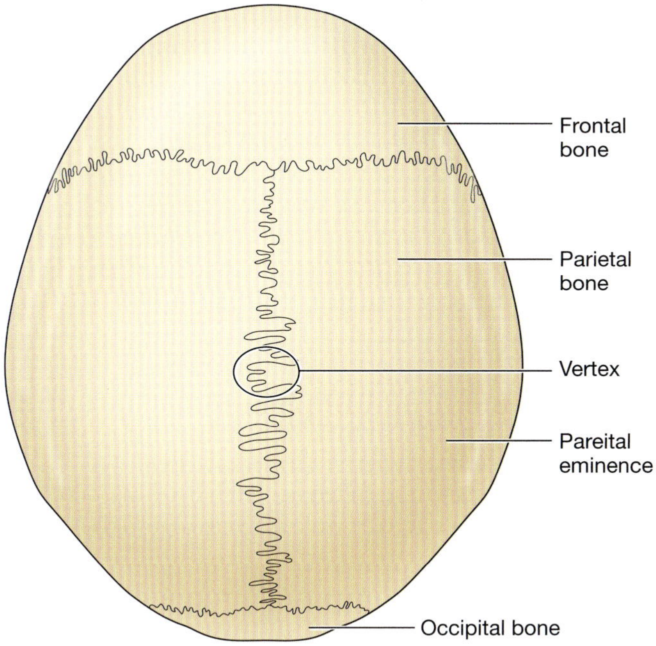

10-27 Superior view of skull.

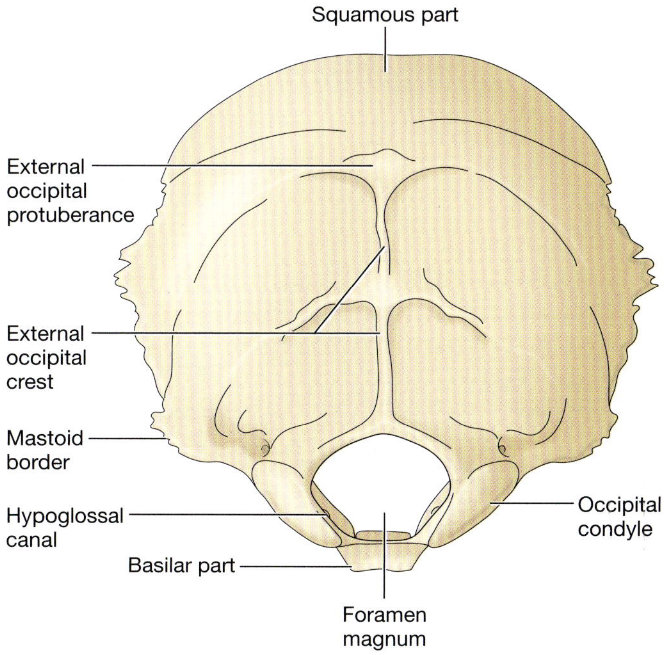

10-29 Occipital bone.

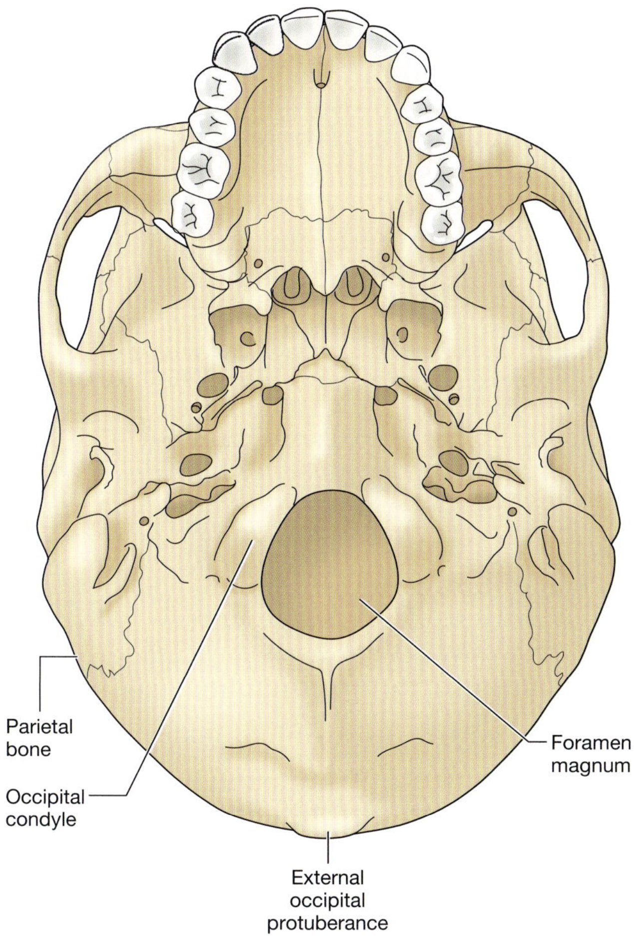

10-28 Inferior view of skull.

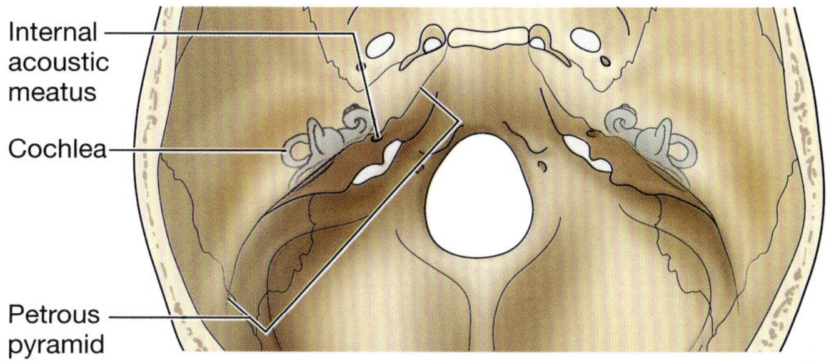

10-30 Petrous pyramids of the temporal bone.

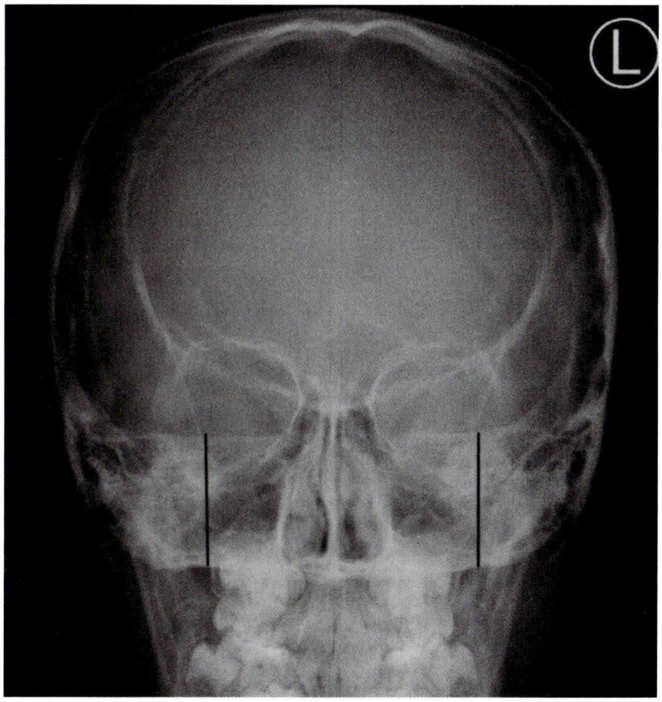

10-31 Black lines denote the right and left petrous pyramids.

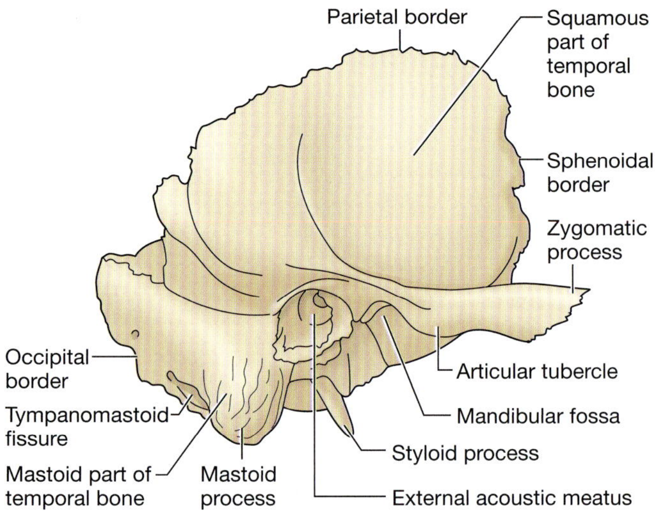

10-32 Lateral view of the external temporal bone.

processes are located on the lesser wings of the sphenoid and are anterior to the midline sella turcica. The posterior clinoid processes sit opposite of the anterior clinoid processes and are located on the dorsum sella. The posterior flattened back of the sella turcica is referred to as the dorsum sella (Fig. 10-34). Posterior to the dorsum sella, the sphenoid travels inferiorly to articulate with the occipital bone. This region is referred to the clivus. The clivus will lead to a suture line formed between sphenoid and occipital bone (Fig. 10-35). This critical location is where a basilar skull fracture can occur and may be obscured when only diagnostic radiography is obtained. A basilar skull fracture may only be revealed with the presence of sphenoidal effusion (pooling of cerebrospinal fluid within the air-filled sphenoid sinus cavity). Sphenoidal effusion will be identified with the use of a horizontal beam lateral, revealing the presence of an air–fluid level.

A greater wing of the sphenoid extends off laterally from the base of the sella turcica on each side. The right and left

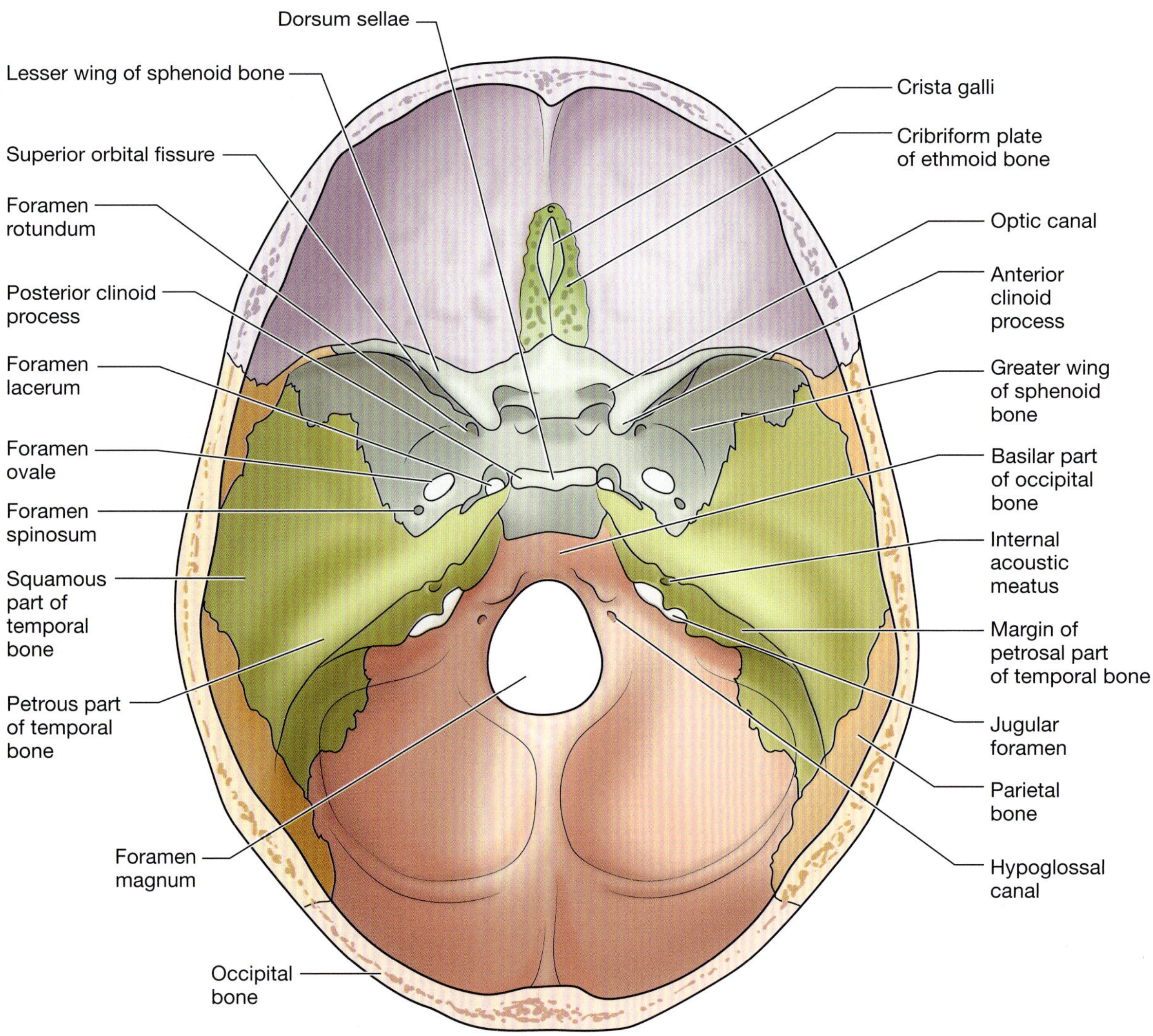

10-33 Sphenoid bone in the base of the skull.

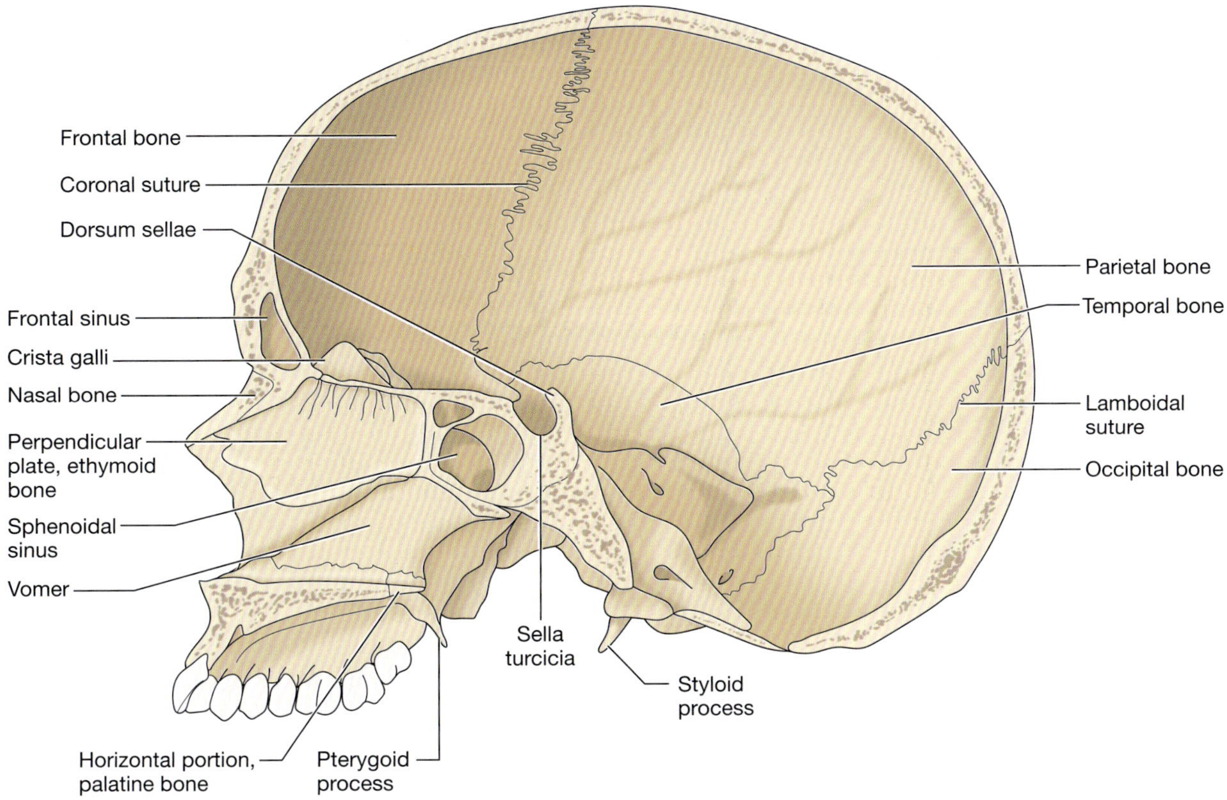

10-34 Sectional midline of the skull.

greater wings, inferior to the lesser wing, contains three foramina on each side foramen rotundum, foramen ovale, and foramen spinosum. Foramen rotundum is round and is the most anteriorly located foramen in the greater wing. Foramen ovale is oval shaped and is the largest of the three foramina in the greater wing. Foramen ovale is located posterior to foramen rotundum. Foramen spinosum is small, round, and located most posteriorly on the greater wing (Fig. 10-33).

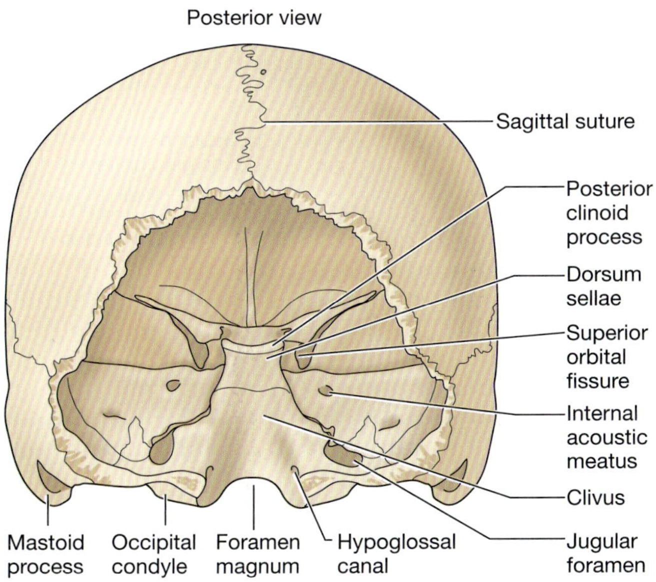

10-35 Posterior view sphenoid bone.

Superior to the greater wing of the sphenoid is the lesser wing of the sphenoid. The lesser wing gives rise to the anterior clinoid processes. Just medial to each anterior clinoid process, the optic groove and optic foramen are located. In between the greater and lesser wings of the sphenoid, the superior orbital fissure (a triangular opening) exists. The superior orbital fissure may be visible radiographically within the medial portions of both orbits when the petrous pyramids are not superimposing (Fig. 10-36).

The pterygoid processes project inferiorly from the sphenoid bone. These long leg–appearing extensions travel inferiorly and posteriorly to the nasal cavity and make contact with the palatine bones. The pterygoid processes each have a medial and lateral side. The medial side of the pterygoid process each contains a hook-like hamulus extension (Figs. 10-34 and 10-36).

Ethmoid Bone

The perpendicular plate drops down midline from the cribriform plate and forms the majority of the bony nasal septum. The perpendicular plate of the ethmoid bone articulates with the vomer (facial bone) to form the entire bony nasal septum (Fig. 10-37). The lateral walls of the nasal cavity are formed by the superior and middle nasal conchae of the ethmoid. The inferior nasal concha are also identified in the lateral nasal cavity, but is a separate facial bone and is not part of the ethmoid bone (Fig. 10-38). The ethmoid air cells compartmentalized into the anterior, middle, and posterior ethmoid sinuses. As air is brought into the nose, the collection of the ethmoid sinuses will filter and warm the air, as it enters the respiratory system (Fig. 10-39).

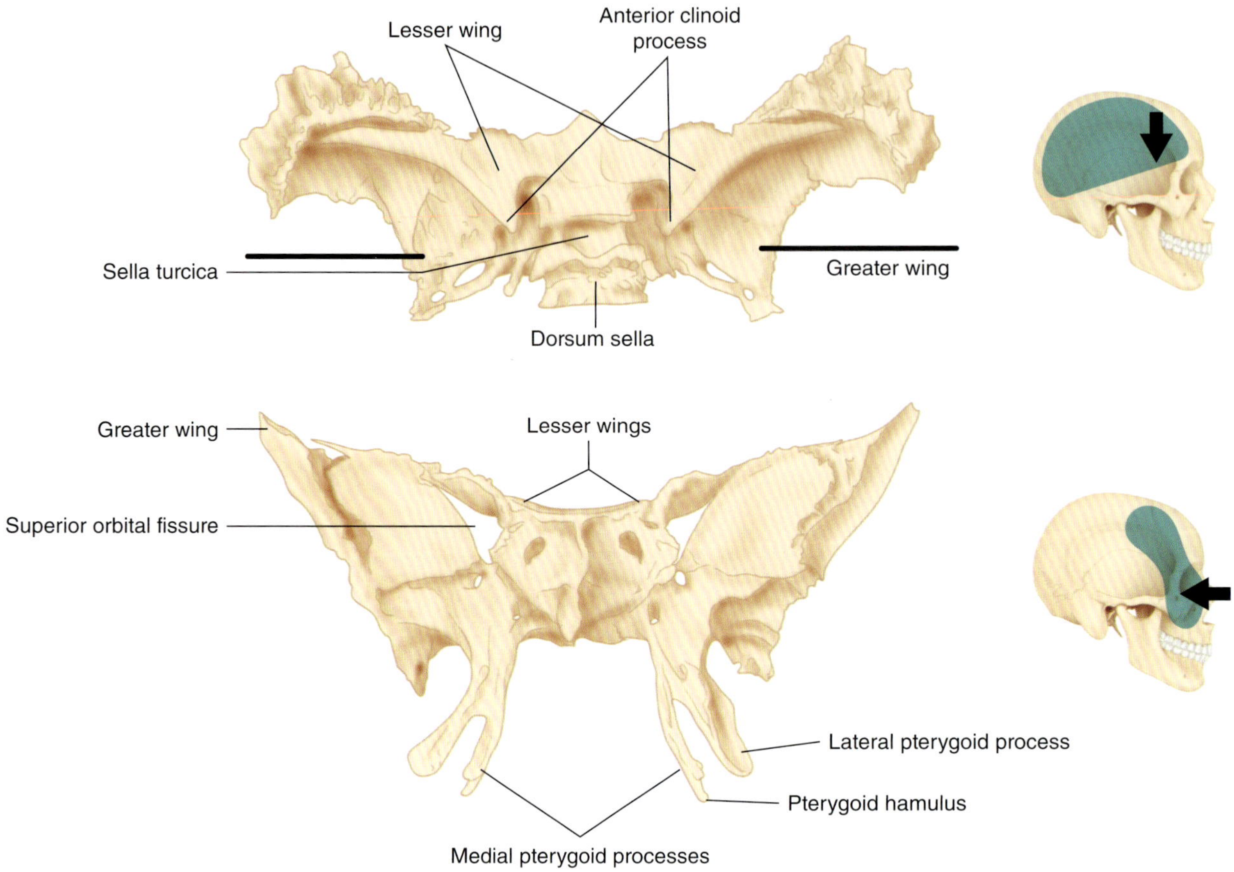

10-36 Sphenoid bone.

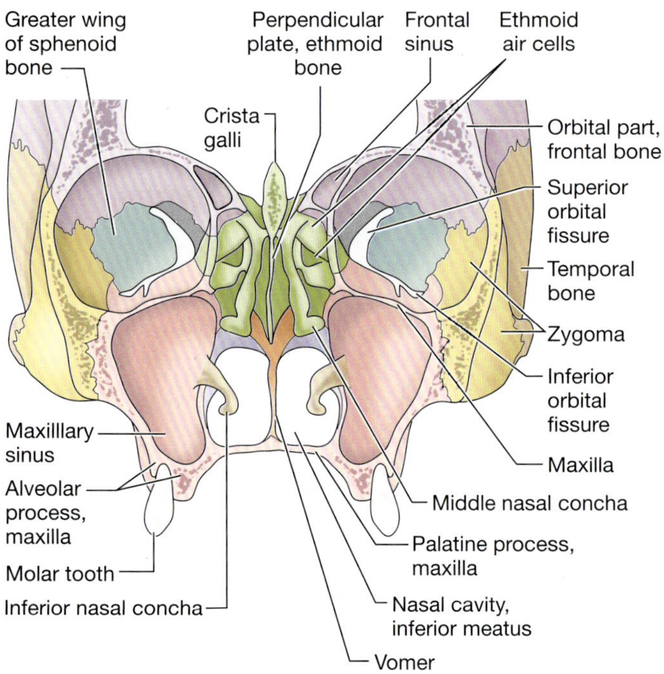

10-37 Coronal view of ethmoid bone.

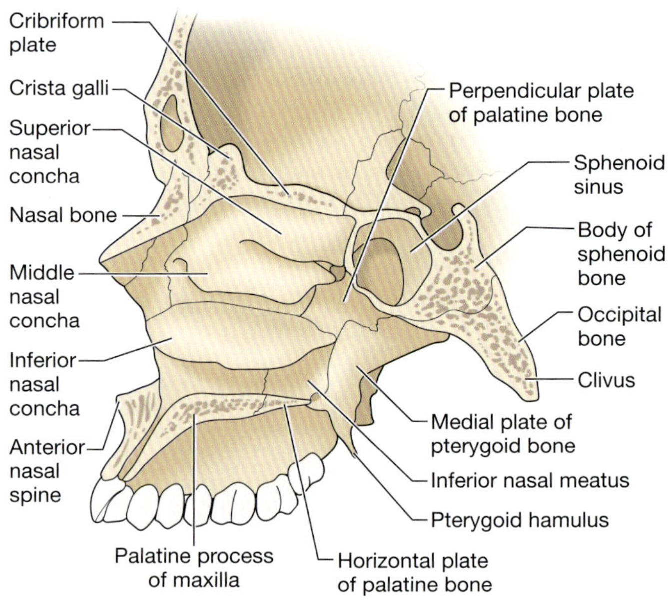

10-38 Sectional midline of the ethmoid bone.

The horizontal portion of the ethmoid fits into the notch on the horizontal portion of the frontal bone that sits between the roofs of the orbits. The horizontal portion of the ethmoid bone is referred to as the cribriform plate. The cribriform plate contains many tiny small openings for the olfactory nerves necessary for smell (Fig. 10-40). The crista galli projects up vertically and resembles the shape of a flame. The crista galli may be identifiable in the region of the glabella, if prominent, on radiographs (Figs. 10-41 and 10-42).

Facial Bones

The majority of the facial bones are paired with the exception of the vomer and the mandible. All of the facial bones are of irregular shape. Imaging the facial bones could entail a protocol

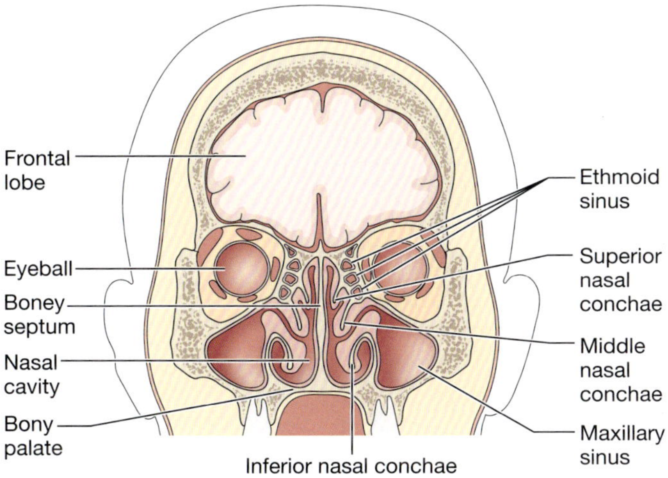

10-39 Nasal cavity.

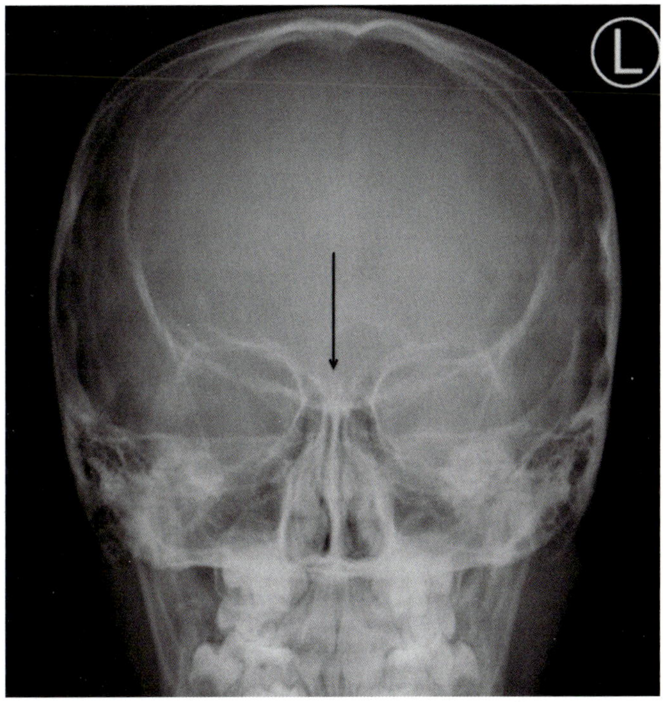

10-42 Arrow denotes crista galli.

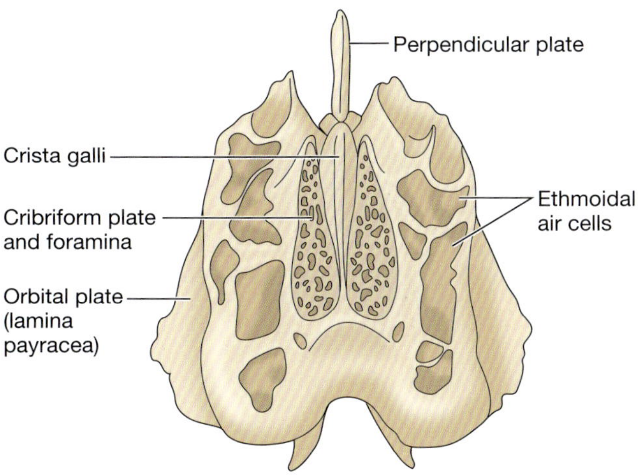

10-40 Superior view of ethmoid bone.

that could provide a general survey of the anatomy or offer improved detail when modified positions, projections, tube angles, and centering are applied.

Maxilla

Each maxilla contributes to the formation of the oral cavity, nasal cavity, and one orbit. The body of the maxilla contains the maxillary sinus cavity. The maxillary sinus cavity is the only cavity developed at birth. The floor of the maxillary sinus is closely positioned to the root system of the upper row of teeth (Fig. 10-43).

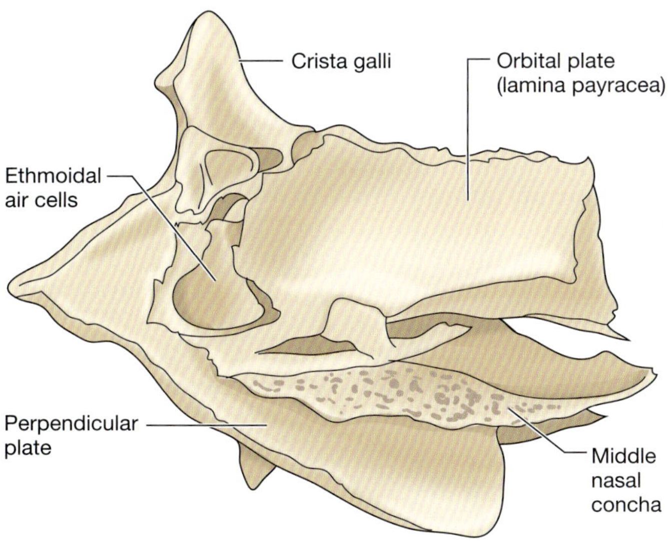

10-41 Lateral view of ethmoid bone.

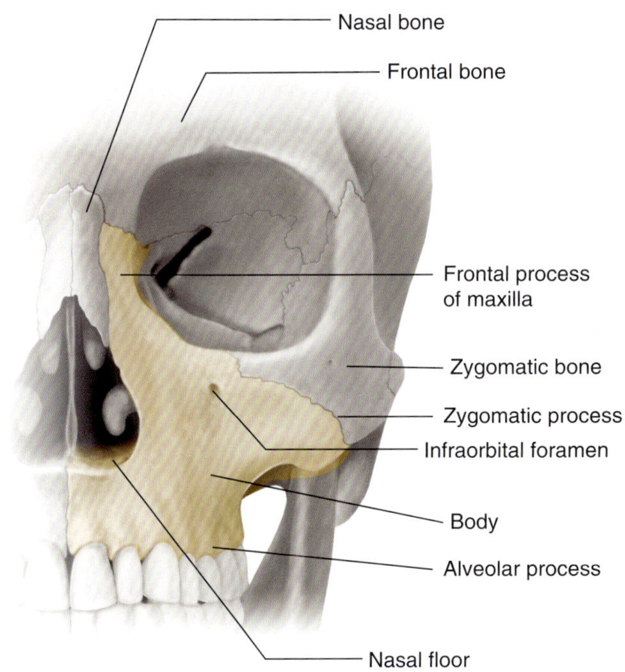

10-43 Maxilla.

The maxilla contributes to the formation of the medial wall of the orbit. The slender frontal process projects superiorly between a nasal bone and a lacrimal bone to articulate with the frontal bone. The maxilla contains a lateral zygomatic process to articulate with the zygoma (Fig. 10-43). Below the body of the maxilla, lie the alveolar processes to support the roots of the upper teeth. The midline anterior fusion of the right and left maxilla forms a small anterior nasal spine which corresponds to the topographical landmark known as the acanthion. The maxilla also contains a fourth process, being the palatine process, not to be misreferenced as the palatine bone. The palatine processes of the right and left maxilla fuse together to form the majority of the bony hard palate (roof) of the oral cavity (Fig. 10-44). Failure of this midline fusion will result in a cleft palate.

Zygoma

The zygoma, (malar) bone, is the cheekbone. The zygoma will articulate with the frontal bone, the maxilla, and the zygomatic process of the temporal bone. The zygoma will contribute to the formation of the lateral wall of the orbit. In instances, in which the zygoma breaks away from its three articulations, a tripod fracture will result (Fig. 10-45).

Nasal Bones

The nasal bones are small. The right and left nasal bones will fuse and junction with the frontal bone to form the bridge of the nose, represented topographically by the nasion (Fig. 10-46). Each nasal bone is imaged separately in a lateral position to place each side closer to the image receptor (Figs. 10-47 and 10-48).

Lacrimal Bones

The lacrimal bones are positioned on the medial side of the orbit but do not contribute to the formation of the base of the

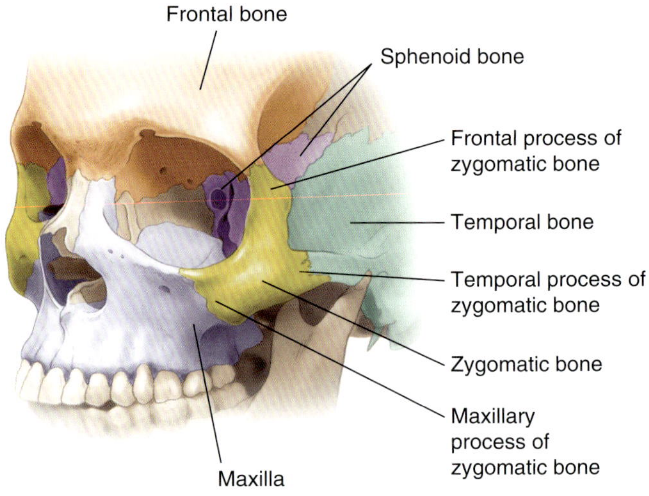

10-45 Zygoma.

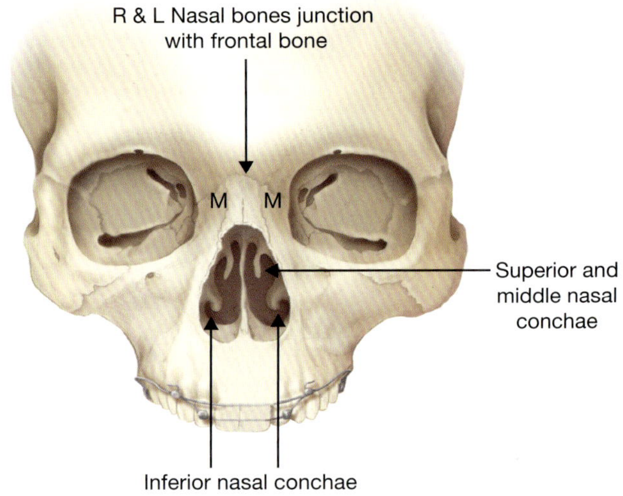

10-46 Frontal view of nasal bones and nasal conchae.

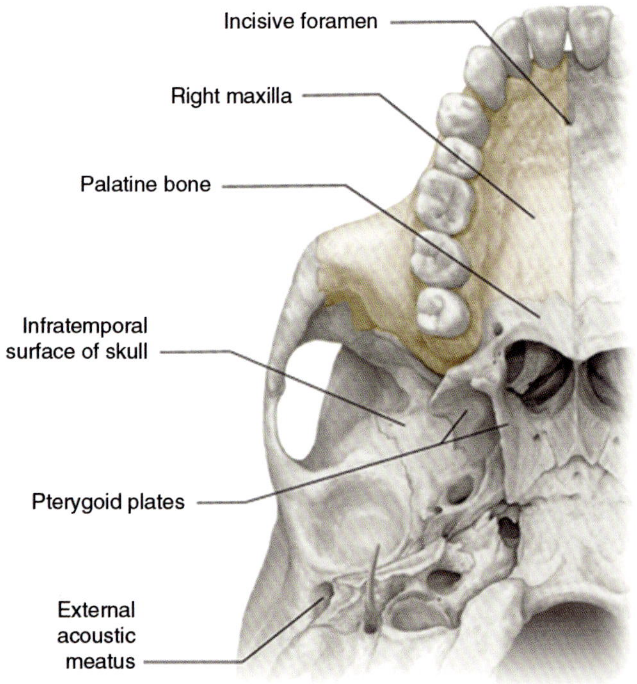

10-44 Inferior view of maxilla.

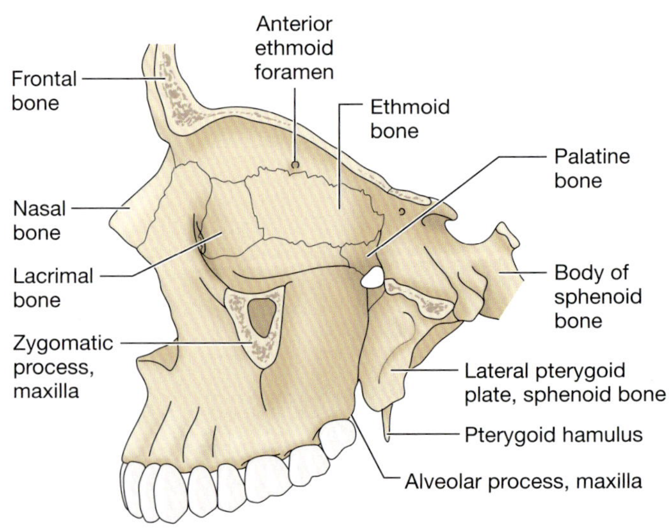

10-47 Sectional view of nasal bones.

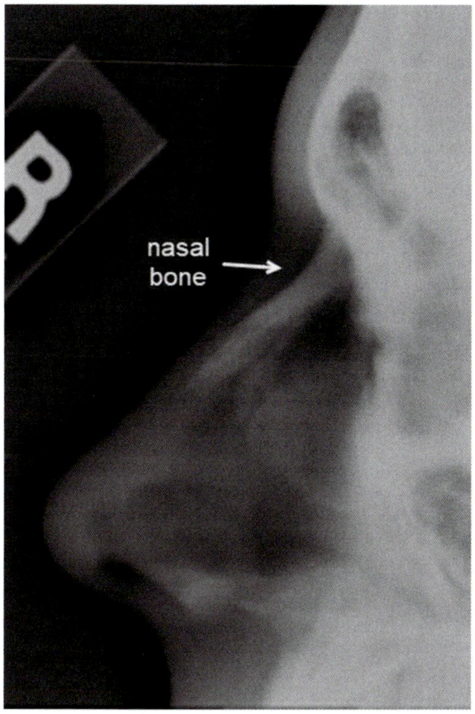

10-48 Lateral nasal bone.

orbit. The tear duct is associated with the lacrimal bone. Visualization of the foramen for the lacrimal duct may be possible on examination of a dry skull (Fig. 10-49).

Palatine Bones

The palatine bones are small and shaped like the letter "L" and are internally located on the skull. The horizontal portion contributes to the formation of the posterior hard palate (Fig. 10-50). The vertical portion of the palatine bone extends superiorly between the pterygoid processes, vomer, and the nasal concha. The palatine bones are not visualized with skull radiography (Fig. 10-51).

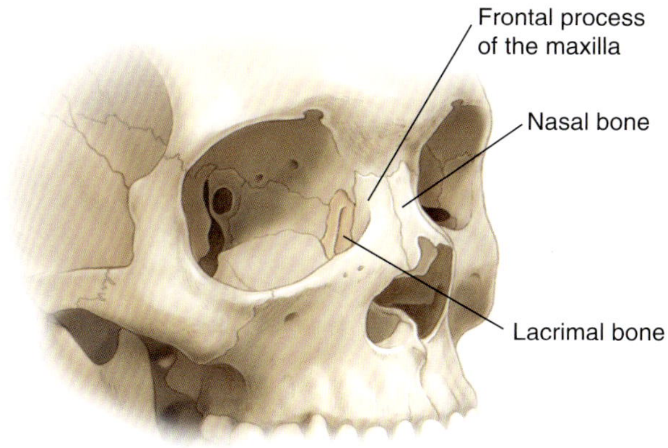

10-49 Lacrimal bone.

Vomer

The vomer is a thin, midline, flat bone. The vomer articulates with the perpendicular plate of the ethmoid bone and forms the inferior and posterior portion of the bony nasal septum (Fig. 10-52).

Inferior Nasal Concha

The inferior nasal conchae are paired and are facial bones. The inferior nasal conchae are separate from the superior and middle nasal conchae of the ethmoid bone, but serves the same purpose that of the superior and middle nasal conchae, to filter and warm the air as it enters the respiratory system (Figs. 10-46 and 10-50).

Orbit

The orbit is composed of the base most anteriorly and the apex most posteriorly. The orbit is shaped like a cone. The apex of the orbit projects toward midline at 37° and 30° superiorly (Fig. 10-53). The optic foramen enters the orbit through the apex of the orbit. Considering the placement of the orbital apex, this influences the positioning necessary to project the optic foramen into the visible lower outer quadrant of the orbit on an image (Fig. 10-54).

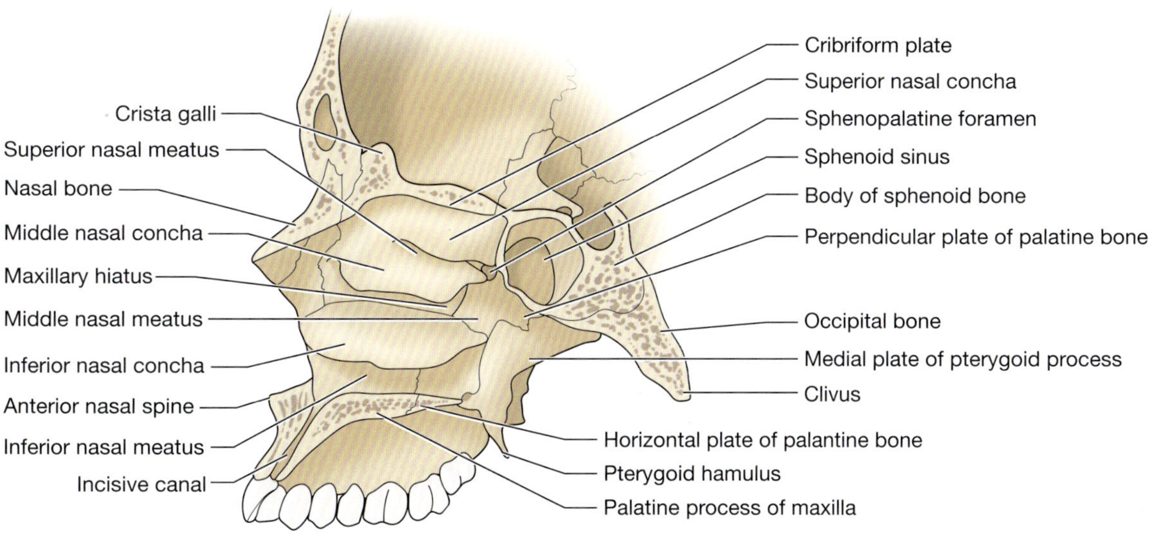

10-50 Palatine bone.

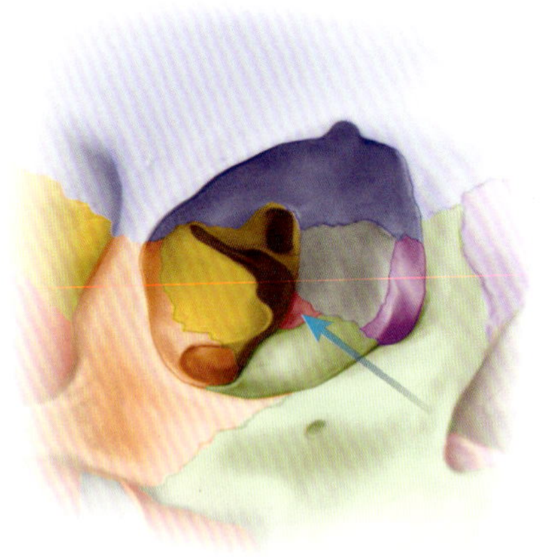

10-51 Arrow denotes superior most end of palatine bone.

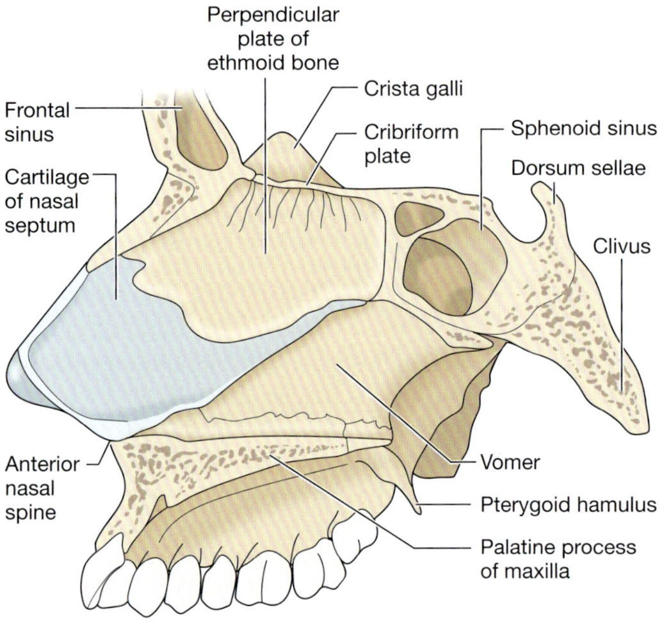

10-52 Vomer.

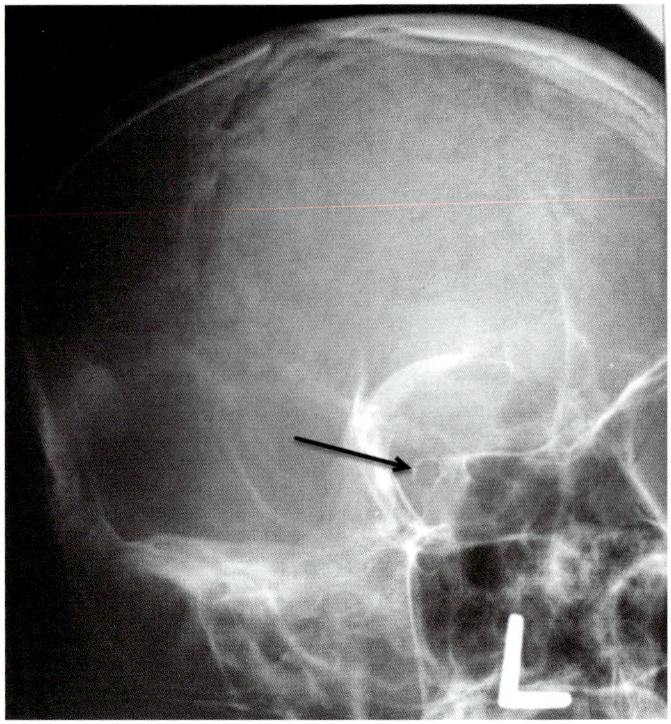

10-54 Optic foramen in the lower outer quadrant of the orbit.

The base of the orbit is formed by the frontal bone, the maxilla, and the zygoma. The frontal bone forms the superior orbit. The zygoma forms the lateral orbit and the maxilla forms the floor and medial portion of the orbit (Fig. 10-55). In instances in which an individual sustains a direct blow to the entire base of the orbit, the direct force may cause the floor of the orbit to "blowout" down into and perforate the maxillary sinus cavity (Fig. 10-56). The posterior and medial portions of the orbit are composed of the ethmoid bone. The posterior and lateral portions of the orbit are composed of the sphenoid bone (Fig. 10-55).

There are three openings into the orbit. The optic foramen enters at the apex of the orbit. There is a small section of bone in between the optic foramen and the superior orbital fissure, referred

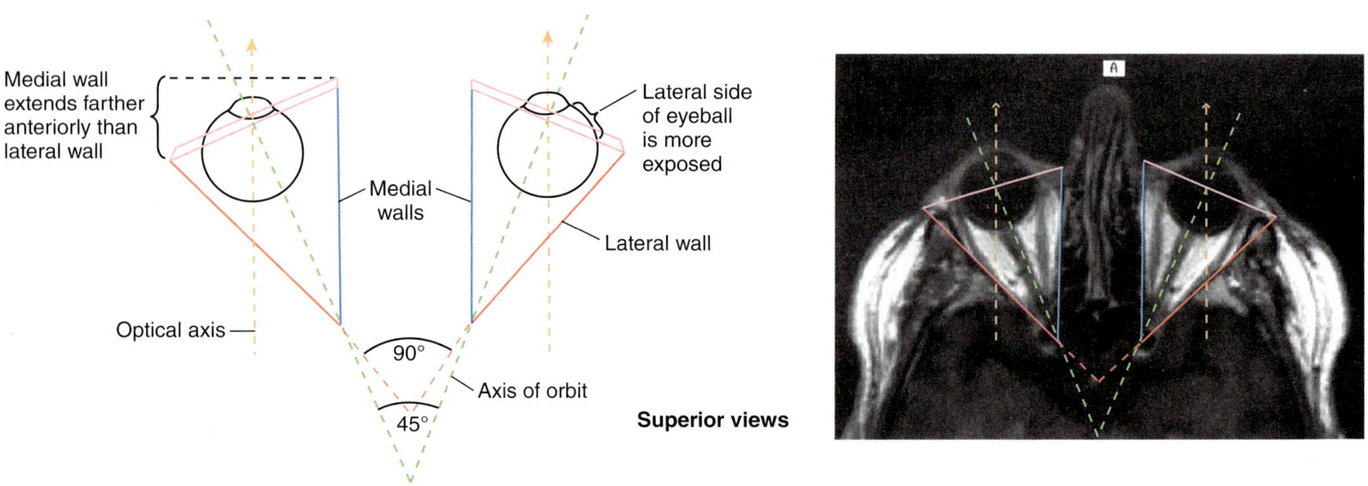

10-53 Position of the orbit.

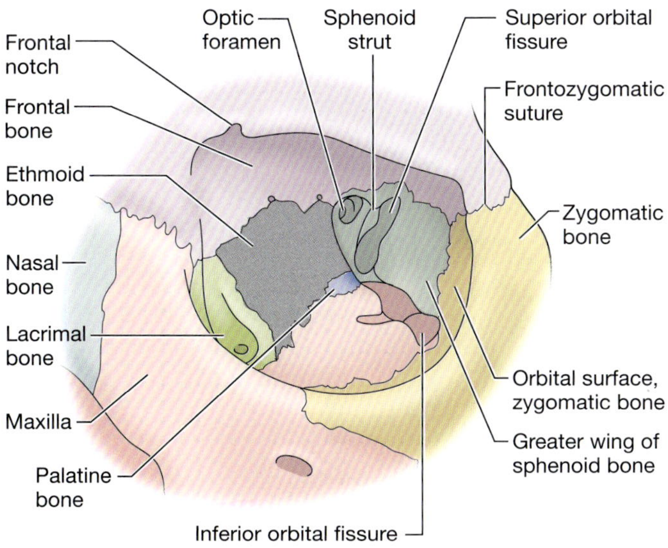

10-55 Orbit.

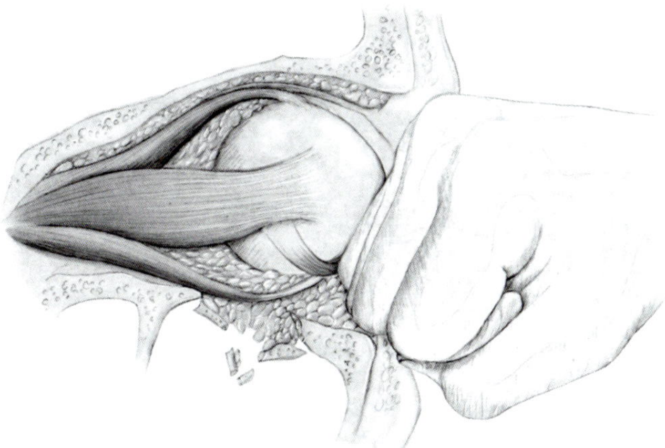

10-56 Direct blow to the base of the orbit.

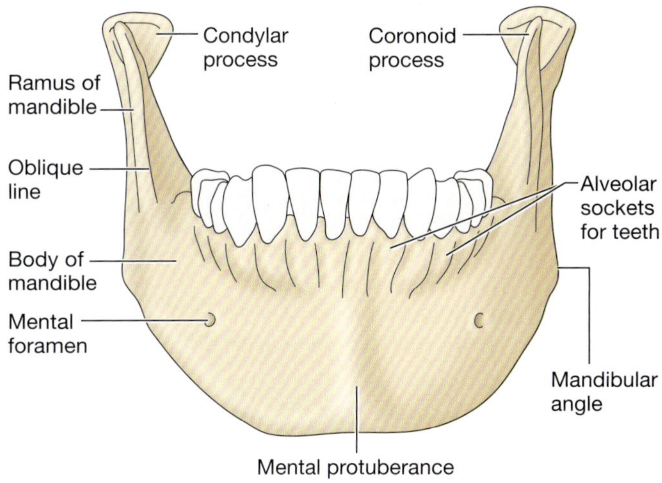

10-57 Frontal view of mandible.

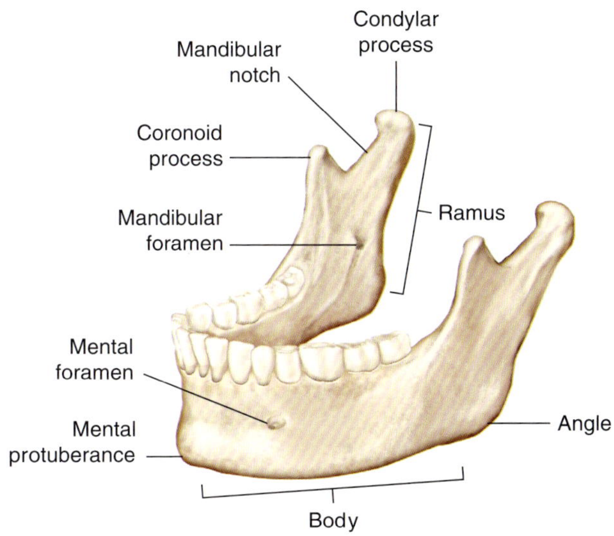

10-58 Anterolateral view of mandible.

to as the sphenoid strut. The superior orbital fissure is a triangular opening between the greater and lesser wings of the sphenoid. The superior orbital fissure may be visible on skull radiographs if the petrous pyramids are not filling the orbits to superimpose this fissure. The inferior orbital fissure, also triangular, is positioned between the sphenoid bone and the maxilla (Fig. 10-55).

Mandible

The mandible is the only facial bone with movement. The mandible is shaped like a "U." Anteriorly, the right and left halves of the mandible fuse at the mandibular symphysis, in the region of the mentum. Located lateral to the mandibular symphysis, on each side, is a small mental foramen to provide for nerve passageway (Fig. 10-57).

The body of the mandible travels posteriorly to the mandibular angle. At the point of the angle or gonion, the ramus travels superiorly. The ramus ends in the mandibular notch that gives rise to two processes. The coronoid process is located anteriorly to the mandibular notch and the condyloid process posteriorly (Fig. 10-58). The condylar head articulates with the temporomandibular fossa to form the TMJ (Fig. 10-59). This

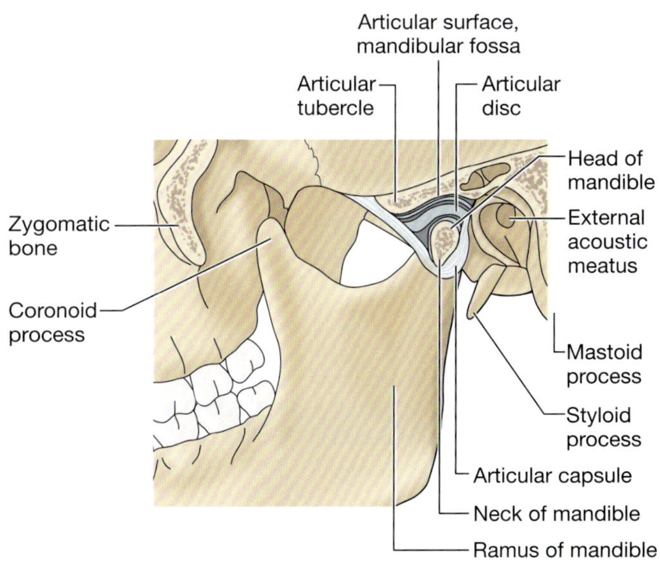

10-59 Temporomandibular joint.

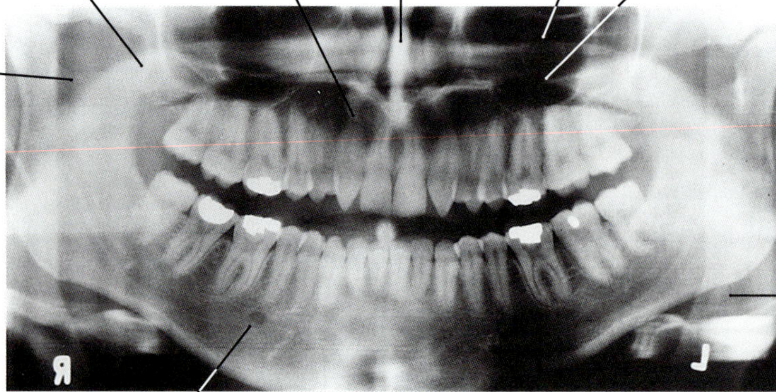

10-60 Panoramic view of the maxilla and mandible.

joint must be included in all mandible images. Just distal to the condylar head is the narrowed region of the neck. Finally, similarly to the maxilla, the mandible possesses alveolar processes to support the roots of the lower teeth (Figs. 10-57 and 10-60).

KEY SUMMATION POINTS OF ANATOMY

- Sutures are considered fibrous joints that are immovable or synarthrodial in their movement in the adult patient.
- The TMJ is the only synovial joint within the skull. The joint has a gliding or bicondylar type movement (Table 10-1).
- The vertex is the most superior point of the skull and must be visualized on all *skull* images.
- The widest portion of the skull exists between the two parietal eminences. The parietal bones form the superior and lateral portions of the skull.
- The frontal bone contributes to the formation of the superior orbits and the forehead.
- The occipital bone forms the posterior, inferior portion of the skull.
- The sphenoid is the anchor bone for all other cranial bones to articulate with.
- The sphenoid bone contains a large number of foramina and fissures.
- The petrous pyramids contain and protect the organs of the inner ear.
- The petrous pyramids are the densest portion of the skull making them identifiable on images. The petrous pyramids provide a means to evaluate images for proper positioning. The petrous ridge is the superior most point of the petrous pyramids and corresponds to the level of the TEA.
- The perpendicular plate of the ethmoid forms the majority of the bony nasal septum. The perpendicular plate of the ethmoid and the vomer articulate to form the entire bony nasal septum.
- The orbital base sits most anteriorly, while the apex sits posteriorly. The optic foramen enters through the apex of the orbit.
- The base of the orbit is composed of the maxilla, frontal, and zygoma. A blowout fracture occurs from direct force to the orbital base causing pressure on the floor of the orbit. A blowout fracture will show a communication between the orbit and the maxillary sinus.
- A tripod fracture is a result of the zygoma breaking free of its three points of articulation: the frontal bone, the maxilla, and the zygomatic arch.
- The superior and middle nasal conchae are part of the ethmoid bone. The inferior nasal conchae are facial bones. Nasal conchae is responsible for filtering and warming air before the air enters into the nasopharynx.
- The majority of the hard palate (roof the mouth) is formed when right and left palatine processes of the maxilla fuse together. Failure of fusion of the palatine processes results in a cleft palate. The most posterior portion of the hard palate is formed by the horizontal portions of the right and left palatine bones.
- The maxillary sinuses are the only present cavity at birth. The maxillary sinuses sit within the body of the maxilla and are the largest sinus cavity (Figs. 10-61 and 10-62).
- The ethmoid sinuses are contained within the lateral masses of the ethmoid bone and sit together as a collection of three sets that communicate: anterior, middle, and posterior (Figs. 10-61 and 10-62).
- The frontal sinuses sit between the inner and outer skull table directly posterior to the glabella (Figs. 10-61 and 10-62).
- The body of the sphenoid, just below the sella turcica, contains the sphenoid sinuses (Figs. 10-61 to 10-63).

10-1 Joints of the Skull

Joint	Classification	General Movement	Specific Movement
Skull sutures (adult)	Fibrous	Synarthrodial	–
Temporomandibular joints	Synovial	Diarthrodial	Bicondylar
Alveolar processes	Fibrous	Synarthrodial	–

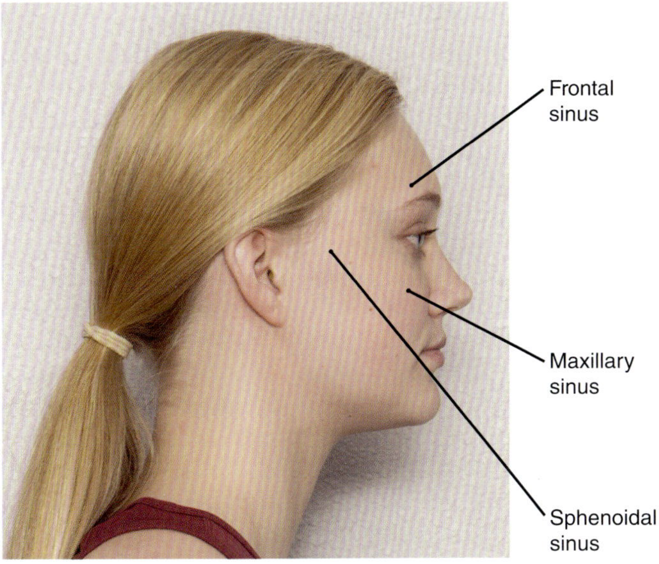

10-61 Sinus placement from lateral perspective.

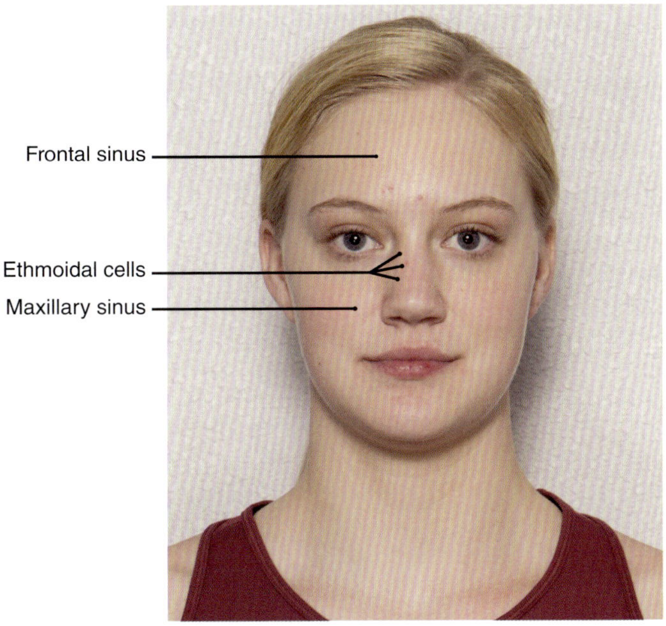

10-62 Sinus placement from frontal perspective.

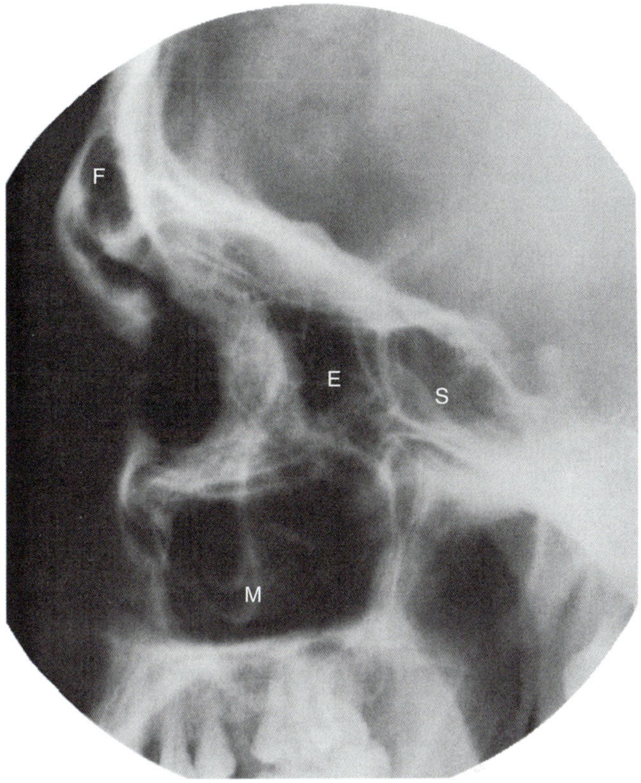

10-63 Lateral sinuses. M, maxillary sinus; F, frontal sinus; E, ethmoid sinus; S, sphenoid sinus.

POSITIONING CONSIDERATIONS

Patient Part Size and Suggested IR Orientation

Imaging the head most commonly includes imaging a part size over 10 cm in thickness, therefore requiring grid imaging. Imaging smaller parts such as nasal bones or pediatric patients may be imaged with nongrid settings.

Centering and Collimation

The central ray should be directed to the proper and suggested centering locations. With proper centering, four-sided collimation can be applied to allow radiation safety practices and ensure all essential anatomy is included.

Breathing Instructions

Specific breathing instructions for all headwork will be to suspend respiration to prevent motion on the image.

Identification between Nontrauma Versus Trauma Situations

Patients with head trauma must be carefully monitored and the technologist must pay special attention to any change in their level of consciousness while in the imaging department. Patients may have spinal precautions as well; therefore, the technologist must use safe approaches during image acquisition. Patients with head trauma will undergo a more basic approach to imaging if ordered, but more commonly CT will allow for a quicker, detailed overall evaluation of head and brain structures. However, it is possible that two-view trauma projections could precede CT imaging.

TECHNICAL CONSIDERATIONS

Setting a Manual Technique

Manual technique is defined when the radiographer sets the kVp and mAs values. Manual techniques are typically set for head imaging, but automatic exposure cells (AEC) could be considered for certain projections.

Tabletop imaging requires the use of manual technique. Kilovoltage is set to penetrate the part thickness and affects the scale of contrast seen on the image. A small focal spot setting is encouraged with skull imaging in an effort to improve the detail of the small bones.

The exposure time should be set as short as possible to minimize any possibility of motion. Patients of any age will struggle to hold still for necessary projections, but especially geriatric and pediatric patients. The technologist should consider measures to properly immobilize a patient if necessary. The best way to reduce the possibility of voluntary patient motion is to give a clear explanation and instructions to the patient.

Source-to-Image Distance

A 40" source-to-image distance (SID) is used for the majority of head imaging. A 72" SID is only necessary for situations where increased object-to-image distance is increased in nonroutine positioning (Fig. 10-64).

Exposure Index

With each exposure, the digital system will produce a numerical value, taking into account the kVp, mAs, part centering, anatomy, and collimation. The exposure index is typically a range established by the manufacturer and aids the technologist in determining if the image was acquired with proper exposure. In instances in which insufficient radiation has reached the image receptors, indicated by the exposure index, the technologist must repeat the image, as often the image will appear grainy or mottled. The goal of the repeat image is to appropriately increase the exposure to produce a diagnostic quality image when displayed on the radiologist's monitor. In instances in which overexposure is numerically indicated, the image may not need to be reacquired to achieve the image within range, as this will again expose the patient to additional and unnecessary radiation in this case. However, the technologist should take note of the lowered technical settings to adjust accordingly for future patient exposures. With digital imaging, the wider latitude of systems lessens the exact science of setting kVp and mAs for each exposure. With the flexibility these wider latitude systems offer, technologists should strive to apply appropriate combinations of technical settings necessary to acquire diagnostic images within acceptable ranges to avoid unnecessary radiation exposure to patients.

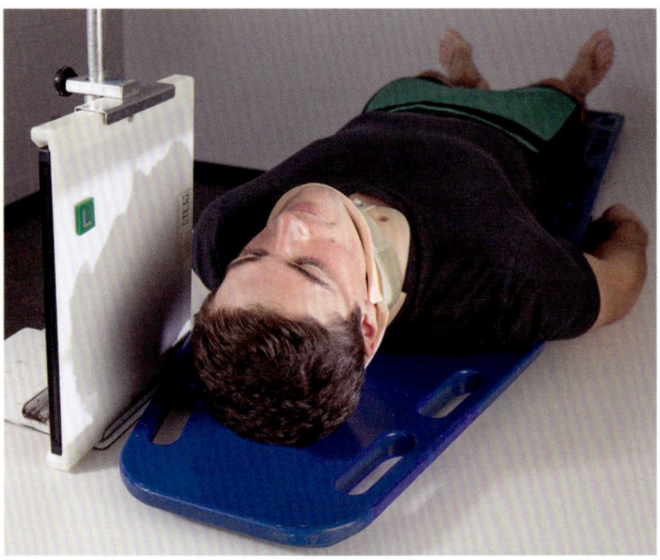

10-64 Increased object-to-image distance calls for an increased SID.

Image Postprocessing

There are a variety of postprocessing options that are available on digital workstations. These options range from windowing, smoothing, subtraction, edge enhancement, black bordering, and annotation. Technologists must realize that the monitor resolution at their workstation will be lower compared to the radiologist's high-resolution monitor for interpretation. Additionally, if a technologist postprocesses an image and pushes it over to the department picture archiving and communications systems (PACS) system, this will prevent the radiologist from being able to make any image adjustments for their purpose of interpretation. Therefore, postprocessing by the technologist is not advised. The most common tool of postprocessing the technologist may utilize is the annotation function. The annotation function should be utilized to add only additional information useful to document and should not replace the use of standardized minimum Right and Left markers that should be positioned within the collimated exposure field. Digital annotations will not uphold in legal litigation cases of malpractice.

Shielding

Acceptable shielding practices include a lap shield at minimum, but a full lead shield could also be considered. With restricted beam use, a thyroid shield is not necessary, and certainly cannot be utilized in instances, where it may superimpose essential anatomy.

Marking the Image

When marking the AP, PA, or axial projections of the head, the anatomic right or left marker should be placed within the collimated exposure field on the corresponding side (Fig. 10-65).

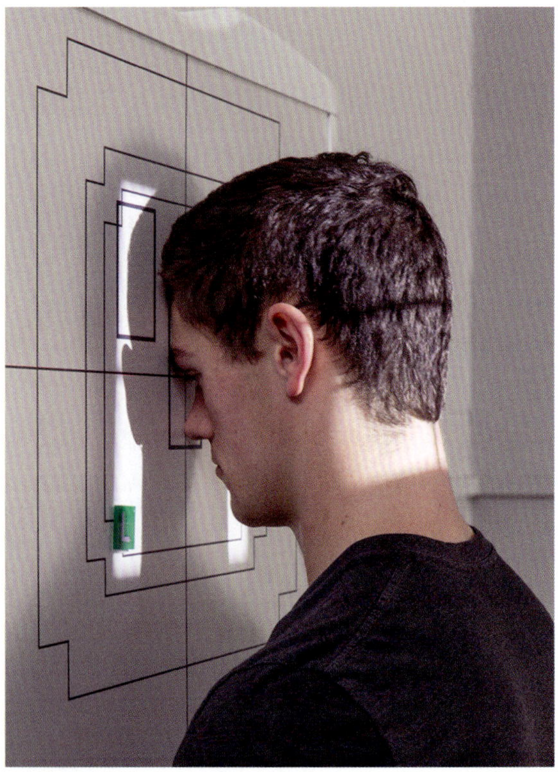

10-65 Proper marking for PA projection.

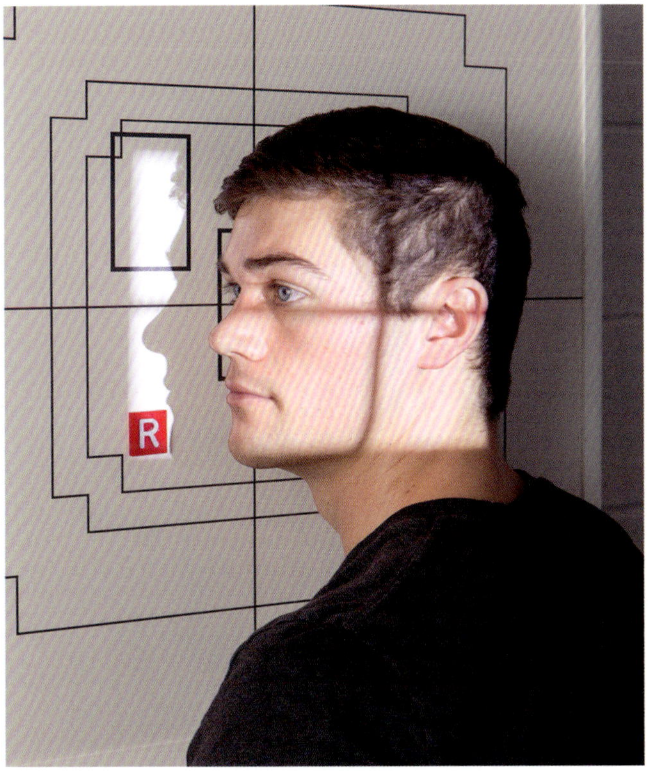

10-66 Proper marking for lateral projection.

When marking the lateral position, the anatomic marker of the side of the head closest to the IR is placed along the anterior surface of the part or "in front" of the part and within the collimated exposure field (Fig. 10-66).

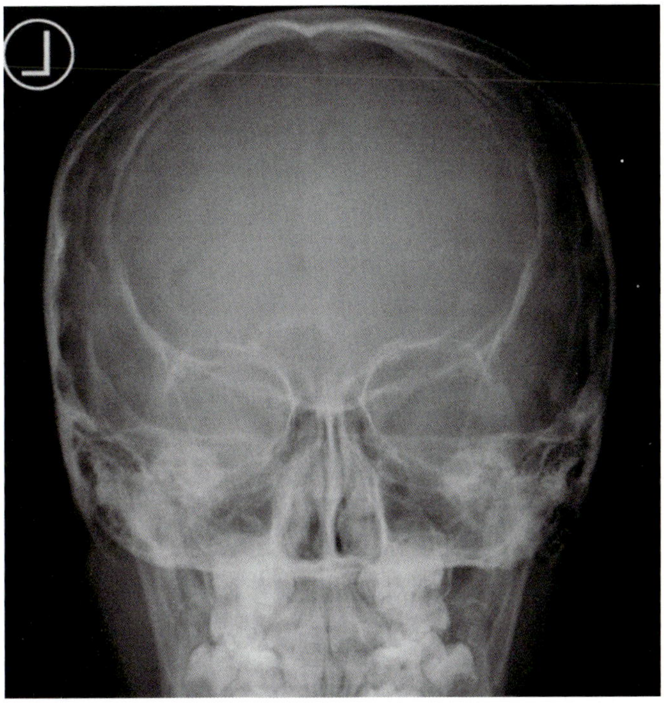

10-68 Incorrect image display for PA projection.

Viewing the Image

When viewing the images of the head, the image is displayed to represent anatomic position. The images are displayed opposite of the viewer facing it, as though the image is in anatomic position. Therefore, in these cases, the side of the image marked "Right," or "Left" is opposite of the viewer's right or left (Figs. 10-67 to 10-69).

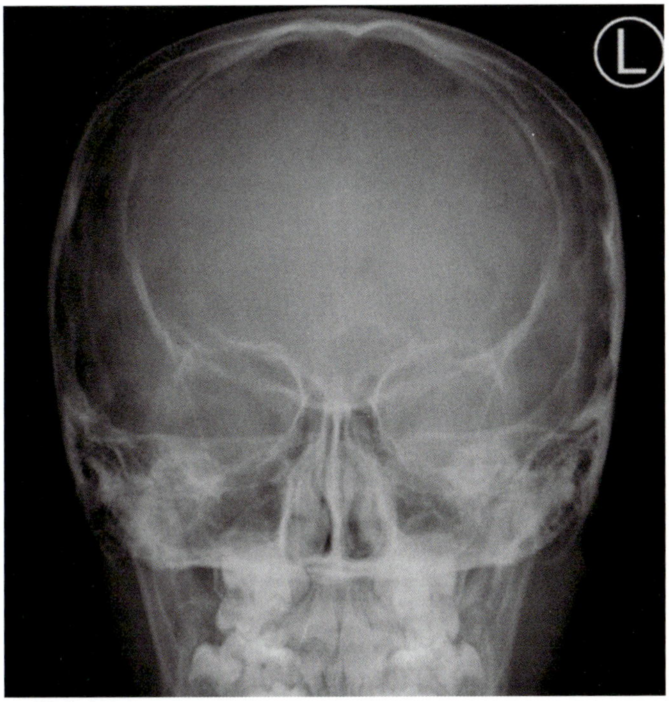

10-67 Correct image display for PA projection.

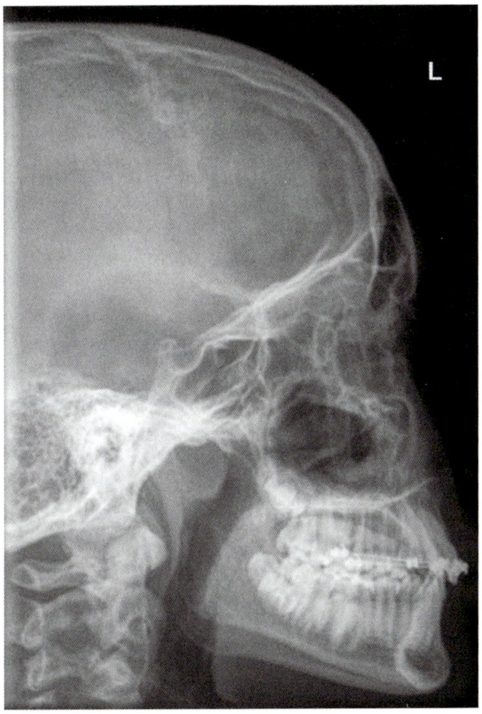

10-69 Correct image display for Lateral projection.

Headwork

- Projection: PA
- PA is part of numerous exam protocols as outlined in Tables 10-2(skull), 10-6(orbits), and 10-7(mandible)

Technical Considerations
- kVp 70–80
- mAs set manually or AEC center cell
- 40" SID

Exposure Field Size
- 10 × 12 lengthwise

Patient Position (Fig. 10-70)
- Seated on a stool or chair at the upright Bucky
- Encourage good patient posture
- Position the patient's forehead and nose in contact with the upright Bucky and adjust the flexion or extension of the neck until the OML is perpendicular to the IR
- Stand behind the patient and ensure the MSP is perpendicular to the IR

Centering
- The centering will be directed according to the part imaged. Set the upright Bucky to the level of the centering location and then adjust the height of the tube to align with the upright Bucky
  - *Skull:* The central ray is set to exit the glabella (Figs. 10-71, 10-73, and 10-74)
  - *Mandible:* The central ray is set to exit the junction of the lips (Figs. 10-72, 10-75, and 10-76)
  - *Orbits:* The central ray is set to exit the nasion

Marking of IR
- Anatomic side marker R or L placed furthest from the patient's midline to the corresponding side

Breathing
- Suspend respiration and instruct the patient to hold still
- Ensure you watch the patient the entire time while walking away to make the exposure

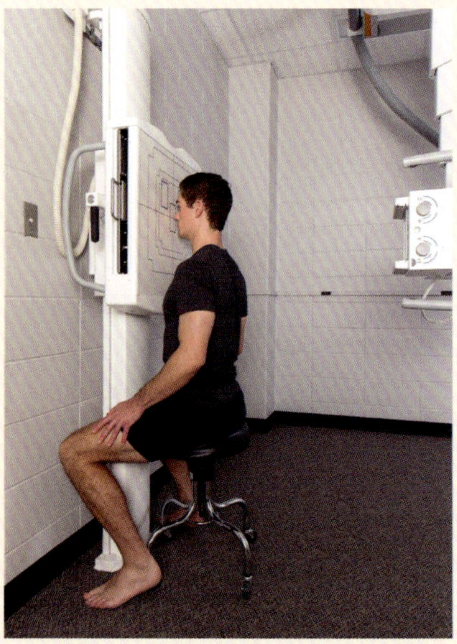

10-70 Upright positioning with good posture.

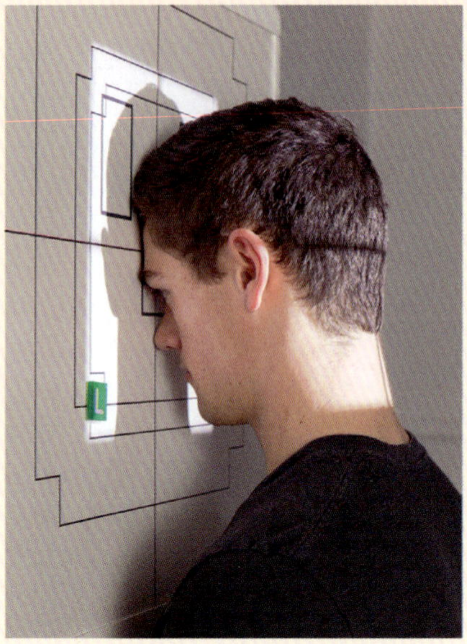

10-71 PA skull.

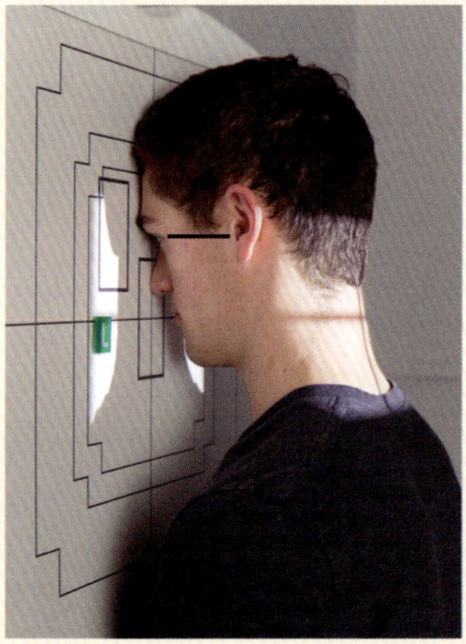

10-72 PA mandible.

(continued)

Headwork (*Continued*)

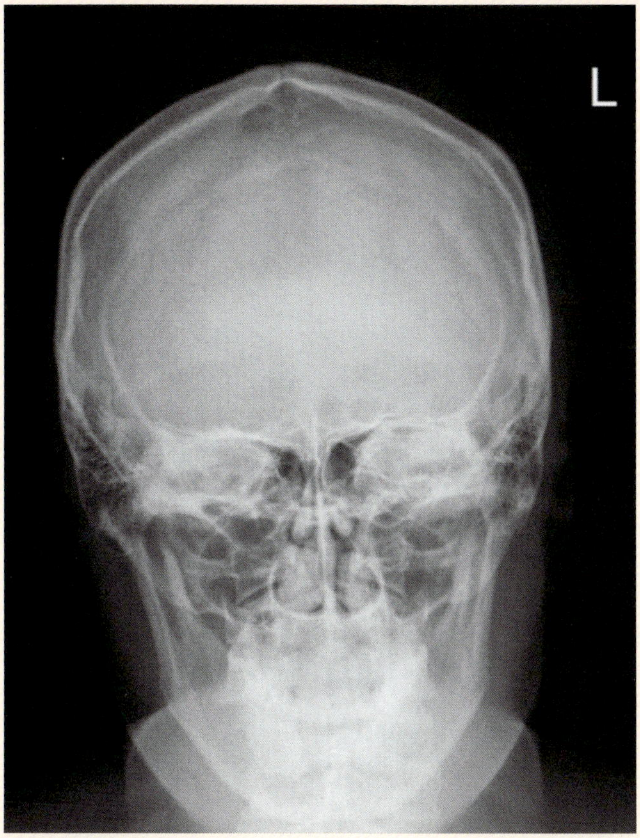

10-73 PA skull.

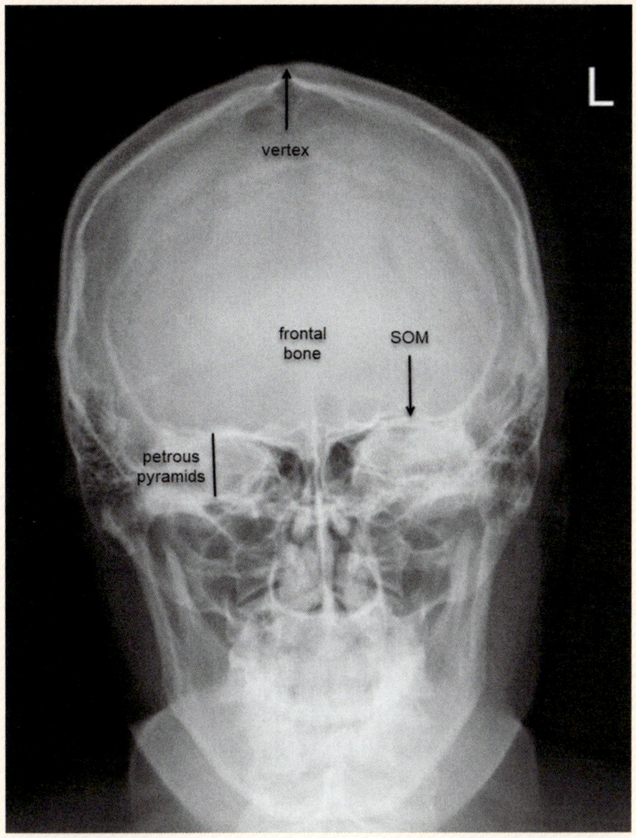

10-74 PA skull.

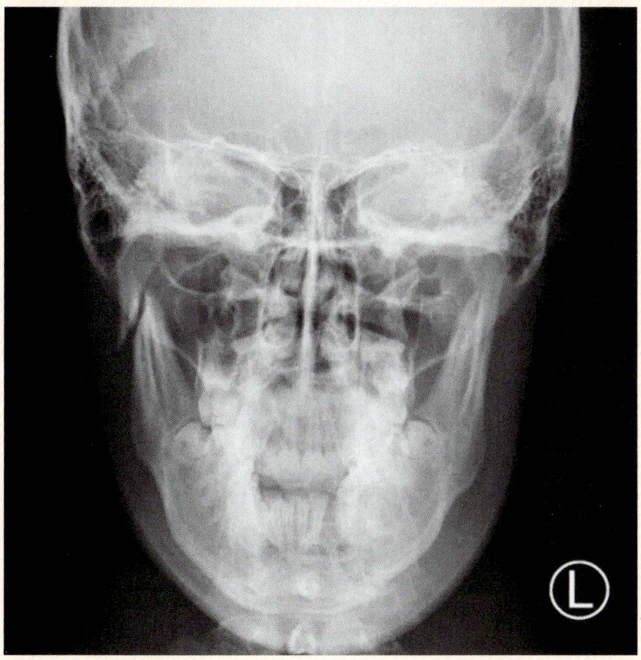

10-75 PA mandible.

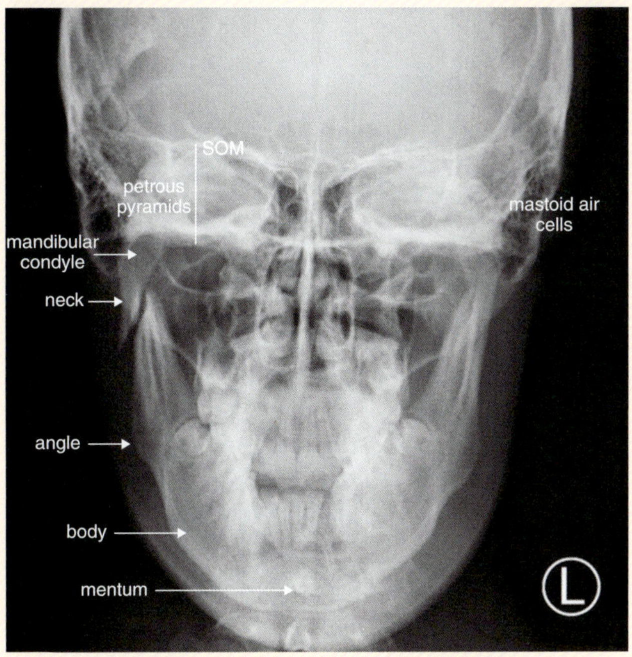

10-76 PA mandible.

IMAGE CRITIQUE

- Proper positioning criteria for the PA:
  - The height of the petrous pyramids fills the orbits entirely. The petrous ridge will correspond to the SOM. The height placement of the petrous pyramids is determined by the OML placement. If the petrous ridge (superior most point of the petrous pyramids) lies above the SOM, the patient's chin was depressed too much (Fig. 10-77). If the petrous pyramids fill the orbits less than full, the patient did not have the chin depressed enough (Fig. 10-78)

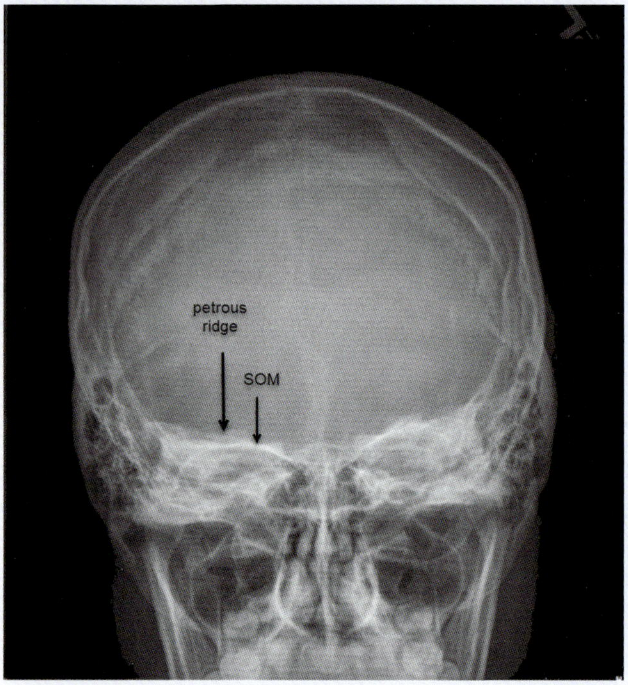

10-77 PA with petrous pyramids to high.

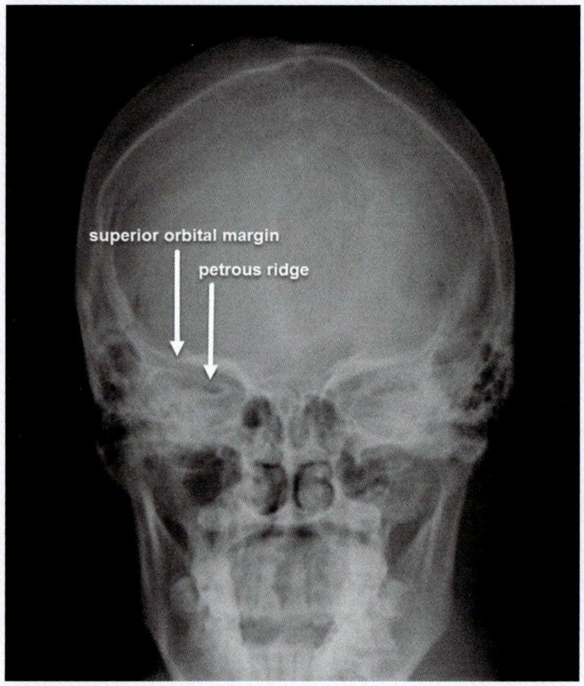

10-78 PA with petrous pyramids to low.

  - The petrous pyramids are symmetrical in comparison of their height. If one petrous pyramid is higher than the opposite, or one SOM is higher than the opposite, this indicates the patient's vertex was tilted to either the right or left side. If the patient's head is tilted to the right, the left SOM or petrous pyramid will appear higher than the right (Fig. 10-79)
  - Equal distance between the orbital oblique line or lateral orbital margin to the lateral margin of the skull. Unequal distance indicates rotation of the skull indicating the MSP was not perpendicular to the IR. Identifying the side of less distance between the orbital oblique line and the lateral margin of the skull indicates the side the face is rotated toward (Fig. 10-80)
- Anatomy of interest is what is positioned closest to the IR
  - PA skull: Frontal bone. Vertex must be included
  - PA mandible: Mentum and portions of the mandibular body
- Properly centered with attempted four-sided collimation

(continued)

IMAGE CRITIQUE *(Continued)*

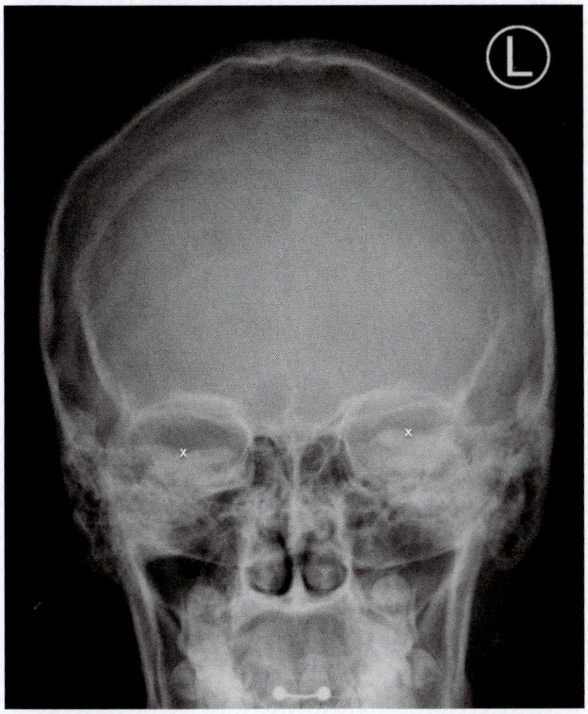

10-79 PA with tilt.

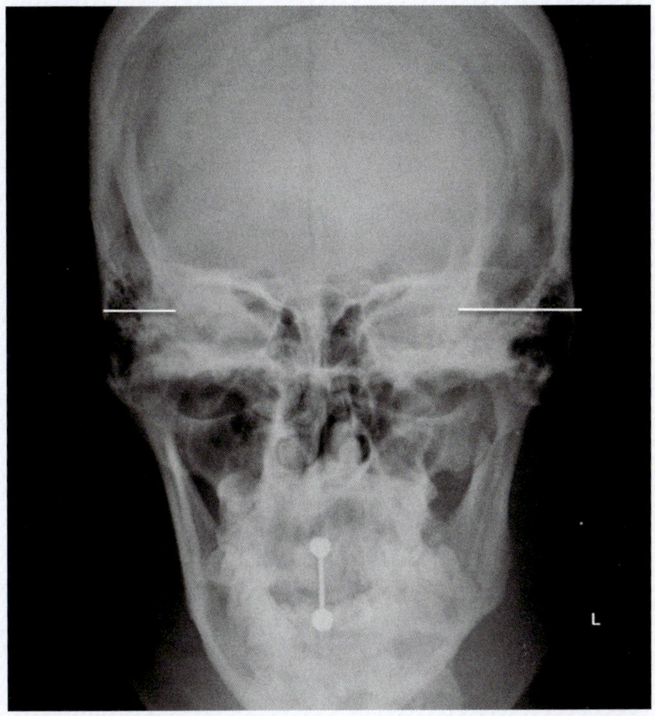

10-80 PA with rotation.

POSITION VARIATION AP (FIG. 10-81)

If PA projection is not possible, the AP projection could be substituted. This would be less preferred due to the magnification of the anatomy of most interest. The patient is positioned with the OML perpendicular to the IR or the tube angled caudally (1°–15°) to match the OML. The central ray will enter the glabella. Evaluation criteria are the same as it is for PA projection. Orbit magnification will aid in distinguishing between the AP and the PA projection.

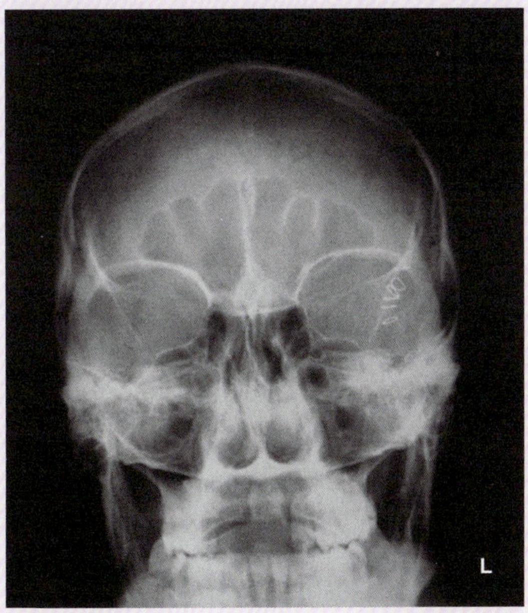

10-81 AP skull.

Headwork

- Projection: AP Axial
- Method: Towne method
- AP Axial is part of numerous exam protocols as outlined in Tables 10-2 (skull), 10-7 (mandible), 10-8 (zygomatic arches), 10-9 (TMJs)

Technical Considerations

- kVp 65–80 (based on exam ordered)
- mAs set manually or AEC center cell
- 40" SID

Exposure Field Size

- 10 × 12 lengthwise

Patient Position (Figs. 10-82 and 10-83)

- Seated on a stool or chair at the upright Bucky
- Encourage good patient posture
- Patient will face the tube
- Position the patient's posterior surface of the head in contact with the upright Bucky
- While trying to have the patient keep the back of their head in contact with the Bucky, depress the patient's chin until OML or IOML is perpendicular to the IR
- Stand in front of the patient and ensure the MSP is perpendicular to the IR

Centering

- The tube will be angled 30° caudal if OML was aligned perpendicular to the IR
- The tube will be angled at 37° caudal if IOML was aligned perpendicular to the IR (Remember the 7° difference that exists between OML and IOML)
- The centering will be directed according to the part imaged
  - *Skull:* The central ray is set to enter approximately the hairline and exiting approximately the inion. Ensure centering includes the vertex of the skull (Figs. 10-84, 10-88, and 10-89)
  - *Mandible:* The central ray is set to enter the nasion or slightly below and ensure the mandibular mentum is included (Figs. 10-85, 10-90, and 10-91)
  - *Zygomatic Arches:* The central ray is set to enter 1" superior to the glabella. Kilovoltage is decreased to 60–70 with a manual mAs set to help avoid overpenetration of the thin zygomatic arches. This axial will produce a view of bilateral arches (Fig. 10-86)
  - *TMJs:* The Towne method will be altered by increasing the tube angle by an additional 5° caudal. If OML is perpendicular, a 35° caudal angle is applied, and if IOML is perpendicular, a 42° caudal tube angle is applied. The central ray is set to enter 1" superior to the glabella. Bilateral TMJs will be acquired with the mouth in closed position (Fig. 10-87)

Marking of IR

- Anatomic side markers R or L placed furthest from the patient's midline to the corresponding side

Breathing

- Suspend respiration and instruct the patient to hold still
- Ensure you watch the patient the entire time while walking away to make the exposure

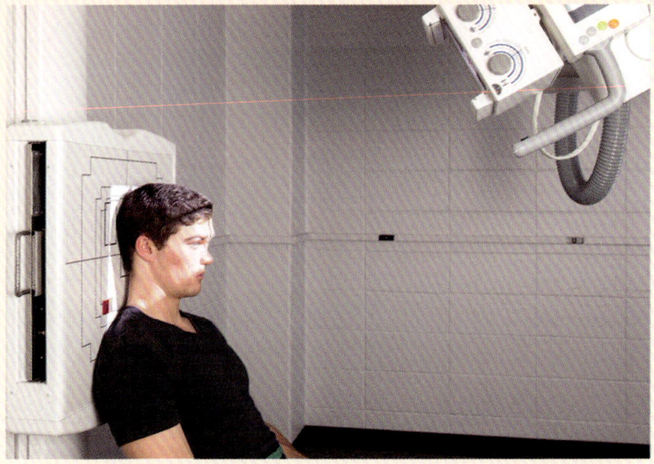

10-82 AP Axial Towne method.

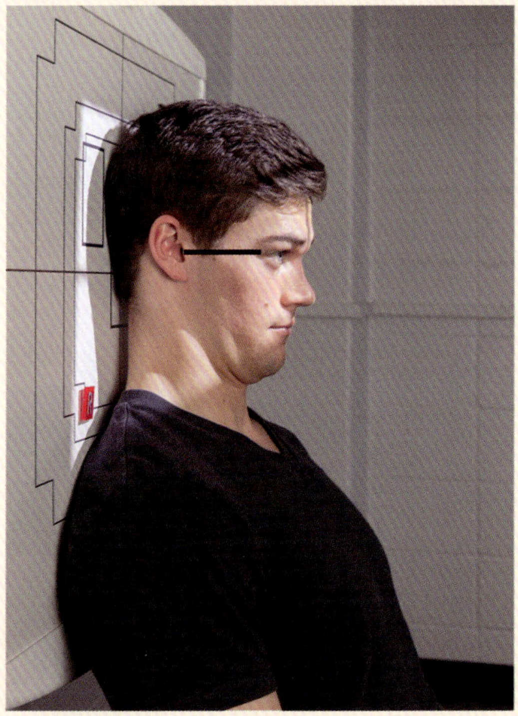

10-83 AP Axial Towne method with OML perpendicular.

(continued)

Headwork (*Continued*)

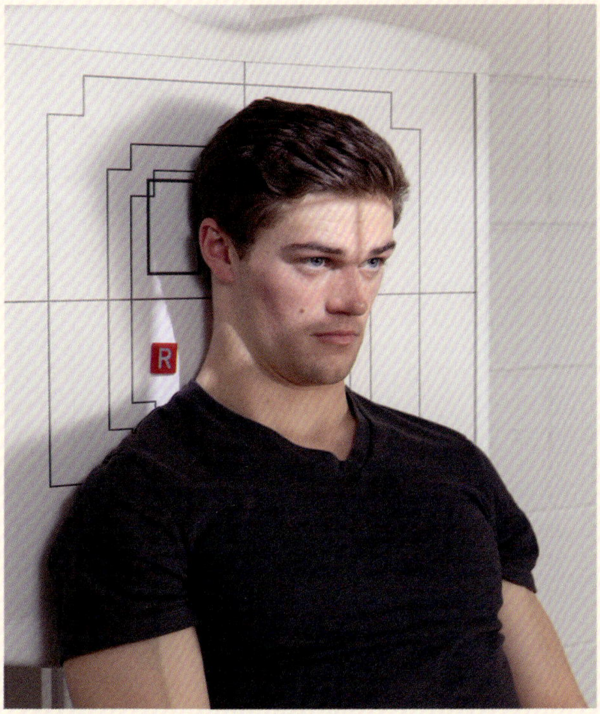

10-84 AP Axial Towne method skull.

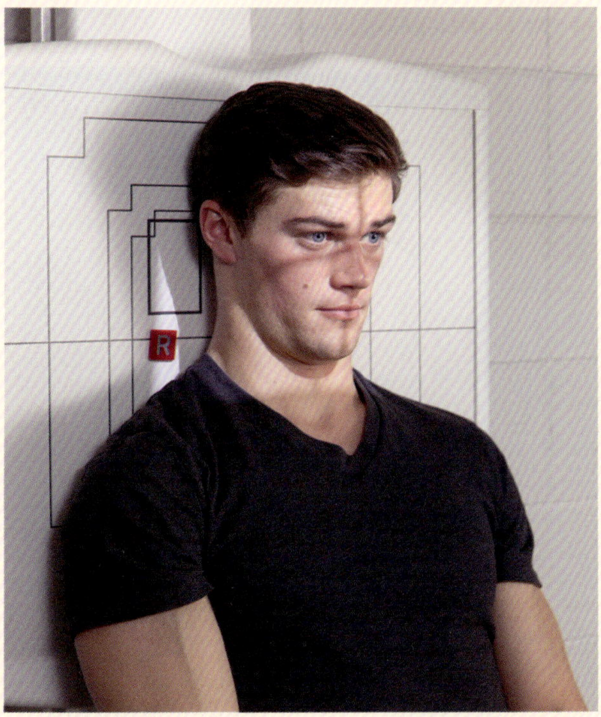

10-85 AP Axial Towne method mandible.

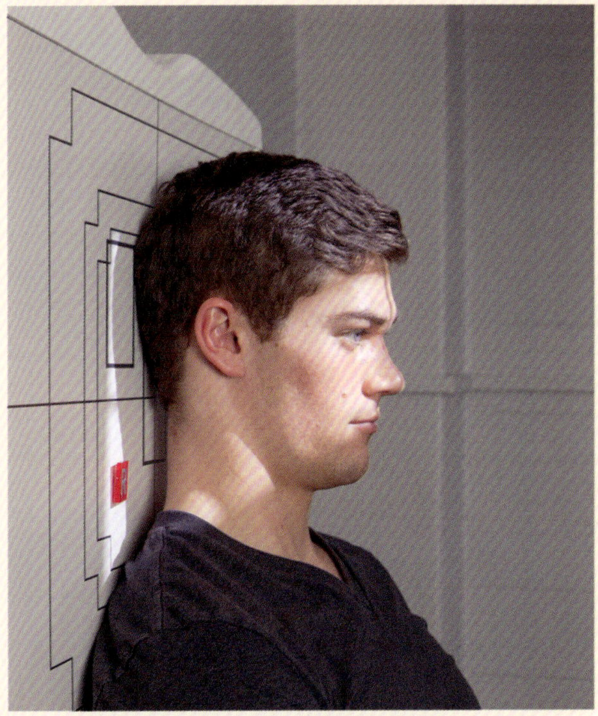

10-86 AP Axial Towne method zygomatic arches.

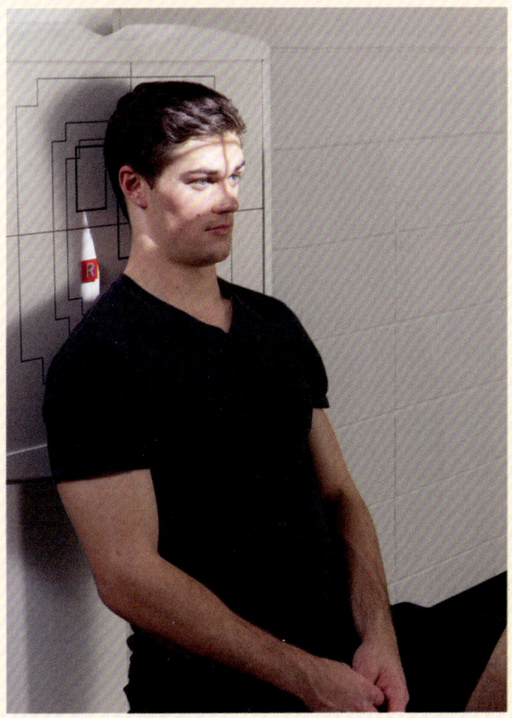

10-87 AP Axial modified Towne method for TMJs.

(*continued*)

POSITION VARIATION TRAUMA AP AXIAL

If an AP Axial is requested in a trauma circumstance, the technologist must apply an additional 30° caudal to the tube angle that was applied to the trauma AP. For instance, if an 8° caudal tube angle was applied to the trauma AP to match up to the OML, 30 additional degrees are applied for a total of 38° for the AP Axial. The caudal tube angle should not exceed 45° due to the extreme distortion of the anatomy. Central ray still enters approximately the hairline and must ensure the vertex is included.

POSITION VARIATION PA AXIAL—HAAS METHOD

If AP Axial projection is not possible for the skull (perhaps only considered in a case of extreme patient condition of kyphosis), the PA Axial projection could be substituted, although it is less desired due to the magnification of the anatomy of interest. The patient is positioned with the OML perpendicular to the IR and the tube angled 25° cephalic to enter the inion and exit approximately at the hairline. The established image criteria as for the AP Axial skull apply in terms of the dorsum sella placement and the vertex inclusion. The tube angle will aid in the elongation of the occipital bone (Fig. 10-94).

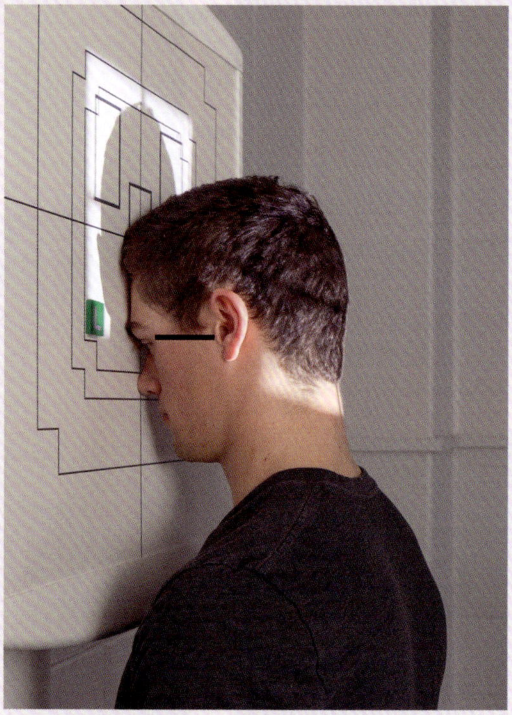

10-94 PA Axial Haas method.

Headwork

- Projection: Lateral
- Lateral is part of numerous exam protocols as outlined in Tables 10-2 (skull), 10-3 (sinuses), 10-4 (nasal bones), 10-5 (facial bones), 10-6 (orbits), and 10-9 (TMJs)

Technical Considerations

- kVp 65–75 (based on exam ordered)
- mAs set manually or AEC center cell
- 40" SID

Exposure Field Size

- 10 × 12 crosswise

Patient Position

- Seated on a stool or chair at the upright Bucky
- Encourage good patient posture
- Patient will face the upright Bucky and then adjusted into a slight anterior oblique allowing the lateral side of the head closer to the IR. For instance, if the right side of the head is of interest, the patient should be positioned into a right anterior oblique (RAO) position (Fig. 10-95)
- Depress the patient's chin until IOML is parallel to the IR. This helps prevent superimposition of the mandibular rami or base of the skull on the cervical spine
- Adjust the vertex of the skull (tilt), until the IPL is perpendicular to the IR (Fig. 10-96)
- Evaluate the MSP and ensure is parallel with the IR (rotation) (Fig. 10-96)

Centering

- The centering will be directed according to the part imaged
  - *Skull:* The central ray set to superior to 1"–2" superior to the EAM. Ensure centering includes the vertex and the base of the skull (Figs. 10-97, 10-104, and 10-105)
  - *Sinuses:* The central ray is set to enter midway between the EAM and the outer canthus (Fig. 10-98)
  - *Facial Bones:* The central ray is set to enter midway between the EAM and the outer canthus (Fig. 10-98)
  - *Orbits:* The central ray is set to exit the outer canthus of the affected side (Fig. 10-99)
  - *Nasal Bones:* The central ray is set to enter ½" inferior to the nasion (Figs. 10-100 and 10-101)
  - *Lateral TMJs:* A true lateral with the need for a 25°–30° caudal tube (*Schuller method*) angle applied set to enter 2" superior to the upside EAM and ½" anterior to upside EAM. Both right and left axiolateral must be acquired for comparison and each side will be acquired with the patient's mouth closed and another with the mouth open. Another variation, the *Modified Law method*, the patient's MSP from a true lateral is rotated 15° toward the plane of the IR. A 15° caudal tube angle is applied with the central ray to enter 2" superior to the upside EAM (Figs. 10-102 and 10-103)

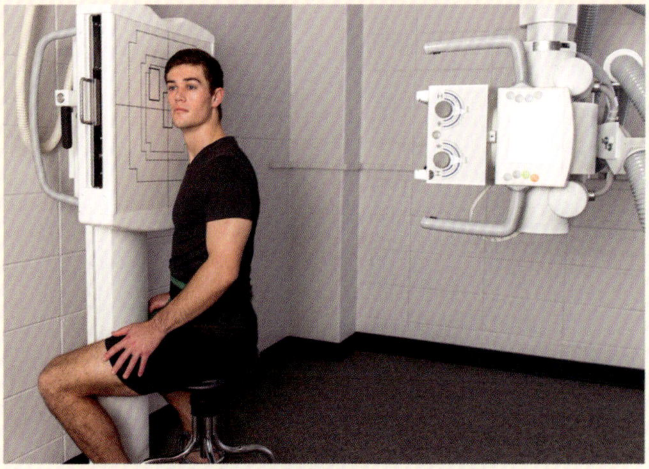

10-95 Lateral headwork position.

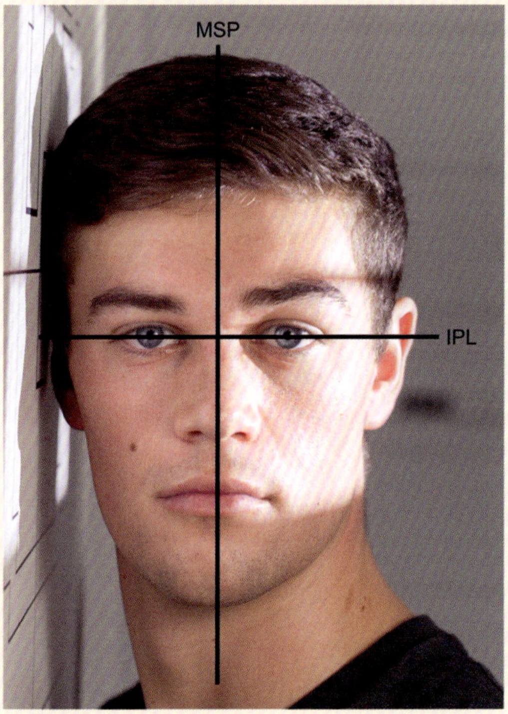

10-96 MSP and IPL for lateral positioning.

(continued)

Headwork (*Continued*)

Marking of IR

- Anatomic side markers R or L placed anterior to the part indicating the side closest to the IR

Breathing

- Suspend respiration and instruct the patient to hold still
- Ensure you watch the patient the entire time while walking away to make the exposure

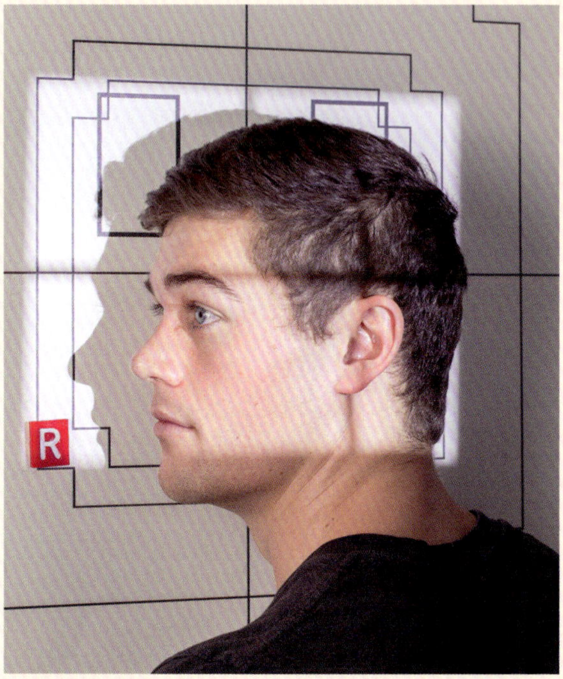

10-97 Lateral skull CR.

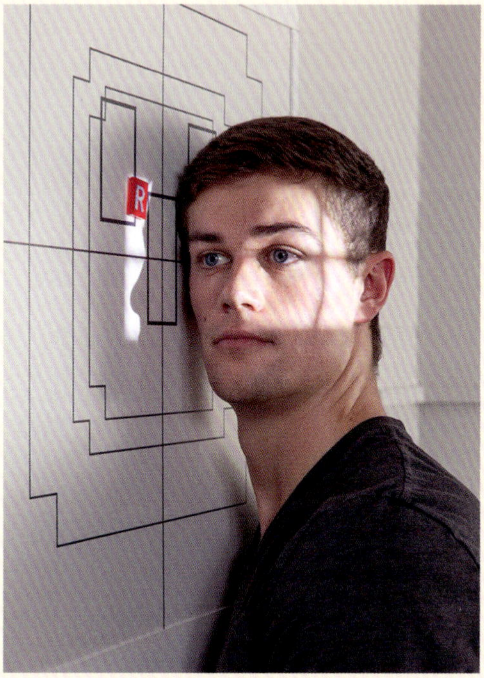

10-99 Lateral orbit CR.

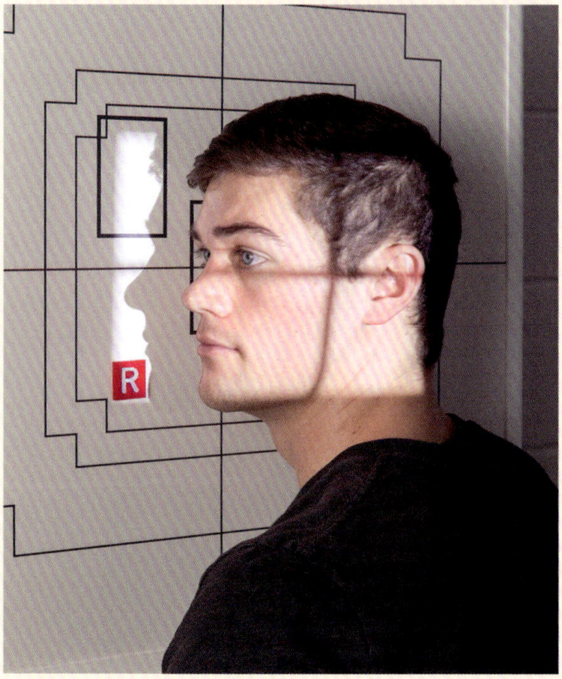

10-98 Lateral sinus and facial bone CR.

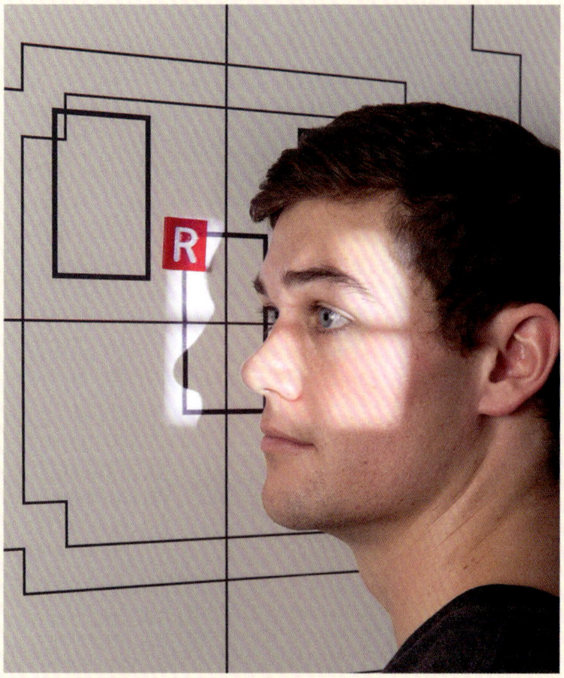

10-100 Lateral nasal bone CR.

(*continued*)

Headwork (*Continued*)

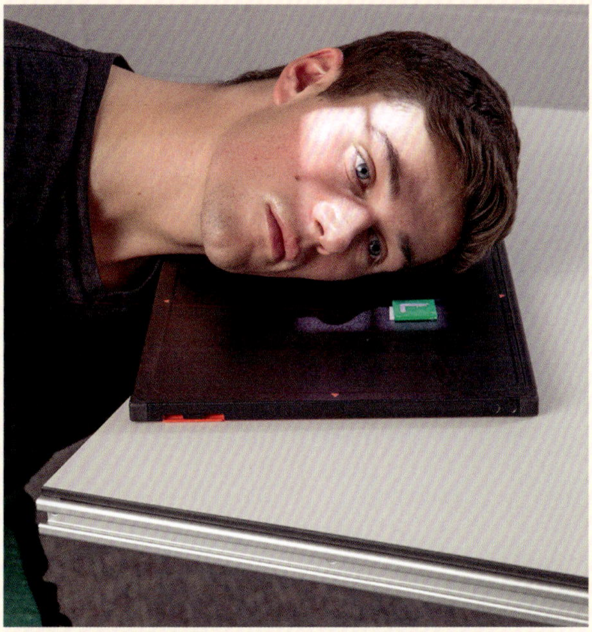

10-101 Lateral nasal bone CR.

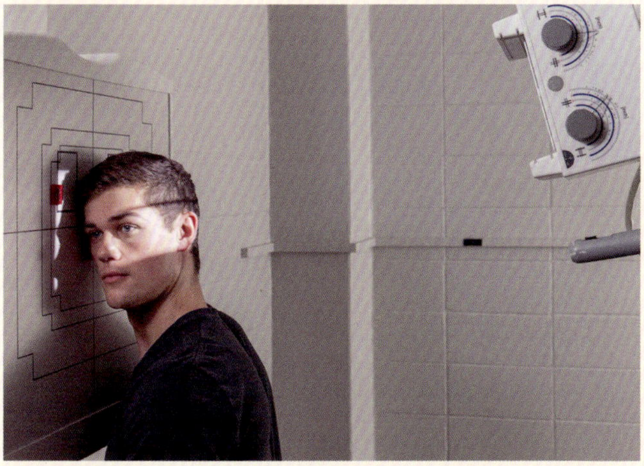

10-102 Lateral TMJ—Schuller method mouth closed.

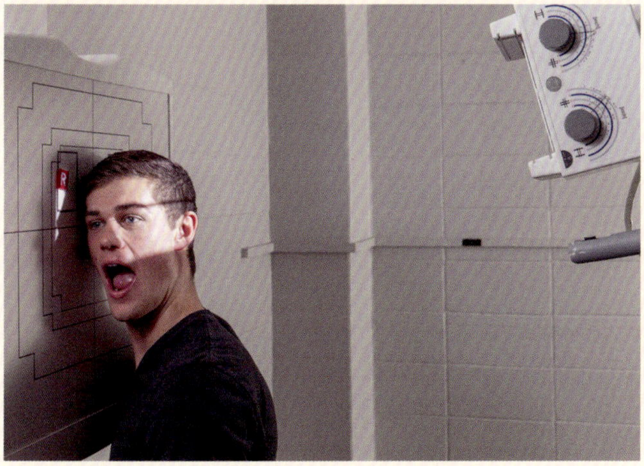

10-103 Lateral TMJ—Schuller method mouth open.

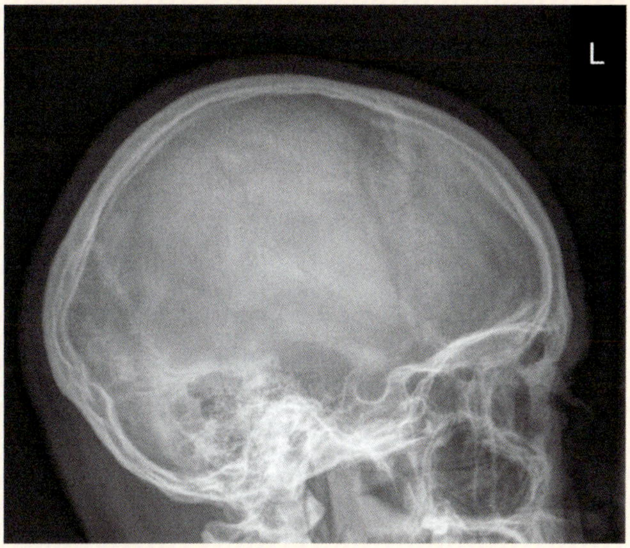

10-104 Lateral skull.

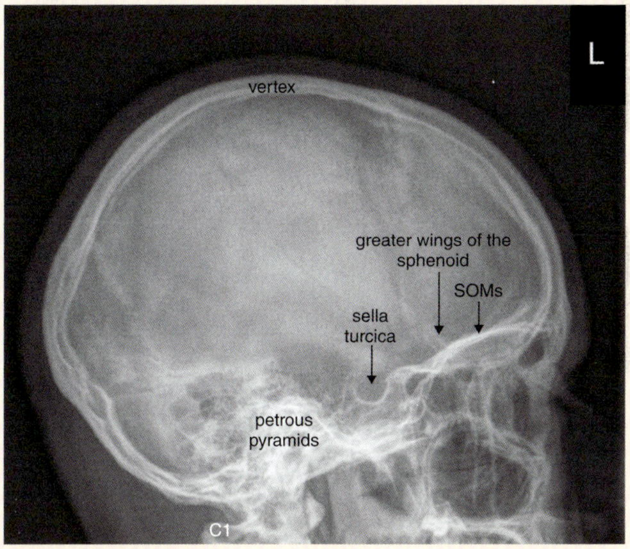

10-105 Lateral skull.

IMAGE CRITIQUE

- Proper positioning criteria for the Lateral:
    - Rotation of the part is determined by evaluating the greater wings of the sphenoid. The greater wings of the sphenoid should be nearly superimposed. Slight separation is not unusual when considering the increased OID of greater wing of the sphenoid furthest from the IR. The mandibular rami would also be an option to evaluate for rotation. Anterior to posterior displacement of the greater wings or the mandibular rami indicates rotation. Rotation results when the MSP was not aligned parallel to the IR (Fig. 10-106)
    - Tilt of the part is determined by evaluating the superior orbital rims. Superior to inferior displacement of the SOMs indicates tilt. Tilt results when IPL was not aligned perpendicular to the IR (Fig. 10-106)

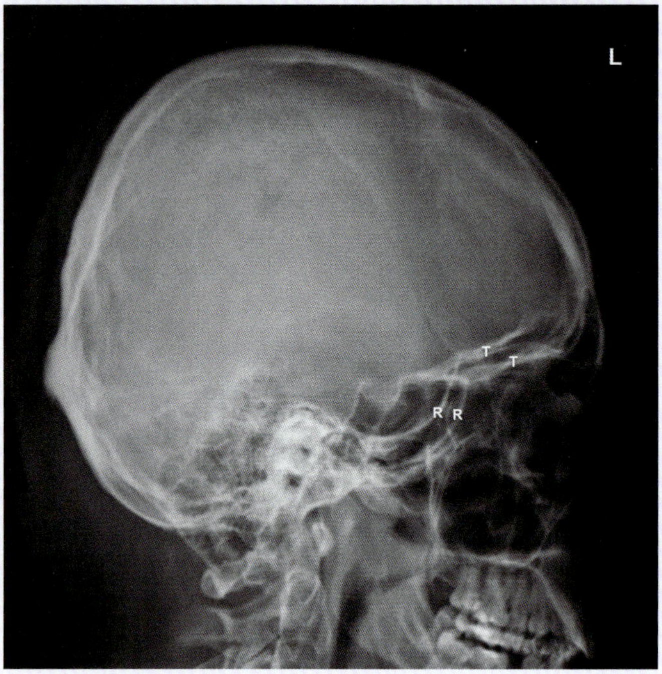

10-106 Lateral skull with rotation and tilt.

(continued)

IMAGE CRITIQUE *(Continued)*

- Anatomy of interest is what is positioned closest to the IR
  - Lateral Skull: Parietal bone closest to the IR (both laterals may be acquired)
  - Lateral Sinuses: All four sinus groups (Fig. 10-107)
  - Lateral Facial Bones: Zygoma of interest and closest to the IR (Fig. 10-108)
  - Lateral Orbits: Anterior to posterior displacement of orbital base

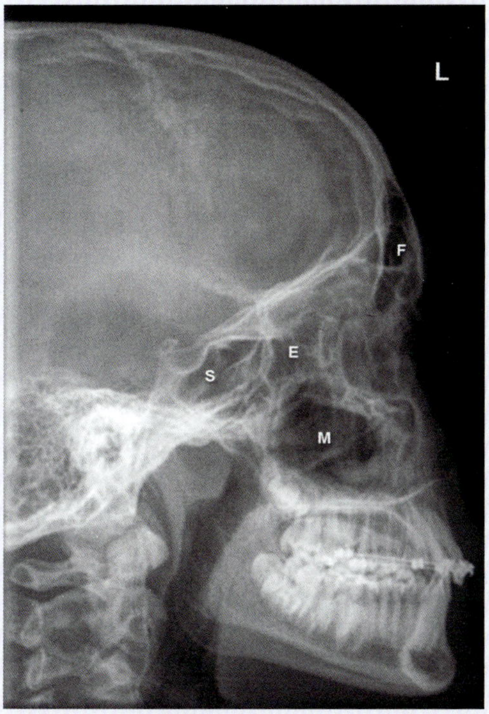

10-107 Lateral sinuses.

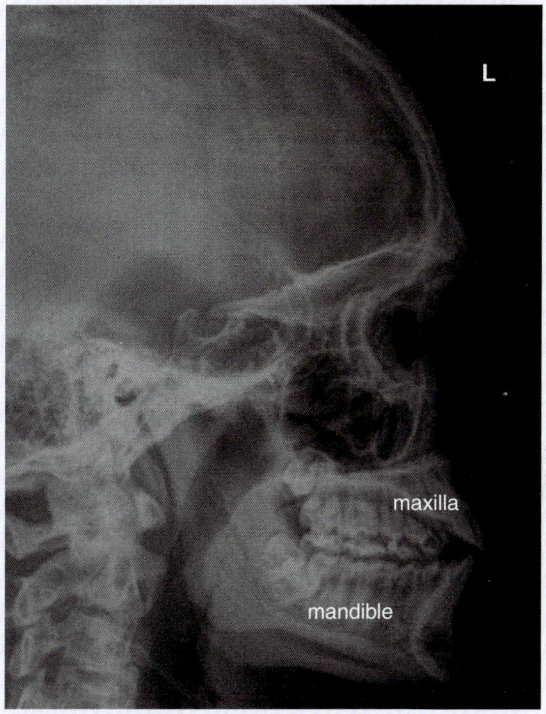

10-108 Lateral facial bones.

  - Lateral Nasal Bones: Nasal bone closest to the IR (both laterals acquired) (Figs. 10-109 and 10-110)
  - Lateral TMJs: Relationship of the mandibular condyle to the temporomandibular fossa (Figs. 10-111 and 10-112)
- Properly centered with attempted four-sided collimation

(continued)

IMAGE CRITIQUE (*Continued*)

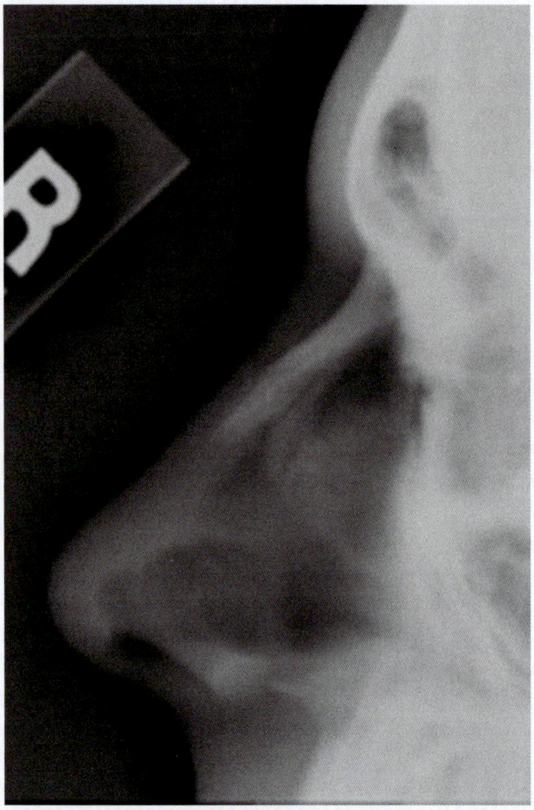

10-109 Lateral nasal bones.

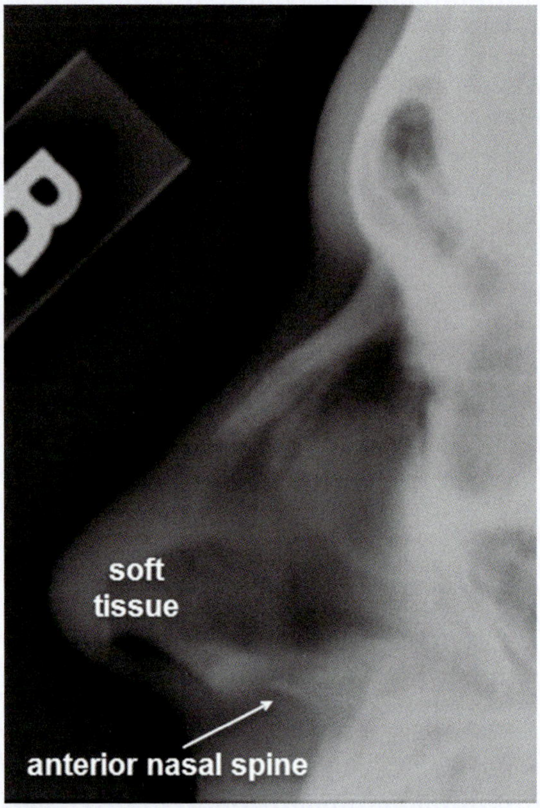

10-110 Lateral nasal bones.

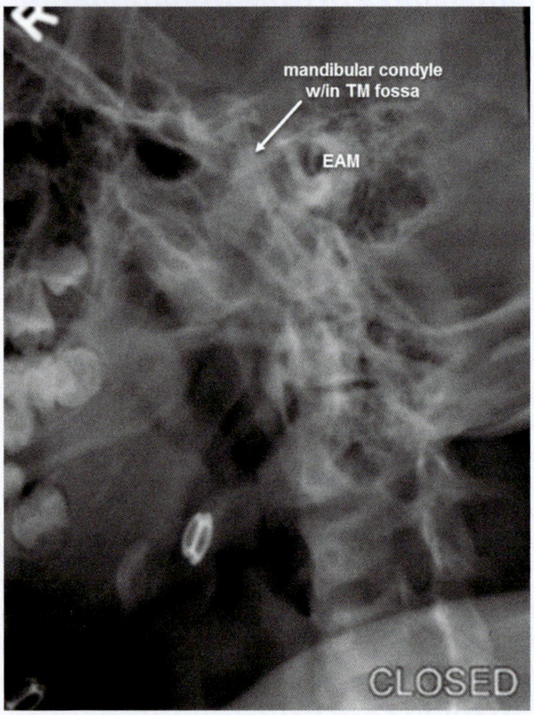

10-111 Lateral TMJ—Schuller method mouth closed.

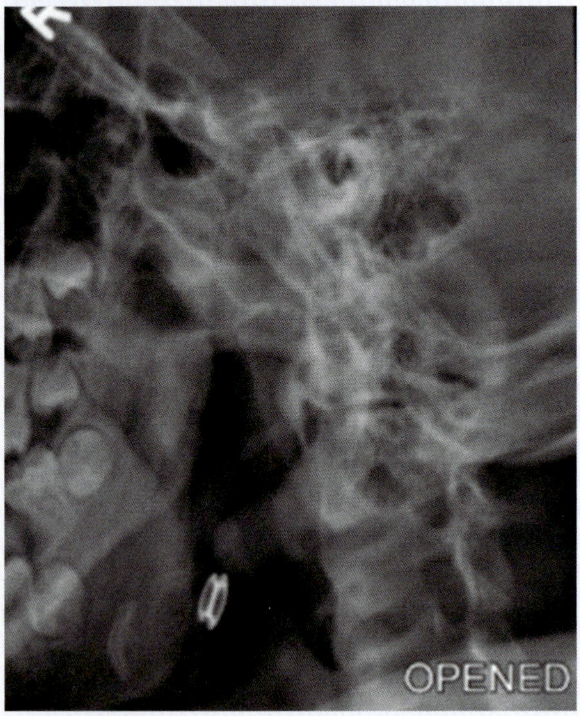

10-112 Lateral TMJ—Schuller method mouth open.

POSITION VARIATION HORIZONTAL BEAM LATERAL FOR TRAUMA SKULL

If an erect right and/or left lateral is not possible for the patient, a horizontal beam may be used. If the patient is able to adjust their head, the back of the head must be built up off the table and then IPL and MSP can be adjusted. The central ray is still directed superior to the EAM to include entire vertex. Source-to-image distance must be considered. If the patient's head can be built up and the IR is close to the parietal bone, a 40" SID can be set. If there is significant OID between the parietal bone and the IR, the SID should be increased to 72" (Figs. 10-113 to 10-115).

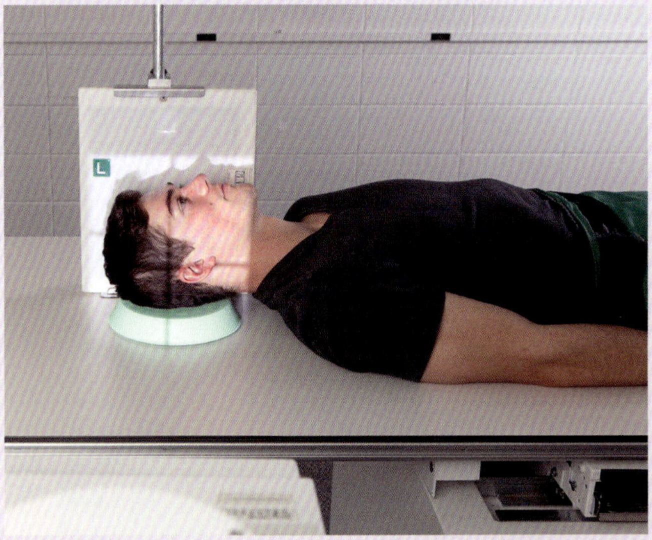

10-113 Horizontal beam lateral skull.

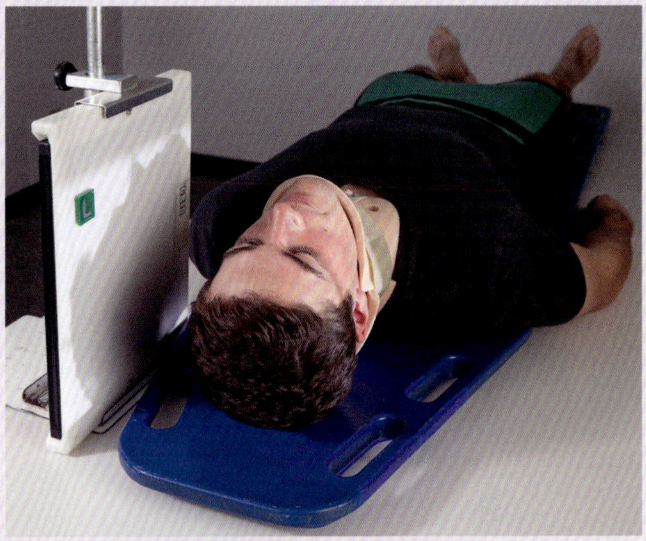

10-114 Horizontal beam lateral trauma skull.

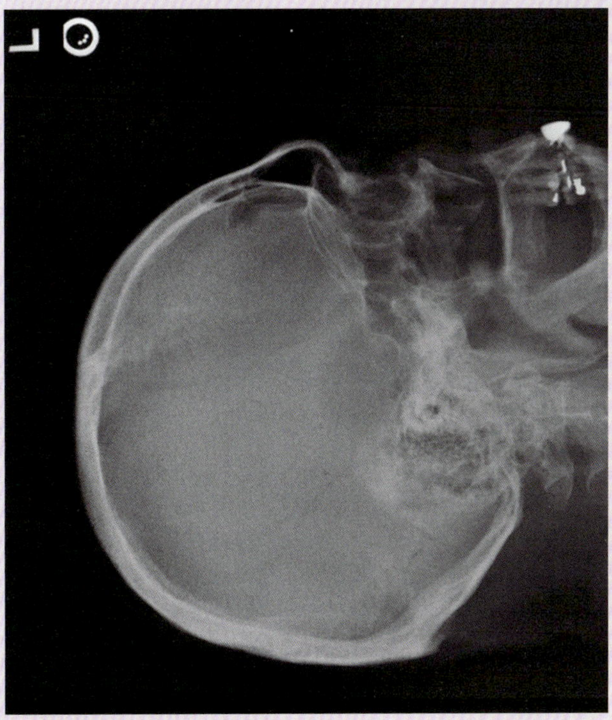

10-115 Horizontal beam lateral skull.

Headwork

- Projection: Submentovertex (SMV)
- SMV is part of numerous exam protocols as outlined in Tables 10-2 (skull), 10-3 (sinuses), and 10-7 (mandible)

Technical Considerations
- kVp 65–80 (based on exam ordered)
- mAs set manually or AEC center cell
- 40" SID

Exposure Field Size
- 10 × 12 lengthwise

Patient Position
- Seated on a stool or chair (with a low back) at the upright Bucky. Extremely important the stool is locked and secured to avoid patient injury. Some patients may require a technologist to support and secure the patient
- Encourage good patient posture
- Support the patient's upper back and guide them back while they hyperextend to look up at the ceiling and place the vertex in contact with the IR
- IOML must be aligned parallel to the IR
- MSP must be aligned perpendicular to the IR
- Expedite the adjustment of positioning lines and ensure patient is stable enough to hold the position while the technologist makes the exposure

Centering
- The centering will be directed according to the part imaged
  - *Skull:* The central ray is set to enter midway between the mandibular angles (Figs. 10-116, 10-118, and 10-119)
  - *Sinuses:* The central ray is set to enter 1" posterior to the mandibular symphysis (Figs. 10-117 and 10-120)
  - *Mandible:* The central ray is set to enter midway between the mandibular angles (Figs. 10-116 and 10-121)

Marking of IR
- Anatomic side markers R or L placed on the corresponding side and anteriolateral to the part

Breathing
- Suspend respiration and instruct the patient to hold still
- Ensure you watch the patient the entire time while walking away to make the exposure

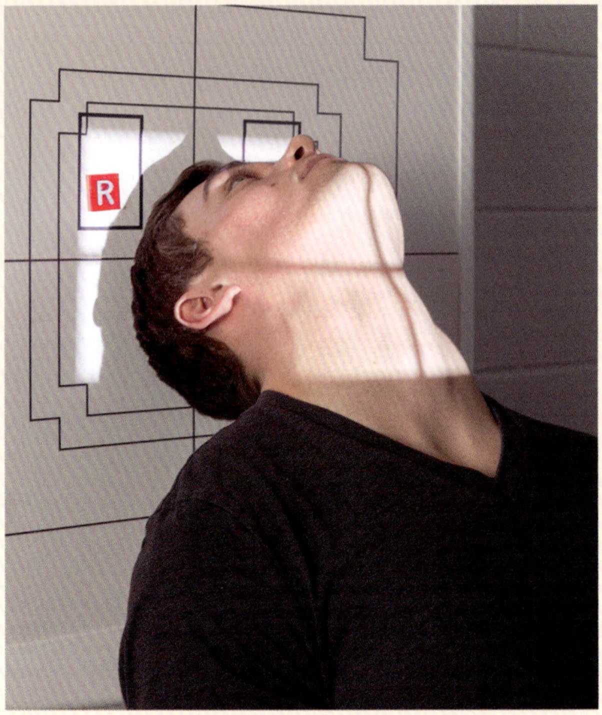

10-116 SMV skull and mandible.

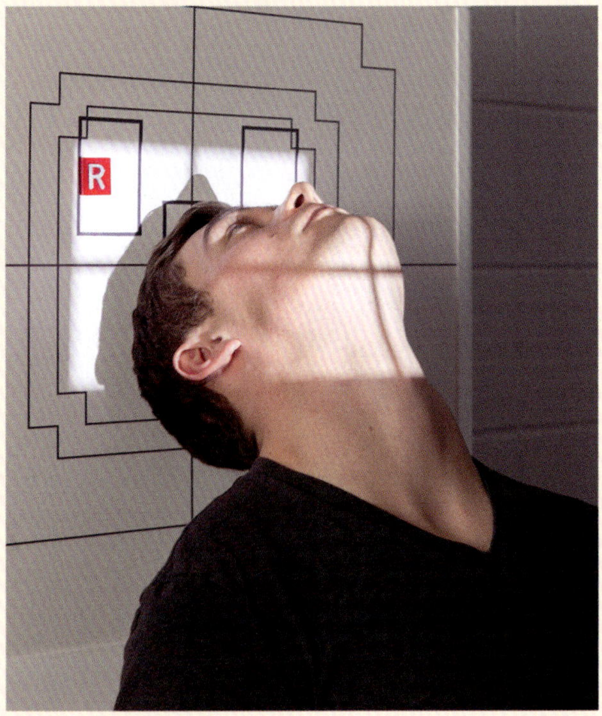

10-117 SMV sinuses.

(continued)

Headwork (*Continued*)

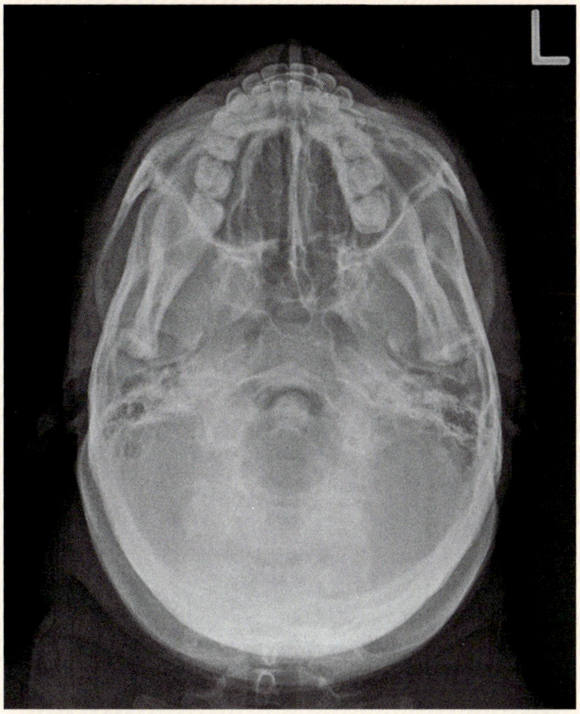

10-118 SMV skull.

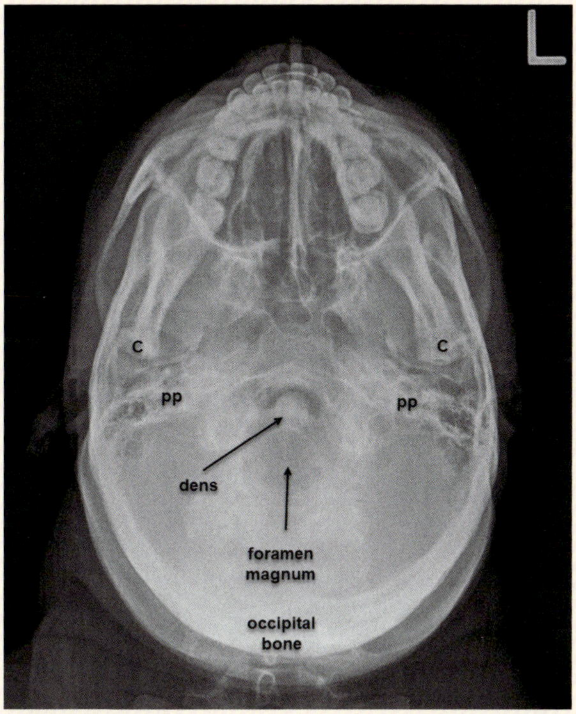

10-119 SMV skull.

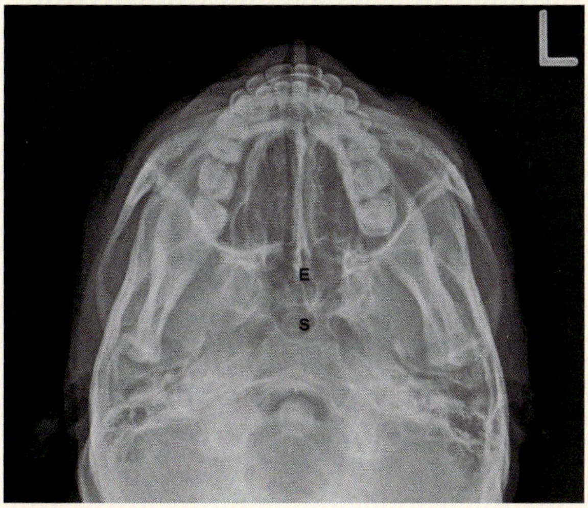

10-120 SMV sinuses.

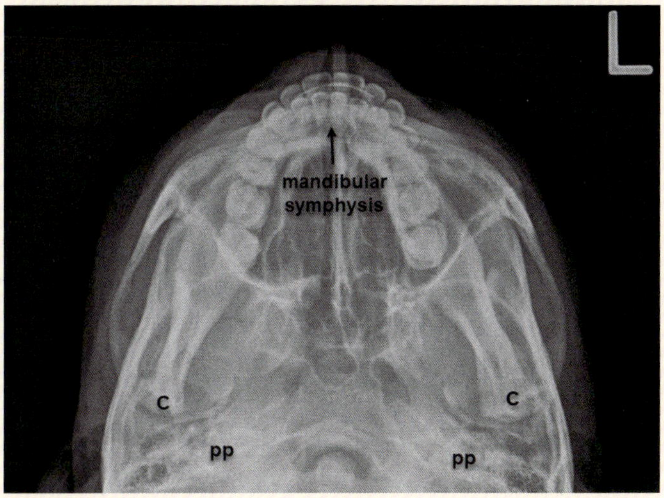

10-121 SMV mandible.

IMAGE CRITIQUE

- Proper positioning criteria for the SMV:
    - The mandibular condyles are anterior to the petrous pyramids. This indicates that the IOML was aligned parallel to the IR. When the mandibular angles are positioned within the petrous pyramids this indicates the head was not hyperextended back far enough; IOML was not parallel to the IR (Fig. 10-122). In instances a patient is unable to hyperextend to allow the IOML parallel to the IR, a cephalic tube angle could be applied. The central ray must intersect perpendicularly with the IOML
    - Rotation of the part is indicated when one mandibular condyle sits more anterior or posterior to the opposite condyle (Fig. 10-123)

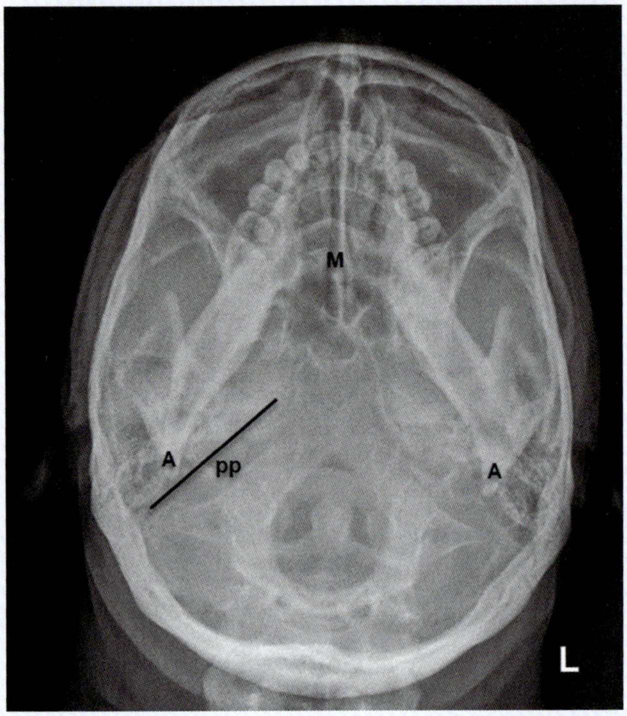

10-122 SMV with insufficient hyperextension of head and neck.

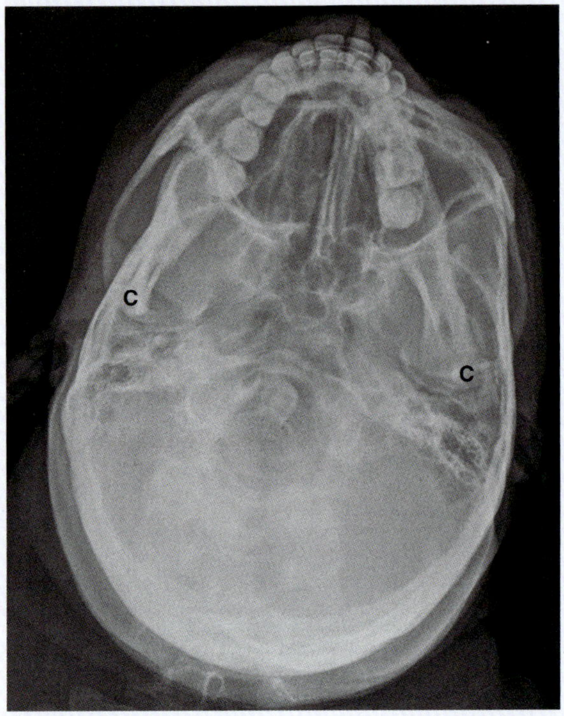

10-123 SMV with rotation.

(continued)

IMAGE CRITIQUE (*Continued*)

- Tilt of the part is indicated when the distance between the mandibular condyles to the lateral margin of the skull are unequal. The side with greater distance indicates the side the chin was tilted toward. For example, if the left condyle had a greater distance than the right, the chin was tilted toward the left side (Fig. 10-124)
- Anatomy of interest is what is positioned closest to the IR
  - *Skull:* Full basal view (base of the skull). Ensure the entire occipital bone is within the collimated exposure field
  - *Sinuses:* Sphenoid and ethmoid sinuses
  - *Mandible:* Entire mandible
- Properly centered with attempted four-sided collimation

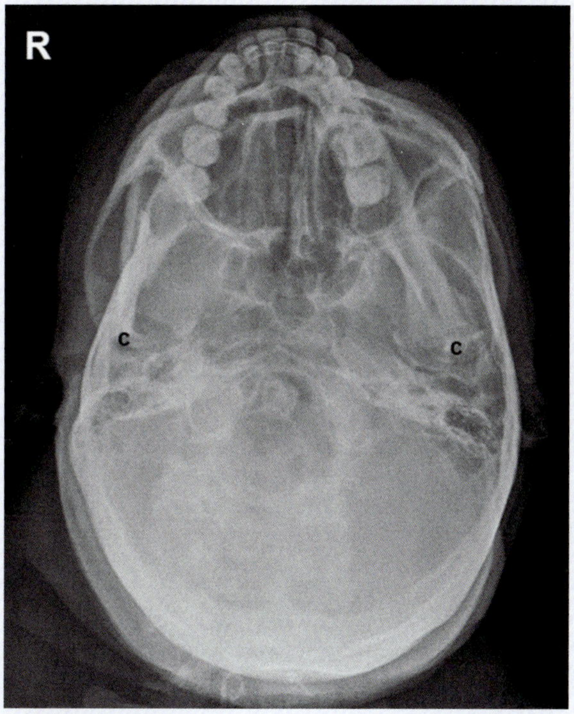

10-124 SMV with tilt.

POSITION VARIATION INFEROSUPERIOR OBLIQUE TANGENTIAL FOR ZYGOMATIC ARCHES

An individual zygomatic arch can be better imaged with a slight variation of the SMV. Once the patient's head is in position for the SMV, the patient's chin is tilted 15° toward the affected arch and then the MSP is rotated 15° toward the affected side. The central ray will skim the zygomatic arch of interest. Typically, a tangential projection of each zygomatic arch is acquired for comparison (Figs. 10-125 to 10-127).

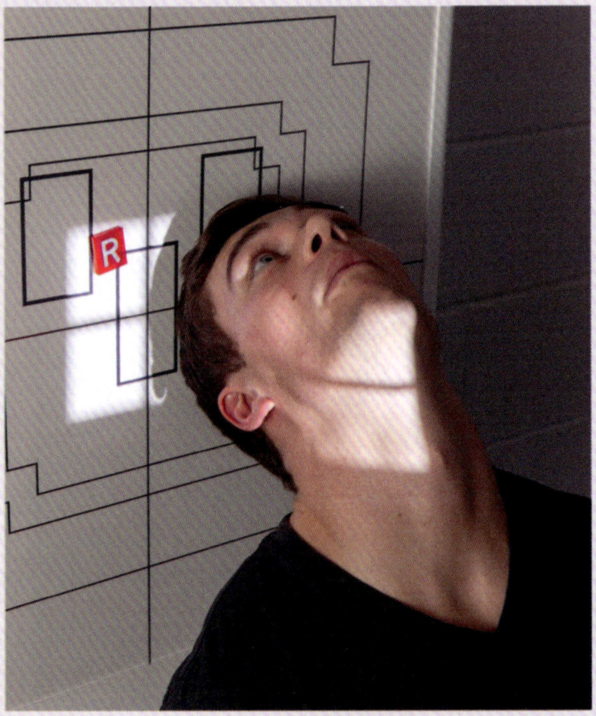

10-125 Inferosuperior oblique tangential—zygomatic arch.

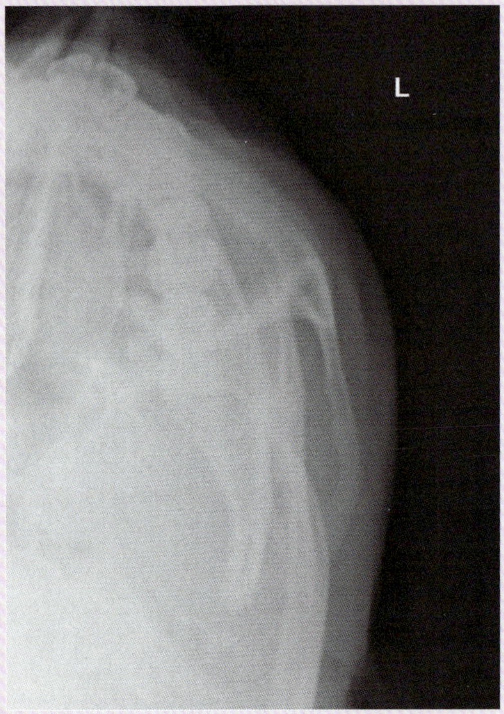

10-126 Inferosuperior oblique tangential—zygomatic arch.

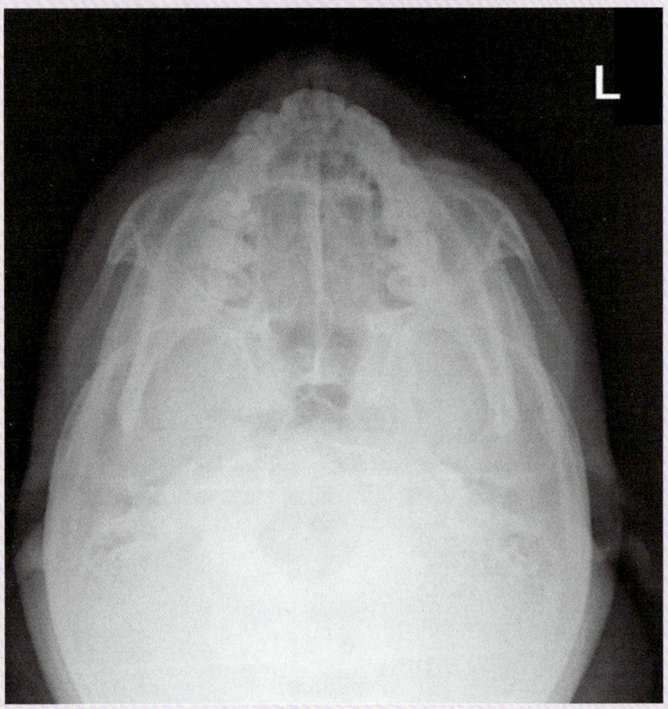

10-127 SMV for bilateral zygomatic arches.

Headwork

- Projection: PA Axial
- Method: Caldwell method
- PA Axial is part of numerous exam protocols as outlined in Tables 10-2 (skull), 10-3 (sinuses), and 10-5 (facial bones)

Technical Considerations

- kVp 70–80
- mAs set manually or center AEC cell
- 40" SID

Exposure Field Size

- 10 × 12 lengthwise

Patient Position

- Seated on a stool or chair at the upright Bucky
- Encourage good patient posture
- Position the patient's forehead and nose on the upright Bucky and adjust the flexion or extension of the neck until the OML is perpendicular to the IR (Fig. 10-128)
- Stand behind the patient and ensure the MSP is perpendicular to the IR

Centering (Figs 10-128 and 10-129)

- A 15° caudal angle
- The centering will be directed according to the part imaged
    - *Skull:* The central ray is set to exit the nasion
    - *Sinuses:* The central ray is set to exit the nasion
    - Facial Bones: The central ray is set to exit the nasion

Marking of IR

- Anatomic side markers R or L placed furthest from the patient's midline to the corresponding side

Breathing

- Suspend respiration and instruct the patient to hold still
- Ensure you watch the patient the entire time while walking away to make the exposure

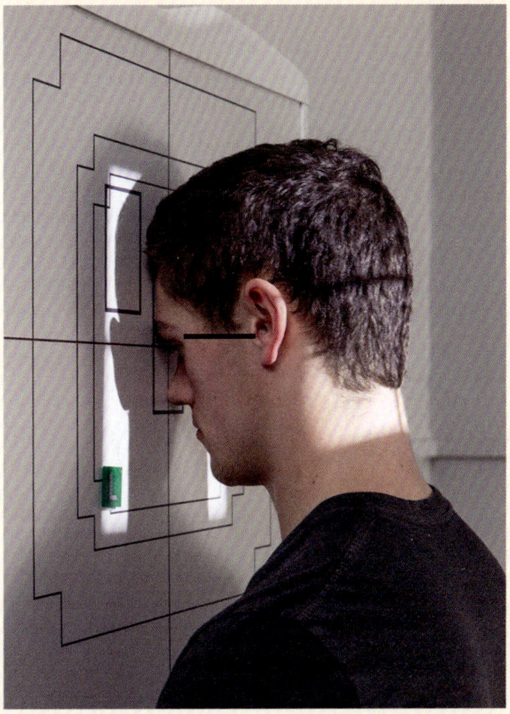

10-128 PA Axial Caldwell method.

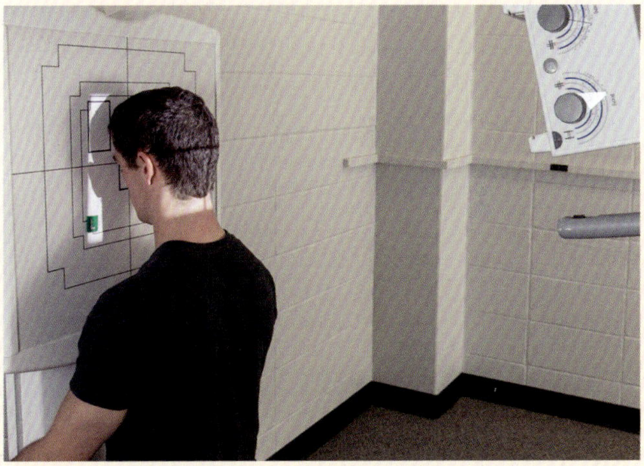

10-129 PA Axial Caldwell method CR for skull and sinuses.

IMAGE CRITIQUE

- Proper positioning criteria for the PA Axial
  - The petrous pyramids fill the lower one-third of the orbits (Figs 10-130 and 10-131). The petrous ridge will correspond with the SOM when OML is adjusted perpendicular. The height placement of the petrous pyramids for the Caldwell method is determined by the OML placement accuracy paired with the 15° caudal tube angle. If the petrous pyramids fall closer to the inferior orbital margin or IOM or below, the likely error was the patient's OML was not truly perpendicular to the IR before the 15° caudal tube angle was applied. Or, if the OML was truly perpendicular to the IR receptor, perhaps a mistakenly >15° caudal tube angle was applied (Fig. 10-132)
  - The petrous pyramids are symmetrical in comparison of their height. If one petrous pyramid is higher than the opposite, or one SOM is higher than the opposite, this indicates the patient's vertex was tilted to either the right or left side. If the patient's head is tilted to the right, the left SOM or petrous pyramid will appear higher (Fig. 10-133)
  - Equal distance between the orbital oblique line or lateral orbital margin to the lateral margin of the skull. Unequal distance indicates rotation of the skull indicating the MSP was not perpendicular to the IR. Identifying the side of less distance between the orbital oblique line and the lateral margin of the skull indicates the side the patient's face is rotated toward (Fig. 10-134)
- Anatomy of interest is the anatomy positioned closest to the IR
  - *Skull:* Frontal bone. Must include vertex
  - *Sinuses:* Frontal Sinuses
- Properly centered with attempted four-sided collimation

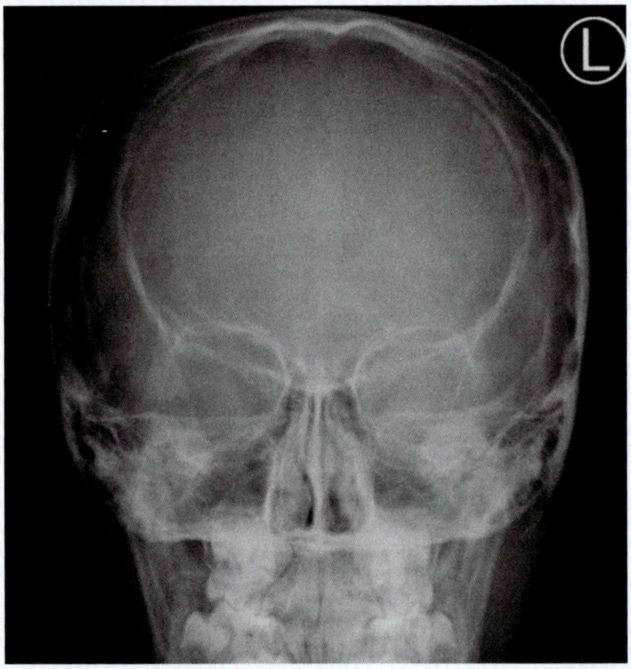

10-130 PA Axial Caldwell method.

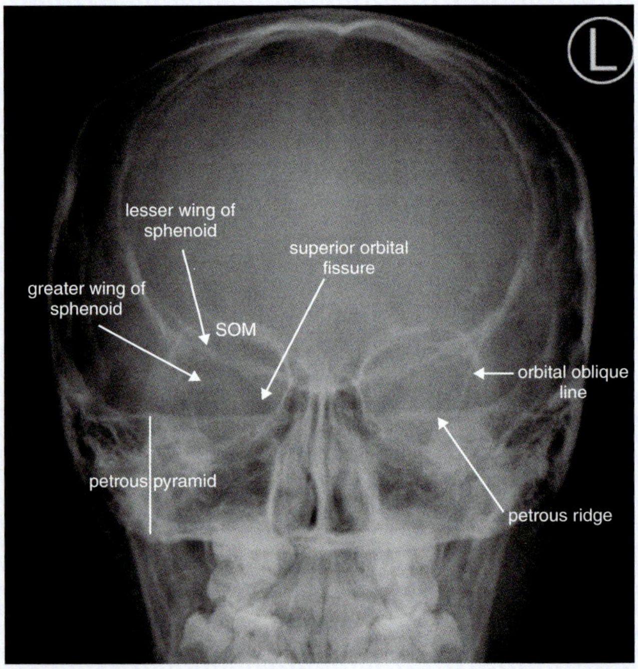

10-131 PA Axial Caldwell method.

(continued)

IMAGE CRITIQUE (*Continued*)

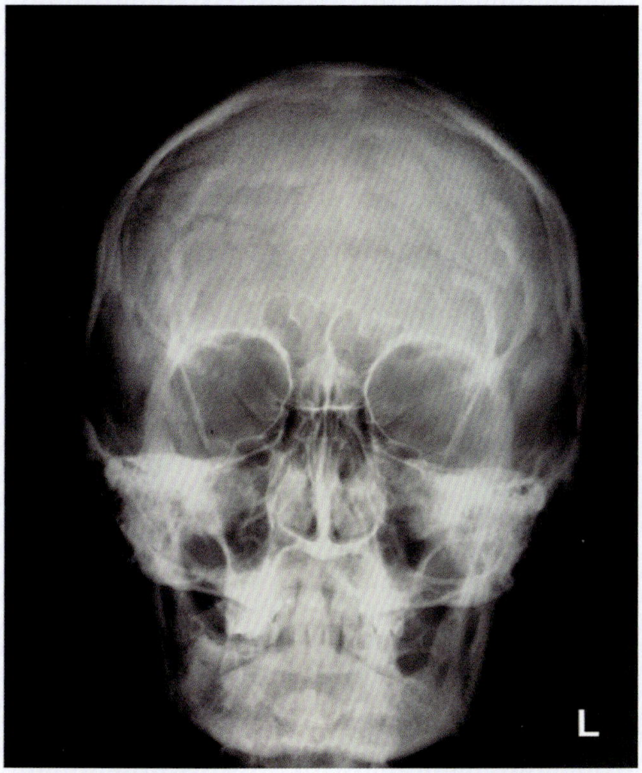

10-132 PA Axial Caldwell method—petrous pyramids at or below IOM.

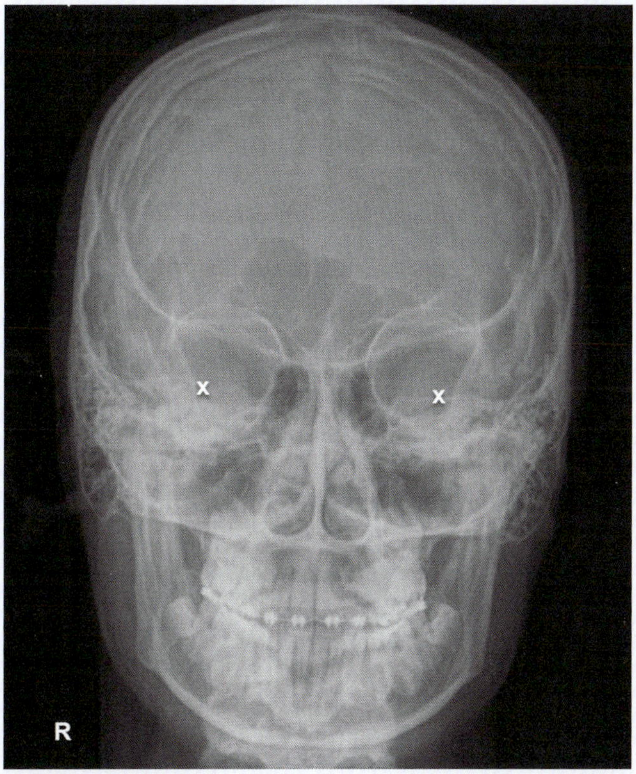

10-133 PA Axial Caldwell method—slight tilt.

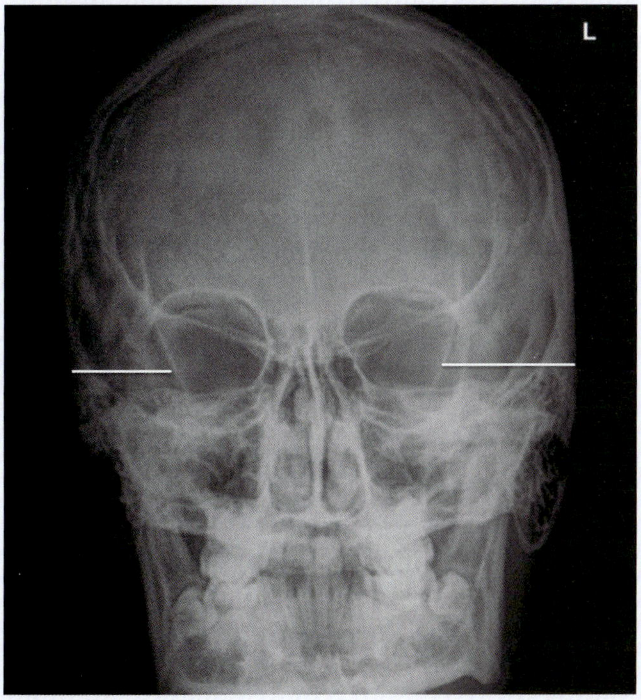

10-134 PA Axial Caldwell method—rotation.

Headwork

- Projection: Parietoacanthial
- Method: Waters method
- Parietoacanthial is part of numerous exam protocols as outlined in Tables 10-3 (sinuses), 10-4 (nasal bones), 10-5 (facial bones),10-6 (orbits), and 10-8 (zygomatic arches)

Technical Considerations

- kVp 70–80
- mAs set manually or center AEC cell
- 40" SID

Exposure Field Size

- 10 × 12 lengthwise

Patient Position (Figs. 10-135, 10-136, and 10-137)

- Seated on a stool or chair at the upright Bucky
- Encourage good patient posture
- Extend the patient's chin up to rest on the upright Bucky. Adjust the MML perpendicular to the IR
- Stand behind the patient and ensure the MSP is perpendicular to the IR

Centering

- The centering will be directed to exit the acanthion

Marking of IR

- Anatomic side marker R or L placed furthest from the patient's midline to the corresponding side

Breathing

- Suspend respiration and instruct the patient to hold still
- Ensure you watch the patient the entire time while walking away to make the exposure

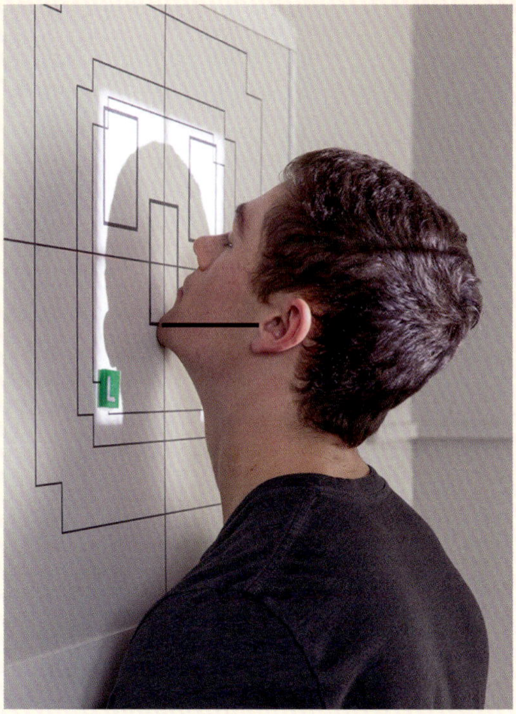

10-135 Parietoacanthial projection—Waters method.

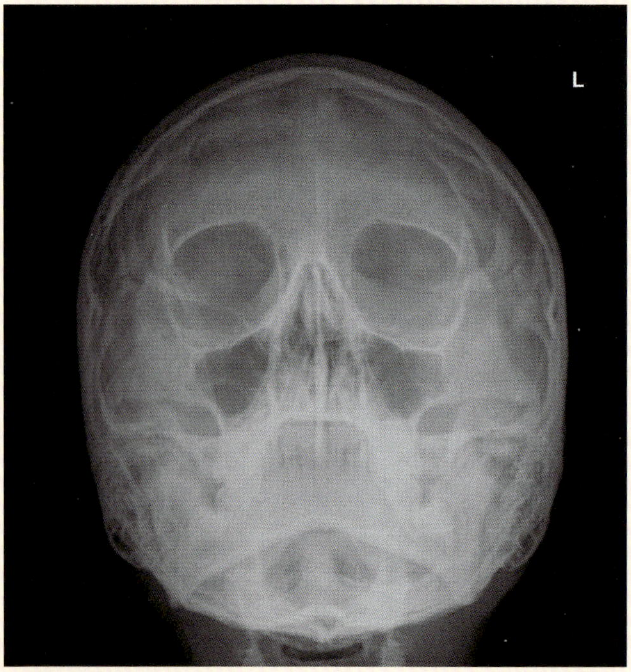

10-136 Parietoacanthial projection—Waters method.

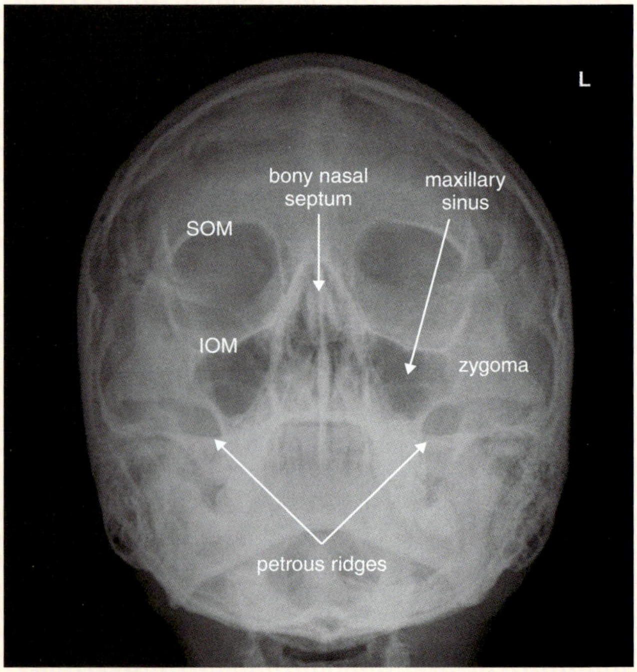

10-137 Parietoacanthial projection—Waters method.

IMAGE CRITIQUE

- Proper positioning criteria for the parietoacanthial projection:
  - The petrous pyramids must drop below the maxillary sinuses. If the petrous pyramids appear within the maxillary sinuses, the patient's chin was not extended enough; MML was not perpendicular (Fig. 10-138)
  - The petrous pyramids are symmetrical in comparison of their height. If one petrous pyramid is higher than the opposite or one SOM is higher than the opposite, this indicates the patient's vertex was tilted to either the right or left side. If the patient's head is tilted to the right, the left SOM or petrous pyramid will appear higher (Fig. 10-139)

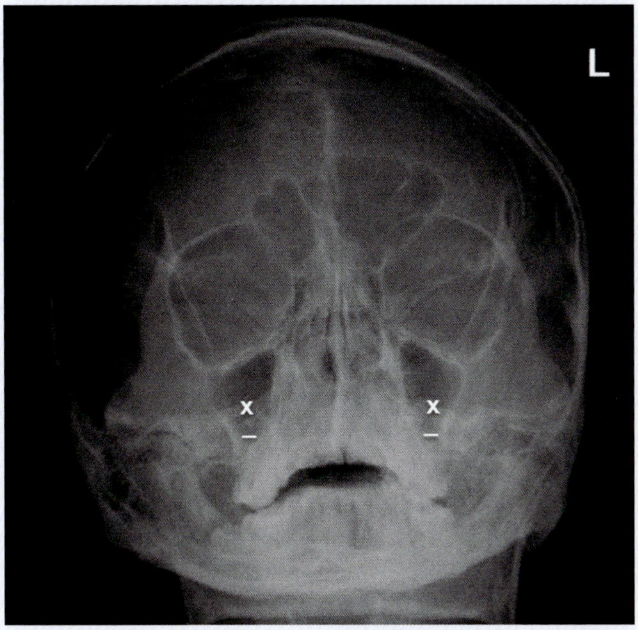

10-138 Waters method—MML not perpendicular.

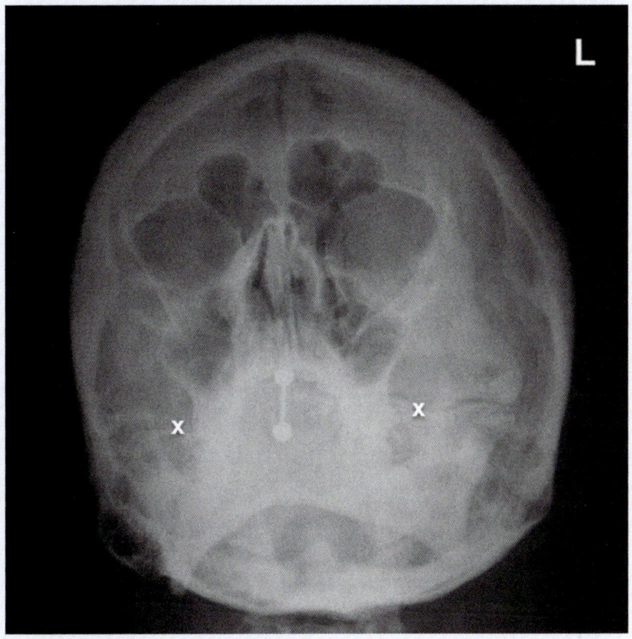

10-139 Waters method—tilt and rotation

(continued)

IMAGE CRITIQUE (*Continued*)

    - Equal distance between the orbital oblique line or lateral orbital margin to the lateral margin of the skull. Unequal distance indicates rotation of the skull indicating the MSP was not perpendicular to the IR. Identifying the side of less distance between the orbital oblique line and the lateral margin of the skull indicates the side the face patient's is rotated toward (Fig. 10-140)
- Anatomy of interest is the anatomy positioned closest to the IR
    - *Sinuses:* Maxillary sinuses
    - *Facial Bones:* IOM of the orbit and zygoma(s)
    - *Orbits:* IOM and orbital base entirely (free of petrous pyramids)
    - *Nasal Bones:* Bony nasal septum
- Properly centered with attempted four-sided collimation

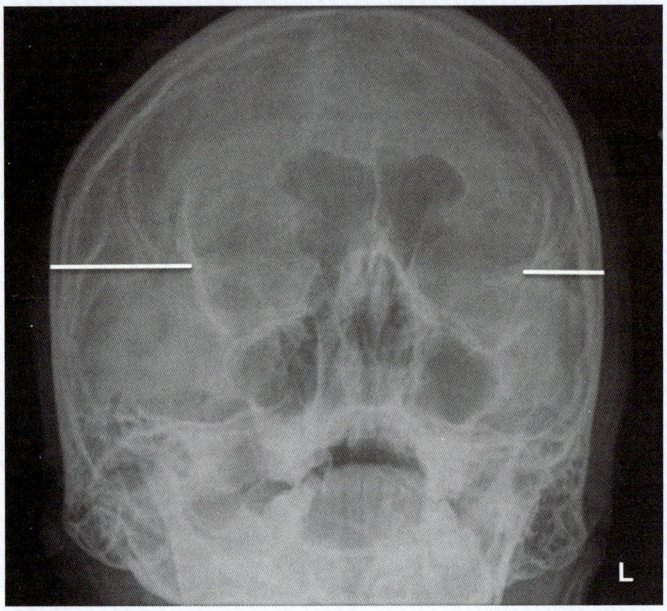

10-140 Waters method—rotation.

POSITION VARIATION MODIFIED WATERS METHOD

If the orbital base is of specific interest in cases of a blowout fracture, the entire orbital base will be positioned closer to the IR by adjusting the lip meatal line (LML) perpendicular to the IR rather than the MML. With the modified method, the petrous pyramids will appear half filling the maxillary sinuses rather than entirely below the maxillary sinuses. The Modified Waters method will demonstrate the entire orbital base (Figs. 10-141 to 10-143).

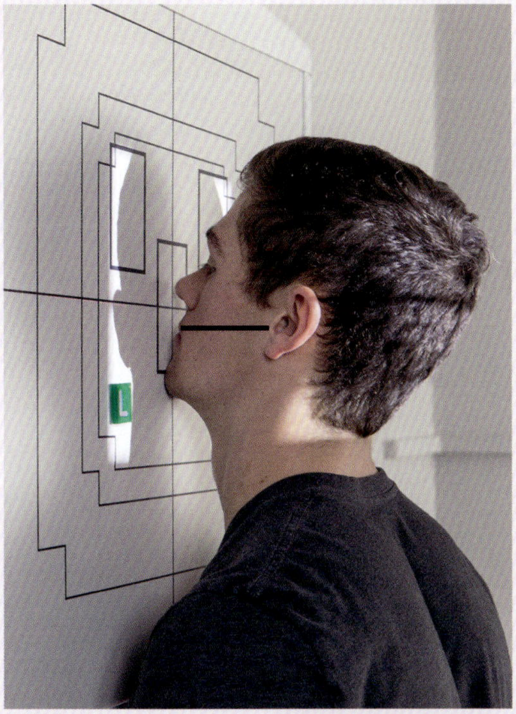

10-141 Modified Waters method.

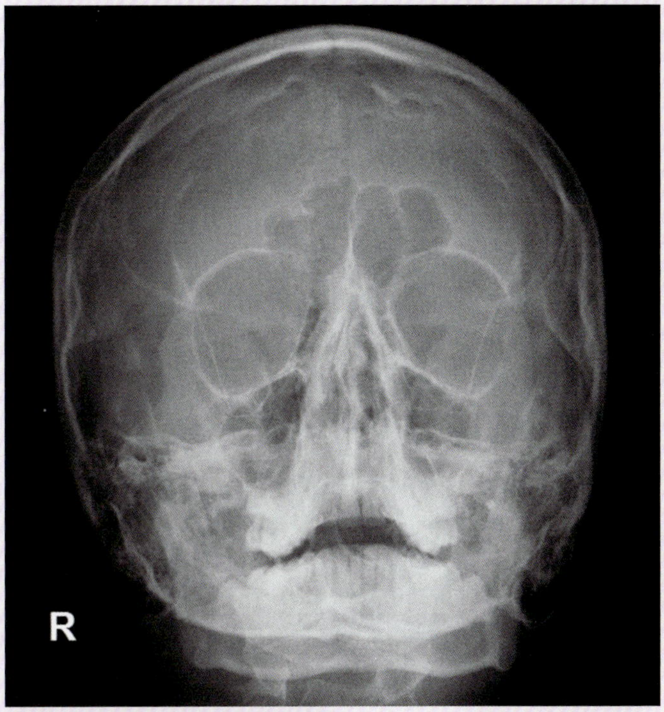

10-142 Modified Waters method.

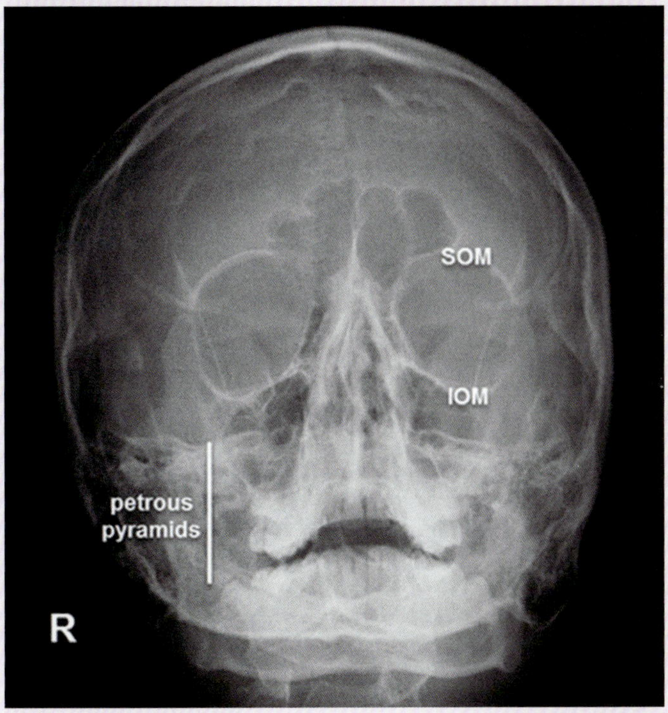

10-143 Modified Waters method.

Headwork

- Projection: Axiolateral Mandible
- Axiolateral is part mandible protocol as outlined in Table 10-7

Technical Considerations

- kVp 65–70
- mAs set manually
- 40" SID

Exposure Field Size

- 10 × 12 lengthwise

Patient Position (Fig. 10-144)

- Seated on a stool or chair at the upright Bucky
- Encourage good patient posture
- Patient will face the upright Bucky and then adjusted into a slight anterior oblique allowing the lateral side of the head closer to the IR. For instance, if the right side of the head is of interest, the patient should be positioned into a right anterior oblique (RAO) position. Both a right and left axiolateral will be applied to visualize each mandibular body
- Have the patient relax the shoulder closest to the tube down. It is helpful for patients with a shorter neck, to slightly shrug up the shoulder closest to the Bucky to help relax the opposite shoulder down
- A variation of a true lateral with rotation of the MSP toward the IR could provide focus on a more specific part of the mandible. A true lateral will demonstrate the ramus. A 30° rotation toward the IR will demonstrate the mandibular body. A 45° rotation toward the IR will demonstrate the mentum

Centering

- Tube angle
  - 20°–25° cephalic tube. CR is directed along the inferior margin of the mandibular body. The tube angle will project the midmandibular body furthest from the IR superiorly (Fig. 10-144)
- Head tilt
  - From a true lateral position, tilt the vertex toward the IR about 25°–30°. The CR will be directed perpendicular toward the midmandibular body closest to the IR (Fig. 10-145)

Marking of IR

- Anatomic side marker R or L is placed anterior to the part indicating the side closest to the IR

Breathing

- Suspend respiration and instruct the patient to hold still
- Ensure you watch the patient the entire time while walking away to make the exposure

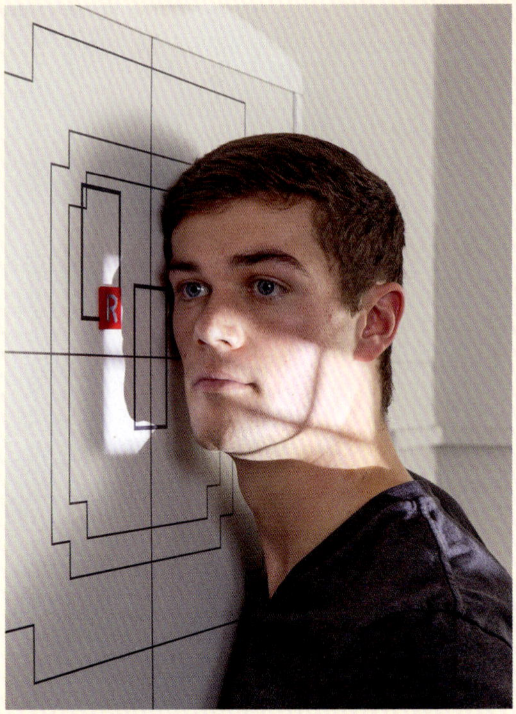

10-144 Axiolateral mandible.

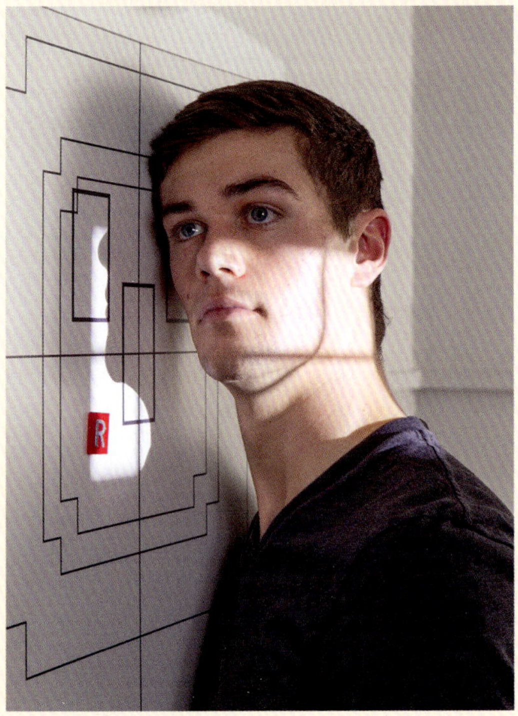

10-145 Axiolateral mandible.

IMAGE CRITIQUE (FIGS. 10-146 and 10-147)

- Proper positioning criteria for the axiolateral projection:
  - Mentum, mandibular angle, ramus, condyle, and condyloid process all included within the collimated exposure field
  - The mandibular body should be free of superimposition of the opposite mandibular body
  - Inadequate extension of the chin will result in superimposition of the posterior ramus upon the C-spine
  - Ensure TMJ is included
- Properly centered with attempted four-sided collimation

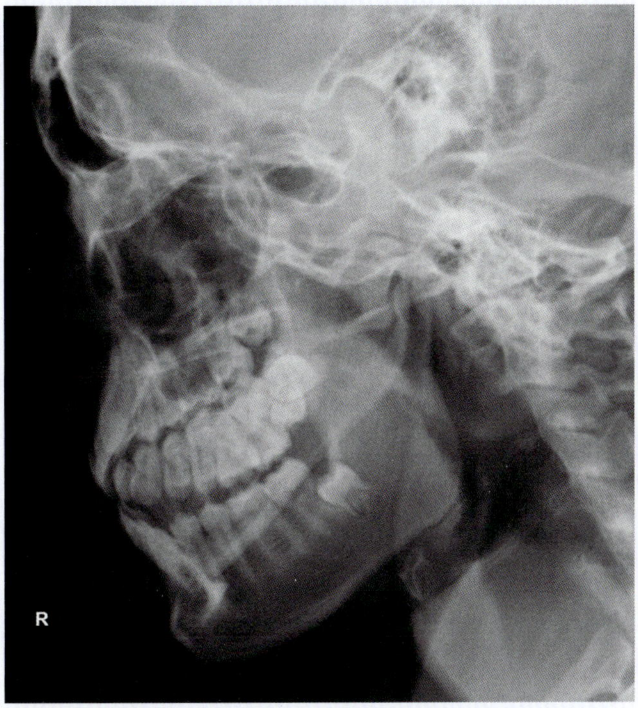

10-146 Axiolateral mandible.

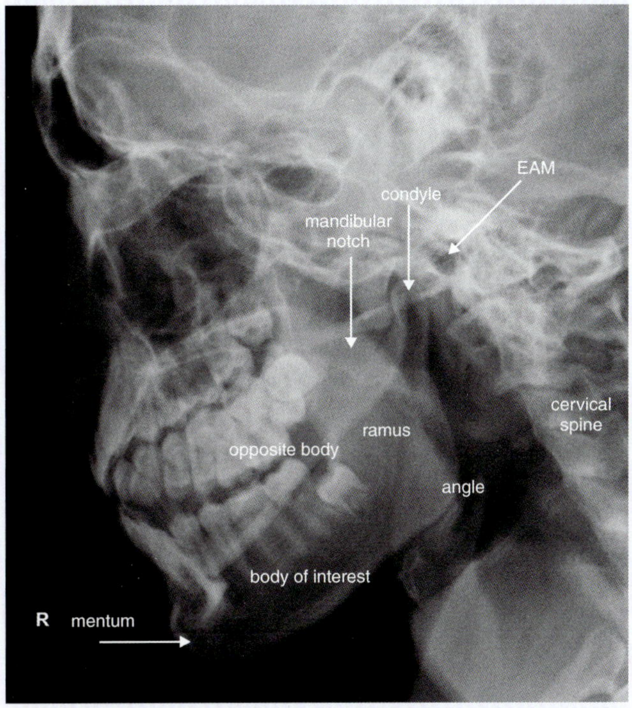

10-147 Axiolateral mandible.

Headwork

- Projection: Parieto-orbital Oblique
- Method: Rhese method
- Parieto-orbital oblique is part orbit protocol as outlined in Table 10-6

Technical Considerations

- kVp 75–80
- mAs set manually or center AEC cell
- 40" SID

Exposure Field Size

- 10 × 12 lengthwise

Patient Position (Fig. 10-148)

- Seated on a stool or chair at the upright Bucky
- Encourage good patient posture
- Have patient face the upright Bucky. Place the chin, cheek, and nose of the affected side in contact with the Bucky. The MSP should form a 53° angle with the surface of the IR (Fig. 10-148). *The MSP is rotated 37° from perpendicular* toward *the affected side*
- Adjust AML (acanthiomeatal line) perpendicular to the IR. This may cause the chin or nose to pull away from the Bucky (Fig. 10-149)

Centering (Figs. 10-148 to 10-152)

- The centering will be directed to exit the affected orbit at the outer canthus
- With proper positioning of the three facial landmarks (chin, cheek, and nose) and the MSP at 53° angle with the IR, the CR will enter the parietal bone (approximately 1½" -2" posterior to the upside TEA)

Marking of IR

- Anatomic side marker R or L placed to denote the orbit of interest

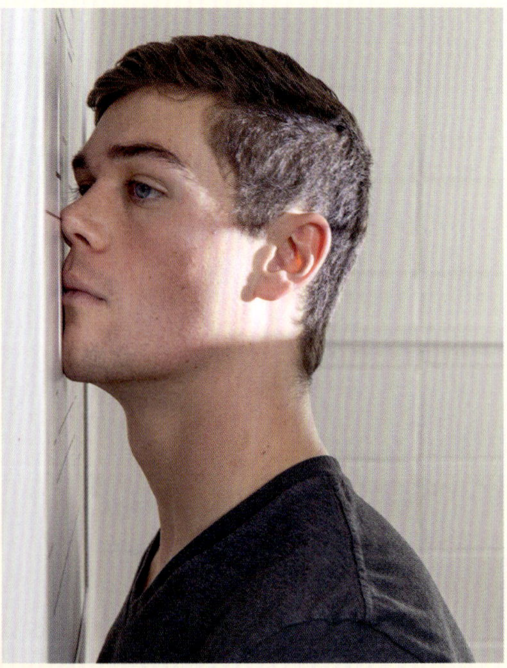

10-148 Parieto-orbital oblique projection—Rhese method.

Breathing

- Suspend respiration and instruct the patient to hold still
- Ensure you watch the patient the entire time while walking away to make the exposure

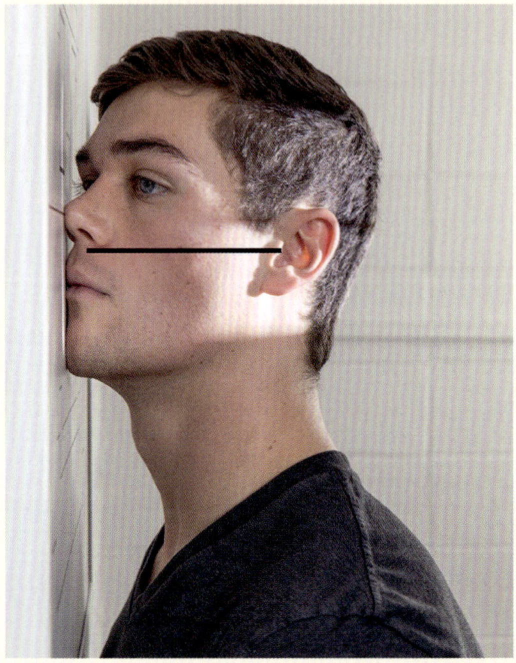

10-149 Parieto-orbital oblique projection—Rhese method.

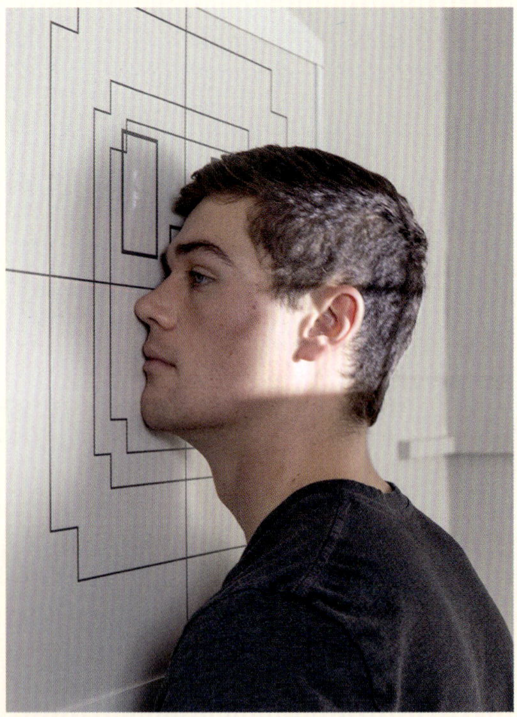

10-150 Parieto-orbital oblique projection—Rhese method.

(continued)

Headwork (*Continued*)

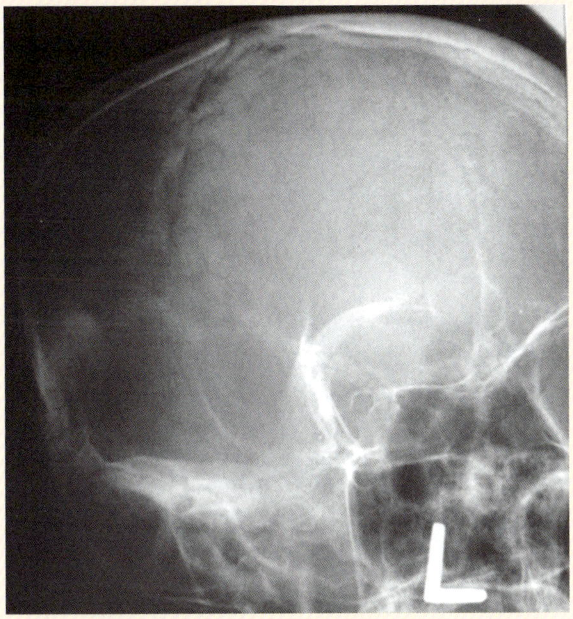

10-151 Parieto-orbital oblique projection—Rhese method with correct positioning.

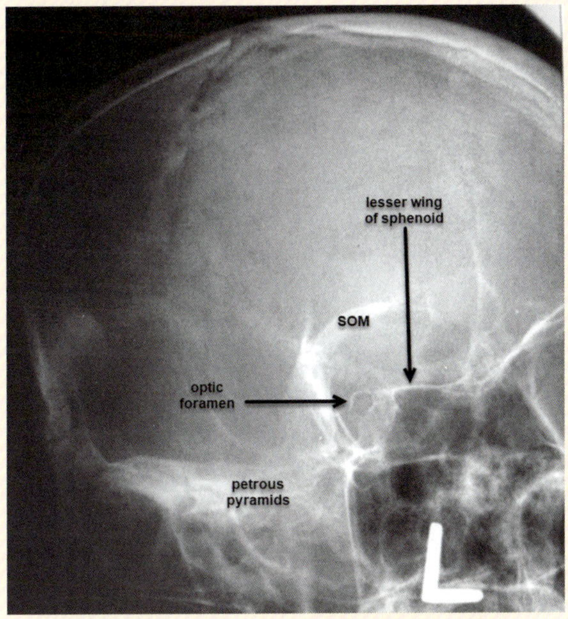

10-152 Parieto-orbital oblique projection—Rhese method.

IMAGE CRITIQUE

- Proper positioning criteria for the parieto-orbital oblique projection:
  - Optic foramen visualized in the lower outer quadrant (LOQ) of the affected orbit indicating the MSP was correctly rotated to form the 53° angle with the IR. More or less angle of rotation will cause the optic foramen to shift medial or lateral in the orbit (Fig. 10-153)
  - The petrous pyramids should be below the IOM if the AML was adjusted to intersect perpendicular with the IR. Too much depression or extension of the chin will cause the optic foramen to shift more superior or inferior in the orbit (Fig. 10-154)
- Properly centered with attempted four-sided collimation

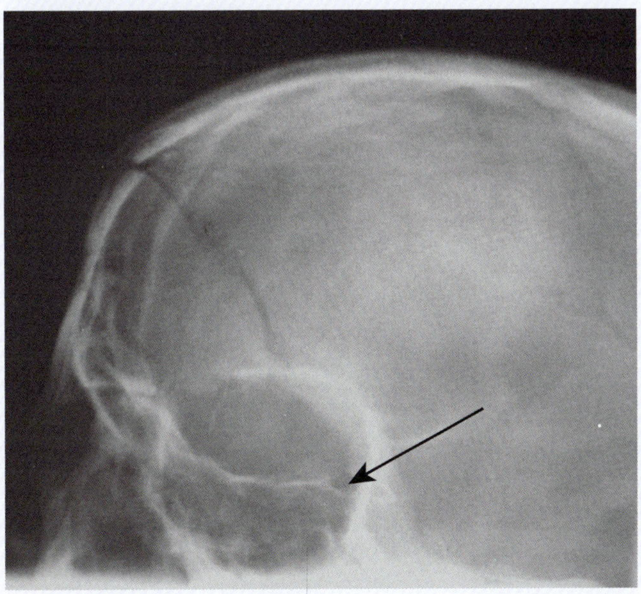

10-153 Rhese method—greater than 53° angle with IR.

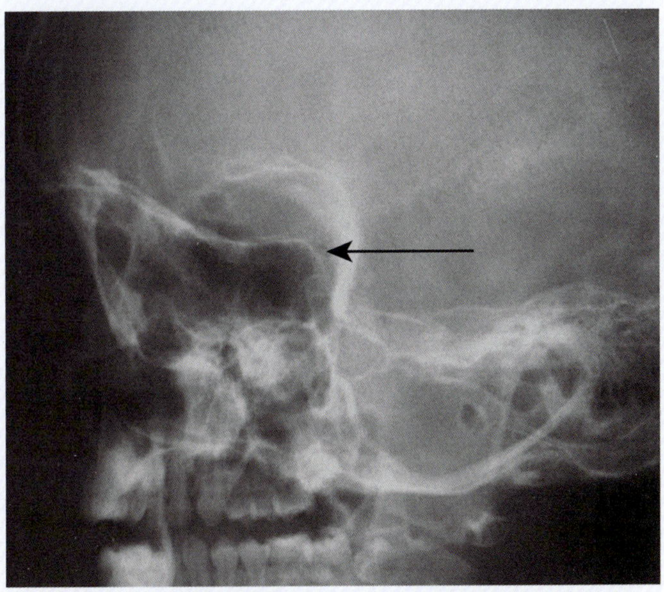

10-154 Rhese method—chin needs slight extension, optic foramen superior to lower outer quadrant.

SKULL PROTOCOL (TABLE 10-2)

10-2

Projection	Positioning Lines	Central Ray	Anatomy of Interest	Evaluation Criteria
PA (PA Axial Caldwell may replace PA) 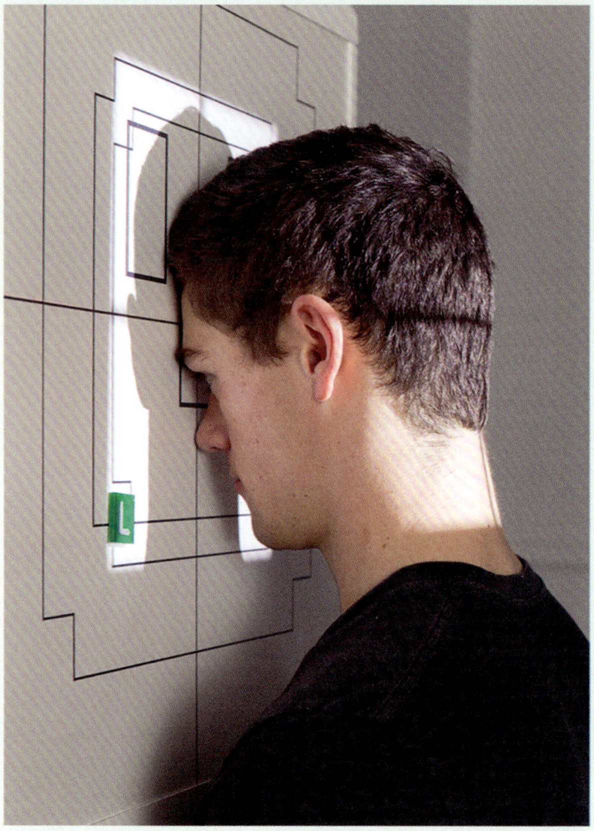	OML ⊥ MSP ⊥	Exits glabella	Frontal Bone	Petrous pyramids fills the entire orbits. Symmetrical height of the superior orbital margins and petrous pyramids indicating no tilt. Symmetrical distance between orbital oblique line and lateral margin of skull indicating no rotation. Vertex included.
AP Axial (Towne method) 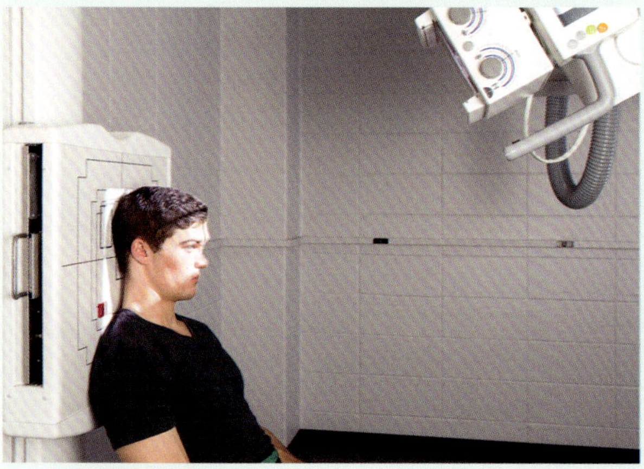	OML ⊥ IOML ⊥ MSP ⊥	OML = 30° caudal angle IOML = 37° caudal angle Enters the hairline	Occipital bone	Dorsum sella centered within the foramen magnum. Symmetrical height of the petrous pyramids indicating no tilt. Symmetrical distance between lateral margin of foramen magnum and lateral margin of skull. Vertex included.

Projection	Positioning Lines	Central Ray	Anatomy of Interest	Evaluation Criteria
Lateral RT and LT lateral may applied 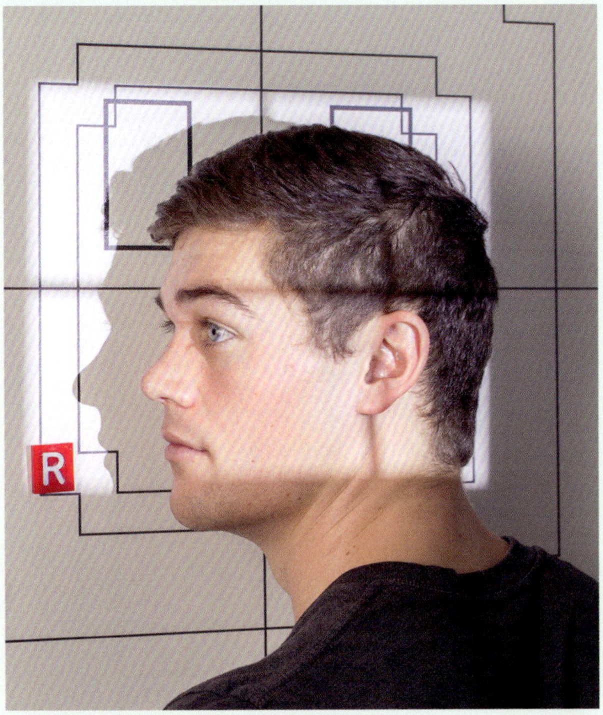 	IOML II IPL ⊥ MSP II	1"–2" superior to the EAM to include vertex	Parietal bone closest to the IR	Sella turcica in profile. Greater wings of the sphenoid nearly superimposed indicating no significant rotation. Superior orbital margins are superimposed indicating no tilt. Vertex included.
Submentovertex (SMV) 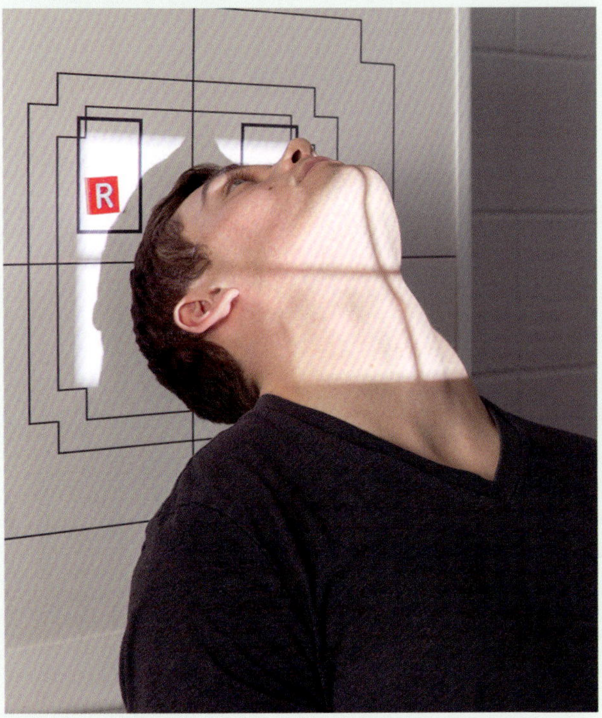 	IOML II MSP ⊥	Midway between the gonions and MSP	Basilar view of the skull	Mandibular condyles anterior to petrous pyramids indicating IOML was parallel. Symmetrical height of the mandibular condyles indicating no rotation. Even distance between the mandibular condyles to the lateral margin of the skull indicating no tilt.

SINUSES (TABLE 10-3)

10-3

Projection	Positioning Lines	Central Ray	Anatomy of Interest	Evaluation Criteria
PA Axial (Caldwell method) 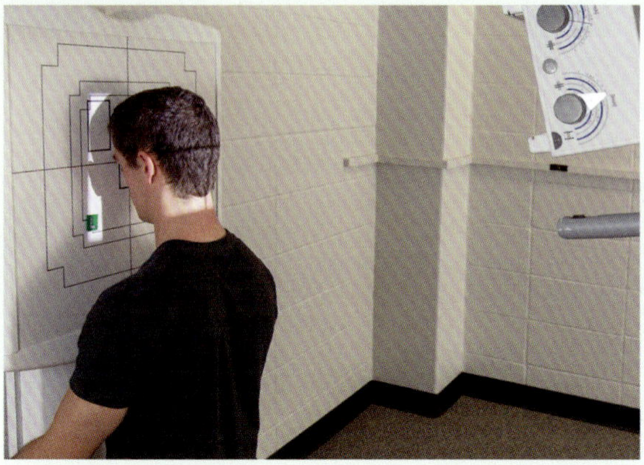	OML ⊥ MSP ⊥	Exits nasion	Frontal sinuses	Petrous pyramids fill the lower one-third of the orbits. Symmetrical height of the superior orbital margins and petrous pyramids indicating no tilt. Symmetrical distance between orbital oblique line and lateral margin of skull indicating no rotation.
Parietoacanthial (Waters method) 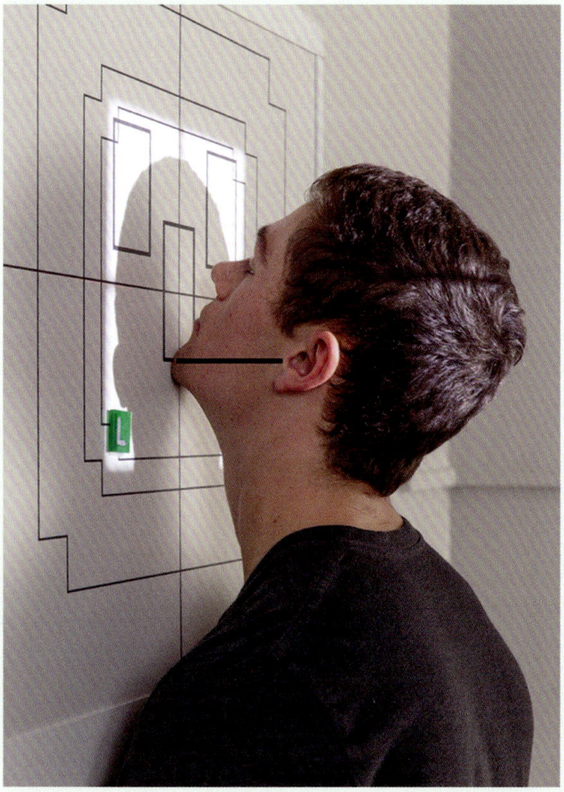	MML ⊥ MSP ⊥	Exits the acanthion	Maxillary sinuses	Petrous pyramids drop below the maxillary sinuses. Symmetrical height of the superior orbital margins and petrous pyramids indicating no tilt. Symmetrical distance between orbital oblique line and lateral margin of skull indicating no rotation.

Projection	Positioning Lines	Central Ray	Anatomy of Interest	Evaluation Criteria
Lateral 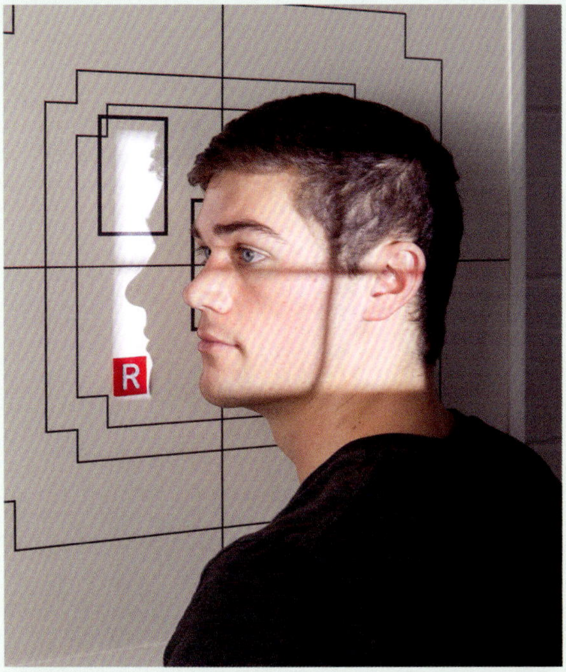 	IOML II IPL ⊥ MSP II	Midway between the EAM and outer canthus	All four sinus sets	Greater wings of the sphenoid nearly superimposed indicating no significant rotation. Superior orbital margins are superimposed indicating no tilt.
SMV 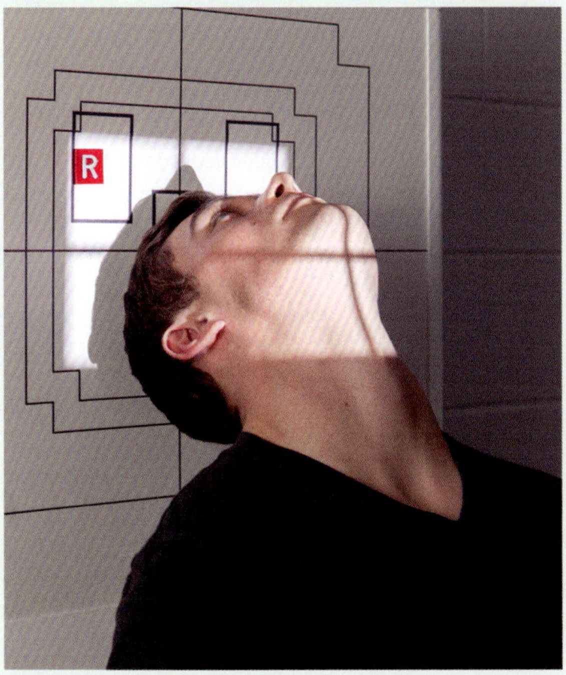 	IOML II MSP ⊥	1" posterior to the mandibular symphysis	Ethmoid and sphenoid sinuses	Mandibular condyles anterior to petrous pyramids indicating IOML parallel. Symmetrical height of the mandibular condyles indicating no rotation. Even distance between the mandibular condyles to the lateral margin of the skull indicating no tilt.

NASAL BONES (TABLE 10-4)

10-4

Projection	Positioning Lines	Central Ray	Anatomy of Interest	Evaluation Criteria
Parietoacanthial (Waters method) 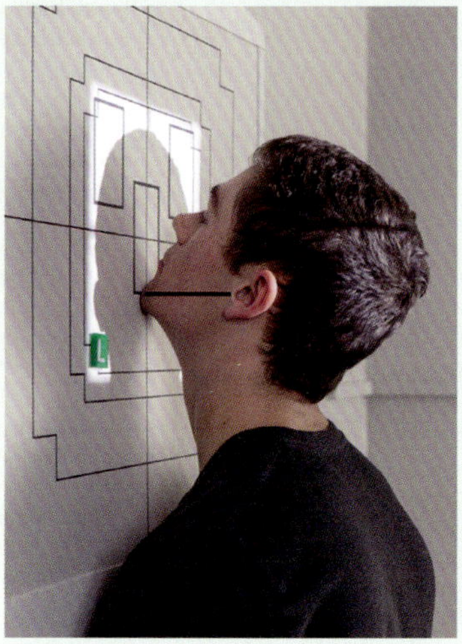	MML ⊥ MSP ⊥	Exits the acanthion	Bony nasal septum	Petrous pyramids drop below the maxillary sinuses. Symmetrical height of the superior orbital margins and petrous pyramids indicating no tilt. Symmetrical distance between orbital oblique line and lateral margin of skull indicating no rotation.
Lateral(s) Both Rt and Lt lateral are acquired 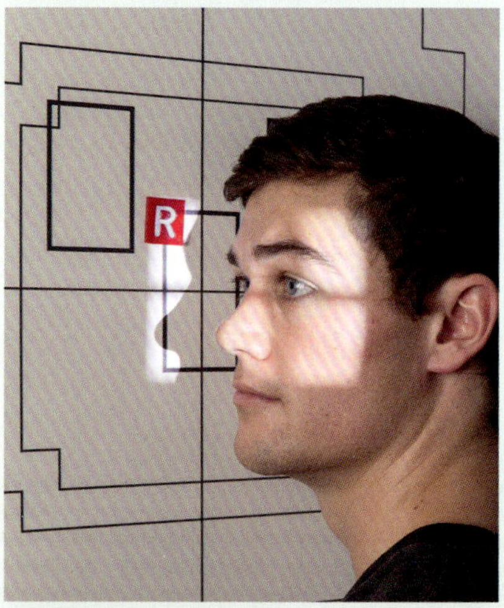 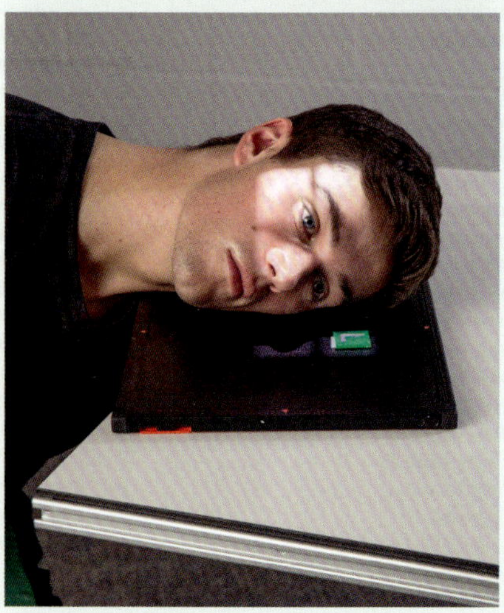	IOML II IPL ⊥ MSP II	½" inferior to the nasion	Nasal bone closest to the IR	Greater wings of the sphenoid superimposed indicating no significant rotation. Superior orbital margins are superimposed indicating no tilt. *With good collimation, rotation and tilt will be difficult to evaluate for.*

FACIAL BONES (TABLE 10-5)

10-5

Projection	Positioning Lines	Central Ray	Anatomy of Interest	Evaluation Criteria
PA axial (Caldwell method) 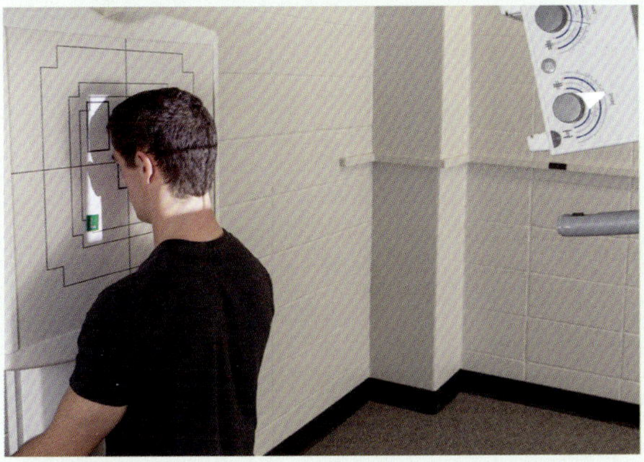	OML ⊥ MSP ⊥	Exits nasion	Superior orbital margins	Petrous pyramids fill the lower one-third of the orbits. Symmetrical height of the superior orbital margins and petrous pyramids indicating no tilt. Symmetrical distance between orbital oblique line and lateral margin of skull indicating no rotation.
Parietoacanthial (Waters method) 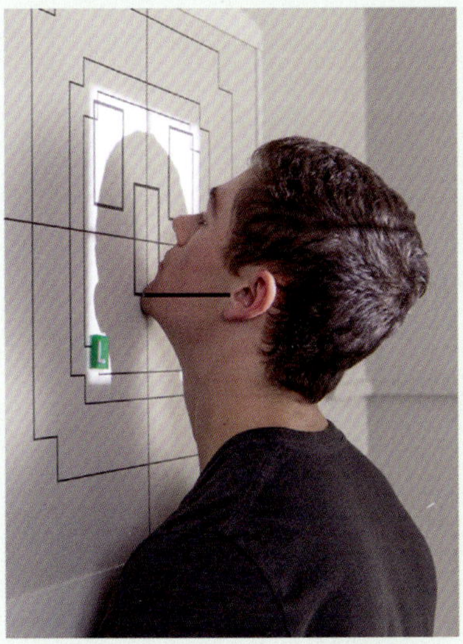	MML ⊥ MSP ⊥	Exits the acanthion	Inferior orbital margins Zygoma(s)	Petrous pyramids drop below the maxillary sinuses. Symmetrical height of the superior orbital margins and petrous pyramids indicating no tilt. Symmetrical distance between orbital oblique line and lateral margin of skull indicating no rotation.
Lateral Affected side 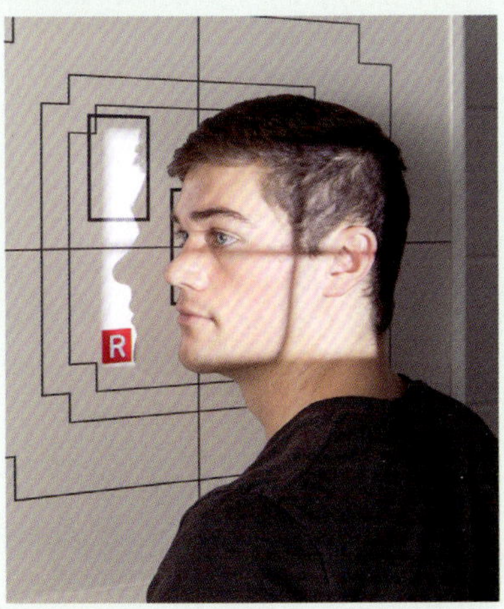	IOML II IPL ⊥ MSP II	Zygoma	Lateral orbital margin and displays anterior/posterior displacement	Greater wings of the sphenoid superimposed indicating no significant rotation. Superior orbital margins are superimposed indicating no tilt. *Good collimation may not reveal rotation and tilt locations for evaluation.*

ORBITS (TABLE 10-6)

10-6

Projection	Positioning Lines	Central Ray	Anatomy of Interest	Evaluation Criteria
PA 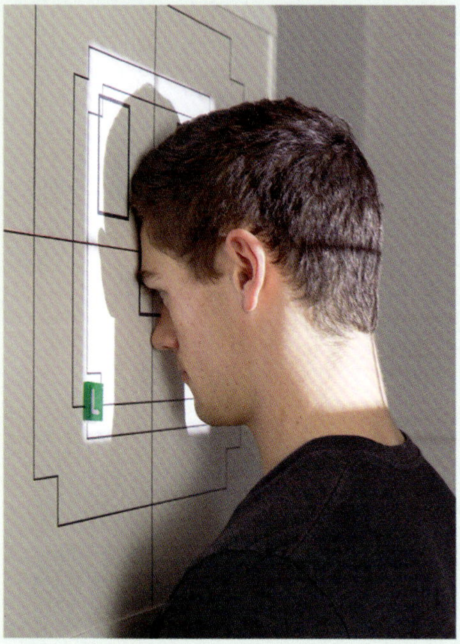 *Protocol may use the PA Axial Caldwell in the place of the PA*	OML ⊥ MSP ⊥	Exits nasion	Superior orbital margins	Petrous pyramids fills the entire orbits. Symmetrical height of the superior orbital margins and petrous pyramids indicating no tilt. Symmetrical distance between orbital oblique line and lateral margin of skull indicating no rotation.
Parietoacanthial (Waters method) 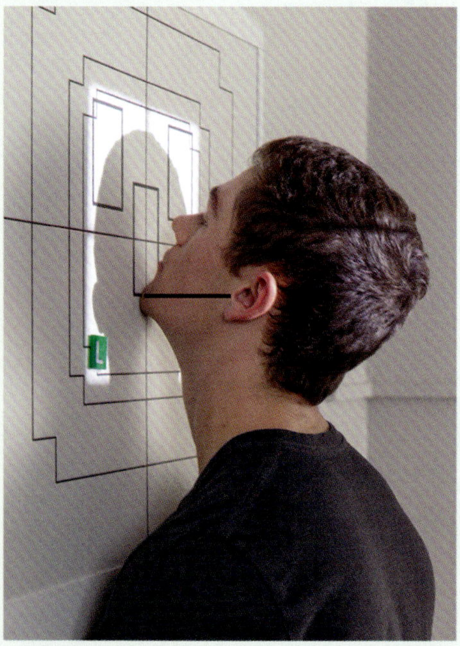	MML ⊥ MSP ⊥	Exits the acanthion	Inferior orbital margins	Petrous pyramids drop below the maxillary sinuses. Symmetrical height of the superior orbital margins and petrous pyramids indicating no tilt. Symmetrical distance between orbital oblique line and lateral margin of skull indicating no rotation. *Modified Waters method will better image the entire orbital base.*

Projection	Positioning Lines	Central Ray	Anatomy of Interest	Evaluation Criteria
Lateral Affected orbit 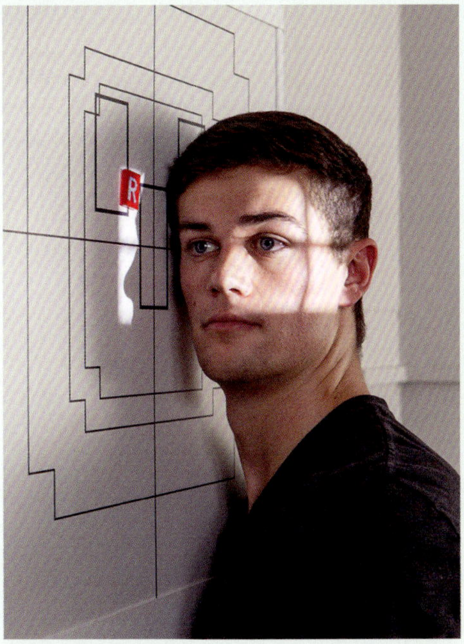	IOML ॥ IPL ⊥ MSP ॥	Midway between the EAM and outer canthus	Lateral orbital margin and displays anterior/posterior displacement	Sella turcica in profile. Greater wings of the sphenoid superimposed indicating no significant rotation. Superior orbital margins are superimposed indicating no tilt.
Parieto-orbital oblique Rhese method 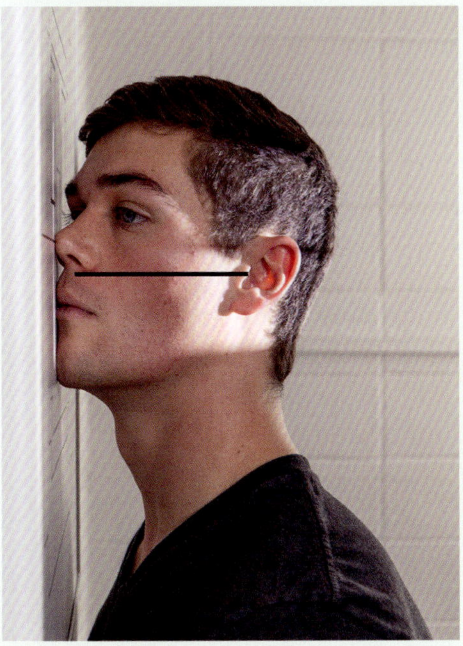	AML ⊥ MSP forms a 53° angle with the IR	1½ -2″ posterior to the upside TEA	Optic foramen in the lower outer quadrant of the orbit	Optic foramen in the LOQ indicate the MSP was correctly rotated and the AML adjusted. More or less angle of rotation will cause the optic foramen to shift medial or lateral in the orbit. Too much flexion or extension of the chin will cause the optic foramen to shift more superior or inferior in the orbit. The petrous pyramids should be below the IOM.

MANDIBLE (TABLE 10-7)

10-7

Projection	Positioning Lines	Central Ray	Anatomy of Interest	Evaluation Criteria
PA 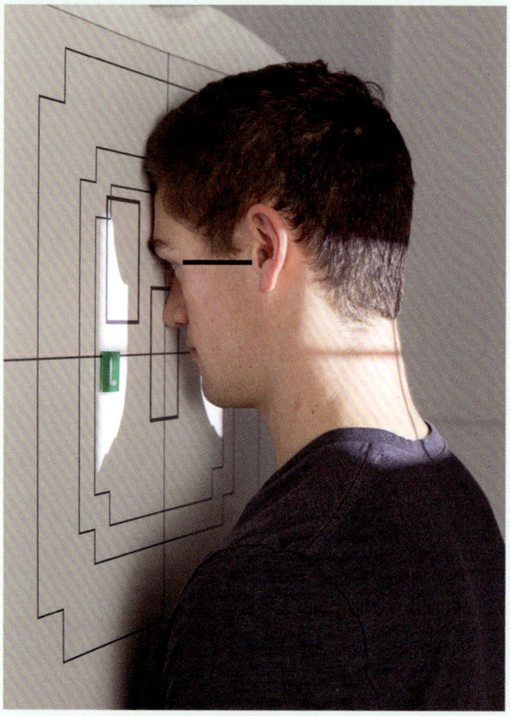	OML ⊥ MSP ⊥	Exits the junction of the lips	Mentum and mandibular bodies	Petrous pyramids fills the entire orbits. When petrous pyramids do not fill the orbits, the petrous pyramids will obscure the mandibular condyles. Symmetrical height of the superior orbital margins and petrous pyramids indicating no tilt. Symmetrical distance between orbital oblique line and lateral margin of skull indicating no rotation.
AP Axial (Towne method) 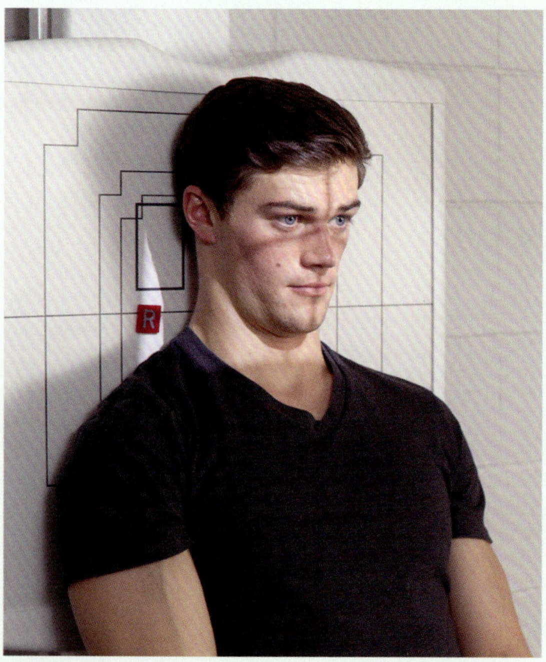	OML ⊥ IOML ⊥ MSP ⊥	OML = 30° caudal angle IOML = 37° caudal angle Enters the hairline	Mandibular rami	Dorsum sella centered within the foramen magnum. Symmetrical height of the petrous pyramids indicating no tilt. Symmetrical distance between lateral margin of foramen magnum and lateral margin of skull. Mandibular rami elongated and mentum is included.

Projection	Positioning Lines	Central Ray	Anatomy of Interest	Evaluation Criteria
Axiolateral Both Rt and Lt are acquired 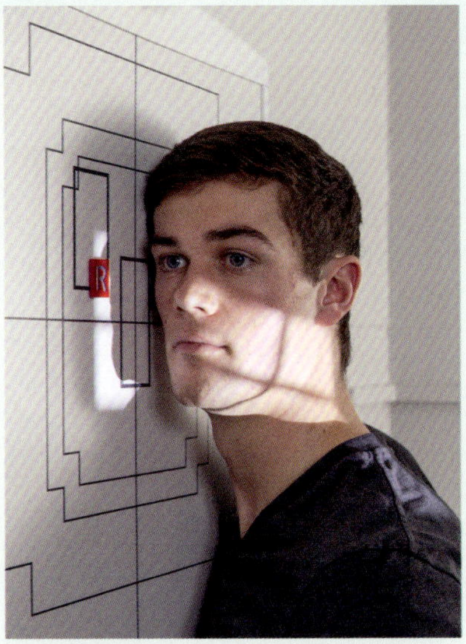 True lateral with 20°–25° cephalic angle 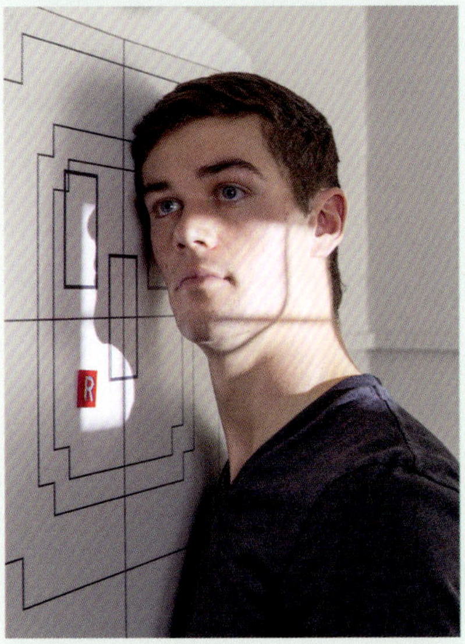 Vertex tilt with perpendicular CR	IOML II IPL ⊥ MSP II	20°–25° cephalic tube angle to enter the mid mandibular body furthest from the IR	Mandibular body closest to the IR	Mentum, mandibular angle, ramus, condyle, and condyloid process all included. The mandibular body should be free of superimposition of the opposite mandibular body. Watch for superimposition of the posterior ramus and the C-spine. Ensure TMJ is included.
SMV 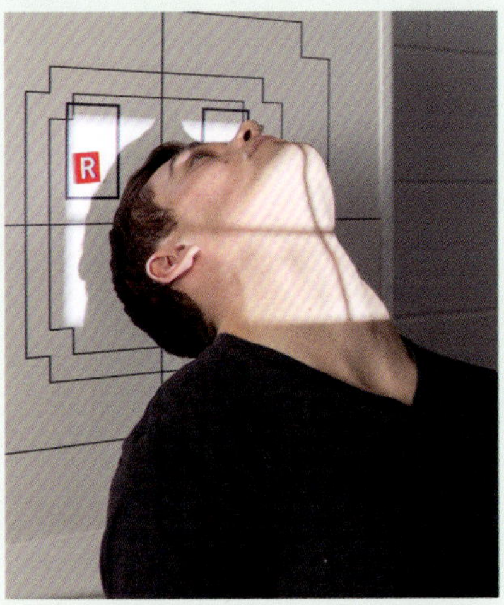	IOML II MSP ⊥	Midway between the gonions and MSP	Entire mandible	Mandibular condyles anterior to petrous pyramids indicating IOML parallel. Symmetrical height of the mandibular condyles indicating no rotation. Even distance between the mandibular condyles to the lateral margin of the skull indicating no tilt.

ZYGOMATIC ARCHES (TABLE 10-8)

10-8

Projection	Positioning Lines	Central Ray	Anatomy of Interest	Evaluation Criteria
SMV 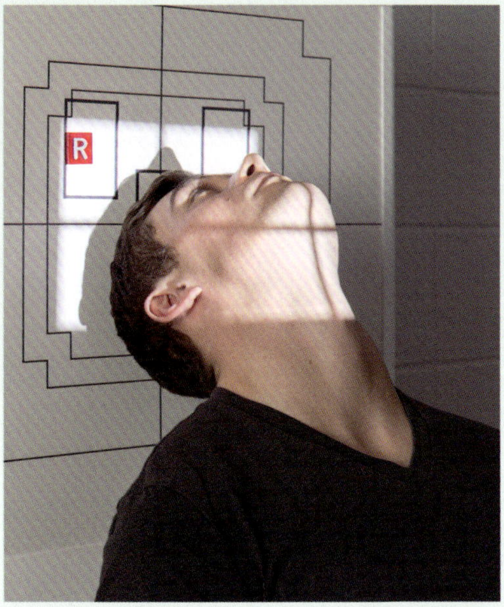	IOML II MSP ⊥	1" posterior to mandibular symphysis and MSP	Bilateral arches	*Same criteria for SMV as before but maybe difficult to appreciate due to technical settings set for arches.* Mandibular condyles anterior to Petrous pyramids indicating IOML was parallel. Symmetrical height of the mandibular condyles indicating no rotation. Even distance between the mandibular condyles to the lateral margin of the skull indicating no tilt.
AP Axial (Towne method) 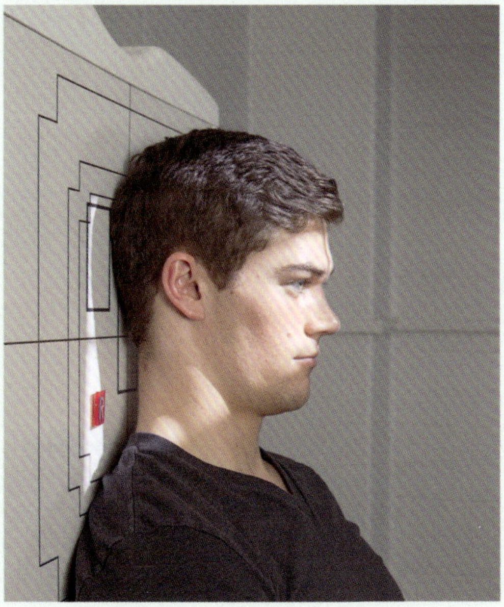	OML ⊥ IOML ⊥ MSP ⊥	OML = 30° caudal angle IOML = 37° caudal angle Enters 1" superior to glabella	Bilateral arches	*Same criteria for AP Axial as before, but maybe difficult to appreciate due to technical settings set for arches.* Dorsum sella centered within the foramen magnum. Symmetrical height of the petrous pyramids indicating no tilt. Symmetrical distance between lateral margin of foramen magnum and lateral margin of skull. Mandibular rami elongated and mentum is included.

Projection	Positioning Lines	Central Ray	Anatomy of Interest	Evaluation Criteria
Parietoacanthial (Waters method) 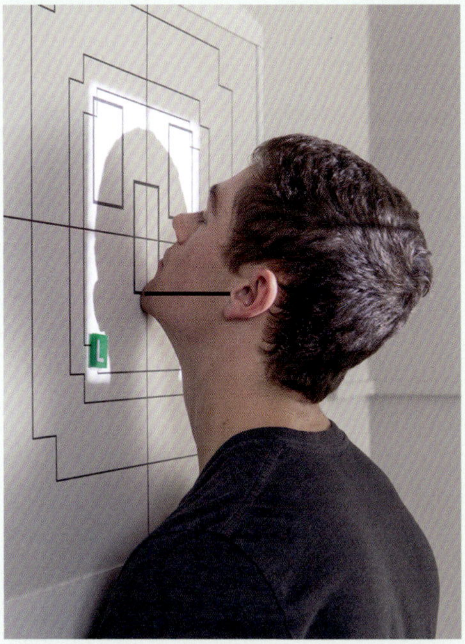	MML ⊥ MSP ⊥	Exits the acanthion	Bilateral arches	*Same criteria for Waters method before but maybe difficult to appreciate due to technical settings set for arches.* Petrous pyramids drop below the maxillary sinuses. Symmetrical height of the superior orbital margins and petrous pyramids indicating no tilt. Symmetrical distance between orbital oblique line and lateral margin of skull indicating no rotation.
Inferosuperior oblique tangential 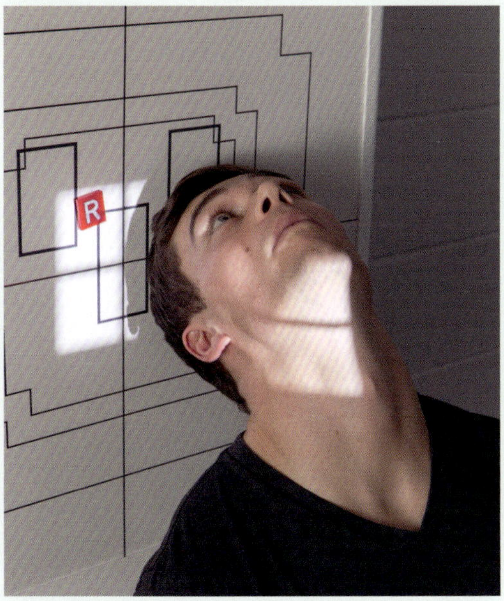	Begin with IOML II MSP ⊥ Proceed to tilt patient's chin 15° toward the affected side and rotate MSP 15° toward affected side	Tangential beam to skim the arch of interest	Unilateral arch	Unilateral arch is free of superimposition from the mandible or skull.

TEMPOROMANDIBULAR JOINTS (TABLE 10-9)

10-9

Projection	Positioning Lines	Central Ray	Anatomy of Interest	Evaluation Criteria
AP Axial (Towne method) 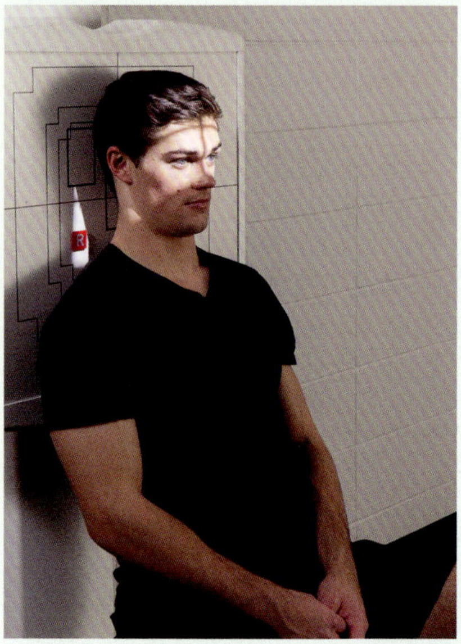 *Departments may acquire closed and open mouth positions.*	OML ⊥ IOML ⊥ MSP ⊥	OML = 35° caudal angle IOML = 42° caudal angle Enters glabella	Bilateral mandibular condyles seated within the TMJ fossa	Dorsum sella centered within the foramen magnum. Symmetrical height of the petrous pyramids indicating no tilt. Symmetrical distance between lateral margin of foramen magnum and lateral margin of skull. Mandibular rami elongated and mentum is included.
Axiolateral of affected side (place closest to the IR) Projection is taken twice. Once with mouth closed and then again with mouth open. (Schuller method) 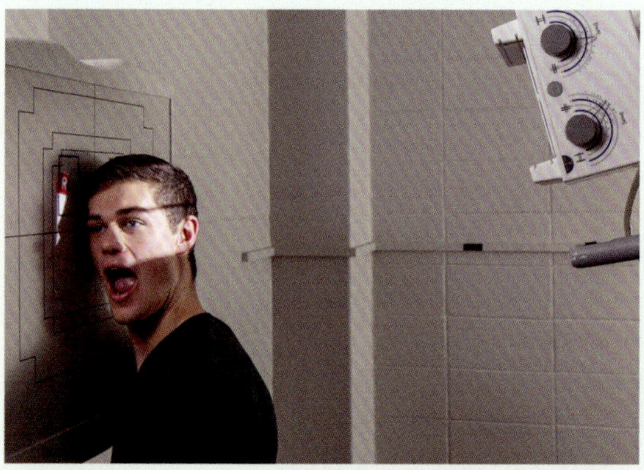 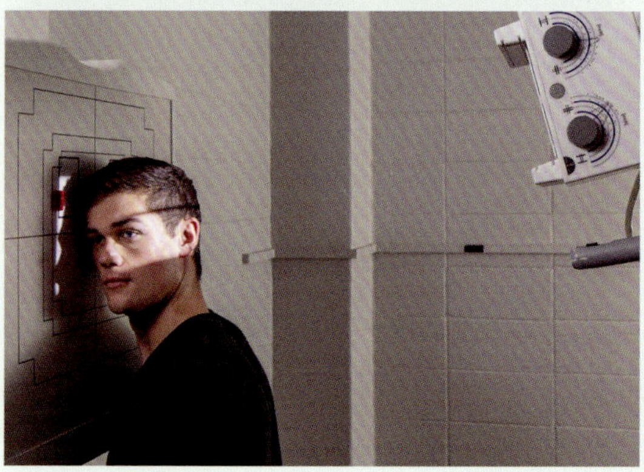	IOML ‖ IPL ⊥ MSP ‖	25°–30° caudal angle to enter 2" superior to upside EAM and slightly anterior to upside EAM	Closed mouth demonstrates the mandibular condyle within the TMJ fossa. Open mouth demonstrates the mandibular condyle anteriorly within the fossa	TM Joint is evaluated for range of motion between the closed and open mouth projections. True lateral representation of the skull and TMJ.

Projection	Positioning Lines	Central Ray	Anatomy of Interest	Evaluation Criteria
Axiolateral oblique of affected side (place closest to the IR) Projection is taken twice. Once with mouth closed and then again with mouth open. (Modified Law method)	From a true lateral skull position, rotate the MSP 15° toward the IR	15° caudal to enter 2" above the upside EAM	Closed mouth demonstrates the mandibular condyle within the TMJ fossa. Open mouth demonstrates the mandibular condyle anteriorly within the fossa	Temporomandibular Joint is evaluated for range of motion between the closed and open mouth projections. TMJ of interest is free of superimposition from opposite TMJ. TMJ is free of cervical spine superimposition.

THE FINAL STEP IMAGE REVIEW

The technologist must take time to review acquired images to ensure image quality is acceptable. The technologist must have the knowledge within their role to not only acquire the images and care for the patient but to also know how to review the images to ensure diagnostic quality has been attained. In certain instances, a projection may need to be repeated. This is to the discretion of the radiologic technologist. The technologist must acquire images that are of diagnostic quality for the radiologist to interpret the images. Technologists must be aware of acceptance standards established by the radiologist and department. The technologist should review each image for the following.

1. Is all of the necessary anatomy included on the image?
   - Was the central ray properly directed to the part? An "X" can be drawn to intersect within the collimated exposure field to determine if the central ray (CR) was directed to the correct location.
   - Was essential anatomy in the collimated exposure field?
   - Is the area free of artifact(s)?
2. Is the anatomy well demonstrated?
   - Did the technologist properly position the patient to adequately demonstrate the anatomy?
   - Can the technologist recognize the anatomy best demonstrated with the use of different projections?
3. Does the image reflect proper image markings?
   - Did the technologist correctly use a lead marker to identify the right or left side?
   - What additional markings or annotations could be helpful to the radiologist interpreting the exam?
   - Is the image properly displayed?
4. Does the image prove to be technically acceptable?
   - Does the exposure index fall within acceptable range for the operating system? Images that are technically insufficient may appear of good quality if just slightly insufficient or "mottled or pixelated" if severely insufficient. Images that are underexposed according to the exposure index for the operating system should be repeated. Images that appear beyond optimal exposure due to higher technique may display high quality, but the patient has received excessive radiation dose.

Zenker's Diverticulum: A weakening of the wall in the proximal esophagus resulting in a large outpouching that causes the patient to experience symptoms such as dysphagia and regurgitation of food or fluid back into the oral cavity.

Emesis: Vomiting. Vomiting with the presence of blood is hematemesis.

Gastritis: Inflammation of the stomach mucosa. Acute gastritis—sudden onset. Chronic gastritis—long-term condition (Fig. 11-4)

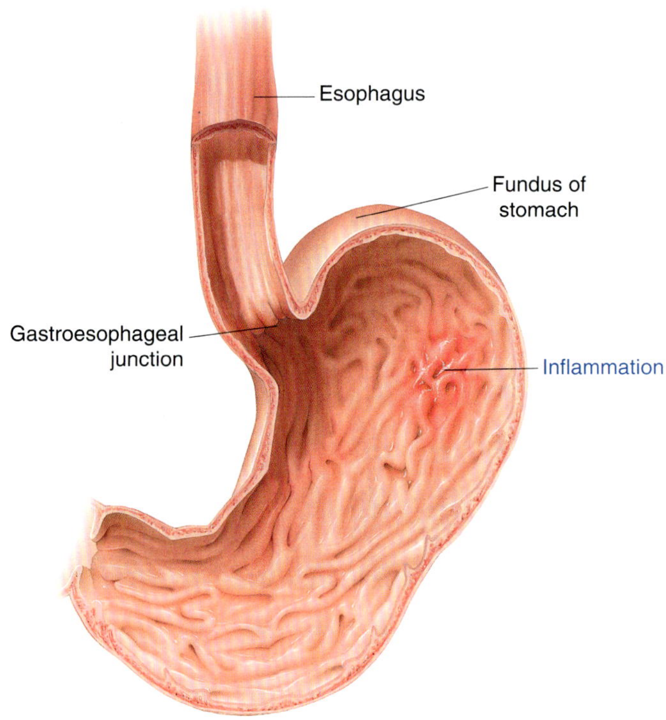

11-4 Gastritis.

Hiatal Hernia: A defect in the diaphragm allows a portion of the stomach to move into the thoracic cavity. A hernia may be demonstrated during the GI procedure by altering the patient into a Trendelenburg position from a supine position or by having the patient perform the Valsalva maneuver (Figs. 11-5 and 11-6).

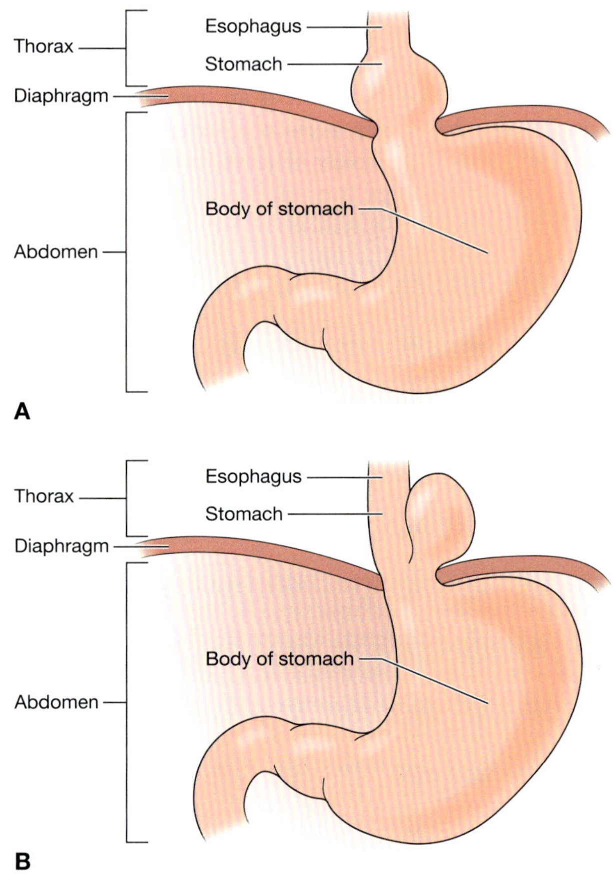

11-5 **A:** Sliding hiatal hernia. **B:** Paraesophageal hiatal hernia.

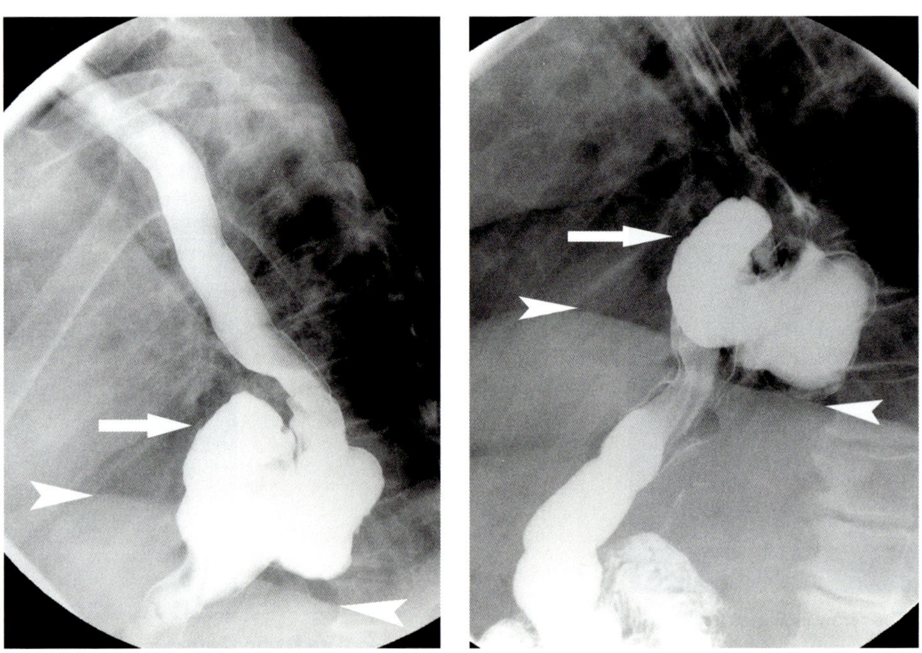

11-6 Arrowheads denote the diaphragm. Large arrow reveals a portion of the stomach above the diaphragm.

Hypertrophic Pyloric Stenosis: The sphincter muscle at the pyloric orifice is underdeveloped creating an obstruction. This affects infants (males more often than females) and clinically presents with abdominal distention and projectile vomiting after feeding (Fig. 11-7).

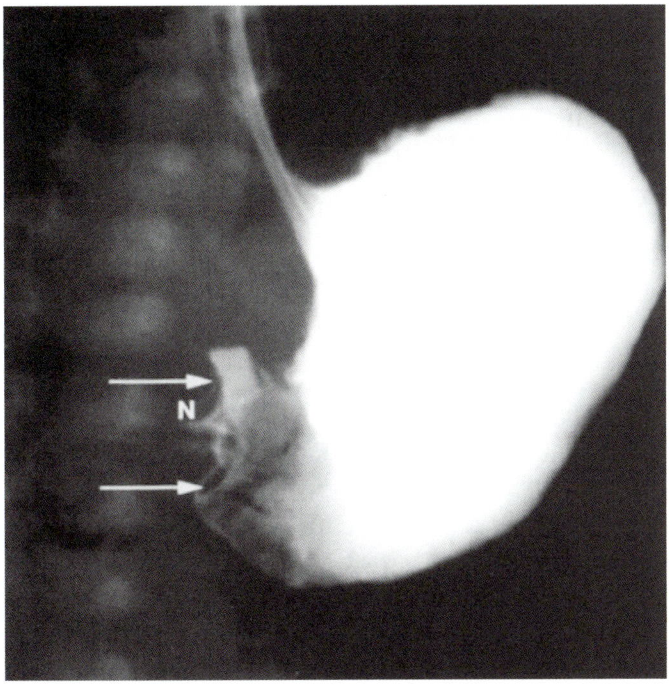

11-7 N represents pyloric narrowing with a dilated stomach antrum consistent with hypertrophic pyloric stenosis.

Ulcer: Damage to the mucosa that can further erode the muscular layer. This can be a result of gastric acids and the use of nonsteroidal antiinflammatory drugs (NSAIDs). A majority of ulcers are benign. Ulcers may occur within the stomach or duodenum. Perforation or hemorrhage is of concern (Fig. 11-8).

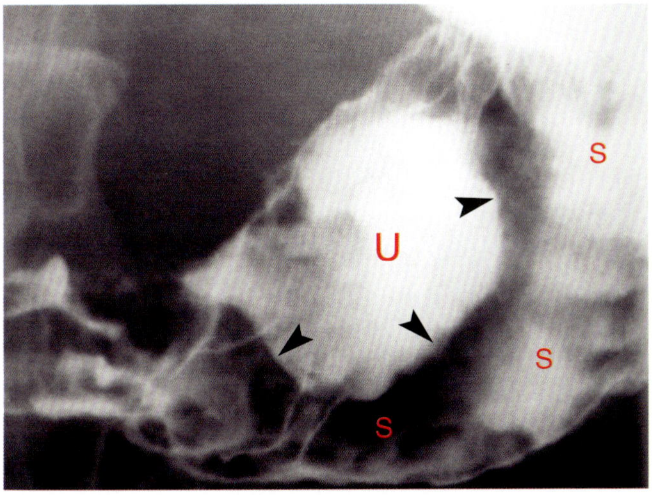

11-8 U denotes the center of a gastric ulcer bordered by arrows.

GERD: Gastroesophageal reflux is chronic disease that affects the distal esophagus. Acid reflux clinically presents with heartburn and epigastric pain (Fig. 11-9).

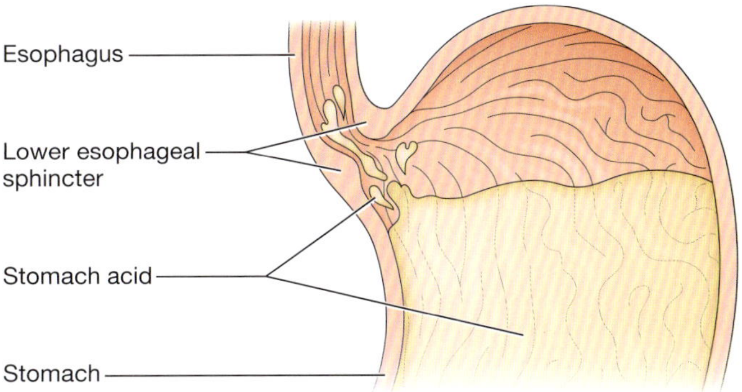

11-9 GERD.

Bezoar: Indigestible material, (certain foods, hair, fingernails) that is collected in the stomach, is unable to pass through the pyloric orifice. The patient may experience a full feeling even before having a meal. The presence of a bezoar can potentially lead to chronic gastritis or obstruction if left untreated (Fig. 1-10).

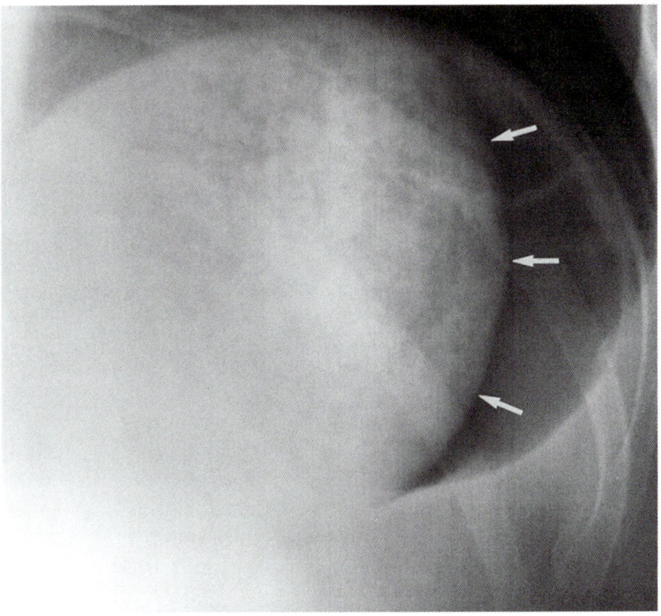

11-10 Bezoar.

Crohn Disease: A form of regional enteritis that chronically inflames the small intestines, specifically the terminal ileum, and may advance into the cecum. The bowel mucosa will thicken and potentially narrow the bowel lumen (Fig. 11-11).

Celiac Disease: A malabsorption syndrome in which the GI tract is unable to absorb particular nutrients. A sensitivity is developed to gluten present in cereal grains.

Ileus: Obstruction that presents with abdominal distention and appearance of dilated bowel loops on a radiograph. The obstruction could also be a result of bowel inactivity (adynamic ileus), associated with postsurgical patients or with certain medications (Fig. 11-12).

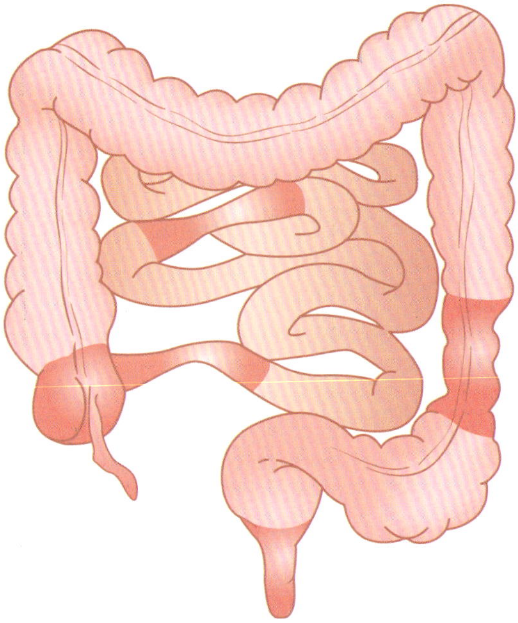

11-11 Crohn disease.

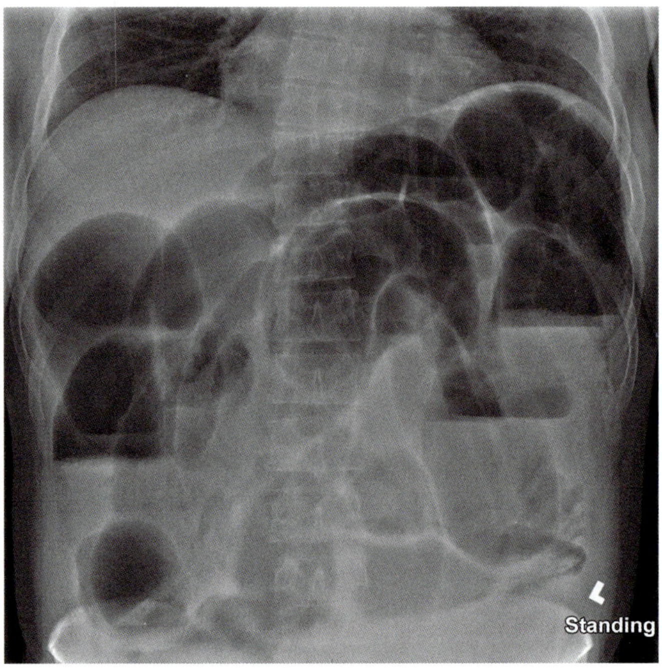

11-12 Ileus.

Colitis: Inflammation of the colon. One cause may stem from a case of regional enteritis seen in the terminal ileum. Ulcerative colitis is an autoimmune disease that affects the rectosigmoid portion (majority) or the ileum. Patients with long-term ulcerative colitis may be at risk for the development of colon cancer (Fig. 11-13).

Diverticulum: Weakening of the wall resulting in an outpouching. Diverticulum can be present within the stomach, small intestines, or large intestines. The condition of diverticulosis in the large bowel is the presence of many diverticula. Diverticulitis is the inflammatory condition of the diverticulum (Fig. 11-14).

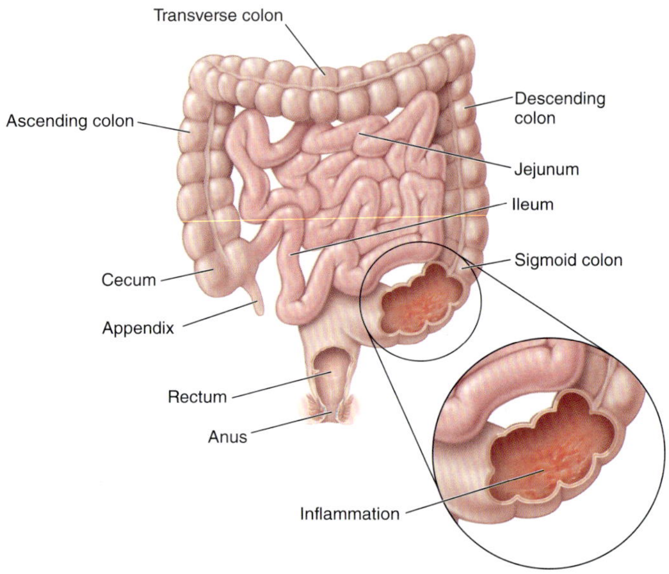

11-13 Colitis.

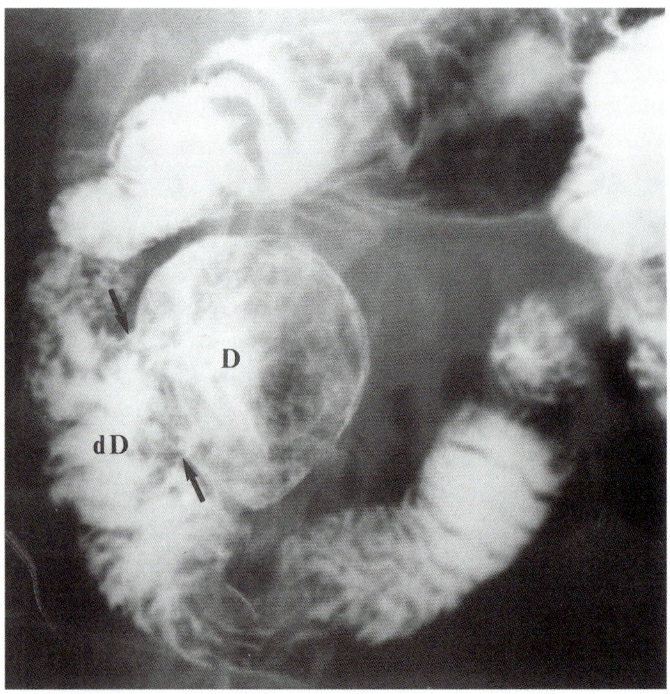

11-14 Diverticulum.

Volvulus: Twisting of bowel that may cause a mechanical obstruction. It is more commonly seen within the most mobile segment of bowel which is often the sigmoid portion of the colon, but could occur elsewhere as well. This condition can also affect the small bowel (Fig. 11-15).

Intussusception: A telescoping effect of the bowel when a more proximal portion of bowel projects into a more distal portion. More commonly seen in children and often is a spontaneous event that causes an obstruction. The barium enema could serve as a diagnostic and therapeutic tool for this condition. This condition can also affect the small bowel (Fig. 11-16).

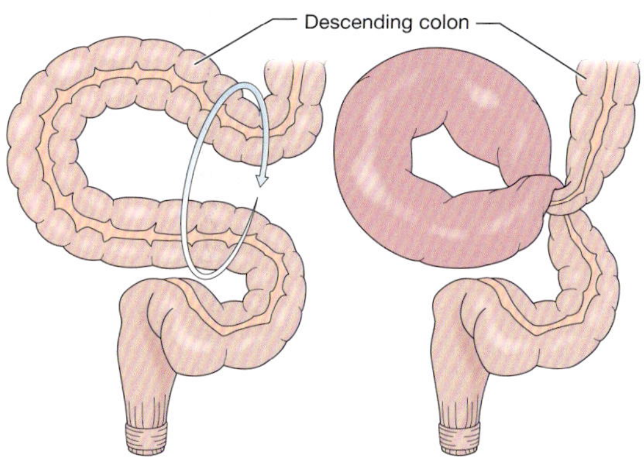

11-15 Volvulus.

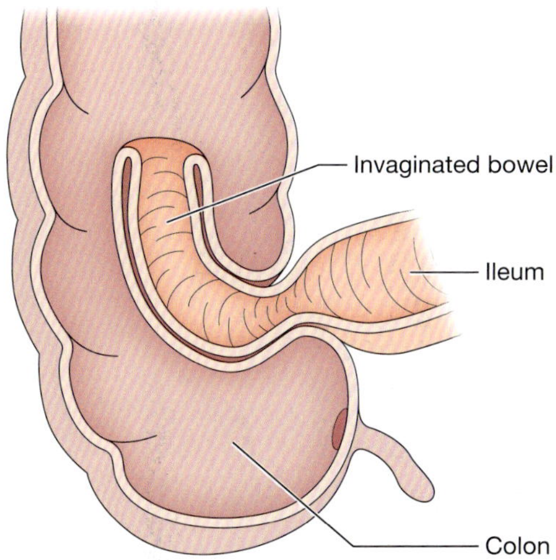

11-16 Intussusception.

Polyp: A form of a neoplasm that is an internal sac (unlike diverticulum that project outward) that has a pedicle vascular supply. Although frequently benign, they do have malignant potential (Figs. 11-17 and 11-18).

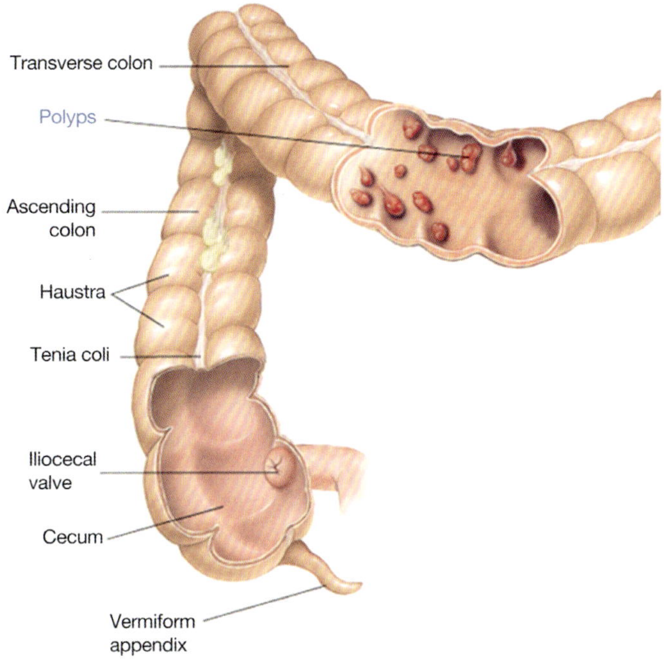

11-17 Polyps.

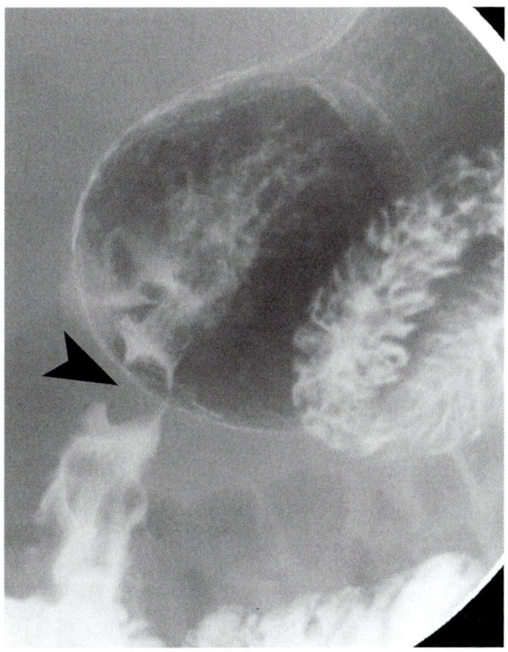

11-18 Filling defect within the duodenum reveals a polyp (arrow).

IMAGING CONSIDERATIONS

Patient Dress

Patient will need to remove clothing and jewelry from the area of ordered imaging. Elastic bands in pants, while not possessing metal components, can create distracting skin lines and creases on the image. Female patients should be instructed to remove their bra. The patient should be dressed in a gown. It should be realized that placement of GI organs cannot always be assumed by just looking at the patient, so removal of all clothing that could interfere with visualization is recommended. Additionally, consider that by changing the patient into a gown, this will allow the patient to leave the facility in their own dry clothes if there were an incident of a barium spill or soiling during the procedure.

Artifacts

Artifacts are unwanted objects that appear on the image superimposing pertinent anatomy. This includes snaps, buttons, bras, and jewelry. Many times, GI exams are scheduled outpatient procedures, so it is essential to ensure the patient is properly dressed into a hospital gown. With inpatient procedures, other artifacts that may appear could be IV lines, ECG patches, oxygen tubing, or safety pins that may secure a line to the patient's gown. The radiographer should assess the patient's lines and tubing, pins, snaps, and try to reposition to avoid obscuring GI anatomy.

Patient Position

Supine—patient lies on their posterior surface.

Prone—patient lies on their anterior surface.

Recumbent Lateral—patient lies on their right or left lateral surface.

Upright—position will allow demonstration of abdominal air–fluid levels (Fig. 11-19).

Decubitus—serves to demonstrate air–fluid levels. Left or right lateral decubitus positions and ventral decubitus positions are used in double-contrast imaging of the large intestines (Figs. 11-20 and 11-21).

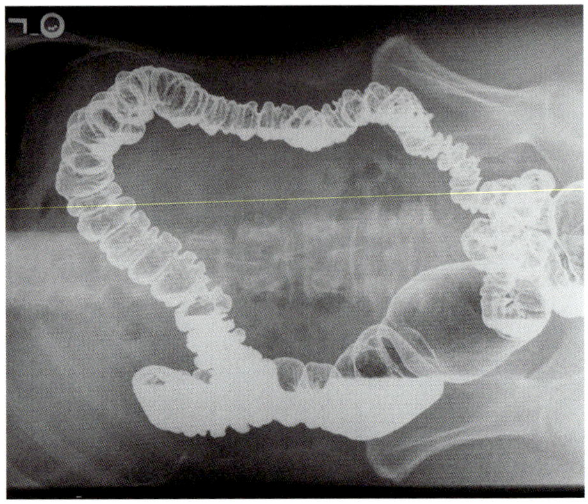

11-20 Right lateral decubitus—double-contrast barium enema.

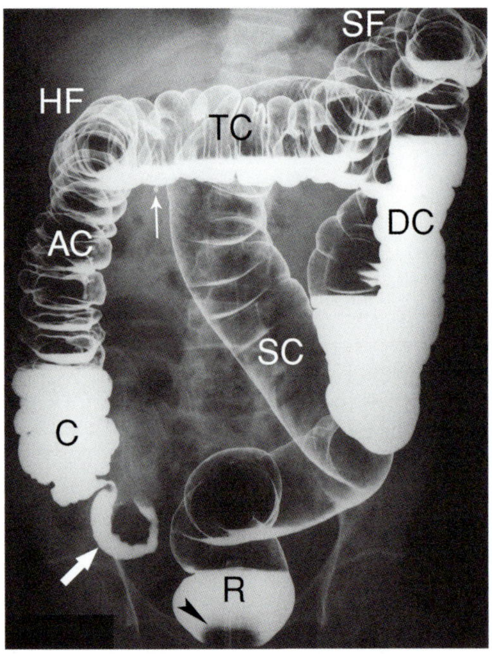

11-19 Double-contrast barium enema—upright position. C, cecum; AC, ascending colon; HF, hepatic flexure; TC, transverse colon; SF, splenic flexure; DC, descending colon; SC, sigmoid colon; R, rectum; white arrow, appendix; black arrow, air-filled balloon on enema tip. Small white arrow, diverticulum.

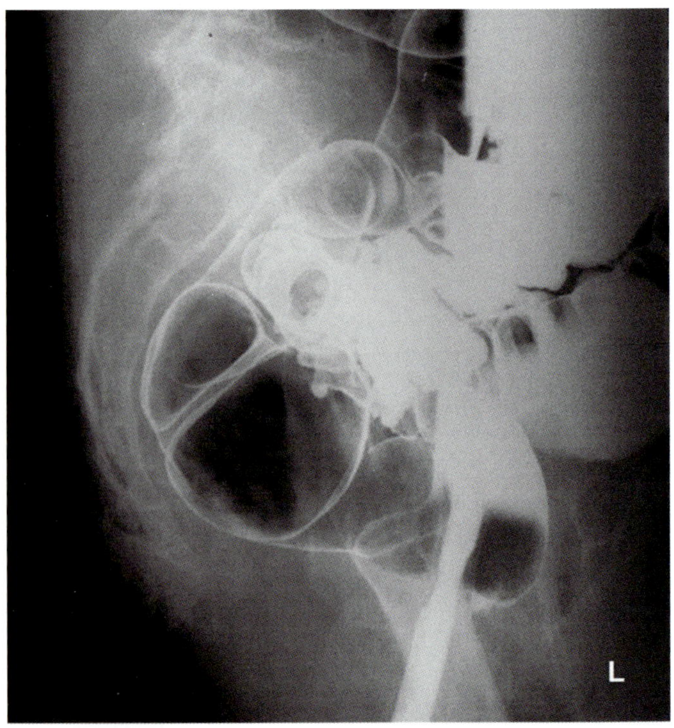

11-21 Double-contrast barium enema—ventral decubitus.

Ambulatory Patient Imaging

An ambulatory patient is one who can maneuver themselves and bear weight with little to no assistance. Ambulatory patients may be able to move between recumbent and upright positions often required for GI imaging, but may still need assistance from the radiologic technologist to expedite the procedural requests of the radiologist.

Nonambulatory Patient Imaging

Patients unable to ambulate and bear weight will need to have exam protocols modified. A patient, who cannot assume an upright position, may not be a candidate for a double-contrast imaging procedure. It is not safe to attempt to position a patient into an upright position if they cannot support their own weight. Certain exams of the GI system will require different involvement levels of the radiologic technologist with the patient, ultimately the technologist should aim for delivery of the highest degree of patient care.

Pediatric Imaging

Pediatric patients may undergo GI exams that may use barium sulfate as prepared for adult patients, but lessened in amount/volume used. Patients must be prepped similarly to adults for a diagnostic outcome to be achieved. Exams that require fasting will be lessened compared to adult patients. Infants for upper GI studies will ingest barium through a bottle. If retrograde barium is necessary, then modification to the enema tip will be sought. With infant patients and toddlers, silicone catheters will be used to introduce contrast rectally. The decision on rectal tip size for an older pediatric patient may be based on their overall size.

Geriatric Imaging

With age, naturally, these patients will experience a loss of hearing, vision, mobility, and reactive times. The technologist needs to be aware of the assistive aids a patient has and accommodate them. Geriatric patients will need assistance getting on and off the table but also with assuming the various body positions a GI procedure entails. Geriatric patients will experience a loss of physical security with the potential fear to fall. This patient population requires the technologist to be more hands-on with the patient, explain the specifics and requirements of the exam in a manner that allows them to process and respond, and patiently assist them with exam positions.

Obese Patient Imaging

Scout and postprocedural imaging will require the use of multiple images to overlap high and low on the abdomen and in other cases more of a four-quadrant approach if necessary. It is key that the technologist be observant during the fluoroscopic components of the exam while performed with the radiologist. During this time, the technologist should identify where the major anatomy of interest lies and to correlative landmarks that may be helpful for centering.

Patient Imaging

Gastrointestinal tract imaging will depend on physician orders. The imaging approach will be influenced by patient ability and the radiologist's decision on contrast use.

Projection(s)

- AP (anteroposterior) or PA (posteroanterior) projection with the patient recumbent in position
- Lateral with the patient recumbent or upright in position
- AP with the patient upright in position
- AP or PA with the patient in a decubitus position
- AP or PA Oblique with the patient recumbent or upright in position

Contrast Media Preparation

Contrast media or the combination of two types of media are needed to visualize the shape, location, mucosal lining, and function of the GI tract. To best image the mucosal lining, a double-contrast effect is created by combining radiopaque and radiolucent contrast mediums. Barium sulfate is the most common form of radiopaque contrast. It is nontoxic, as there are few known to have a sensitivity to this purer form of contrast and it is eliminated naturally from the body's system days after use. With the high atomic number of barium sulfate, a higher kilovoltage is necessary. The radiolucent form of contrast is typically air or carbon dioxide crystals. Air or carbon dioxide will distend the organ and allow the barium sulfate to adhere to the mucosal lining.

Barium Sulfate

Oral Contrast

Different consistencies of barium are used for oral ingestion. The thickest type will be applied to a spoon for the patient to ingest. This consistency represents a bolus of food (Fig. 11-22). There are also two different consistencies of liquid barium. A higher density, thicker barium, similar to a milkshake, uses a ratio of water mixed with the barium sulfate powder (Fig. 11-23). This thicker barium cannot be ingested through a straw and the

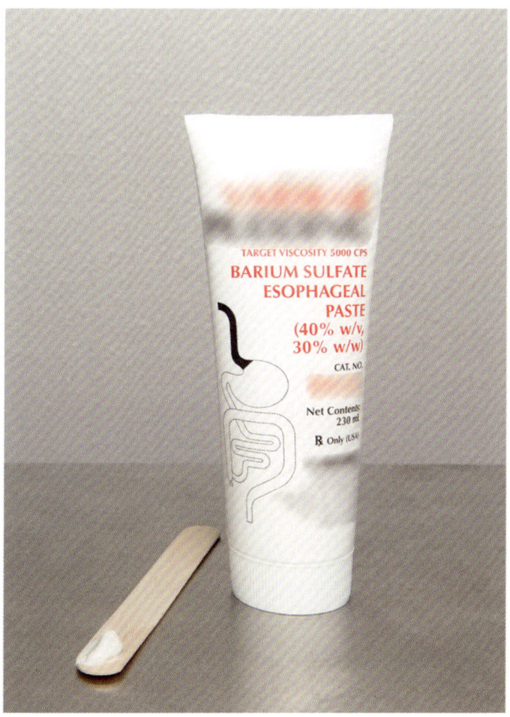

11-22 Barium paste.

patient needs to be in an upright position to drink it from a cup (Figs. 11.23). The barium sulfate powder will not dissolve in the water when mixed and will settle and separate if allowed to sit for a period of time. A thinner form of ingestible barium may come in a premixed jug and will be marked for oral ingestion. This thinner barium can be ingested with the use of a straw; therefore, it can be administered to the patient while in recumbent positions, but also upright if needed or requested Figs. 11-24

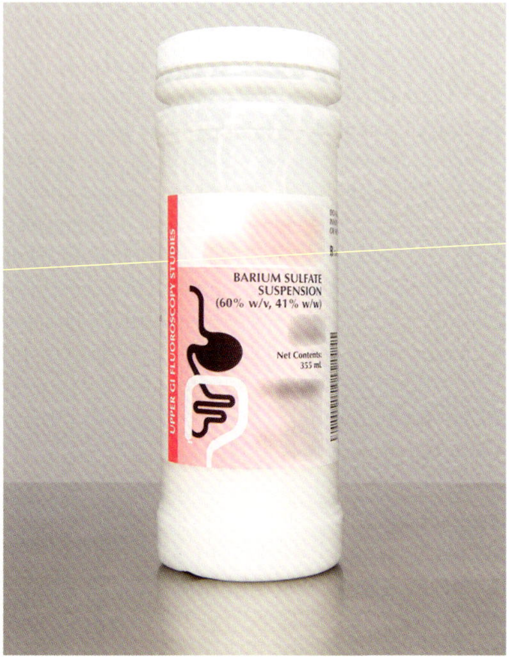

11-23 Thicker oral contrast powder—add water to dilute to radiologist preference.

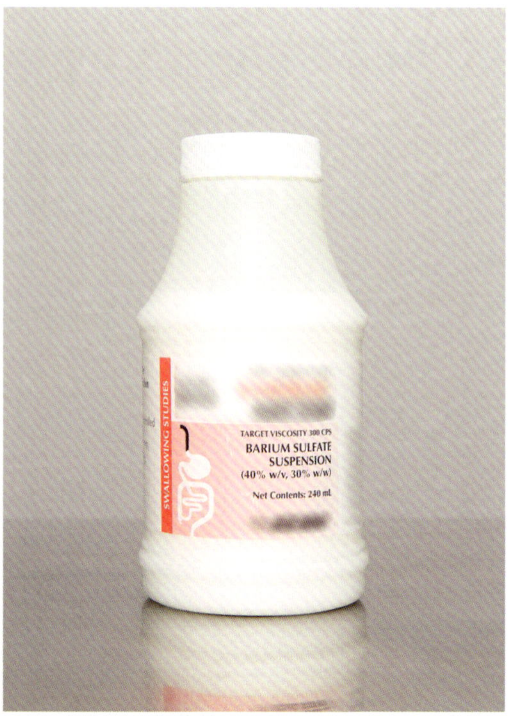

11-24 Thinner oral contrast solution.

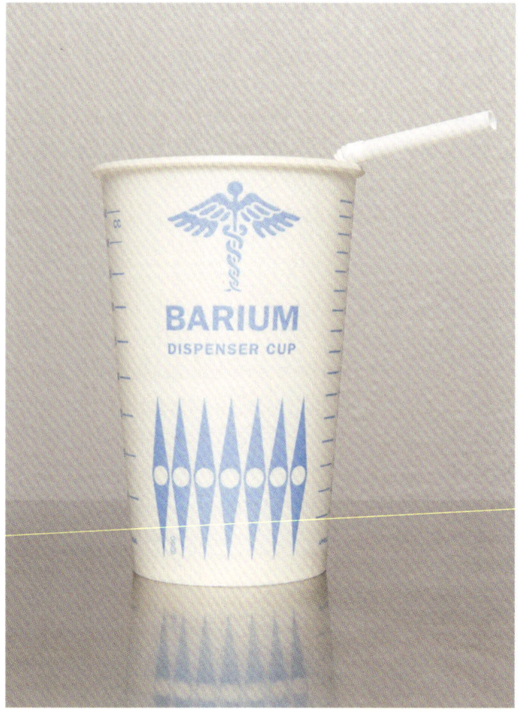

11-25 Thin oral contrast solution can be administered with a straw.

and 11-25. It is not uncommon for the patient to ingest anywhere from 8 to 16 oz of this barium consistency, and it is more tolerable if the substance is served cold.

Retrograde Contrast

Barium sulfate is also used to retrograde fill the large intestines. The amount and consistency of this barium sulfate are dependent upon if the study is a single or double-contrast study. If a single-contrast study is ordered, it is possible that 1,500–2,000 cc of barium sulfate is prepared with tepid water temperature and introduced into the colon (Fig. 11-26). A single-contrast study will be able to evaluate large bowel obstruction, form, and size. In some cases, a single-contrast study will serve as a therapeutic means for a patient's condition, such as with large bowel obstruction. If a double-contrast study is ordered, it is possible that 600–800 cc is prepared with water and introduced into the colon along with air (Fig. 11-27). Again, the air will distend the colon and then the more concentrated barium is introduced to coat only the lining of the mucosa, not to fill the entire colon lumen. Regardless, if the study is single or double contrast, the barium sulfate is recommended predominantly to be mixed with "tepid" temperature water. A tepid temperature means the temperature of the solution is warm or lukewarm and it is vital to avoid scalding the mucosa, which could be the risk of using hot water. Colonic spasms, may result when barium sulfate is mixed with cold water and introduced into the colon.

Carbon Dioxide/Air

Air, with a low atomic number and easily penetrated, is introduced into a cavity to create distention of stomach, small intestine, or large intestine. Patients are expected to have some

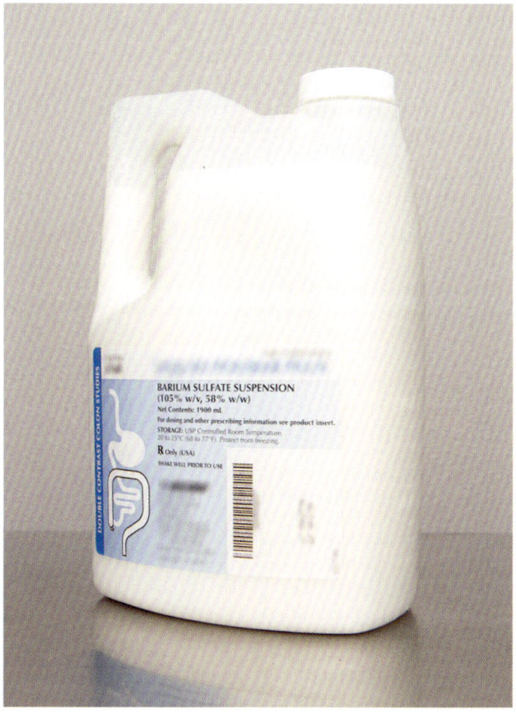

11-26 Barium contrast for a double-contrast study is a liquid and comes in a jug. Barium contrast for a single-contrast study comes as a powder already in the barium bag.

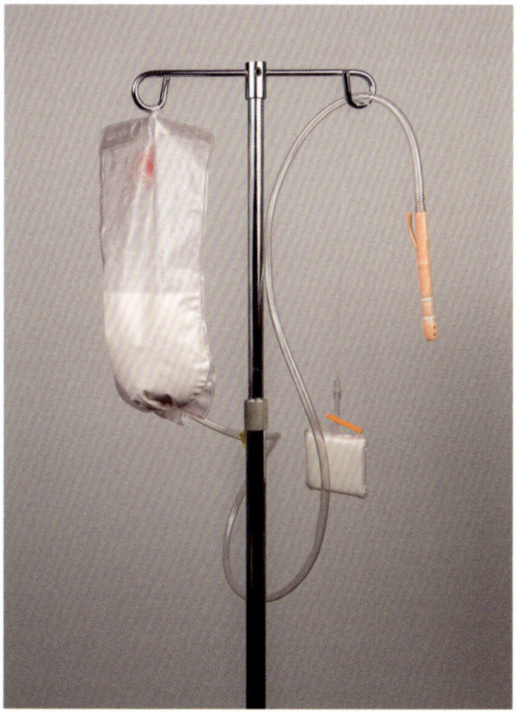

11-27 Barium contrast solution prepared.

discomfort with the organ distention, but should not be overly painful. Carbon dioxide may be introduced into the stomach by having the patient ingest the carbon dioxide crystals with a small amount of water (Fig. 11-28). When in the small or large intestine, air is introduced into the cavity through a catheter placed into the small bowel or through an enema tip for the large bowel (Fig. 11-29).

Iodinated Contrast Media

Iodinated contrast media is administered to a patient who may have a possible organ perforation. Iodinated contrast media is water-soluble contrast and can be reabsorbed by the body if an instance of perforation is present, unlike barium sulfate (Fig. 11-30). Iodinated contrast media has a lower atomic number than barium sulfate and the radiographic appearance will not offer the same diagnostic quality as barium sulfate. In cases of suspected perforation, this contrast media should not be combined with a radiolucent contrast to form a double-contrast effect. An organ with suspected perforation should not be purposely overdistended with air. Finally, it is important to screen the patient with a questionnaire to identify any risk factors. Patients identified to have a sensitivity to iodine should not receive iodinated contrast orally or intravenously.

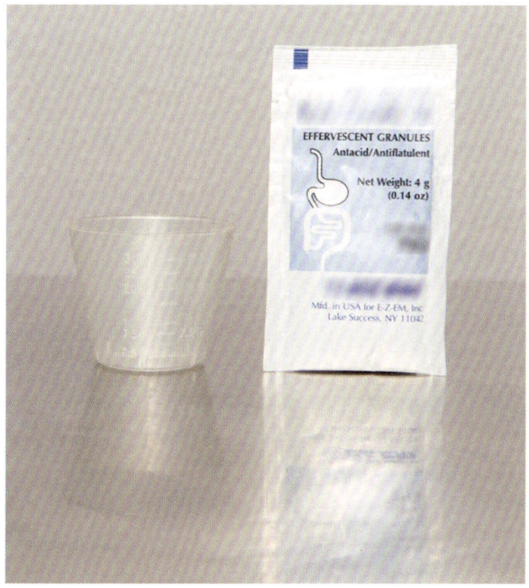

11-28 Carbon dioxide crystals.

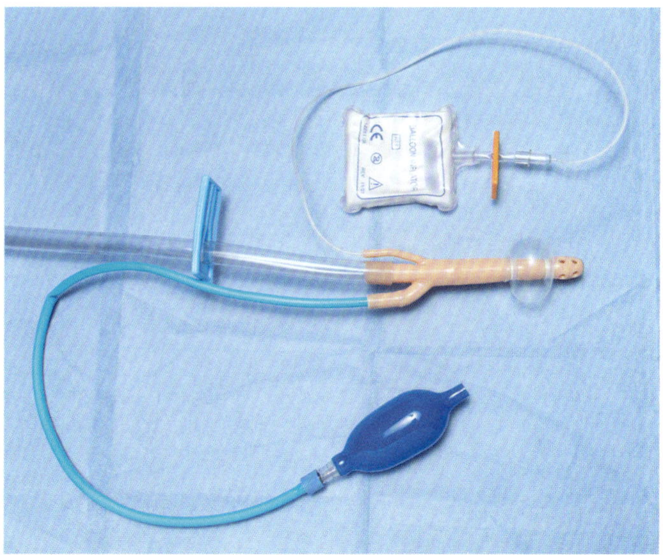

11-29 Double-contrast enema tip. Blue port allows for air to be introduced into the colon.

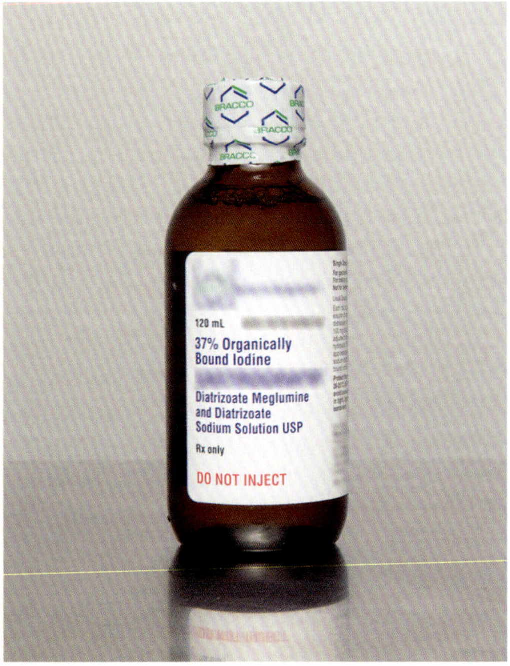

11-30 Water-soluble iodinated contrast.

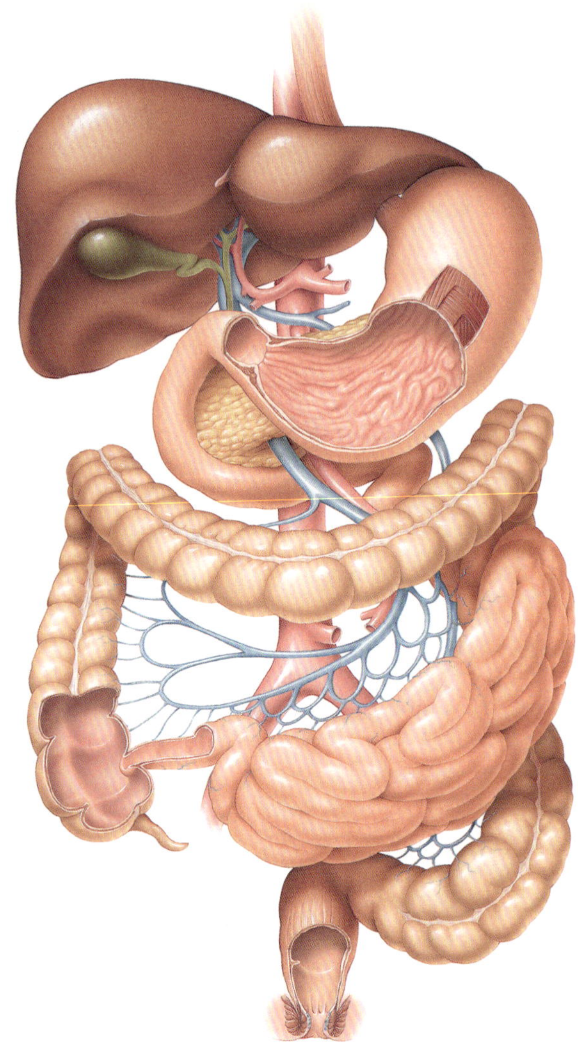

11-31 Alimentary canal.

ANATOMY

The digestive system involves the movements of food through the alimentary canal paired with the assistance the accessory organs provide. The alimentary canal begins with the mouth and continues with pharynx, esophagus, stomach, small intestines, large intestines, and terminates with the anus (Fig. 11-31). The accessory organs of the liver, gallbladder, and pancreas (discussed in Chapter 4), and salivary glands assist with the digestive process through the release of digestive enzymes (Fig. 11-32). The digestive system functions to take food in, digest it, absorb essential nutrients, and to eliminate waste.

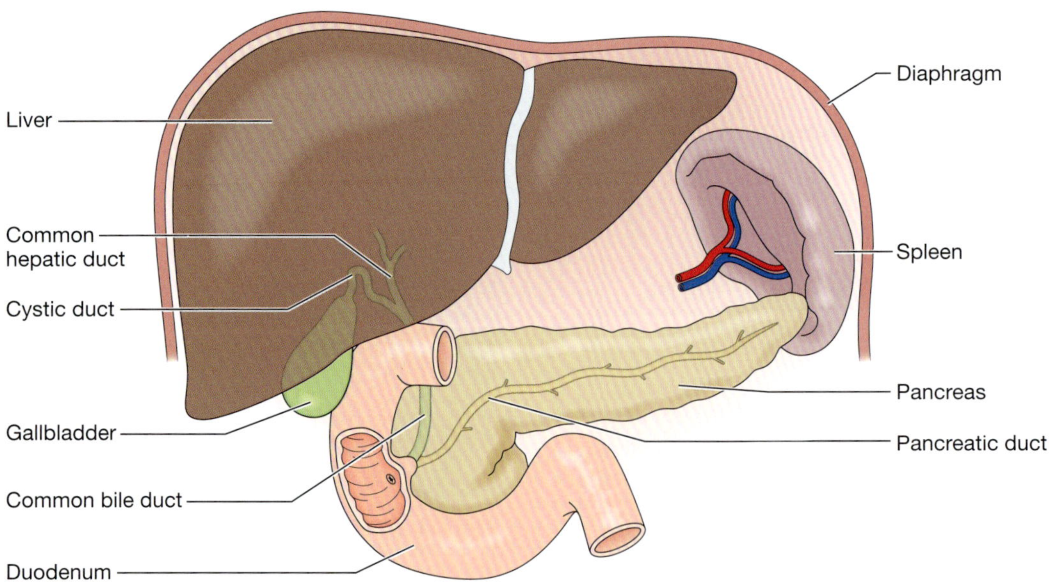

11-32 Accessory organs.

GASTROINTESTINAL SYSTEM

Oral Cavity and Esophagus

The digestive system begins with the mouth or the oral cavity. As food is brought into the mouth, the mechanical chewing motion or *mastication* begins to break down the food particles. The three pairs of salivary glands (sublingual, parotid, and submandibular) secrete chemical enzymes to begin the breakdown of food and mucus is secreted to form a bolus of food (Fig. 11-33). With the event of swallowing or *deglutition*, the uvula (soft palate/tissue that extends off the posterior border of the hard palate), flips up to seal off the nasopharynx, and the epiglottis flips down to seal off the trachea to prevent aspiration into the proper respiratory system (Fig. 11-34). The oropharynx division is positioned in between the uvula and epiglottis (Fig. 11-35). The esophagus begins at cervical vertebra, C5/6, passes through the mediastinum, and projects through the left hemidiaphragm at about 10th thoracic vertebra level, T10. The esophagus is positioned posterior to the trachea. When empty, the esophagus, which is a hollow tube, collapses. With deglutition, fluid passes easily to the stomach with gravity and a solid bolus will rely on the assistance of gravity and peristaltic action of the muscular walls to propel food toward the stomach (Fig. 11-36).

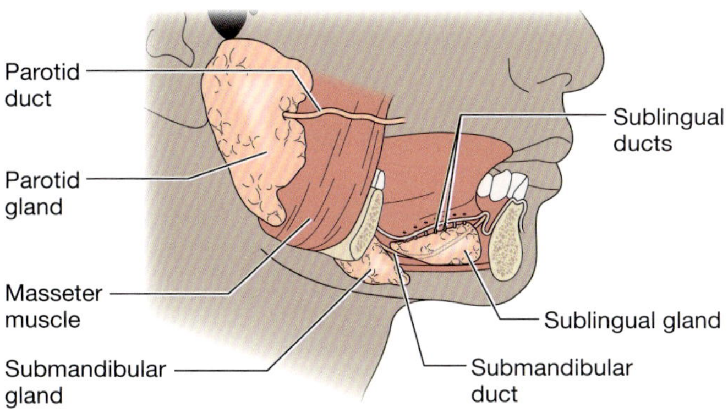

11-33 Salivary glands.

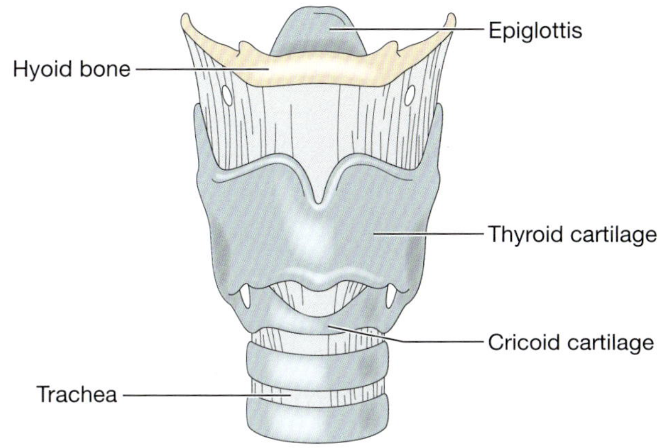

11-34 Posterior view of larynx, which is suspended from the hyoid bone. Note the epiglottis.

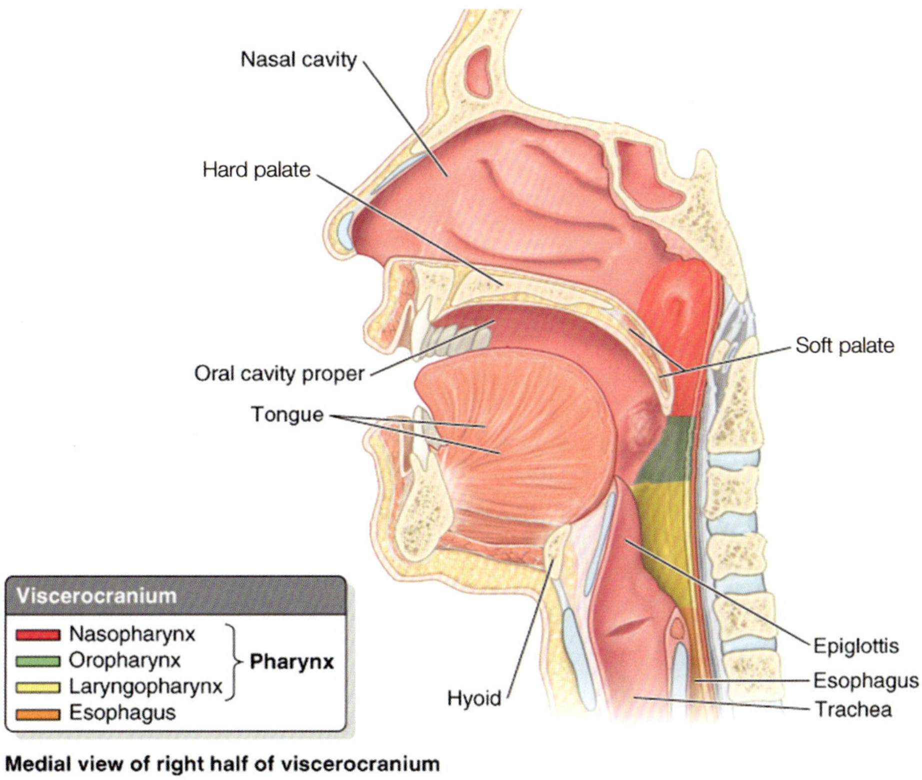

11-35 Oral cavity and divisions of the pharynx.

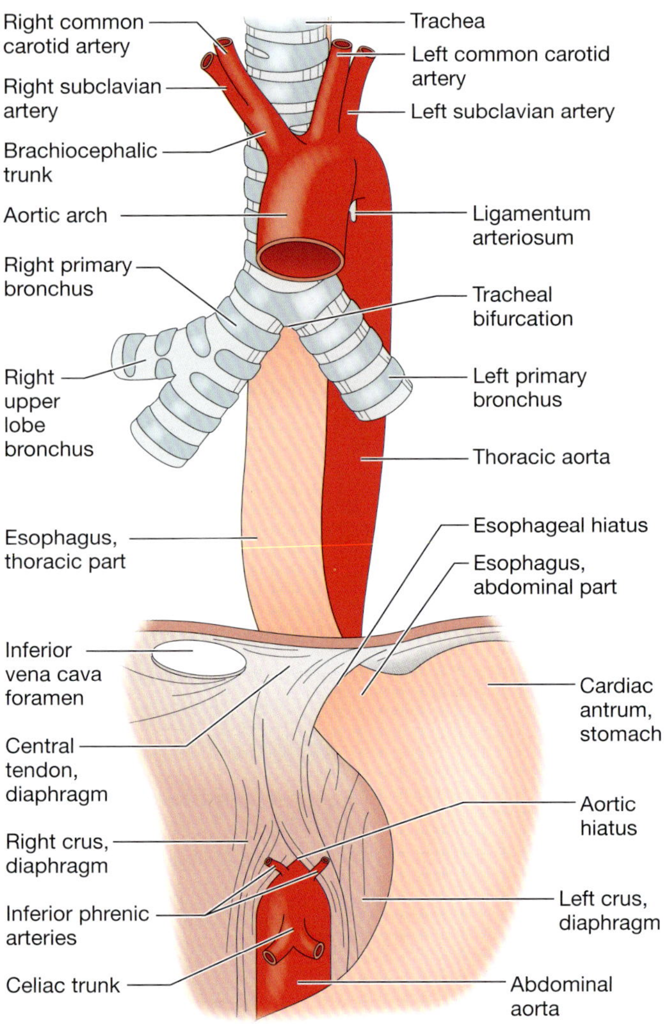

11-36 Esophagus.

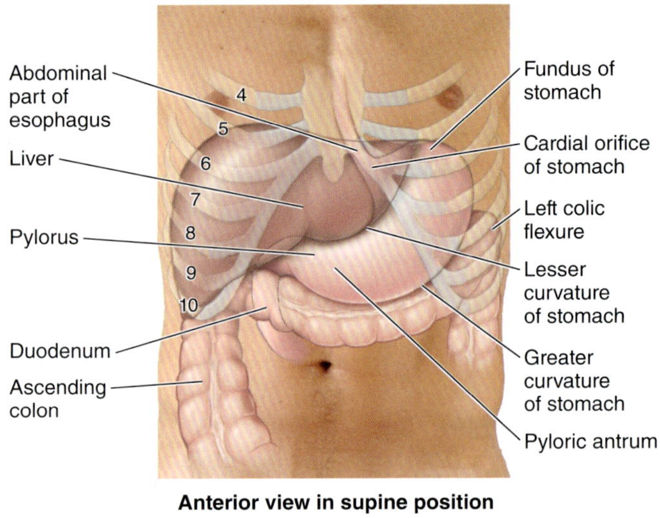

11-37 Stomach shape and position that is affected by body habitus.

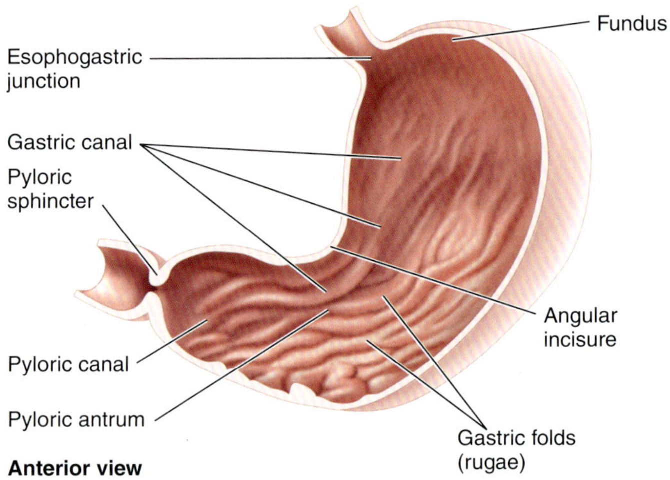

11-38 Stomach.

Stomach

The stomach is described generally as being "J" shaped in the average-type patient and is positioned in the left upper quadrant. The stomach may take on a variable shape and location dependent on the patient's body habitus (Fig. 11-37). When the stomach is empty, the longitudinal folds or "rugae," collapse (Fig. 11-38). As contents enter the stomach, they are exposed to gastric juices and a churning action that continues to break food down eventually into a substance called *chyme.*

The stomach has two openings, the cardiac orifice (esophagogastric junction) proximally and the pyloric orifice distally. Both of these openings have a sphincter muscle present. At the junction of the distal esophagus and the proximal stomach, the cardiac orifice is located. This opening is referenced by its close proximity to the heart and functions to prevent reflux of stomach contents back into the distal esophagus. Above the cardiac orifice is the cardiac notch. The pyloric orifice regulates the passage of chyme from the stomach into the C-loop of the duodenum (Fig. 11-38).

The stomach is divided into three divisions. The fundus is most superior and positioned most posteriorly compared with the other two divisions. There is always a small gastric air bubble often seen present within the fundus when the patient is in an upright position. The body is the largest division (Fig. 11-39). It is confined by the greater and lesser curvatures.

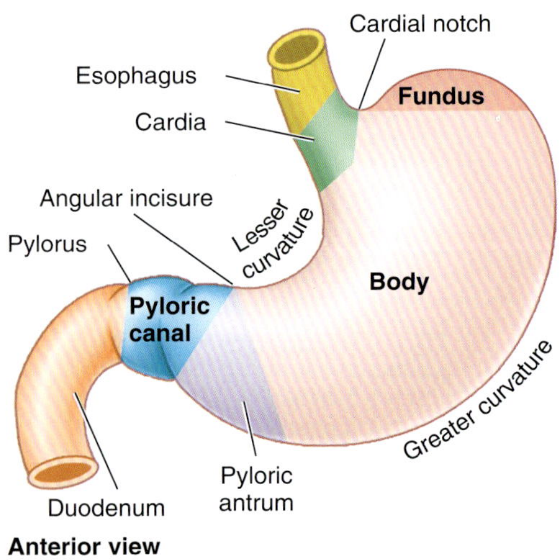

11-39 Three divisions of the stomach.

The greater curvature is located on the left lateral side of the stomach, while the lesser curvature is located on the right lateral side of the stomach closer to the midline. Longitudinal folds of the stomach referred to as rugae run in the region of the greater curvature and define the gastric canal in the region of the lesser curvature. When the stomach is not fully distended, these folds may be noted radiographically (Fig. 11-38). The body is the most anterior division of the stomach. The third division of the stomach is the pylorus. The pylorus can in some instances be identified by the presence of the angular notch (incisure) seen on the lesser curvature side of the stomach. Distal to this notch marks the pyloric antrum, which is the most dilated portion of the pylorus. The pylorus narrows into the pyloric canal leading to the pyloric orifice. The pylorus division is positioned, in reference to anterior and posterior, between the fundus and the body (Fig. 11-40).

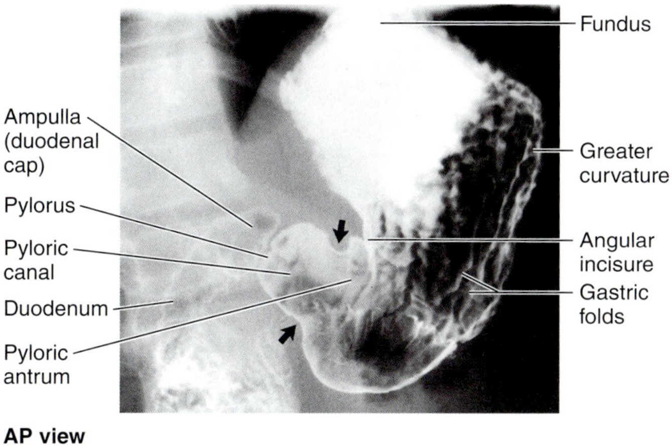

11-40 AP view of the stomach.

The significance of the anterior to posterior location of each of the three divisions of the stomach factors in when using air–barium distribution to determine patient position. Patient position on a radiograph can be determined by recognizing the air–barium distribution and position/appearance of the spine. From the evaluation of the spine, the general symmetry seen with the pedicles and spinous processes can indicate a prone or supine position (Fig. 11-41). The visualization of the "Scottie Dog" indicates a prone or supine oblique position (Fig. 11-42). The lateral position of the spine with visualization the intervertebral disk spaces and intervertebral foramen indicates a lateral patient position; however, air–barium distribution is not significant in this position (Fig. 11-43).

A patient can be determined to be in a supine position or supine oblique position by looking at the spine and then observing that the barium will gravitate to the most posterior division of the stomach; the fundus (Fig. 11-41). A patient can be determined to be in a prone position or a prone oblique position by looking at the spine and then observing that the air will rise to the highest point in the stomach which will be the fundus in this position; the fundus is most posterior in its anatomic placement (Fig. 11-42).

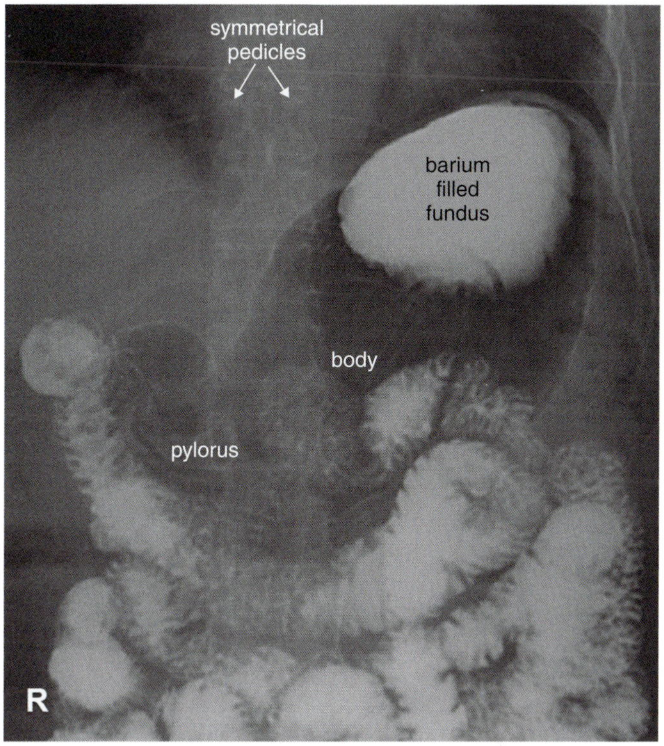

11-41 AP projection—supine position. Barium gravitates to the most posterior portion of the stomach being the fundus.

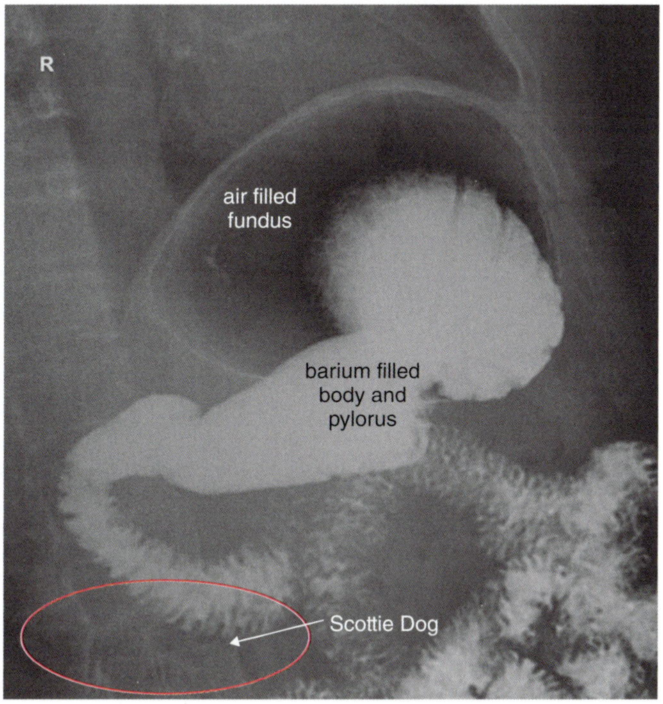

11-42 PA Oblique projection—RAO position. Air rises to the most posterior portion of the stomach being the fundus. The "Scottie Dog" in the lumbar spine aids in determining patient position.

Body Habitus and Stomach Position

The body habitus of a patient will influence the shape appearance of the stomach and its position. The sthenic patient will represent the slight "J" stomach positioned in the left upper

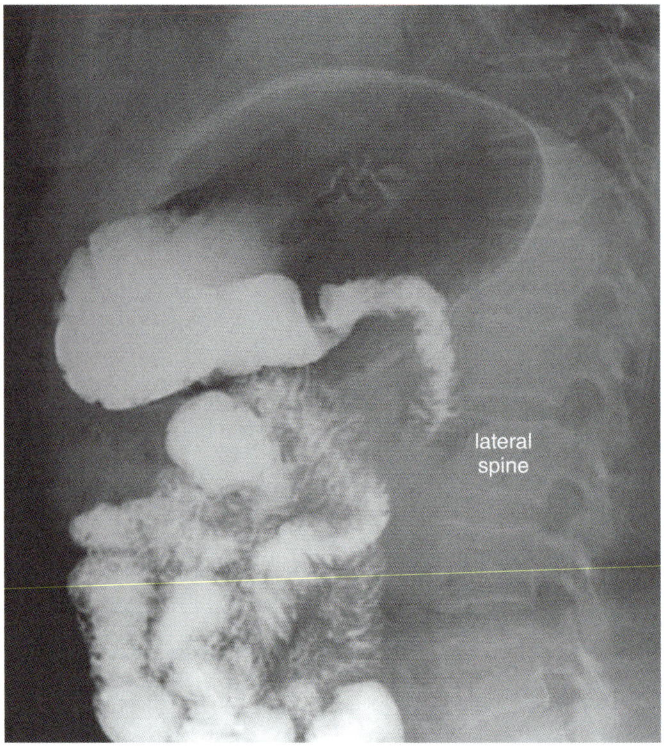

11-43 Lateral projection—lateral position. Note the appearance of the true lateral spine.

quadrant. The hypersthenic patient's stomach will be high and transverse in its orientation. The hyposthenic/asthenic patient will have an elongated "J" shape which could dip down into the pelvis. If the radiographer is to acquire postfluoroscopic images, it is helpful for the radiographer to pay close attention to the shape and position of the stomach during fluoroscopy with the radiologist to aid with the identification of topographical landmarks that would be helpful with centering postfluoroscopy images (Fig. 11-44).

Small Intestines

The small intestines continue to assist with the digestion and absorption of essential nutrients into the system. The small intestines are divided into three divisions: duodenum, jejunum, and ileum. The first segment, the duodenum, is the shortest, widest division and is characterized as having a "C" shape positioned in the right upper quadrant (Fig. 11-37). Evaluation of the duodenum concludes the radiographic exam of the upper GI system. The C-loop of the duodenum surrounds the head of the pancreas. Within the C-loop, the hepatopancreatic ampulla (opening), controlled by the hepatopancreatic sphincter, regulates bile from the biliary tree and pancreatic digestive enzymes into the duodenum. The most proximal portion of the C-loop, closest to the pyloric orifice is the duodenal bulb. Distal duodenum and at its junction point with the jejunum, the ligament of Treitz secures this portion of the bowel to the posterior abdominal wall. This is the most secure point of the small intestine (Fig. 11-45). The second division of the small intestine, the jejunum, occupies the left upper quadrant (LUQ) and moves down into the left lower quadrant (LLQ) (Fig. 11-46). The mucosal lining in this division contains an increased number of muscular folds to aid with absorption. With the increased number of muscular folds, this division is identifiable on radiographs because of its

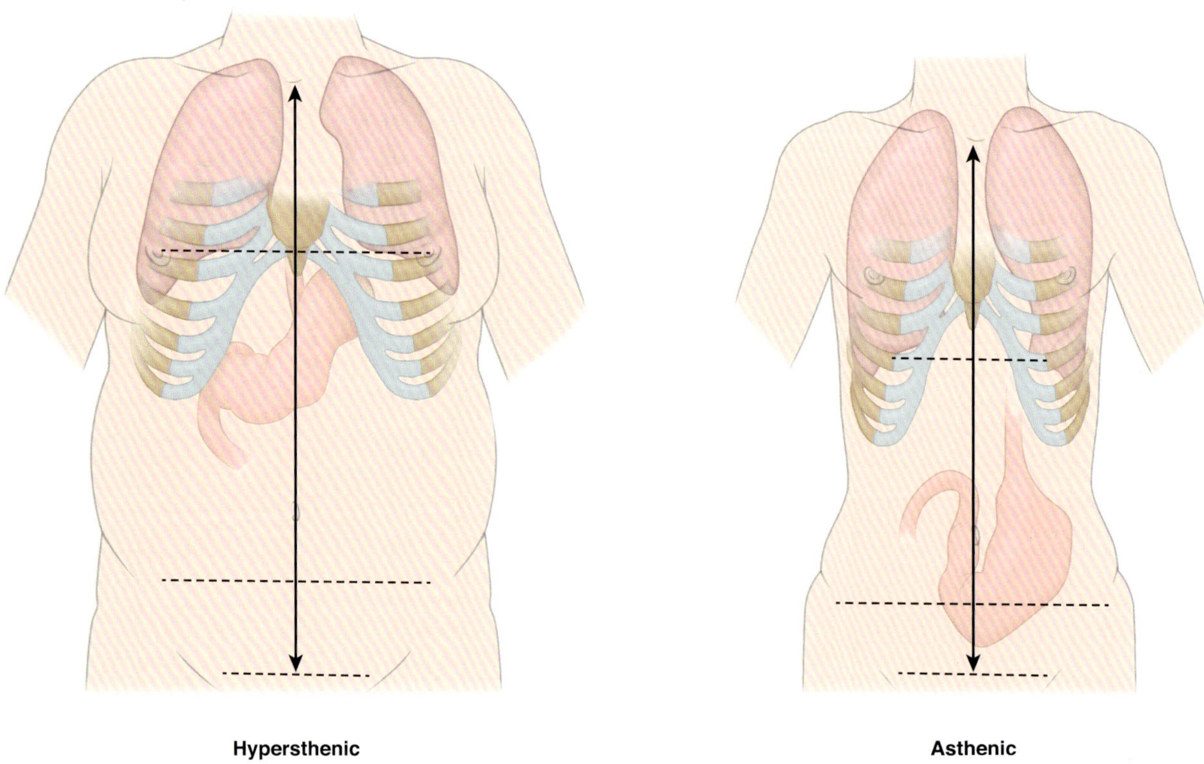

11-44 Body habitus influences stomach placement.

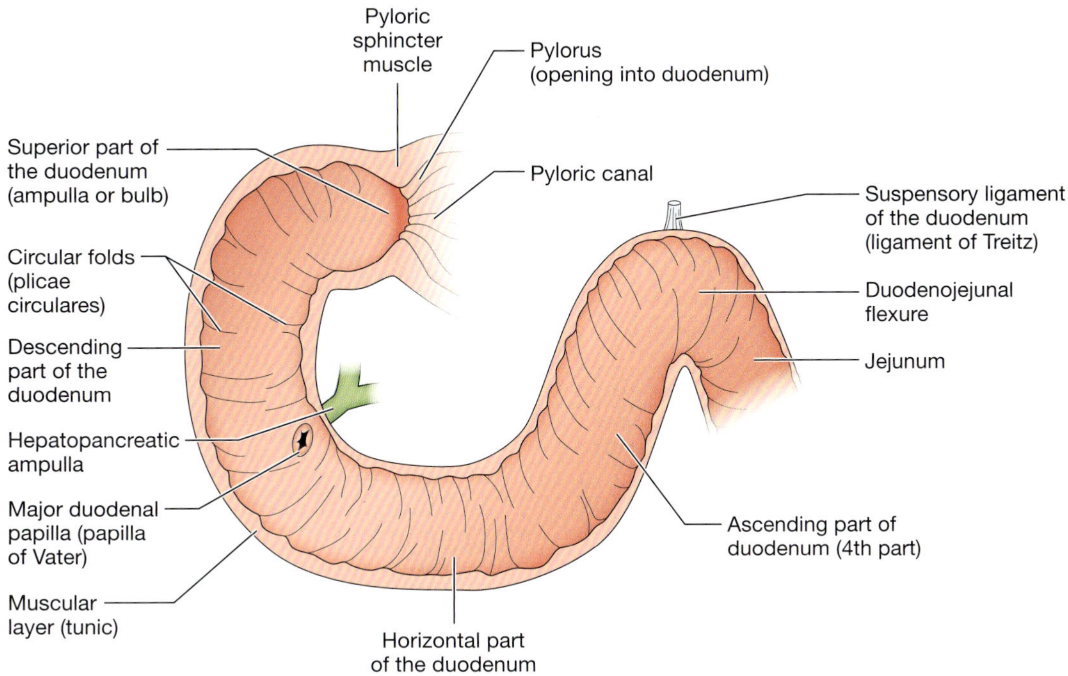

11-45 Duodenum.

change of appearance when filled with barium (Fig. 11-47). The third division and longest division is the ileum. It occupies the central abdomen and right lower quadrant (RLQ). The terminal ileum decreases in diameter and possesses fewer muscular folds creating a change in its barium appearance. The ileocecal valve regulates contents from the small intestines into the proximal portion of the large intestine—the cecum (Figs. 11-48 to 11-50).

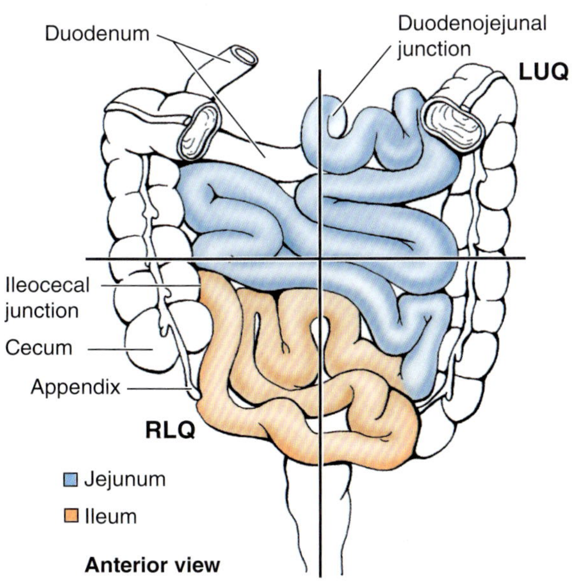

11-46 Placement of the jejunum and ileum.

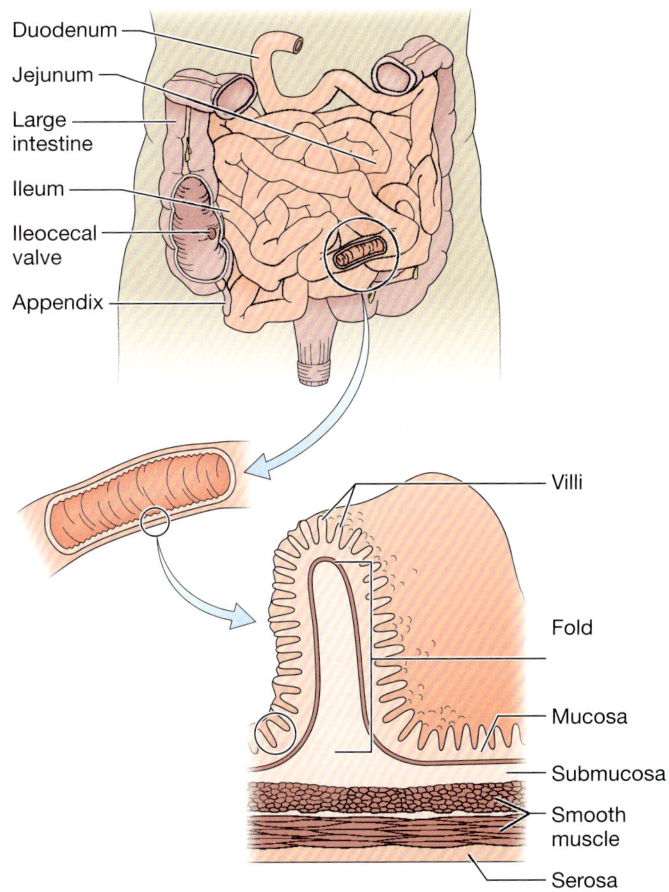

11-47 Mucosal lining.

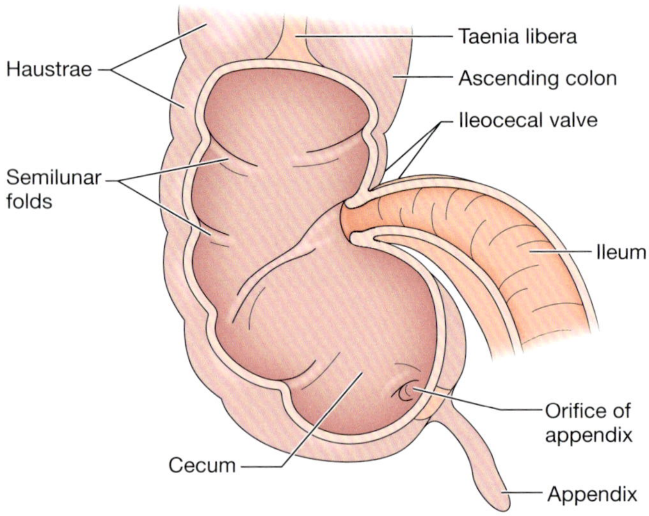

11-48 Terminal ileum and cecum.

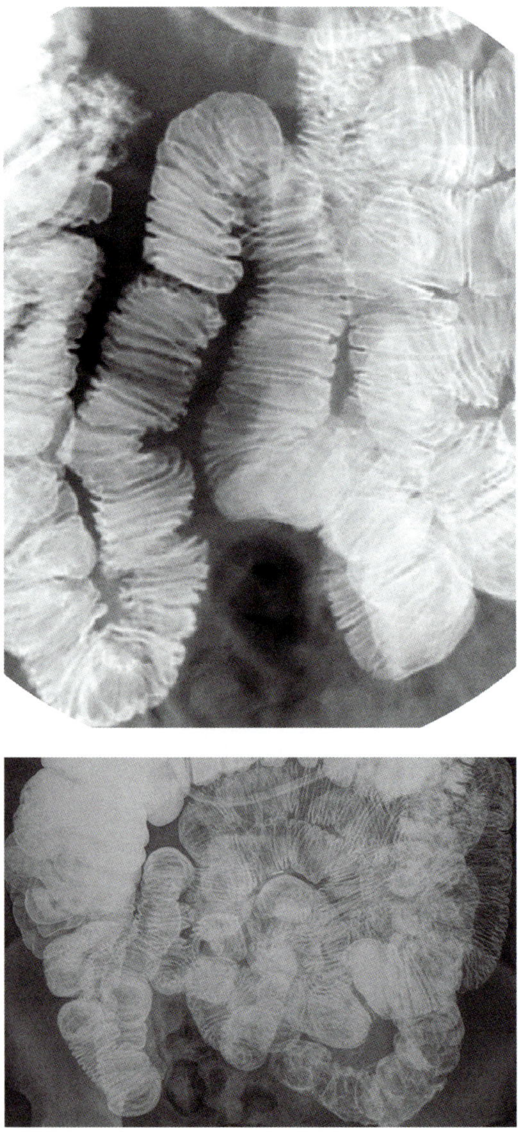

11-49 CT enteroclysis small bowel study.

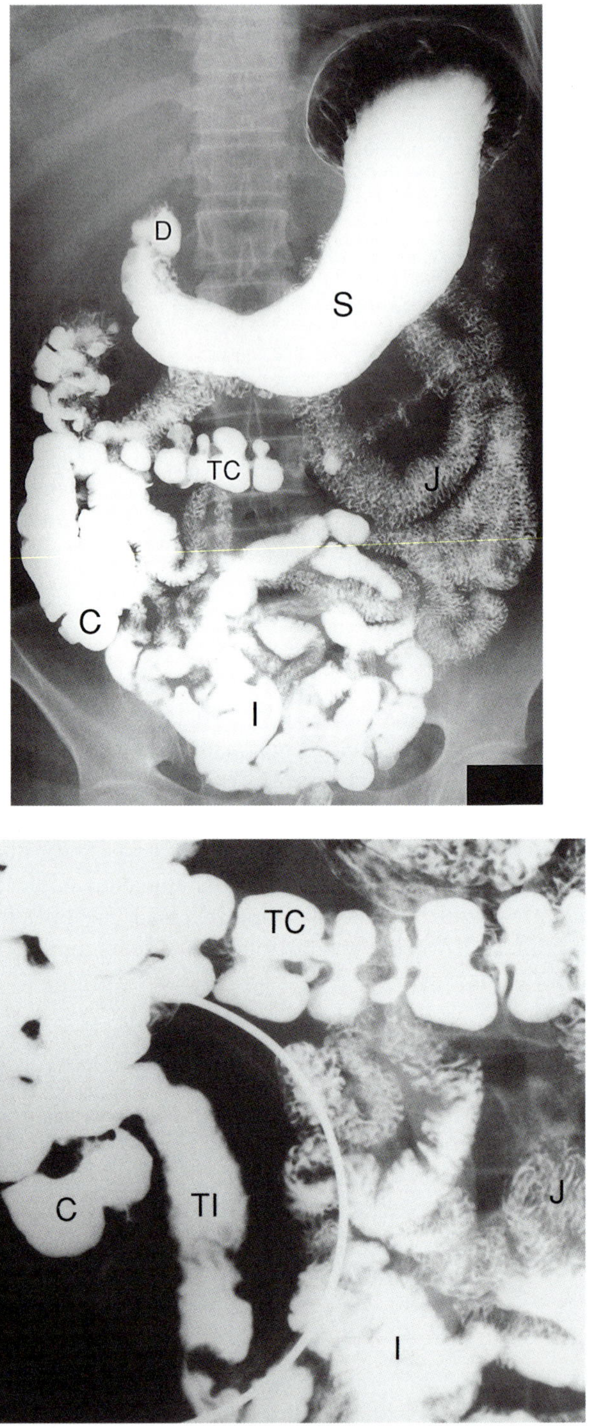

11-50 Small bowel series with a spot image for the terminal ileum and cecum. Note the change in barium appearance from the jejunum to the ileum. Image A has anatomy depicted (C) cecum; (I) ileum; (J) jejunum; (S) stomach; (D) duodenum; (TC) transverse colon. Image B anatomy depicted (C) cecum; (TI) terminal ileum; (I) ileum; (J) jejunum; (TC) transverse colon.

Large Intestine

The large intestines refer to the cecum, colon, rectum, and anus. The large intestine primarily functions to eliminate waste and reabsorb water and electrolytes. The large intestine is positioned around the small intestine at the periphery of the abdomen (Fig. 11-51). Within the large intestine, longitudinal muscular fibers known as the taenia coli creates compartmentalized sacs (*haustrum*) that function to propel waste toward the rectum (Fig. 11-52). The proximal portion of the large intestine begins in the right lower quadrant. The cecum is a dilated proximal portion of the large intestine and receives contents from the ileocecal valve. The appendix (vermiform process) is suspended from the posteromedial surface of the cecum (Fig. 11-48). The ascending colon courses up the right lateral side of the abdomen. The colon will bend beneath the liver and is referenced as the right colic flexure or hepatic flexure. The transverse colon moves across the midline and toward the left upper quadrant. The transverse colon will bend beneath the spleen and is referenced as the left colic flexure or splenic flexure. The splenic flexure, beneath the spleen, is typically positioned more superiorly in the abdomen than the hepatic flexure. The size of the liver in the right upper quadrant occupies more space than the spleen does in the left upper quadrant. The descending colon descends down the left lateral side of the abdomen toward the iliac crest. In the region of the iliac crest, the sigmoid colon courses back to midline, which may be recognized by its “S” shape which then becomes rectum (Fig. 11-52). The rectum follows the curvature of the sacrum and finally the colon terminates with the anus. *Defecation* or bowel movement is the primary function of the rectum (Figs. 11-53 and 11-54).

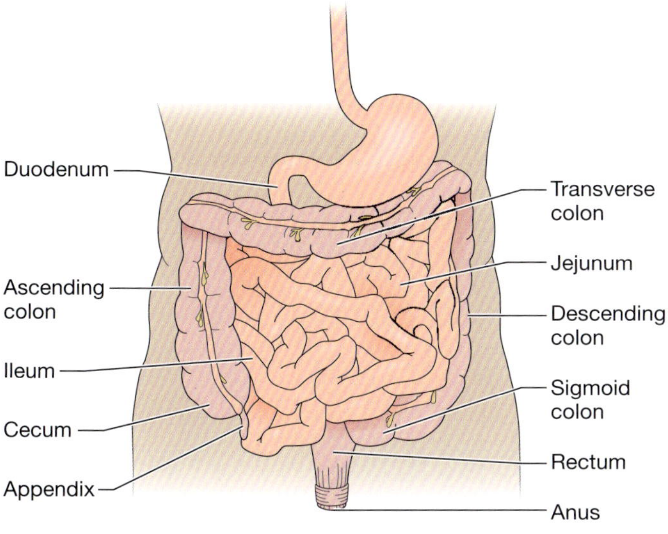

11-51 Large intestines.

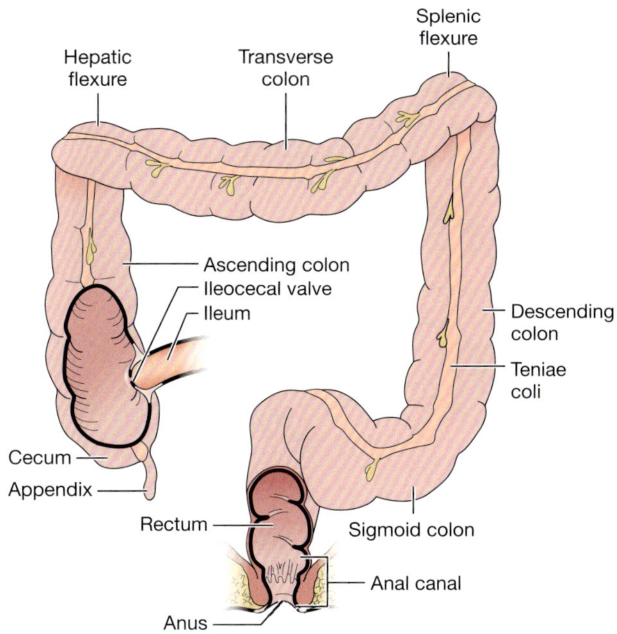

11-52 Divisions of the large intestines.

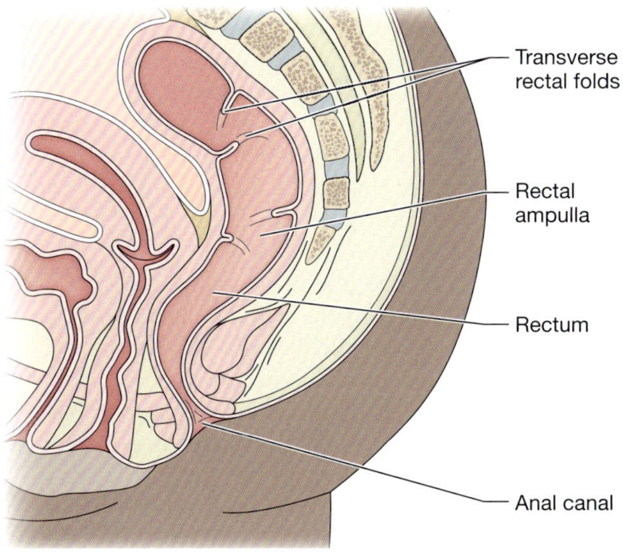

11-53 Rectum.

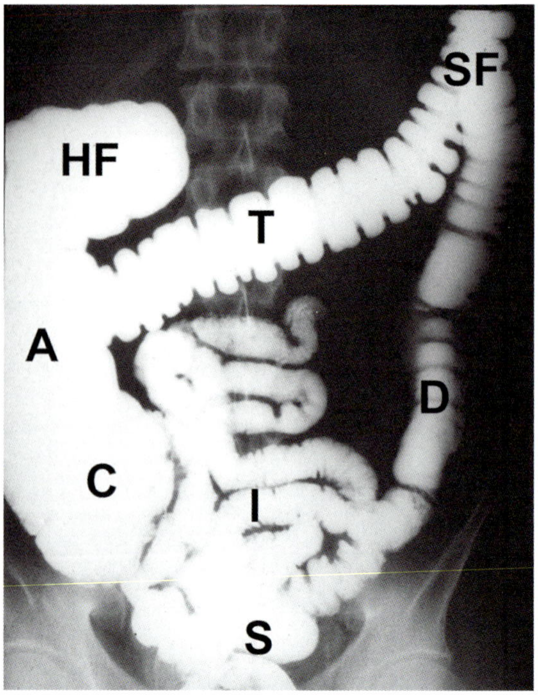

11-54 Divisions of the large intestines.

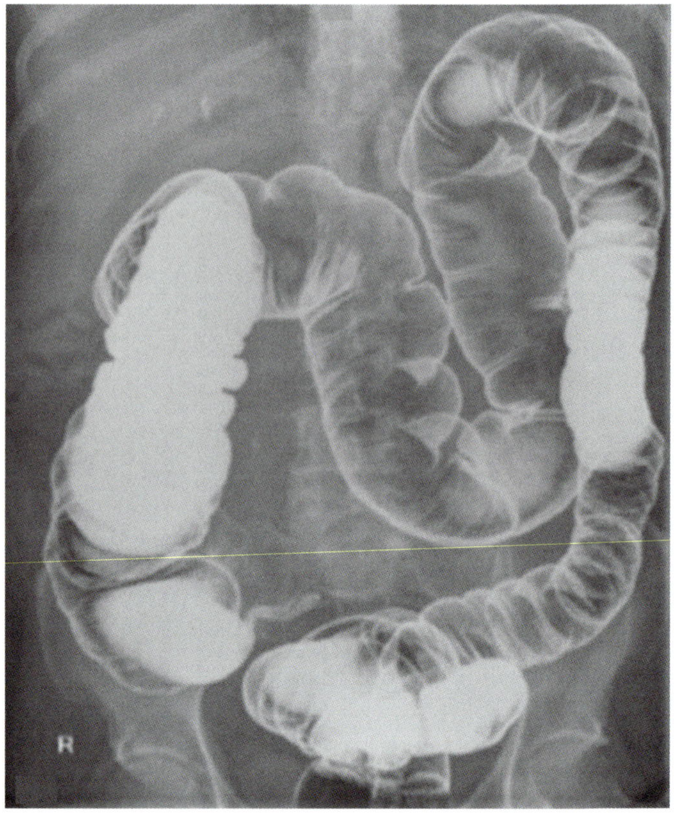

11-55 AP projection—supine position. Air rises to fill the most anterior divisions of the large intestines to be the transverse and sigmoid colon.

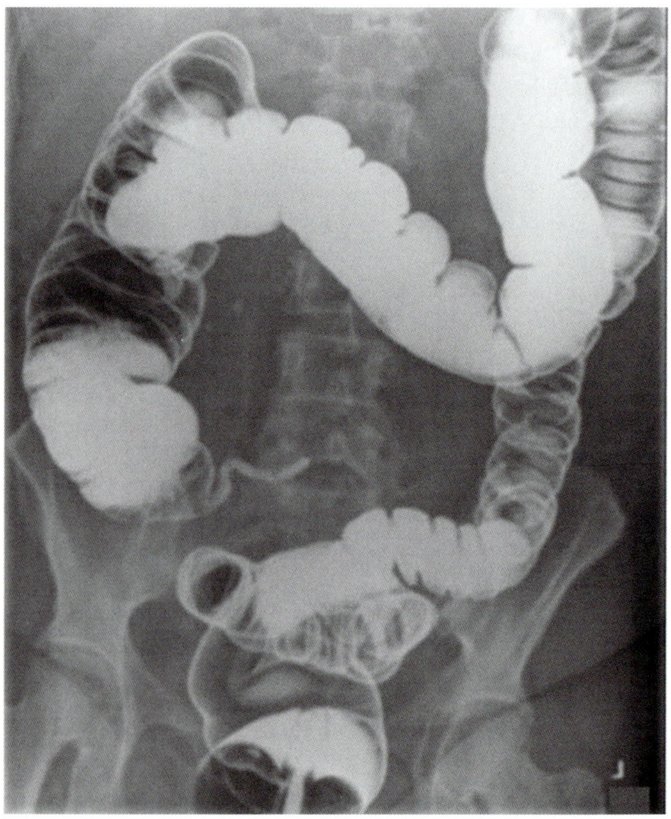

11-56 PA projection—prone position. Air rises to fill the most posterior divisions of the large intestines to be the ascending and descending colon. Barium gravitates to the most anterior divisions to be the transverse and sigmoid colon.

Radiographically, the ascending, descending, transverse, and sigmoid segments of the colon may be distinguished when air–fluid levels are created within. The ascending and descending segments lie posterior to the transverse and sigmoid segments. If a patient lays supine, barium will gravitate into the ascending and descending portions (because of their more posterior placement), while air will rise to the more anterior segments of the transverse and sigmoid colon (Figs. 11-55 and 11-56). If a patient lays prone, barium will gravitate into the anterior-most portions being the transverse and sigmoid colon while air will rise the highest or most posterior segments of the ascending and descending colon.

Imaging of the large intestines will also involve oblique positions to help open up the natural superimposition that occurs at splenic and hepatic flexures. The lumbar spine will visually show the "Scottie Dog" to represent an oblique position (Fig. 11-57). Decubitus positions are utilized to demonstrate portions of the ascending and descending colon with an air–barium distribution. The technologist can determine the right or left lateral decubitus patient position by identifying the hepatic from the splenic flexure and the distribution of the air and barium. Barium will gravitate to the lowest point within the patient or toward the downside. Air will rise to the highest point or toward the upside within the loops of bowel (Fig. 11-58).

Body Habitus and Large Intestines

The large intestines may take on a variable position based on body habitus that should be considered by the technologist when centering. Again, as mentioned previously, the technologist should be observant during the fluoroscopic procedure while with the

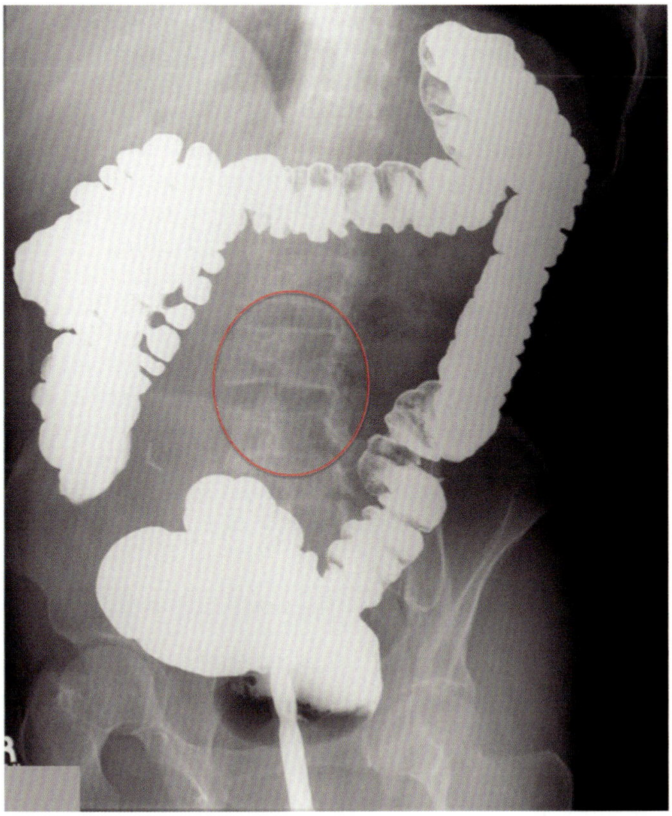

11-57 AP Oblique projection—RPO position. Note the appearance of the "Scottie Dog."

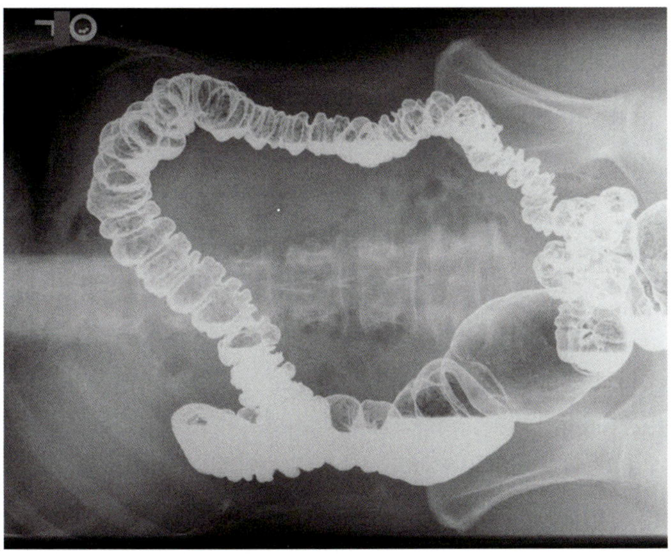

11-58 RLD double-contrast barium enema.

radiologist to note location of the bowel within the abdomen and identify potential topographical landmarks to assist with more accurate centering when postfluoroscopy images are acquired. The hypersthenic patient tends to have a high and transverse stomach and a transverse colon that lies high within the abdominal cavity. The asthenic patient tends to have an elongated stomach that drops down toward the pelvis and a transverse colon that sits lower toward the pelvis (Fig. 11-59).

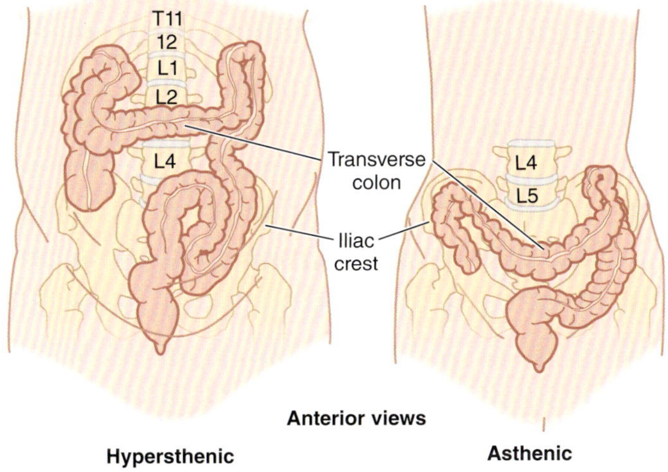

11-59 Large intestines placement according to body habitus.

KEY SUMMATION POINTS OF ANATOMY

- Pharynx serves as part of the respiratory system and digestive system. The oropharynx division is positioned in between the uvula and the epiglottis.
- Mechanical digestion begins in the mouth with mastication (chewing) while the salivary glands release initial enzymes and mucous to begin chemical digestion and aid in the formation of a bolus. Mechanical and chemical digestion continues in the stomach and within the small bowel.
- Esophagus is a collapsible tube that begins about C5, passes through the mediastinum, and passes through the left hemidiaphragm at T10.
- Stomach has two openings: cardiac and pyloric orifice. Stomach has three divisions: fundus, body, and pylorus. The fundus is the most posterior division while the body is the most anterior division. The location of the stomach divisions influences air and barium distribution when the patient is in different positions.
- The C-loop of the duodenum surrounds the head of the pancreas. The duodenal bulb is the most dilated division of the duodenum.
- The hepatopancreatic ampulla is the opening into the C-loop of the duodenum that is surrounded by the hepatopancreatic sphincter. The sphincter regulates the release of biliary and pancreatic enzymes into the small intestines.
- The ligament of Treitz secures the proximal portion of the jejunum of to the posterior abdominal wall creating the most fixed portion of the small intestines.
- The C-loop is the shortest and widest division of the small intestine. The jejunum occupies the left upper and lower quadrants. The ileum occupies the majority of the central component of the small intestine and terminates in the right lower quadrant with the ileocecal valve opening into the cecum.
- The small intestine is more central in location while the large intestine is located around its periphery of the abdominal cavity.
- The small intestine is primarily responsible for the absorption of nutrients and reabsorption of water while the large intestine is responsible for waste elimination and reabsorption of water and electrolytes.
- The large intestine has two flexures: the hepatic (right colic) flexure and the splenic (left colic) flexure. The splenic flexure typically sits 1″–2″ superior to the level of the hepatic flexure. The flexure heights are influenced by the organ sizes of the

liver and spleen in the RUQ (right upper quadrant) and LUQ (left upper quadrant).

- The two most anterior portions of the colon are the transverse and sigmoid divisions. The two most posterior portions of the colon are the ascending and descending divisions. The location of the colon divisions influences air and barium distribution when the patient is in different positions.

POSITIONING AND TECHNICAL CONSIDERATIONS

Body Habitus and Suggested Image Receptor Orientation

Sthenic Patient: This patient represents the most average size dimension in the population. Patient is of modest height and weight. Abdominal organs are located in their predictable quadrants. Patients will easily fit to a lengthwise image receptor.

Hypersthenic Patient: This patient is broad through the chest and abdomen. The stomach typically sits high and underneath the diaphragm in a transverse orientation. Due to the placement of the stomach, it may be necessary to center 1″–2″ superior to the centering location for a sthenic patient and in some cases set the exposure field to crosswise to match the stomach's orientation. The large intestines are found at the periphery of the abdomen. To adequately image the entire abdomen, two 14 × 17 crosswise images set to overlap are recommended.

Asthenic/Hyposthenic Patient: This patient is long and lean through the thorax and abdomen. Abdominal structures, such as stomach and bowel, tend to sit lower in the abdomen and extend down into the pelvis. Due to the placement of the stomach, it may be necessary to center 1″–2″ inferior to the centering location for a sthenic patient. Lengthwise image receptor orientation will be the best fit for the patient. Certain patients may need two images set to overlap to include all necessary anatomy.

Centering for Gastrointestinal Tract

When acquiring post images the GI tract, the centering may need to be modified to include necessary anatomy when considering different body types. The radiologic technologist can identify topographical landmarks to best accommodate a patient's anatomy while paying attention to the fluoroscopic component of the exam performed by the radiologist.

KEY ANATOMIC LANDMARKS (FIG. 11-60)

- Xiphoid tip corresponds to thoracic vertebral level of T9–T10.
- Iliac crest corresponds to lumbar vertebral level of L4–L5.
- Jugular notch, xiphoid tip, and spine would all be landmarks for midsagittal plane (MSP).
- Symphysis pubis
- Greater trochanter may serve as an alternative landmark for the symphysis pubis.

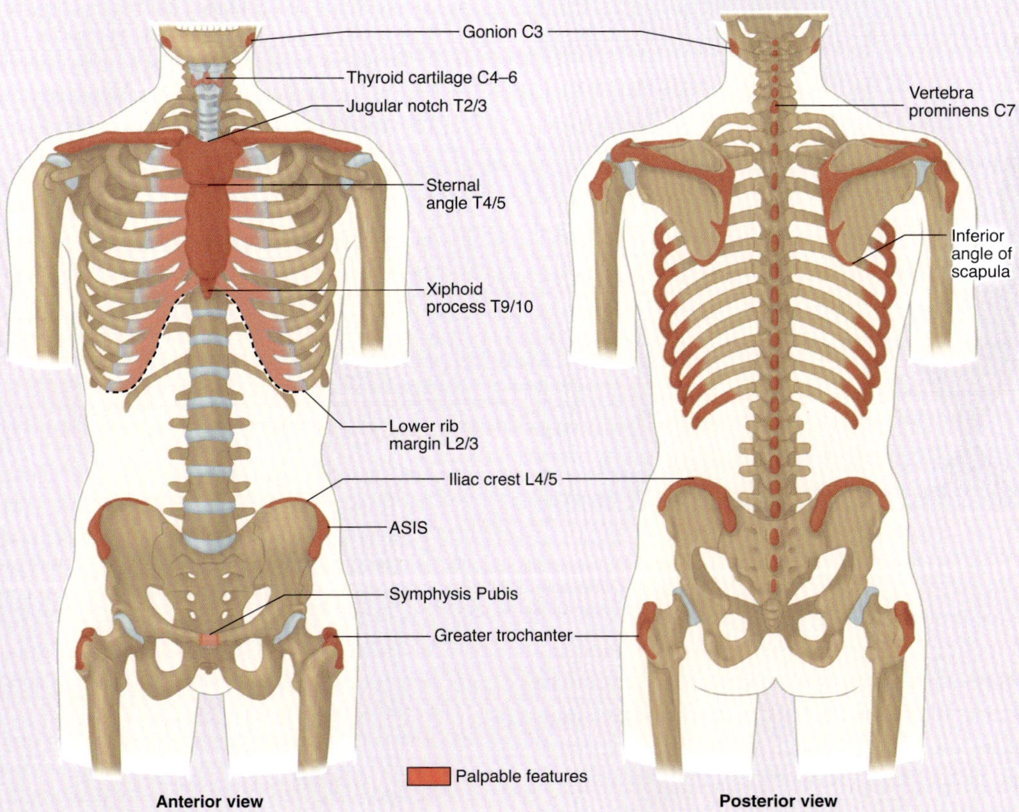

11-60 Topographical landmarks.

Breathing Instructions for Gastrointestinal Exams

Breathing instructions will vary depending on which portion of the GI tract is being studied. When imaging the esophagus, breathing instructions are not necessary to give because breathing less likely during active swallowing. With proper function of the swallowing mechanism, aspiration into the airway is mostly prevented. When imaging the stomach, to avoid displacement of the stomach by the position of the diaphragm, images should be acquired after the patient exhales. When imaging the small or large intestines, suspension of breath to avoid motion on the image is advised.

TECHNICAL CONSIDERATIONS

Setting a Manual Technique

With single-contrast imaging with barium sulfate, the kilovoltage is set high to penetrate the barium-filled structure. Kilovoltage higher than 110 is very likely. With double contrast imaging, such as with air and barium sulfate, kilovoltage is lowered to avoid overpenetration of the mucosal lining and air-filled areas. Kilovoltage may be closer to 90.

Setting Technique With Automatic Exposure Control

Automatic exposure control (AEC) may be an option in the imaging department even with barium studies. With AEC, the technologist will set the kVp value, will not set a mAs, but rather must select which exposure cell(s) correspond to the anatomy centered and anatomy coverage over the cell(s) according to the projection. The kilovoltage level selected will still be based on if the study is single or double contrast. The exposure cell(s) selected will determine when an adequate exposure has been reached according to the part thickness and composition and then the exposure is terminated. After the exposure terminates, the radiographer can then see the mAs value displayed on the control panel. With higher kilovoltage levels set, mAs readouts will be lower.

Source-to-Image Distance

40″ source-to-image distance (SID) is employed for all GI studies.

Shielding of the Patient

With fluoroscopy and post imaging, shielding can be difficult and limited. The shield placement may superimpose essential anatomy on certain exams. For instance, a patient having a study of the esophagus would still allow the waist apron shield to be applied. The decision on shielding is left to the discretion of the technologist. The technologist should consider the exam, patient age, and placement of the patient's GI anatomy. In addition to efforts on shielding, the technologist must question all reproductive-aged patients regarding the possibility of pregnancy. It is important to rule out pregnancy with the increased exposure times to the abdominal and pelvic area with fluoroscopic imaging. Post the fluoroscopic procedure the technologist is required to record the fluoroscopy exposure time at the end of the procedure, the number of images acquired, number of live (cine) runs, and the patient dose received in the patient exam notes.

Shielding of the Technologist

Radiologic technologists play an active role in fluoroscopic procedures. They are required to assist the patient and the radiologist to expedite a procedure. During fluoroscopic exams, the technologist needs to practice personal protection and dress in an appropriately sized lead apron and a thyroid shield (Fig. 11-61). The technologist's dosimeter should be worn at the collar level on the outside of their lead shield. The technologist should stand at a 90° angle from the source and not directly at the head or foot of the radiographic table unless absolutely necessary (Fig. 11-62). The technologist should also consider increasing their distance from the source of radiation whenever possible while minimizing their time exposed. In other words, if the technologist is not needed for different aspects of a procedure by the patient or the radiologist, they should maximize their distance or even consider standing a distance behind the radiologist or completely behind the primary barrier. It is also the technologist's responsibility to advocate personal safety and provide protective garments to others that are present within the imaging suite (Fig. 11-63).

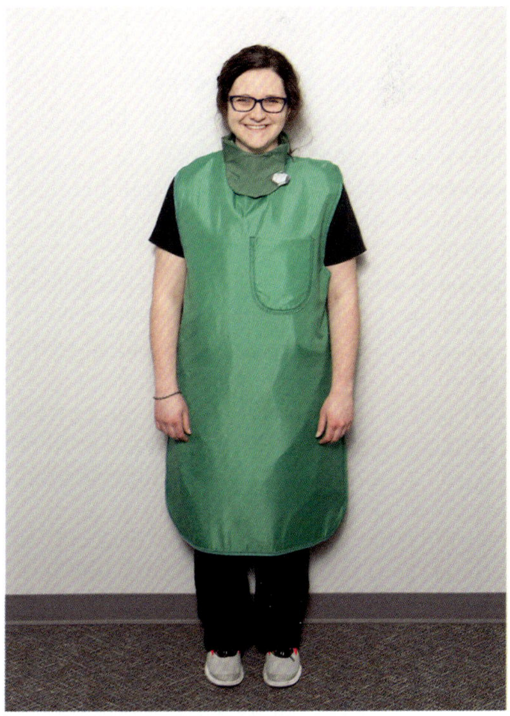

11-61 Technologist personal radiation protection.

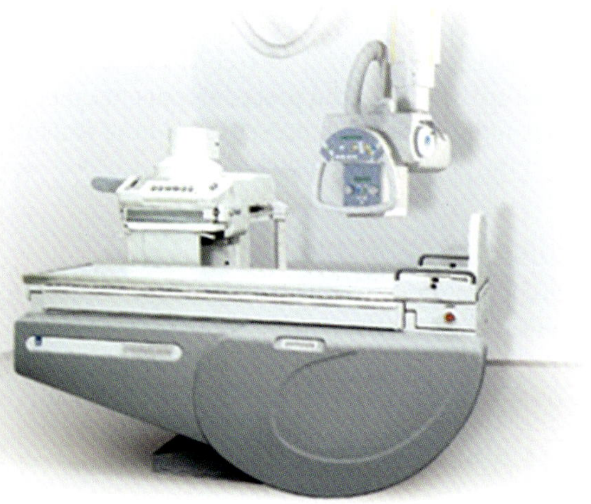

11-62 Radiography and fluoroscopy unit.

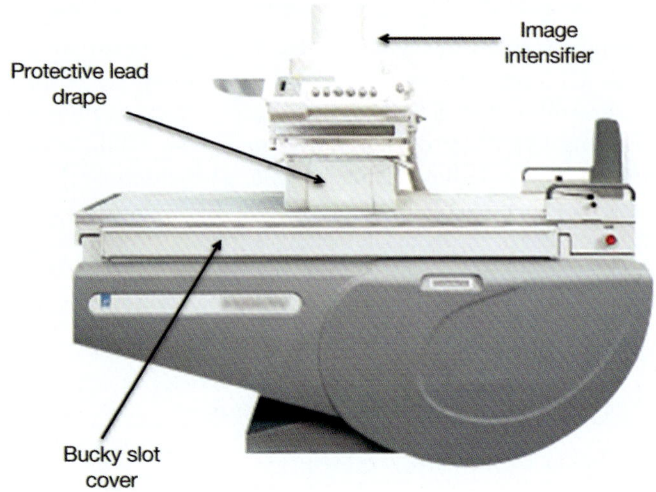

11-64 Fluoroscopy unit radiation safety measures.

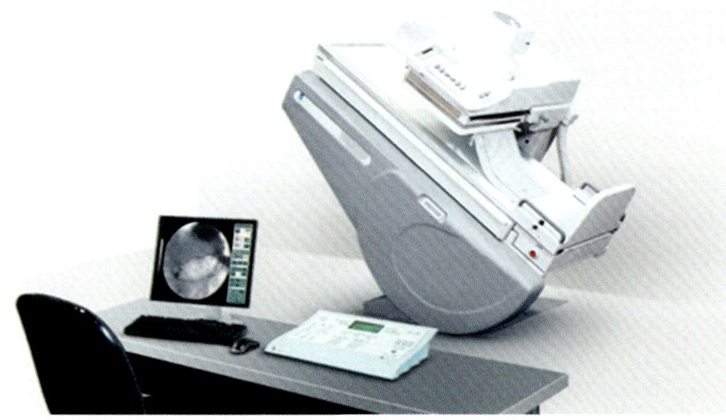

11-63 Fluoroscopy suite.

Other Radiation Safety Measures

Intermittent Fluoroscopy: Pulsed use of fluoroscopy rather than continuous viewing.

Beam Restriction: Reducing the overall fluoroscopy field size will reduce scatter radiation and the patient area of radiation exposure.

Bucky Slot Cover: By moving the table Bucky to the foot of the table, a protective piece will be allowed to flip up to shield the waist area from scatter and leakage radiation that occurs directly below the tabletop (Fig. 11-64).

Lead Drape: A series of flexible lead pieces attach to the front of the fluoroscopic tower and provide an additional barrier means between the patient and the imaging professional (Fig. 11-64).

Protective Garments: Properly fitted lead aprons will reduce personal exposure during procedures. Additional shielding for the thyroid is strongly encouraged. Reducing extremity exposure by using a compression cone, paddle, or lead gloves is best practice.

Tower Distance: Scatter radiation emitted may be reduced when the fluoroscopy tower is positioned closer to the patient. The alteration of this distance will be highly influenced by the patient's size (Fig. 11-64).

Digital Radiography and Fluoroscopic (R&F) Suites and Post Imaging

A digital fluoroscopic and radiographic system is becoming more of the standard for imaging of the gastrointestinal (GI) tract. The radiologist is able to observe the dynamics of the GI tract while acquiring cine loop captures (rapid succession of a function event in motion) of the procedure and digital spot images. With the advent of digital fluoroscopic capabilities, GI exam times have reduced and the need for the technologist to acquire additional post procedural images or "overheads" has lessened and even become obsolete. Comparable to digital radiography, digital fluoroscopy provides the radiologist with the manipulation features such as edge enhancement, digital subtraction, window and leveling, and contrast inversion.

Marking the Image

When marking flat abdominal images, the right or left anatomic side lead marker should be placed down toward the hip or in area that will least interfere with the position of the GI anatomy of interest. When marking an oblique position, the lead marker should be placed within the collimated exposure field indicating the side closest to the IR on that anatomic side. For example, with a right posterior oblique position, the right marker is placed lateral to the patient's right side. When marking decubitus positions, generally it is easiest to mark the "side up" as it visually assessable. Additional markers or digital annotations should be considered to indicate functional and timed exams, such as with a small bowel series. Positional markers such as "side up" or an arrow are encouraged for decubitus and upright positions (Fig. 11-65). Preprocedural images or "scout" images may be marked or annotated as so. A "scout" image provides the radiologist with insight on the patient's exam preparation, an initial look at their anatomy, and rules out gross pathology (Fig. 11-66).

Viewing the Image

Assuming the abdomen image was correctly marked, the image is displayed opposite of the viewer facing it, as though the

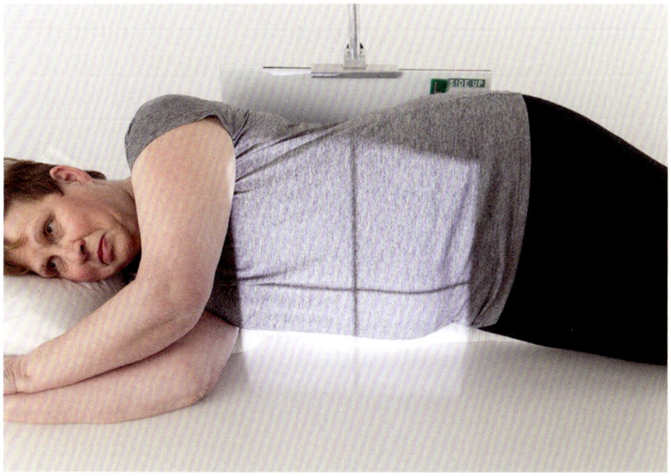

11-65 Decubitus marking.

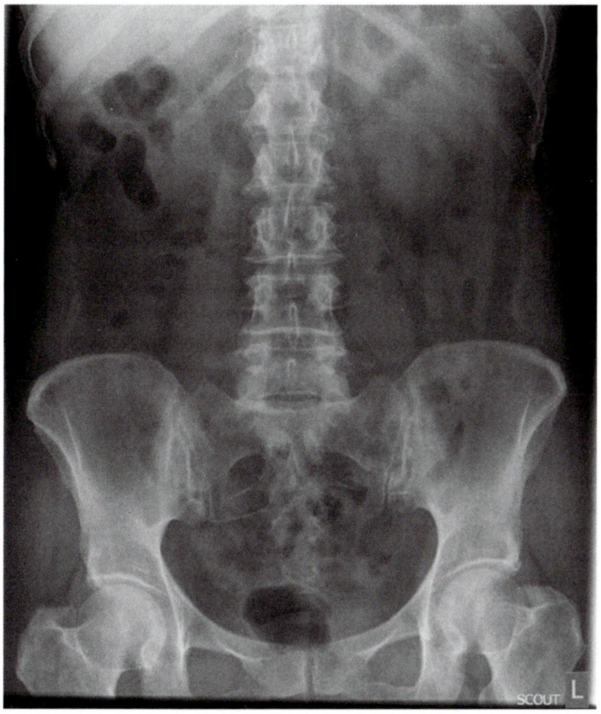

11-66 Scout radiograph.

image is in anatomic position. Therefore, the side of the image marked "Right" or "Left" is opposite of the viewer's right or left (Figs. 11-67 and 11-68).

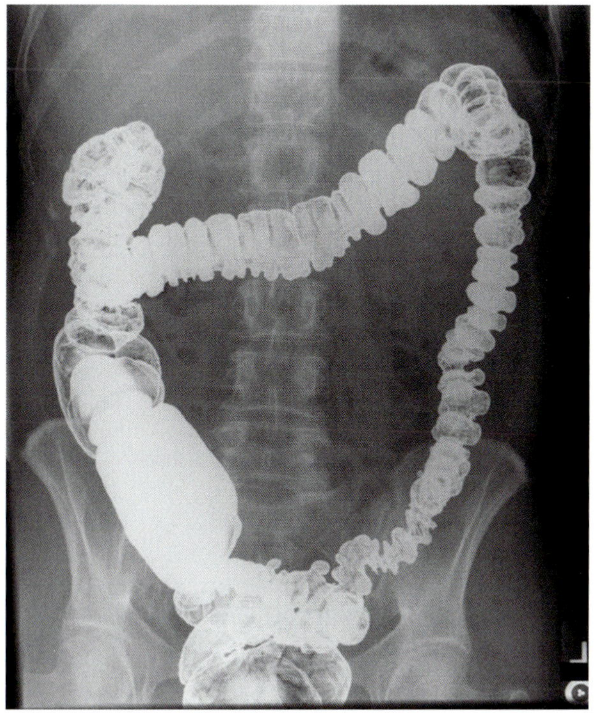

11-67 Correct image display.

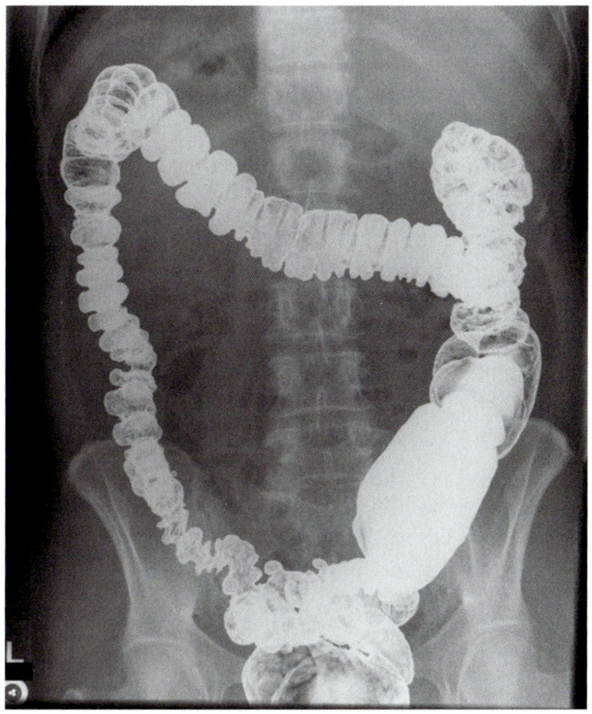

11-68 Incorrect image display.

BARIUM SWALLOW OR ESOPHAGRAM

- Radiographic study of the oropharynx, swallowing mechanism, and entire esophagus.

Indications

- Achalasia, dysphagia, esophageal varices, GERD, foreign bodies

Contraindications

- Contrast sensitivity

Patient Prep

- No prep, unless an upper gastrointestinal (UGI) is considered to follow.

Contrast Prep (Highly Dependent on Radiologist Preference)

- High-density thick barium paste (Fig. 11-22).

- 8 oz thin liquid barium sulfate to drink through a straw (Fig. 11-25).
- This study may be modified to better evaluate the swallowing mechanism of a patient suffering recent stroke. In these cases, a modified swallowing dysfunctional study may also involve different food consistencies (applesauce, pudding, crackers) mixed with barium. The patient will sit in a special designed chair of a particular width to fit in between the imaging table and x-ray tube. The entire exam will keep the patient in the upright position. Postexam images are not acquired in these cases.

Room Setup

- Control panel switched to fluoroscopy with time zeroed and kVp set at desired kVp level for a single contrast study at the facility (potential 110+ kVp).
- Footboard attached to imaging table and table stood up vertically (footboard is not attached if the exam is a modified study for the patient in the stroke imaging chair).
- Table Bucky positioned to the foot of the table.
- Viewing monitor and fluoroscopy foot pedal arranged for radiologist.

Procedure

- Radiologist will begin exam with initial scout assessment of the chest and abdominal area with fluoroscopy in an upright position.
- Radiologist will position the upright patient in the starting position of their preference. This could be flat, oblique, or lateral.
- Radiologist will watch with fluoroscopy the patient swallow and examine the form and function of the esophagus.
- Radiologist may decide to lay the radiographic table horizontal and observe the patient ingesting barium in different positions. This may include the Trendelenburg position.
- The radiologist will capture digital fluoroscopic images or cine loops (live clips) throughout the exam. This may limit the number of postfluoroscopic images acquired by the technologist.
- If postfluoroscopic images are requested by the radiologist, the technologist would proceed with those.

POST IMAGING

- All post images of the esophagus should be acquired recumbent if possible. Recumbent imaging will slow the effect of gravity on the barium passing through the esophagus. In cases of severe aspiration and post images are desired, upright imaging can be implemented.
- Images should display the majority of the esophagus distended and filled with barium. This is best accomplished by administering a bolus of thick barium paste to the patient followed with thin barium. The patient will swallow down the barium paste by drinking the thin liquid barium. The bolus will help distend the esophagus and the thin barium will back fill behind it and distend the esophagus.
- To acquire a barium-filled esophagus, the technologist will want to watch the patient and take the exposure after the patient has consumed three or four big swallows of the barium liquid. This process will happen with each post image requested.
- If acquiring post images for the radiologist, ensure that the radiologist reviews the images before the patient is dismissed.
- With dismissal of the patient, the patient should be given postexam instructions to increase clear fluid to help move the barium sulfate through the GI tract.

MODIFIED BARIUM SWALLOW

A modified version of a barium swallow is a common procedure performed with patients who have suffered a stroke. This exam provides an evaluation of the swallowing mechanism that may be impaired by a stroke and assists specialists in making recommendations regarding what type of restrictions the patient should be on for food and fluid intake. The technologist's role in this exam is to transport the patient and prepare for the procedure. The patient will sit in a specific type of chair that supports the patient properly and can fit in between the imaging table and the fluoroscopy tower. The technologist will assist with gathering the barium liquid and paste. The patient will be observed by the speech pathologist while drinking thick barium through a straw and may progress to eating different consistencies of food (applesauce, pudding, crackers) mixed with barium. The radiologist is present to evaluate the swallowing mechanism of the patient. Cine loop captures are typically acquired. Postexam imaging is not necessary.

Barium Swallow or Esophagram—Supine

- Projection: AP

Technical Considerations

- 110+ kVp
- Center AEC cell or manual mAs
- 40″ SID

Exposure Field Size

- 14 × 17 lengthwise collimated in side-to-side

Patient Position

- Patient preferred supine with no rotation of the chest and abdomen
- Patient will have to turn head to the side to be able to drink the barium from the cup through a straw

Centering

- CR directed to T5–T6 and MSP. The top of the 14 × 17 exposure field should be at the bottom of the chin (Fig. 11-69)

Marking of IR

- Anatomic side marker R or L within the collimated exposure field

Breathing

- The patient will be instructed on drinking the barium necessary for the image. Administration of the barium paste just prior to drinking may improve filling of the esophagus
- Breathing function during deglutition (swallowing) is suppressed; specific breathing instructions are not necessary

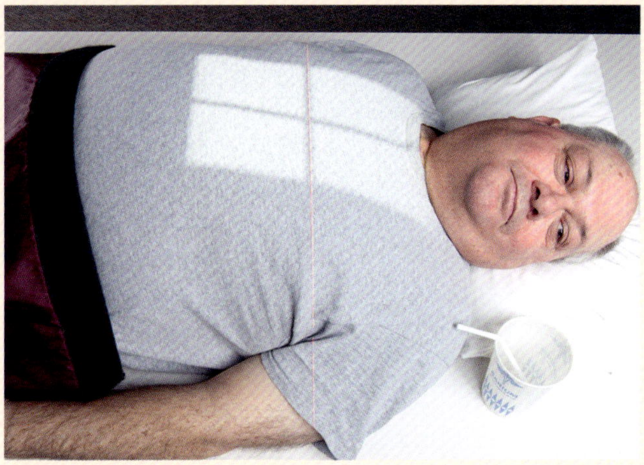

11-69 AP esophagus.

IMAGE CRITIQUE (FIGS. 11-70 and 11-71)

- The majority of the esophagus is distended and filled with barium
- The esophagus is demonstrated from C5 to include the junction with the stomach
- AP esophagus will demonstrate esophagus superimposed on the thoracic spine, which may limit diagnostic information
- Asymmetry of the sternoclavicular (SC) joints will suggest rotation of the thorax

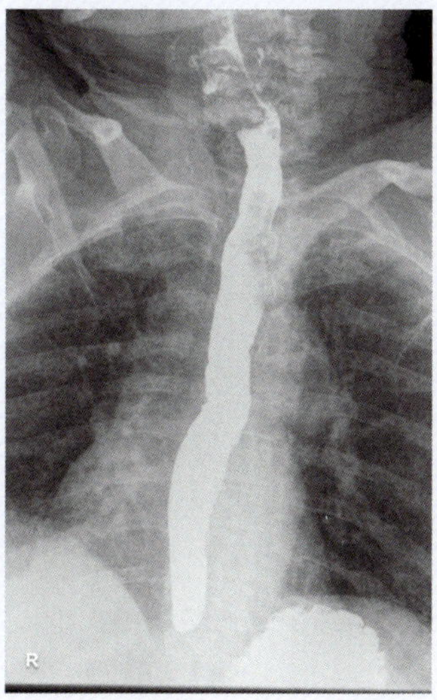

11-70 AP esophagus.

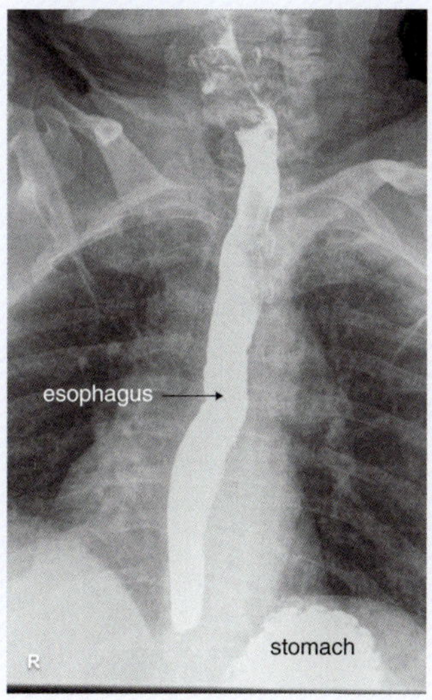

11-71 AP esophagus.

Barium Swallow or Esophagram—Lateral

- Projection: Lateral

Technical Considerations

- 110+ kVp
- Center AEC cell or manual mAs
- 40″ SID

Exposure Field Size

- 14 × 17 lengthwise collimated in anterior to posterior

Patient Position (Fig. 11-72)

- Patient is preferably in a recumbent lateral position. It is encouraged to position the patient in the lateral position that allows you to watch them swallowing for the exposure
- True lateral position with shoulders and hips stacked and aligned

Centering

- CR directed to T5–T6 and posterior to MCP. The top of the 14 × 17 exposure field should be at the bottom of the chin
- Anterior to posterior collimation is encouraged

Marking of IR

- Anatomic side marker R within the collimated exposure field anterior to the patient

Breathing

- The patient will be instructed on drinking the barium necessary for the image. Administration of the barium paste just prior to drinking may improve filling of the esophagus
- Breathing function during deglutition (swallowing) is suppressed; specific breathing instructions are not necessary

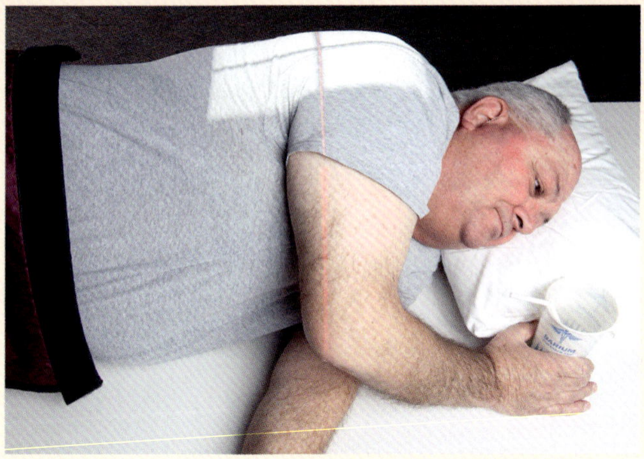

11-72 Lateral esophagus.

IMAGE CRITIQUE (FIGS. 11-73 and 11-74)

- The majority of the esophagus is distended and filled with barium
- The esophagus is demonstrated from C5 to include the junction with the stomach
- Lateral esophagus will demonstrate the esophagus between the heart and the thoracic spine. It is likely that due to the thickness of the shoulders, the esophagus will not be well visualized. If it is necessary to better visualize this area, a swimmer's lateral could be considered

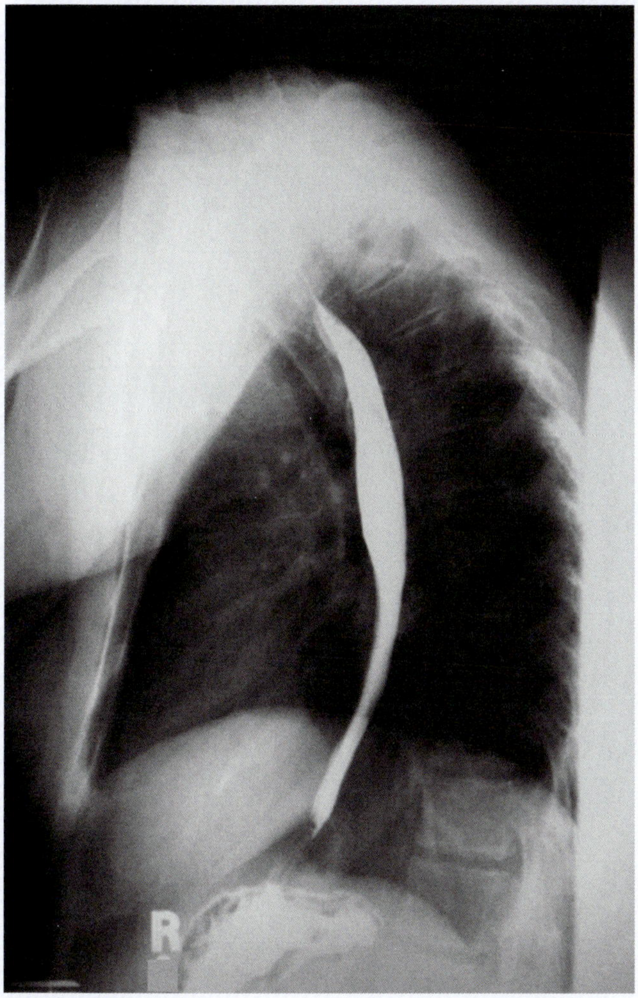

11-73 Lateral esophagus.

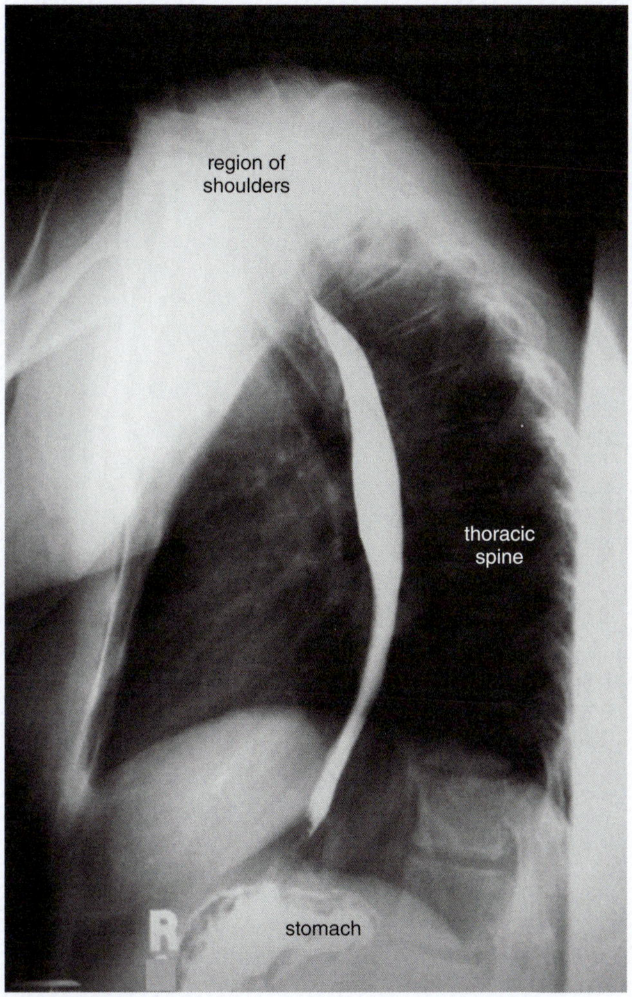

11-74 Lateral esophagus.

Barium Swallow or Esophagram—Right Anterior Oblique or Left Anterior Oblique

- Projection: PA Oblique or alternate AP oblique

Technical Considerations

- 110+ kVp
- Center AEC cell or manual mAs
- 40″ SID

Exposure Field Size

- 14 × 17 lengthwise collimated in side-to-side

Patient Position

- Patient is preferably positioned into a 40° recumbent right anterior oblique (RAO). This obliquity aims to position the esophagus between the heart and the thoracic spine
  - If patient is unable to assume the RAO position, an left posterior oblique (LPO) could be substituted as the reverse position to acquire an identical image
- Patient may also be positioned into a 40° recumbent left anterior oblique

Centering

- RAO
  - CR directed to T5–T6 and 2″ left of the thoracic spine (Fig. 11-75)
- LAO
  - CR directed to T5–T6 and 2″ right of the thoracic spine
- LPO
  - CR directed to T5–T6 and 2″ right of the thoracic spine (Fig. 11-76)

Marking of IR

- Anatomic R or L side marker placed on the corresponding side of the patient, indicating the side was closest to the IR

Breathing

- The patient will be instructed on drinking the barium necessary for the image. Administration of the barium paste just prior to drinking may improve filling of the esophagus
- Breathing function during deglutition (swallowing) is suppressed; specific breathing instructions are not necessary

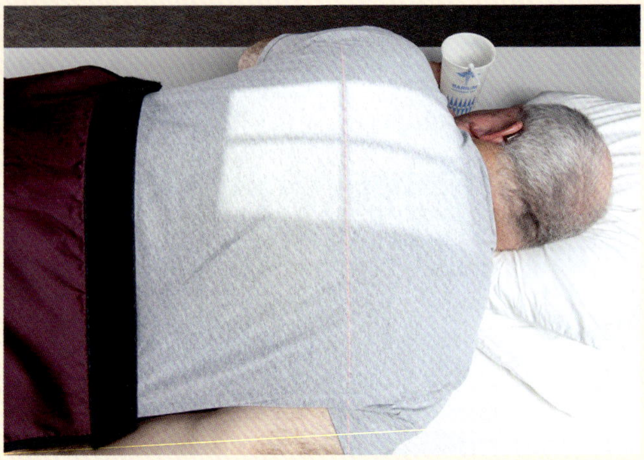

11-75 PA Oblique projection—RAO position.

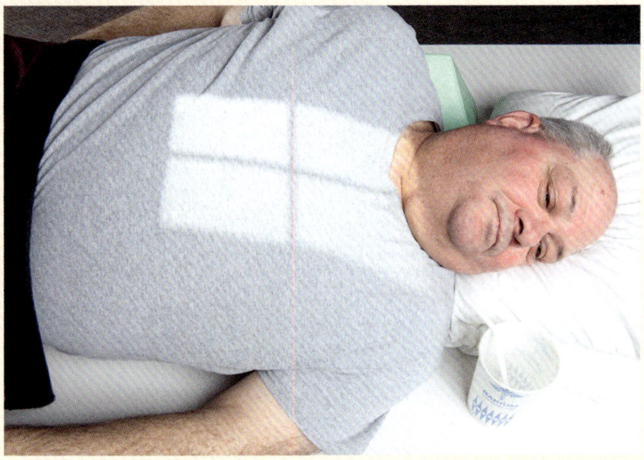

11-76 AP Oblique projection—LPO position.

IMAGE CRITIQUE (FIGS. 11-77 and 11-78)

- The majority of the esophagus is distended and filled with barium
- The esophagus is demonstrated from C5 to include the junction with the stomach
- RAO and LPO esophagus will show the esophagus between the heart and the thoracic spine. Under-rotation of the patient will display the esophagus superimposed on the thoracic spine. Over-rotation of the patient will display the esophagus superimposed on the heart shadow
- LAO esophagus will show the esophagus between the thoracic spine and medial margin of the lung

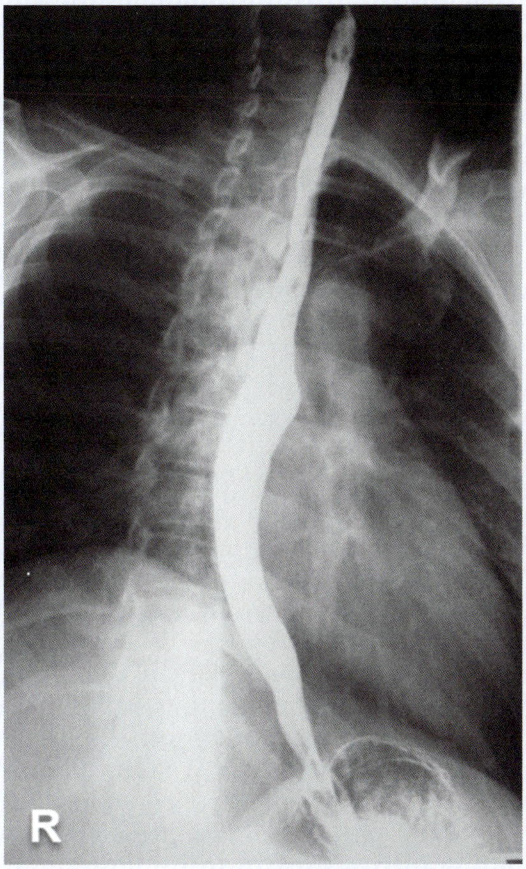

11-77 Esophagus PA Oblique projection—RAO position.

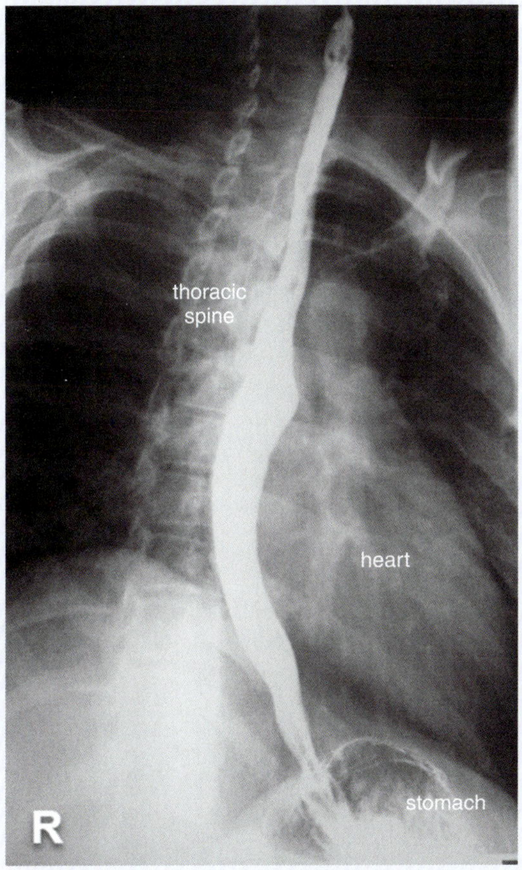

11-78 Esophagus PA Oblique projection—RAO position.

UPPER GASTROINTESTINAL (GI) STUDY

- Radiographic study of the distal esophagus, stomach, and duodenum.

Indications

- Reflux, ulcers, potential perforating ulcer, gastritis, hiatal hernia, gastric carcinoma, gastric diverticula, and emesis

Contraindications

- Contrast sensitivity.
- Suspected perforation to the stomach or bowel. Perforation would require the contrast media to be altered to the iodinated contrast media. A double-contrast study will not be possible with suspected perforation.

Patient Prep

- Patient NPO (nothing passed orally) 8 hours before exam. Patient is instructed not to chew gum or smoke before the exam as this stimulates gastric juices and may interfere with barium adhering to the mucosal lining.

Contrast Prep (Highly Dependent on Radiologist Preference)

- Single Contrast
  - Barium sulfate according to radiologist.
- Double Contrast
  - Carbon dioxide crystals poured into a medicine cup. A second medicine cup filled with water will be needed (Fig. 11-28).
  - High-density thick barium (milkshake consistency)—no straw (Fig. 11-23)
  - 8 oz thin liquid barium sulfate to drink through a straw (Figs. 11-24 and 11-25)

Room Setup

- Control panel switched to fluoroscopy with time zeroed and kVp set according to the needs of a single or double-contrast study. Single contrast is likely 110+ kVp. Double-contrast study is likely around 90 kVp.
- Footboard attached to imaging table and table stood up vertically.
- Table Bucky positioned to the foot of the table.
- Viewing monitor and fluoroscopy foot pedal arranged for radiologist.

General Procedure

- Radiologist will begin exam with initial scout assessment of the chest and abdominal area with fluoroscopy in an upright position.
- Radiologist will position the upright patient in the starting position of their preference. This could be flat, oblique, or lateral.
- Radiologist will have the patient ingest the carbon dioxide crystals with only a small amount of water to help the patient swallow down. These crystals will create air and distend the stomach.
- Radiologist will next have the patient drink the thicker barium solution from the cup. The radiologist will watch with fluoroscopy the patient swallowing and examine the form and function of the esophagus, cardiac sphincter, and the stomach.
- Radiologist will lay the radiographic table recumbent. The radiologist may have the patient roll from back to stomach and back around a couple of times. This helps the thick barium to coat the mucosa of the stomach.
- Radiologist may have the patient ingest the thin liquid barium through a straw to add additional barium volume to the stomach.
- The radiologist needs to see the barium move from the stomach into the duodenum before the exam will be a complete study. In certain instances, this is slow to happen with the patient, the radiologist may have the patient move into a RAO position and have them think about a favorite food to stimulate the stomach to empty.
- Patients with potential esophageal reflux or hiatal hernia may undergo these additional measures during the procedure with the radiologist.
  - Valsalva Maneuver: The patient will be instructed to take in a big deep breath, hold it, and bear down as they would when having a bowel movement. This increased change in pressure on the abdominal cavity may help stimulate an event of reflux or a sliding hiatal hernia.
  - Trendelenburg Position: The patient may undergo a slight Trendelenburg position on while on the recumbent table. Again, this attempted to stimulate an event of reflux or sliding hiatal hernia.
  - Toe Touch Technique: With the imaging table set up vertically, the patient bends over to touch their toes. Again, this change in position may stimulate the event of reflux or a hiatal hernia.
  - Compression Paddle: The radiologist may use the compression paddle to apply pressure directly to points on the abdomen to create a potential event (Fig. 11-79).

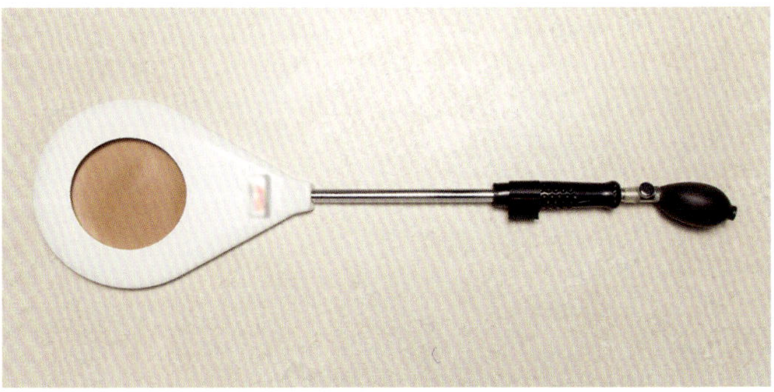

11-79 Compression paddle.

- The radiologist will capture digital fluoroscopic images or cine loops (live clips) throughout the exam. This may limit the number of post images acquired by the technologist.
- If postfluoroscopic images are requested by the radiologist, the technologist would proceed with those.

POST IMAGING

- All images should be organized in a sequence that is efficient and easy for the patient. The patient does not drink additional barium for post images for an upper GI study.
- Images should display the entire stomach.
- If the upper GI study is combined with an esophagram, the technologist *must* acquire the stomach postfluoroscopy images first to preserve the air–barium effect created by the radiologist for the stomach. After confirming those images to be acceptable, post images of the esophagus can then be acquired.
- If acquiring post images for the radiologist, ensure that the radiologist reviews the images before the patient is dismissed.
- With dismissal of the patient, the patient should be given postexam instructions to increase clear fluid intake to help facilitate the barium sulfate through the GI tract.

Upper GI—Prone

- Projection: PA

Technical Considerations

- 90 kVp for double contrast
- 110+ kVp for single contrast
- Center AEC cell or manual mAs
- 40″ SID

Exposure Field Size

- 14 × 17 lengthwise collimated to radiologist preference size

Patient Position

- Patient is positioned prone. Ensure the patient is flat and without rotation

Centering

- It is highly recommended that the technologist be observant to the stomach position and relative landmarks while the radiologist is performing fluoroscopy. During this observation, the technologist can identify topographical landmarks to assist with better centering that may be necessary for postfluoroscopy imaging
- CR directed to L1 and 1″–2″ left of the thoracic spine (Fig. 11-80)
- It may be necessary to alter from the above centering location if the patient has an asthenic/hyposthenic or hypersthenic body habitus. The asthenic/hyposthenic patient will most likely need the CR directed 1″–2″ inferior from the sthenic patient. The hypersthenic patient will most likely need the CR directed 1″–2″ superior from the sthenic (Fig. 11-81)

Marking of IR

- Anatomic R or L side marker placed on the corresponding right or left side of the patient

Breathing

- Breathing is suspended after expiration

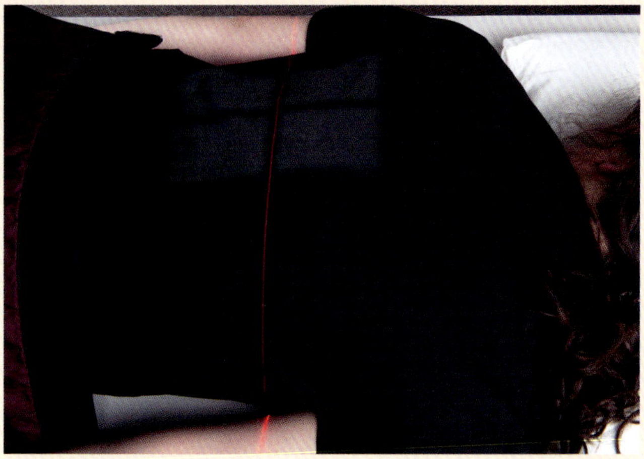

11-80 PA projection stomach—sthenic patient.

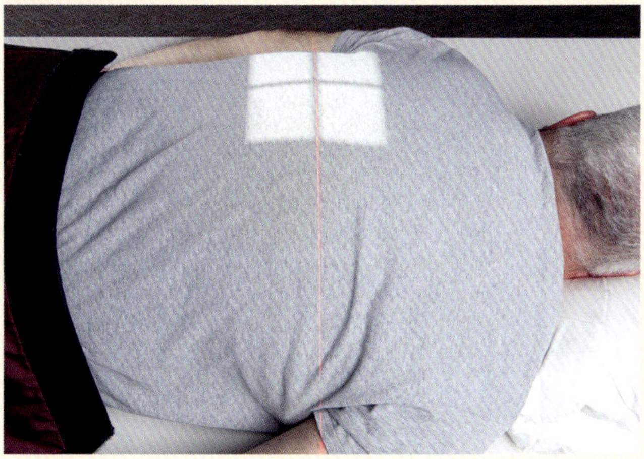

11-81 PA projection stomach—hypersthenic patient.

IMAGE CRITIQUE (FIGS. 11-82 and 11-83)

- With a patient prone and free of rotation, the spine pedicles should appear symmetrical
- The entire stomach is visible. The duodenum or portion of the duodenum may be barium filled dependent on peristalsis of the bowel
- With a double-contrast study, the fundus will appear air filled while the body will be barium filled

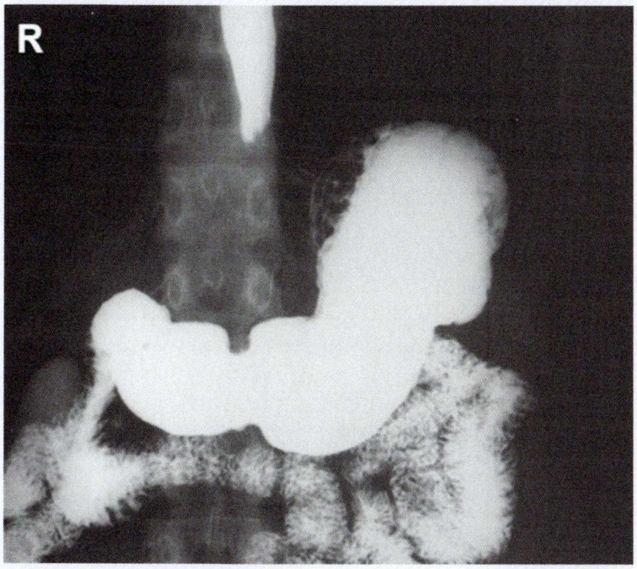

11-82 PA projection stomach—prone position.

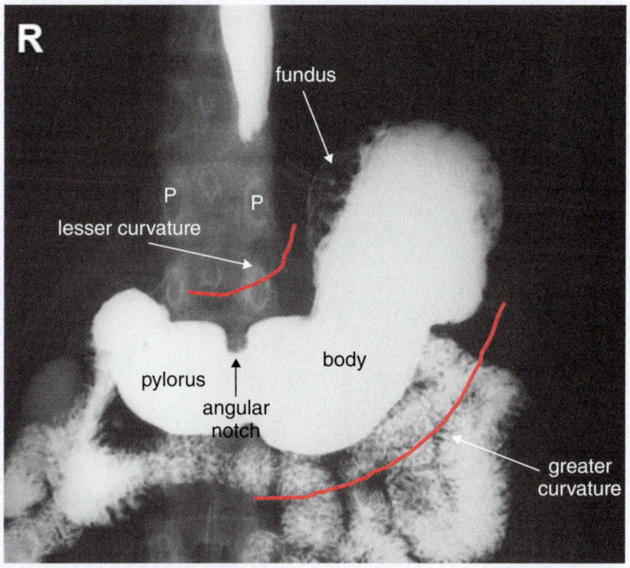

11-83 PA projection stomach—prone position. (P) represents the pedicles of the vertebra.

POSITION VARIATION SUPINE

A patient unable to assume a prone position for the PA projection, could be reversed to a supine position and the image acquired with an AP projection. The central ray is still directed to L1 and 1″–2″ left of the MSP. Radiographically the air–barium distribution will be opposite of the appearance seen with the patient in the prone position. With the patient supine, the barium will fill the fundus as it is most posterior and closer to the spine, while air will rise to the highest or most anterior point being the gastric body (Fig. 11-84).

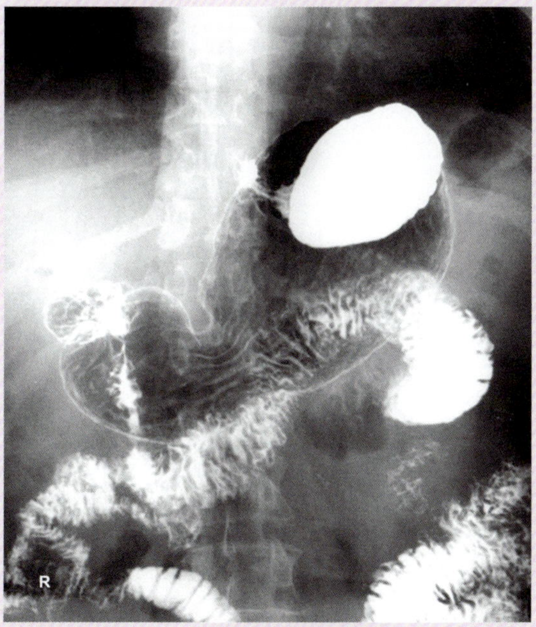

11-84 Alternate AP projection stomach—supine position.

Upper GI—Right Anterior Oblique

- Projection: PA Oblique

Technical Considerations

- 90 kVp for double contrast
- 110+ kVp for single contrast
- Center AEC cell or manual mAs
- 40″ SID

Exposure Field Size

- 14 × 17 lengthwise collimated to radiologist preference size

Patient Position

- Patient is positioned into prone oblique—RAO. The average patient will be in a 45° oblique. The hypersthenic patient will need a steeper oblique position to achieve the desired internal placement of stomach anatomy and duodenal bulb

Centering

- It is highly recommended that the technologist be observant to the stomach position and relative landmarks while the radiologist is performing fluoroscopy. During this observation, the technologist can identify topographical landmarks to assist with better centering
- CR directed to L1 and midway between MSP and left lateral margin of the patient. The CR must enter on the "upside" or left side of the patient (Fig. 11-85)
- It may be necessary to alter from the above centering location if the patient has an asthenic/hyposthenic or hypersthenic body habitus. The asthenic/hyposthenic patient will most likely need the CR directed 1″–2″ inferior from the sthenic patient. The hypersthenic patient will most likely need the CR directed 1″–2″ superior from the sthenic patient (Fig. 11-86)

Marking of IR

- Anatomic R side marker placed on the corresponding right side of the patient, indicating the right side was closest to the IR

Breathing

- Breathing is suspended after expiration

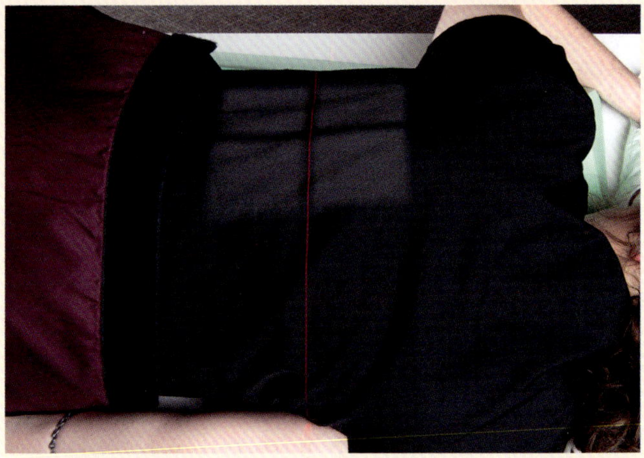

11-85 PA Oblique projection stomach—RAO position. Sthenic patient.

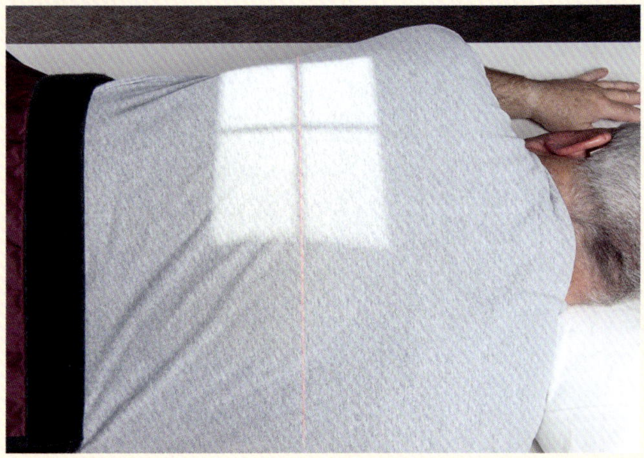

11-86 PA Oblique projection stomach—RAO position. Hypersthenic patient.

IMAGE CRITIQUE (FIGS. 11-87 and 11-88)

- With a patient in a 45° oblique, the "Scottie Dog" should help reveal the oblique position of the patient
- The entire stomach is visible. With the position obliquity, the duodenum should ideally be free of superimposition from the pylorus. The duodenum or portion of the duodenum may be barium filled dependent on peristalsis of the bowel
- With a double-contrast study, the fundus will appear air filled while the body will be barium filled. By observing the appearance of the spine and the air–barium distribution, the technologist should be able to determine the patient position

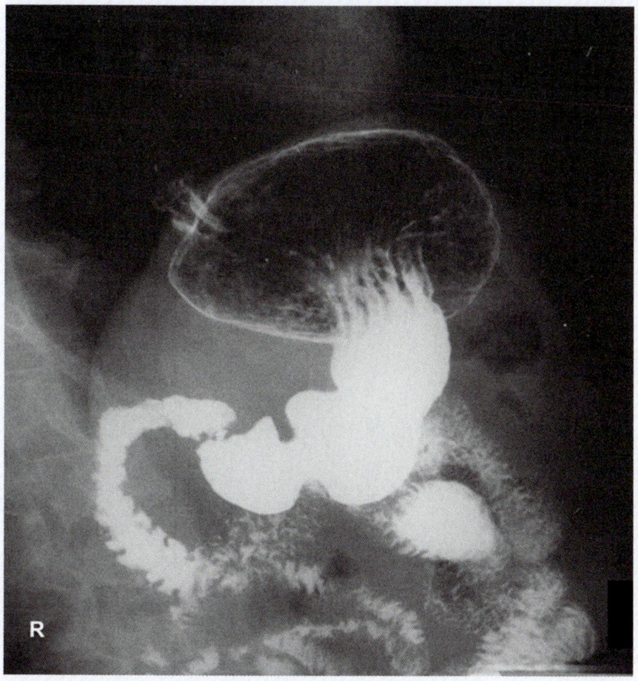

11-87 PA Oblique projection stomach—RAO position.

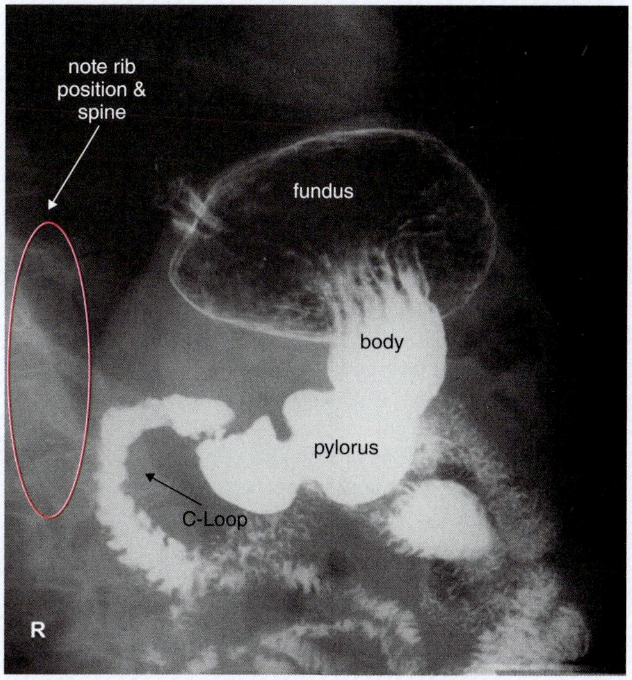

11-88 PA Oblique projection stomach—RAO position.

Upper GI—Lateral

- Projection: Lateral

Technical Considerations
- 90 kVp for double contrast
- 110+ kVp for single contrast
- Center AEC cell or manual mAs
- 40″ SID

Exposure Field Size
- 14 × 17 lengthwise collimated to radiologist preference size

Patient Position
- Patient in a lateral position
- True lateral position with shoulders and hips stacked and aligned

Centering (Fig. 11-89)
- It is highly recommended that the technologist be observant to the stomach position and relative landmarks while the radiologist is performing fluoroscopy. During this observation, the technologist can identify topographical landmarks to assist with better centering
- CR directed to L1 and 1″–2″ anterior to MCP
- Anterior to posterior collimation is encouraged
- It may be necessary to alter from the above centering location if the patient has an asthenic/hyposthenic or hypersthenic body habitus. The asthenic/hyposthenic patient will most likely need the CR directed 1″–2″ inferior from the sthenic patient. The hypersthenic patient will most likely need the CR directed 1″–2″ superior from the sthenic patient

Marking of IR
- Anatomic side closest to the image receptor is marked and placed within the collimated exposure field anterior to the patient

Breathing
- Breathing is suspended after expiration

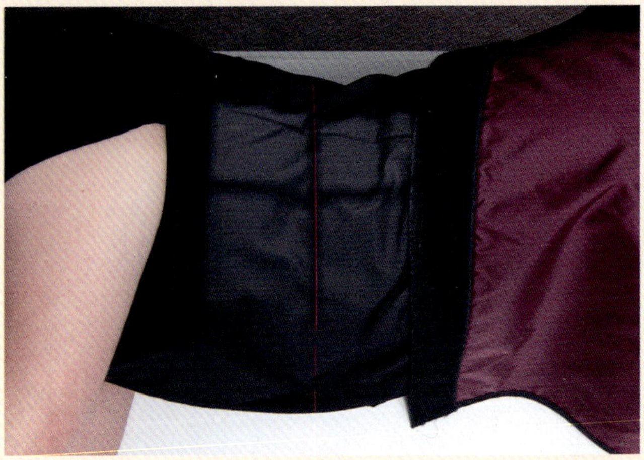

11-89 Lateral projection stomach.

IMAGE CRITIQUE (FIGS. 11-90 and 11-91)

- With a patient in a true lateral, the vertebral column should display the alignment of the vertebral bodies, intervertebral disk spaces, and intervertebral foramina
- The entire stomach is visible. The retrogastric space is of interest. The retrogastric space is located posterior to the stomach and anterior to the spine. This projection allows a stomach mass to be ruled out from the posterior aspect of the stomach
- With a double contrast study, the air–barium distribution in the stomach is not of importance for this position

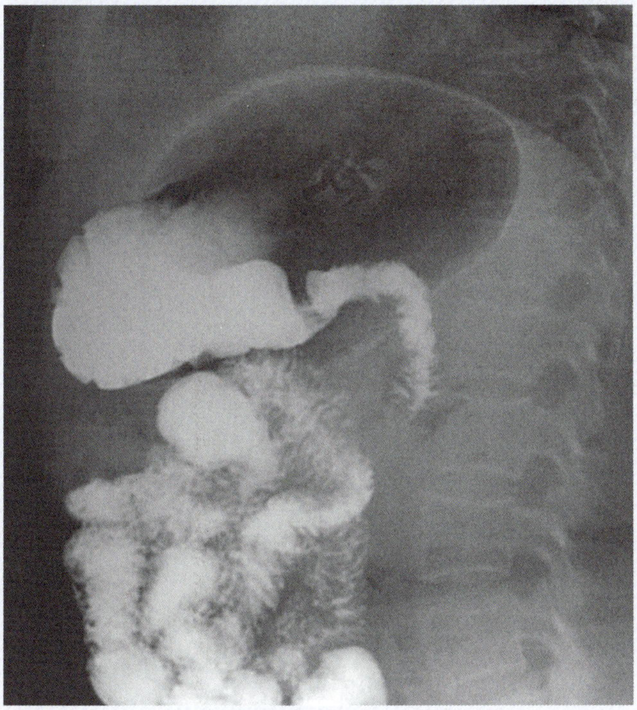

11-90 Lateral projection stomach.

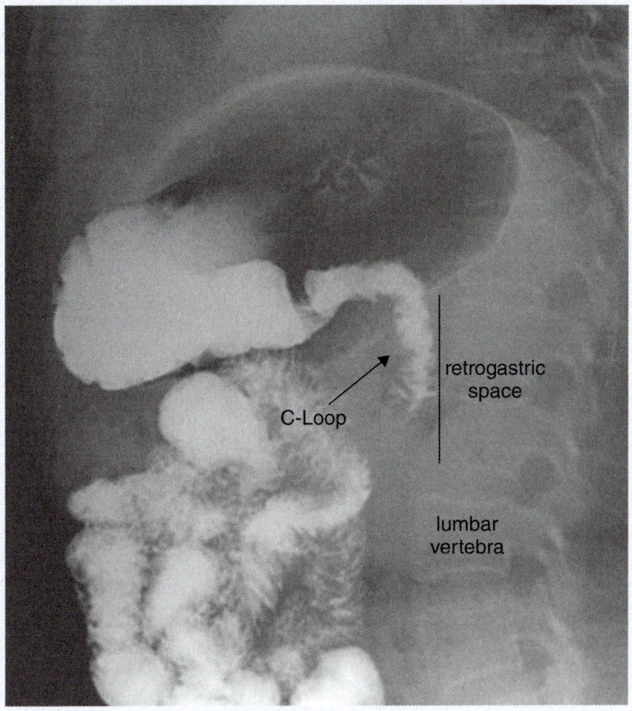

11-91 Lateral projection stomach.

Upper GI—Left Posterior Oblique

- Projection: AP Oblique

Technical Considerations

- 90 kVp for double contrast
- 110+ kVp for single contrast
- Center AEC cell or manual mAs
- 40″ SID

Exposure Field Size

- 14 × 17 lengthwise collimated to radiologist preference size

Patient Position

- Patient is positioned into supine oblique—LPO. The average patient will be in a 45° oblique. The hypersthenic patient in a steeper oblique position to achieve the desired internal placement of stomach anatomy and duodenal bulb

Centering (Fig. 11-92)

- It is highly recommended that the technologist be observant to the stomach position and relative landmarks, while the radiologist is performing fluoroscopy. During this observation, the technologist can identify topographical landmarks to assist with better centering
- CR directed to L1 and midway between MSP and left lateral margin
- It may be necessary to alter from the above centering location if the patient has an asthenic/hyposthenic or hypersthenic body habitus. The asthenic/hyposthenic patient will most likely need the CR directed 1″–2″ inferior from the sthenic patient. The hypersthenic patient will most likely need the CR directed 1″–2″ superior from the sthenic patient

Marking of IR

- Anatomic L side marker placed on the corresponding left side of the patient, indicating the left side was closest to the IR

Breathing

- Breathing is suspended after expiration

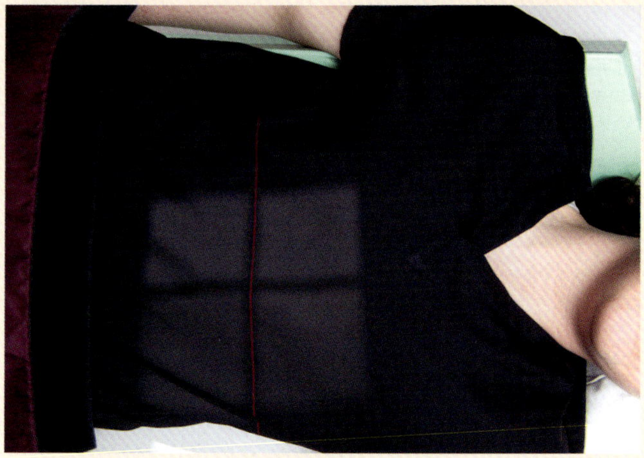

11-92 AP Oblique projection stomach—LPO position.

IMAGE CRITIQUE (FIGS. 11-93 and 11-94)

- With a patient in a 45° oblique, the "Scottie Dog" should reveal the oblique position of the patient
- The entire stomach is visible. With obliquity the duodenum should ideally be free of superimposition from the pylorus. The duodenum or portion of the duodenum may be barium filled dependent on peristalsis of the bowel
- With a double-contrast study, the fundus will appear barium filled while the body will be air filled. By observing the appearance of the spine and the air–barium distribution, the technologist should be able to determine the patient position

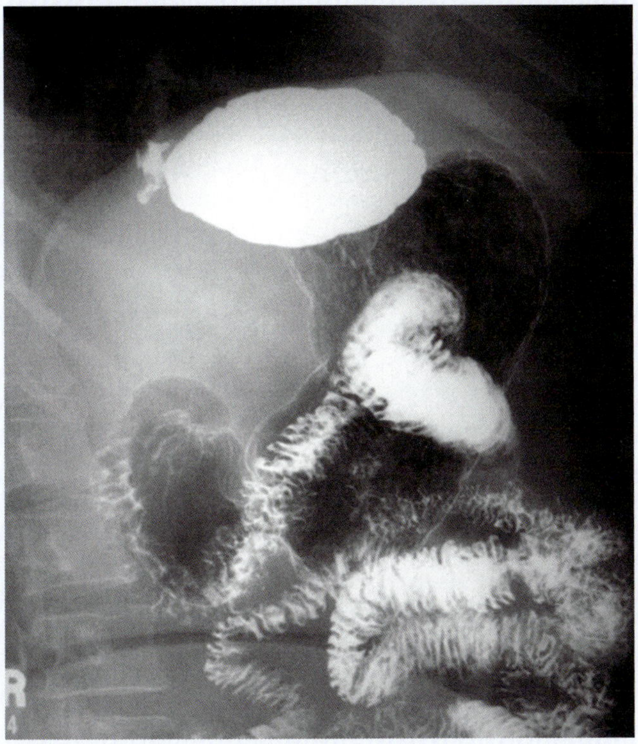

11-93 AP Oblique projection stomach—LPO position.

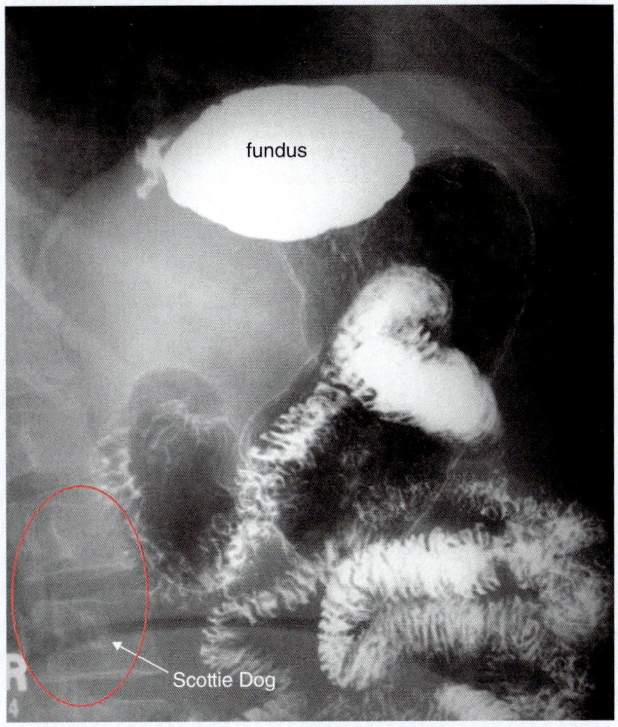

11-94 AP Oblique projection stomach—LPO position.

SMALL BOWEL SERIES

- Radiographic study of the duodenum, jejunum, and ileum.

Indications

- Enteritis, regional enteritis (i.e., Crohn disease), mechanical obstruction, ileus

Contraindications

- If bowel perforation is suspected, the contrast media is altered to the iodinated contrast media.
- Patients with a large bowel obstruction should not ingest barium.

Patient Prep

- Patient NPO 8 hours before exam along with a low residue diet the day preceding the procedure. Patient is instructed not to chew gum or smoke before the exam as this stimulates gastric juices and may interfere with barium adhering to the mucosal lining.

Contrast Prep (Highly Dependent on Radiologist Preference)

- 16 oz thin liquid barium sulfate. Serving the thin barium cold may allow the patient to ingest quicker. This is a functional study, so the study is timed. The timer begins on the *completion* of ingestion of 16 oz of barium.

Room Setup

- The room is not set up in the typical fluoroscopic arrangement.
- At the end of the procedure, the radiologist may use fluoroscopy to study the ileocecal valve.

General Procedure

- The patient will have a scout supine abdominal image (KUB - kidneys, ureters, bladder). This image provides an overall look at the abdominal cavity and bowel prep. This image is shared with the radiologist. The radiologist will determine if the procedure will move forward.
- The patient will ingest 16 oz of thin barium as quickly as possible. The stomach should fill will barium and the barium should begin to empty into the duodenum. If a patient is having this exam and has a nasogastric tube (NG) placed, the technologist will syringe push the 16 oz of barium through the NG tube. The technologist needs to ensure saline is used to flush the NG tube after the barium.
- 30 minutes after ingestion of the barium, a prone abdominal image centered 2″ above the crest is acquired. The higher centering will include the stomach on the image. The prone position is preferred if it is possible for the patient. Prone position will allow the patient's weight to separate the loops of bowel apart and will be closer to the image receptor.
- 1 hour after ingestion of the barium, a prone abdominal image is acquired centered at the level of the iliac crest. Each time an abdominal image is acquired, the radiologist should review the image.
- The patient will undergo a prone abdominal image every 30 minutes up to 2 hours. If at 2 hours, the barium has not passed through the ileocecal valve, it is possible the radiologist will ask that an image be acquired every hour or longer until the barium passes through the ileocecal valve. For most outpatients, a small bowel series (SBS) is attainable within 2 hours or less. For inpatients, this exam can get rather lengthy. Images of the abdomen may at this point be acquired with the mobile unit depending on the mobility of the patient.
- The small bowel series (SBS) is not a complete study until the barium passes through the ileocecal valve into the cecum.
- Once the barium has passed through the ileocecal valve, the final images acquired are of the ileocecal valve. This is done with fluoroscopy. Spot images are typically acquired of this area. The terminal ileum is a common site of occurrence for Crohn disease.
- To evaluate the terminal ileum and the ileocecal valve, the patient is often rotated into oblique positions to help separate bowel loops apart. Additionally, the compression paddle can apply pressure on the right lower quadrant to separate bowel loops to identify the ileocecal valve.

Post Imaging

- Acquired images begin 30 minutes after the patient finishes ingesting the 16 oz of barium.
- Prone abdominal images are acquired every 30 minutes up to the 2-hour mark. If the patient is unable to assume a prone position, a supine position can be substituted.
- If the SBS is combined with a UGI realize that the patient ingested about 8 oz of barium for the UGI. If post images of the UGI are requested by the radiologist, these images must be acquired and cleared by the radiologist. Then, the patient will ingest the remaining 8 oz of barium needed for the SBS. Then, the image sequence aligns with the standard SBS.
- With dismissal of the patient, the patient should be given postexam instructions to increase clear fluid intake to help facilitate the barium sulfate through the GI tract.

Small Bowel Series—Prone Abdomen

- Projection: PA of the abdomen is preferred

Technical Considerations

- 110+ kVp
- All three AEC cells or manual mAs
- 40″ SID

Exposure Field Size

- 14 × 17 lengthwise or two 14 × 17 overlapping crosswise if necessary for the patient

Patient Position (Fig. 11-95)

- If the patient is capable, prone position is most desirable to place the small bowel closer to the IR and create pressure on the abdomen to help separate the loops of bowel apart
- If the patient is unable to assume a prone position, a supine abdomen can be substituted
- For imaging of the ileocecal valve, the patient will be supine or into a slight supine oblique

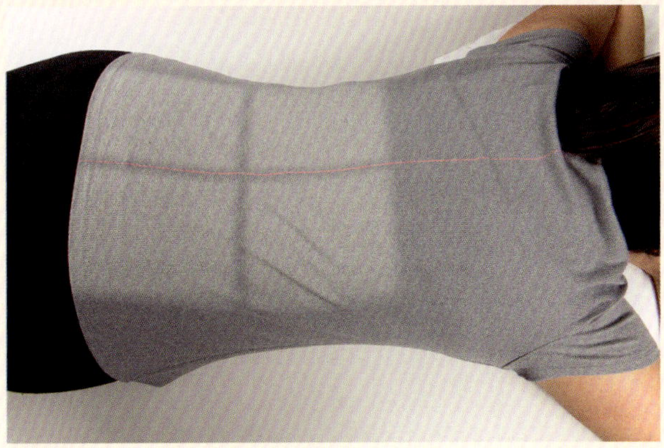

11-95 Prone position—abdomen.

Centering

- The 30-minute image is acquired with the CR directed 2″ above the crest and with MSP. The higher centering will include the stomach to display the volume of barium within the stomach
- The 1-hour image and moving forward, the CR is directed to the level of the iliac crest and MSP

Marking of IR

- Anatomic R or L side marker placed on the corresponding right or left side of the patient
- A time annotation needs to be on each image

Breathing

- Breathing is suspended after expiration

IMAGE CRITIQUE (FIGS. 11-96 to 11-100)

- Inclusion of all the small bowel. The three divisions of the small bowel can be distinguished by their radiographic appearance when filled with barium and by location
  - Duodenum will display its C-loop shape in the RUQ
  - Jejunum will appear in the LUQ and LLQ
  - Ileum will appear smooth and with smaller diameter in the central and RLQ of the abdomen

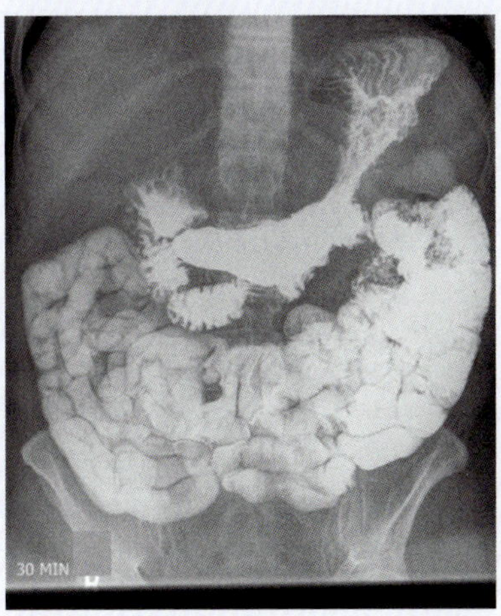

11-96 SBS—30 minutes.

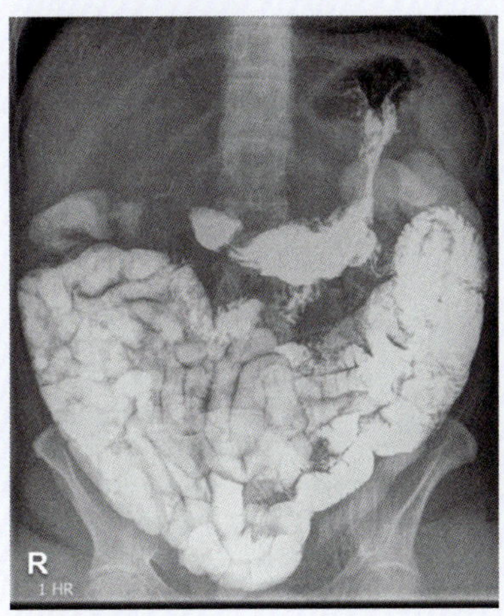

11-97 SBS—1 hour.

(Continued)

IMAGE CRITIQUE (*Continued*)

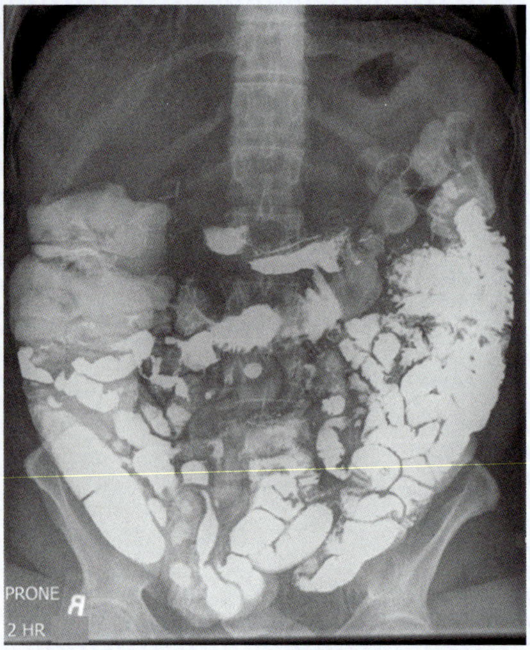

11-98 SBS—2 hours.

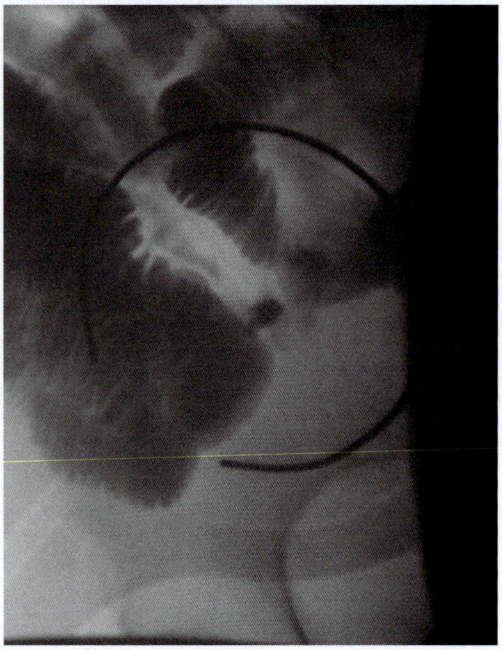

11-99 SBS—ileocecal spot.

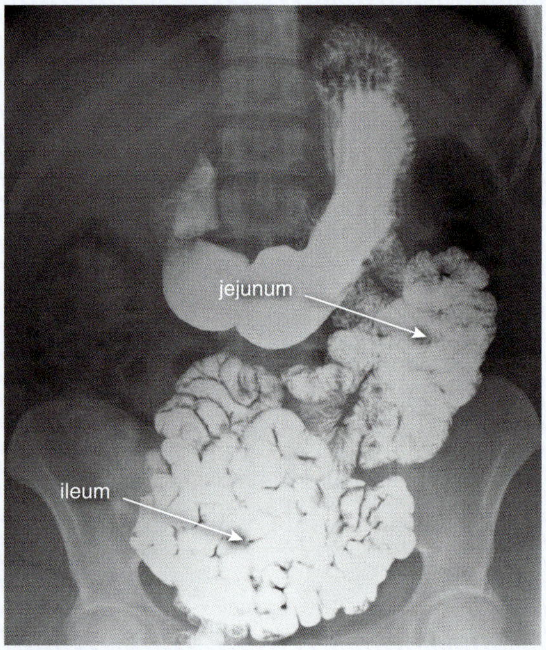

11-100 SBS—jejunum and ileum.

ENTEROCLYSIS

- Double-contrast radiographic study of the duodenum, jejunum, and ileum.

Indications

- Double contrast may provide a more diagnostic means to identify enteritis or regional enteritis.

Contraindications

- If small bowel perforation is suspected, a double-contrast study could not be performed.

Patient Prep

- Patient NPO 8 hours before exam along with a low residue diet the day preceding the procedure. Patient is instructed not to chew gum or smoke before the exam as this stimulates gastric juices and may interfere with barium adhering to the mucosal lining.

Contrast Prep (Highly Dependent on Radiologist Preference)

- 16 oz thin liquid barium sulfate
- Methylcellulose solution or air (serves to create a double-contrast effect)
- The contrast will be introduced into the small bowel through a catheter placed into the small intestine. This is a functional study, so the study is timed. The timer begins on the *completion* of introduction of contrast into the patient.

Room Setup

- Control panel switched to fluoroscopy with time zeroed and kVp set at 90–110 kVp.
- Footboard attached to imaging table so table could be stood up vertically if necessary.
- Table Bucky positioned to the foot of the table.
- Viewing monitor and fluoroscopy foot pedal arranged for radiologist.

General Procedure

- The patient will have a scout supine abdominal image (KUB). This image provides an overall look at the abdominal cavity and bowel prep. This image will be shared with the radiologist. The radiologist will determine if the procedure will move forward.
- Patient consent is acquired after being informed of the procedure and the primary risk of the procedure being potential bowel perforation.
- The patient may gargle with a lidocaine solution or have a lidocaine spray administered to the back of the throat to suppress the gag reflex.
- The radiologist will advance a catheter through the mouth or nose down toward the stomach. The catheter must be advanced through the pyloric orifice and into the duodenum. Typically, the tip of the catheter is placed at the duodenojejunal junction (ligament of Treitz). The end of the catheter is secured there by inflating the balloon at the tip of the catheter. The radiologist will use fluoroscopic guidance as needed to properly position the catheter.
- Once the catheter is in position, a double-contrast effect will be created with barium and the methylcellulose or air. These will be introduced into the small intestine by syringe and through the catheter.
- 30 minutes after introduction of the contrast, a prone abdominal image centered 2″ above the crest is acquired. The higher centering will include the stomach on the image. The prone position is preferred if it is possible for the patient. Prone position will allow the patient's weight to separate the loops of bowel apart and will be closer to the image receptor.
- The patient will undergo a prone abdominal image every 30 minutes up to 2 hours. If at 2 hours, the barium has not passed through the ileocecal valve, it is possible the radiologist will ask that an image be acquired every hour or longer until the barium passes through the ileocecal valve.
- The enteroclysis is not a complete study until the contrast passes through the ileocecal valve into the cecum.
- Once the contrast has passed through the ileocecal valve, the final images acquired are of the ileocecal valve. This is done with fluoroscopy. Spot images may be acquired of the terminal ileum and the ileocecal valve.
- To evaluate the terminal ileum and the ileocecal valve, the patient is often rotated into oblique positions to help separate bowel loops apart. Additionally, the compression paddle can apply pressure on the right lower quadrant to separate bowel loops to identify the ileocecal valve.

Post Imaging

- The images acquired begin 30 minutes post completion of introduction of the contrast media.
- Prone abdominal images are acquired every 30 minutes for up to the 2 hour mark. If the patient is unable to assume a prone position, the supine position can be substituted.
- With dismissal of the patient, the patient should be given postexam instructions to increase clear fluid intake to help move the barium sulfate through the GI tract.

- A barium mixture of barium and tepid water is created according to the radiologist's preferences and mixed in a double-contrast enema bag.
- Barium needs to be ran through the tubing connecting the barium bag to the tip. This is to remove air from the tube before the enema tip is inserted into the rectum. If this air is not removed from the tubing before tip insertion, a volume of air will enter the colon before the barium solution; this potentially could create a vapor lock (wall), which will not allow the barium to pass beyond this point.

Room Setup

- Control panel switched to fluoroscopy with time zeroed and kVp set at 90 for a double-contrast study and 110+ for a single-contrast study.
- Footboard attached to imaging table and so the table could be stood up vertically if desired.
- Table Bucky positioned to the foot of the table.
- Viewing monitor and fluoroscopy foot pedal arranged for radiologist.
- Towels and a trash receptacle close by.

General Procedure

- The patient will have a scout supine abdominal image (KUB). This image provides an overall look at the abdominal cavity and bowel prep. This image will be shared with the radiologist. The radiologist will determine if the procedure will move forward (Figs. 11-106 and 11-107).
- Single or double-contrast barium bag is prepared.
- Barium solution is run through the tubing up to the point of the enema tip. This step is done before the enema tip is inserted into the patient's rectum (Fig. 11-105).
- Patient is positioned into the Sim's position. Patient is recumbent in a left lateral position with the knees flexed slightly. The right leg is dropped in front of the left leg helping to relax the lower abdomen (Fig. 11-108).
- The enema tip is lubricated. The technologist will expose the patient's rectal region, trying to maintain as much patient modesty as possible. The technologist will explain to the patient step by step what is happening during tip insertion into the rectum (Fig. 11-109).
- If the facility allows the technologist to place the enema tip, while wearing gloves, the technologist will lift the upper buttock to visualize the rectum. The rectal tip is first inserted toward the direction of the umbilicus. The rectal tip will advance about 1½″ anteriorly. The rectal tip should then be directed superiorly another approximate 1½.″ Once the tip is initially directed properly anteriorly, the tip will position itself superiorly without resistance.
- A tip should never be forced. If the patient is not relaxed, there may be some resistance with insertion. Forcing a tip could potentially perforate the rectum. Patients expectantly will be nervous and tense through this part of the process. While using the Sim's position for rectal tip insertion, the technologist utilizes the patient's expiratory phase to position the enema tip.

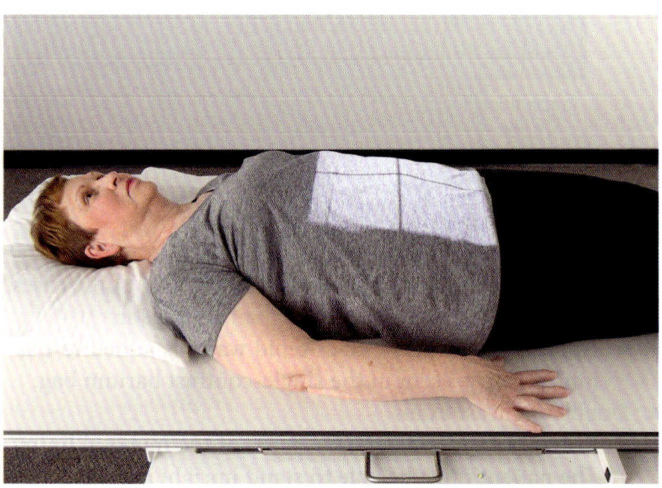

11-106 Supine abdomen.

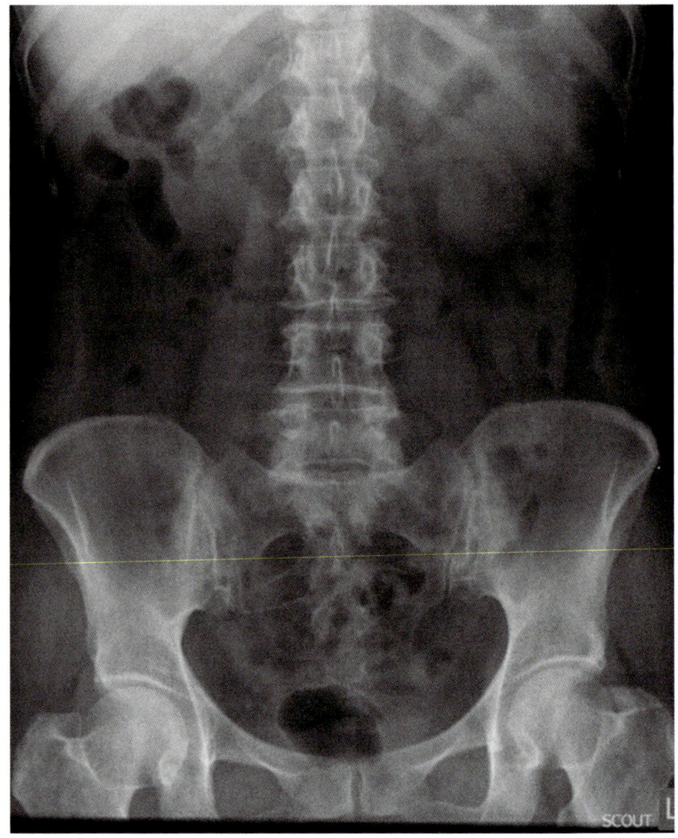

11-107 Scout abdomen.

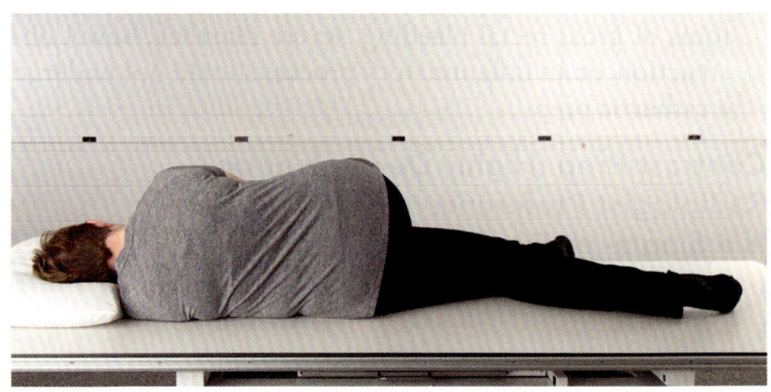

11-108 Sim's position.

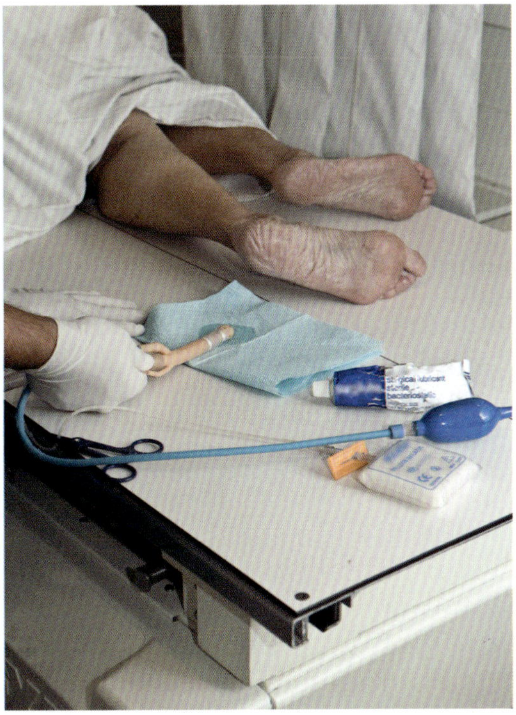

11-109 Enema tip preparation.

- Once the enema tip is positioned, there is a small balloon at the end of the tip that could be inflated. The inflation of this balloon is typically with one puff of air with the cufflator. Some facilities may not allow the technologist to inflate the balloon. If this is the case, the radiologist will do it at the beginning of the procedure. The balloon on the enema tip is positioned within the rectal ampulla (dilated segment of the rectum) to prevent barium from being able to leak out (Fig. 11-110).
- The radiologist will begin the study, with a survey of the patient's abdomen with fluoroscopy.
- The radiologist will loosen the clamp on the tubing allowing the barium solution to enter into the colon. If it is a single-contrast study, a large amount of barium will flow into the colon to help distend and fill it. If it is a double-contrast study, a small amount of barium will flow into the colon and then the radiologist will then introduce air into the colon through the end of the enema tip. This air will cause discomfort to the patient. The bowel will distend, and the barium will adhere to the mucosal lining, thus creating improved detail of the mucosal lining.
- During the procedure, the radiologist will instruct the patient to move into different positions: prone, lateral recumbent, supine, anterior oblique, posterior oblique, and potentially erect (only if the study is double contrast). The technologist will need to be available to assist the patient with these positional changes. Again, the technologist is there to help expedite the procedure. During this entire time, the radiologist will be capturing spot images with the digital fluoroscopy.
- Once the radiologist has completed their part of the study, they will indicate to the technologist if there are any post-fluoroscopy images they want additionally acquired.
- If additional images are acquired by the technologist, the technologist will want to expedite these quickly. It is imperative the technologist efficiently organize and sequence these final images for the patient. With completion of these final images, they must be cleared with the radiologist.
- Once the radiologist has indicated the exam is done, the technologist will first attempt to drain as much barium from the colon back into the enema bag before removing the enema tip. By lowering the barium bag to the floor and opening up the tubing clamp, gravity will help drain the barium back out. This is extremely important to do on the single-contrast studies because these patients have a large volume of barium within the colon.
- Once the barium return to the bag has slowed, the technologist should remove air from the balloon on the end of the tip. This may result in more barium return in the bag from the area of the rectum. Then, the tip is removed. The patient should be assisted to the restroom, and the patient will evacuate as much residual barium as possible.
- Once the patient has relief, they can clean up and dress into a clean gown. A final postevacuation KUB is acquired and shared with the radiologist. If the radiologist has approved the postevacuation image, the patient can dress and be dismissed.
- With dismissal of the patient, the patient should be given postexam instructions to increase clear fluid intake to help facilitate the barium sulfate through the GI tract.

Post Imaging

- If multiple images are requested by the radiologist, the technologist should choose the order of the images that will be most efficient and logical for the patient. The patient should end near or in the left lateral position. Once the radiologist approves all post images and declares the procedure complete, the patient will need to be in the left lateral position for the barium drainage the enema tip removal.
- A technologist may have to consider modification of the facility protocol projections/positions if the patient has limited movement. For example, if the protocol includes a prone abdomen and the patient is unable to roll into a prone position, then a supine abdomen could be the substitute. Another example, if the protocol includes a right anterior oblique and the patient is unable to roll into this prone oblique, a left posterior oblique would be the correct substitute position to demonstrate the same anatomy.

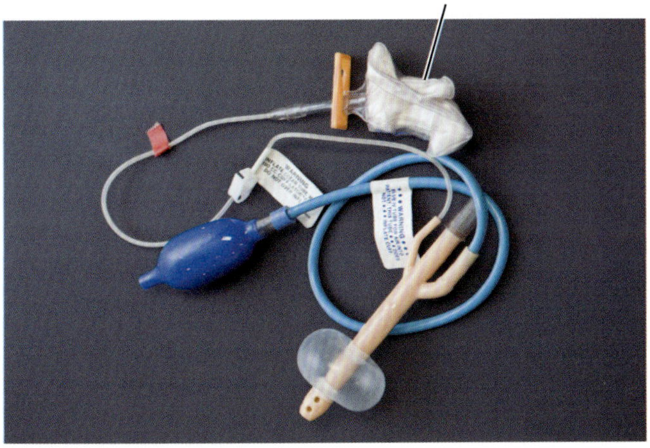

11-110 Balloon inflation.

Barium Enema—Supine and/or Prone Abdomen

- Projection: AP or PA

Technical Considerations

- 90 kVp for double contrast
- 110+ kVp for single contrast
- 80+ kVp for iodinated contrast
- All three AEC cells or manual mAs
- 40″ SID

Exposure Field Size

- 14 × 17 lengthwise or two 14 × 17 overlapping crosswise if necessary for the patient

Patient Position

- Supine. No rotation
- Prone. No rotation

Centering (Figs. 11-111 to 11-114)

- If the entire colon can fit on a single lengthwise IR; the CR is directed to the level of the iliac crest and MSP
- If the entire colon will not fit on a single lengthwise IR; two separate exposures acquired with 2- 14 × 17 IRs orientated crosswise

Marking of IR

- Anatomic R or L side marker placed on the corresponding right or left side of the patient

Breathing

- Breathing is suspended after expiration

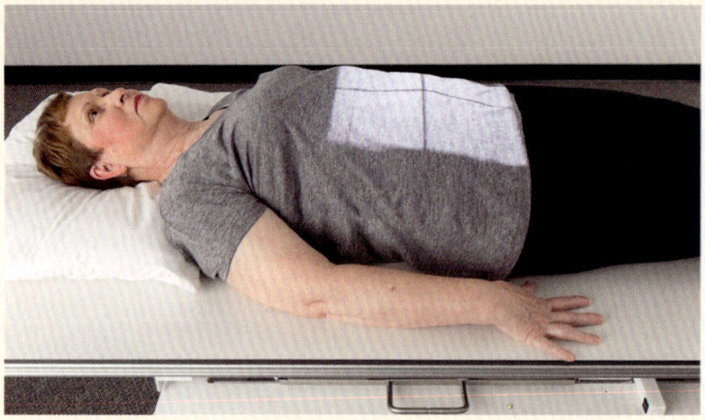

11-111 AP projection—supine abdomen.

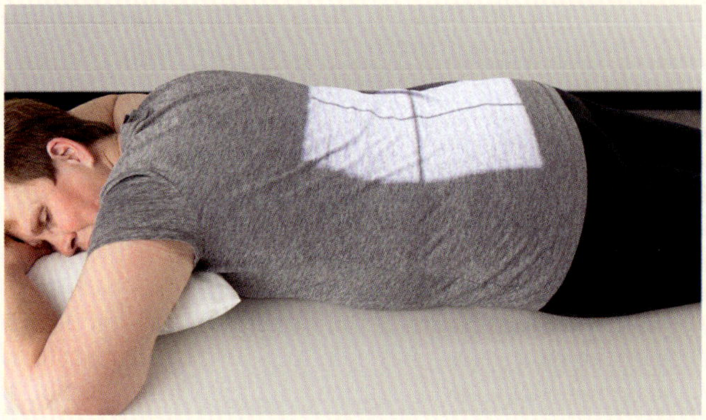

11-112 PA projection—prone abdomen.

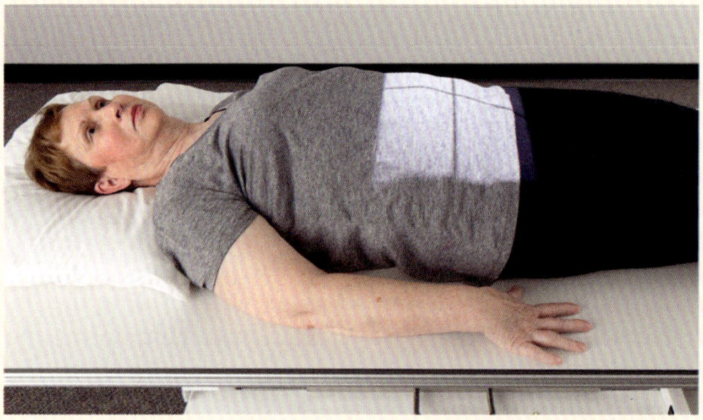

11-113 AP projection—supine abdomen low CW image.

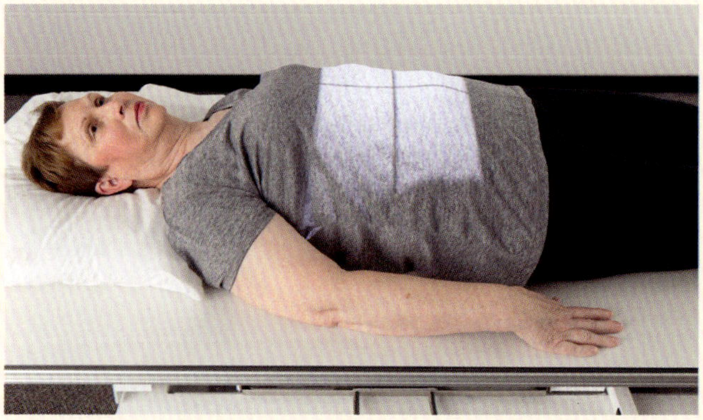

11-114 AP projection—supine abdomen with overlap high CW image.

IMAGE CRITIQUE (FIGS. 11-115 to 11-118)

- Symmetry of the vertebral pedicles and pelvic iliac wings indicate the part was positioned without rotation
- Inclusion of all the large bowel. The enema tip should be included with the symphysis pubis
- A double-contrast study will display air–barium distribution. The transverse and sigmoid colon are positioned more anteriorly in the abdomen than the ascending and descending colon
  - Supine: Air will rise to the highest point (more anterior) within the transverse and sigmoid portions. Barium will gravitate to the lowest points (more posterior) within the ascending and descending portions
  - Prone: Air will rise to the highest point (more posterior) within the ascending and descending portions. Barium will gravitate to the lowest points (more anterior) within the transverse and sigmoid portions
- A single-contrast study will display a distended contrast filled colon

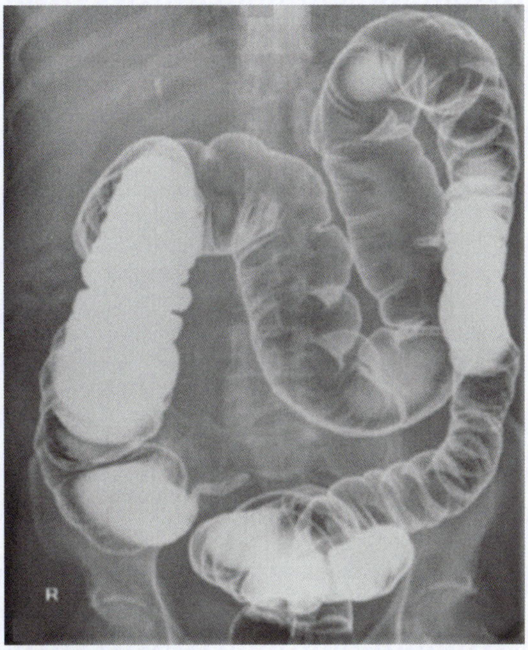

11-115 AP projection—Double Contrast/Air Contrast barium enema.

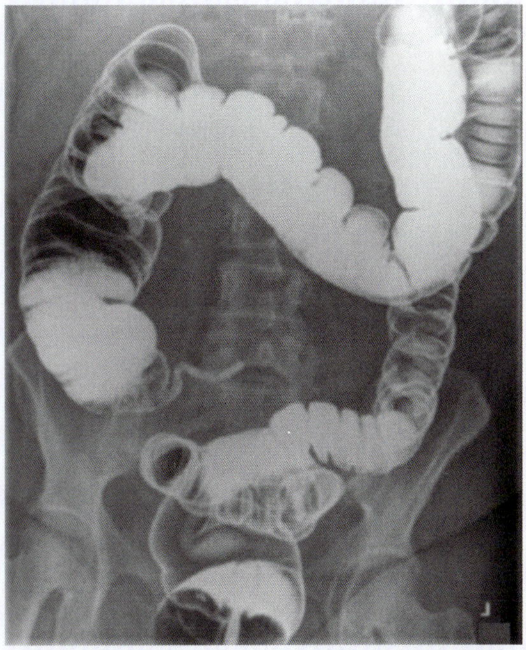

11-116 PA projection—Double Contrast/Air Contrast barium enema.

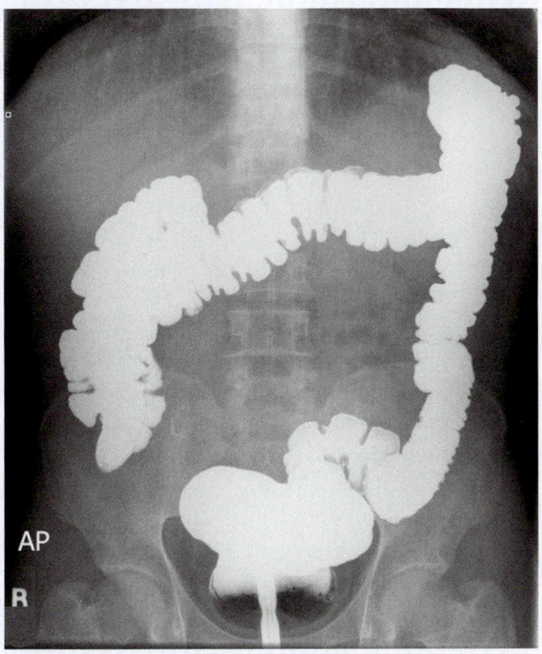

11-117 AP projection—Single Contrast barium enema.

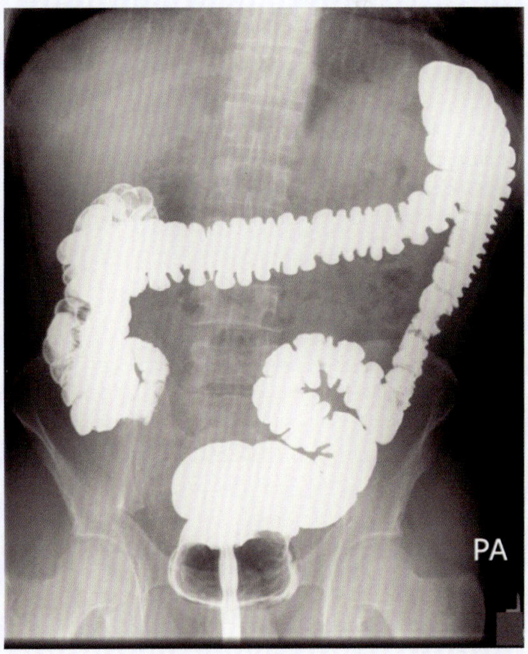

11-118 PA projection—Single Contrast barium enema.

Barium Enema—Posterior or Anterior Obliques

- Projection: AP Obliques or PA Obliques

Technical Considerations
- 90 kVp for double contrast
- 110+ kVp for single contrast
- 80+ kVp for iodinated contrast
- All three AEC cells or manual mAs
- 40″ SID

Exposure Field Size
- 14 × 17 lengthwise or two 14 × 17 overlapping crosswise if necessary for the patient

Patient Position (Figs. 11-119 to 11-122)
- Posterior Oblique with 45° rotation RPO and LPO. Ensure the patient has even oblique rotation between the shoulders and the hips
- Posterior oblique positions demonstrate the upside colic flexure open
  - RPO = Splenic flexure
  - LPO = Hepatic flexure
- Anterior Oblique with 45° rotation RAO and LAO
- Anterior oblique positions demonstrate the downside colic flexure open. Ensure the patient has even oblique rotation between the shoulders and the hips
  - RAO = Hepatic flexure
  - LAO = Splenic flexure

Centering
- Centering is based on which colic flexure is of interest with 45° oblique position
- Splenic Flexure
  - RPO and LAO: The CR is directed 1″–2″ superior to the iliac crest 1″–2″ off MSP toward the upside of the patient
- Hepatic Flexure
  - LPO and RAO: The CR is directed to the level of the iliac crest and 1″–2″ off MSP toward the upside of the patient

Marking of IR
- Anatomic R or L side marker placed on the corresponding right or left side of the patient
- Suggested markings for a torso oblique are to mark the anatomic side closest to the IR on that corresponding side of the IR

Breathing
- Breathing is suspended after expiration

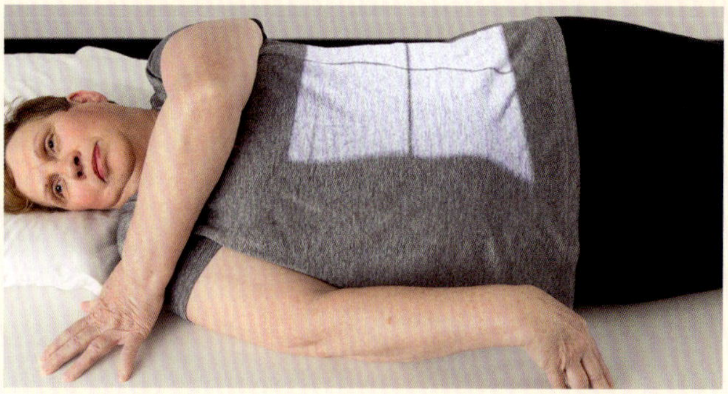

11-119 AP Oblique projection—RPO position. Splenic flexure.

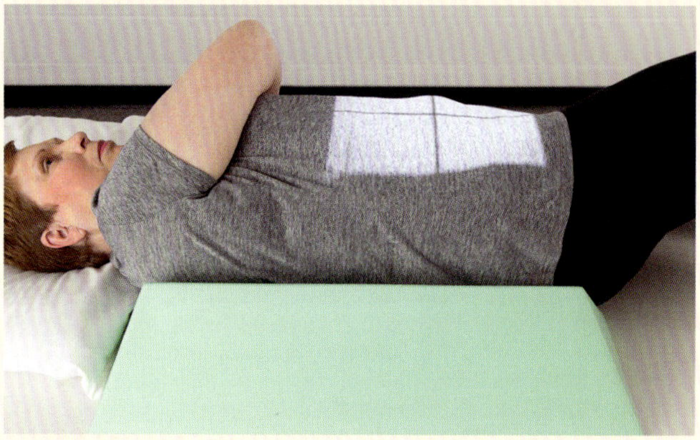

11-120 AP Oblique projection—LPO position. Hepatic flexure.

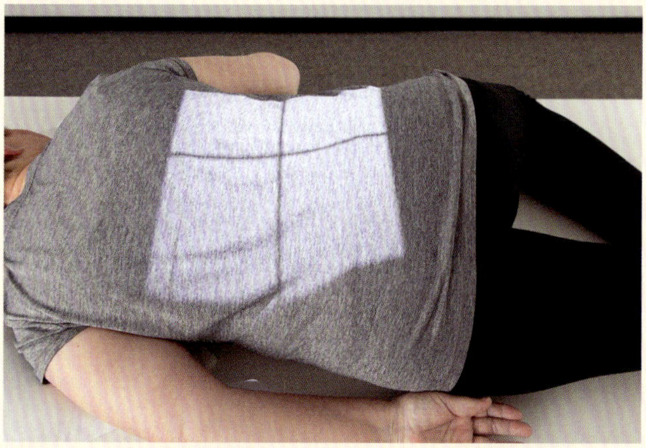

11-121 PA Oblique projection—LAO position. Splenic flexure.

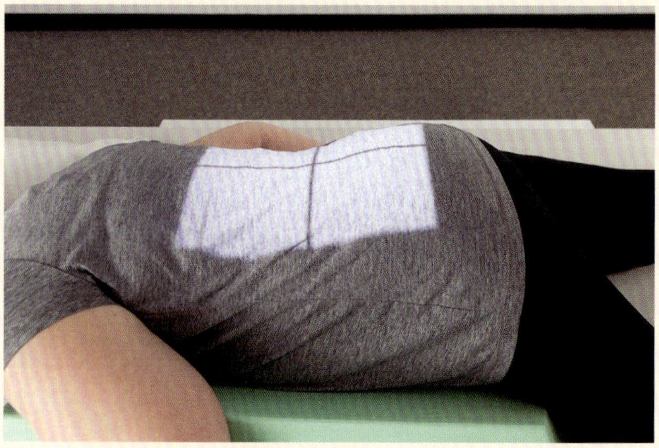

11-122 PA Oblique projection—RAO position. Hepatic flexure.

IMAGE CRITIQUE (FIGS. 11-123 and 11-124)

- Inclusion of the majority of or all of the large bowel
- Obliquity of the patient can be revealed when the "Scottie Dog" is visualized within the lumbar spine
- Obliquity of the patient is to aid in opening up the colic flexures to view free of superimposition from the transverse colon from the ascending or descending colon. Centering must be appropriately directed to image each flexure separately. Generally, both a right and left oblique is attained. Modification from site protocol to accommodate the patient's ability is acceptable
  - RAO and LPO will each demonstrate the hepatic flexure
  - LAO and RPO will each demonstrate the splenic flexure

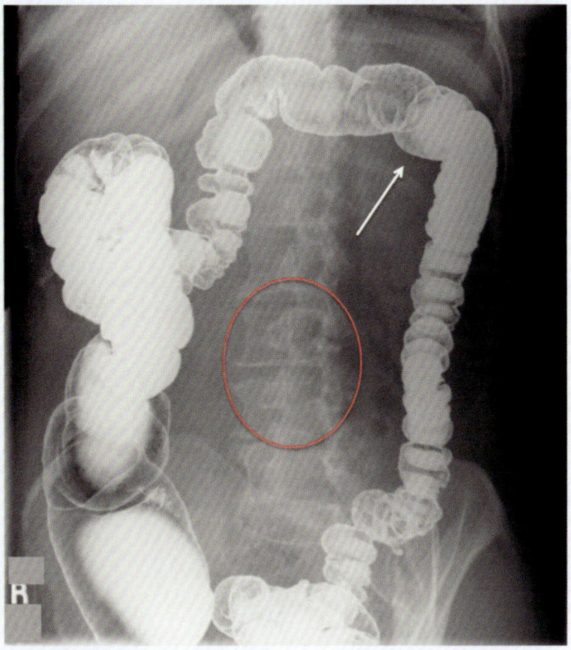

11-123 RPO or LAO position—splenic flexure open. Arrow represents the splenic flexure. Red circle reveals presence of the "Scottie Dog."

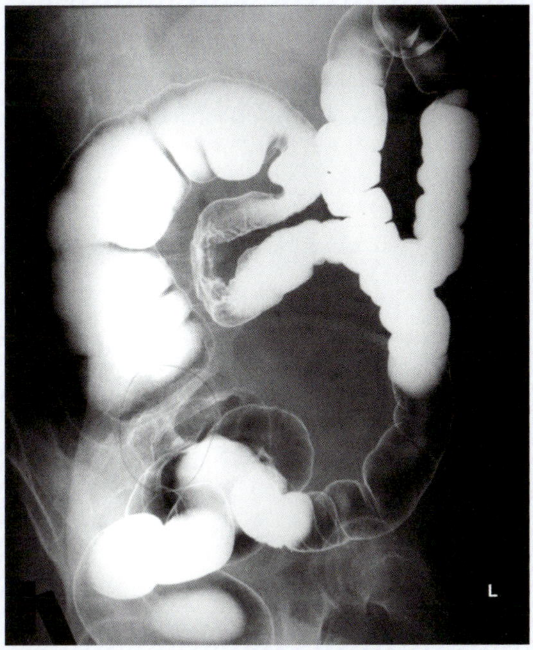

11-124 LPO or RAO position—hepatic flexure open.

Barium Enema

- Projection: PA Axial or alternate AP Axial

Technical Considerations
- 90 kVp for double contrast
- 110+ kVp for single contrast
- Center AEC cell or manual mAs
- 40″ SID

Exposure Field Size
- 14 × 17 lengthwise

Patient Position
- Prone. No rotation. The prone position is preferred as the sigmoid colon is positioned closer to the IR
- Patient unable to assume a prone position, can be left supine

Centering
- Prone position
  - CR is directed 30°–40° caudal to the small curve of the lower most back and MSP (Fig. 11-125)
- Supine position
  - If image must be attained with the patient supine, the CR is directed 30°–40° cephalic midway between the symphysis pubis and ASIS and MSP (Fig. 11-126)

Marking of IR
- Anatomic R or L side marker placed on the corresponding right or left side of the patient

Breathing
- Breathing is suspended after expiration

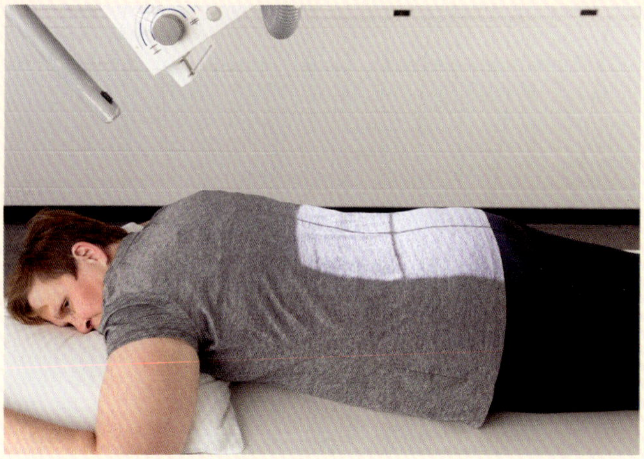

11-125 PA Axial projection.

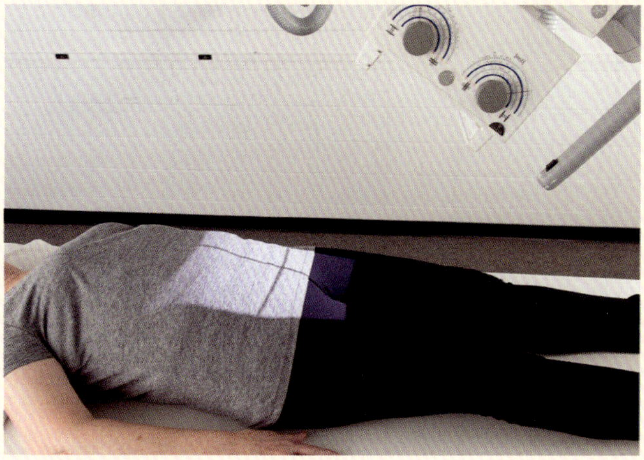

11-126 AP Axial projection.

IMAGE CRITIQUE (FIGS. 11-127 and 11-128)

- Inclusion of the rectum and elongated sigmoid colon. The ascending, descending, transverse, and colic flexures are not of interest and do not need to be entirely included. The tube angle will elongate the tortuosity of the sigmoid colon
- The pelvic bones will appear elongated along with the sigmoid colon
- The enema tip visualized within the rectum

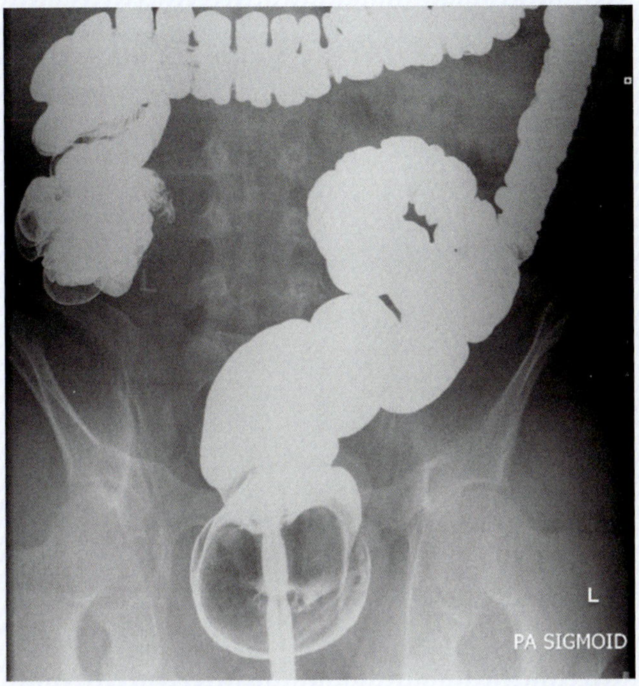

11-127 PA Axial projection.

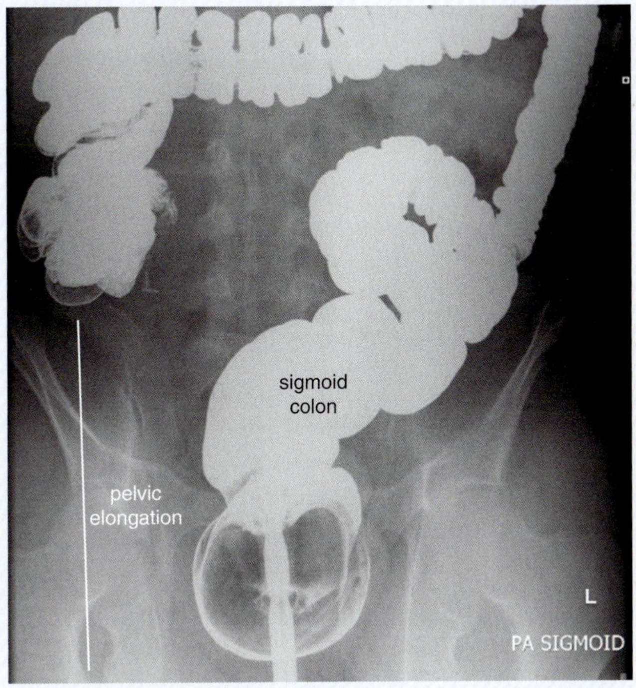

11-128 PA Axial projection.

Barium Enema—Lateral Rectum or Ventral Decubitus

- Projection: Lateral

Technical Considerations
- 90 kVp for double contrast
- 110+ kVp for single contrast
- Center AEC (lateral rectum) or manual mAs (ventral decubitus)
- 40″ SID
- Compensating filter could be applied to the upside portion of the colon for double-contrast studies

Exposure Field Size
- 10 × 12 lengthwise

Patient Position
- Single Contrast—Lateral Rectum (Fig. 11-129)
  - Patient positioned into a true recumbent left lateral position. Ensure the shoulders and hips are lateral and aligned. Flex the knees slightly for patient stability
- Double Contrast—Ventral Decubitus (Fig. 11-130)
  - Patient positioned prone

Centering
- Single Contrast—Lateral Rectum (Fig. 11-129)
  - CR is directed to the level of anterior superior iliac spine (ASIS) and 1″–2″ posterior to the MCP
- Double Contrast—Ventral Decubitus (Fig. 11-130)
  - CR is directed to the level of ASIS and 1″–2″ posterior to the MCP
  - Grid imaging is recommended

Marking of IR
- Anatomic R or L side marker indicating anatomic side closest to the IR

Breathing
- Breathing is suspended after expiration

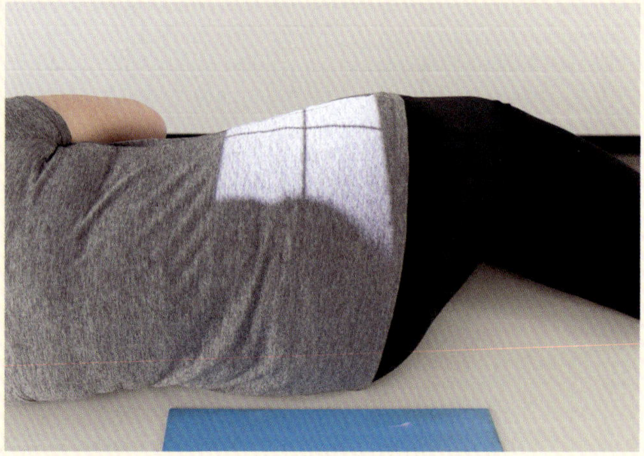

11-129 Lateral rectum.

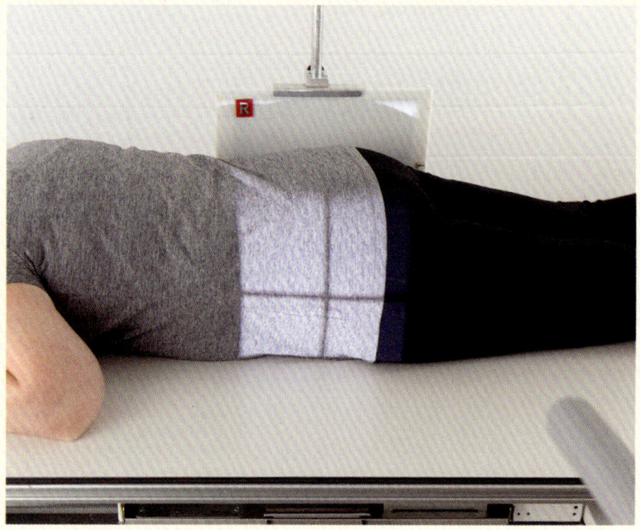

11-130 Ventral decubitus.

IMAGE CRITIQUE (FIGS. 11-131 to 11-133)

- Inclusion of the entire rectum with the enema tip included
- A true lateral sacrum and coccyx visualized
- The ventral decubitus will display an air–fluid distribution. The fluid will gravitate more anterior within the rectum and the air will rise to the highest point (posterior) within the rectum

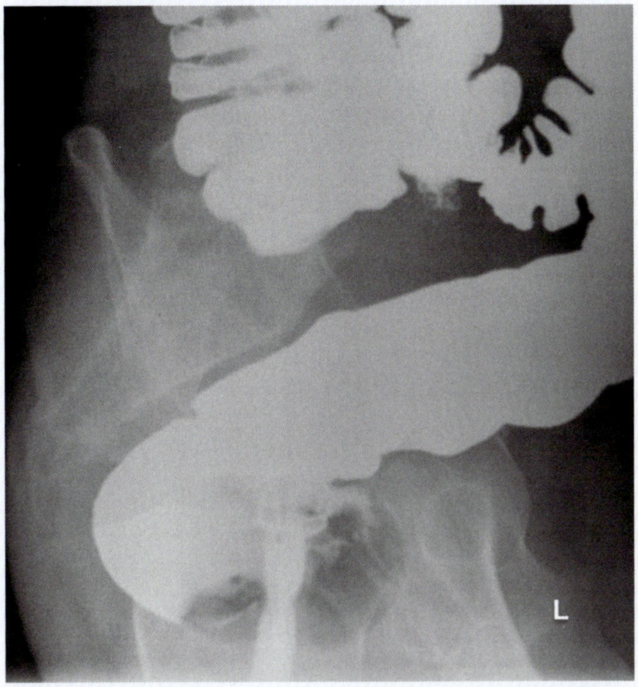

11-131 Lateral rectum. Single Contrast barium enema

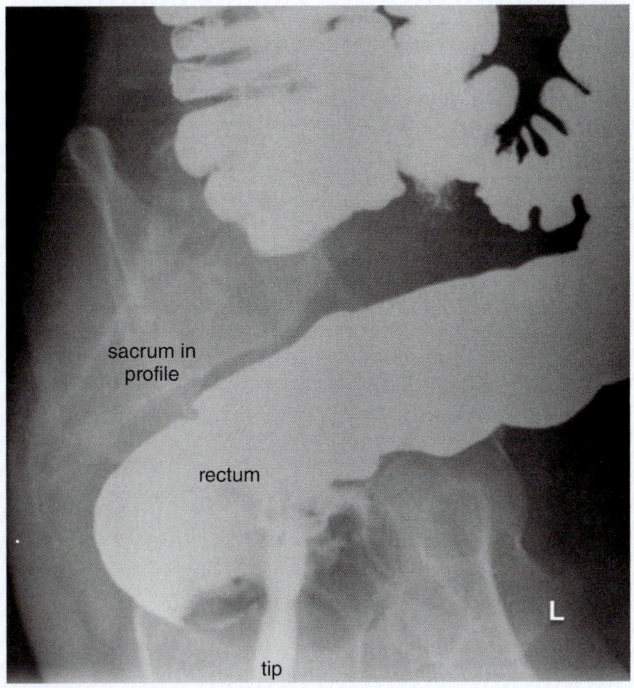

11-132 Lateral rectum. Single Contrast barium enema.

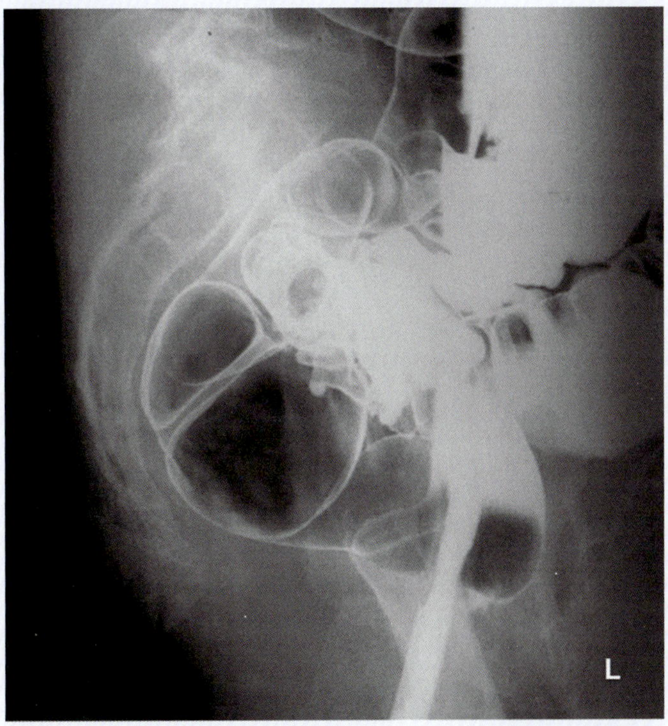

11-133 Ventral decubitus. Double Contrast barium enema.

Barium Enema—Right and Left Lateral Decubitus

- Projection: AP or PA with the patient in both Right Lateral and Left Lateral Decubitus positions. Decubitus positions are only acquired with a double-contrast study

Technical Considerations

- 90 kVp for double contrast
- mAs manually set
- 40″ SID
- Grid

Exposure Field Size

- 14 × 17 lengthwise or two 14 × 17 overlapping crosswise if necessary for the patient

Patient Position

- Right Lateral Decubitus (likely acquired with AP projection)
  - Patient positioned into a true right lateral position. Barium will gravitate into the lateral margin of the ascending and into the medial margin of the descending colon. Air will rise to the medial margin of the ascending colon and into the lateral margin of the descending colon
  - The patient's right side should be slightly elevated off the imaging table to allow the IR to drop below the right lateral margin of the patient
- Left Lateral Decubitus (likely acquired with PA projection)
  - Patient positioned into a true left lateral position. Barium will gravitate into the lateral margin of the descending and into the medial margin of the ascending colon. Air will rise to the medial margin of the descending colon and into the lateral margin of the ascending colon
  - The patient's left side should be slightly elevated off the imaging table to allow the IR to drop below the right lateral margin of the patient

Centering

- Right Lateral Decubitus (RLD) (Fig. 11-134)
  - CR is directed 1″–2″ superior to the crest (to include the splenic flexure) and MSP
- Left Lateral Decubitus (LLD) (Fig. 11-135)
  - CR is directed to the level of iliac crest (to include the hepatic flexure) and MSP

Marking of IR

- Anatomic R or L side marker indicating the correct anatomic side.
- Additional marking or annotation of "side up" or an arrow next to the anatomic side marker

Breathing

- Breathing is suspended after expiration

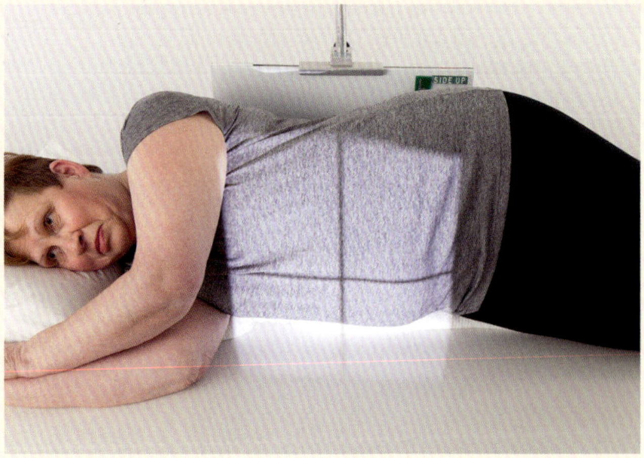

11-134 Right lateral decubitus. Double Contrast barium enema.

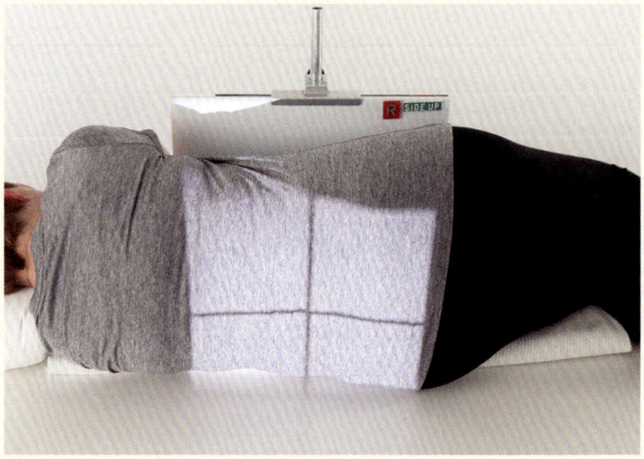

11-135 Left lateral decubitus. Double Contrast barium enema.

IMAGE CRITIQUE (FIGS. 11-136 to 11-139)

- Air–fluid levels demonstrated in the ascending and descending colon. Inclusion of both RLD and LLD in a procedure will alter the distribution of air and fluid, which could be helpful with pathology identification. The colon segment on the "upside" of the image is of most interest
- A patient properly elevated off the imaging table will allow demonstration of both the ascending and descending divisions
- Inclusion of the rectum and symphysis pubis will happen only when centering specifically for the hepatic flexure

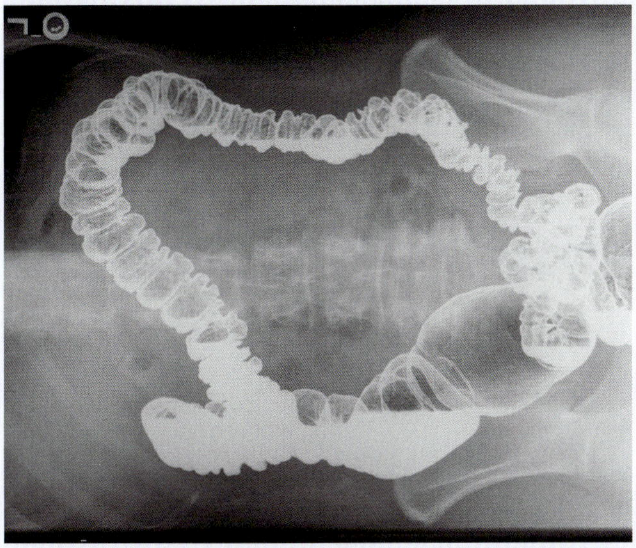

11-136 Right lateral decubitus. Double Contrast barium enema.

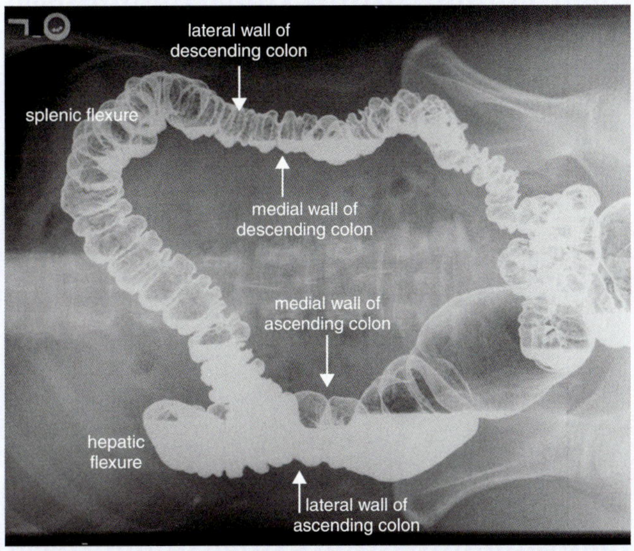

11-137 Right lateral decubitus. Double Contrast barium enema.

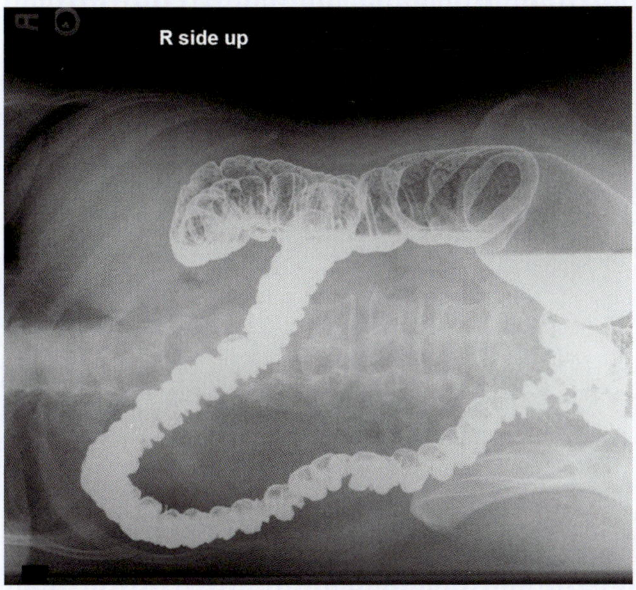

11-138 Left lateral decubitus. Double Contrast barium enema.

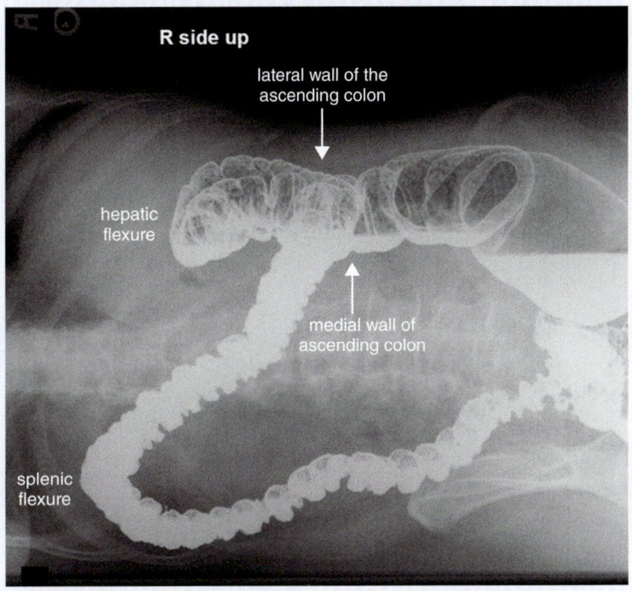

11-139 Left lateral decubitus. Double Contrast barium enema.

Barium Enema—Postevacuation

- Projection: AP

Technical Considerations

- 90–100 kVp
- Center AEC cell or manual mAs
- 40″ SID

Exposure Field Size

- 14 × 17 lengthwise or two 14 × 17 overlapping crosswise if necessary for the patient

Patient Position

- Supine. No rotation

Centering (Fig. 11-140)

- To the level of the iliac crest and MSP

Marking of IR

- Anatomic R or L side marker placed on the corresponding right or left side of the patient

Breathing

- Breathing is suspended after expiration

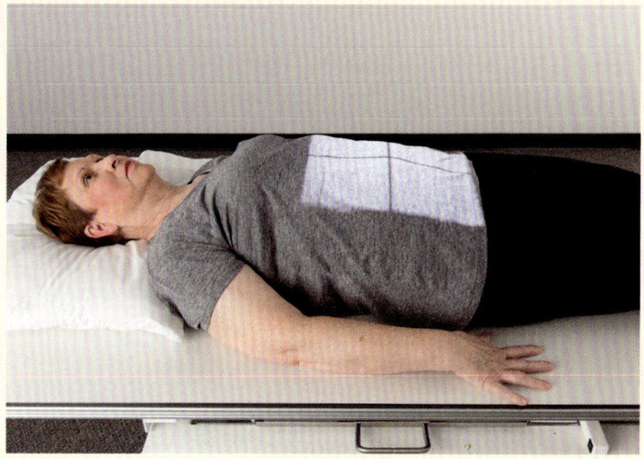

11-140 Supine abdomen (postevacuation).

IMAGE CRITIQUE (FIG. 11-141)

- Inclusion of all the large bowel. This image is acquired after the patient has attempted to evacuate as much barium as possible. This image will demonstrate the amount of residual barium within the bowel. This image must be checked by the radiologist before patient dismissal

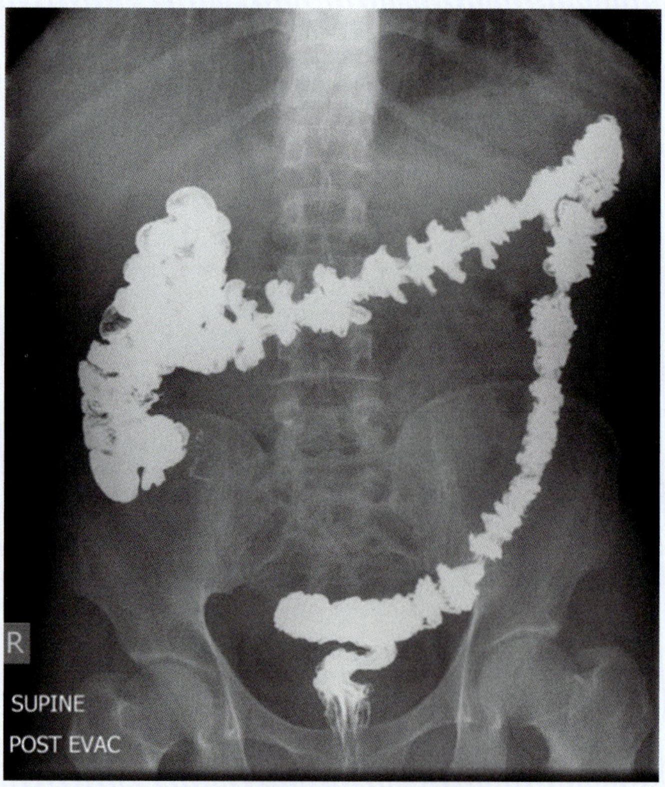

11-141 Supine abdomen (postevacuation).

THE FINAL STEP IMAGE REVIEW

The technologist must take time to review acquired images to ensure image quality is acceptable. The technologist must have the knowledge within their role to not only acquire the images and care for the patient but also to know how to review the images to ensure diagnostic quality has been attained. In certain instances, a projection may need to be repeated. This is to the discretion of the radiologic technologist. The technologist should review each image for the following.

1. Is all of the necessary anatomy included on the image?
   - Was the central ray (CR) properly directed to the part? An "X" can be drawn to intersect within the collimated exposure field to determine if the CR was directed to the correct location.
   - Was essential anatomy in the collimated exposure field?
   - Is the area free of artifact(s)?
2. Is the anatomy well demonstrated?
   - Did the technologist properly position the patient to adequately demonstrate the anatomy?
   - Can the technologist recognize the anatomy best demonstrated with use of different projections?
3. Does the image reflect proper image markings?
   - Did the technologist correctly use a lead marker to identify the right or left side?
   - What additional markings or annotations could be helpful to the radiologist interpreting the exam?
   - Is the image properly displayed?
4. Does the image prove to be technically acceptable?
   - Does the exposure index fall within acceptable range for the operating system? Images that are technically insufficient may appear of good quality if just slightly insufficient or "mottled or pixelated" if severely insufficient. Images that appear "mottled" should be repeated. Images that appear beyond optimal exposure due to higher technique may display high quality, but the patient has received excessive radiation dose.

8. In review of the double-contrast barium enema image (Fig. 11-149), what is the patient's position?
   a. Supine
   b. Prone
   c. AP
   d. PA

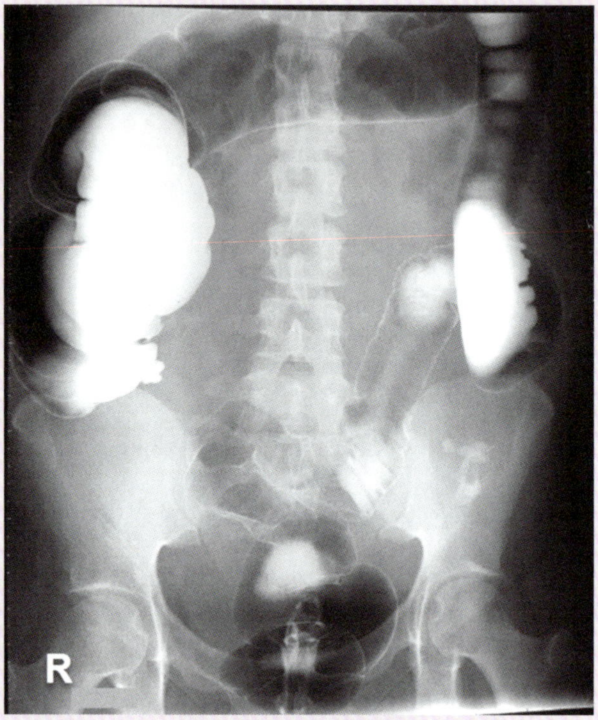

11-149

9. In review of the double-contrast barium enema image (Fig. 11-150), what is the patient's position?
   a. Ventral decubitus
   b. Dorsal decubitus
   c. Right lateral decubitus
   d. Left lateral decubitus

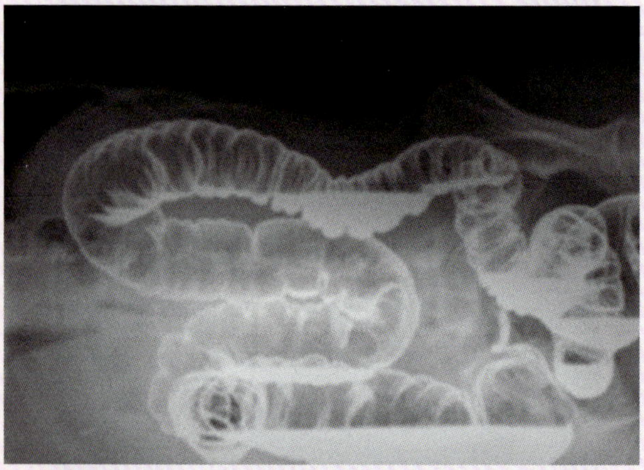

11-150

10. In review of the double-contrast barium enema image (Fig. 11-151), what should the technologist consider?
   a. Pass the image as the descending colon is only of interest and entirely visualized.
   b. Pass the image as the ascending colon is only of interest and entirely visualized.
   c. Repeat the image and build the patient up so the descending colon is entirely visualized.
   d. Repeat the image and build the patient up so the ascending colon is entirely visualized.

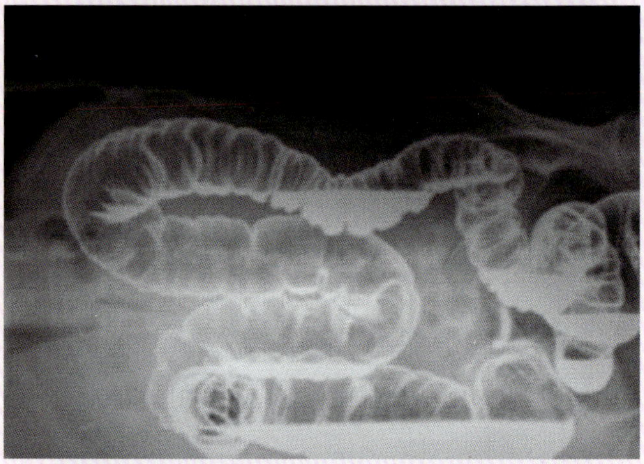

11-151

ANSWERS TO THE CRITICAL THINKING QUESTIONS

1. c
2. b
3. b
4. d
5. c
6. a
7. d
8. a
9. c
10. d

CHAPTER 12 Contrast Media–Assisted Procedures

The visibility of anatomic cavities and certain organs within the body for diagnosis is enhanced with nonionic iodinated contrast media. These procedures will require informed patient consent, may require a sterile field to be established, and the procedure completed with the radiologist. The radiologic technologist will be responsible for the room preparation, sterile tray setup, the patient's preprocedural history, exam explanation, and imaging. Some radiology departments employ a nurse to assist with duties such as sterile tray setup, patient monitoring, urinary catheter placement, administration of medications, and informed patient consent. The radiologic technologist will assist the radiologist or physician to expedite the exam and acquire postcontrast images if requested beyond the acquisition of images taken with digital fluoroscopy during the procedure. Digital fluoroscopic equipment has reduced the number of postcontrast images acquired by the radiologic technologist.

CLINICAL INDICATIONS

Indications and contraindications will be mentioned with each individual procedure in this chapter.

IMAGING CONSIDERATIONS

Patient dress, patient positioning, and imaging will be addressed with each individual exam discussed in this chapter.

IODINATED CONTRAST MEDIA

Nonionic water-soluble iodinated contrast media is administered to patients for contrast media–assisted procedures. Nonionic contrast agents have fewer particles per amount of solution, which reduces the overall toxicity of the media due to its lower osmolality nature (Fig. 12-1). With a lower osmolality solution, side effects and potential contrast reactions decrease. Water-soluble media is easily absorbed and mixes well (miscibility) with bodily fluids or blood. It is important to screen the patient with a questionnaire to identify any risk factors that would place the patient at a higher risk for contrast reaction. A patient with a history of iodine sensitivity or poor renal function should not receive iodinated contrast. On injection of nonionic contrast media into the bloodstream, patients commonly experience a metallic taste in the mouth and a warm flush sensation. While these side effects dissipate quickly, the patient should be informed that they could potentially experience them.

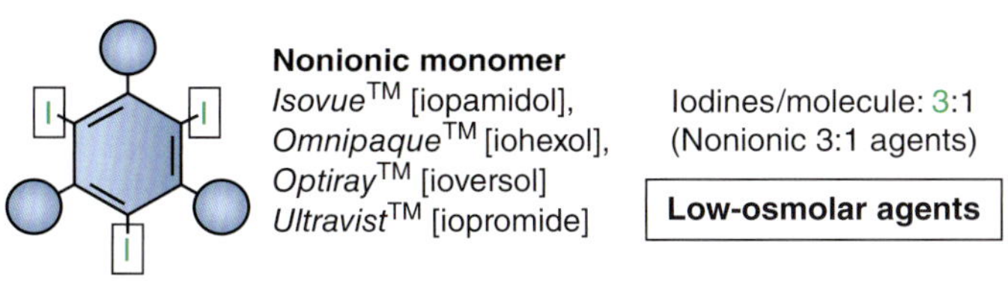

12-1 Lower osmolality agents have fewer particles per solution.

ACQUISITION OF PATIENT HISTORY

When exams involve the administration of contrast media, the technologist will need to make certain to acquire and report patient history. If the technologist discovers something concerning in the patient's history, the technologist should consult the radiologist or patient's physician before the start of the procedure (Fig. 12-2). Facilities typically have a patient history form that the technologist completes prior to the exam. Essential questions are as follows:

- Allergies to food
- Allergies to medications
- Allergies to iodine
- Previous imaging exams in which the contrast media was injected into the bloodstream

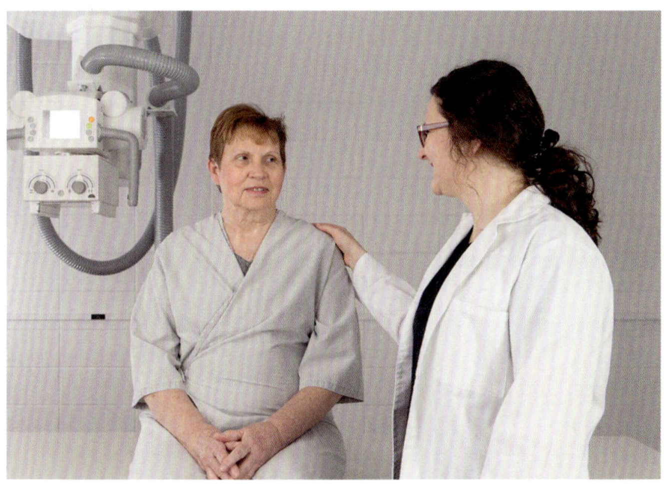

12-2 Acquisition of thorough patient history.

- History of asthma or hives
- History of diabetes
  - Some sites may question diabetic patients on the use of a form of metformin or Glucophage. Patients on metformin must discontinue the use of it for at least 48 hours pre and post the procedure and then only resumed when normal kidney function level returns.
  - It is highly important that blood urea nitrogen (BUN) and creatinine levels are checked by the radiologic technologist and the radiologist informed before the administration of contrast media.
- History of sickle-cell disease, multiple myeloma, or pheochromocytoma

BLOOD CHEMISTRY RESULTS

The radiologic technologist should check the blood results of the BUN and creatinine. These levels reveal the patient's kidney function. These results should be checked before the procedure starts. A patient, who has values outside the normal range, should not have contrast media intravenously injected. Abnormal and questionable laboratory values must be cleared with the radiologist before proceeding with the exam. A glomerular filtration rate (GFR) may also be ordered. The GFR determines the level of kidney function. The value is determined from a creatinine value in the blood, patient's age, race, and gender.

- Normal creatinine range: 0.6–1.5 mg/dL
- Normal BUN range: 8–25 mg/dL
- Normal GFR: 90 or above

CONTRAST MEDIA REACTIONS

With the injection of contrast media, if a reaction were to occur, it will most likely occur in the first 5 minutes of administration. The patient must be closely monitored during the entire procedure. If reaction symptoms do occur, treatment, if any, will be administered. An emergency response cart should be within close vicinity anytime contrast media is injected. It is unknown when instances may require drugs such as epinephrine or cardiopulmonary resuscitation equipment. In addition, quick access to blood pressure equipment and oxygen may be necessary. In some instances, a patient may be premedicated to lessen the effects of contrast media and can reduce the risk of a reaction event if they suffer from food allergies, environmental allergies, or asthma. A common drug utilized for premedication is Benadryl.

Mild reactions can usually be managed by the technologist by providing the patient with reassurance in an effort to keep the patient's anxiety down. Providing the patient with a cool compress and encouraging them to slow down their breathing may help calm the patient. Mild symptoms are listed in the table (Table 12-1).

Moderate reactions are definitely more concerning, and treatment is necessary. The radiologist should be notified immediately. The course of action will require the administration of medications to counter effect the reaction. Moderate symptoms are listed in the table (Table 12-1).

Severe reactions are life threatening, and a rapid medical response is necessary. A code blue call may be initiated. The emergency crash cart should be readily accessible in the exam room. Severe symptoms are listed in the table (Table 12-1).

12-1 Contrast Media Reactions—Symptom Classification

Reaction Level	Possible Symptoms	Recommended Action
Mild	Warm, flushed sensation (hot flash) Metallic taste Nausea Vomiting Itching/mild hives	Reassure patient and closely monitor them. With the identification of hives, it is recommended to notify the physician.
Moderate	Moderate to severe hives Laryngospasms Hypotension Bradycardia or tachycardia	Initiate a medical response
Severe	Hypotension Bradycardia Pulseless Cardiac arrest Respiratory arrest	Call a code

INFORMED PATIENT CONSENT

Before the start of an invasive procedure, even before venipuncture, the procedure must be fully explained to the patient. This includes the steps of the procedure, the common potential side effects they may experience, and risk factors of the procedure. The patient must sign and date the informed consent form. If the patient is a minor, the parent or guardian must be informed of everything aforementioned and will sign on their behalf.

VENIPUNCTURE

A common venipuncture site of access is in the antecubital space of the elbow. The vein must be capable to withstand the injection of the contrast media. Injection of contrast media into central lines or shunts is contraindicated. Intravenous access must be maintained for the entire length of the procedure in the event of a contrast reaction and intravenous medications must be administered. For radiographic procedures, such as the intravenous urogram (IVU), an 18- to 22-gauge needle or over the needle-catheter design is typically sought.

Basic steps to venipuncture:

- Technologist should wash their hands and don gloves.
- Technologist will apply a tourniquet above the elbow and have the patient rotate the palm up. The technologist will locate the vessel.
- The skin should be prepped with an alcohol wipe working in a circular motion from the center out. Allow the skin to dry (Fig. 12-3).
- The technologist will stabilize the vessel and tighten the skin above and below the injection site with their thumb and index finger of their nondominant hand (Fig. 12-4).
- The technologist will use their dominant hand and direct the needle with the bevel up at an angle of 20°–45° to the surface. Once in the vessel, the needle should be directed in a parallel manner with the vein.

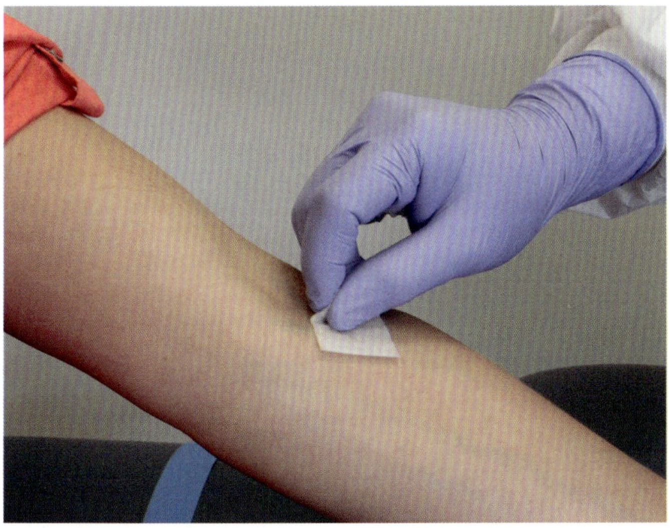

12-3 Antecubital space prepped for venipuncture.

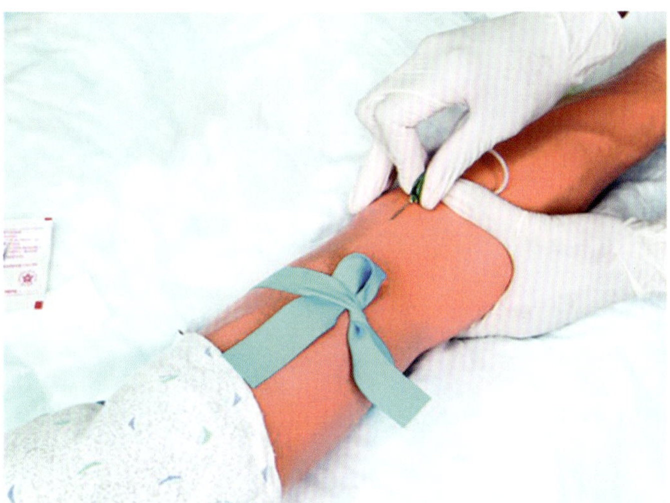

12-4 Establishing vein access for contrast injection.

- Look for a flash of blood return to signify being within the vessel. Once present, the butterfly needle can be secured or advance the catheter and remove the needle if using a needle-catheter device.
- Injection of the contrast media at an appropriate rate. The injection start time should be documented. The time, type, and amount of contrast must be documented. The technologist should look for signs of contrast extravasation. If extravasation (infiltration) occurs, the needle must be removed from the site. After the bleeding has stopped, cold compression is applied to constrict the vessel walls followed by a warm compress to help with reabsorption. This incident must be documented.
- *At the end of the contrast procedure*, the needle or catheter is removed, venipuncture site compressed and then the needle is correctly disposed into the designated sharps container. The intravenous access must be maintained until the end of the contrast procedure in the event of a contrast reaction.

UROLOGIC STUDY INTRAVENOUS UROGRAM (IVU)

Radiographic functional study of the kidney and allows visualization of the ureters and bladder.

INDICATIONS (NUMEROUS, THIS IS NOT AN ALL-INCLUSIVE LIST OF URINARY SYSTEM PATHOLOGIES)

Renal calculi, pyelonephritis, hydronephrosis, congenital anomalies, benign prostatic hyperplasia

CONTRAINDICATIONS

- Patient with known allergy to iodinated contrast media
- History of iodine sensitivity
- Diabetes
- Blood chemistries (BUN, creatinine, GFR) out of normal range
- Pheochromocytoma
- Sickle-cell anemia
- Anuria
- Renal disease
- Congestive heart failure

ANATOMY

The right and left kidneys are located in the retroperitoneal space with the right kidney slightly lower than the left kidney due to liver in the right upper quadrant. The superior poles of the kidneys are positioned slightly closer to the vertebral column than the inferior poles. The kidneys lie within the T12–L3 range. The position of the kidneys will change with respiratory phase as well as by a change in patient position (recumbent versus upright) (Fig. 12-5).

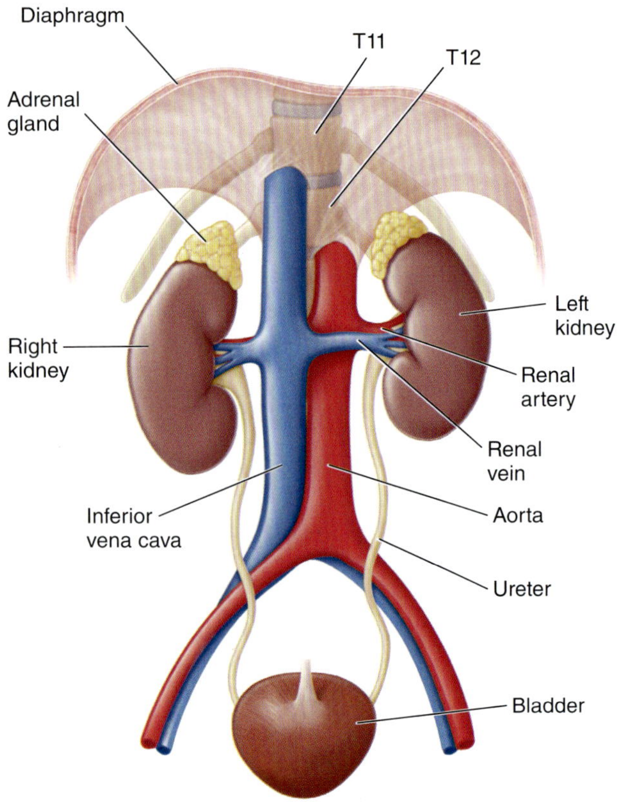

12-5 Urinary system.

KEY ANATOMIC COMPONENTS OF THE KIDNEY (FIG. 12-6)

- Capsule: Outer surface covering of the kidney
- Renal Parenchyma: Functional tissue of the kidney; it includes the cortex and the medullary portion.
  - Cortex: The outermost layer of the renal parenchyma. Contains the microscopic functional anatomy; the nephrons
  - Medullary portion: The functional portion of the renal parenchyma that contains the medullary pyramids. Blood is filtered, and urine is produced.
- Minor and Major Calyces: Medullary pyramids drain into minor calyces (8–20 per kidney) and merge down into 2–3 major calyces (at superior, mid, and inferior divisions of the kidney). Major calyces come together to form the renal pelvis (Fig. 12-7). The renal pelvis funnels into the proximal ureter.
- Renal Hilum: The ureter, renal vein, and renal artery are located at this entrance/exit point of the organ.
- At the ureteropelvic junction (UPJ), the ureter courses inferiorly from the kidney down to the inferior and posterior insertion point on the bladder, the ureterovesical junction (UVJ). As the ureter courses down toward the bladder, it follows the lordotic curvature of the lumbar spine.
- The urethra exits the bladder. The trigone is referenced as the two insertion points of the ureters and the exit point of the urethra (Fig. 12-8).

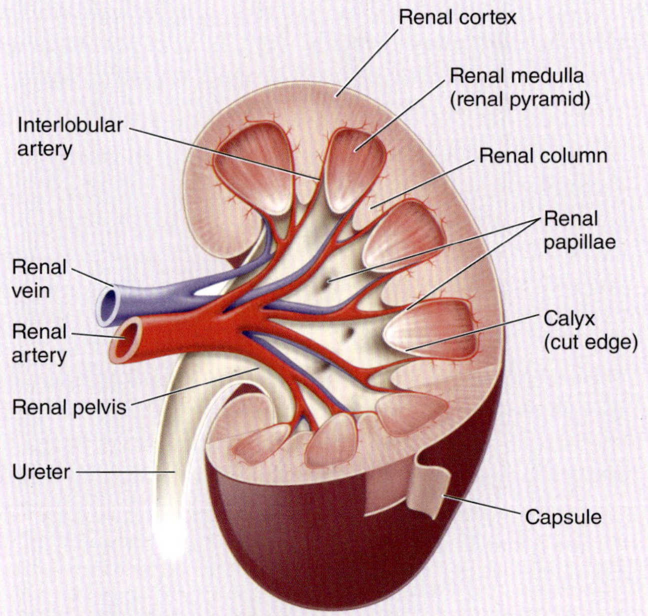

12-6 Kidney.

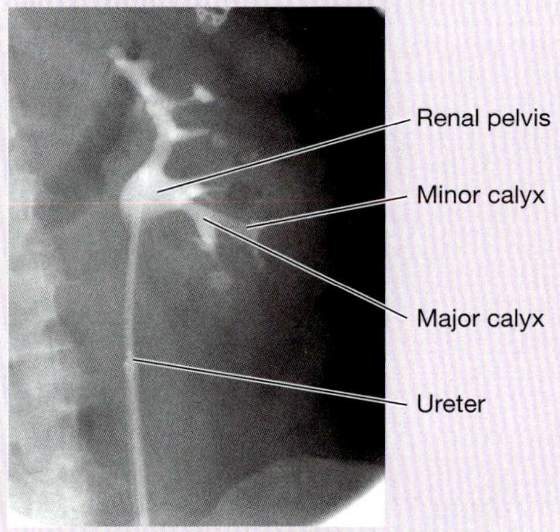

12-7 Radiographic image of kidney filled with contrast.

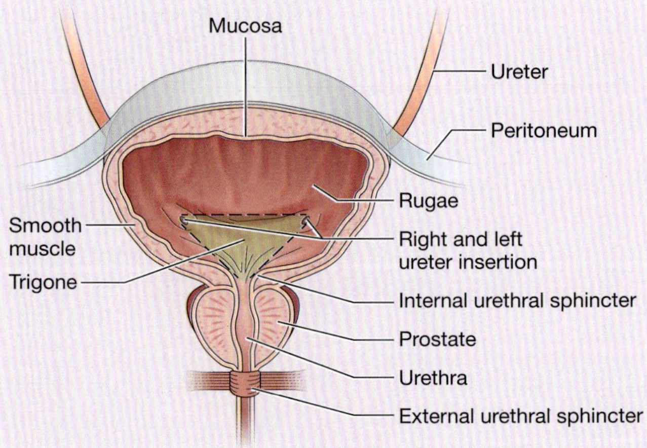

12-8 Bladder.

PATIENT PREP

- Light diet the evening before and nothing passed orally (NPO) after midnight. Ideally, a prep similar to a barium enema would ensure the elimination of overlying bowel gas patterns and fecal material.
- Patient must empty the bladder before procedure to prevent contrast dilution as it collects in the bladder.

CONTRAST MEDIA

Nonionic iodinated contrast is pulled often from a secure medication station and drawn up by syringe according to the patient's weight per the facility's protocol. Ensure the needle and contrast media remain sterile. Contrast injection is typically introduced in the antecubital space (elbow).

PROCEDURE

- Patient dressed in a gown.
- Patient history is acquired and documented on the institutional contrast screening form.
- The exam is explained to the patient and informed consent is acquired. Potential patient pregnancy has been ruled out.
- Scout supine abdomen was acquired and presented to the radiologist. This image will reveal patient preparation, initial read for any pathology, proper technical settings, and positioning (Figs. 12-9 and 12-10).

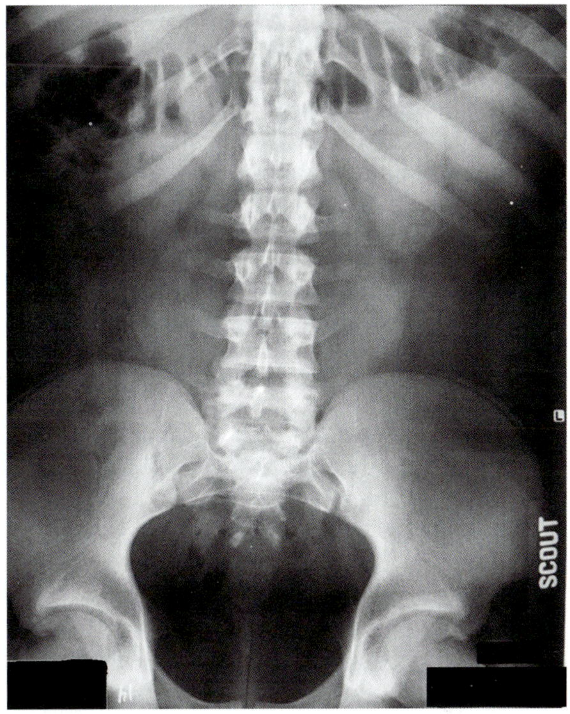

12-10 Scout abdomen.

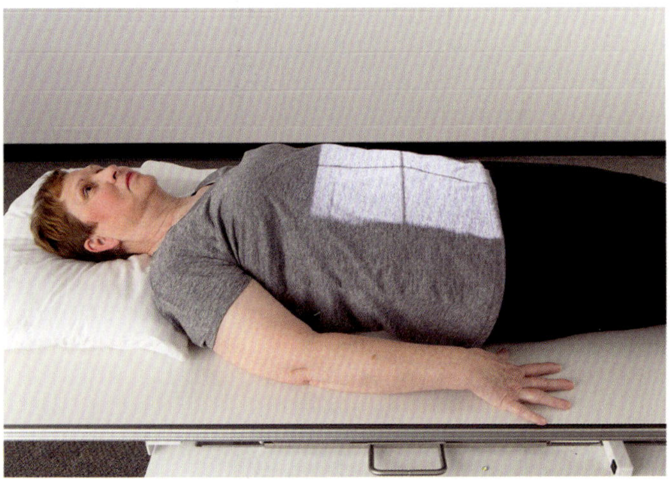

12-9 Supine abdomen—scout image.

- Control panel set correctly to acquire the first image of the kidneys—1-minute postinjection of the contrast media. This is also referred to as the nephrogram.
- Ureteric compression may be applied along the upper pelvic brim to achieve a prolonged filling of the collecting system in the kidneys. Place the lower border of the compression paddles even with and medial to the anterior superior iliac spine (ASIS) on each side, secure with compression band, and inflate. Ureteric compression should not be applied when ureteric stones, abdominal trauma, severe pain, or abdominal aortic aneurysm are of concern. Ureteric compression may not be applied at all clinical facilities. If ureteric compression is desired, but contraindicated, a slight Trendelenburg position could be implemented. If applied, a postrelease radiograph of the abdomen may be acquired (Fig. 12-11).

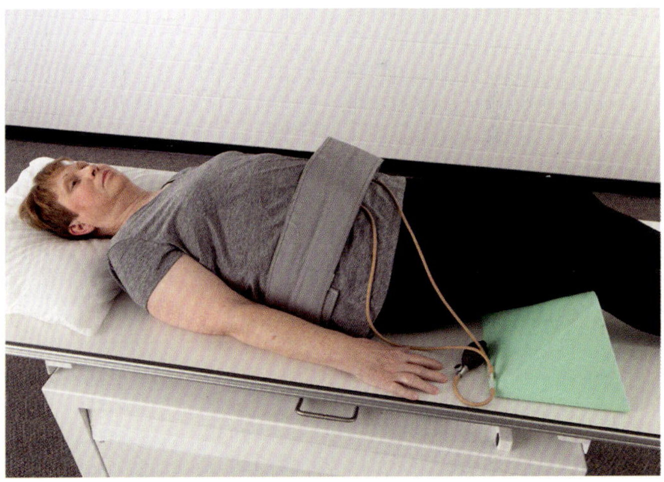

12-11 Application of ureteric compression.

- Skin is prepped for venipuncture, and venipuncture is performed. Venous access must be maintained for the length of the procedure in the event of a contrast reaction.
- The time at which injection of contrast media begins should be noted. The entire amount of contrast is injected for this procedure—a bolus injection. Contrast type and the amount must be documented in the patient's record. This procedure is a functional study; therefore, protocol images will be acquired at timed intervals. All images must be annotated with time.

- The injection of contrast media presents risk for an allergic reaction. Most patients will experience mild symptoms such as a metallic taste, warm, flush feeling, nausea, or vomiting. A patient is at their highest risk to experience a contrast media reaction within the first 5 minutes of contrast injection. The radiologic technologist must stay with the patient the entire exam and initiate emergency procedures if reactions escalate beyond mild symptoms.

POSTCONTRAST INJECTION IMAGING

- All images must have the time annotated moving forward.
- A nephrogram or nephrotomogram is taken immediately following the full injection of contrast media. This image reveals the "blush" of contrast within the nephrons of the kidneys. This image is centered at midsagittal plane (MSP) and midway between the iliac crest and xiphoid tip (Fig. 12-12).

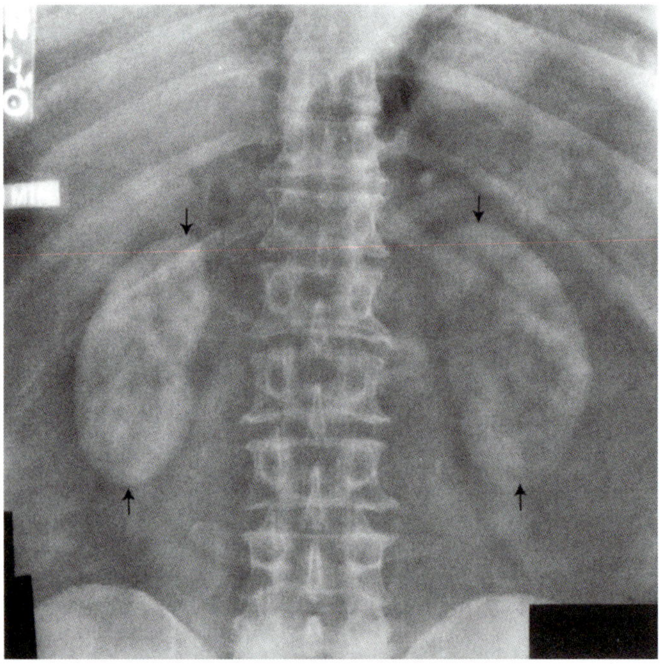

12-12 1-minute nephrogram.

- 5-minute image acquired with the patient supine and centered to include the kidneys only or centered to include the kidneys, ureters, and bladder (Fig. 12-13).
- 10–15 minutes acquired with the patient supine and centered to include the kidneys, ureters, and bladder (Fig. 12-14)
- 20-minute 30° right posterior oblique (RPO) and left posterior oblique (LPO) for each kidney. The upside kidney is positioned parallel to the image receptor and will free the ureter closest to the image receptor of the spine. This image is centered to include the side up kidneys, ureters, and bladder or sometimes this image is centered for the kidneys only (Figs. 12-15 to 12-18).
- Patient voids. Again, urine should be strained to capture potential stone(s).

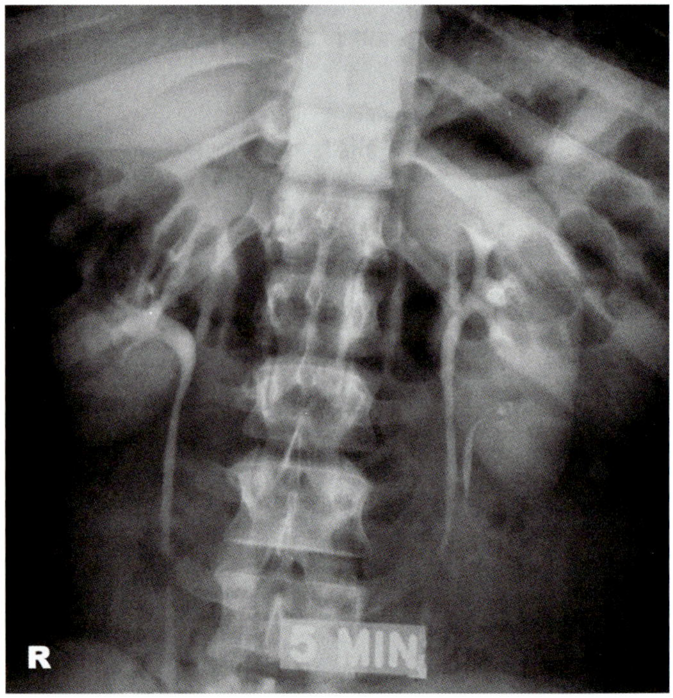

12-13 5-minute nephrogram.

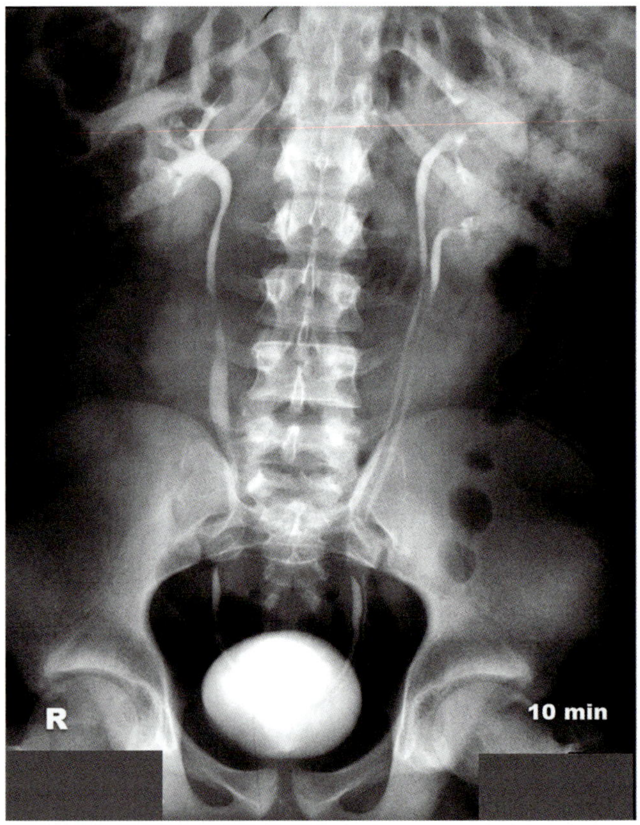

12-14 10- to 15-minute IVU.

- Postvoid acquired with the patient supine, prone or erect. Special attention to inclusion of the entire bladder is required (Fig. 12-19). Upright imaging will also reveal a condition in which a kidney drops downward extremely in its position (nephroptosis).
- All images must be reviewed by the radiologist before the patient is dismissed. In some cases, delayed radiographs may be requested.

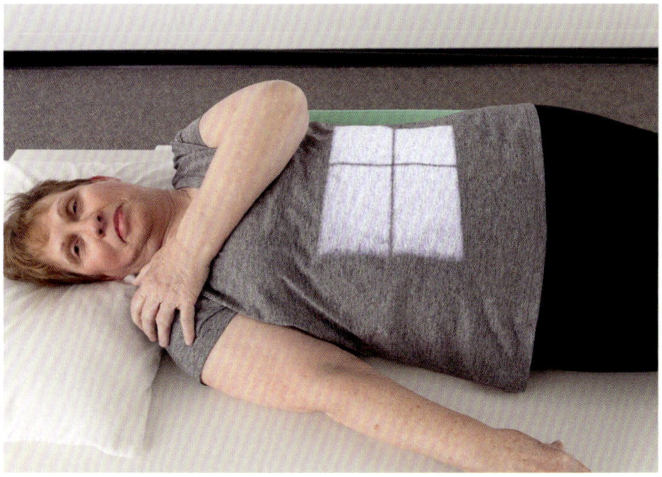

12-15 Posterior oblique position centered to the kidneys.

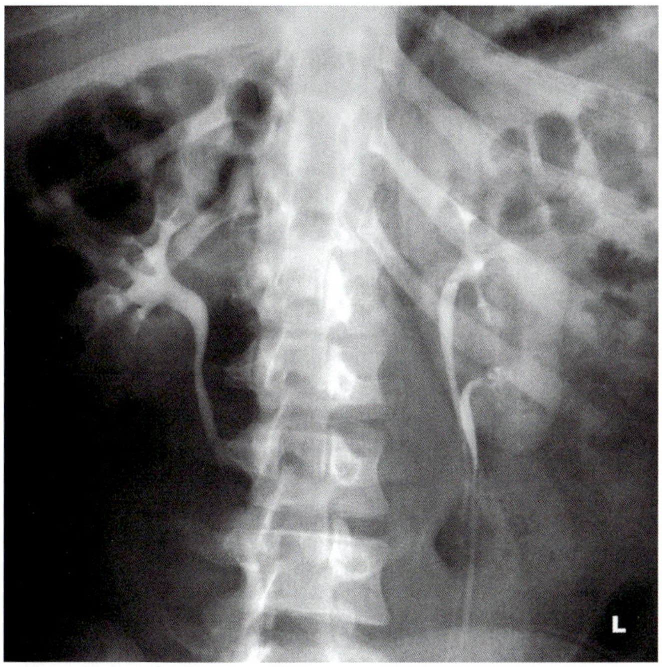

12-16 Posterior oblique centered to the kidneys.

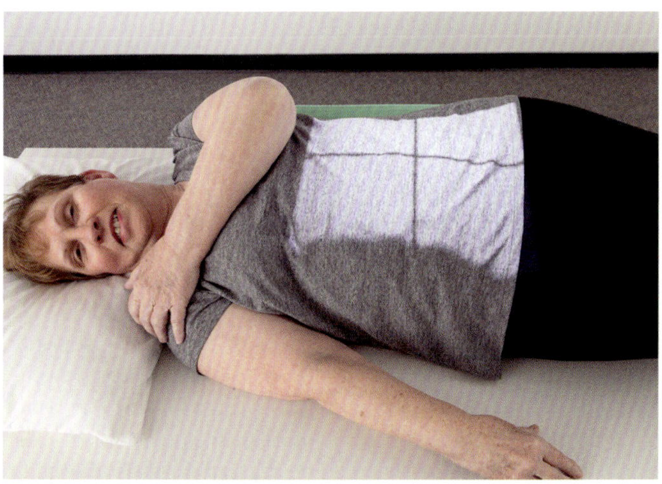

12-17 Posterior oblique position centered to include the entire abdomen for IVU.

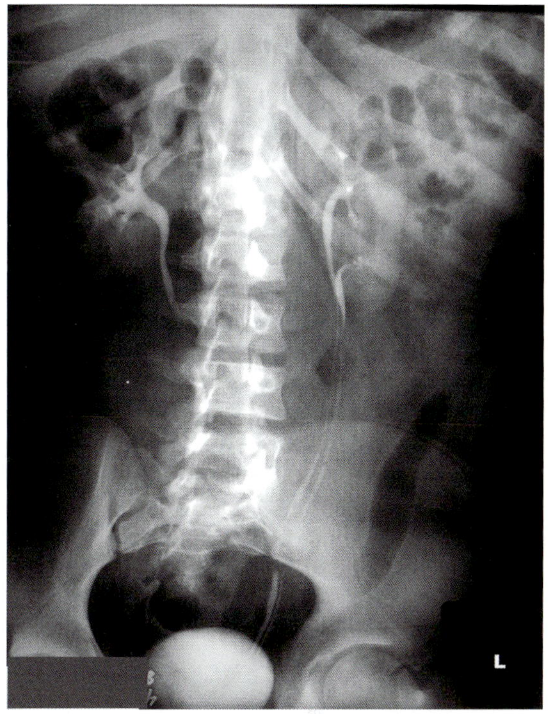

12-18 Posterior oblique abdomen for IVU.

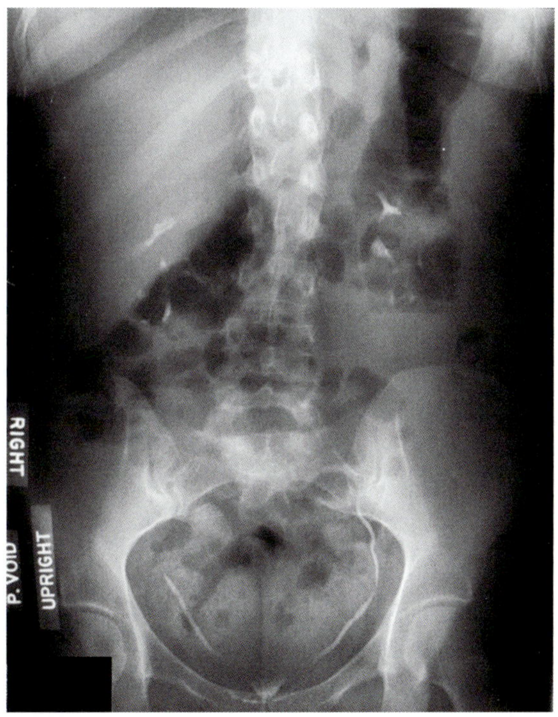

12-19 Postvoid IVU.

POSTPROCEDURAL INSTRUCTIONS

Patient can resume normal diet and activity postprocedure. A patient who self-medicates with a form of metformin may be instructed not to take this medication for 48 hours or longer dependent on the level of their renal function. The discontinuation of medication may be dependent on the facility.

UROLOGIC STUDY RETROGRADE CYSTOGRAM

- A nonfunctional radiographic study of the bladder.

INDICATIONS

- Trauma, bladder calculi, bladder tumors, cystitis, ureteral reflux

CONTRAINDICATIONS

- Recent bladder surgery
- Damage to the urethra

ANATOMY

The bladder is an expandable muscular sac that attaches to the floor of the pelvis and sits posterior to the symphysis pubis. The bladder may have the capacity fullness of 300–500 mL.

KEY ANATOMIC COMPONENTS OF THE BLADDER (FIG. 12-20)

- UVJ: Each ureter junctions with the bladder on the posterior side and inferior on the bladder
- Urethra exits the bladder.
- Trigone defines the triangular area where the two ureters insert into the bladder and the urethra exits the bladder.

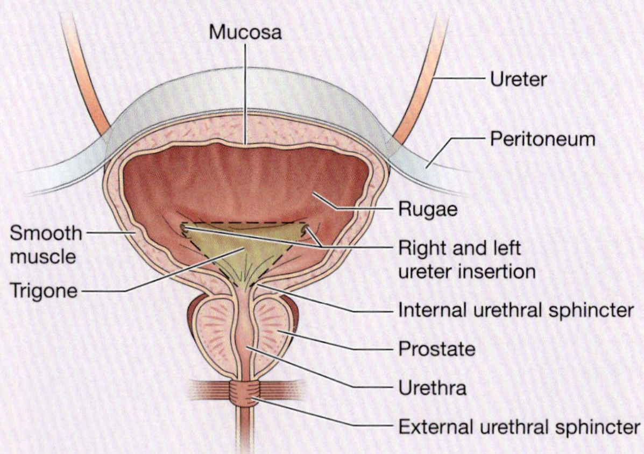

12-20 Bladder.

PATIENT PREP

- Patient must empty bladder before procedure.

CONTRAST MEDIA

Nonionic iodinated contrast will retrograde fill the bladder by gravity. The bladder will be filled with approximately 150–500 mL of contrast (Fig. 12-21)

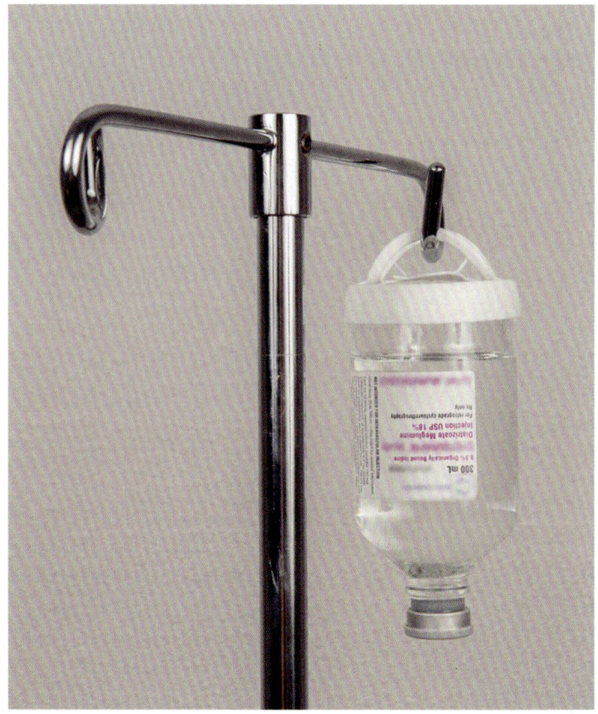

12-21 Nonionic iodinated contrast media.

PROCEDURE

- Patient removes undergarments and dressed in a gown.
- Patient history is acquired and documented on the facility's contrast screening form.
- The exam is explained to the patient and informed consent is acquired. Potential patient pregnancy has been ruled out.
- Scout supine abdomen was acquired and presented to the radiologist. This image will reveal patient preparation, initial read for any pathology, proper technical settings, and positioning (Fig. 12-22).
- The peroneal area is prepped, and a sterile catheter is positioned into the bladder. Urine is drained from the bladder before contrast media is introduced. A balloon on the end of the catheter is inflated. A urine specimen may be sent to the laboratory.
- Control panel set correctly for fluoroscopy to monitor the filling of the bladder.
- Once the bladder is filled with contrast, digital fluoroscopic spot images are acquired by the radiologist. The technologist will assist the patient into different positions from supine and into right and left posterior oblique(s).
    - The supine position is centered midway between ASIS and symphysis pubis and with the midsaggital plane (MSP) (Figs. 12-23 and 12-24). A 10° caudal angle may be applied to project the symphysis pubis below the base of the bladder.
    - 45° posterior oblique position(s) are centered 2″ superior to the symphysis pubis and 1″ medial to the upside anterior superior iliac spine (ASIS). A steeper oblique could be utilized to demonstrate more of the posterior bladder wall, or a true lateral could be utilized if this is of specific interest (Figs. 12-25 to 12-27).

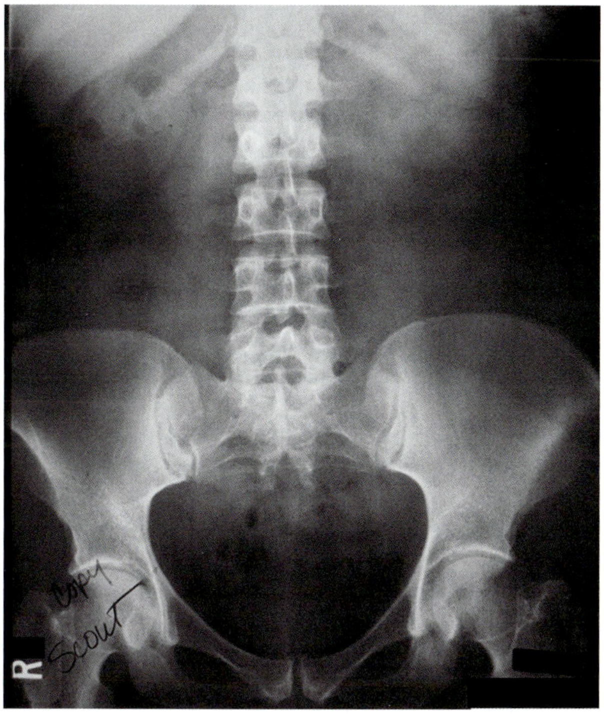

12-22 Supine abdomen—scout image.

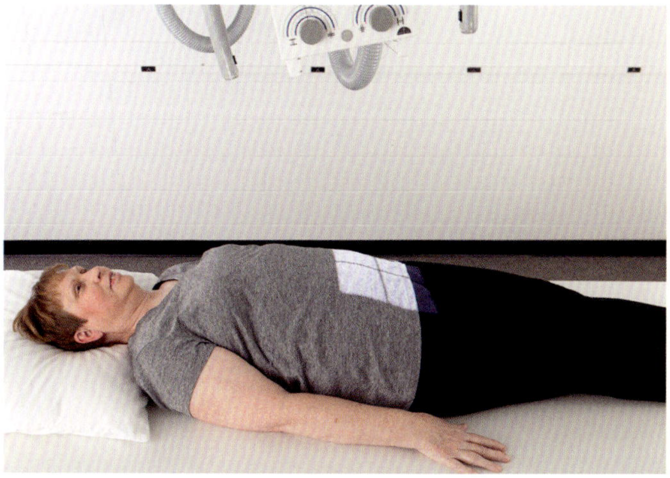

12-23 Supine bladder position and centering.

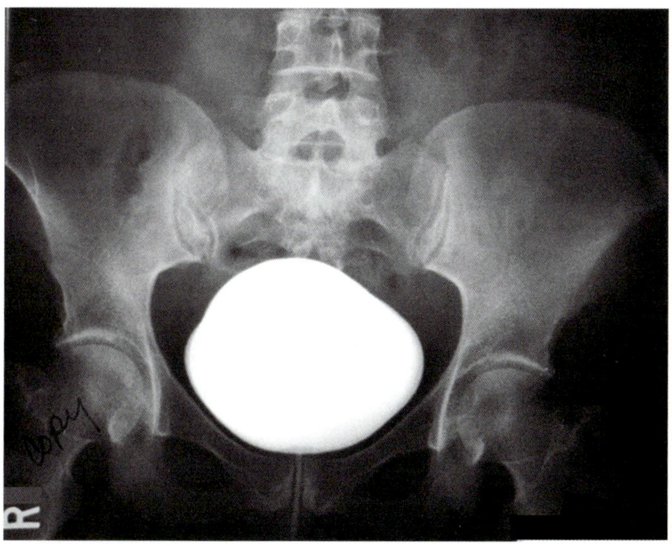

12-24 Supine bladder.

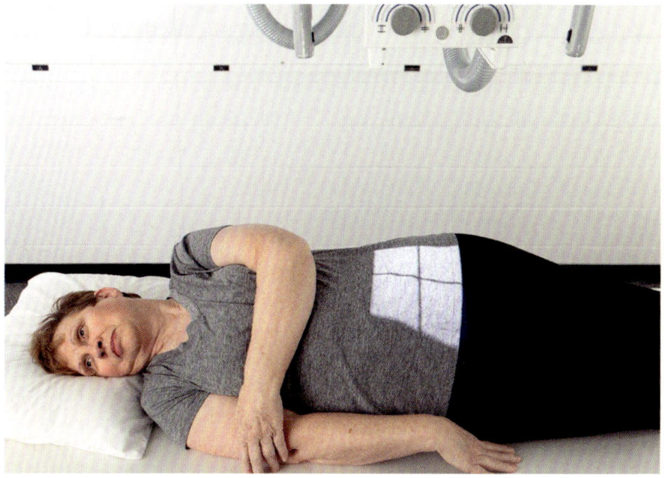

12-25 45° right posterior oblique bladder.

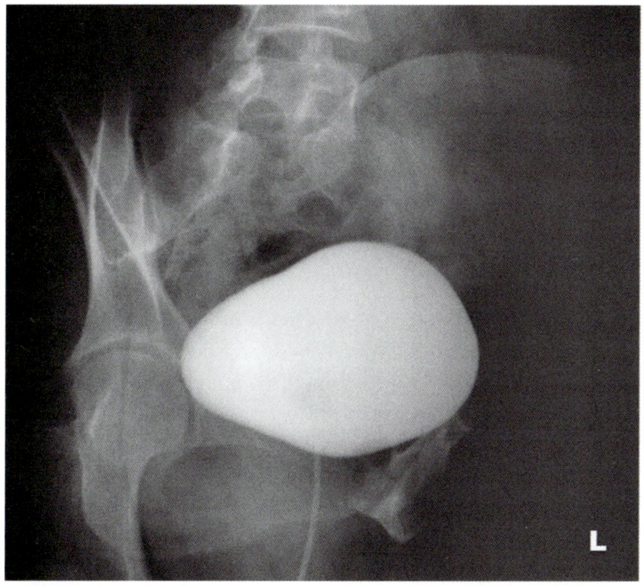

12-26 45° left posterior oblique bladder.

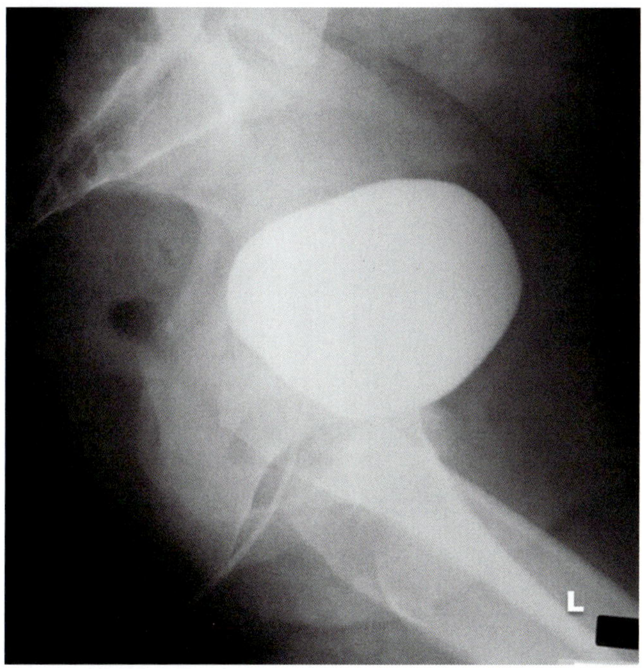

12-27 True lateral bladder.

POSTPROCEDURAL INSTRUCTIONS

- The urinary catheter is removed. The patient can resume normal diet and activity post the procedure.

UROLOGIC STUDY VOIDING CYSTOURETHROGRAPHY

- A functional radiographic study of the bladder and urethra with urination

INDICATIONS

- Trauma, incontinence, ureteral reflux, chronic urinary tract infections

ANATOMY

The bladder is an expandable muscular sac that attaches to the floor of the pelvis and sits posterior to the symphysis pubis. The bladder may have the capacity fullness of 300–500 mL (Fig. 12-28).

KEY ANATOMIC COMPONENTS OF THE BLADDER (FIG. 12-28)

- UVJ: Each ureter junctions with the bladder on the posterior surface and inferiorly on the bladder
- Urethra: Exits the bladder
- Trigone: Defines the triangular area where the two ureters insert into the bladder and the urethra exits the bladder.

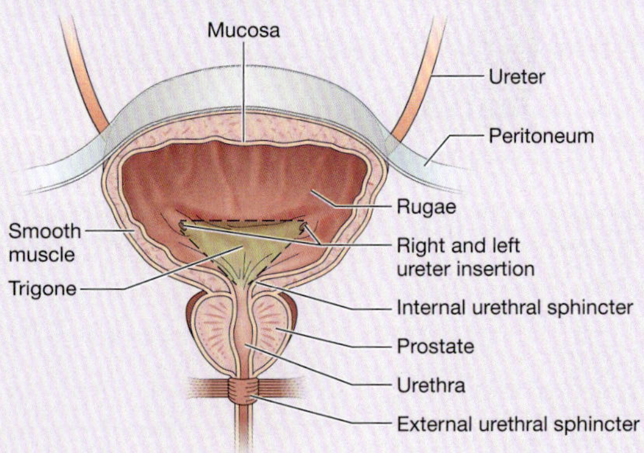

12-28 Bladder.

PATIENT PREP

- Patient must empty bladder before procedure.

CONTRAST MEDIA

Nonionic iodinated contrast will retrograde fill the bladder by gravity. The bladder will be filled with approximately 150–500 mL of contrast. The patient's bladder will be filled until the patient states it is intolerable (Figs. 12-29 and 12-30).

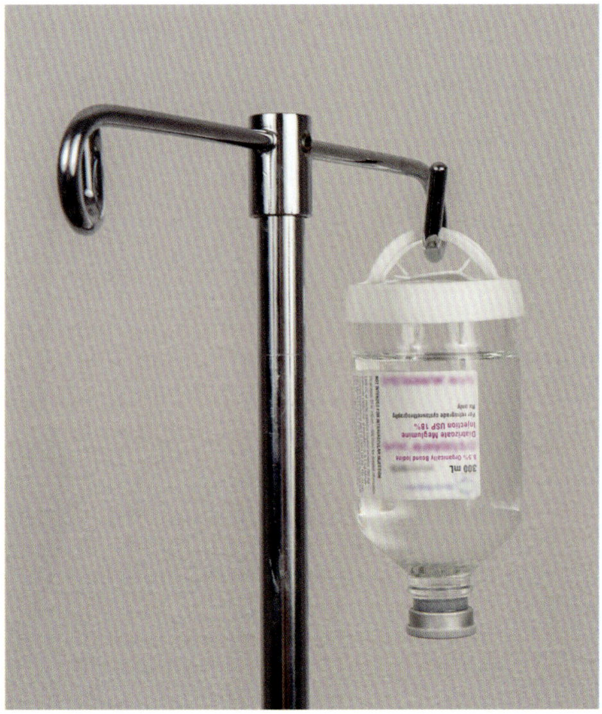

12-29 Nonionic iodinated contrast media.

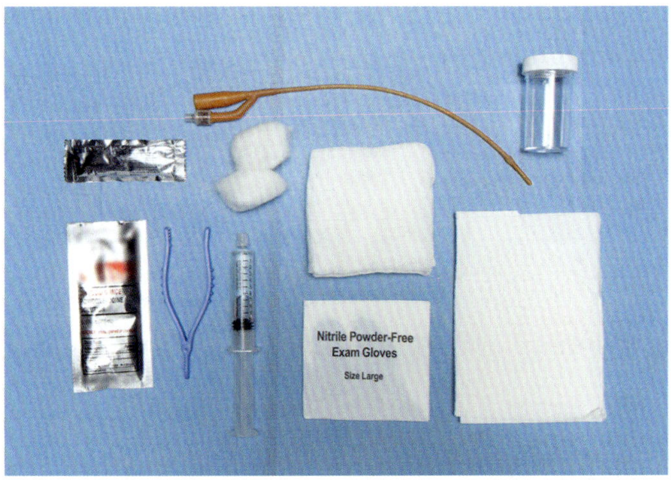

12-30 Example of sterile tray setup for voiding cystourethrography.

PROCEDURE

- Patient dressed in a gown.
- Patient history is acquired and documented on the facility's contrast screening form.
- The exam is explained to the patient and informed consent is acquired. Potential patient pregnancy has been ruled out.
- Scout supine abdomen was acquired and presented to the radiologist. This image will reveal patient preparation, initial read for any pathology, proper technical settings, and positioning (Figs. 12-31 and 12-32).
- Prep the peroneal area and a sterile catheter is positioned into the bladder. Urine is drained from the bladder before contrast media is introduced. A balloon is inflated on the end of the catheter to stabilize its position. A urine specimen may be sent to the laboratory.

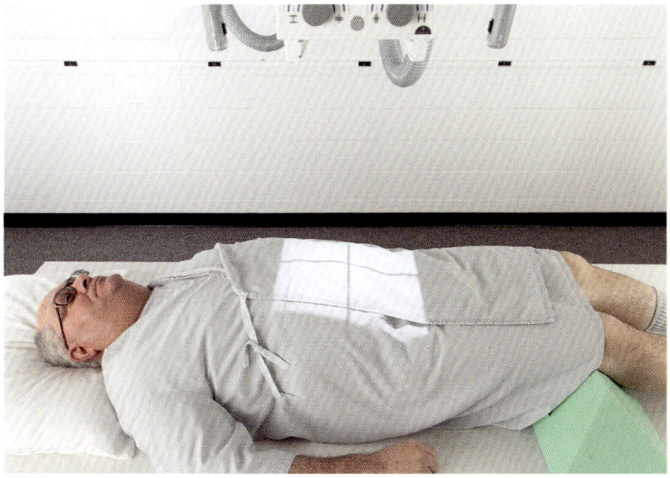

12-31 Scout abdomen.

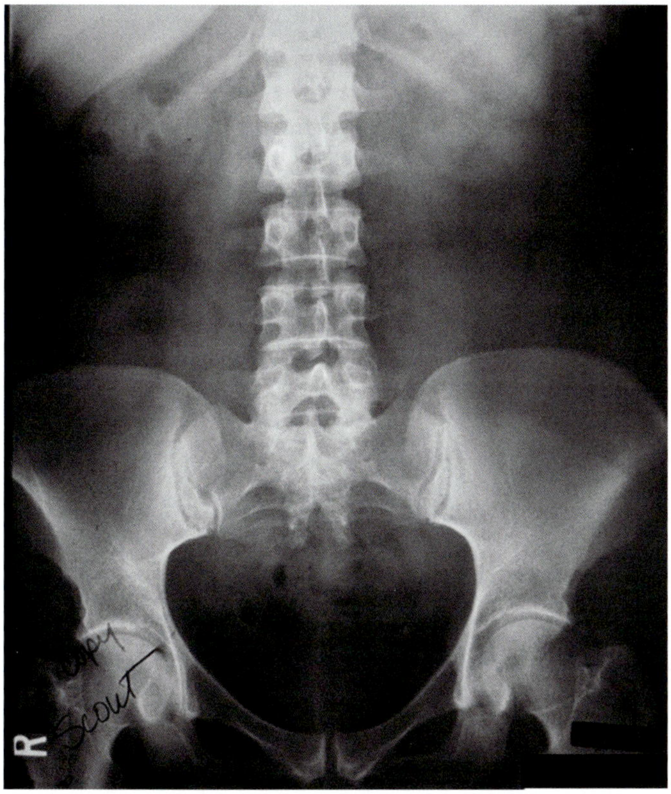

12-32 Supine abdomen—scout image.

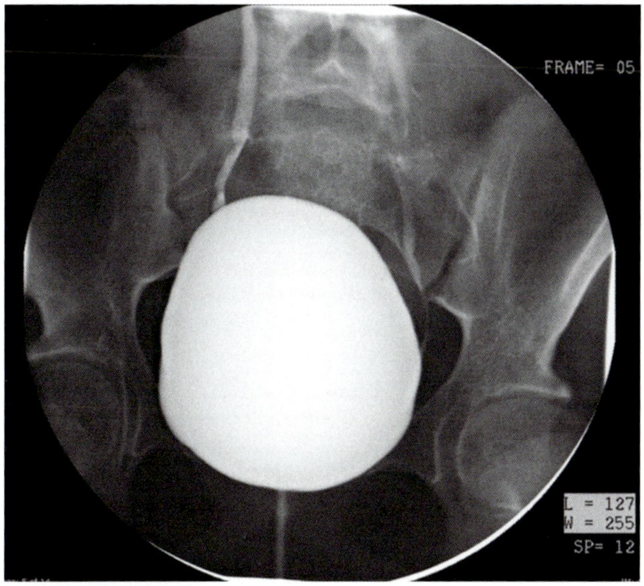

12-33 Supine bladder.

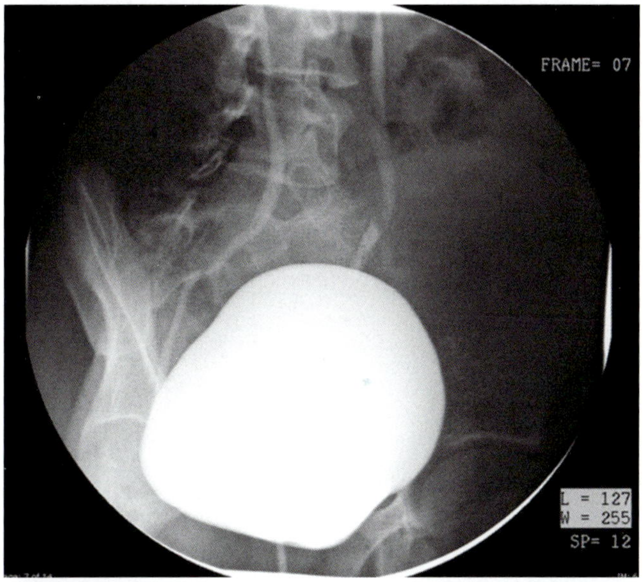

12-34 Left posterior oblique bladder.

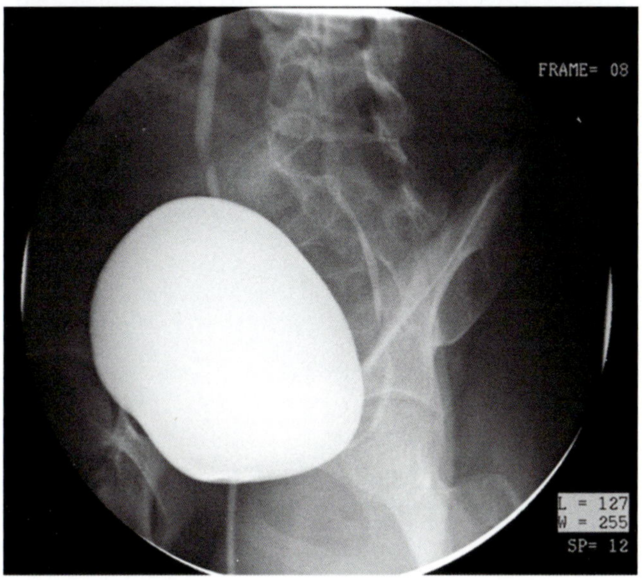

12-35 Right posterior oblique bladder.

- Control panel set correctly for fluoroscopy to monitor filling of the bladder.
- The bladder is filled with contrast. The bladder is imaged distended with contrast (Figs. 12-33 to 12-35).
- Once the bladder is full, the air balloon on the end of the catheter is released and the catheter is carefully removed from the patient's bladder while the patient begins to void.
- While the patient is voiding, the patient may lie in a supine, supine oblique position or positioned erect. A receptacle or absorbent towel is needed to absorb voided contrast. The technologist will assist the patient into different positions from supine and into right and left posterior oblique(s) (Figs. 12-36 and 12-37). While the patient voids, digital fluoroscopic images are acquired by the radiologist (Figs. 12-38 and 12-39).

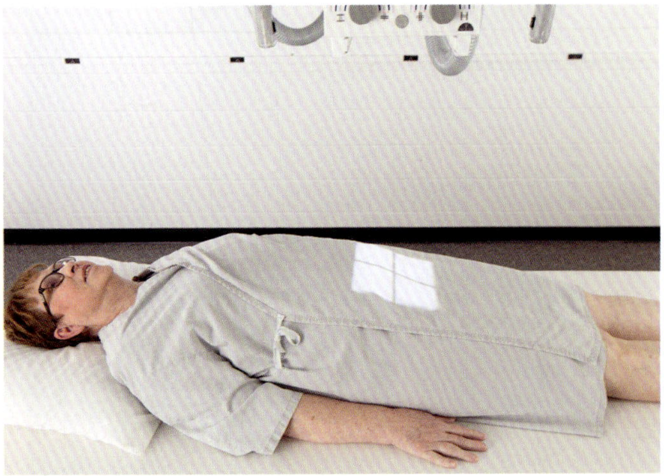

12-36 Supine bladder shot.

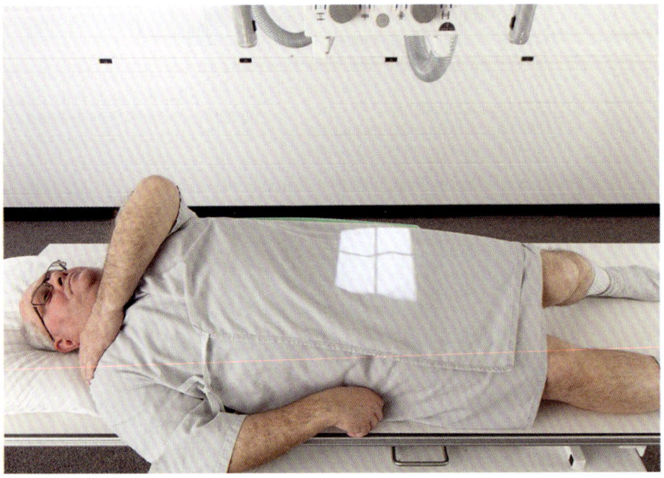

12-37 RPO bladder.

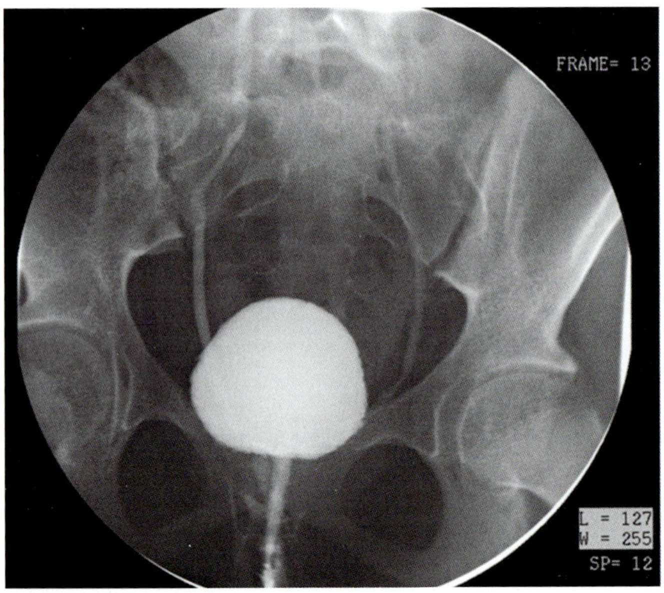

12-38 Supine voiding.

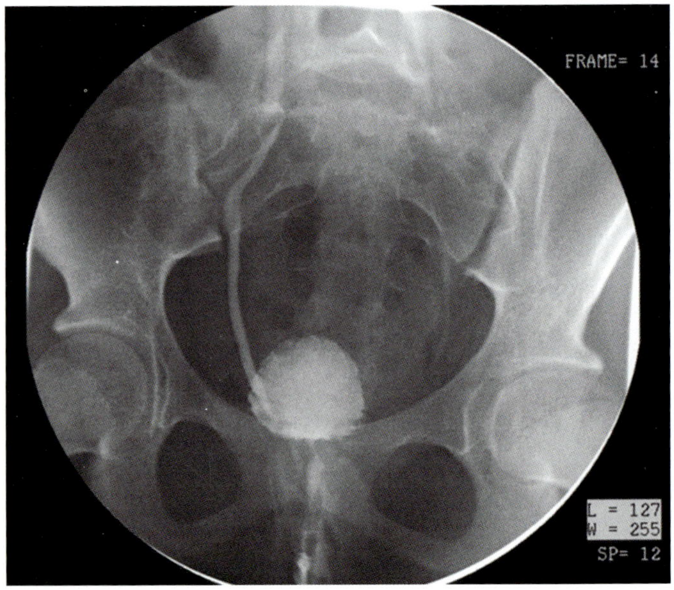

12-39 Supine voiding.

- Females are best evaluated supine or in a slight posterior oblique position while voiding. The central ray is directed to the level of the symphysis pubis (Fig. 12-36).
- Males are best evaluated in a 30° right posterior oblique position while voiding. The urethra should be displayed over the soft tissue of the upper thigh. The central ray is directed to the level of the symphysis pubis (Fig. 12-37).
- An AP post void image may be requested.

POSTPROCEDURAL INSTRUCTIONS

- Patient can resume normal diet and activity postprocedure.

ARTHROGRAPHY

Synovial joints such as the shoulder, knee, wrist, ankle, and hip are traditionally studied with diagnostic radiology with the added enhancement of contrast media introduced into the joint capsule.

INDICATIONS

- Joint capsule tears or other pathologic processes to a joint.

CONTRAINDICATIONS

- Allergy to iodinated contrast media or local anesthetics

ANATOMY

KEY ANATOMIC COMPONENTS OF A JOINT OF A JOINT (FIGS. 12-40 and 12-41)

- Cartilage: Covers the surfaces of the bones to avoid friction building with movement
- Synovial Membrane: Surrounds the joint and secretes synovial fluid
- Ligaments: Elastic tissue that helps to stabilize a joint and attach bone to bone
- Tendons: Elastic tissue that helps control a joint's movement. Tendons attach muscle to bone.
- Bursa: Fluid-filled sacs that help reduce friction in a joint (Fig. 12-42)

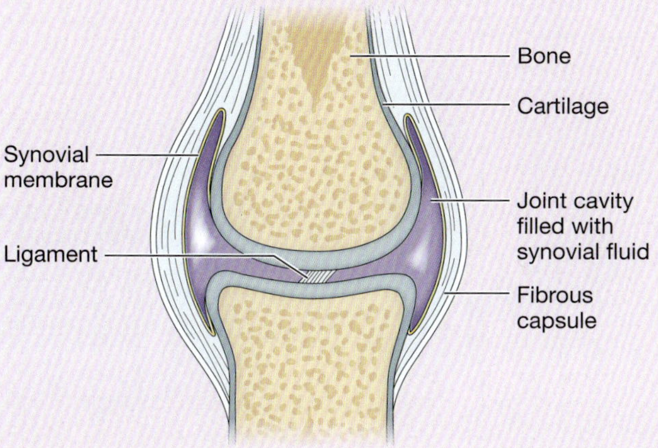

12-40 Components of a synovial joint.

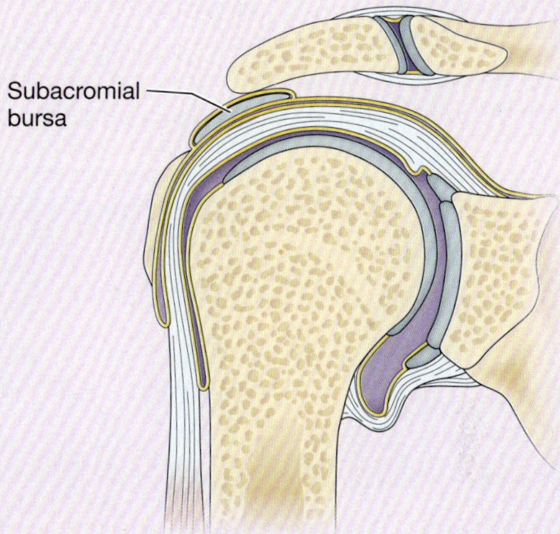

12-42 Bursa.

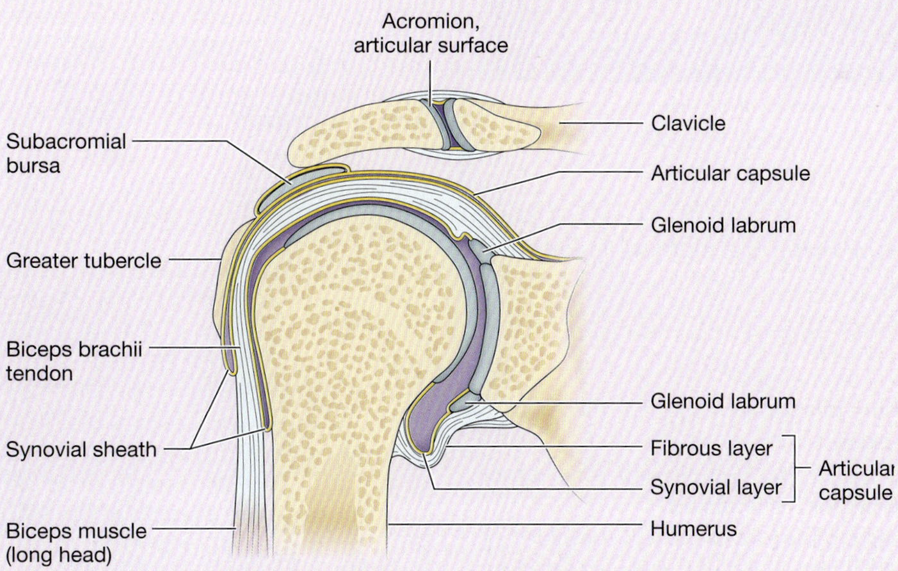

12-41 Shoulder joint anatomy showing essential joint components.

PATIENT PREP

- No prep necessary

STERILE TRAY SETUP (HIGHLY DEPENDENT ON RADIOLOGIST PREFERENCE) (FIG. 12-43)

Disposable tray with basic setup to include betadine or chlorahexidine prep sponges, sterile drape, sterile gloves, various syringe sizes, various needles of different lengths, plastic flexible connector, local anesthetic, 4 × 4 gauze, and bandage. Iodinated contrast would be drawn up from a vial, it is not included in the disposable tray. A hemostat may be requested for the tray to mark the joint after the skin has been prepped.

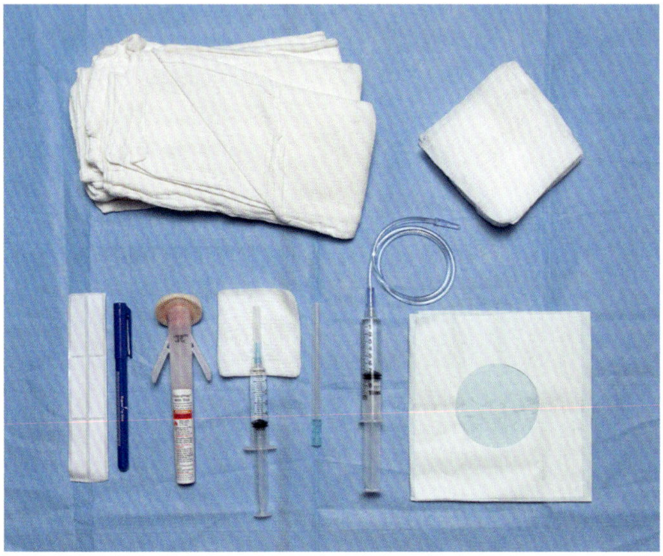

12-43 Example of a sterile tray setup for an arthrogram.

CONTRAST MEDIA

A combination of positive (iodinated contrast) and negative (air) media are utilized.

ROOM SETUP

After preliminary (scout) images are acquired, the room is converted over for the exam.

- Control panel switched to fluoroscopy with time zeroed and kVp set appropriate for the joint size.
- Table Bucky positioned to the foot or head of the table
- Viewing monitor and fluoroscopy foot pedal arranged for radiologist.

PROCEDURE

- Patient dressed in a gown.
- Patient history is acquired and documented on the facility's contrast screening form. If the patient will be imaged with MRI in conjunction with the arthrogram, the MRI screening form must also be completed.
- The exam is explained to the patient and informed consent is acquired. Potential patient pregnancy has been ruled out.
- Precontrast (scout) images of the joint are acquired according to the facility protocol. These images are presented to the radiologist (Fig. 12-44).

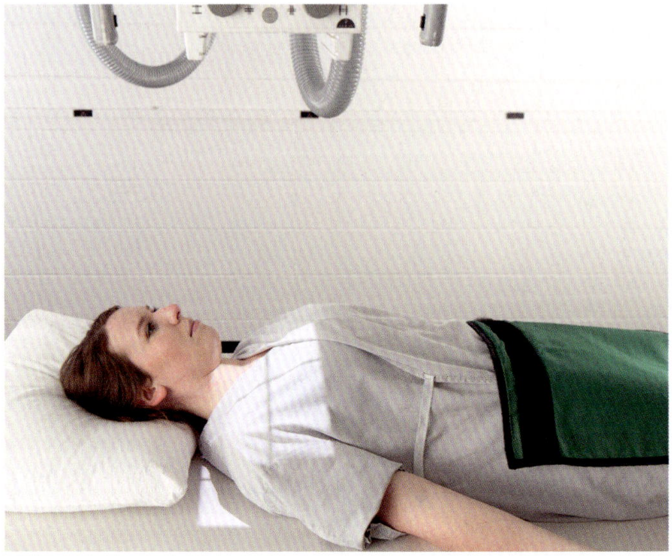

12-44 Preliminary joint imaging.

- The radiologist will prep the area and establish the sterile field (Fig. 12-45).

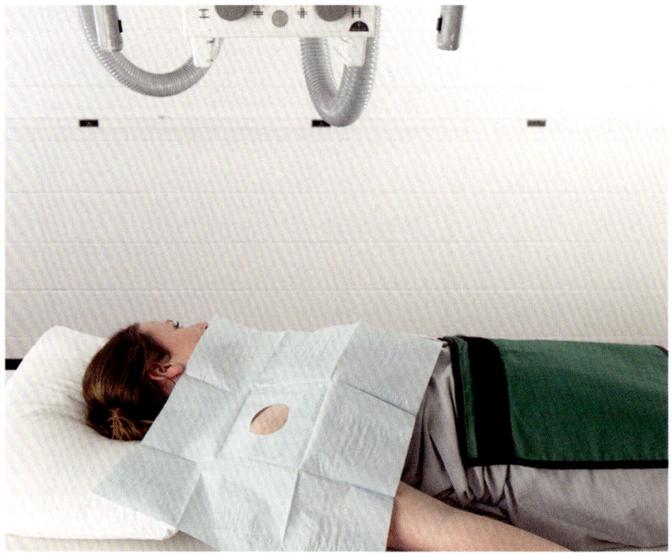

12-45 Patient prepped with sterile field established.

- The radiologist introduces the local anesthetic.
- The radiologist will position the needle in the joint space with the use of fluoroscopic guidance. An image is acquired to document correct needle location (Fig. 12-46).
- The needle will remain in position and the radiologist will connect the contrast syringe with plastic connector tubing

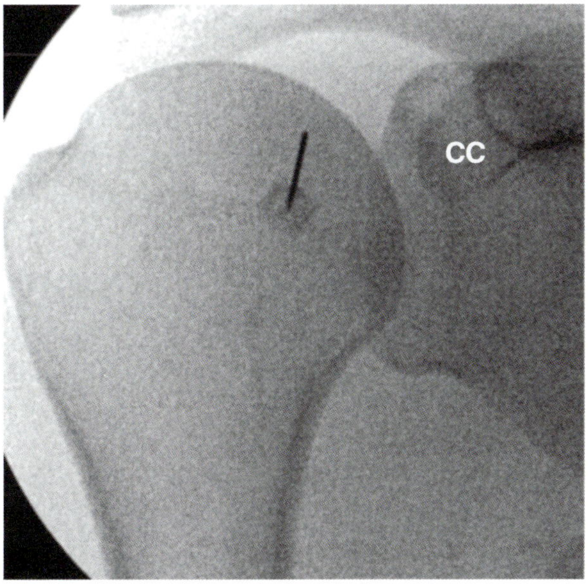

12-46 Needle placement verified.

to the hub of the needle. Iodinated contrast is injected into the joint space. If an MRI will be in conjunction with the arthrogram, gadolinium must be added to the contrast media (Figs. 12-47 and 12-48).

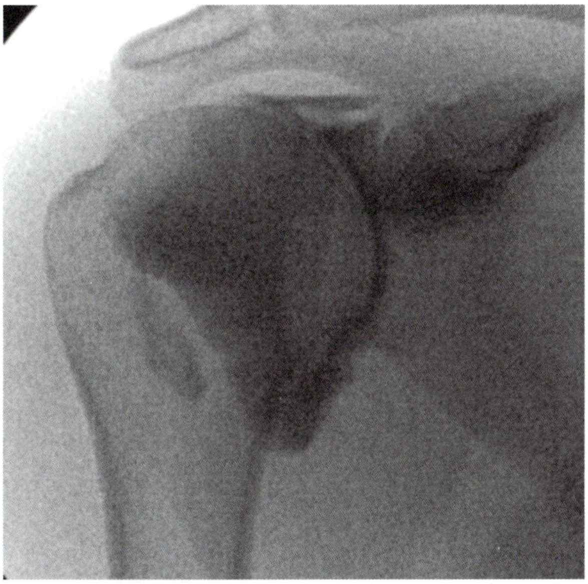

12-47 Contrast injected during fluoroscopic evaluation.

- If a dual contrast study is desired, the radiologist may inject negative contrast (air) into the cavity.
- Following the completion of the radiologist's portion of the exam, the radiologist will remove the needle. The patient's area will be cleaned off and a bandage applied.
- The technologist will acquire the protocol established at the facility for post imaging of the joint (Figs. 12-49, 12-51, and 12-52).

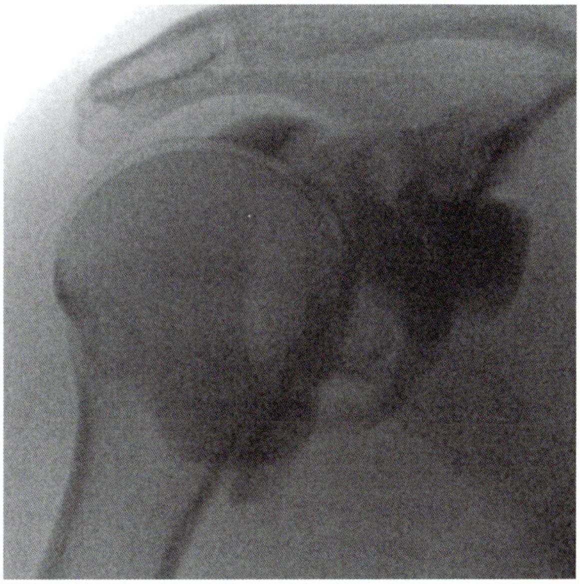

12-48 Fluoroscopic evaluation with the anatomy viewed in different patient positions.

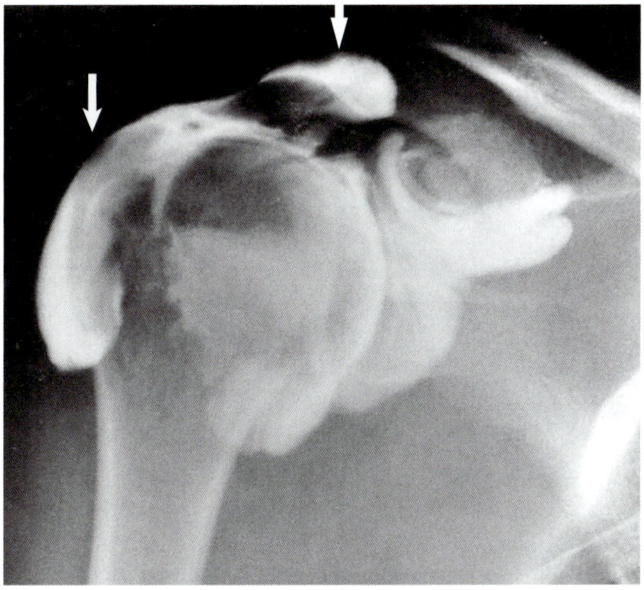

12-49 Postprocedural image of shoulder arthrogram. White arrows reveal a rotator cuff tear.

POSTPROCEDURAL INSTRUCTIONS

- Depending on site protocol, certain facilities may send the patient over for additional imaging in computed tomography (CT) or Magnetic Resonance Imaging (MRI) (Fig. 12-50).
- Patient will be given postprocedural care dismissal instructions.

MYELOGRAPHY

A radiographic contrast study of the spinal cord and its nerve roots to determine the location and the extent of a pathology; most commonly seen in the cervical and lumbar region.

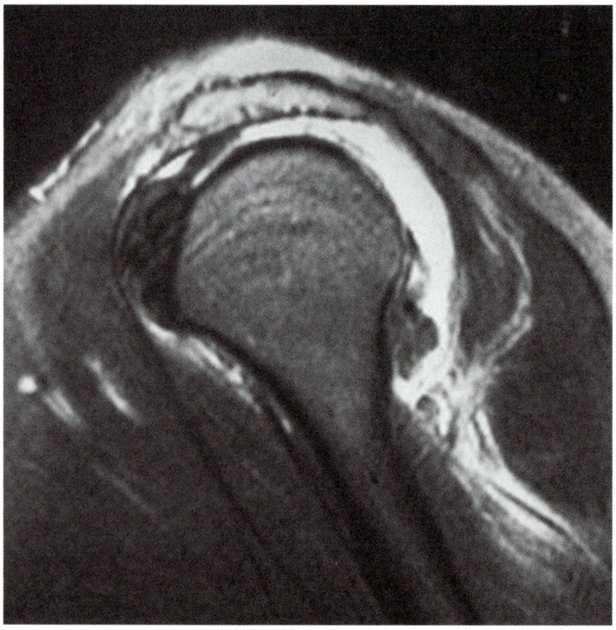

12-50 MRI shoulder arthrogram image.

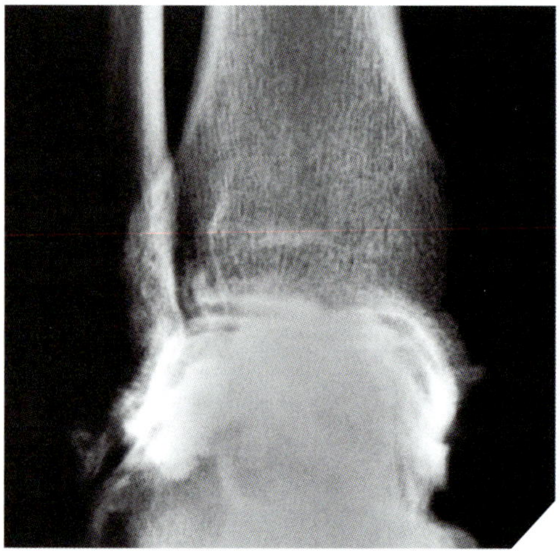

12-51 Ankle arthrogram.

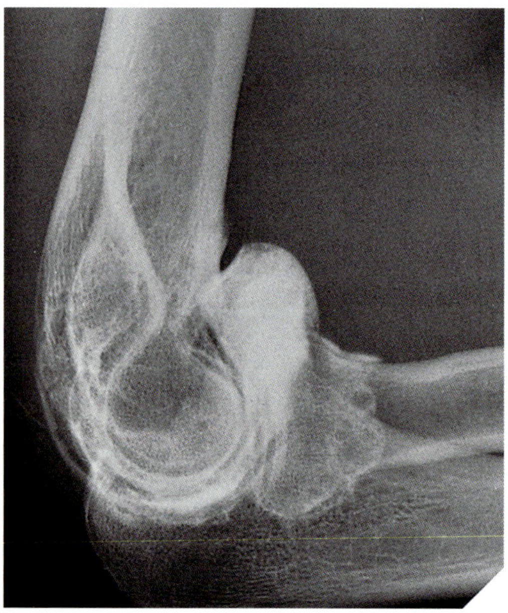

12-52 Elbow arthrogram.

INDICATIONS

Patient who exhibits symptoms such as pain and numbness into extremities caused by potential bone fragments, disk herniation, cyst(s), or tumor impinging on the nerves.

CONTRAINDICATIONS

- Recent lumbar puncture (could cause extravasation of contrast)
- Inflammation of the arachnoid space
- Increased intracranial pressure
- Blood within the cerebrospinal fluid

ANATOMY

KEY ANATOMIC COMPONENTS OF THE SPINAL COLUMN (FIGS. 12-53 TO 12-55)

- Vertebral Column: Succession of many vertebra in a combination of convex and concave curvatures
- Spinal Cord: The cord begins with the medulla oblongata and terminates at approximately L1–L2. The distal end of the cord tapers down into the conus medullaris.

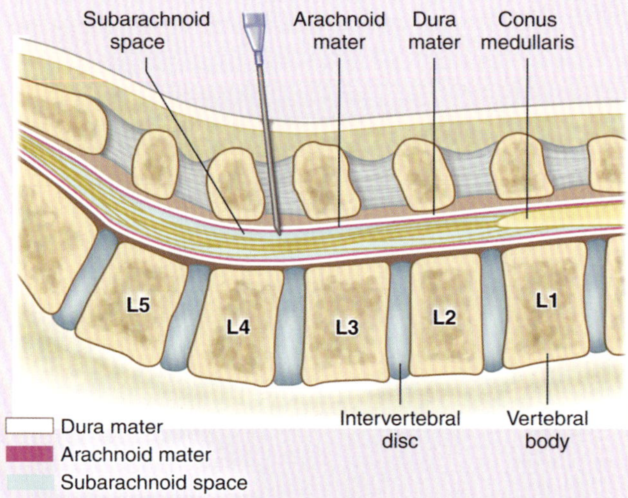

12-53 Conus medullaris.

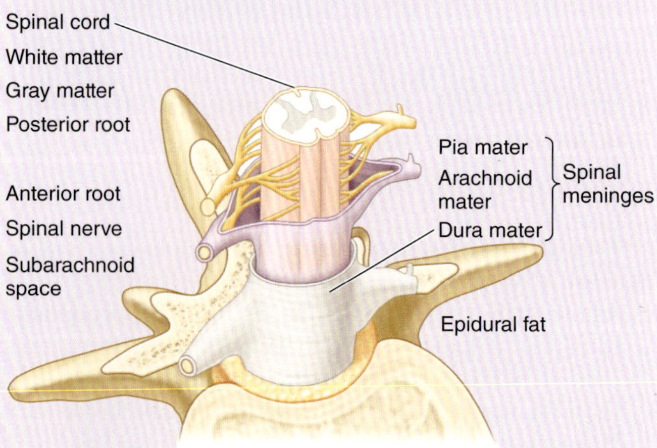

12-54 Meninges.

- Meninges: The pia mater (innermost), subarachnoid mater (middle), and dura mater (outermost) layers cover and protect the spinal cord. Contrast media will be introduced into the subarachnoid space.
- Nerve Roots: The nerves take off from the spinal cord and run outward through the intervertebral foramen.

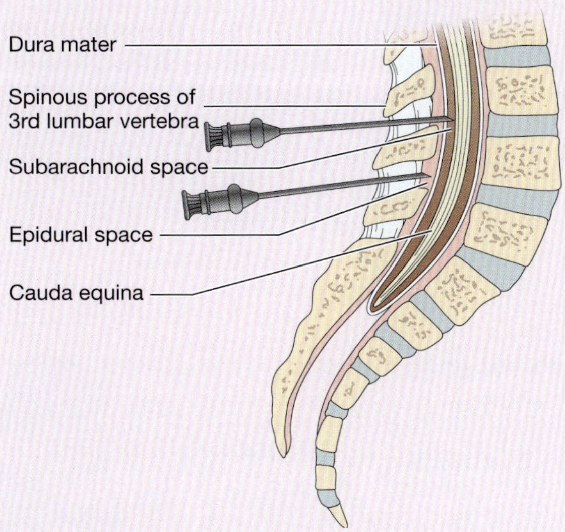

12-55 Meninges.

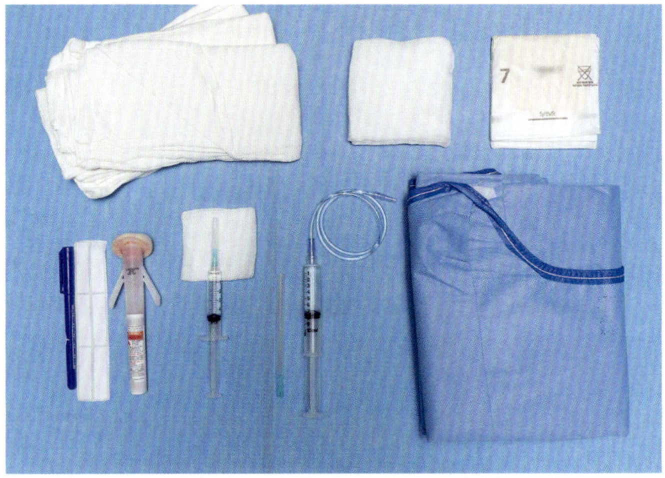

12-56 Example of a sterile tray setup for a myelogram.

PATIENT PREP

- No patient prep. Patients with anxiety may be given a mild sedative before the procedure. Patients on anticoagulant therapy will be recommended to discontinue drugs for a period of time before the scheduled procedure. Patients may also have other laboratory values drawn before the procedure such as International Normalized Ratio (INR), prothrombin time (PT), and partial thromboplastin time (PTT) to determine the amount of time it takes the blood to clot.

STERILE TRAY SETUP (Highly Dependent on Radiologist Preference) (FIG. 12-56)

Disposable myelography tray with basic setup to include betadine or chlorhexidine, prep sponges, sterile drape, sterile gloves, various syringe sizes, various spinal needles, plastic flexible connector, local anesthetic, 4 × 4 gauze, test tubes, and bandage. A hemostat may be requested for the tray to mark the entry location after the skin has been prepped. Iodinated contrast would be drawn up from a vial, it is not included in the disposable tray.

CONTRAST MEDIA

- A nonionic (lower toxicity) water-soluble iodinated contrast.

ROOM SETUP

After scout images are acquired, the room is converted over for the exam.

- Control panel switched to fluoroscopy with time zeroed and kVp set appropriate for the myelogram.
- Table Bucky positioned to the foot or head of the table.
- Footboard must be attached to the table and shoulder braces can be attached as well. The patient will be adjusted from horizontal to Trendelenburg and into upright positions to facilitate the movement of the contrast media.
- Viewing monitor and fluoroscopy foot pedal arranged for radiologist.

PROCEDURE

- Patient dressed in a gown.
- Patient history is acquired and documented on the institutional contrast screening form.
- The exam is explained to the patient and consent is acquired. Potential patient pregnancy has been ruled out.
- Precontrast (scout) images of the vertebral region are acquired. These images are presented to the radiologist.
- The radiologist will prep the area and establish the sterile field. Access to the lumbar region is used most commonly. Cervical access is considered in instances a patient has an obstruction above the lumbar access point that prevents contrast from ascending to the cervical region.
- For the radiologist to place the needle for lumbar access, the patient may be laid prone with a bolster positioned under the hips to flatten out the lumbar curvature or the patient may lay in a left lateral position in flexion to open the spinous process interspaces (Fig. 12-57).
- For the radiologist to place the needle for cervical access, the patient may sit erect or lie prone with neck flexed. Flexion of the neck moves the spinous processes apart to allow access. With cervical access with a patient in the prone position, it is important that the patient remains in a hyperextended position to prevent the contrast media from passing further into the cranial subarachnoid space (Fig. 12-58).

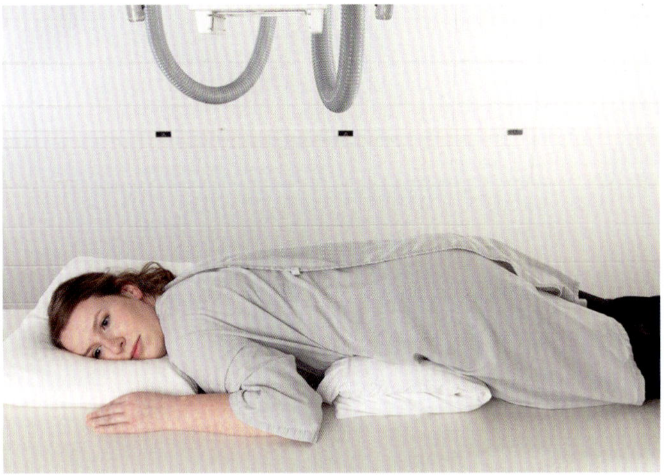

12-57 Lumbar access position.

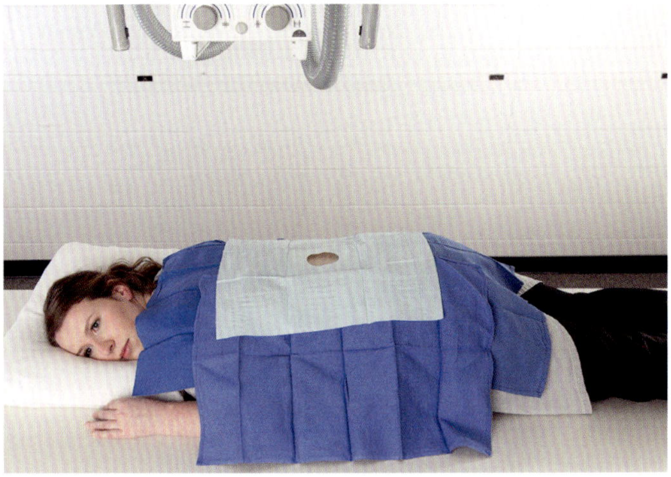

12-59 Patient prepped with sterile field established.

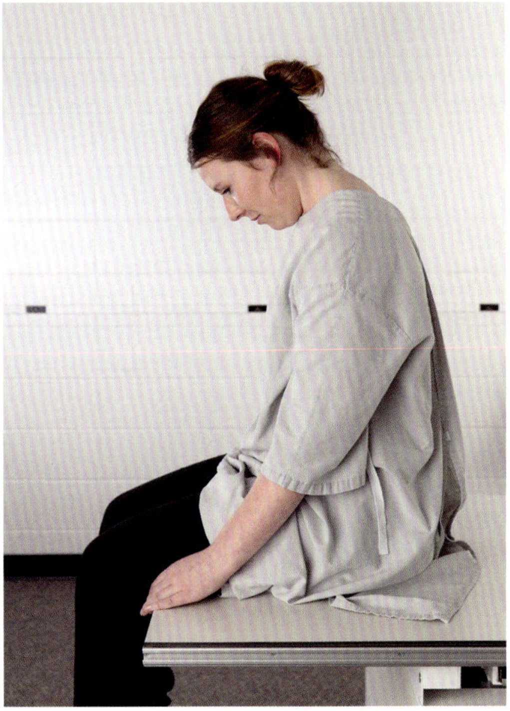

12-58 Cervical access position.

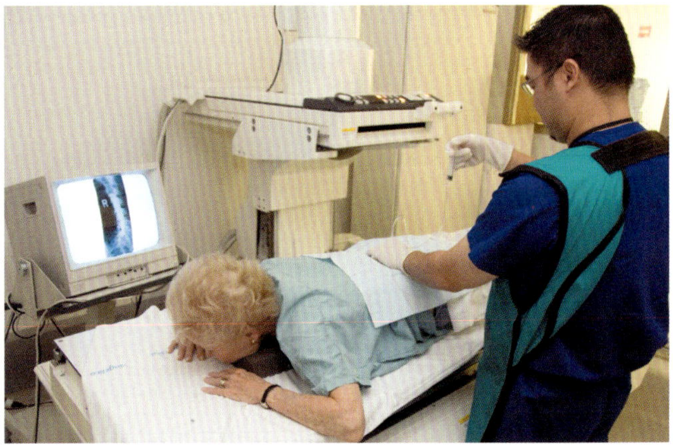

12-60 Radiologist access under fluoroscopic guidance.

- After the patient is in position, the area is prepped and draped, creating a sterile field (Fig. 12-59).
- The radiologist introduces the local anesthetic.
- For a lumbar puncture, the L3–L4 disk location will be accessed. For a cervical puncture, the C1–C2 location will be accessed.
- The radiologist will position the spinal needle in the subarachnoid space. The radiologist determines this location by the return of cerebrospinal fluid (CSF). A sample of the patient's CSF will be sent for laboratory analysis.
- The needle will remain in position, and the radiologist will connect the contrast syringe with plastic connector tubing to the hub of the needle. Nonionic iodinated contrast is injected into the subarachnoid space (Figs. 12-60 and 12-61).
- The patient will be altered in position from Trendelenburg to potentially upright to encourage the distribution of the contrast media (Figs. 12-62 and 12-63).
- Following the completion of the radiologist's portion of the exam, the radiologist will remove the needle. The patient's area will be cleaned off and a bandage applied.
- The technologist will acquire the protocol established at the facility for post imaging, which typically includes prone and horizontal beam imaging (Figs. 12-64 to 12-68).

POSTPROCEDURAL INSTRUCTIONS

- Patient will be monitored postprocedure for approximately 1 hour to monitor for any potential side effects.
- Patient may be sent to CT for a scan after injection.
- Patient will be given postprocedural care dismissal instructions.

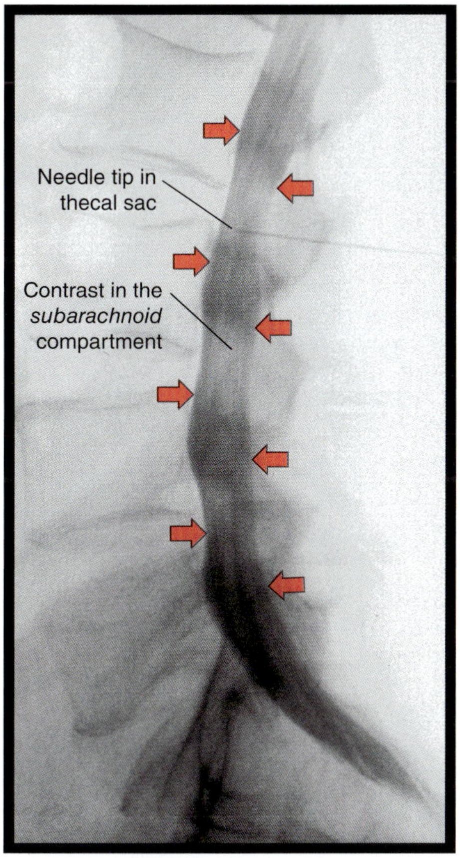

12-61 Contrast media introduced into the subarachnoid space.

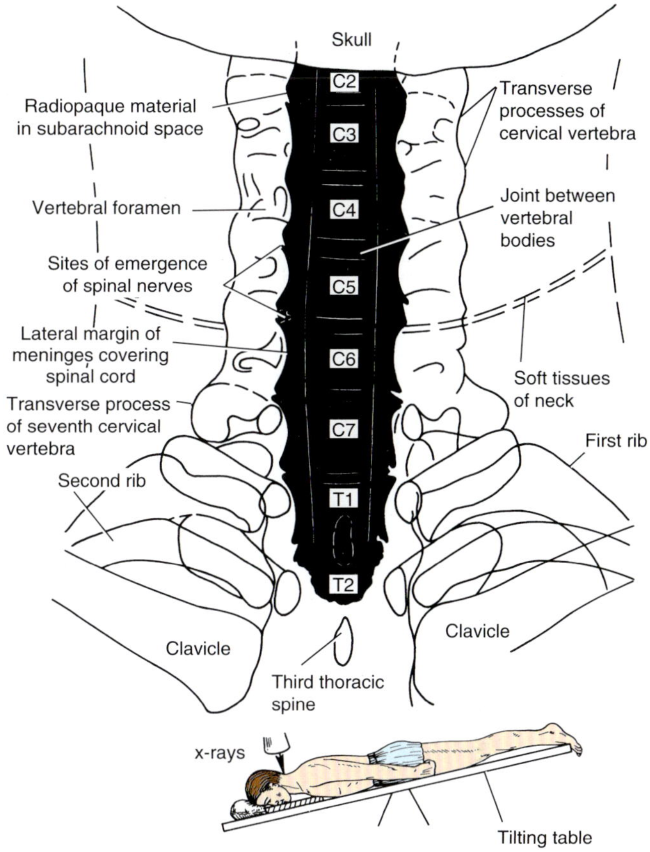

12-63 Alteration of patient position to assist with contrast media distribution.

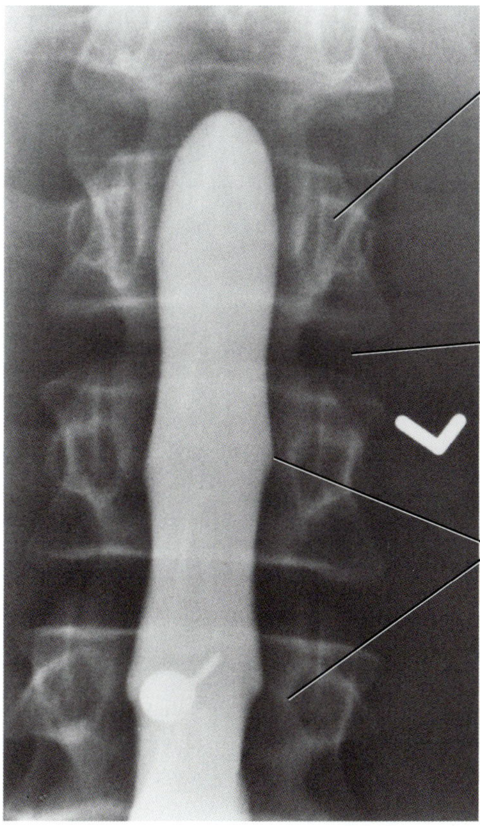

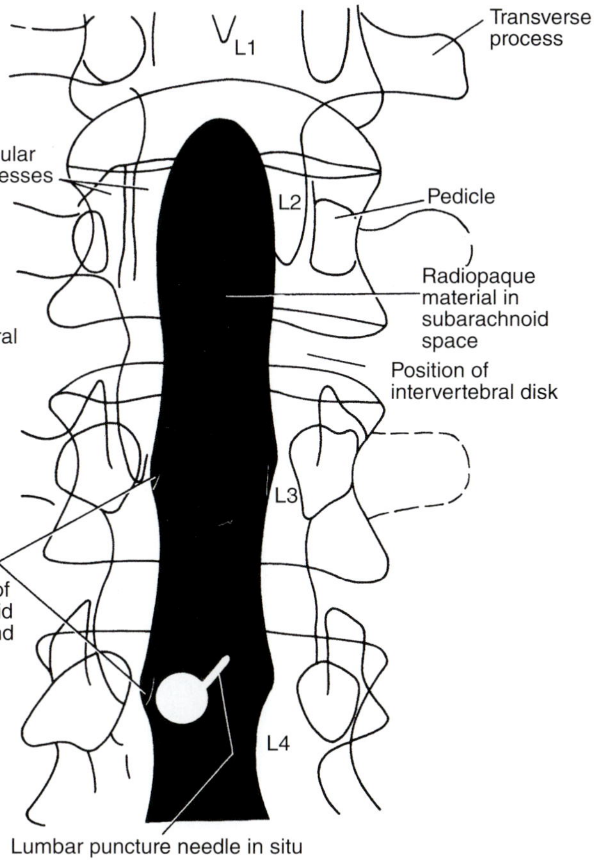

12-62 Radio opaque contrast in subarachnoid space.

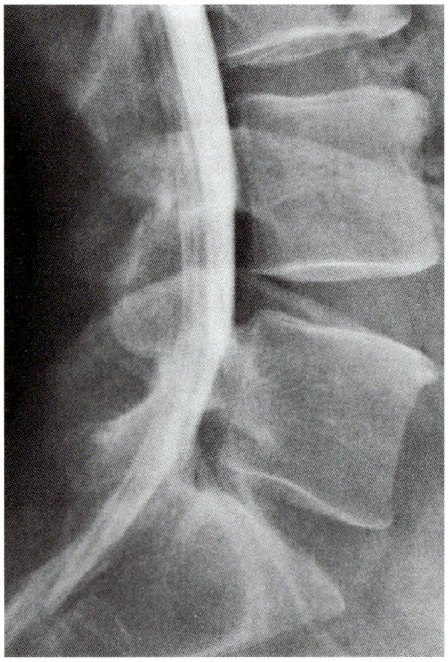

12-64 Post image cross-table lateral lumbar spine.

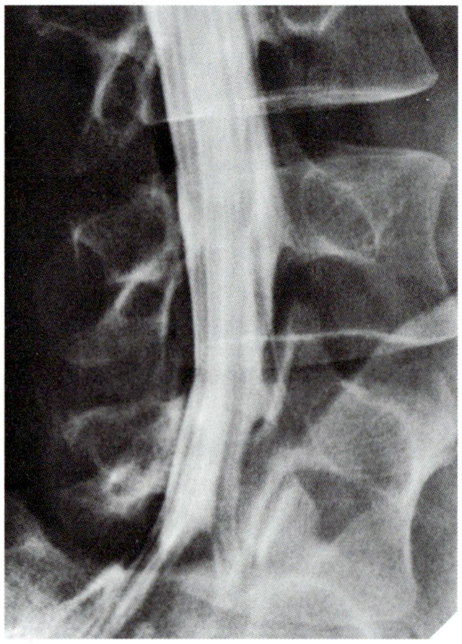

12-66 Post image myelogram lumbar oblique.

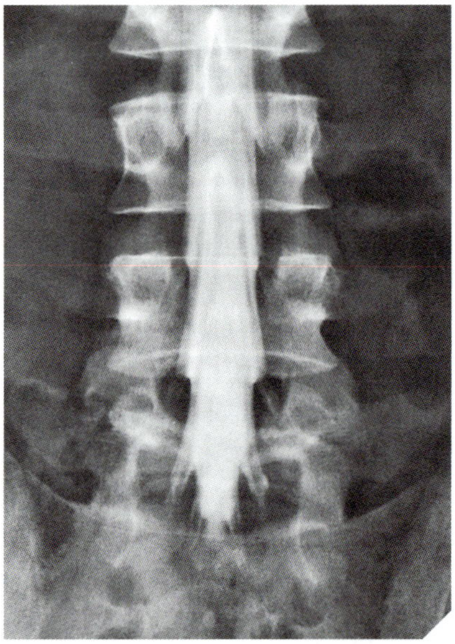

12-65 Post image lumbar myelogram.

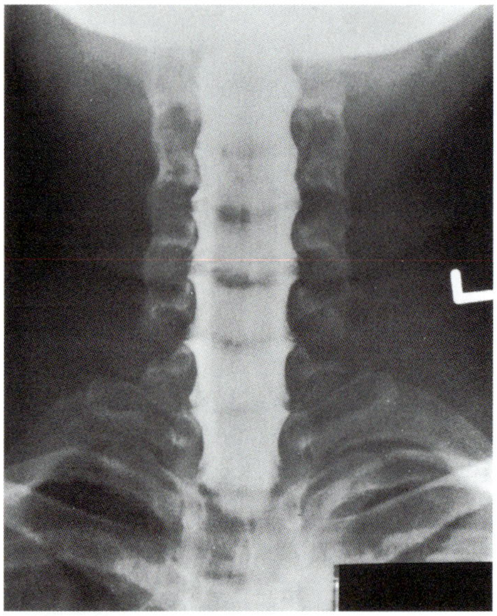

12-67 Post image cervical myelogram.

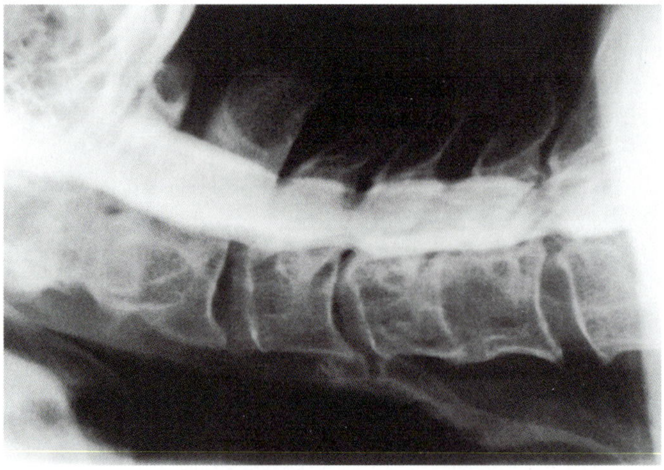

12-68 Post image cross-table lateral cervical spine.

HYSTEROSALPINGOGRAPHY (HSG)

Radiographic study of the uterine cavity and fallopian tubes. This exam may serve as therapeutic study to the patient as well.

INDICATIONS

- Uterine cavity defects (congenital anomalies, adhesions, polyps, fibroids), fallopian tube obstruction, to evaluate competency of tubal ligation.

CONTRAINDICATIONS

- Pelvic inflammatory disease
- Confirmed pregnancy

ANATOMY

The female reproductive uterus undergoes monthly physiologic cyclic changes influenced by different hormones released by the body. The inner most layer of the uterus, the endometrium, lines the uterine cavity and will undergo changes alongside the ovaries during the 28 day menstrual cycle. The endometrium and the ovaries are influenced by sequential hormones in order to achieve pregnancy. The uterine cavity will hold and provide for the fetal environment. The uterus is comprised of muscular layers that are essential to the delivery process of a fetus.

KEY ANATOMIC PARTS OF THE FEMALE REPRODUCTIVE SYSTEM (FIG. 12-69)

- The subdivisions of the uterus are: cervix, isthmus, body, and fundus.
- The uterine cavity communicates with the fallopian tubes. The fallopian tubes insert at the uterine fundus.
- The fallopian tubes are 7-10 centimeter in length and 1/2 centimeter in diameter.
- The divisions of the fallopian tubes from proximal to distal are: interstitial, isthmus, ampulla, and the infundibulum.
- The distal most end of the infundibulum contain fimbria (finger-like extensions) that open up to the peritoneal cavity. The fimbrae are adjacent to the ovary which function to capture the egg as it is released from the ovary at ovulation and draws it up into the fallopian tube where it awaits fertilization.
- The ovary is positioned lateral to the uterus and secured by the ovarian ligament.

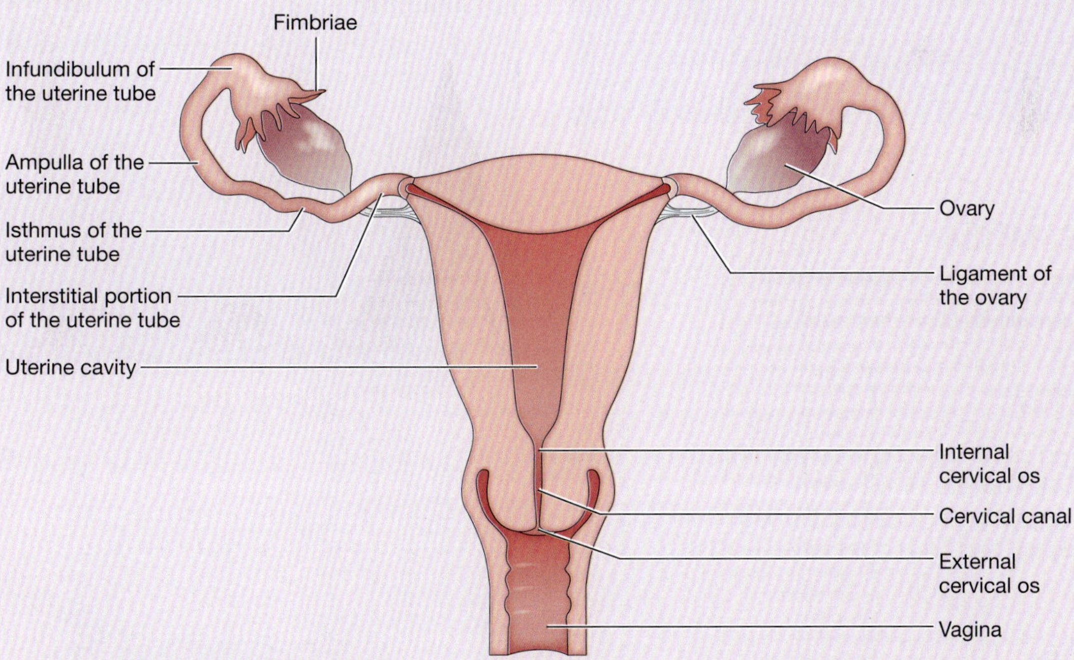

12-69 Female reproductive system.

PATIENT PREP

- No prep unless the ordering physicians prefer a bowel prep; patient must have a negative pregnancy test 24 hours before the procedure.
- Patient should empty her bladder before the procedure.

STERILE TRAY SETUP (Highly Dependent on Radiologist or Physician Preference)

Disposable hysterosalpingography (HSG) tray provides basic setup to include: vaginal speculum, cotton balls, betadine, sterile gauze and drape, forceps, syringes, extension tubing, balloon catheter, lubricating jelly, and sterile gloves. Iodinated contrast will be drawn up (not included in the tray). At the additional request of the physician, a tenaculum (instrument to secure tissues or a structure) can be added to the sterile tray (Fig. 12-70).

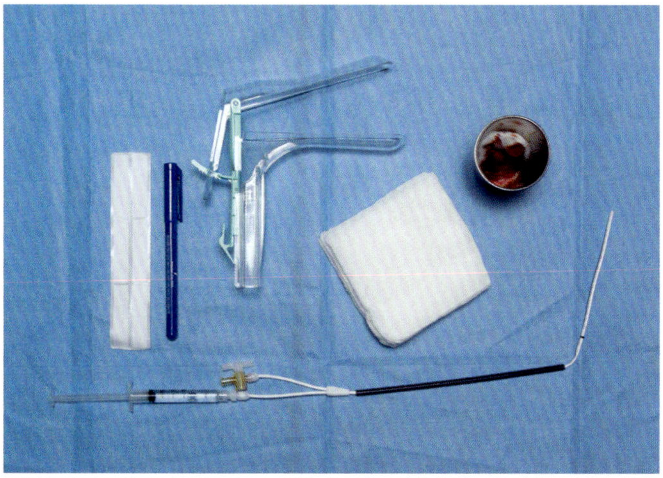

12-70 Example of a sterile tray setup for an HSG.

CONTRAST MEDIA

- Iodinated water-soluble contrast is drawn up. The volume may be determined by the physician.

ROOM SETUP

- Control panel switched to fluoroscopy with time zeroed and kVp set appropriate for the pelvis.
- Table Bucky positioned to the foot or head of the table.
- Viewing monitor and fluoroscopy foot pedal arranged for physician.

PROCEDURE

- The exam is explained and the patient's informed consent acquired. Potential patient pregnancy has been ruled out. Scout image may be acquired (Fig. 12-71).
- Patient is positioned in a lithotomy position on top of an absorbent pad (Fig. 12-72). The peroneal area is prepped for sterile procedure.
- Physician will need additional focused lighting to place the speculum to visualize the cervix and then to prep the cervix. A small catheter will be directed through the cervical canal and into the lower uterine segment (Fig. 12-73).
- Once the catheter is in place, a balloon is distended to hold it into position. The patient is positioned on the table for the introduction of the contrast media.
- Under fluoroscopy, contrast media will be introduced into the uterine cavity. Once the uterine cavity is filled with contrast, the contrast moves to fill the fallopian tubes. The contrast media will course from the ends of the fallopian tubes and into the peritoneal cavity if there is not a tubal obstruction. The patient will experience cramping during this portion of the procedure (Figs. 12-74 and 12-75).
- Digital fluoroscopic images or cine loops are acquired throughout the administration of the contrast media. This may limit the number of post images acquired by the technologist.
- The patient is assisted off the table to clean up and try to allow removal of some contrast from the uterine cavity.

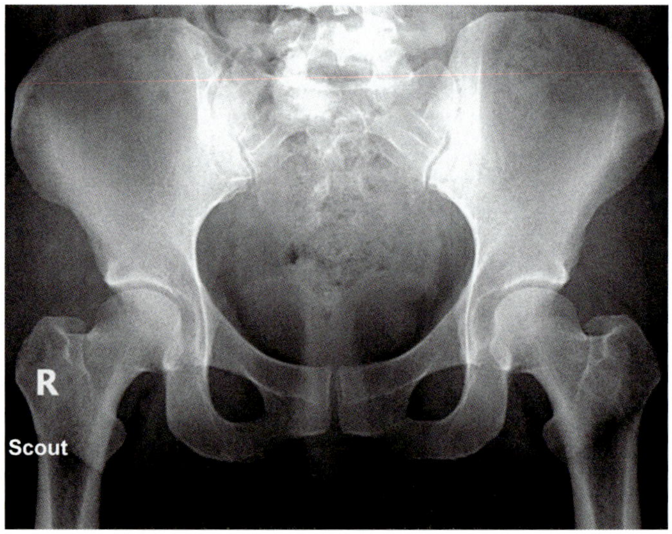

12-71 Scout pelvis.

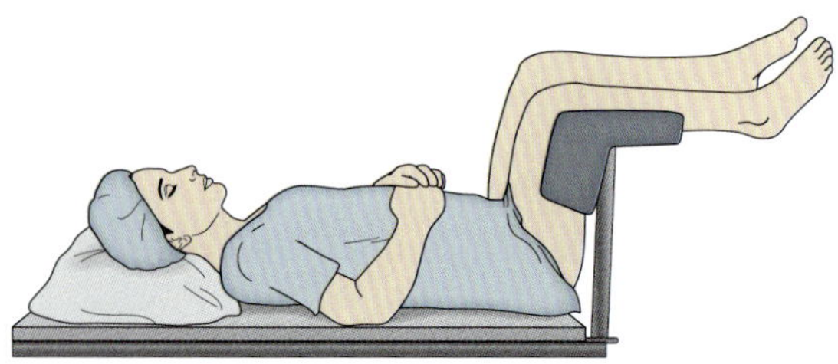

12-72 Lithotomy position.

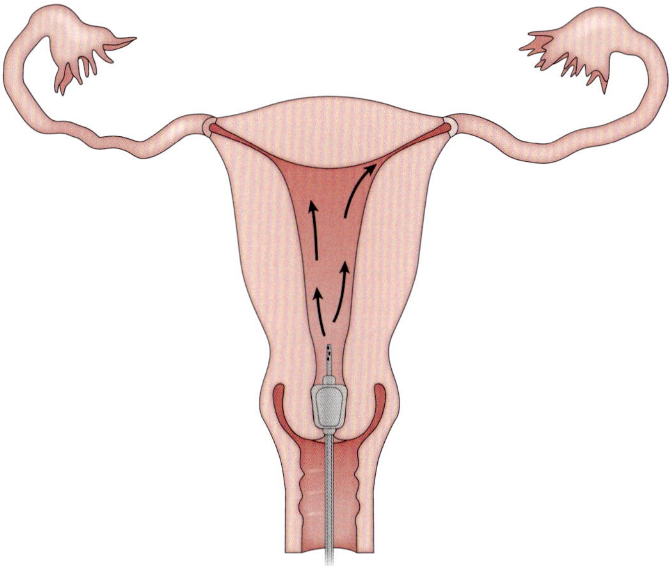

12-73 HSG catheter placement.

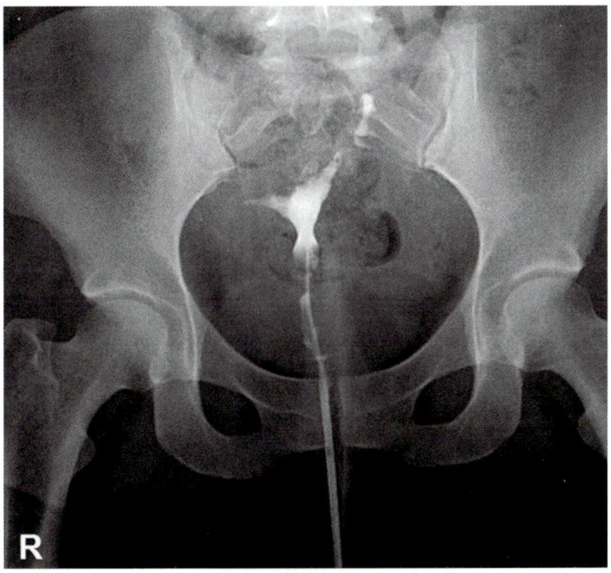

12-74 Contrast filling of the uterus.

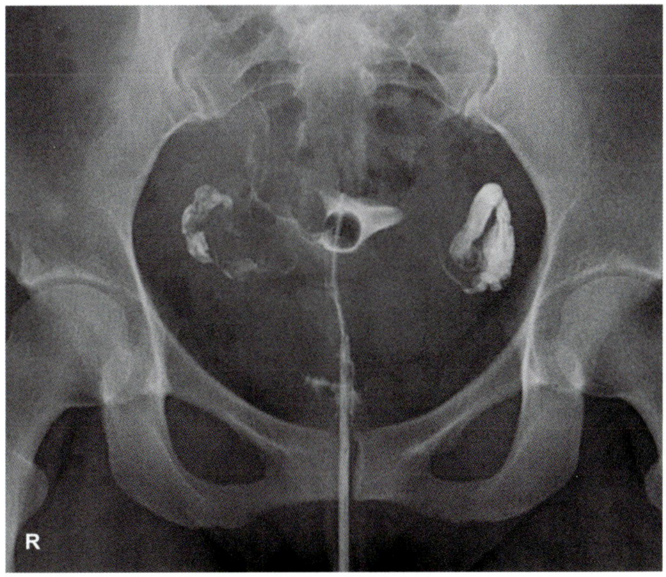

12-75 Contrast coursing from the fallopian tubes into the peritoneum.

POST IMAGING

- A post image spot of the pelvis is acquired to document the residual amount of contrast media.

POSTPROCEDURAL INSTRUCTIONS

- Patient will be given postprocedural care dismissal instructions.

CHAPTER 13 Operative Radiography

Radiologic technologists are called to the operative suite to image the patient with either the mobile unit or a C-arm or O-arm unit. Technologists are expected to be efficient and confident within this environment to expedite the surgeon's requests with minimal to no error. The technologist must respond to the surgeons' request(s), while respecting the sterile field. In addition, the technologist must be proficient at creatively maneuvering the equipment into necessary positions. Once the technologist works with a surgeon on multiple cases, the technologist is better able to anticipate the surgeon's preferences. The radiologic technologist plays an important role during the surgical procedure by not only providing imaging, but ensuring a safe radiation environment.

OPERATIVE SUITE ENVIRONMENT

The surgical suite will have several on the team necessary to coordinate the surgery (Fig. 13-1). The surgical suite will consist of sterile and nonsterile areas and personnel. When working within this suite, it is imperative to identify the sterile and nonsterile areas and personnel. The sterile personnel will consist of the surgeon(s), scrub nurse, and surgical assistant. The nonsterile personnel will include the radiologic technologist, circulating nurse, and the anesthesiologist.

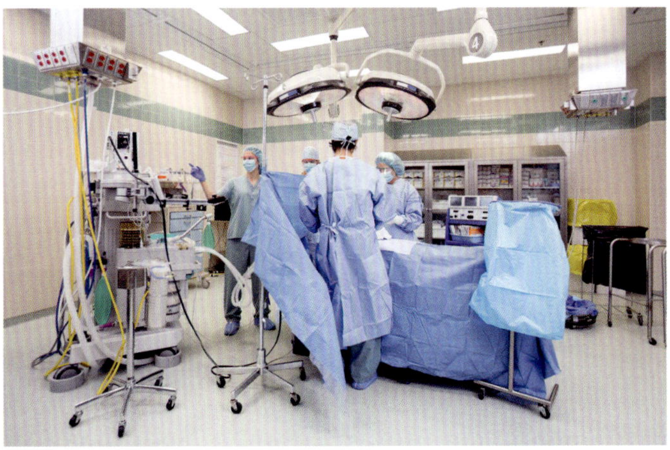

13-1 Surgical suite with the surgical team.

Surgical Attire for the Nonsterile Personnel

Clean surgical scrub attire is supplied by the surgical department. The technologist will change before a surgical procedure and should change out of surgical scrubs at the end of their shift. If scrubs were to become soiled during a surgical procedure, the technologist must change into a new set of scrubs before the next surgical procedure. Surgical scrubs should not be worn home and personally laundered (Fig. 13-2).

- Shoe covers should cover closed-toe shoes. Covers should be replaced when soiled and before entering another surgical suite or when leaving the surgical corridor.
- Hair cover over the top of the head. Covers should be removed and changed with each new surgical case. Facial hair must also be covered.
- Masks are worn to reduce the spread of microorganisms dispersed by the technologist and reduce the risk of the technologist breathing in any pathogens during a procedure. Masks should be removed and replaced with a new one for each surgical case.
- Protective eyewear should be considered in cases where patient blood and bodily fluids may be dispersed during the procedure.
- Nonsterile gloves are necessary for the technologist to wear when exchanging image receptors or cleaning equipment that may have been contaminated with blood or body fluids.

Surgical Attire for the Sterile Personnel

In addition to the surgical attire for the nonsterile personnel, the sterile personnel will undergo a proper surgical hand and arm scrub. A sterile gown and gloves are put on. The gown is sterile from the waist up on the front (Figs. 13-3 and 13-4). Sterile gloves must remain above the waist (Fig. 13-5). A technologist, even though not sterile, should keep their hands above waist level. The level of the surgical table and above is considered sterile (Fig. 13-6).

Surgical Drapes

Blue surgical drapes will designate where an aseptic technique is required. Sterile drapes provide an additional barrier to prevent microorganisms from entering the surgical site. The sterile area will include the surgical table, surgical team, surgical stands, surgical equipment, and the imaging equipment. Only sterile personnel can touch sterile items.

Mobile Imaging Equipment

Mobile equipment designated for the surgical suites is typically stored in the surgical department to allow for quick access if needed. Equipment such as the mobile unit, C-arm, O-arm or image receptors must be disinfected regularly and any time after a unit or image receptor is contaminated with blood or bodily fluids. C-arms or O-arms are typically setup and powered up before the start of a surgical procedure. The technologist can bring the unit and viewing monitor into the surgical suite according to the suite design and power it up to ensure

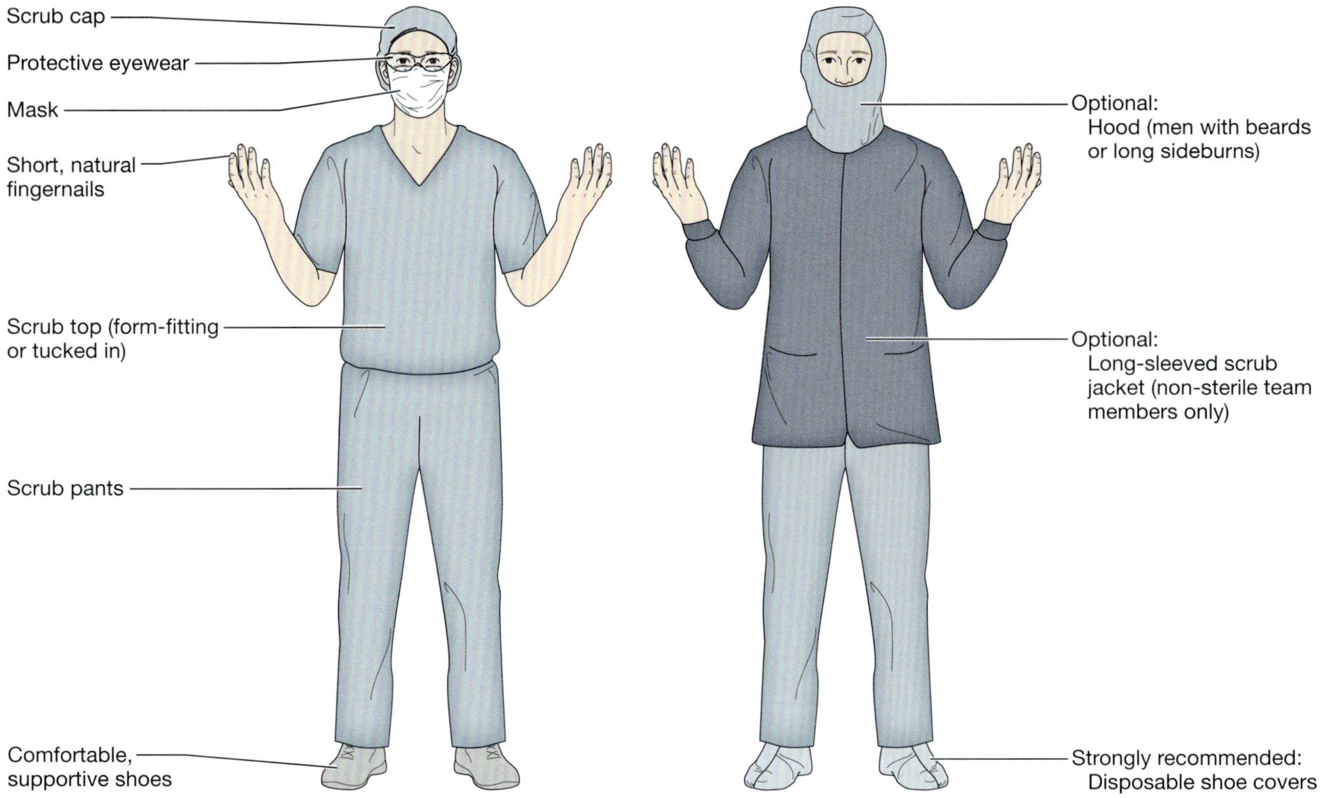

13-2 Surgical attire for the nonsterile personnel.

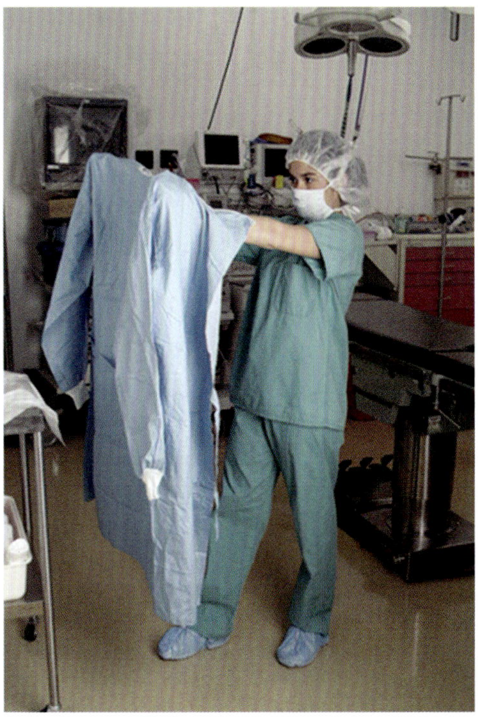

13-3 Sterile gown.

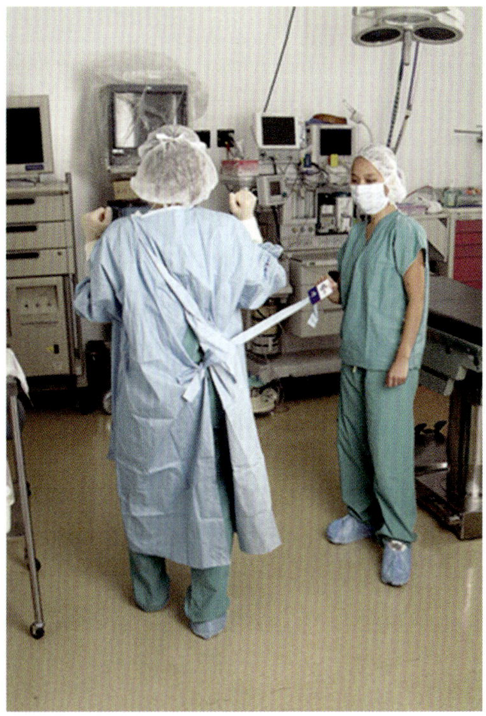

13-4 Sterile gown.

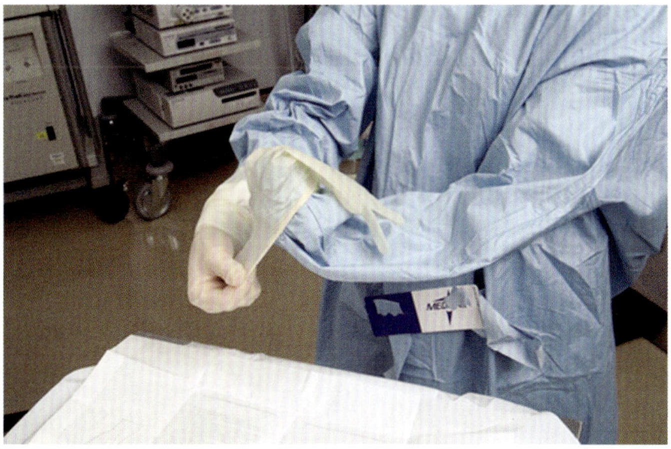

13-5 Sterile gloves.

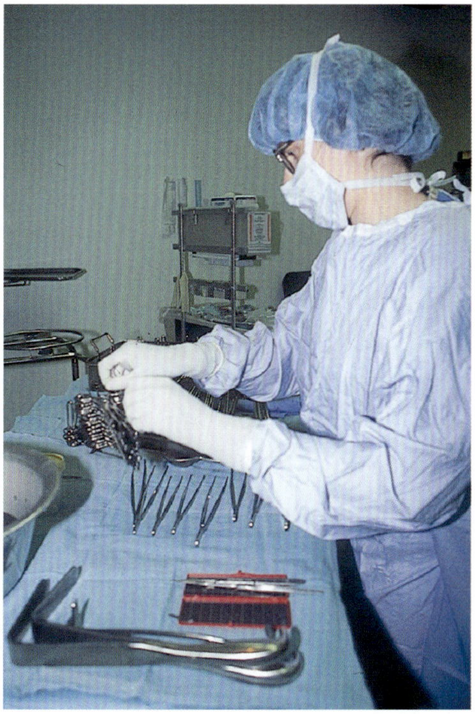

13-6 Surgical table.

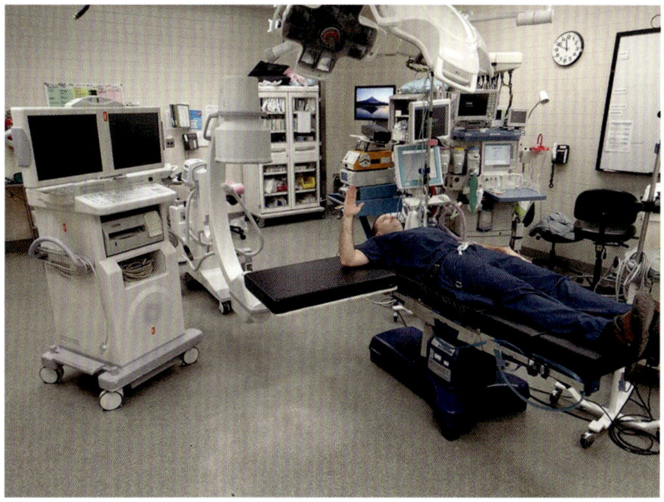

13-7 C-arm equipment.

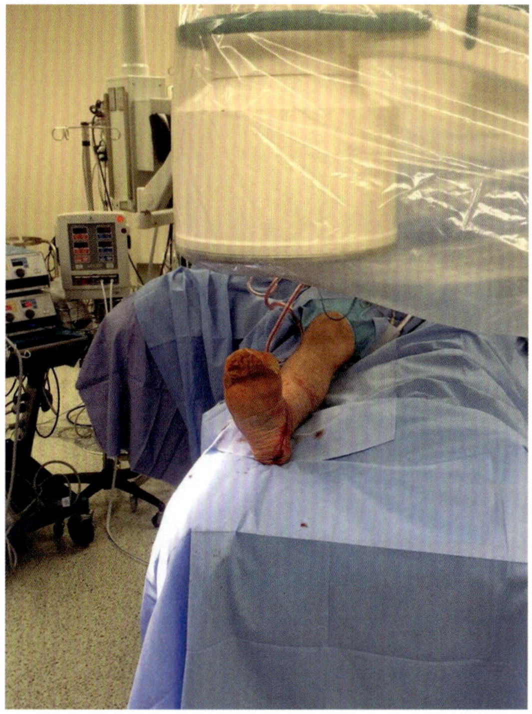

13-8 C-arm within the sterile field.

it is functioning when the technologist is called to the room for the procedure (Fig. 13-7). Once the sterile field is in place, imaging equipment will be wrapped or bagged (Fig. 13-8). The technologist will adjust the position of the monitor for viewing, the foot pedal for operating, and ensure image orientation is set before procedural images begins.

Basic C-arm Components

C-arm Control Panel: Displays exposure time, kVp and mA setting, image orientation, contrast, collimation, image capture, and the technologist will be able to raise and lower the height of the C-arm (Fig. 13-10).

C-arm Monitor Controls: Patient information, image review, image inversion, and zoom (Fig. 13-9)

Tube: Produces the x-ray beam. To reduce the entrance dose to the patient and to reduce dose overall to personnel, the tube should be positioned beneath the surgical table (Fig. 13-11).

Image Intensifier: Converts the beam exiting the patient to the image displayed on the monitor. The image intensifier should ideally be positioned at a height that is as close to the patient as possible to reduce personnel exposure, reduce image magnification, and will produce a brighter and more detailed image (Fig. 13-11).

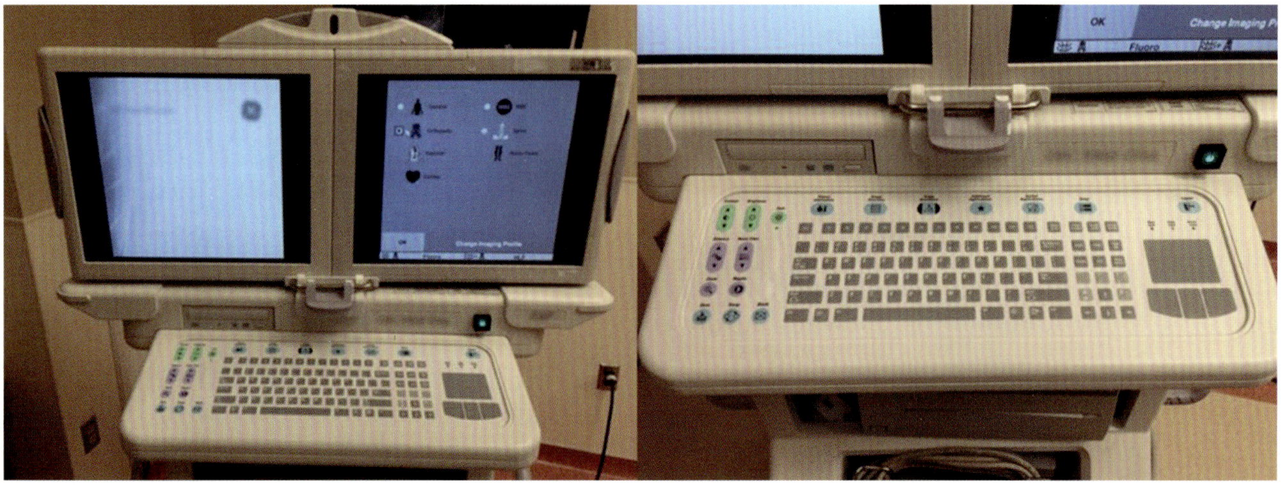

13-9 C-arm monitor controls.

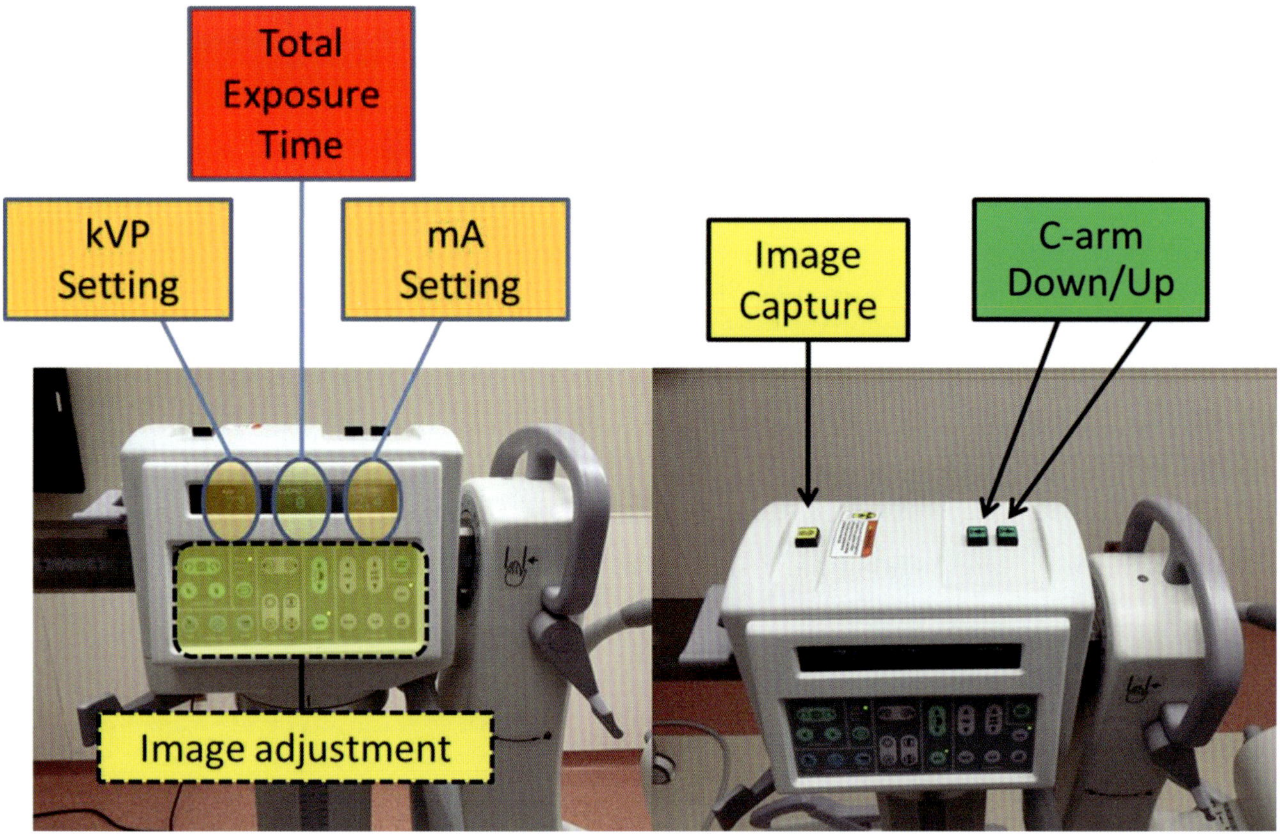

13-10 C-arm control panel.

Basic C-arm Movements

- Push/Pull: Moving the unit in and out of the surgical field
- Raise/Lower: The height of the C-arm adjusted to fit below the table and the ensure the image intensifier is high enough to avoid contact with the instruments in the sterile field.
- Wag: With the C-arm base stationary, the C-arm moves to the right or left (Fig. 13-12).
- Angle: The C-arm can be adjusted from perpendicular to angle toward the head or feet as requested by the surgeon (Fig. 13-13).
- Inversion: The C-arm can be inverted to place the image intensifier beneath the surgical table and the tube above the surgical table.
- Rollover or Rollunder (Rainbow): From vertical position of the C-arm, the image intensifier can "rollover" the area of interest or "rollback" to provide a lateral view of a part if anteroposterior (AP)/posteroanterior (PA) was acquired with the C-arm vertical (Fig. 13-14).

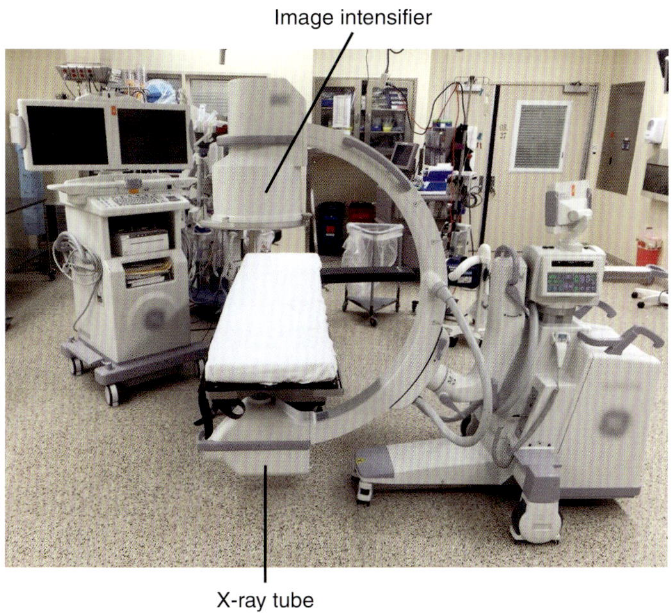

13-11 C-arm x-ray tube and image intensifier.

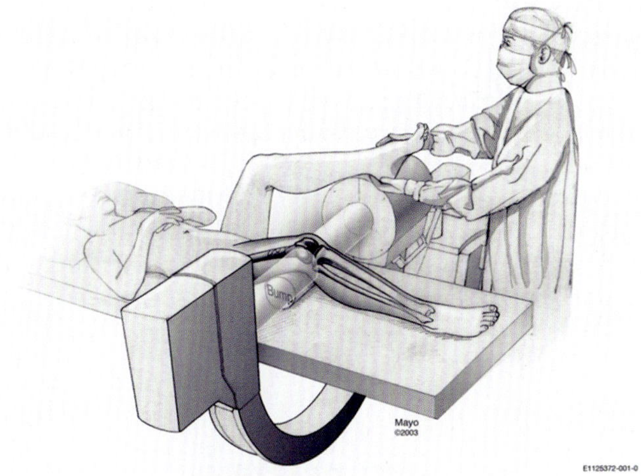

13-14 C-arm "rollunder" movement.

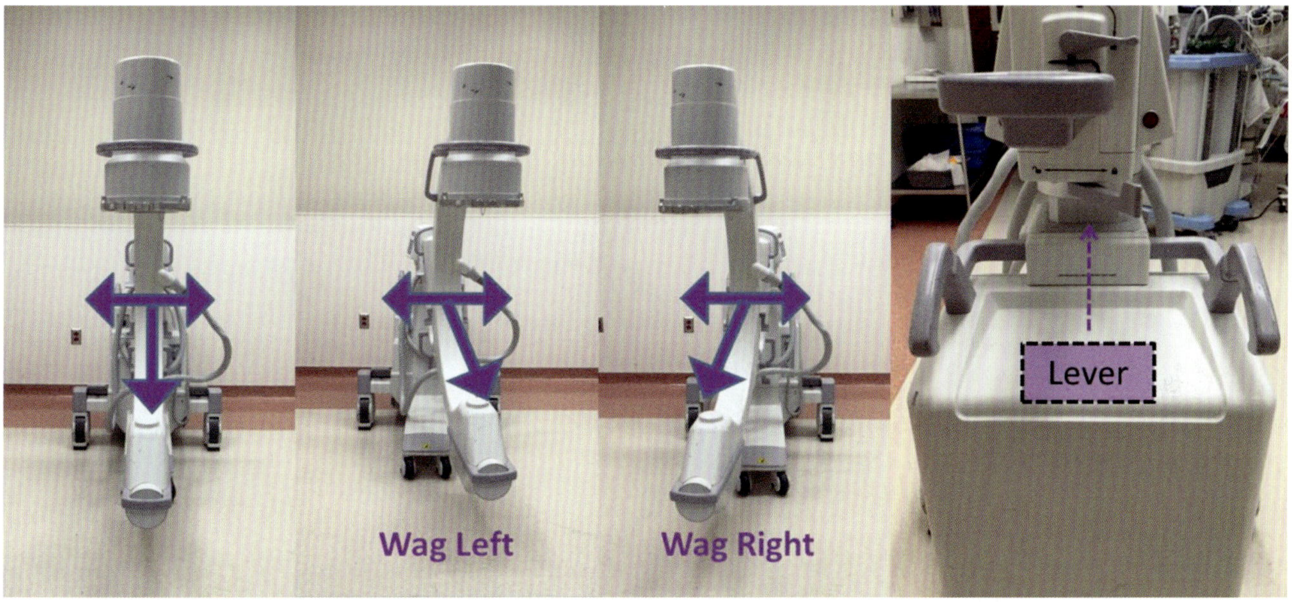

13-12 C-arm "wag" movement.

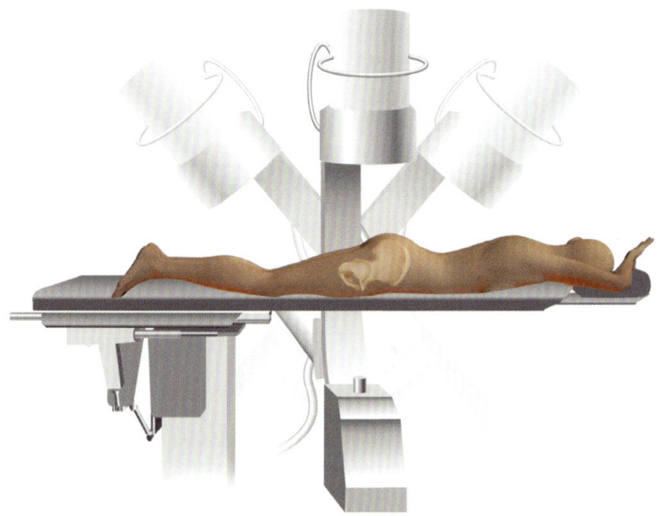

13-13 C-arm "angle" movement.

RADIATION PROTECTION CONSIDERATIONS

A technologist should always consider the basic rules of shielding, time, and distance while in professional practice. The technologist is responsible for ensuring their own personal *protection* (such as lead apron or wrap around shield and thyroid shield), but also protecting everyone in the suite. The surgeon planning to use imaging during a procedure will typically wear lead under their sterile attire. It is possible that portable lead shields may also be available in the suite. If necessary, the technologist should supply lead apron *shielding* to the individual on the surgical team that has no protection and cannot briefly step out for the exposure. These same practices hold true in the recovery room, but oftentimes, health care personnel are able to achieve a minimum 6-foot *distance* for mobile equipment exposure; therefore, no personal protection is required. The technologist must be aware and ensure the safety of everyone in the vicinity. The radiologic technologist must vocalize when the use of x-ray is "on" or "off" to allow health care workers to temporarily vacate the area. Personnel that work within the radiation field must wear a personal radiation monitoring device. When wearing a lead apron rated at the recommended 0.5 mm lead equivalent for fluoroscopic procedures, the radiation monitoring device must be worn at the collar level and on the outside of the apron. The technologist has the responsibility to ensure that any personnel in the operative suite are wearing protective lead during the exposure or procedure.

Exposure *time* is limited when intermittent fluoroscopy is employed during a procedure. This reduces exposure to the health care personnel and to the patient. Another effort to reduce personnel exposure is to reduce the *distance* between the image intensifier and the patient. Exposure is reduced to the health care professionals when the C-arm tube is positioned vertically with the tube under the table and the image intensifier is above the patient (Fig. 13-15). A vertical position of the C-arm with a patient positioned supine on the surgical table will produce a posteroanterior projection with the x-ray tube positioned below the table. A vertical position of the C-arm with the patient positioned prone on the surgical table will produce an anteroposterior projection with the x-ray tube under the table. With the image intensifier positioned above the patient, this reduces exposure levels to the head and neck (Figs. 13-15 and 13-16). When the C-arm is positioned horizontally, personnel exposure is reduced if the operator or health care professionals stand directly behind the x-ray tube (Fig. 13-17).

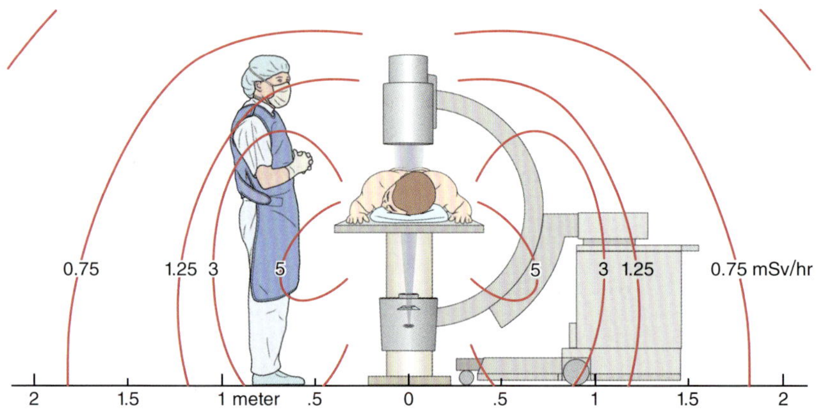

13-15 Radiation exposure is reduced to personnel's head and neck region when the x-ray tube is positioned beneath the table.

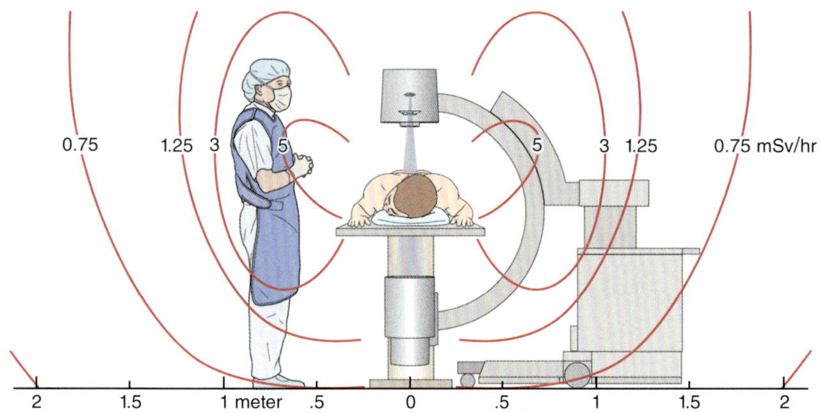

13-16 Radiation exposure is increased to personnel's head and neck region when the x-ray tube is inverted and positioned above the table.

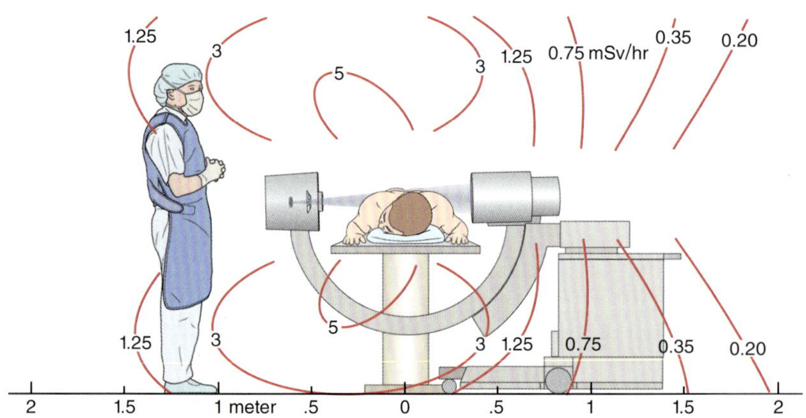

13-17 To reduce radiation exposure during a lateral approach the personnel should stand behind the x-ray tube.

STERILE ASEPSIS AND STERILE FIELDS

The technologist will stand in the nonsterile field along with the anesthesiologist and the circulating nurse. If a technologist ever questions where they can be within the suite or what items can be touched, he/she should ask for clarification to avoid contamination of the sterile field. If the sterile field is contaminated or even potentially contaminated, the technologist should report this so new sterile drapes and instruments are implemented. The C-arm will have to be covered to enter into the sterile field. The surgeon will guide the technologist as to where to position the C-arm within the sterile field. The technologist must be aware of the height of the image intensifier to clear contact with the surgical instruments. If the mobile radiography unit is needed for imaging, the image receptor must be placed into a sterile covering. The technologist will hold onto the nonsterile image receptor and slide it into the sterile covering held by sterile personnel. The technologist may have contact with the nonsterile image receptor and only ever touch the inside of the sterile covering. The open end of the sterile covering is secured by the sterile person and positions it for imaging by the instructions given by the surgeon or the technologist. The technologist will position the mobile unit over the patient while respecting the sterile field and center and collimate according to the surgeon's instruction. After the exposure, the image receptor (IR) will be carefully pulled from the sterile cover. The technologist should be ready to receive the covered image receptor with gloves on to reduce exposure to bodily fluids. In some instances, surgical tables are designed to have an image receptor tray that lies just beneath the tabletop (Fig. 13-18).

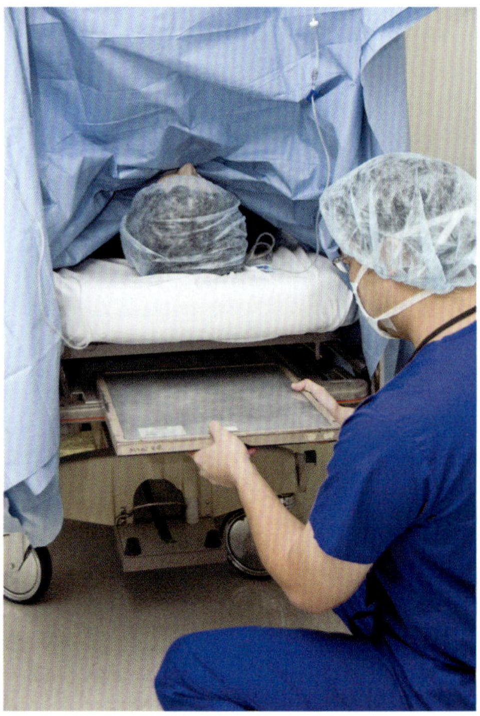

13-18 Image receptor may be placed in a sterile covering if making direct contact with the patient. The image receptor may also slide into an IR tray beneath the surgical table.

ENDOSCOPIC RETROGRADE CHOLANGIOGRAPHIC PANCREATOGRAPHY

A study of the biliary tree with the use of an endoscope. The endoscope is inserted through the mouth and navigated down the esophagus, through the stomach, and into the duodenum. Once positioned in the duodenum, a cannula accesses the hepatopancreatic sphincter into the common bile duct. Contrast media is introduced to retrograde fill the biliary tree. This procedure is performed by a gastroenterologist with a team to assist with the procedure.

Indications

- Potential biliary stones or strictures within the biliary tree that may be causing patient symptoms

Contraindications

- Iodine sensitivity
- Biliary tree infection
- Elevated kidney function levels (GFR or glomerular filtration rate, BUN or blood urea nitrogen, and creatinine)

ANATOMY

KEY ANATOMIC COMPONENTS OF THE BILIARY TREE (FIG. 13-19)

- Liver: Responsible for production of bile
- Right and Left Hepatic Ducts: Drain bile produced in the respective right and left lobes of the liver
- Common Hepatic Duct: A junction of the right and left hepatic ducts proximal to the gallbladder
- Gallbladder: Storage organ to concentrate bile. The gallbladder will distend when full and contract with the stimulation of the cholecystokinin (CCK) hormone.
- Cystic Duct: Small duct that connects the neck of the gallbladder into the biliary tree
- Common Bile Duct: Duct formed when the cystic duct and the common hepatic duct anastomose. It courses down through the head of the pancreas.
- Main Pancreatic Duct: Duct that drains the digestive enzymes produced by the pancreas. The main pancreatic duct and the common bile duct join together.
- Hepatopancreatic Ampulla: Opening into the C-loop of the duodenum
- Hepatopancreatic Sphincter: Sphincter muscle that relaxes and contracts to regulate the flow of bile into the duodenum

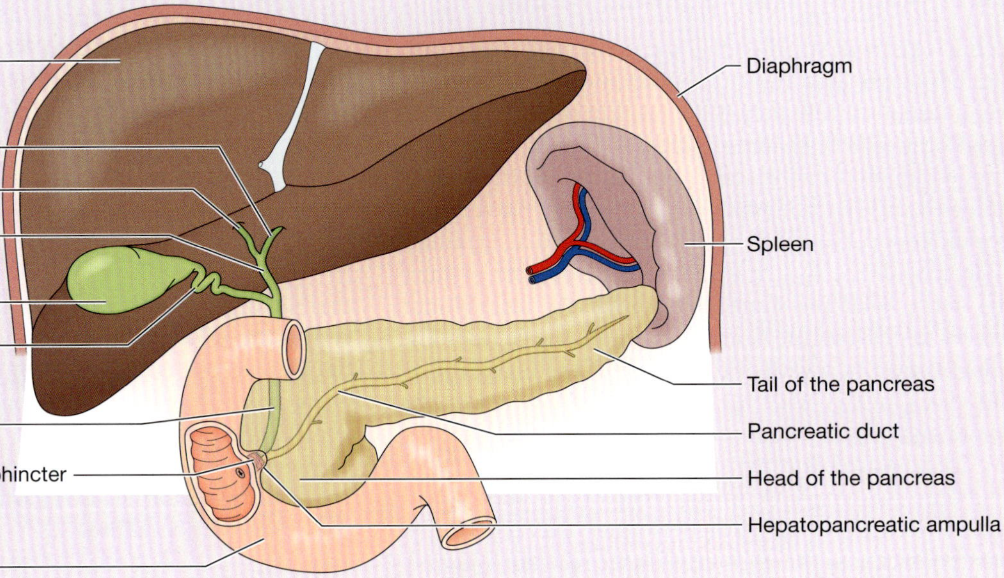

13-19 Biliary system.

Patient Prep

- Patient should be NPO for a minimum of 8 hours. Patients will receive sedation for the procedure.

Sterile Tray Setup (Highly Dependent on Physician Preference)

- Surgical team will prepare the endoscope and sterile setup desired by the gastroenterologist.

Contrast Media

- A nonionic (lower toxicity) water-soluble iodinated contrast. Iodinated contrast would be drawn up and potentially diluted to prevent the visualization of a potential biliary stone.

Room Setup

- Typically, the exam is performed in a GI surgical suite. Fluoroscopy will be needed for the procedure. Fluoroscopic guidance will show the endoscope, the position of the catheter within the biliary duct, and filling of the biliary tree with contrast.

Procedure

- Patient was dressed in a gown.
- Patient history is acquired. In addition, the institutional contrast screening form is utilized.
- The exam is explained to the patient and informed consent is acquired. Potential patient pregnancy has been ruled out.
- Patient will receive a local anesthetic to the throat as well as an intravenous sedative.
- The endoscope is advanced through the mouth, down the esophagus, in and out of the stomach, and into the C-loop of the duodenum. The hepatopancreatic duct is cannulated, and a catheter is advanced into the biliary tree (Fig. 13-20).
- Precontrast images spot images of the right upper quadrant (RUQ) are acquired once the endoscope is in place and the catheter is positioned.
- Contrast media is injected into the biliary tree under fluoroscopic guidance. Spot images will be acquired to document the sequence and findings of the procedure (Figs. 13-21 and 13-22).
- Biliary stent placement or biliary stone retraction may occur.

Postprocedural Instructions

- Post the procedure, the patient will move into recovery phase. The patient should have food or fluids withheld for approximately 1 hour post the procedure in an effort to avoid aspiration.
- Patient will be given postprocedural care dismissal instructions.

OPERATIVE CHOLANGIOGRAM

A study of the biliary tree with the injection of contrast media either before or after the gallbladder is removed. A catheter is placed within the common bile duct and while contrast is being injected the surgeon is able to observe biliary tree filling and drainage into the duodenum.

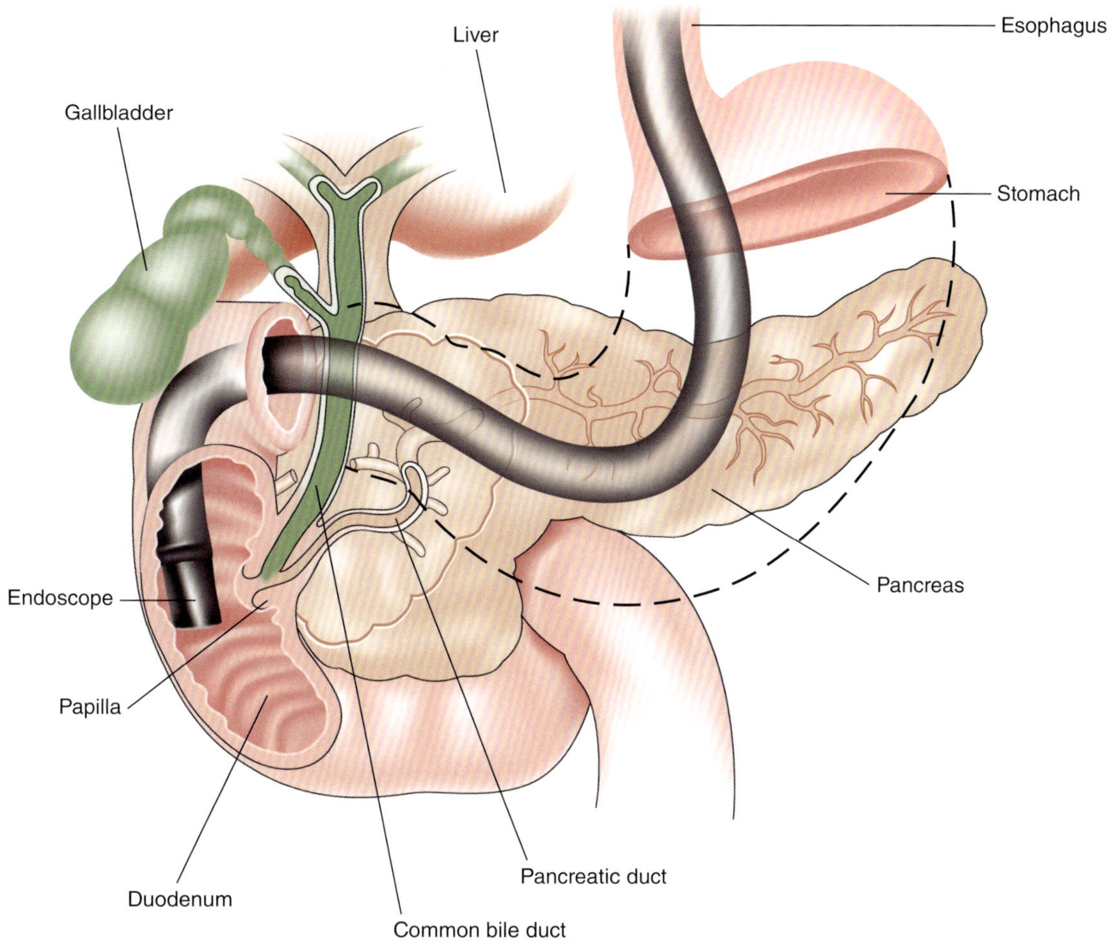

13-20 Endoscope placement for the endoscopic retrograde cholangiographic pancreatography.

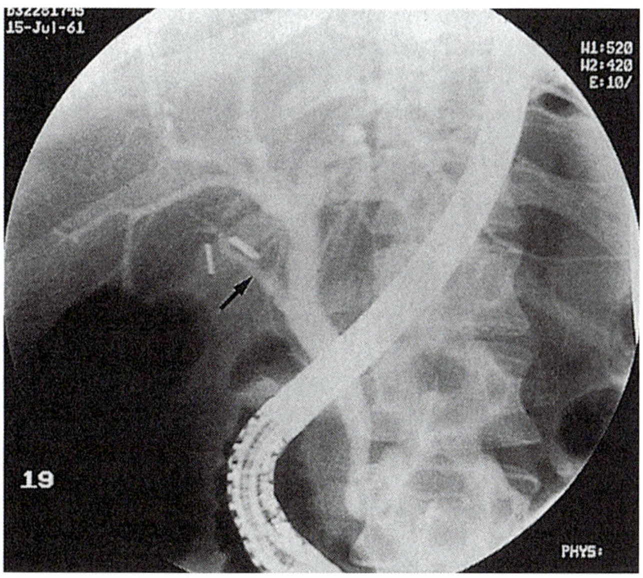

13-21 Endoscope placement with contrast injection to interrogate the biliary tree.

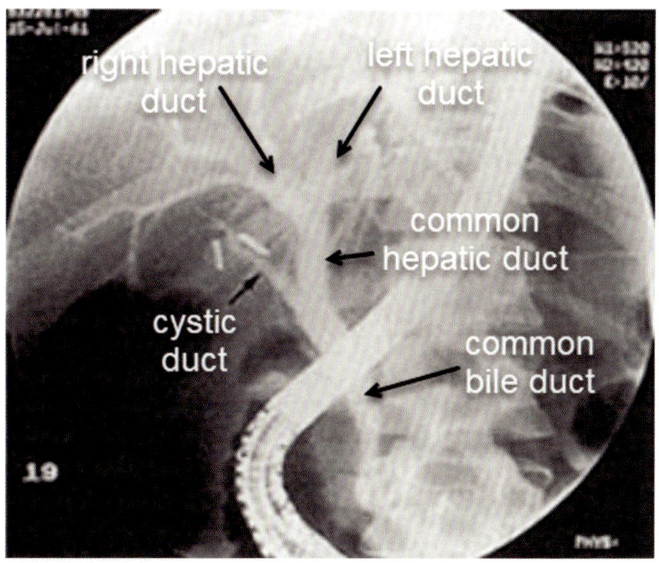

13-22 Biliary tree filled with contrast. Surgical clips confirm a cholecystectomy.

INDICATIONS

- Poorly or nonfunctioning gallbladder, cholelithiasis (gallstones), cholecystitis (gallbladder inflammation) that are causing gastrointestinal (GI) symptoms or pain

CONTRAINDICATIONS

- Iodine sensitivity
- Biliary tree infection
- Elevated kidney function levels (GFR, BUN, or creatinine)

ANATOMY

KEY ANATOMIC COMPONENTS OF THE BILIARY TREE (FIG. 13-23)

- Liver: Responsible for production of bile
- Right and Left Hepatic Ducts: Drain bile produced in the respective right and left lobes of the liver
- Common Hepatic Duct: A junction of the right and left hepatic ducts proximal to the gallbladder
- Gallbladder: Storage organ and concentrates bile. The gallbladder will distend when full and contract with the stimulation of the CCK hormone.
- Cystic Duct: Small duct that connects the neck of the gallbladder into the biliary tree.
- Common Bile Duct: Duct formed when the cystic duct and the common hepatic duct anastomose. It courses down through the head of the pancreas.
- Main Pancreatic Duct: Duct that drains the digestive enzymes produced by the pancreas. The main pancreatic duct and the common bile duct join together
- Hepatopancreatic Ampulla: Opening into the C-loop of the duodenum
- Hepatopancreatic Sphincter: Sphincter muscle that relaxes and contracts to regulate the flow of bile into the duodenum

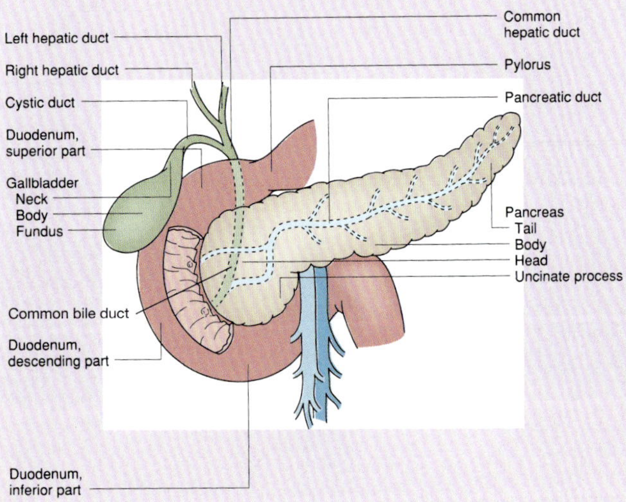

13-23 Biliary system.

Patient Prep

- Patient should be NPO for a minimum of 8 hours. Patients will receive anesthesia for the procedure.

Sterile Tray Setup

- Surgical team will prepare the laparoscope (less invasive over full-open RUQ incision) and sterile setup desired by the surgeon.

Contrast Media

- A nonionic (lower toxicity) water-soluble iodinated contrast. Iodinated contrast would be drawn up and potentially diluted to prevent the visualization of a potential biliary stone.

Room Setup

The exam is performed in a surgical suite. Typically, fluoroscopy will be administered with the C-arm during the procedure. The C-arm may be brought into the surgical suite for initial setup before the patient being brought in and prepped. Mobile radiography is an option for this procedure. A scout image will be acquired before the contrast is injected. Once the contrast is injected, the radiographer will take images on cue from the surgeon. The patient's respiration will be temporarily halted by the anesthesiologist to prevent motion on the image.

Procedure

- Patient history is acquired. In addition, the institutional contrast screening form is utilized.
- The surgical procedure exam is explained to the patient and informed consent is acquired. Potential patient pregnancy has been ruled out.
- Patient is brought into the surgical suite, anesthesia is administered, and the patient's skin is surgically prepped, and the sterile field is established by the surgical team.
- The C-arm specifically the image intensifier is covered with a sterile drape. When the surgeon is ready, the technologist will position the C-arm. The technologist must be aware of the height of the C-arm to ensure the image intensifier clears contact with surgical instruments.
- Precontrast images fluoroscopic spot image may be acquired to determine correct placement of the C-arm over the essential anatomy.
- Contrast media is injected into the biliary tree under fluoroscopic guidance. Cine loop function is predominantly used. The surgeon should be able to clearly view the fluoroscopic monitor during this part of the procedure (Fig. 13-24).
- PA (posteroanterior) and oblique views of the biliary tree may be acquired to provide better visualization.

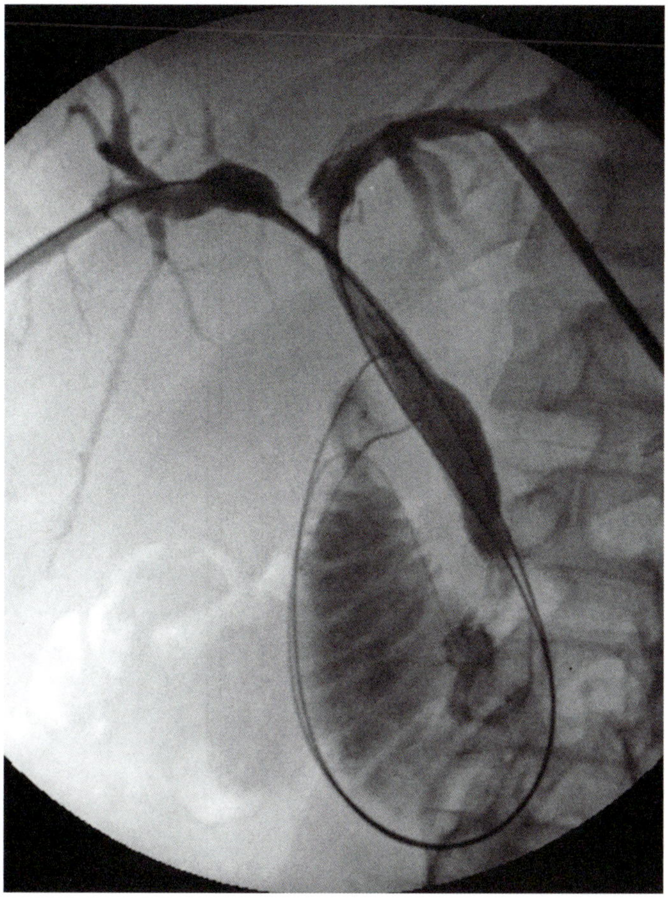

13-24 Cholangiogram.

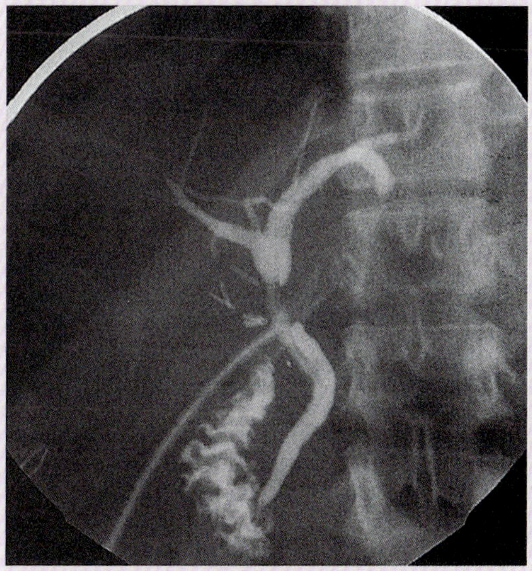

13-25 T-Tube cholangiogram.

Postprocedural Instructions

- Post the procedure, the patient will move to into recovery phase.
- Patient will be given postprocedural care dismissal instructions.

T-TUBE CHOLANGIOGRAPHY

In an instance in which the surgeon has concern for potential residual stones within the biliary system during an operative cholecystectomy or with concern of biliary stricture, a T-Tube can be inserted into the biliary tree. A "T" shaped catheter is placed in the common bile duct and the then catheter allows external access. The external portion of the catheter is clamped off. The biliary system is later assessed in the radiology department by injecting iodinated contrast into the T-Tube to interrogate for potential stones under fluoroscopy. Before contrast media being injected into the T-Tube, the catheter is unclamped, and bile from the biliary tree is allowed to drain. Iodinated contrast can then be injected (Fig. 13-25). If a potential stone(s) is identified, the radiologist may choose to retrieve them. Patients evaluated with a T-Tube must be NPO for a minimum of 8 hours before the procedure, have normal renal lab values, and no history of iodine sensitivity.

UROLOGICAL STUDY: RETROGRADE UROGRAPHY

A nonfunctional radiographic study through retrograde filling of a ureter, renal pelvis, and renal calyces through access of the bladder.

INDICATIONS

- Obstruction such as renal calculi or other obstruction, anatomical defect, or infection

CONTRAINDICATIONS

- Urinary tract infection
- Recent bladder surgery
- Iodine sensitivity
- Renal failure
- Severe dehydration

ANATOMY

KEY ANATOMIC COMPONENTS OF THE URINARY SYSTEM (FIGS. 13-26 and 13-27)

- Urethra: Exits the bladder
- Ureterovisceral Junction (UVJ): Each ureter junctions with the bladder on the posterior side and inferior surface
- Ureter: Hollow tube that connects the kidney to the bladder
- Renal Pelvis: Dilated portion of the collecting system that narrows into the proximal ureter
- Ureteropelvic Junction (UPJ): The proximal ureter junctions with the kidney at the renal pelvis
- Calyces: Minor calyces collect the production of urine from the renal pyramids and drain into the two to three major calyces, which form the renal pelvis.

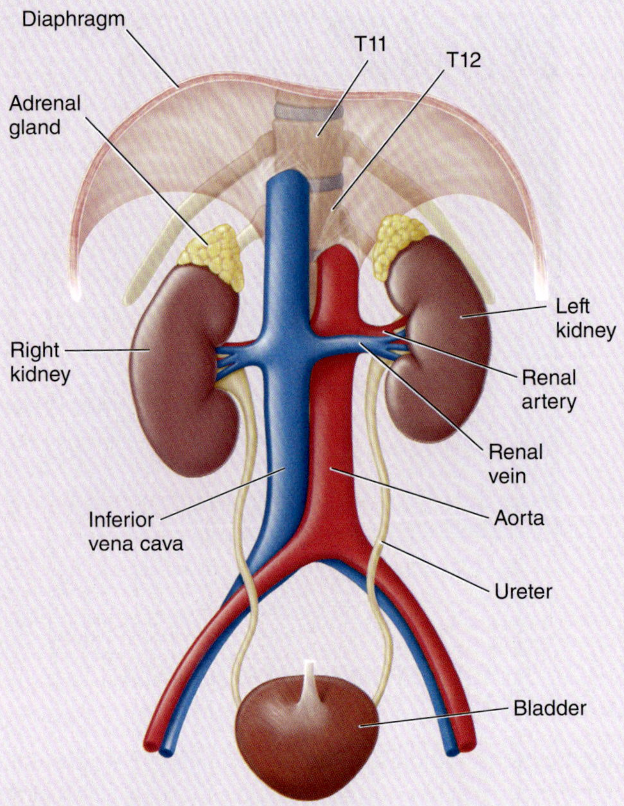

13-26 Urinary system.

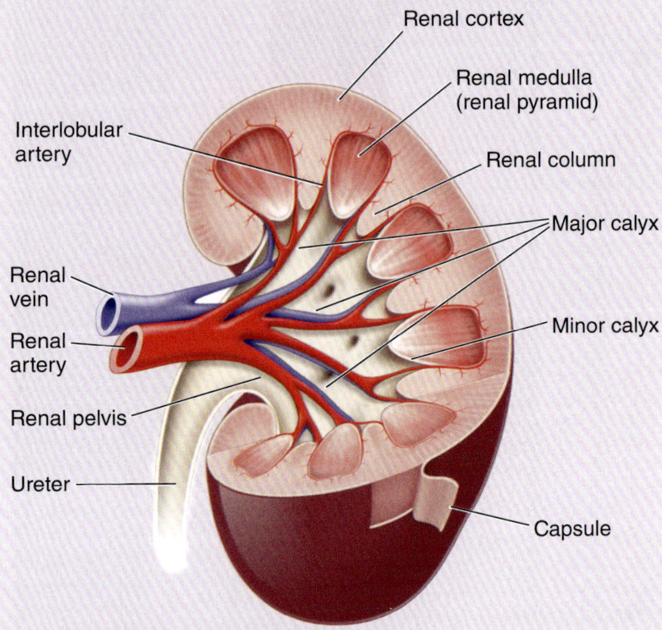

13-27 Kidney anatomy.

Patient Prep

- Patient must empty bladder before procedure. A specimen collected may be sent for a urine analysis.
- Patient should be NPO for a minimum of 8 hours. Patients may undergo a bowel prep to clear out overlying gas and fecal matter.
- Patients will receive anesthesia for the procedure.

Contrast Media

- Nonionic-iodinated contrast will retrograde fill the ureter and renal pelvis and calyces.

Room Setup

The exam is performed in a surgical suite, typically a designated urography room. This type of room will likely contain a cystoscopy table, which abducts the thighs and elevates the legs and feet into the lithotomy position. The C-arm may be brought into the surgical suite for initial setup before the patient being brought in and prepped. Mobile radiography is an option for this procedure. A scout image will be acquired before the contrast is injected. Once the contrast is injected, the radiographer will take images on cue from the surgeon. The patient's respiration will be temporarily halted by the anesthesiologist to prevent motion on the image.

Procedure

- Patient admitted for the surgical procedure
- Preprocedural instructions and patient assessment are performed by the nurse.
- Patient history is acquired and documented on the institutional contrast screening form.
- The exam is explained to the patient and informed consent is acquired. Potential patient pregnancy has been ruled out.
- Patient is brought into the surgical suite, patient positioned in lithotomy position, anesthesia is administered, and the patient's peroneal area is surgically prepped, and the sterile field is established by the surgical team (Fig. 13-28).
- The surgeon will introduce the cystoscope through the urethra and into the bladder. One or both ureters will have a catheter introduced. The catheter may be advanced to the level of the renal pelvis.
- When the surgeon is ready, the technologist will position the C-arm not to compromise the sterile field.
- Precontrast images fluoroscopic spot image may be acquired to determine correct placement of the C-arm to demonstrate the catheter placement.
- Contrast media is injected into the kidney through the catheter. This is observed under fluoroscopic guidance. Cine loop function is predominantly used. The surgeon should be able to clearly view the fluoroscopic monitor during this part of the procedure (Figs. 13-29 and 13-30).

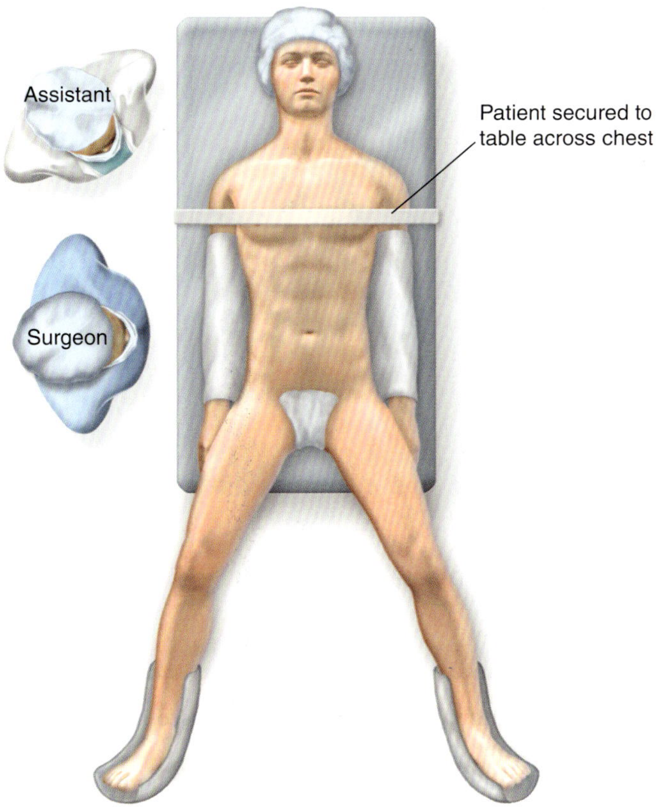

13-28 Lithotomy position.

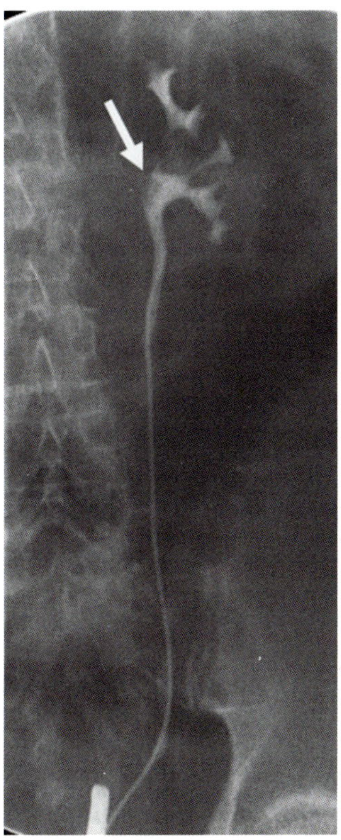

13-29 Retrograde urogram.

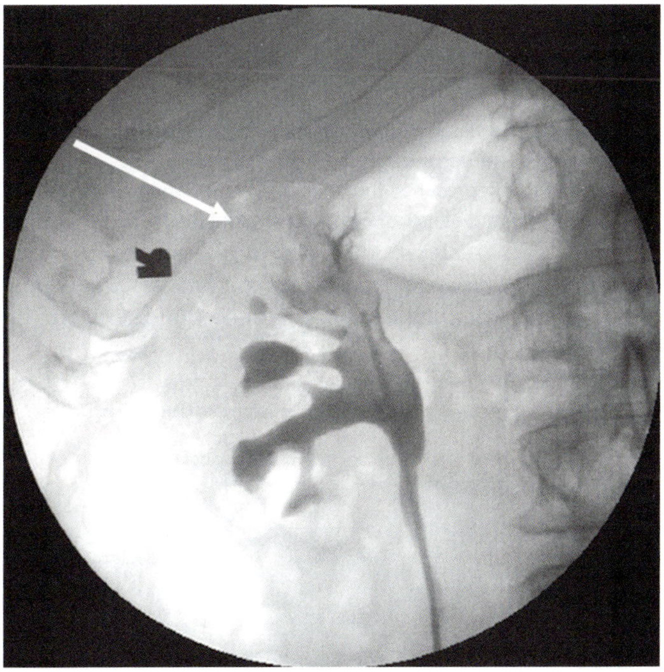

13-30 Spot image of a kidney to reveal a filling defect in the upper pole.

Postprocedural Instructions

- Post the procedure, the patient will move to into recovery phase.
- Patient will be given postprocedural care dismissal instructions.

ORTHOPEDIC PROCEDURES

A surgical procedure is considered to reduce and align a fracture, surgically repair a fracture site with fixation device(s) or replace joints to improve joint mobility.

INDICATIONS

- Fracture, surgical device implantation, joint replacement, or removal of surgical hardware

CONTRAINDICATIONS

- Patient not cleared for surgical procedure due to a medical condition or risk of anesthesia

ANATOMY

KEY ANATOMIC COMPONENTS OF BONE (FIG. 13-31)

- Cortex: The outermost hard shell of the bone. The cortex tends to be thicker toward the body of the bone.
- Medullary Cavity: The hollow portion of the bone located in the body that contains the yellow bone marrow.
- Cancellous Bone (Spongy): Cancellous bone is porous, contains the red bone marrow, and is located between the cortex and medullary cavity.

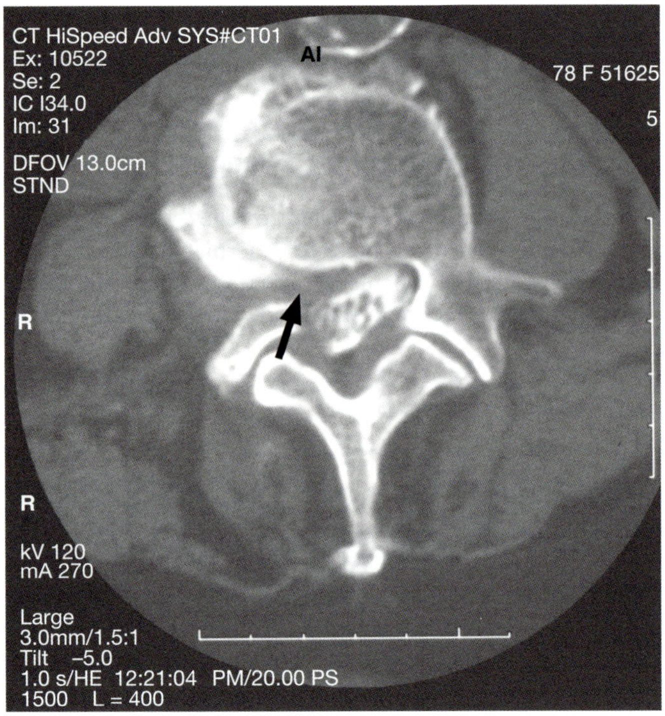

13-38 Axial CT displaying right lateral stenosis.

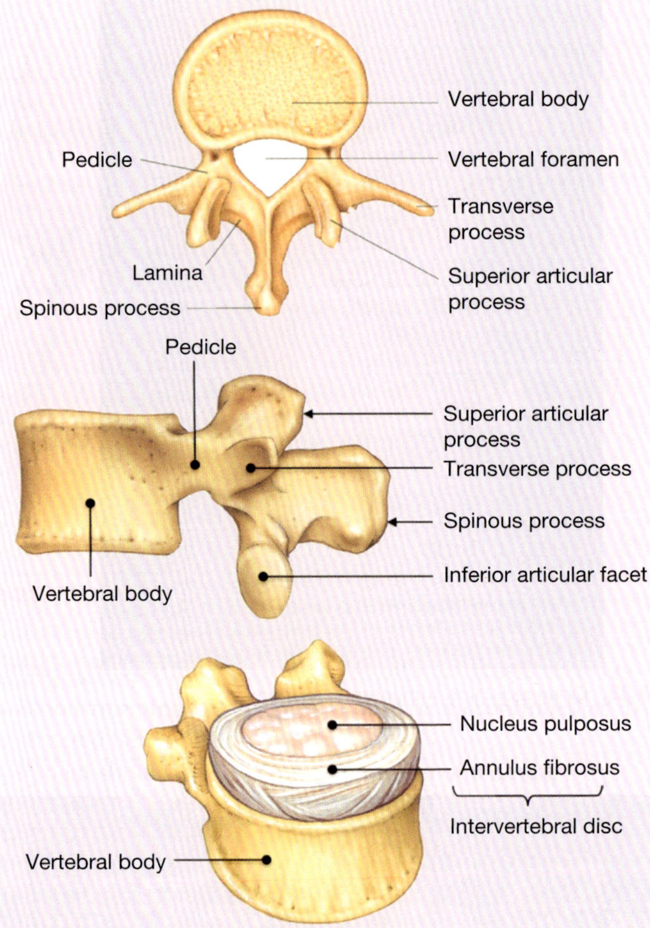

13-39 Key anatomic parts of a vertebra.

INDICATIONS

- Nerve pain caused from impingement of nerves or cord from stenosis, bone spurs, or herniated disk.

CONTRAINDICATIONS

- Instability of the spine or severe abnormal curvatures of the spine

ANATOMY

KEY ANATOMIC COMPONENTS OF THE VERTEBRA (FIG. 13-39)

- Vertebral Body: Weight-bearing, anterior most structure. The vertebral arch extends off the posterior aspect of the vertebral body.
- Vertebral Arch: The vertebral arch consists of the pedicles laterally and the lamina posteriorly. The vertebral arch extends off the vertebral body and creates the vertebral foramen for the spinal cord.
- Vertebral Foramen: The spinal cord passes through the vertebral foramen.
- Intervertebral Disk: Above and below each vertebral body is an intervertebral disk to serve as a cushion or shock absorber.

Patient Prep

- Blood-thinning medications should be discontinued as instructed before the procedure.
- Patient should be NPO for a minimum of 8 hours.
- Patients will receive anesthesia for the procedure.

Room Setup

The exam is performed in a surgical suite. The C-arm may be brought into the surgical suite for initial setup before the patient being brought in and prepped. Some facilities may have O-arm that may be used in these types of cases over a C-arm. The O-arm provides a 360° view of the anatomy, much like what a computed tomography (CT) scan would provide. Mobile radiography is also an option for this procedure (Fig. 13-40).

Procedure

- Patient admitted for the surgical procedure
- Preprocedural instructions and patient assessment performed by the nurse.

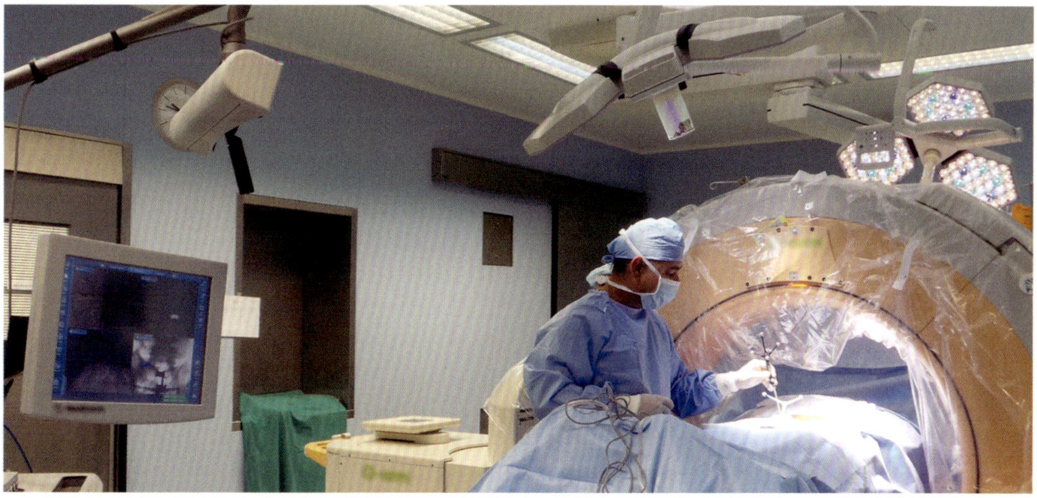

13-40 Use of the O-arm to navigate internal fixation placement.

- Patient history is acquired and documented.
- The exam is explained to the patient and informed consent is acquired. Potential patient pregnancy has been ruled out.
- Patient is brought into the surgical suite, patient positioned prone for a lumbar procedure, and supine for a cervical procedure. Anesthesia is administered, the patient's area is surgically prepped, and the sterile field is established by the surgical team.
- When the surgeon is ready, the technologist will position the C-arm not to compromise the sterile field. The technologist will be expected to manipulate the C-arm from vertical and rainbow it into a horizontal position.
- The technologist will provide fluoroscopy for the surgeon to determine correct vertebral location as well as to guide the placement of any orthopedic hardware (screws, plates, rods) (Fig. 13-41).

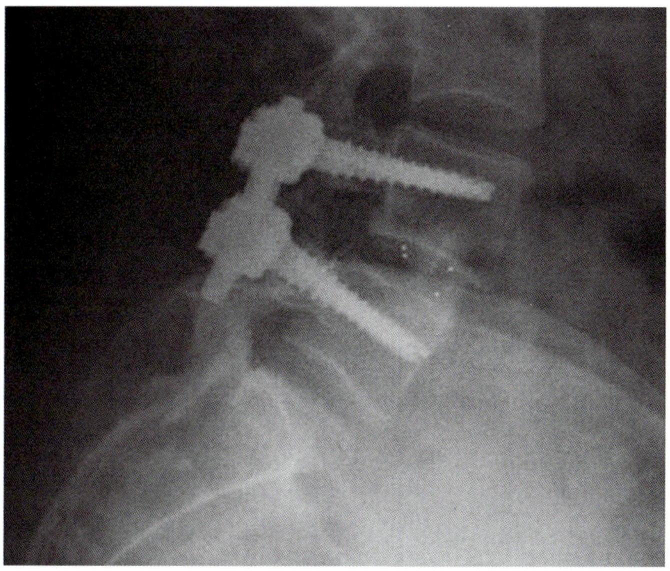

13-41 L4–L5 laminectomy to reduce spondylolisthesis.

Postprocedural Instructions

- Post the procedure, the patient will move to into recovery phase.
- Patient will be given postprocedural care dismissal instructions.

SPINAL PROCEDURES: VERTEBROPLASTY OR KYPHOPLASTY

A surgical procedure considered to relieve pain caused by compression of the vertebral body, commonly a secondary result of osteoporosis (Fig. 13-42).

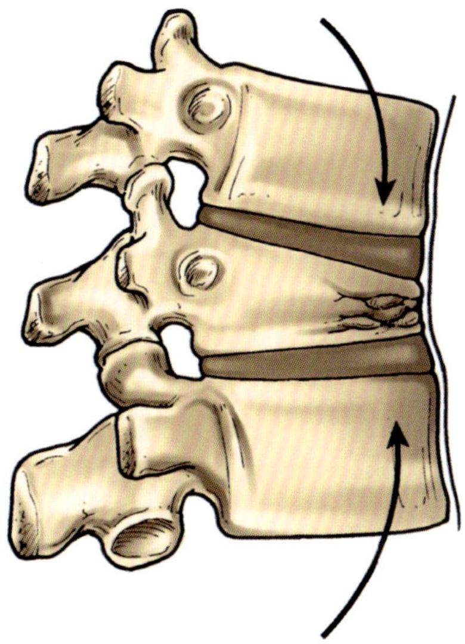

13-42 Compression of the vertebral body.

INDICATIONS

- To relieve back pain caused by compression fracture of the vertebral body(ies)

CONTRAINDICATIONS

- Bleeding disorder, iodinated contrast sensitivity, unstable fracture

ANATOMY

KEY ANATOMIC COMPONENTS OF THE VERTEBRA (FIG. 13-43)

- Vertebral Body: Weight-bearing, anterior most structure. The vertebral arch extends off the posterior aspect of the vertebral body.
- Vertebral Arch: The vertebral arch consists of the pedicles laterally and the lamina posteriorly. The vertebral arch extends off the vertebral body and creates the vertebral foramen for the spinal cord.
- Vertebral Foramen: The spinal cord passes through the vertebral foramen.
- Intervertebral Disk: Above and below each vertebral body is an intervertebral disk to serve as a cushion or shock absorber.

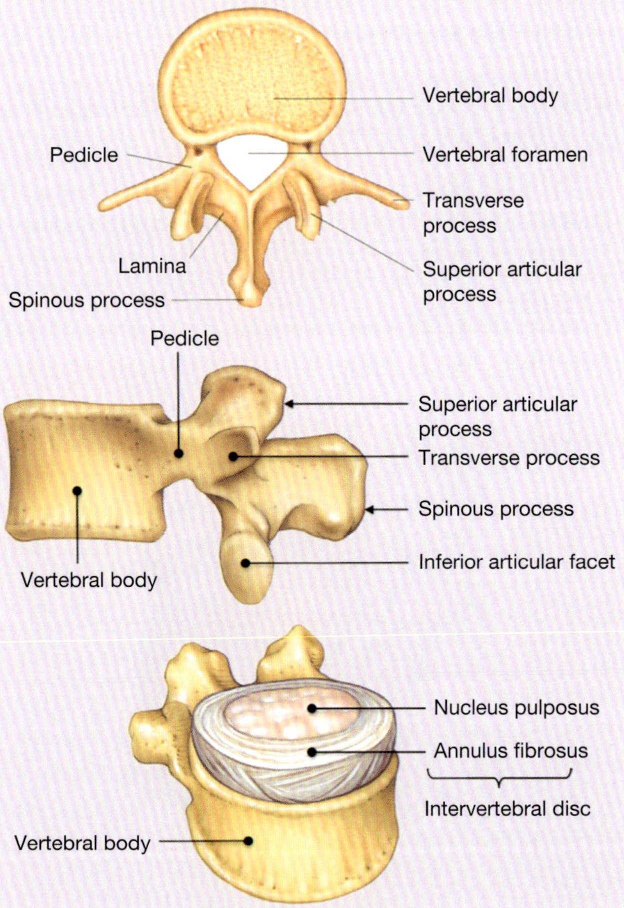

13-43 Key anatomic parts of a vertebra.

Patient Prep

- Blood-thinning medications should be discontinued as instructed before the procedure.
- Patient should be NPO for a minimum of 8 hours.
- Patients will receive moderate sedation for the procedure.

Room Setup

The exam is performed in an interventional or neurologic suite. The C-arm may be brought into the surgical suite for initial setup before the patient being brought in and prepped.

Procedure

- Typically, it is an outpatient procedure.
- Preprocedural instructions and patient assessment performed by the nurse.
- Patient history is acquired and documented.
- The exam is explained to the patient and informed consent is acquired.
- Patient will lay prone for the procedure. The skin is prepped for the procedure. Local anesthetic is given.
- A small incision is made in the skin. A trocar is introduced into the vertebral body of interest. A small amount of iodinated contrast may be introduced to confirm trocar placement. Imaging will be key in this step of the procedure (Figs. 13-44 to 13-46).
- For vertebroplasty, after the site is localized with the trocar, an orthopedic cement will be injected to strengthen the bone and fuse bone fragments that may be causing pain.
- For kyphoplasty, a balloon is introduced first through the trocar into the vertebral body and inflated to create a cavity. The balloon is deflated and removed. The orthopedic cement is then injected.
- Patient may remain prone for after the completion of the procedure. The patient will then lay supine while allowing the orthopedic cement to harden. Postimaging may be ordered to verify cement dispersal.
- Patient will recover and typically be dismissed that same day.

Postprocedural Instructions

- Post the procedure, the patient will move to into recovery phase.
- Patient will be given postprocedural care dismissal instructions

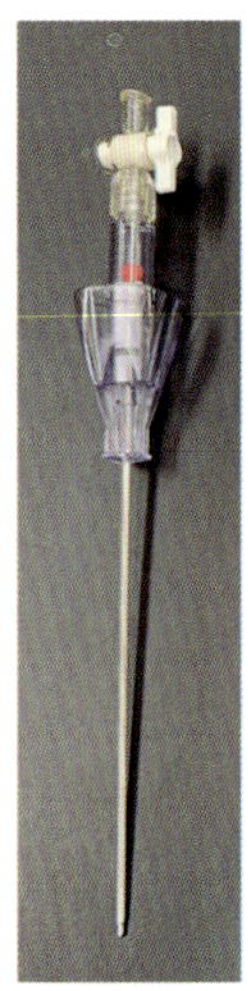

13-44 Trocar.

SPINAL PROCEDURES: THERAPEUTIC INJECTION

An injection to provide pain management to patients who suffer acute or chronic back pain.

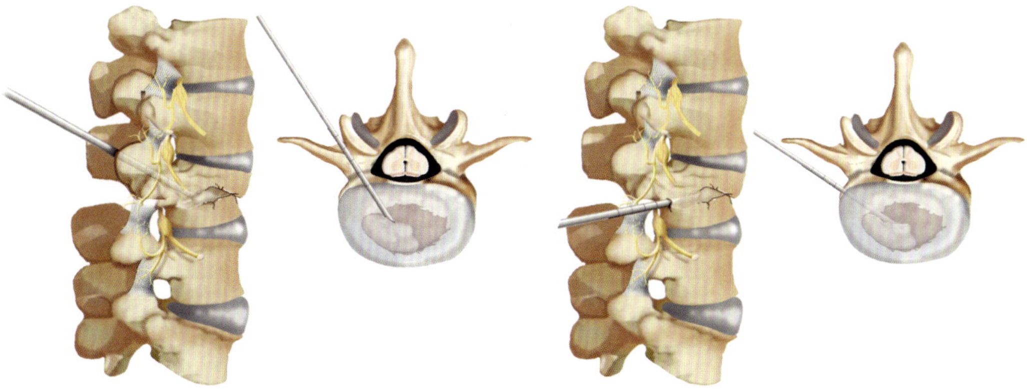

13-45 Trocar placement.

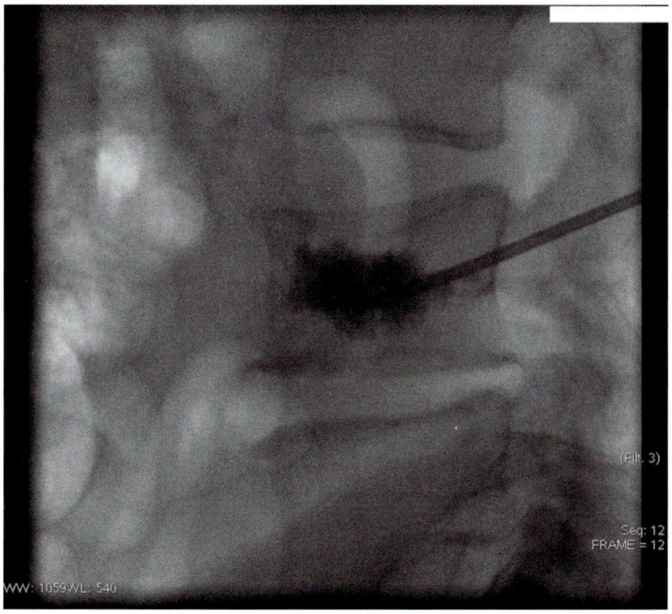

13-46 Contrast introduction.

INDICATIONS

- To relieve back pain caused by spinal stenosis, herniated disk, degenerative disk, sciatica, inflammation, or spondylolisthesis before a surgical option is considered.

CONTRAINDICATIONS

- Infection at the site or a systemic infection
- Bleeding disorder
- Iodinated contrast sensitivity
- Allergy to corticosteroid

ANATOMY

KEY ANATOMIC COMPONENTS OF THE VERTEBRA (FIG. 13-47)

- Vertebral Body: Weight-bearing, anterior most structure. The vertebral arch extends off the posterior aspect of the vertebral body.
- Vertebral Arch: The vertebral arch consists of the pedicles laterally and the lamina posteriorly. The vertebral arch extends off the vertebral body and creates the vertebral foramen for the spinal cord.
- Vertebral Foramen: The spinal cord passes through the vertebral foramen
- Intervertebral Disk: Above and below each vertebral body is an intervertebral disk to serve as a cushion or shock absorber.

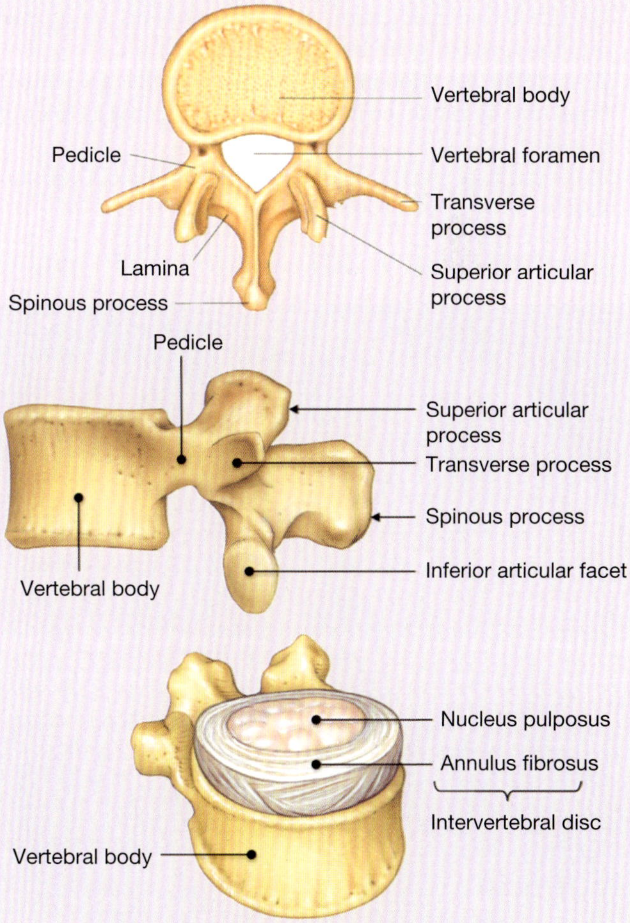

13-47 Key anatomic parts of a vertebra.

Patient Prep

- Blood-thinning medications should be discontinued as instructed before the procedure.

Room Setup

The exam is performed in an interventional or neurologic suite. The C-arm may be brought into the surgical suite for initial setup before the patient being brought in and prepped.

Procedure

- Typically, it is an outpatient procedure.
- Preprocedural instructions and patient assessment performed by the nurse.
- Patient history is acquired and documented.
- The exam is explained to the patient and informed consent is acquired. Potential patient pregnancy has been ruled out.
- Patient will lay prone for the procedure. The skin is prepped for the procedure. Local anesthetic is given.
- With fluoroscopic guidance, the physician will insert the needle between the vertebra and into the epidural space (the space between the spinal cord and the vertebral canal). Once the needle is in the correct position, a small amount of contrast media is injected to ensure the correct location in which the medication will be administered to (Figs. 13-48 to 13-50).
- Corticosteroid medication and an anesthetic are injected into the space to surround the nerve roots.
- A single site injection may occur or right and left side injections may be made, or injections may be made at multiple levels.
- Patient will recover and typically be dismissed that same day.

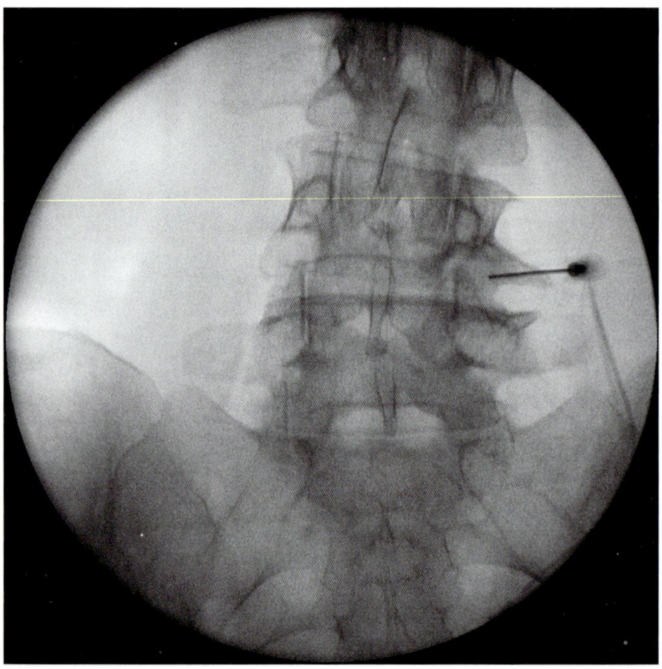

13-48 Needle placement.

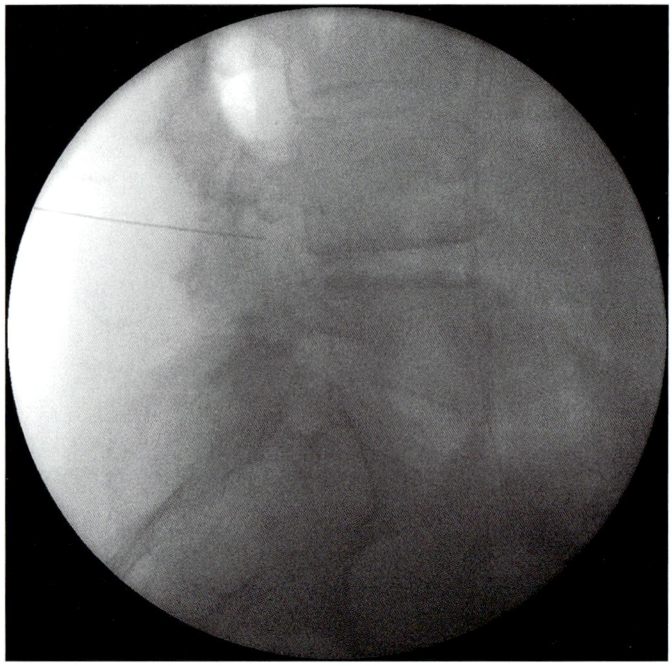

13-49 Needle placement.

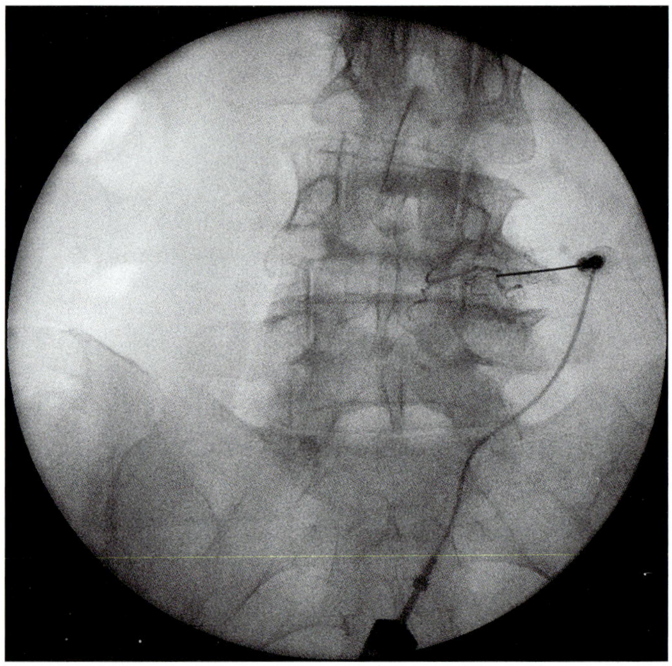

13-50 Contrast introduction.

Postprocedural Instructions

- Patient will be given postprocedural care dismissal instructions.

CENTRAL VENOUS LINE PLACEMENT OR PORT-A-CATH PLACEMENT

A catheter or a catheter and port are positioned within a vein to provide venous access or to administer treatment.

INDICATIONS

- A temporary or permanent site of access to administer medications such as chemotherapy, blood withdrawal, administer nutrition, or to perform dialysis.

CONTRAINDICATIONS

- Poor clotting ability of the blood
- Iodinated contrast sensitivity
- Vessel trauma
- Vein thrombus

ANATOMY

KEY ANATOMIC COMPONENTS OF UPPER VASCULAR ANATOMY (FIG. 13-51)

- Antecubital Space: Space anterior to the elbow joint where major vessels can be accessed
- Basilic Vein: Large vein that travels up the medial aspect of the humerus from the antecubital space toward the axilla. This vein is not accompanied by an artery.
- Axillary Vein: Large vein formed when the paired brachial veins and basilic vein anastomose near the axilla. The vein continues across the anterior, superior bony thorax.
- Cephalic Vein: Singular vein that runs up the lateral forearm and humerus. It travels up and through the shoulder joint region and continues anteriorly and superior on the bony thorax. The cephalic vein drains into the axillary vein, which then forms the subclavian vein.
- Subclavian Vein: Vein located near the clavicle and the first rib
- Brachiocephalic Vein: Large vein formed when the internal jugular vein and the subclavian vein anastomose. The brachiocephalic vein connects to the superior vena cava.
- Superior Vena Cava: Vein that brings blood into the right atrium of the heart

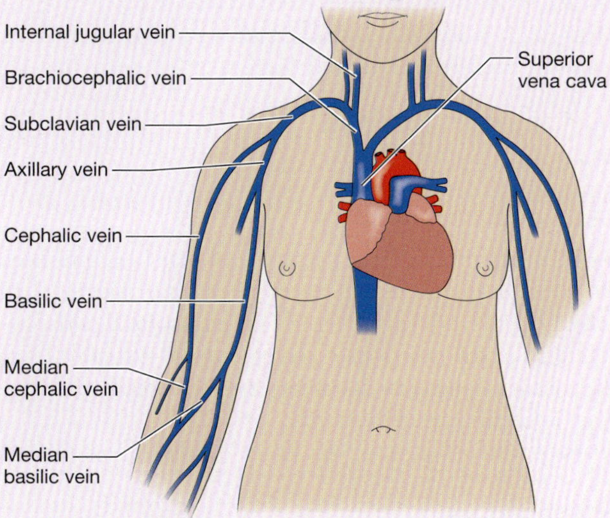

13-51 Key upper vascular anatomy.

ANATOMIC LOCATIONS FOR ACCESS

- Port-a-Cath: Catheter and port placed typically on the right upper chest wall underneath the skin (Figs. 13-52 to 13-55)
- PICC (peripherally inserted central catheter) Line: A peripheral catheter placed in the upper arm and sutured into place (Fig. 13-56 to 13-58).

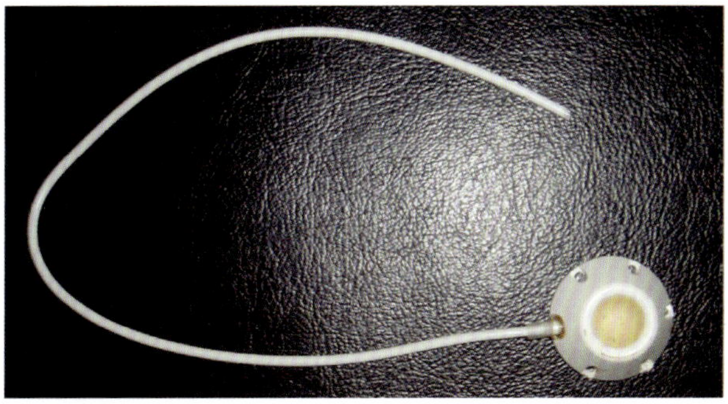

13-52 Port-a-cath.

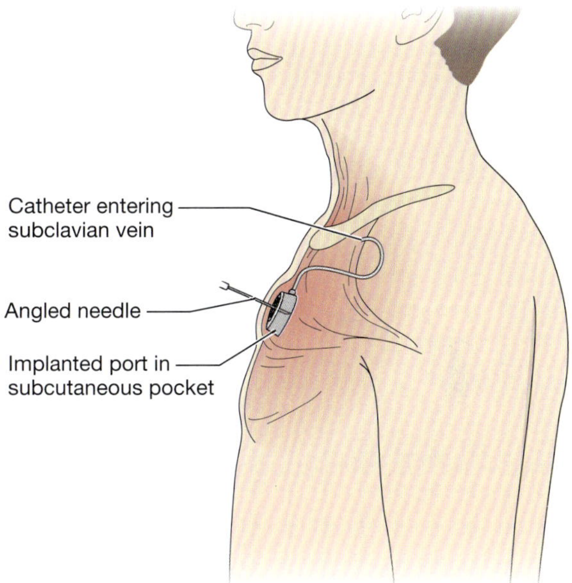

13-53 Port-a-cath placement.

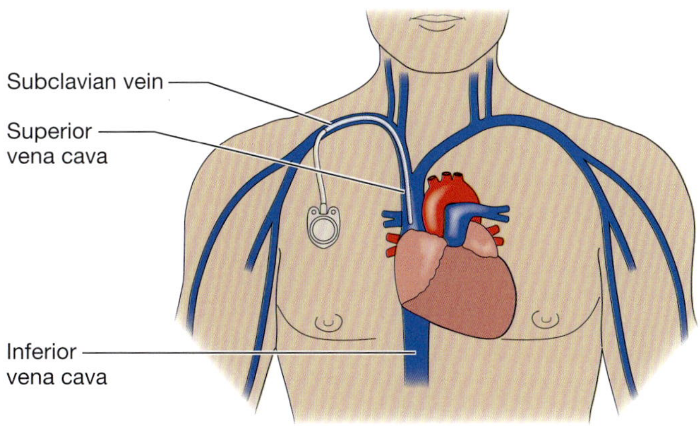

13-54 Port-a-cath placement within vasculature.

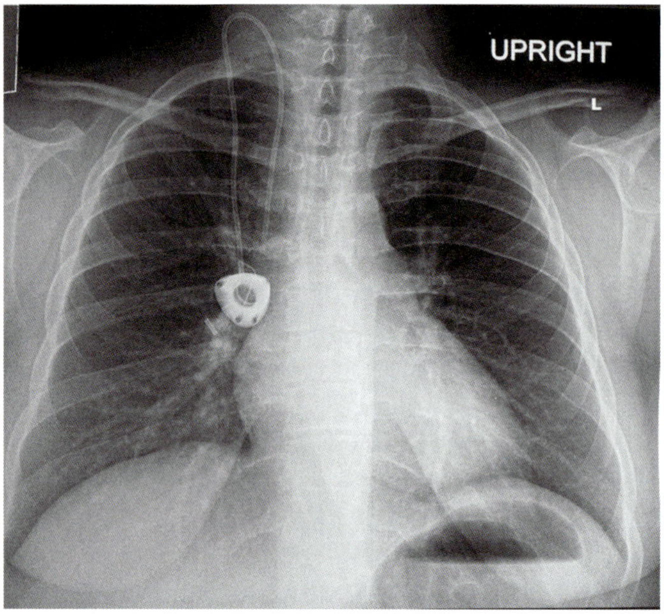

13-55 AP chest revealing port placement.

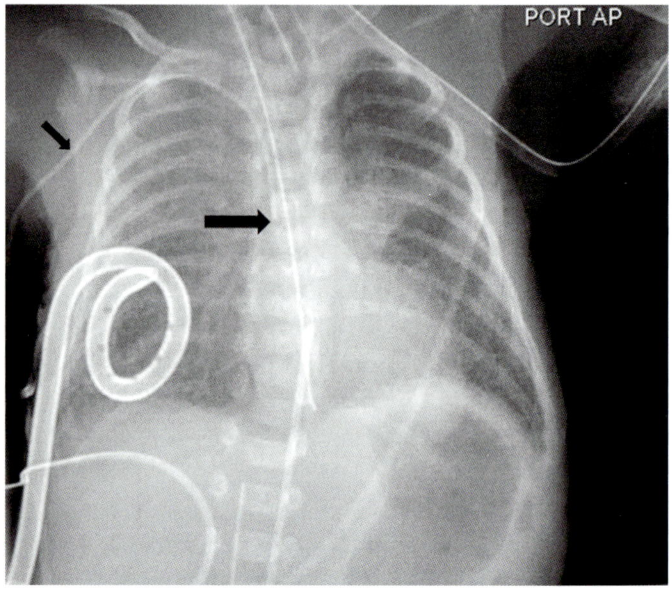

13-58 AP chest revealing PICC line placement.

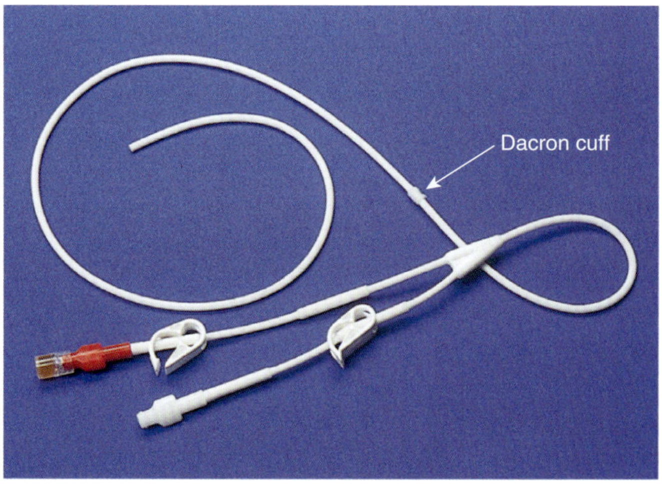

13-56 PICC line.

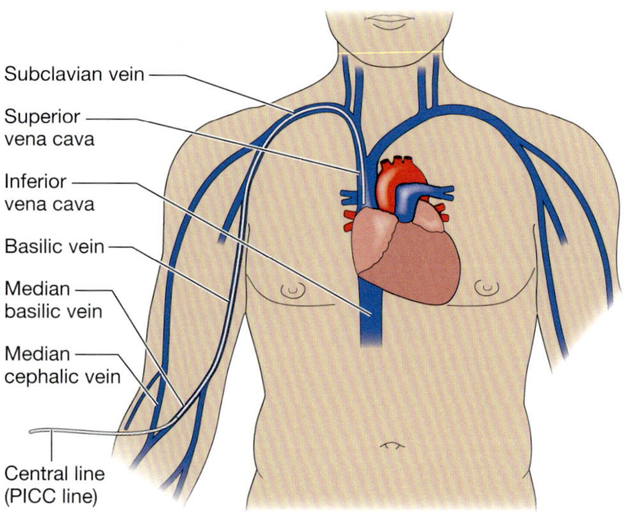

13-57 PICC line placement.

Patient Prep

- Blood-thinning medications should be discontinued as instructed before the procedure.
- Patient may have no prep if sedation is not administered.

Room Setup

The exam is performed in an interventional suite, surgical suite, or the intensive care unit. The C-arm may be brought into the surgical suite for initial setup before the patient being brought in and prepped.

Procedure

- Typically, it is an outpatient or same-day procedure.
- Preprocedural instructions and patient assessment performed by the nurse.
- Patient history is acquired and documented.
- The exam is explained to the patient and informed consent is acquired. Potential patient pregnancy has been ruled out.
- Patient will lay supine for the procedure. The skin is prepped for the procedure. Local anesthetic is given.
- Catheter with or without a port is placed into a large vein. The use of fluoroscopy will assist with catheter placement. A small amount of iodinated contrast may be administered to confirm the correct location. PICC line placement may also be achieved with point of care ultrasound guidance.
- Patients post a port-a-cath placement will typically have an AP chest acquired to document line placement and to rule out a potential pneumothorax.
- Patient will recover and typically be dismissed that same day.

Postprocedural Instructions

- Patient will be given postprocedural care dismissal instructions.

PACEMAKER PLACEMENT

An implanted device with wires (leads) directed into the right ventricular chamber of the heart to stimulate the heart muscle to beat within a range of programmed rates.

INDICATIONS

- The heart has the inability to maintain normal pace and is typically inserted to prevent the heart from beating slower or faster than the determined rate.

CONTRAINDICATIONS

- Poor clotting ability of the blood
- Iodinated contrast sensitivity

ANATOMY

KEY ANATOMIC COMPONENTS OF THE HEART (FIG. 13-59)

- Subclavian Vein: Transports deoxygenated blood from the upper extremities to the heart
- Superior Vena Cava: Is formed by the union of the right and left brachiocephalic veins and drain in to the right atrium
- Atria: Right and left atria are separated by the interatrial septum
- Ventricles: Right ventricle and left ventricle separated by the interventricular septum
- Tricuspid Valve: Located between the right atrium and the right ventricle
- Mitral Valve: Located between the left atrium and the left ventricle

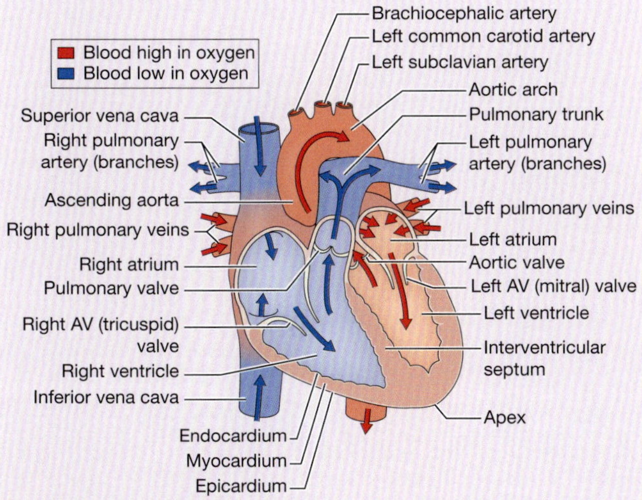

13-59 Heart anatomy.

Patient Prep

- Blood-thinning medications should be discontinued as instructed before the procedure.
- Patient should be NPO for a minimum of 8 hours.
- Patients will receive sedation for the procedure.

Room Setup

The exam is performed in an interventional or surgical suite. The C-arm may be brought into the surgical suite for initial setup before the patient being brought in and prepped.

Procedure

- Typically, it is an outpatient procedure, but a patient may be kept overnight.
- Preprocedural instructions and patient assessment performed by the nurse.
- Patient history is acquired and documented.
- The exam is explained to the patient and informed consent is acquired. Potential patient pregnancy has been ruled out.
- Patient will lay supine for the procedure. The skin is prepped for the procedure. Local anesthetic is given. A sedative is administered.
- A sheath is introduced into a vein beneath the collarbone. The pacer wire lead will be advanced through the sheath and into the vein and then into the heart. Once in the right atrium, it is advanced through the tricuspid valve and into the right ventricle to the point of the heart apex (Fig. 13-60).

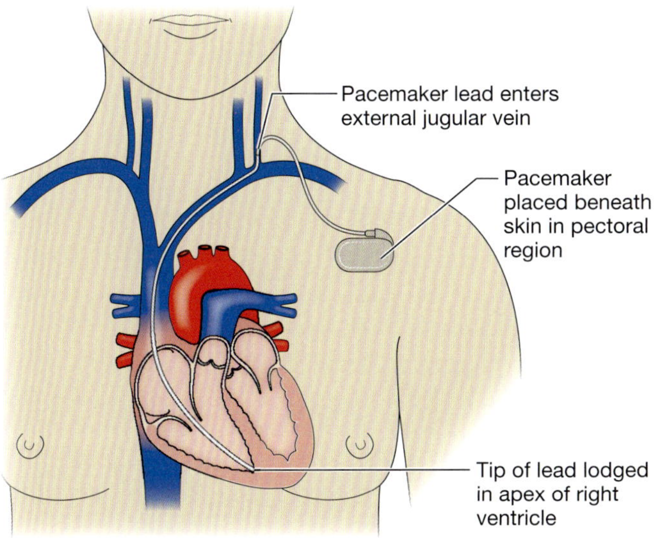

13-60 Pacemaker placement.

- The lead wire(s) is attached to the battery, which is positioned beneath the skin and the incision site is sutured closed.
- While in recovery, an AP chest is acquired to document wire placement and to rule out a potential pneumothorax. The patient's arm on the insertion side of the pacemaker will be immobilized. The arm should not be moved from position to avoid displacement of the wire leads that are not yet embedded into the heart muscle (Fig. 13-61).

Postprocedural Instructions

- Patient will be given postprocedural care dismissal instructions.

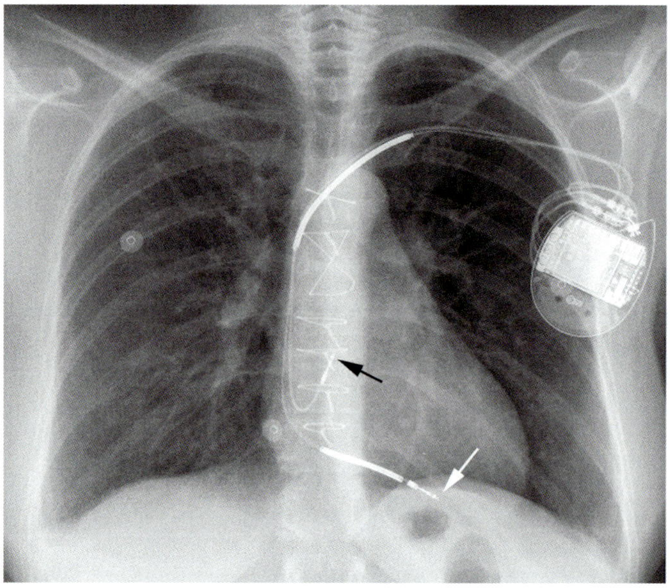

13-61 PA chest revealing pacemaker lead placement. White arrow reveals lead placement within the right ventricle. The black arrow to reveal lead placement within the right atrium.

Figure Credits

CHAPTER 1

Figure 1-1. Reprinted with permission from Moorcroft C. *Myology and Kinesiology for Massage Therapists.* Wolters Kluwer; 2012:16. Figure 2-2A.

Figure 1-5. Modified with permission from Wineski LE. *Snell's Clinical Anatomy by Regions.* 10th ed. Wolters Kluwer; 2018:14. Figure 1-10.

Figure 1-6. Reprinted with permission from Moore KL, Dalley AF, Agur AMR. *Clinically Oriented Anatomy.* 7th ed. Wolters Kluwer; 2013:27. Figure I-17.

Figure 1-8. Modified with permission from Moore KL, Dalley AF, Agur AMR. *Clinically Oriented Anatomy.* 8th ed. Wolters Kluwer; 2017:290.

Figure 1-9. Modified with permission from Skaggs D, Flynn JM. *Staying Out of Trouble in Pediatric Orthopaedics.* 2nd ed. Wolters Kluwer; 2020:233. Figure 14-12.

Figure 1-11. Modified with permission from Moore KL, Dalley AF, Agur AMR. *Clinically Oriented Anatomy.* 8th ed. Wolters Kluwer; 2017:25. Figure 1-16.

Figure 1-12. Modified with permission from Moore KL, Dalley AF, Agur AMR. *Clinically Oriented Anatomy.* 8th ed. Wolters Kluwer; 2017:25. Figure 1-16.

Figure 1-14. Modified with permission from Moore KL, Dalley AF, Agur AMR. *Clinically Oriented Anatomy.* 8th ed. Wolters Kluwer; 2017:7. Figure 1-4.

Figure 1-28. Reprinted with permission from Wingerd B. *Human Body.* 3rd ed. Wolters Kluwer; 2014:150. Figure 6-36J.

Figure 1-38. Modified with permission from Moore KL, Dalley AF, Agur AMR. *Clinically Oriented Anatomy.* 8th ed. Wolters Kluwer; 2017:6. Figure 1-2.

Figure 1-67. Modified with permission from Moore KL, Dalley AF, Agur AMR. *Clinically Oriented Anatomy*, 8th Ed. Wolters Kluwer, 2017: 454. Figure 5-36. Based on Grant JCB. *Grant's Method of Anatomy: By Regions, Descriptive and Deductive*, 9th ed. Williams & Wilkins, 1975.

CHAPTER 2

Figure 2-2. Reprinted with permission from Daffner RH, Hartman M. *Clinical Radiology.* 4th ed. Wolters Kluwer; 2013:84. Figure 4-11b.

Figure 2-3. Reprinted with permission from Brit LD, Peitzman AB, Barie PS, Jurkovich GJ. *Acute Care Surgery.* 2nd ed. Wolters Kluwer; 2018:444. Figure 35-3a.

Figure 2-4. Reprinted with permission from Brant WE, Helms CA. *Brant and Helms Solution.* Wolters Kluwer; 2006:522. Figure 18-13.

Figure 2-5. Reprinted with permission from Frendl G, Urman RD. *Pocket ICU.* 2nd ed. Wolters Kluwer; 2017:RI 48-6. Figure 48-5.

Figure 2-7. Reprinted with permission from Webb WR, Higgins CB. *Thoracic Imaging.* 3rd ed. Wolters Kluwer; 2016:397. Figure 11-41a.

Figure 2-8. Reprinted with permission from Collins J, Stern EJ. *Chest Radiology: The Essentials.* 3rd ed. Wolters Kluwer; 2015:91. Figure 5-36.

Figure 2-9. Reprinted with permission from Herzog E. *Herzog's CCU Book.* Wolters Kluwer; 2017:564. Figure 48-27.

Figure 2-10. Reprinted with permission from Smith WL. *Radiology 101.* 4th ed. Wolters Kluwer; 2013:391. Figure 12-19.

Figure 2-11. Reprinted with permission from Gupta A, Jones DB. *Surgery Boot Camp Manual.* Wolters Kluwer; 2019:97. Figure 11-5.

Figure 2-12. Reprinted with permission from Collins J, Stern EJ. *Chest Radiology: The Essentials.* 3rd ed. Wolters Kluwer; 2014:81. Figure 5-11.

Figure 2-13. Reprinted with permission from Waldman S. *Comprehensive Atlas of Ultrasound-Guided Pain Management Injection Techniques.* 2nd ed. Wolters Kluwer; 2019:654. Figure 92-1.

Figure 2-15. Reprinted with permission from Brant WE, Helms C. *Fundamentals of Diagnostic Radiology.* 4th ed. Wolters Kluwer; 2012:494. Figure 18-11.

Figure 2-16. Reprinted with permission from Frendl G, Urman RD. *Pocket ICU.* 3rd ed. Wolters Kluwer; 2024:RI 10-7. Figure 10-7.

Figure 2-18. Reprinted with permission from Braun MB. *Introduction to Massage Therapy.* 3rd ed. Wolters Kluwer; 2013:90. Figure 3-27.

Figure 2-19. Modified with permission from Agur AMR, Dalley AF. *Moore's Essential Clinical Anatomy.* 6th ed. Wolters Kluwer; 2019:187. Figure 4-5A.

Figure 2-20. Modified with permission from Moore KL, Dalley AF, Agur AMR. *Clinically Oriented Anatomy.* 7th ed. Wolters Kluwer; 2013:75. Figure 1-3.

Figure 2-21. Modified with permission from Agur AMR, Dalley AF. *Moore's Essential Clinical Anatomy.* 6th ed. Wolters Kluwer; 2019:187. Figure 4-4.

Figure 2-27. Reprinted with permission from McArdle WD, Katch FI, Katch VL. *Exercise Physiology.* 8th ed. Wolters Kluwer; 2014:256. Figure 12-3.

Figure 2-29. Modified with permission from Pawlina W, Ross MH. *Histology: A Text and Atlas.* 8th ed. Wolters Kluwer; 2018:704. Figure 19-2.

Figure 2-33. Reprinted with permission from Moore KL, Agur AM, Dalley AF. *Essential Clinical Anatomy.* 5th ed. Wolters Kluwer; 2014:66. Figure 1-17.

Figure 2-35. *Asset provided by the Anatomical Chart Company.*

Figure 2-36. Reprinted with permission from Iyer R, Chapman T. *Pediatric Imaging: The Essentials.* Wolters Kluwer; 2015:55. Figure 6-1c.

Figure 2-38. Modified with permission from Agur AMR, Dalley AF. *Moore's Essential Clinical Anatomy.* 6th ed. Wolters Kluwer; 2019:242. Figure 4-44b.

Figure 2-39. Modified with permission from Moore KL, Dalley AF, Agur AMR. *Clinically Oriented Anatomy.* 8th ed. Wolters Kluwer; 2017:451. Figure 5-33a.

Figure 2-40. Modified with permission from Moore KL, Dalley AF, Agur AMR. *Clinically Oriented Anatomy.* 8th ed. Wolters Kluwer; 2017:451. Figure 5-33c.

Figure 2-49. Modified with permission from Linn-Watson, TA. *Radiographic Pathology.* 2nd ed. Wolters Kluwer; 2014:72. Figure 3-19.

Figure 2-89. Reprinted with permission from Mansoor A. *Frameworks for Internal Medicine*; Wolters Kluwer; 2018:647. Figure 48-3.

Figure 2-95. Reprinted with permission from Torres LS, Dutton AG, Linn-Watson TA. *Patient Care in Imaging Technology.* 7th ed. Wolters Kluwer; 2009:192. Figure 10-8a.

Figure 2-96. Reprinted with permission from Torres LS, Dutton AG, Linn-Watson TA. *Patient Care in Imaging Technology.* 7th ed. Wolters Kluwer; 2009:192. Figure 10-8b.

Figure 2-99. Reprinted with permission from Torres LS, Dutton AG, Linn-Watson TA. *Patient Care in Imaging Technology.* 7th ed. Wolters Kluwer; 2009:193. Figure 10-8c.

CHAPTER 3

Figure 3-1. Reprinted with permission from Yochum TR, Rowe LJ. *Essentials of Skeletal Radiology.* 3rd ed. Wolters Kluwer; 2004:888. Figure 9-152.

Figure 3-2. Reprinted with permission from Waldman S. *Comprehensive Atlas of Ultrasound-Guided Pain Management Injection Techniques.* 2nd ed. Wolters Kluwer; 2019:654. Figure 92-1.

Figure 3-3. Reprinted with permission from Webb WR, Higgins CB. *Thoracic Imaging.* 2nd ed. Wolters Kluwer; 2010:650. Figure 26-44a.

Figure 3-4. Reprinted with permission from Lippincott, Williams, and Wilkins. *Steadman's Medical Dictionary*, 28th Ed. Wolters Kluwer; 2005: 847.

Figure 3-5. Reprinted with permission from Fleisher GR, Ludwig S, Baskin MN. *Atlas of Pediatric Emergency Medicine.* Wolters Kluwer; 2003. Figure 21-6a.

Figure 3-9. Reprinted with permission from Braun MB. *Introduction to Massage Therapy.* 3rd ed. Wolters Kluwer; 2013:90. Figure 3-27.

Figure 3-10. Reprinted with permission from Agur AMR, Dalley AF. *Moore's Essential Clinical Anatomy.* 6th ed. Wolters Kluwer; 2019:187. Figure 4-5.

Figure 3-11. Reprinted with permission from Moore KL, Dalley AF, Agur AMR. *Clinically Oriented Anatomy.* 8th ed. Wolters Kluwer; 2017:300. Figure 4-9.

Figure 3-18. Reprinted with permission from McArdle WD, Katch FI, Katch VL. *Exercise Physiology.* 8th ed. Wolters Kluwer; 2014:256. Figure 12-3.

CHAPTER 4

Figure 4-1. Reprinted with permission from Brant WE, Helms C. *Fundamentals of Diagnostic Radiology.* 4th ed. Wolters Kluwer; 2012:674. Figure 25-8b.

Figure 4-2. Reprinted with permission from Chi D, Berchuck A, Dizon DS, Yashar CM. *Principles and Practice of Gynecologic Oncology.* 7th ed. Wolters Kluwer; 2017:809. Figure 28-6a.

Figure 4-3. Reprinted with permission from Shaffner DH, Nichols DG. *Rogers' Textbook of Pediatric Intensive Care.* 5th ed. Wolters Kluwer; 2015:1678. Figure 102-4.

Figure 4-4. Reprinted with permission from Chi D, Berchuck A, Dizon DS, Yashar CM. *Principles and Practice of Gynecologic Oncology.* 7th ed. Wolters Kluwer; 2017:809. Figure 28-6b.

Figure 4-5. Reprinted with permission from Penny SM. *Introduction to Sonography and Patient Care.* Wolters Kluwer; 2015:351. Figure 13-2.

Figure 4-6. Reprinted with permission from Mullholland MW. *Greenfield's Surgery.* 6th ed. Wolters Kluwer; 2016:800. Figure 49-14.

Figure 4-7. *Asset provided by the Anatomical Chart Company.*

Figure 4-8. Reprinted with permission from Moore KL, Dalley AF, Agur AMR. *Clinically Oriented Anatomy*, 8th Ed. Wolters Kluwer, 2018: 485. Figure B5.18. Based on Cohen BJ, DePetris A. *Medical Terminology: An Illustrated Guide*, 8th ed. Wolters Kluwer; 2017.

Figure 4-9. Reprinted with permission from Lawrence PF. *Essentials of General Surgery and Surgical Specialties.* 6th ed. Wolters Kluwer; 2018:229. Figure 15-14.

Figure 4-11. Reprinted with permission from Fleisher GR, Ludwig S, Baskin MN. *Atlas of Pediatric Emergency Medicine.* Wolters Kluwer; 2003. Figure 21-6a.

Figure 4-12. Reprinted with permission from Eisenberg RL. *Clinical Imaging.* 5th ed. Wolters Kluwer; 2009:520. Figure GI 36-15.

Figure 4-13. Reprinted with permission from Daffner RH, Hartman M. *Clinical Radiology.* 4th ed. Wolters Kluwer; 2013:243. Figure 7-36a.

Figure 4-15. Modified with permission from Dutton AG, Linn-Watson TA, Torres LS. *Torres' Patient Care in Imaging Technology.* 8th ed. Wolters Kluwer; 2012:249. Figure 13-3.

Figure 4-16. Reprinted with permission from Wolfson AB, Hendey GW, Ling LJ, Rosen CL, Schaider JJ, Sharieff GQ. *Harwood-Nuss' Clinical Practice of Emergency Medicine.* 5th ed. Wolters Kluwer; 2009:657. Figure 126-1.

Figure 4-17. Reprinted with permission from Bear MF, Connors BW, Parasido MA. *Neuroscience: Exploring the Brain*, 4th ed. Wolters Kluwer; 2016:187. Box 7.1, Figure A.

Figure 4-18. Reprinted with permission from Daffner RH, Hartman M. *Clinical Radiology.* 4th ed. Wolters Kluwer; 2013:219. Figure 7-5a.

Figure 4-27. Reprinted with permission from Daffner RH, Hartman M. *Clinical Radiology.* 4th ed. Wolters Kluwer; 2013:248. Figure 7-43a.

Figure 4-30. Modified with permission from Moore KL, Dalley AF, Agur AMR. *Clinically Oriented Anatomy.* 7th ed. Wolters Kluwer; 2013:232. Figure 2-36b.

Figure 4-31. Reprinted with permission from Wingerd B. *Human Body.* 3rd ed. Wolters Kluwer; 2013:395. Figure 15-12.

Figure 4-33. Reprinted with permission from Britt LD, Peitzman A, Barie P, Jurkovich G. *Acute Care Surgery.* Wolters Kluwer; 2012:57. Figure 5-16.

Figure 4-34. Reprinted with permission from Arnold C, Lam-himlin D, Montgomery EA. *Atlas of Gastrointestinal Pathology: A Pattern Based Approach to Neoplastic Biopsies.* Wolters Kluwer; 2018:234. Figure 3-143.

Figure 4-37. Modified with permission from Moore KL, Dalley AF, Agur AMR. *Clinically Oriented Anatomy.* 7th ed. Wolters Kluwer; 2013:253. Figure 2-57.

Figure 4-38. *Asset provided by the Anatomical Chart Company.*

Figure 4-39. Reprinted with permission from Pawlina W, Ross MH. *Histology: A Text and Atlas.* 8th ed. Wolters Kluwer; 2018:680. Figure 18-14.

Figure 4-40. *Asset provided by the Anatomical Chart Company.*

Figure 4-41. *Asset provided by the Anatomical Chart Company.*

Figure 4-44. Reprinted with permission from Wingerd B. *Human Body.* 3rd ed. Wolters Kluwer; 2013:386. Figure 15-3A,B.

Figure 4-45A. Reprinted with permission from Wingerd B. *Human Body.* 3rd ed. Wolters Kluwer; 2013:386. Figure 15-3C.

Figure 4-74. Modified with permission from White AJ. *The Washington Manual of Pediatrics.* 3rd ed. Wolters Kluwer; 2022:600. Figure 25-5b.

Figure 4-75. Reprinted with permission from Dutton A, Ryan TA. *Torres' Patient Care in Imaging Technology.* 9th ed. Wolters Kluwer; 2018:160. Figure 7-10a.

CHAPTER 5

Figure 5-1. *Asset provided by the Anatomical Chart Company.*

Figure 5-2. Reprinted with permission from Tornetta P, Ricci W. Court-Brown CM, McQueen MM, McKee M. *Rockwood and Green's Fractures in Adults.* 9th ed. Wolters Kluwer; 2019:283. Figure 9-45.

Figure 5-3. *Asset provided by the Anatomical Chart Company.*

Figure 5-4. Reprinted with permission from Greenberg MI, Hendrickson RG, Silverberg M, Campbell C, Morocco A, Salvaggio CA, Spencer MT. *Greenberg's Text-Atlas of Emergency Medicine.* Lippincott Williams & Wilkins; 2004:483. Figure 15-27.

Figure 5-5. Reprinted with permission from Klein J, Vinson EN, Brant WE, Helms CA. *Brant and Helms' Fundamentals of Diagnostic Radiology.* 5th ed. Wolters Kluwer; 2018:1326. Figure 50-31.

Figure 5-6. *Asset provided by the Anatomical Chart Company.*

Figure 5-7. Reprinted with permission from Yochum TR, Rowe LJ. *Essentials of Skeletal Radiology.* 3rd ed. Wolters Kluwer; 2004:906. Figure 9-188.

Figure 5-8. Modified with permission from Farrell TA. *Radiology 101.* 5th ed. Wolters Kluwer; 2019:206. Figure 6-33b.

Figure 5-9. Reprinted with permission from Iyer R, Chapman T. *Pediatric Imaging: The Essentials.* Wolters Kluwer; 2015:290. Figure 25-16.

Figure 5-10. *Asset provided by the Anatomical Chart Company.*

Figure 5-11. Reprinted with permission from Hunt TR, Wiesel SW. *The Johns Hopkins High-Yield Review for Orthopaedic Surgery.* Wolters Kluwer; 2016:411. Figure Tech Fig 1A.

Figure 5-19. *Asset provided by the Anatomical Chart Company.*

Figure 5-20. *Asset provided by the Anatomical Chart Company.*

Figure 5-23. Modified with permission from Moore KL, Dalley AF, Agur AMR. *Clinically Oriented Anatomy.* 7th ed. Wolters Kluwer; 2013:679. Figure 6-9b.

Figure 5-26. Modified with permission from Greenspan A, Beltran J. *Orthopaedic Imaging: A Practical Approach.* 7th ed. Wolters Kluwer; 2020:278. Figure 7-35b.

Figure 5-27. Modified with permission from Greenspan A, Beltran J. *Orthopaedic Imaging: A Practical Approach.* 7th ed. Wolters Kluwer; 2020:279. Figure 7-38.

Figure 5-28. Modified with permission from Agur AM, Dalley AF. *Grant's Atlas of Anatomy.* 16th ed. Wolters Kluwer; 2024:139. Figure 2-58.

Figure 5-29. Reprinted with permission from Gest TR, *Lippincott Atlas of Anatomy*, 2nd ed. Wolters Kluwer; 2019:38. Plate 204.

Figure 5-30. Modified with permission from Agur AM, Dalley AF. *Grant's Atlas of Anatomy.* 16th ed. Wolters Kluwer; 2024:70. Figure 2-3c.

Figure 5-31. Modified with permission from Agur AM, Dalley AF. *Grant's Atlas of Anatomy*, 16th ed. Wolters Kluwer; 2024:70. Figure 2-3c.

Figure 5-34. Modified with permission from Agur AM, Dalley AF. *Grant's Atlas of Anatomy.* 16th ed. Wolters Kluwer; 2024:70. Figure 2-3c.

Figure 5-35. Modified with permission from Agur AM, Dalley AF. *Grant's Atlas of Anatomy.* 16th ed. Wolters Kluwer; 2024:70. Figure 2-3g.

Figure 5-37. Modified with permission from Agur AM, Dalley AF. *Grant's Atlas of Anatomy.* 16th ed. Wolters Kluwer; 2024:141. Figure 2-60.

Figure 5-38. Modified with permission from Smith WL. *Radiology 101.* 4th ed. Wolters Kluwer; 2013:172. Figure 6-3.

Figure 5-39. Modified with permission from Koval KJ, Zuckerman JD. *Atlas of Orthopaedic Surgery: A Multimedia Reference.* Wolters Kluwer; 2003:52. Figure 5-1a.

Figure 5-42. Reprinted with permission from Yochum TR, Rowe LJ. *Essentials of Skeletal Radiology.* 3rd ed. Wolters Kluwer; 2004:893. Figure 9-163.

Figure 5-43. *Asset provided by the Anatomical Chart Company.*

Figure 5-44. *Asset provided by the Anatomical Chart Company.*

Figure 5-45. *Asset provided by the Anatomical Chart Company.*

Figure 5-114. Reprinted with permission from Greenspan A, Beltran J. *Orthopaedic Imaging: A Practical Approach.* 7th ed. Wolters Kluwer; 2020:279. Figure 7-38bc.

Figure 5-150. Modified with permission from Waters PM, Bae DS. *Pediatric Hand and Upper Limb Surgery.* Wolters Kluwer; 2012:380. Figure 32-1a.

Figure 5-153. Reprinted with permission from Swiontkowski MF. *Manual of Orthopaedics.* 7th ed. Wolters Kluwer; 2012:329. Figure 19-3b.

Figure 5-154. Reprinted with permission from Swiontkowski MF. *Manual of Orthopaedics.* 7th ed. Wolters Kluwer; 2012:330. Figure 19-3a.

CHAPTER 6

Figure 6-1. Reprinted with permission from Greenspan A, Beltran J. *Orthopaedic Imaging: A Practical Approach.* 7th ed. Wolters Kluwer; 2020:179. Figure 5-46.

Figure 6-2. *Asset provided by the Anatomical Chart Company.*

Figure 6-3. *Asset provided by the Anatomical Chart Company.*

Figure 6-4. Reprinted with permission from Daffner RH, Hartman M. *Clinical Radiology.* 4th ed. Wolters Kluwer; 2013:371. Figure 11-26.

Figure 6-5. Reprinted with permission from Bridgeforth GM. *Lippincott's Primary Care Musculoskeletal Radiology.* Wolters Kluwer; 2010:160. Figure 32-3c,d.

Figure 6-6. Reprinted with permission from Greenspan A, Gershwin ME. *Imaging in Rheumatology.* Wolters Kluwer; 2017:171. Figure 5-53.

Figure 6-7. Reprinted with permission from Greenspan A, Gershwin ME. *Imaging in Rheumatology.* Wolters Kluwer; 2017:210. Figure 6-7.

Figure 6-12. Modified with permission from Koval KJ, Zuckerman JD. *Atlas of Orthopaedic Surgery: A Multimedia Reference.* Wolters Kluwer; 2003:52. Figure 5-1a.

Figure 6-13. Reprinted with permission from Wingerd B. *Human Body.* 3rd ed. Wolters Kluwer; 2013:138. Figure 6-23.

Figure 6-14. Reprinted with permission from Yochum TR, Rowe LJ. *Essentials of Skeletal Radiology.* 3rd ed. Wolters Kluwer; 2004:893. Figure 9-163.

Figure 6-15. *Asset provided by the Anatomical Chart Company.*

Figure 6-16. *Asset provided by the Anatomical Chart Company.*

Figure 6-17. Modified with permission from Moore KL, Dalley AF, Agur AMR. *Clinically Oriented Anatomy.* 8th ed. Wolters Kluwer; 2017:145. Figure 3-4.

Figure 6-18. Modified with permission from Moore KL, Dalley AF, Agur AMR. *Clinically Oriented Anatomy.* 8th ed. Wolters Kluwer; 2017:263. Figure 3-90.

Figure 6-19. *Asset provided by the Anatomical Chart Company.*

Figure 6-20. Modified with permission from Moore KL, Dalley AF, Agur AMR. *Clinically Oriented Anatomy.* 8th ed. Wolters Kluwer; 2017:145. Figure 3-5a.

Figure 6-21. Modified with permission from Moore KL, Dalley AF, Agur AMR. *Clinically Oriented Anatomy.* 8th ed. Wolters Kluwer; 2017:145. Figure 3-5a.

Figure 6-22. Modified with permission from Moore KL, Dalley AF, Agur AMR. *Clinically Oriented Anatomy.* 8th ed. Wolters Kluwer; 2017:145. Figure 3-5d.

Figure 6-24. Modified with permission from Harris JH. *Imaging Handbook for Physical Therapists.* Wolters Kluwer; 2014:23. Figure 3-8a.

Figure 6-26. Modified with permission from Harris JH. *Imaging Handbook for Physical Therapists.* Wolters Kluwer; 2014:23. Figure 3-8b.

CHAPTER 7

Figure 7-1. Modified with permission from Greenspan A, Gershwin ME. *Imaging in Rheumatology.* Wolters Kluwer; 2017:277. Figure 7-12b.

Figure 7-2. Modified with permission from Greenspan A, Gershwin ME. *Imaging in Rheumatology.* Wolters Kluwer; 2017:97. Figure 3-9a.

Figure 7-3. Modified with permission from Greenspan A, Beltran J. *Orthopaedic Imaging: A Practical Approach.* 7th ed. Wolters Kluwer; 2020:519. Figure 10-103.

Figure 7-4. Modified with permission from Greenspan A, Beltran J. *Orthopaedic Imaging: A Practical Approach.* 7th ed. Wolters Kluwer; 2020:474. Figure 10-29.

Figure 7-5. Modified with permission from Klein J, Vinson EN, Brant WE, Helms CA. *Brant and Helms' Fundamentals of Diagnostic Radiology.* 5th ed. Wolters Kluwer; 2018:1350. Figure 58-20.

Figure 7-6. Modified with permission from Klein J, Vinson EN, Brant WE, Helms CA. *Brant and Helms' Fundamentals of Diagnostic Radiology.* 5th ed. Wolters Kluwer; 2018:1306. Figure 56-14.

Figure 7-7. *Asset provided by the Anatomical Chart Company.*

Figure 7-8. Reprinted with permission from Tornetta P, Ricci W, Court-Brown CM, McQueen MM, McKee M. *Rockwood and Green's Fractures in Adults.* 9th ed. Wolters Kluwer; 2018:92. Figure 4-4.

Figure 7-9. Reprinted with permission from Iyer R, Chapman T. *Pediatric Imaging: The Essentials.* Wolters Kluwer; 2015:318. Figure 27-10a.

Figure 7-14. Reprinted with permission from Bittle MM, Gunn ML, Gross JA, Stern EJ. *Trauma Radiology Companion.* 2nd ed. Wolters Kluwer; 2011:409. Figure 5-53a.

Figure 7-18. Reprinted with permission from Olinger AB. *Human Gross Anatomy*. Wolters Kluwer; 2015:216. Figure 4-1.

Figure 7-19. Modified with permission from Seffinger, M. *Foundations of Osteopathic Medicine*. 4th ed. Wolters Kluwer; 2018:674. Figure 28H.1, lower right.

Figure 7-20. Modified with permission from Seffinger, M. *Foundations of Osteopathic Medicine*. 4th ed. Wolters Kluwer; 2018:674. Figure 28H.1, upper right.

Figure 7-21. Modified with permission from Tank PW, Gest TR. *Lippincott Atlas of Anatomy*, 2nd ed. Wolters Kluwer; 2019:138. Figure Plate 340A.

Figure 7-22. Modified with permission from Tank PW, Gest TR. *Lippincott Atlas of Anatomy, 2nd ed.* Wolters Kluwer; 2019:138. Figure Plate 340B.

Figure 7-30. Modified with permission from Moore KL, Dalley AF, Agur AMR. *Clinically Oriented Anatomy*. 8th ed. Wolters Kluwer; 2017:815. Figure 7-105A,B.

Figure 7-31. Modified with permission from Moore KL, Dalley AF, Agur AMR. *Clinically Oriented Anatomy*. 8th ed. Wolters Kluwer; 2017:815. Figure 7-105C.

Figure 7-32. *Asset provided by the Anatomical Chart Company.*

Figure 7-37. Reprinted with permission from Wiesel SW, Albert T. *Operative Techniques in Orthopaedic Surgery*. 3rd ed. Wolters Kluwer; 2021:1453. Figure 1B.

Figure 7-40. Reprinted with permission from Greenspan A, Beltran J. *Orthopaedic Imaging: A Practical Approach*. 7th ed. Wolters Kluwer; 2020:462. Figure 10-6c.

Figure 7-49. Modified with permission from Clemente CD. *Anatomy*. 6th ed. Elsevier; 2010:Plate 495. Figure 495.4.

Figure 7-50. Modified with permission from Moore KL, Dalley AF, Agur AMR. *Clinically Oriented Anatomy*. 8th ed. Wolters Kluwer; 2017:793. Figure 7-86.

Figure 7-89. Reprinted with permission from Easley ME, Wiesel SW. *Operative Techniques in Foot and Ankle Surgery*. 3rd ed. Wolters Kluwer; 2021:450. Figure Tech Fig 21D.

Figure 7-91. Reprinted with permission from Easley ME, Wiesel SW. *Operative Techniques in Foot and Ankle Surgery*. 3rd ed. Wolters Kluwer; 2021:134. Figure Tech Fig 6C.

Figure 7-118. Modified with permission from Thordarson D. *Foot & Ankle*. 2nd ed. Wolters Kluwer; 2012:326. Figure 14-7.

Figure 7-145. Modified with permission from Berry DJ, Pagnano MW. *Illustrated Tips and Tricks in Hip and Knee Reconstructive and Replacement Surgery*. Wolters Kluwer; 2019:333. Figure 44-2A,B.

Figure 7-171. Reprinted with permission from Flynn JM, Weinstein S. *Lovell and Winter's Pediatric Orthopaedics*. 8th ed. Wolters Kluwer; 2020:1541. Figure 30-2.

Figure 7-174. Modified with permission from Berry DJ, Pagnano MW. *Illustrated Tips and Tricks in Hip and Knee Reconstructive and Replacement Surgery*. Wolters Kluwer; 2019:333. Figure 44-2D.

CHAPTER 8

Figure 8-1. Reprinted with permission from Greenspan A, Gershwin ME. *Imaging in Rheumatology*. Wolters Kluwer; 2017:148. Figure 5-5D.

Figure 8-2. Reprinted with permission from Vigorita VJ. *Orthopaedic Pathology*. 3rd ed. Wolters Kluwer; 2015:124. Figure 3-7C.

Figure 8-3. Reprinted with permission from Farrell TA. *Radiology 101*. 5th ed. Wolters Kluwer; 2019:231. Figure 6-71.

Figure 8-4. Modified with permission from Berry DJ, Pagnano MW. *Illustrated Tips and Tricks in Hip and Knee Reconstructive and Replacement Surgery*. Wolters Kluwer; 2019:85. Figure 13-8B.

Figure 8-5. Reprinted with permission from Greenspan A, Gershwin ME. *Imaging in Rheumatology*. Wolters Kluwer; 2017:156. Figure 5-19B.

Figure 8-6. Reprinted with permission from Greenspan A, Beltran J. *Orthopaedic Imaging: A Practical Approach*. 7th ed. Wolters Kluwer; 2020:1373. Figure 32-22A.

Figure 8-7. Modified with permission from Flynn JM, Wiesel SW. *Operative Techniques in Pediatric Orthopaedics*. Wolters Kluwer; 2010:528. Figure 74-2A.

Figure 8-8. *Asset provided by the Anatomical Chart Company.*

Figure 8-11. Modified with permission from Moore KL, Dalley AF, Agur AMR. *Clinically Oriented Anatomy*. 8th ed. Wolters Kluwer; 2017:558. Figure 6-4A.

Figure 8-13. Modified with permission from Moore KL, Dalley AF, Agur AMR. *Clinically Oriented Anatomy*. 8th ed. Wolters Kluwer; 2017:673. Figure 7-6A.

Figure 8-15. Modified with permission from Moore KL, Dalley AF, Agur AMR. *Clinically Oriented Anatomy*. 8th ed. Wolters Kluwer; 2017:673. Figure 7-6A.

Figure 8-17. Modified with permission from Moore KL, Dalley AF, Agur AMR. *Clinically Oriented Anatomy*. 8th ed. Wolters Kluwer; 2017:673. Figure 7-6A.

Figure 8-18. *Asset provided by the Anatomical Chart Company.*

Figure 8-20. Modified with permission from Moore KL, Dalley AF, Agur AMR. *Clinically Oriented Anatomy*. 8th ed. Wolters Kluwer; 2017:675. Figure 7-7B.

Figure 8-22. Modified with permission from Moore KL, Dalley AF, Agur AMR. *Clinically Oriented Anatomy*. 8th ed. Wolters Kluwer; 2017:557. Figure 6-3.

Figure 8-23. Reprinted with permission from Wineski LE. *Snell's Clinical Anatomy by Regions*. 11th ed. Wolters Kluwer; 2024:474, 475. Figure 6-49 and 6-51.

Figure 8-24. Reprinted with permission from Wineski LE. *Snell's Clinical Anatomy by Regions*. 10th ed. Wolters Kluwer; 2018:471. Figure 9-30.

Figure 8-25. Reprinted with permission from Wineski LE. *Snell's Clinical Anatomy by Regions*. 10th ed. Wolters Kluwer; 2018:472. Figure 9-32.

Figure 8-28. Modified with permission from Moore KL, Dalley AF, Agur AMR. *Clinically Oriented Anatomy*. 8th ed. Wolters Kluwer; 2017:558. Figure 6-4A.

Figure 8-69. Courtesy of Marc R. Safran, MD.

Figure 8-70. Courtesy of Marc R. Safran, MD.

Figure 8-83. Reprinted with permission from Greenspan A, Beltran J. *Orthopaedic Imaging: A Practical Approach*. 7th ed. Wolters Kluwer; 2020:338. Figure 8-5B.

Figure 8-84. Reprinted with permission from Greenspan A, Beltran J. *Orthopaedic Imaging: A Practical Approach*. 7th ed. Wolters Kluwer; 2020:337. Figure 8-4B.

Figure 8-86. Reprinted with permission from Pope TL, Harris JH. *Harris & Harris' The Radiology of Emergency Medicine*. 5th ed. Wolters Kluwer; 2012:750. Figure 17-3b.

Figure 8-88. Reprinted with permission from Pope TL, Harris JH. *Harris & Harris' The Radiology of Emergency Medicine*. 5th ed. Wolters Kluwer; 2012:750. Figure 17-3a.

CHAPTER 9

Figure 9-1. Modified with permission from Wineski LE. *Snell's Clinical Anatomy by Regions*. 11th ed. Wolters Kluwer; 2024:68. Figure 2-26D.

Figure 9-2. Modified with permission from Wineski LE. *Snell's Clinical Anatomy by Regions*. 11th ed. Wolters Kluwer; 2024:68. Figure 2-26E.

Figure 9-3. Modified with permission from Wineski LE. *Snell's Clinical Anatomy by Regions*. 11th ed. Wolters Kluwer; 2024:68. Figure 2-26B.

Figure 9-4. Modified with permission from Wineski LE. *Snell's Clinical Anatomy by Regions*. 11th ed. Wolters Kluwer; 2024:68. Figure 2-26C.

Figure 9-5. Reprinted with permission from Yochum TR, Rowe LJ. *Essentials of Skeletal Radiology*. 3rd ed. Wolters Kluwer; 2004:837. Figure 9-63.

Figure 9-6. Modified with permission from Koopman WJ, Moreland LW. *Arthritis and Allied Conditions*. 15th ed. Wolters Kluwer; 2004. Figure 110-7.

Figure 9-7. Modified with permission from Koopman WJ, Moreland LW. *Arthritis and Allied Conditions*. 15th ed. Wolters Kluwer; 2004. Figure 63-3.

Figure 9-8. Reprinted with permission from Klein J, Vinson EN, Brant WE, Helms CA. *Brant and Helms' Fundamentals of Diagnostic Radiology*. 5th ed. Wolters Kluwer; 2018:1319. Figure 57-11.

Figure 9-9. Reprinted with permission from Benzel EC. *Cervical Spine*. 5th ed. Wolters Kluwer; 2013:845. Figure 62-3a,b.

Figure 9-10. Modified with permission from Capriotti T. *Pathophysiology Made Incredibly Visual*. 3rd ed. Wolters Kluwer; 2016. Figure 6-Sciatica.

Figure 9-11. Modified with permission from Yochum TR, Rowe LJ. *Essentials of Skeletal Radiology*. 3rd ed. Wolters Kluwer; 2004:311. Figure 3-77D.

Figure 9-18. Modified with permission from Agur AMR, Dalley AF. *Moore's Essential Clinical Anatomy*. 6th ed. Wolters Kluwer; 2019:46. Figure 2-1A-C.

Figure 9-20. Reprinted with permission from Agur AMR, Dalley AF. *Moore's Essential Clinical Anatomy*. 6th ed. Wolters Kluwer; 2019:46. Figure 2-1D,E.

Figure 9-21. *Asset provided by the Anatomical Chart Company.*

Figure 9-22. Modified with permission from Moore KL, Dalley AF, Agur AMR. *Clinically Oriented Anatomy*. 8th ed. Wolters Kluwer; 2017:74. Figure 2-2A.

Figure 9-23. Modified with permission from Moore KL, Dalley AF, Agur AMR. *Clinically Oriented Anatomy*. 8th ed. Wolters Kluwer; 2017:74. Figure 2-2C,D.

Figure 9-24. Modified with permission from Moore KL, Dalley AF, Agur AMR. *Clinically Oriented Anatomy*. 8th ed. Wolters Kluwer; 2017:74. Figure 2-2B.

Figure 9-25. *Asset provided by the Anatomical Chart Company.*

Figure 9-26. Modified with permission from Hamill J, Knutzen K, Derrick T. *Biomechanical Basis of Human Movement*. 4th ed. Wolters Kluwer; 2014:247. Figure 7-8.

Figure 9-27. Reprinted with permission from Pansky B, Gest TR. *Lippincott Concise Illustrated Anatomy*. Wolters Kluwer; 2014:55. Figure 1-9C.

Figure 9-28. Reprinted with permission from Pansky B, Gest TR. *Lippincott Concise Illustrated Anatomy*. Wolters Kluwer; 2014:55. Figure 1-9D.

Figure 9-30. Reprinted with permission from Pansky B, Gest TR. *Lippincott Concise Illustrated Anatomy*. Wolters Kluwer; 2014:55. Figure 1-9E.

Figure 9-32. Reprinted with permission from Greenspan A, Beltran J. *Orthopaedic Imaging: A Practical Approach*. 7th ed. Wolters Kluwer; 2020:538. Figure 11-9.

Figure 9-34. *Asset provided by the Anatomical Chart Company.*

Figure 9-35. Reprinted with permission from Oatis CA. *Kinesiology*. 3rd ed. Wolters Kluwer; 2017:498. Figure 26-7A.

Figure 9-36. Modified with permission from Gest TR. *Lippincott Atlas of Anatomy*. 2nd ed. Wolters Kluwer; 2019:8. Figure 1-04E.

Figure 9-38. Reprinted with permission from Gest TR. *Lippincott Atlas of Anatomy*. 2nd ed. Wolters Kluwer; 2019:9. Figure 1-05.

Figure 9-39. Modified with permission from Achar S, Taylor KS. *5-Minute Sports Medicine Consult*. 3rd ed. Wolters Kluwer; 2019:635. Figure 50e.

Figure 9-40. *Asset provided by the Anatomical Chart Company.*

Figure 9-41. *Asset provided by the Anatomical Chart Company.*

Figure 9-43. Modified with permission from Gest TR. *Lippincott Atlas of Anatomy*. 2nd ed. Wolters Kluwer; 2019:11. Figure 1-07.

Figure 9-46. *Asset provided by the Anatomical Chart Company.*

Figure 9-48. Reprinted with permission from Gest TR. *Lippincott Atlas of Anatomy*. 2nd ed. Wolters Kluwer; 2019:12. Figure 1-08.

Figure 9-49. Modified with permission from Greenspan A. Beltran J. *Orthopaedic Imaging: A Practical Approach*. 7th ed. Wolters Kluwer; 2020:567. Figure 11-54c.

Figure 9-50. Modified with permission from Smith WL. *Radiology 101*. 4th ed. *Wolters* Kluwer; 2013:295. Figure 9-10A.

Figure 9-52. *Asset provided by the Anatomical Chart Company.*

Figure 9-57. Reprinted with permission from Greenspan A. Gershwin ME. *Imaging in Rheumatology*. Wolters Kluwer; 2017:36. Figure 2-20B.

Figure 9-67. Reprinted with permission from Benzel EC. *Cervical Spine*. 5th ed. Wolters Kluwer; 2012:279. Figure 23-2.

Figure 9-70. Reprinted with permission from Harris JH. *Imaging Handbook for Physical Therapists*. Wolters Kluwer; 2014:12. Figure 2-7a.

Figure 9-72. Reprinted with permission from Harris JH. *Imaging Handbook for Physical Therapists*. Wolters Kluwer; 2014:12. Figure 2-7b.

Figure 9-77. Reprinted with permission from Achar S, Taylor KS. *5-Minute Sports Medicine Consult*. 3rd ed. Wolters Kluwer; 2019:635. Figure 50e.

Figure 9-78. Modified with permission from Achar S, Taylor KS. *5-Minute Sports Medicine Consult*. 3rd ed. Wolters Kluwer; 2019:635. Figure 50e.

Figure 9-92. Reprinted with permission from Greenspan A, Beltran J. *Orthopaedic Imaging: A Practical Approach*. 7th ed. Wolters Kluwer; 2020:553. Figure 11-29C.

Figure 9-98. Reprinted with permission from Greenspan A, Gershwin ME. *Imaging in Rheumatology*. Wolters Kluwer; 2017:33. Figure 2-16C.

Figure 9-99. Reprinted with permission from Greenspan A, Beltran J. *Orthopaedic Imaging: A Practical Approach*. 7th ed. Wolters Kluwer; 2020:538. Figure 11-10B.

Figure 9-117. Reprinted with permission from Greenspan A, Beltran J. *Orthopaedic Imaging: A Practical Approach*. 7th ed. Wolters Kluwer; 2020:538. Figure 11-10B.

Figure 9-170. Reprinted with permission from Bridwell KH, DeWald RL. *Textbook of Spinal Surgery*. 3rd ed. Wolters Kluwer; 2011:1494. Figure 138-7A2.

Figure 9-172. Reprinted with permission from Bridwell KH, DeWald RL. *Textbook of Spinal Surgery*. 3rd ed. Wolters Kluwer; 2011:1494. Figure 138-7A1.

CHAPTER 10

Figure 10-1. Reprinted with permission from Farrell TA. *Radiology 101*. 5th ed. Wolters Kluwer; 2020:298. Figure 8-4.

Figure 10-2. Reprinted with permission from Bittle MM, Gunn ML, Gross JA, Stern EJ. *Trauma Radiology Companion*. 2nd ed. Wolters Kluwer; 2011:71. Figure 2-26B.

Figure 10-3. Reprinted with permission from Yochum TR, Rowe LJ. *Essentials of Skeletal Radiology*. 3rd ed. Wolters Kluwer; 2004:809. Figure 9-24.

Figure 10-4. Reprinted with permission from Pope TL, Harris JH. *Harris & Harris' The Radiology of Emergency Medicine*. 5th ed. Wolters Kluwer; 2012:129. Figure 4-55.

Figure 10-5. Reprinted with permission from Anderson MK, Barnum M. *Foundations of Athletic Training*. 7th ed. Wolters Kluwer; 2021:808. Figure 24-13.

Figure 10-6. Reprinted with permission from Pope TL, Harris JH. *Harris & Harris' The Radiology of Emergency Medicine.* 5th ed. Wolters Kluwer; 2012:5. Figure 1-4.

Figure 10-7. Reprinted with permission from Sanelli P, Schaefer P, Loevner L. *Neuroimaging: The Essentials.* Wolters Kluwer; 2015:57. Figure 3-25a.

Figure 10-8. Modified with permission from Agur AM, Dalley AF. *Moore's Essential Clinical Anatomy.* 6th ed. Wolters Kluwer; 2020:557. Figure 8-46d,e.

Figure 10-19. Reprinted with permission from DiGiovanna E, Amen C, Burns D. *An Osteopathic Approach to Diagnosis and Treatment.* 4th ed. Wolters Kluwer; 2020:486. Figure 103-117.

Figure 10-20. Reprinted with permission from DiGiovanna E, Amen C, Burns D. *An Osteopathic Approach to Diagnosis and Treatment.* 4th ed. Wolters Kluwer; 2020:480. Figure 103-6B.

Figure 10-21. Reprinted with permission from DiGiovanna E, Amen C, Burns D. *An Osteopathic Approach to Diagnosis and Treatment.* 4th ed. Wolters Kluwer; 2020:486. Figure 103-117.

Figure 10-22. Reprinted with permission from DiGiovanna E, Amen C, Burns D. *An Osteopathic Approach to Diagnosis and Treatment.* 4th ed. Wolters Kluwer; 2020:483. Figure 103-113.

Figure 10-23. Reprinted with permission from DiGiovanna E, Amen C, Burns D. *An Osteopathic Approach to Diagnosis and Treatment.* 4th ed. Wolters Kluwer; 2020:480. Figure 103-6B.

Figure 10-24. Reprinted with permission from DiGiovanna E, Amen C, Burns D. *An Osteopathic Approach to Diagnosis and Treatment.* 4th ed. Wolters Kluwer; 2020:486. Figure 103-18.

Figure 10-36. Reprinted with permission from DiGiovanna E, Amen C, Burns D. *An Osteopathic Approach to Diagnosis and Treatment.* 4th ed. Wolters Kluwer; 2020:481. Figure 103-8.

Figure 10-43. Modified with permission from Chung KC, Disa JJ, Gosain A, Lee G, Mehrara B, Thorne CH, van Aalst J. *Operative Techniques in Plastic Surgery.* Wolters Kluwer; 2019:1011. Figure 1A.

Figure 10-46. Modified with permission from Chung KC, Disa JJ, Gosain A, Lee G, Mehrara B, Thorne CH, van Aalst J. *Operative Techniques in Plastic Surgery.* Wolters Kluwer; 2019:587. Figure Tech Fig 2D.

Figure 10-49. Modified with permission from Chung KC, Disa JJ, Gosain A, Lee G, Mehrara B, Thorne CH, van Aalst J. *Operative Techniques in Plastic Surgery.* Wolters Kluwer; 2019:866. Figure 1A.

Figure 10-51. Modified with permission from Chung KC, Disa JJ, Gosain A, Lee G, Mehrara B, Thorne CH, van Aalst J. *Operative Techniques in Plastic Surgery.* Wolters Kluwer; 2019:848. Figure 3.

Figure 10-53. Modified with permission from Moore KL, Dalley AF, Agur AMR. *Clinically Oriented Anatomy.* 8th ed. Wolters Kluwer; 2017:897. Figure 8-44A.

Figure 10-56. Modified with permission from Bailey BJ, Johnson JT, Newlands SD, et al. *Head and Neck Surgery—Otolaryngology.* 4th ed. Wolters Kluwer; 2006:979. Figure 70-6.

Figure 10-58. Modified with permission from Chung KC, Disa JJ, Gosain A, Lee G, Mehrara B, Thorne CH, van Aalst J. *Operative Techniques in Plastic Surgery.* Wolters Kluwer; 2019:399. Figure 1A.

Figure 10-60. Reprinted with permission from Daffner RH, Hartman M, *Clinical Radiology,* 4th ed. Wolters Kluwer; 2014:4.35. Figure 12-7.

Figure 10-63. Reprinted with permission from Snell R. *Clinical Anatomy.* 7th ed. Wolters Kluwer; 2003. Figure 11-103.

CHAPTER 11

Figure 11-1. Reprinted with permission from Singh A. *Gastrointestinal Imaging: The Essentials.* Wolters Kluwer; 2016:14. Figure 2-7.

Figure 11-3. Reprinted with permission from Lee E. *Pediatric Radiology: Practical Imaging Evaluation of Infants and Children.* Wolters Kluwer; 2017:861. Figure 16-93A.

Figure 11-4. Reprinted with permission from Stewart J. *Anatomical Chart Company Atlas of Pathophysiology.* 4th ed. Wolters Kluwer; 2017:195. Figure unfig 11.

Figure 11-6. Reprinted with permission from Farrell TA. *Radiology 101.* 5th ed. Wolters Kluwer; 2019:82. Figure 3-20.

Figure 11-7. Reprinted with permission from Mulholland MW. *Greenfield's Surgery.* 6th ed. Wolters Kluwer; 2016:1904. Figure 103-37.

Figure 11-8. Reprinted with permission from Klein J, Vinson EN, Brant WE, Helms CA. *Brant and Helms' Fundamentals of Diagnostic Radiology.* 5th ed. Wolters Kluwer; 2019:1060. Figure 44-21.

Figure 11-10. Reprinted with permission from Pope TL, Harris JH. *Harris & Harris' The Radiology of Emergency Medicine.* 5th ed. Wolters Kluwer; 2013:632. Figure 14-90.

Figure 11-11. Modified with permission from Whalen K. *Lippincott Illustrated Reviews: Pharmacology.* 7th ed. Wolters Kluwer; 2018:551. Figure 40-16A.

Figure 11-12. Reprinted with permission from Herzog E. *Herzog's CCU Book.* Wolters Kluwer; 2017:536. Figure 47-1b.

Figure 11-13. Reprinted with permission from Braun C, Anderson C. *Applied Pathophysiology.* 3rd ed. Wolters Kluwer; 2016:66. Figure 3-28.

Figure 11-14. Reprinted with permission from Brant WE, Helms CA. *Brant and Helms Solution.* Wolters Kluwer; 2007:828. Figure 30-21.

Figure 11-17. *Asset provided by the Anatomical Chart Company.*

Figure 11-18. Reprinted with permission from Singh A. *Gastrointestinal Imaging: The Essentials.* Wolters Kluwer; 2016:74. Figure 4a-17.

Figure 11-19. Reprinted with permission from Brant WE, Helms CA. *Brant and Helms Solution.* Wolters Kluwer; 2006:849. Figure 32-1.

Figure 11-20. Reprinted with permission from Daffner RH, Hartman M. *Clinical Radiology.* 4th ed. Wolters Kluwer; 2014:227. Figure 7-13a.

Figure 11-21. Reprinted with permission from Erkonen W, Smith WL. *Radiology 101.* 2nd ed. Wolters Kluwer; 2004. Figure 3-60.

Figure 11-31. *Asset provided by the Anatomical Chart Company.*

Figure 11-35. Reprinted with permission from Moore KL, Dalley AF, Agur AMR. *Clinically Oriented Anatomy.* 8th ed. Wolters Kluwer; 2017:943. Figure 8-83.

Figure 11-37. Reprinted with permission from Moore KL, Dalley AF, Agur AMR. *Clinically Oriented Anatomy.* 8th ed. Wolters Kluwer; 2017:454. Figure 5-36A.

Figure 11-38. Reprinted with permission from Moore KL, Dalley AF, Agur AMR. *Clinically Oriented Anatomy.* 8th ed. Wolters Kluwer; 2017:455. Figure 5-37B.

Figure 11-39. Reprinted with permission from Moore KL, Dalley AF, Agur AMR. *Clinically Oriented Anatomy.* 8th ed. Wolters Kluwer; 2017:456. Figure 5-38A.

Figure 11-40. Reprinted with permission from Moore KL, Dalley AF, Agur AMR. *Clinically Oriented Anatomy.* 8th ed. Wolters Kluwer; 2017:456. Figure 5-38B.

Figure 11-46. Modified with permission from Moore KL, Dalley AF, Agur AMR. *Clinically Oriented Anatomy.* 8th ed. Wolters Kluwer; 2017:465. Figure 5-47.

Figure 11-49. Reprinted with permission from Singh A. *Gastrointestinal Imaging: The Essentials.* Wolters Kluwer; 2016:49. Figure 1-5.

Figure 11-50. Reprinted with permission from Brant WE, Helms CA. *Brant and Helms Solution.* Wolters Kluwer; 2006:833. Figure 31-1.

Figure 11-54. Reprinted with permission from Daffner RH, Hartman M. *Clinical Radiology.* 4th ed. Wolters Kluwer; 2013:221. Figure 7-8B.

Figure 11-59. Modified with permission from Moore KL, Dalley AF, Agur AMR. *Clinically Oriented Anatomy.* 8th ed. Wolters Kluwer; 2017:476. Figure 5-57.

Figure 11-62. Courtesy of Browns Medical Imaging.

Figure 11-63. Courtesy of Browns Medical Imaging.

Figure 11-64. Courtesy of Browns Medical Imaging.

Figure 11-100. Reprinted with permission from Singh A. *Gastrointestinal Imaging: The Essentials*. Wolters Kluwer; 2016:78. Figure 4b-1a.

Figure 11-101. Reprinted with permission from Farrell TA. *Radiology 101*. 5th ed. Wolters Kluwer; 2019:84. Figure 3-24.

Figure 11-102. Reprinted with permission from Singh A. *Gastrointestinal Imaging: The Essentials*. Wolters Kluwer; 2016:4. Figure 1-5b.

Figure 11-105. Reprinted with permission from Dutton A, Ryan TA. *Torres' Patient Care in Imaging Technology*. 9th ed. Wolters Kluwer; 2018:239. Figure 12-5.

Figure 11-109. Reprinted with permission from Dutton A, Ryan TA. *Torres' Patient Care in Imaging Technology*. 9th ed. Wolters Kluwer; 2018:239. Figure 12-6.

Figure 11-110. Reprinted with permission from Dutton A, Ryan TA. *Torres' Patient Care in Imaging Technology*. 9th ed. Wolters Kluwer; 2018:238. Figure 12-3.

CHAPTER 12

Figure 12-1. Modified with permission from Kern MJ. *SCAI Interventional Cardiology Review*. 3rd ed. Wolters Kluwer; 2018:71. Figure 6-7.

Figure 12-3. Reprinted with permission from McCall R. *Phlebotomy Exam Review*. 7th ed. Wolters Kluwer; 2019:194. Figure 8-8.

Figure 12-4. Reprinted with permission from Lynn P. *Taylor's Clinical Nursing Skills*. 5th ed. Wolters Kluwer; 2018:1072. Figure Skill 18-9, Fig 4.

Figure 12-5. Modified with permission from Braun C, Anderson C. *Applied Pathophysiology*. 3rd ed. Wolters Kluwer; 2016:462. Figure 18-1A.

Figure 12-6. Modified with permission from Braun C, Anderson C. *Applied Pathophysiology*. 3rd ed. Wolters Kluwer; 2016:462. Figure 18-1B.

Figure 12-7. Reprinted with permission from Farrell TA. *Radiology 101*, 5th Ed. Wolters Kluwer, 2019: 104. Figure 3-51.

Figure 12-12. Reprinted with permission from Farrell TA. *Radiology 101*. 5th ed. Wolters Kluwer; 2019:106. Figure 3-54.

Figure 12-20. Reprinted with permission from Cohen BJ, Hull K. *Memmler's The Human Body in Health and Disease*. 14th ed. Wolters Kluwer; 2018:502. Figure 21-8.

Figure 12-28. Reprinted with permission from Cohen BJ, Hull K. *Memmler's The Human Body in Health and Disease*. 14th ed. Wolters Kluwer; 2018:502. Figure 21-8.

Figure 12-46. Reprinted with permission from Chew FS. *Musculoskeletal Imaging: The Essentials*. Wolters Kluwer; 2018:482. Figure 29-2a.

Figure 12-47. Reprinted with permission from Chew FS. *Musculoskeletal Imaging: The Essentials*. Wolters Kluwer; 2018:482. Figure 29-2b.

Figure 12-48. Reprinted with permission from Chew FS. *Musculoskeletal Imaging: The Essentials*. Wolters Kluwer; 2018:482. Figure 29-2c.

Figure 12-49. Reprinted with permission from Greenspan A, Beltran J. *Orthopaedic Imaging: A Practical Approach*. 7th ed. Wolters Kluwer; 2020:24. Figure 2-7.

Figure 12-50. Reprinted with permission from Wiesel SW. *Operative Techniques in Orthopaedic Surgery*. 2nd ed. Wolters Kluwer; 2015:3650. Figure Fig 1F.

Figure 12-51. Reprinted with permission from Greenspan A, Beltran J. *Orthopaedic Imaging: A Practical Approach*. 6th ed. Wolters Kluwer; 2014:380. Figure 10-12B.

Figure 12-52. Reprinted with permission from Greenspan A, Beltran J. *Orthopaedic Imaging: A Practical Approach*. 7th ed. Wolters Kluwer; 2020:226. Figure 6-16C.

Figure 12-54. Reprinted with permission from Moore KL, Dalley AF, Agur AMR. *Clinically Oriented Anatomy*. 8th ed. Wolters Kluwer; 2017:132. Figure 2-42.

Figure 12-60. Reprinted with permission from Ryan TA. *Torres' Patient Care in Imaging Technology*. 10th ed. Wolters Kluwer; 2024:349. Figure 14-26.

Figure 12-62. Reprinted with permission from Wineski LE. *Snell's Clinical Anatomy by Regions*. 10th ed. Wolters Kluwer; 2018:81. Figure 2-33.

Figure 12-63. Reprinted with permission from Splittgerber R. *Snell's Clinical Neuroanatomy*. 9th ed. Wolters Kluwer; 2024:174. Figure 4-37.

Figure 12-64. Reprinted with permission from Greenspan A, Gershwin ME. *Imaging in Rheumatology*. Wolters Kluwer; 2017:47. Figure 2-37c.

Figure 12-65. Reprinted with permission from Greenspan A, Gershwin ME. *Imaging in Rheumatology*. Wolters Kluwer; 2017:47. Figure 2-37a.

Figure 12-66. Reprinted with permission from Greenspan A, Gershwin ME. *Imaging in Rheumatology*. Wolters Kluwer; 2017:47. Figure 2-37b.

Figure 12-67. Reprinted with permission from Splittgerber R. *Snell's Clinical Neuroanatomy*. 8th ed. Wolters Kluwer; 2018:173. Figure 4-36.

Figure 12-68. Modified with permission from Benzel EC. *Cervical Spine*. 5th ed. Wolters Kluwer; 2012:304. Figure 24-12A.

CHAPTER 13

Figure 13-1. Photo Credit: Tyler Olson/Shutterstock.

Figure 13-3. Reprinted with permission from *Lippincott's Visual Encyclopedia of Clinical Skills*. Wolters Kluwer; 2008:499. Figure NA.

Figure 13-4. Reprinted with permission from *Lippincott's Visual Encyclopedia of Clinical Skills*. Wolters Kluwer; 2008:500. Figure 4th Image.

Figure 13-5. Reprinted with permission from *Lippincott's Visual Encyclopedia of Clinical Skills*. Wolters Kluwer; 2008:500. Figure 3rd Image.

Figure 13-6. Modified with permission from Craven RF, Hernle CJ, Henshaw CM. *Fundamentals of Nursing*. 8th ed. Wolters Kluwer; 2016:560. Figure 22-2B.

Figure 13-7. Reprinted with permission from Gardner MJ. *Illustrated Tips and Tricks for Intraoperative Imaging in Fracture Surgery*. Wolters Kluwer; 2017:87. Figure 10-10.

Figure 13-8. Reprinted with permission from Gardner MJ. *Illustrated Tips and Tricks for Intraoperative Imaging in Fracture Surgery*. Wolters Kluwer; 2017:293. Figure 27-11.

Figure 13-9. Reprinted with permission from Gardner MJ. *Illustrated Tips and Tricks for Intraoperative Imaging in Fracture Surgery*. Wolters Kluwer; 2017:310. Figure A1-3.

Figure 13-10. Reprinted with permission from Gardner MJ. *Illustrated Tips and Tricks for Intraoperative Imaging in Fracture Surgery*. Wolters Kluwer; 2017:310. Figure A1-2.

Figure 13-11. Reprinted with permission from Gardner MJ. *Illustrated Tips and Tricks for Intraoperative Imaging in Fracture Surgery*. Wolters Kluwer; 2017:279. Figure 26-7.

Figure 13-12. Reprinted with permission from Gardner MJ. *Illustrated Tips and Tricks for Intraoperative Imaging in Fracture Surgery*. Wolters Kluwer; 2017:312. Figure A1-7.

Figure 13-13. Modified with permission from Brinker MR. *Review of Orthopaedic Trauma.* 2nd ed. Wolters Kluwer; 2013:221. Figure 15-14.

Figure 13-14. Reprinted with permission from Pagnano MW. *Master Techniques in Orthopedic Surgery: Knee Arthroplasty.* Wolters Kluwer; 2018:413. Figure 33-17A.

Figure 13-15. Reprinted with permission from Rathmell JP. *Atlas of Image-Guided Intervention in Regional Anesthesia and Pain Medicine.* 2nd ed. Wolters Kluwer; 2011:14. Figure 2-6A.

Figure 13-16. Reprinted with permission from Rathmell JP. *Atlas of Image-Guided Intervention in Regional Anesthesia and Pain Medicine.* 2nd ed. Wolters Kluwer; 2011:14. Figure 2-6D.

Figure 13-17. Reprinted with permission from Rathmell JP. *Atlas of Image-Guided Intervention in Regional Anesthesia and Pain Medicine.* 2nd ed. Wolters Kluwer; 2011:14. Figure 2-6C.

Figure 13-18. Reprinted with permission from Dutton A, Ryan TA. *Torres' Patient Care in Imaging Technology.* 9th ed. Wolters Kluwer; 2018:280. Figure 14-21.

Figure 13-20. Reprinted with permission from Jaffe RA. *Anesthesiologist's Manual of Surgical Procedures.* 5th ed. Wolters Kluwer; 2014:1513. Figure 13.1-7.

Figure 13-21. Reprinted with permission from Swanstorm LL, Soper NJ. *Mastery of Endoscopic and Laparoscopic Surgery.* 4th ed. Wolters Kluwer; 2013:373. Figure 35-6.

Figure 13-22. Modified with permission from Swanstorm LL, Soper NJ. *Mastery of Endoscopic and Laparoscopic Surgery.* 4th ed. Wolters Kluwer; 2013:373. Figure 35-6.

Figure 13-23. Reprinted with permission from Mulholland MW, Lillemoe KD, Doherty GM, Maier RV, Simeone DM, Upchurch GR. *Greenfield's Surgery.* 5th ed. Wolters Kluwer; 2010:800. Figure 51-1.

Figure 13-24. Reprinted with permission from Mulholland MW, Lillemoe KD, Doherty GM, Maier RV, Simeone DM, Upchurch GR. *Greenfield's Surgery.* 5th ed. Wolters Kluwer; 2010:1010. Figure 62-8C.

Figure 13-25. Reprinted with permission from Swanstorm LL, Soper NJ. *Mastery of Endoscopic and Laparoscopic Surgery.* 4th ed. Wolters Kluwer; 2013:374. Figure 34-8.

Figure 13-26. Modified with permission from Braun C, Anderson C. *Applied Pathophysiology.* 3rd ed. Wolters Kluwer; 2016:462. Figure 18-1a.

Figure 13-27. Modified with permission from Braun C, Anderson C. *Applied Pathophysiology.* 3rd ed. Wolters Kluwer; 2016:462. Figure 18-1b.

Figure 13-28. Modified with permission from Albo D. *Operative Techniques in Colon and Rectal Surgery.* Wolters Kluwer; 2015:224. Figure 27-3.

Figure 13-29. Modified with permission from Scardino PT, Linehan WM, Zelefsky MJ, et al. *Comprehensive Textbook of Genitourinary Oncology.* 4th ed. Wolters Kluwer; 2011:354. Figure 20-12c.

Figure 13-30. Modified with permission from Scardino PT, Linehan WM, Zelefsky MJ, et al. *Comprehensive Textbook of Genitourinary Oncology.* 4th ed. Wolters Kluwer; 2011:353. Figure 20-9a.

Figure 13-32. Reprinted with permission from Strickland JW, Graham TJ. *Master Techniques in Orthopaedic Surgery: The Hand.* 2nd ed. Wolters Kluwer; 2004:129. Figure 9-5B.

Figure 13-33. Reprinted with permission from Cooney WP. *Wrist.* 2nd ed. Wolters Kluwer; 2010:308. Figure 12-36E-H.

Figure 13-34. Reprinted with permission from Gardner MJ. *Illustrated Tips and Tricks for Intraoperative Imaging in Fracture Surgery.* Wolters Kluwer; 2017:162. Figure 17-3.

Figure 13-35. Reprinted with permission from Gardner MJ. *Illustrated Tips and Tricks for Intraoperative Imaging in Fracture Surgery.* Wolters Kluwer; 2017:170. Figure 17-30.

Figure 13-36. Reprinted with permission from Gardner MJ, Siegel J. *Minimally Invasive Orthopaedic Trauma.* Wolters Kluwer; 2013:107. Figure 9-22.

Figure 13-37. Reprinted with permission from Rhee J. *Emory's Illustrated Tips and Tricks in Spine Surgery.* Wolters Kluwer; 2019:94. Figure 9-4.

Figure 13-38. Reprinted with permission from Koval KL, Zuckerman JD. *Atlas of Orthopaedic Surgery: A Multimedia Reference.* Wolters Kluwer; 2003. Figure 18-4.

Figure 13-39. Reprinted with permission from Pope TL, Harris JH. *Harris & Harris' The Radiology of Emergency Medicine.* 5th ed. Wolters Kluwer; 2012:266. Figure 7-1A-C.

Figure 13-40. Reprinted with permission from Tannoury C. *Minimally Invasive Spine Surgery.* Wolters Kluwer; 2017:21. Figure 4-1.

Figure 13-41. Modified with permission from Zdeblick TA, Albert T. *Master Techniques in Orthopaedic Surgery: The Spine.* 3rd ed. Wolters Kluwer; 2013:331. Figure 26-8C.

Figure 13-42. Reprinted with permission from Dirette D. Gutman SA. *Occupational Therapy for Physical Dysfunction.* 8th ed. Wolters Kluwer; 2020:1017. Figure 49-3.

Figure 13-43. Reprinted with permission from Pope TL, Harris JH. *Harris & Harris' The Radiology of Emergency Medicine.* 5th ed. Wolters Kluwer; 2012:266. Figure 7-1A-C.

Figure 13-44. Reprinted with permission from Handa VL, Ven Le L. *Te Linde's Operative Gynecology.* 13th ed. Wolters Kluwer; 2024:178. Figure 9-7.

Figure 13-45. Reprinted with permission from Tannoury C. *Minimally Invasive Spine Surgery.* Wolters Kluwer; 2017:264. Figure 32-1A,b.

Figure 13-46. Reprinted with permission from Frontera WR, DeLisa JA, Gans BM, Robinson LW, Bockeneck W, Chase J. *DeLisa's Physical Medicine and Rehabilitation: Principles and Practice.* 6th ed. Wolters Kluwer; 2019:708. Figure 31-4B.

Figure 13-47. Reprinted with permission from Pope TL, Harris JH. *Harris & Harris' The Radiology of Emergency Medicine.* 5th ed. Wolters Kluwer; 2012:266. Figure 7-1A-C.

Figure 13-48. Reprinted with permission from Rathmell JP. *Atlas of Image-Guided Intervention in Regional Anesthesia and Pain Medicine.* 2nd ed. Wolters Kluwer; 2011:78. Figure 6-13A.

Figure 13-49. Reprinted with permission from Rathmell JP. *Atlas of Image-Guided Intervention in Regional Anesthesia and Pain Medicine.* 2nd ed. Wolters Kluwer; 2011:78. Figure 6-13B.

Figure 13-50. Reprinted with permission from Rathmell JP. *Atlas of Image-Guided Intervention in Regional Anesthesia and Pain Medicine.* 2nd ed. Wolters Kluwer; 2011:78. Figure 6-13C.

Figure 13-52. Photograph courtesy of Wikimedia Commons user: Tristanb, Public Domain.

Figure 13-56. Reprinted with permission from Rosdahl CB, Kowalski MT. *Textbook of Basic Nursing.* 11th ed. Wolters Kluwer; 2016:981. Figure 64-13D.

Figure 13-58. Modified with permission from Kline-Tilford AM, Haut C. *Lippincott Certification Review: Pediatric Acute Care Nurse Practitioner.* Wolters Kluwer; 2015:84. Figure 3-50.

Figure 13-61. Modified with permission from Webb WR, Higgins CB. *Thoracic Imaging.* 3rd ed. Wolters Kluwer; 2016:397. Figure 11-41A.

Index

Note: Page numbers followed by "*f*" and "*t*" denote figures and tables, respectively.

D

E

F

G

H

R

S

T

U

QUADM0725